NUTRITION AND IMMUNOLOGY

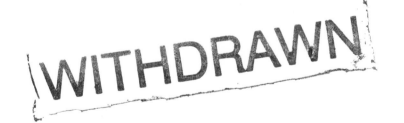

NUTRITION AND IMMUNOLOGY

PRINCIPLES AND PRACTICE

EDITED BY

M. ERIC GERSHWIN, MD

DIVISION OF RHEUMATOLOGY/ALLERGY AND CLINICAL
IMMUNOLOGY, DEPARTMENT OF INTERNAL MEDICINE
UNIVERSITY OF CALIFORNIA AT DAVIS, DAVIS, CA

J. BRUCE GERMAN, PhD

DEPARTMENT OF FOOD SCIENCE AND TECHNOLOGY
UNIVERSITY OF CALIFORNIA AT DAVIS, DAVIS , CA

CARL L. KEEN, PhD

DEPARTMENT OF NUTRITION
UNIVERSITY OF CALIFORNIA AT DAVIS, DAVIS, CA

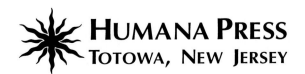

HUMANA PRESS
TOTOWA, NEW JERSEY

Dedications

The editors and authors write this book in the hope that the knowledge it provides will help to achieve the day when no child on this planet will go to bed hungry. Wish it were so.

This book is also dedicated by MEG in the memory of the late Dr. Orval L. Hamm, a farm boy from western Kansas who spent his life sharing his knowledge of medicine and his love of people in Sialkot, Pakistan.

© 2000 Humana Press Inc.
999 Riverview Drive, Suite 208
Totowa, New Jersey 07512

For additional copies, pricing for bulk purchases, and/or information about other Humana titles, contact Humana at the above address or at any of the following numbers: Tel.: 973-256-1699; Fax: 973-256-8341; E-mail:humana@humanapr.com; http://humanapress.com

Cover design by Patricia F. Cleary

This publication is printed on acid-free paper. ∞
ANSI Z39.48-1984 (American National Standards Institute) Permanence of Paper for Printed Library Materials.

Printed in the United States of America.   10 9 8 7 6 5 4 3 2 1

Nutrition and immunology : principles and practice / edited by M. Eric
  Gershwin, J. Bruce German, Carl L. Keen
        p.   cm.
    Includes bibliographical references
    ISBN 0-89603-719-3 (alk. paper)
    1.Nutrition. 2. Immunity--Nutritional aspects. I. German, Bruce
II. Gershwin, M. Eric, 1946- . III. Keen, Carl L.
    [DNLM: 1. Nutrition. 2. Nutritional Requirements. 3. Immunity.
  QU 145 N97172 1999]
  QP141.N7767 1999
  612.3'9--dc21
  DNLM/DLC   99-10901
    for Library of Congress   CIP

Foreword

It is a pleasure to write the foreword to *Nutrition and Immunology: Principles and Practice*. In fact, this book comes at a timely moment, when the impact of nutrition and immunology is being widely felt because of the AIDS epidemic. This is particularly of note in Africa, where large sums of money are being spent on nutritional intervention programs in the hopes of improving immune responsiveness. We should not forget, however, early advances in our understanding of protein energy malnutrition (PEM). PEM can be used as a model to understand the nutritional basis of immunity, as well as the immunological influences on nutritional status. Despite advances in agricultural production, PEM continues to affect hundreds of millions of the world's population. The functional impact of undernutrition varies from mild morbidity to life-threatening infection. The preface to the classic World Health Organization monograph on Interactions of Nutrition and Infection (*1*) stated, "That malnutrition increases susceptibility to infectious disease seems a reasonable assumption, and clinical observation in areas where malnutrition is common has generally lent support to this belief. Equally reasonable is the supposition that infectious diseases have an adverse effect on the nutritional state." It is only recently, however, that the pathogenetic and casual role of impaired immunity has been examined in systematic studies (*2*). Since the early 1970s, there has been a geometric increase in the interest in nutritional immunology and a corresponding plethora of original articles, reviews, and monographs on the subject (*3–12*).

HETEROGENEITY OF SYNDROMES AND MULTIFACTORIAL CAUSALITY

In laboratory animals, it is possible to produce isolated nutrient deficiencies. In contrast, human malnutrition is almost always a syndrome of multiple nutrient deficiencies compounded by genetic influences, age, gender, and the superadded effect of infection.

Also, distinct dietary habits in various parts of the world may play an additional role. Furthermore, the timing and duration of nutritional deprivation has a significant impact on the extent and duration of immunological impairment.

It is important to state at the outset that the results of controlled animal experiments have great scientific impor-

Table 1
Nutritional Status and Outcome of Infection

Definite adverse outcome
Measles, diarrhea, tuberculosis
Probable adverse outcome
HIV, malaria, pneumonia
Little or no effect
Poliomyelitis, tetanus, viral encephalitis

Note: HIV= human immunodeficiency virus

tance. However, both in vitro studies and tests in laboratory animals may have little resemblance to what is experienced in humans under field conditions.

INFECTIONS IN PROTEIN-ENERGY MALNUTRITION

The enormous collection of clinical and epidemiologic data now available suggest that PEM is associated with an increase in the severity and duration of most infectious diseases. In some cases, incidence and prevalence are also increased. Only rarely has an antagonism between PEM and infection been reported. **Table 1** gives a few examples of the interactions between nutritional status and infection.

IMMUNOLOGICAL CHANGES

Beisel has provided a historical account of successive findings in this area (*6*). From early historical accounts and anecdotal observations, there have been comprehensive systemic studies in humans and laboratory animals. These have led to many clinical and public health applications. Lymphoid atrophy is a prominent feature in PEM. Anatomical changes in lymphoid tissues in malnutrition have been described for decades. The term "nutritional thymectomy" illustrates the profound changes that occur in the thymus in malnutrition. The size and weight of the thymus are reduced. Histologically, there is a loss of corticomedullary differentiation, there are fewer lymphoid cells, and the Hassal bodies are enlarged, degenerated, and, occasionally, calcified. These changes are easily differentiated from findings in primary immunity deficiency, such as DiGeorge's syndrome. In the spleen, there is a loss of lymphoid cells around

Table 2
Delayed Cutaneous Hypersensitivity Responses
in Young Children with PEM

	Candida	Trichophyton	Tetanus	DNCB
Baseline	38	29	43	68
After 8 wk of nutrition Support	63	59	78	92

Note: DNCB= 2,4 dimitrochlorobenzene. Figures refer to percent positive responses.

Table 3
Complement System

	Healthy	Protein-energy malnutrition
Total hemolytic complement activity CH50 (kU/L)	116 ± 19	67 ± 12
C3 (g/L)	1.43 ± 0.15	0.61 ± 0.09
C5 (g/L)	0.081 ± 0.003	0.049 ± 0.002
Factor B (g/L)	2.29 ± 0.17	1.21 ± 0.11

Note: Values are shown as mean ± standard deviation.

small blood vessels. In lymph nodes, the thymus-dependent paracortical areas show depletion of lymphocytes.

Protein-energy malnutrition (PEM) is associated with an impairment of most of the host barriers. Delayed cutaneous hypersensitivity responses both to recall and new antigens are indicators of in vivo cell-mediated immunity and are markedly depressed in PEM (**Table 2**). These changes are observed in moderate deficiencies as well. Findings in patients with kwashiorkor are more striking than findings in patients with marasmus. The skin reactions are restored after appropriate nutritional therapy for several weeks and months (**Table 2**). One possible reason for reduced cell-mediated immunity in PEM is the reduction in mature fully differentiated T lymphocytes. The reduction in serum thymulin activity observed in primary PEM may underlie the impaired maturation of T lymphocytes. There is an increase in the amount of deoxynucleotidyl transferase activity in leukocytes, a feature of immaturity. The proportion of helper and/or inducer T lymphocytes recognized by the presence of the CD4+ antigen on the cell surface is markedly decreased. There is a slight reduction in the number of suppressor and/or cytotoxic CD8+ cells. Thus, the ratio CD4+:CD8+ is significantly decreased compared with that in well-nourished control subjects. Moreover, coculture experiments showed a reduction in the number of antibody-producing cells and in the amount of immunoglobulin secreted. This is largely because of the decreased help provided by T lymphocytes. Lymphocyte proliferation and synthesis of DNA are reduced, especially when the autologous plasma from a patient is used in cell cultures. This may be the result of inhibitory factors as well as deficiency of essential nutrients lacking in the patient's plasma. Another aspect of lymphocyte function that changes in PEM is the traffic and homing pattern. For example, lymphocytes derived from mesenteric lymph nodes of immunized rodents revert back to the intestine in large numbers, whereas this homing is reduced in malnutrition.

Serum antibody responses are generally intact in PEM, particularly when antigens in adjuvant are administered or for materials that do not evoke T-cell response. Rarely, the antibody response to some organisms, such as *Salmonella typhi*, may be decreased. However, before impaired antibody response can be attributed to nutritional deficiency, one must carefully rule out infection as a confounding factor. Antibody affinity is decreased in patients who are mal-

nourished. This may provide an explanation for a higher frequency of antigen–antibody complexes found in such patients. As opposed to serum antibody responses, secretory immunoglobulin A (sIgA) antibody concentrations are decreased after immunization with viral vaccines; there is a selective reduction in sIgA concentrations. This may have several clinical implications, including an increased frequency of septicemia commonly observed in undernourished children.

Phagocytosis is also affected in PEM. Complement is an essential opsonin and the concentrations and activity of most complement components are decreased. The best documented is a reduction in complement C3, C5, factor B, and total hemolytic activity (**Table 3**). There is a reduction in opsonic activity of plasma when tests are run using plasma diluted 1:10 or more. Although the ingestion of particles by phagocytes is intact, subsequent metabolic activation and destruction of bacteria is reduced. Finally, recent work in humans and animals demonstrated that the production of several cytokines, including interleukins 2 and 6 and γ-interferon, is decreased in PEM. Moreover, malnutrition alters the ability of T lymphocytes to respond appropriately to cytokines. There is some work on the effect of malnutrition on the integrity of physical barriers, quality of mucus, or several other innate immune defenses. For example, lysozyme concentrations are decreased, largely the result of reduced production by monocytes and neutrophils increased excretion in the urine. Adherence of bacteria to epithelial cells is a first step before invasion and infection can occur. The number of bacteria adhering to respiratory epithelial cells is increased in PEM fetal malnutrition.

FETAL MALNUTRITION

Any insult during the critical developmental period is likely to have a greater and more prolonged impact on physiological functions. The immune system is no exception.

Preterm appropriate-for-gestation low-birth-weight (LBW) infants have reduced levels of IgG, largely a result of the shorter time available for mother-to-infant transfer. The number of T lymphocytes is decreased but this responds dramatically to small supplements of zinc.

Small-for-gestational age (SGA) LBW infants have a higher morbidity because of infection in the first 2–3 yr after birth. This correlates with impaired immunity. The majority of SGA infants show atrophy of the thymus and prolonged impairment of cell-mediated immunity. Delayed cutaneous hypersensitivity to a variety of microbial recall antigens is impaired. Serum thymic factor activity is lower in SGA infants tested at age 1 mo or later. In contrast to preterm low-birth-weight infants who recover immunologically by approx 2–3 mo of age, SGA infants continue to exhibit impaired cell-mediated immune responses for up to 12 yr. This is particularly true of those infants whose weight-for-height continues to remain <80% of standard. The prolonged immunosuppression in some SGA infants correlates with clinical experience of infectious illness and, thus, may have considerable biological significance. In animal models of intrauterine nutritional deficiency, PEM results in reduced immune responses in the offspring.

Phagocyte function is deranged in low-birth-weight infants. There is a slight reduction in ingestion of particulate matter and a significant reduction both in metabolic activity and bactericidal capacity.

IgG from the mother, acquired through placental transfer, is the principal immunoglobulin in cord blood. The half-life of IgG is 21 d, thus all infants show physiological hypo-immunoglobulinemia between ages 3 and 5 mo. This is pronounced and prolonged in low-birth-weight infants because their concentration of IgG at birth is significantly lower than that of full-term infants. In SGA low-birth-weight infants the cord blood concentrations of IgG1 are reduced much more than those of other subclasses. Thus the ratio of infant to maternal concentrations is significantly low for IgG1 but not for IgG2. The number of immunoglobulin-producing cells and the amount of immunoglobulin secreted is decreased in SGA infants who are symptomatic (i.e., those who have recurrent infections). In the second year of life, SGA infants show a marked reduction in IgG2 concentrations and often show infections with organisms that have a polysaccharide capsule. The SGA group is also at risk of developing infection with opportunistic microorganisms, such as *Pneumocystis carinii*, as observed in postnatal malnutrition also.

Clearly, protein-energy malnutrition is not a paradigm for all of the areas covered in *Nutrition and Immunology: Principles and Practice*. However, it is perhaps the best studied and the most understood. There are a number of novel areas treated in this book that illustrate the changing tides and the great need to understand the molecular basis of interactions, in addition to understanding and performing simple dietary assessment. A goal for all of us should be to recruit more researchers into this area and especially to increase the dialog between nutritional and food scientists and immunologists.

Ranjit Kumar Chandra, DSc, PhD, MD

REFERENCES

1. Scrimshaw NS, Taylor CE, Gordon JE. Interactions of Nutrition and Infection. WHO, Geneva; 1968.
2. Chandra RK. Immunocompetence in undernutrition. J Pediatr 1972;81:1194–200.
3. Chandra RK, Newberne PM. Nutrition, immunity and infection. In: Mechanisms of Interactions. Plenum, New York; 1977.
4. Victora CG, Barros FC, Kirkwood BR, Vaughan JP. Pneumonia, diarrhea, and growth in the first 4 y of life: a longitudinal study of 5914 urban Brazilian children. Am J Clin Nutr 1990; 52:391–6.
5. Gershwin ME, Beach RS, Hurley LS. Nutrition and Immunity. Academic, New York; 1984.
6. Beisel WR. The history of nutritional immunology. J Nutr Immunol 1991;1:16–24.
7. Chandra RK, ed. Nutrition and immunology. Alan R. Liss, New York, 1988.
8. Kirby DF. Enteral nutrition in immunocompromised patients. Nutr Clin Prac 1997;12:S25–7.
9. Pomeroy C, Mitchell J, Eckert E, Raymond N, Crosby R, Dalmasso AP. Effect of body weight and caloric restriction on serum complement proteins, including Factor D/adipsin: studies in anorexia nervosa and obesity. Clin Exper Immunol 1997;108: 507–15.
10. Zaman K, Baqui AH, Yunus M, Sack RB, Bateman OM, Chowdhury HR, et al. Association between nutritional status, cell-mediated immune status and acute lower respiratory infections in Bangladeshi children. Eur Clin Nutr 1996;50:309–14.
11. Marcos A, Varela P, Toro O, Lopez-Vidriero I, Nove E, Madruga D, et al. Interactions between nutrition and immunity in anorexia nervosa: a 1-y follow-up study. Am J Clin Nutr 1997;66: 485S–490S.
12. Scrimshaw NS, SanGiovanni JP. Synergism of nutrition, infection, and immunity: an overview. Am J Clin Nutr 1997;66:464S–477S.

Preface

Nutrition and immunology are at the focus of a scientific revolution. The food supply as a source of nutrients has evolved dramatically over the past two centuries, but never before has there been such a promise for innovation. The genetic revolution has provided the promise to truly change the food supply as never before imagined. Plant geneticists and physiologists are providing the capability, and agribusiness is poised to dramatically change the chemical makeup of food commodities. With this capability has come the compelling question: To what should it be changed? Unquestionably, if the food supply is to be improved nutritionally, the needs of the immune system need to be a major target of that improvement. Establishing the framework to direct this new revolution is a considered goal of *Nutrition and Immunology: Principles and Practice,* and we have thus brought together experts from around the world in nutrition and immunology to provide the consensus state-of-the-art in these fields.

The first great nutritional age of this century brought the sciences of biochemistry, physiology, chemistry, and medicine together to define in molecular terms the essential nutrients for humans. This triumph of scientific discovery was primarily completed before 1950 when most vitamins and essential minerals and major diseases associated with their respective nutritional deficiencies had been described. A valuable outcome of this chemical approach was the capability to produce vitamins synthetically, which made it possible to implement a true solution to the problem of nutrient deficiency in the Western world and, in particular, the United States, through aggressive food fortification. Interestingly, this "first" nutritional revolution addressed only those nutrients that were essential for growth and reproduction. This perspective failed to address either optimal nutrition or the specific requirements of particular tissues during aging, including the varying and specific needs of the growing and functioning immune system. Some of the reasons for not addressing immunology directly lay in the relative state of knowledge of molecular immunology, but were also in part a consequence of the decision to limit the definitions of nutrient requirements to normal development, neglecting the increased nutrient needs attributable to stress and the increased demands of a stimulated immune response. Over the past half century, these knowledge gaps have been addressed and it is now possible to more closely assess the nutritional requirements of various aspects of immunity. Assembling this information is a second important goal of *Nutrition and Immunology: Principles and Practice.*

Appreciating the nutritional requirements of the immune system has been gained from various directions. Overt dietary deficiency of virtually all nutrients compromises the quality, speed, and integrity of the immune response, leading most obviously to increases in susceptibility to infectious disease. The insights gained from the quality of the immune response associated with nutrient deficiencies are the subject of several chapters in *Nutrition and Immunology: Principles and Practice.* Intriguingly, in the context of infectious disease, microbial pathogens themselves are sensitive to the nutritional status of the host, and chapters address this burgeoning issue including the influence of nutrition on viral evolution. The immune system, however, is not simply affected by overt nutrient deficiencies, but both the elaboration of the multitissue immune system through life and the mounting of an aggressive immune response place specific metabolic demands on the organism, many of which are directly related to increased needs for specific dietary nutrients. The last 20 years have seen an explosion in research, expanding on the molecular requirements of the immune system. From the role of minerals and cofactors in transcriptional regulation of immune maturation, through the specific protein, vitamin, and lipid needs of immune responses, to the increased demand for antioxidant protection and tissue repair created by the consequences of immune activation, these fields of the molecular nutrition of the immune system are the focus of multiple chapters in the text.

By defining only nutrient essentiality as the subject for public health, the role of nutrient imbalances, especially as they relate to the gradual development of chronic and degenerative diseases in maturity, was largely ignored in the first revolution of nutrition research. Thus, in modern Western societies, the successful elimination of nutritional deficiencies through nutrient fortification has not eliminated the diet as a contributor to disease, but rather delayed the consequences of suboptimal diets to the diseases that develop during adulthood. More insidiously, by solving nutrient deficiencies by fortification, the food supply has evolved in the second half of the century without sound nutritional intervention, but rather under soft, educational guidance. Ironically, the first nutritional revolution that eliminated nutrient deficiencies and promoted a significantly greater fraction of the population into old age also allowed an evolution of the food supply toward lower nutritional density (*1,2*). This lower nutrient density of diets permitted nutritional imbalances that are now emerging epidemiologically as a greater risk of chronic and degenerative disease during aging (*3*). Equally ironic, although the fortification of foods was implemented as a public health program in the United States with genuinely spectacular benefits to public health, the important nutritional improvements warranted by chronic disease prevention (i.e., cholesterol reduction) have been left largely to individual discretionary choice (*4*). The strategy to improve nutritional status beyond simple essentiality has been to implement diet change via individual education (*5*), which has led to competition within the food marketplace in, as one example, targeted cholesterol-lowering foods, and the emergence of a large food supplement industry. An obvious consequence of recruiting such vested interests as the food and supplement industries into the nutritional educational process is a substantial disaffection of the public with nutrition education in general and the credibility of the science underlying it as well. Additionally, the focus of attention has shifted from molecules and scientific mechanisms to specific commodities or products as purportedly superior in a competitive marketplace. A valuable asset of *Nutrition and Immunology: Principles and Practice* is an effort to refocus this attention on the science issues and to provide clear, understandable summaries of the state of science at the present time nutritional immunologic.

The now recognized role of diet in health has led to a nutritional revolution in the second half of the century addressing the larger role of diet in optimal health and disease prevention (*6–8*). Within this context, the role of diet in immunological status has emerged as important, if not piv-

otal. It is possible to redesign the food supply because of the technological advances of genetic manipulation. If this manipulation is to improve long-term health, the specific nutritional needs of the immune system, throughout life and importantly, during immunologic challenge, must be defined in molecular terms. With this improved food supply in mind, *Nutrition and Immunology* should serve as a strong blueprint for that design.

M. Eric Gershwin, MD
J. Bruce German, PhD
Carl L. Keen, PhD

REFERENCES

1. Steven, A.M. and Sieber, G.M. Trends in individual fat consumption in the UK 1900–1985. Brit J Nutr 1994; 71.
2. Drewnowski, A. and Popkin, B.M. 1997. The Nutrition Transition: New Trends in the Global Diet. Nutr Rev 55 (2): 31–44.
3. Shetty, P.S. Diet, lifestyle and chronic disease: lessons from contrasting worlds. In: Diet, Nutrition and Chronic Disease: Lessons from Contrasting Worlds. Shetty P.S. and McPherson, K., eds. John Wiley and Sons, NY, 1997.
4. James WPT. Where do we go from here in public health? In: Diet Nutrition and Chronic Disease: Lessons from Contrasting Worlds. Shetty, P.S. and McPherson, K., eds., John Wiley and Sons, NY, 1997.
5. Foerster, S.B., Heimendinger, J., DiSogra, L.K. and Pivonka, E. 1997. The national 5 a day for better health program: an American nutrition and cancer prevention initiative. In: Implementing Dietary Guidelines for Healthy Eating. Wheelock, V., ed. Chapman & Hall, London, 1997.
6. Gombs, G.F. Should intakes with beneficial actions often requiring supplementation be considered for RDA's? Am J Clin Nutr 1996; 126:2373S–2376S.
7. Hambidge, K.M. Overview and purpose of the work shop on new approaches, endpoints and paradigms for RDA's of mineral elements. Am J Clin Nutr 1996; 126:2301S–2303S.
8. Metz W. Food fortification in the United States. Nutr Rev 1997; 55(2):44–9.

Contents

Contributors

MANUEL E. BALDEÓN, MD, PhD, *Combined Program in Pediatric Gastroenterontology and Nutrition, Massachusetts General Hospital, Charlestown, MA*

RONALD R. BARBOSA, MD, *Department of Surgery, University of California at Davis, Sacramento Medical Center, Sacramento, CA*

MELINDA A. BECK, PhD, *Departments of Pediatrics and Nutrition, Frank Porter Graham Child Development Center, University of North Carolina at Chapel Hill, Chapel Hill, NC*

WILLIAM R. BEISEL, MD, *Department of Molecular Immunology and Infection, School of Hygiene and Public Health, The Johns Hopkins University, Baltimore, MD*

MAURO BERNARDI, MD, *Semeiotica Medica, Dipartimento di Medicina Interna, Cardioangiologia Epatologia, Universita di Bologna, Bologna, Italy*

TIFFANY L. BIERER, BS, PhD, *Waltham USA, Vernon, CA*

STEPHANIE BLUM, PhD, *Nestle Research Center, Lausanne, Switzerland*

GILBERT A. BOISSONNEAULT, PhD, *Department of Clinical Sciences, University of Kentucky, Lexington, KY*

ANDREA T. BORCHERS, PhD, *Division of Rheumatology/Allergy and Clinical Immunology, University of California at Davis, Davis, CA*

KENNETH H. BROWN, MD, *Department of Nutrition, University of California at Davis, Davis, CA*

MARY C. CANTRELL, PhD, *Division of Gastroenterology, University of California at Davis, Davis, CA*

RANJIT K. CHANDRA, MD, PhD, *Memorial University of Newfoundland, Janeway Child Health Centre, Newfoundland, Canada*

CHRISTOPHER CHANG MD, PhD, *Division of Rheumatology/Allergy and Clinical Immunology, University of California at Davis, Davis, CA*

ROBERT S. CHAPKIN, PhD, *Molecular and Cell Biology Group, Faculty of Nutrition, Texas A & M University, TX*

KATI CHEVAUX, MS, *Fundamental Research Group, M&M/Mars, Hackettstown, NJ*

FRANCESCO CHIAPPELLI, PhD, *Section of Diagnostic Sciences, Orofacial Pain, and Occlusion, School of Dentistry and Dental Research Institute, University of California at Los Angeles, Los Angeles, CA*

CAROLYN K. CLIFFORD, PhD, *Division of Cancer Prevention, National Cancer Institute, Bethesda, MD*

PAUL A. DAVIS, PhD, *Division of Clinical Nutrition and Metabolism, University of California at Davis, Davis, CA*

YVES DELNESTE, PhD, *Nestle Research Center, Lausanne, Switzerland*

ANNE DONNET, PhD, *Nestle Research Center, Lausanne, Switzerland*

GABRIEL FERNANDES, PhD, *Division of Clinical Immunology, Department of Medicine, University of Texas Health Science Center at San Antonio, San Antonio, TX*

FRANCESCO GIUSEPPE FOSCHI, MD, *Semeiotica Medica, Dipartimento di Medicina Interna, Cardioangiologia Epatologia, Universita di Bologna, Bologna, Italy*

PAM FRAKER, PhD, *Department of Biochemistry, Michigan State University, East Lansing, MI*

CLAUDIO GALPERIN, MD, *Hospital do Cancer, Sao Paulo, Brazil*

H. REX GASKINS, PhD, *Department of Animal Sciences, University of Illinois as Urbana-Champaign, Urbana, IL*

J. BRUCE GERMAN, PhD, *Food Science and Technology, University of California at Davis, Davis, CA*

M. ERIC GERSHWIN, MD, *Division of Rheumatology/Allergy and Clinical Immunology, University of California at Davis, Davis, CA*

MARI S. GOLUB, PhD, *California Regional Primate Research Center, University of California at Davis, Davis, CA*

CECILIA GORREL, MA, Vet MB, DDS, *Division of Rheumatology, Department of Medicine, University of Florida, Gainesville, FL*

GEORGE K. GRIMBLE, BSc, PhD, *Roehampton Institute, School of Life Sciences, Whitelands College, London, UK*

KATHERINE GUNDLING, MD, *Department of Internal Medicine, University of California at Davis, Sacramento Medical Center, Sacramento, CA*

CHARLES H. HALSTED, MD, *Division of Clinical Nutrition and Metabolism, University of California at Davis, Davis, CA*

BERNHARD HENNIG, PhD, *Department of Nutrition and Food Science, University of Kentucky, Lexington, KY*

CHRISTOPHER A. JOLLY, PhD, *Department of Clinical Immunology, University of Texas Health Science Center at San Antonio, TX*

STEVEN KATZNELSON, MD, *Department of Transplantation, California Pacific Medical Center, San Francisco, CA*

CARL L. KEEN, PhD, *Department of Nutrition, University of California at Davis, Davis, CA*

GERALD T. KEUSCH, MD, *Fogarty International Center, National Institutes of Health, Bethesda, MD*

JANET C. KING, PhD, *Western Human Nutrition Research Center, USDA/ARS, Presidio of San Francisco, CA*

KIRK C. KLASING, PhD, *Department of Avian Sciences, University of California at Davis, Davis, California*

MICHELLE A. KUNG, DDS, *Section of Diagnostic Sciences, Orofacial Pain, and Occlusion, School of Dentistry and Dental Research Institute, University of California at Los Angeles, Los Angeles, CA*

TATIANA V. LESHCHINSKY, PhD, *Department of Animal Science, University of California at Davis, Davis, CA*

JOHN K. LODGE, PhD, *Department of Molecular and Cell Biology, University of California at Berkeley, Berkeley, CA*

BO LÖNNERDAL, PhD, *Department of Nutrition, University of California at Davis, Davis, CA*

LORENZO MARSIGLI, *Divisione di Geriatria, Arcispedale S. Maria Nuova, Italy*

DAVID N. MCMURRAY, MD, PhD, *Department of Medical Microbiology and Immunology, Texas A&M University, School of Medicine, College Station, TX*

SIMIN NIKBIN MEYDANI, DVM, PhD, *Nutritional Immunology Laboratory, Department of Nutrition, Jean Mayer USDA Human Nutrition Research Center on Aging at Tufts University, Boston, MA*

RICARDO M. OLIVEIRA, MD, *Division of Clinical Pathology, Sao Paulo University, School of Medicine and Cancer Hospital, Sao Paulo, Brazil*

LESTER PACKER, MD, *Department of Molecular and Cell Biology, University of California at Berkeley, Berkeley, CA*

RICHARD V. PEREZ, MD, *Division of Transplantation, Department of Surgery, University of California at Davis, Davis, CA*

JONATHAN POWELL, MD, *Division of Rheumatology/Allergy and Clinical Immunology, University of California at Davis, Davis, CA*

THOMAS P. PRINDIVILLE, MD, *Division of Gastroenterology, University of California at Davis, Sacramento Medical Center, Sacramento, CA*

LINDA RASOOLY, PHD, *Department of Molecular Microbiology and Immunology, The Johns Hopkins University, Baltimore, MD*

NOEL R. ROSE, MD, PHD, *Departments of Pathology and of Molecular Microbiology, and Immunology, The Johns Hopkins University, Baltimore, MD*

ROBERT RUCKER, PhD, *Department of Nutrition, University of California at Davis, Davis, CA*

MICHELLE SCHELSKE SANTOS, PhD, *School of Family Ecology and Nutrition, University of Puerto Rico, Rio Piedras Campus, San Juan, Puerto Rico*

EDUARDO JORGE SCHIFFRIN, MD, *Nestle Research Center, Lausanne, Switzerland*

HAROLD SCHMITZ, PhD, *Fundamental Research Group, M&M/Mars, Hackettstown, NJ*

NOEL W. SOLOMONS, PhD, *CESSIAM Hospital de Ojos-Oidos, Dr. Rodolfo Robles V, Guatemala City, Guatemala*

GIUSEPPE FRANCESCO STEFANINI, MD, *Divisione di Medicina Interna, Ospedale di Faenza, Faenza (Ravenna), Italy*

JUDITH S. STERN, ScD, *Department of Nutrition, University of California at Davis, Davis, CA*

MICHAL TOBOREK, MD, *Department of Surgery, University of Kentucky, Lexington, KY*

DEAN A. TROYER, MD, *Department of Pathology, University of Texas Health Science Center at San Antonio, San Antonio, TX*

OLWYN M. R. WESTWOOD, PhD, BSc, *Roehampton Institute, School of Life Sciences, Whitelands College, London, UK*

BRUCE M. WOLF, MD, *Department of Surgery, University of California at Davis, Davis, CA*

STEVEN YOSHIDA, PhD, *Division of Rheumatology, Allergy and Clinical Immunology, University of California at Davis, Davis, CA*

VERNON R. YOUNG, PhD, DSc, *Laboratory of Human Nutrition, School of Science, Massachusetts Institute of Technology, Cambridge, MA*

VINCENT A. ZIBOH, PhD, *Department of Dermatology, University, of California at Davis, Davis, CA*

NUTRITIONAL ASSESSMENT

I

1 Application and Interpretation of Commonly Used Nutritional Assessment Techniques

Kenneth H. Brown, MD

INTRODUCTION

Nutritional assessment can be defined as the collection and interpretation of information on tissue nutrient reserves (i.e., nutritional status), dietary factors that affect these reserves, and health and functional performance in relation to these nutrient stores. Whereas direct or indirect measurements of tissue nutrient reserves can be considered as true indicators of nutritional status, dietary intake data reflect only the likelihood of low (or high) intake and the consequent risk of undernutrition (or overnutrition). Thus, dietary data are *not* indicators of nutritional status *per se*. For example, dietary intake may appear to be "inadequate" relative to theoretical nutrient requirements, but nutritional status may still be satisfactory if the individual's actual requirements are low, the nutrient can be stored in the body and previous intake had been sufficient, or supplements or other sources of nutrients are consumed in addition to the diet. On the other hand, dietary intake may appear to be "adequate," yet nutritional status may be depleted if an individual's actual requirements are relatively high, malabsorption is present, or other nutrients, food components, or drugs interfere with nutrient utilization. Thus, other nutritional assessment techniques must be combined with dietary measurements to provide information on current nutritional status.

This chapter will provide a general overview of the objectives of nutritional assessment, the range of available assessment techniques, and the factors that should be considered in selecting any particular method or combination of methods. Emphasis will be given to dietary and anthropometric assessment, both because these are the simplest and most easily completed methods for assessing nutritional status and because a detailed treatment of the intricacies of clinical and biochemical assessment is beyond the limitations of this introductory section. A considerable amount of scientific research has been devoted to the topic of nutritional assessment; more detailed information is available in existing textbooks (*1*) and specific references on individual assessment techniques.

From: *Nutrition and Immunology: Principles and Practice* (ME Gershwin et al. eds.), © Humana Press, Inc., Totowa, NJ

OBJECTIVES OF NUTRITIONAL ASSESSMENT Nutritional assessment is carried out clinically and in public health practice to identify those individuals or population groups that might benefit from some form of nutritional (or other therapeutic) intervention; the same techniques can also be used to evaluate the success of these interventions. In the context of research studies, nutritional status may be assessed, on the one hand, to explore relationships between risk factors of interest and particular nutritional deficiencies or excess and, on the other hand, to examine relationships between nutritional status and human health and function. In relation to the main topic of this book, for example, nutritional assessment techniques can be applied to examine the relationships between nutritional status and immune function. Finally, nutritional assessment of populations is frequently used not only to characterize nutritional conditions *per se* but also to describe social development in general.

TYPES AND SELECTION OF ASSESSMENT TECHNIQUES Traditionally, nutritional assessment techniques have been divided into four or five categories, including dietary, anthropometric, clinical, biochemical, and (sometimes) functional assessment. Anthropometric assessment provides general information on nutritional status, but it is not specific for any particular nutrient. The other forms of assessment offer both general information on the adequacy of the diet and tissue reserves and, in some cases, more specific data with regard to the status of individual nutrients. Each of these techniques will be explained in somewhat more detail in the following sections; but, first, several considerations that might be used in the selection of individual techniques will be reviewed.

Issues that should be contemplated in selecting a particular nutritional assessment technique include the ability of the technique to portray an individual's or population's true nutritional status with an acceptably small margin of error, its responsiveness to recent changes in conditions that influence nutritional status, and its cost, ease of implementation, and acceptability to the patient or client. Each of these items will be reviewed briefly.

Validity, Accuracy, and Precision The validity of an assessment technique refers to its ability to reflect the true nutritional status of an individual or population under the conditions that the test is applied. For example, serum ferritin concentration is a valid

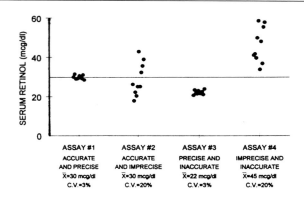

Fig. 1. Examples of different levels of accuracy and precision in measurement of plasma retinol concentration to assess vitamin A status.

indicator of iron status under usual circumstances, because it is strongly correlated with tissue (bone marrow) iron reserves. However, because serum ferritin is an acute-phase protein, its concentration increases dramatically in the presence of systemic infection or inflammation. Thus, in infected individuals, serum ferritin is no longer a valid indicator of iron status. Similarly, quantitative dietary records may be a valid indicator of the amount of food consumed by an individual during a particular period of observation, but they may not necessarily indicate the usual food consumption by that individual during other times. Thus, this technique may or may not be a valid indicator of the person's usual, or habitual, dietary intake. It is essential that the person carrying out nutritional assessment think critically about the appropriate application of a particular test and understand its physiological basis to be sure that the technique is applied and interpreted correctly in any given circumstance.

The accuracy of an assessment technique is the extent to which its results approximate the true value of what is being measured. If a test systematically under- or over-estimates the true value, it is considered biased. Precision, on the other hand, indicates the extent to which repeated measurements of the same samples provide the same results. Precision is also referred to as the reproducibility or repeatability of a test result, and is usually expressed in terms of the coefficient of variation (SD * 100/mean) of repeated measurements of the same sample. The concepts of accuracy and precision are summarized in Fig. 1.

Sources of variability in assessment of nutritional status include true biological variability (minute-to-minute or day-to-day changes in nutritional status indicators, as occurs, for example, with changes in body weight or plasma lipoprotein concentrations in relation to a meal), instrument error or analytic error (as produced, for example, by fluctuations in electrical current when reading a spectrophotometric assay, miscalibration of the instrument, or underconcentration or overconcentration of an analytic reagent), and interobserver and intraobserver error (as may occur during anthropometry if one observer positions the subject differently from another observer or from one subject to another). Whereas analytic error and observer error can be controlled or minimized by careful attention to detail and frequent training and standardization of observers, biological variability must be accepted as inevitable. Nevertheless, even biological variability can be reduced by standardizing the timing of measurements

(e.g., in relation to meals or physical activity) and other test conditions.

Time Frame There is a typical progression of signs of depletion with regard to most nutritional deficiencies. Thus, the selection of appropriate assessment tools also depends on whether the investigator prefers an indicator of the current nutritional condition or possible risk of future depletion or deficiency. In general, nutritional deficiency is preceded by a period of low dietary intake, which leads to decreased tissue reserves and lower circulating nutrient levels in body fluids (1,2). These early stages of low intake and tissue depletion can be assessed by dietary and biochemical methods, respectively. In most cases, disturbances in enzyme function, tissue morphology, and physical growth or status occur only after full or partial depletion of nutrient reserves. Thus, anthropometric, clinical, and some forms of biochemical assessment may be less sensitive to early stages of nutritional inadequacy. An exception to this usual sequence of events may occur with the so-called "type-2 nutrients," such as zinc and phosphorus, in which impaired physical growth may be the first evidence of nutritional deficiency (3).

Even among anthropometric indicators of nutritional status, some tests respond more rapidly to recent nutritional disturbances than others. Stature, for example, reflects the cumulative nutritional situation during periods of active growth, both *in utero* and during childhood. Because negative changes in stature generally do not occur (except with compression of the spine during aging), stature or height-for-age does not respond rapidly to recent nutritional deprivation. On the other hand, indicators of body mass, such as weight-for-age and especially weight-for-height and especially indicators of growth velocity (i.e., change in weight or height per unit time) are relatively good indicators of recent nutritional conditions. For these reasons, the choice of anthropometric indicators depends in part on whether one is interested in the effects of recent or longer-term nutritional conditions.

Cost, Complexity, and Acceptability Other considerations in the selection of appropriate nutritional assessment techniques include their cost, complexity, and acceptability to the patient or client. The cost of an assessment procedure refers not only to the financial expense of the measurement itself but also to the amount of time involved and any necessary capital investment that is required to procure the measurement instruments or other essential infrastructure. The complexity of a procedure may also affect its suitability for different applications. Generally, only simple procedures are suitable for field assessments and more complex techniques can be performed only in clinical settings. The latter techniques are reasonable only when appropriately trained personnel are available to carry out the procedures. Finally, the degree of discomfort and the amount of respondent time required will influence the acceptability of particular techniques in different situations. Whereas patients may be willing to undergo more invasive procedures that are completed to assess their own clinical condition, participants in community-based surveys or research projects may be more resistant to procedures that do not contribute to their own personal well-being or that impose substantial discomforts or burdens of time. Cultural factors may also dictate which procedures are appropriate. In some settings, for example, blood drawing may be unacceptable, so alternative assessment techniques must be applied.

Individual Versus Population Assessment Nutritional assessment techniques can be used to examine individuals or populations. A population refers to a finite aggregation of individuals defined by some common characteristic(s), such as their geographic location or age group. Although the same techniques that are used to characterize individual nutritional status can also be applied in populations, population assessment requires, in addition, the proper selection of a representative sample of the population of interest. The precision and accuracy with which the population's status can be characterized depends on the size and representativity of this sample. A full discussion of sampling design is beyond the limits of this chapter, but appropriate expertise must be sought when carrying out population assessment.

DIETARY ASSESSMENT

Assessment of the adequacy of dietary intake is generally conducted in three stages:

1. Collection of observed or reported information on food intake;
2. Conversion of food intake to nutrient intake; and
3. Comparison of nutrient intake with recommended levels of consumption.

The following sections will briefly describe a selection of the most commonly used techniques to collect dietary information and will then review several key issues concerning the analysis and interpretation of this information.

DIETARY DATA COLLECTION TECHNIQUES Dietary assessment techniques can be categorized by the unit of observation, the period of time covered by the data, and the quantitative or qualitative nature of the information obtained. With regard to the unit of observation, data can be collected for large aggregates of people (e.g., global regions and nations), smaller groups (e.g., households), or individuals. National data are generally summarized for periods of 1 yr, whereas household data are typically collected for 1 wk and individual data for single or multiple periods of 24 h. The recommended number of subjects to include in a study and the appropriate number of study days per individual vary by:

1. Whether group-level or individual-specific data are desired;
2. Factors related to the individuals or setting that is being studied, such as age, physiological status, and culture;
3. The nutrient(s) of interest; and
4. The desired level of precision (4,5).

To describe the typical intake of a group of individuals, it is more efficient to study a greater number of subjects for 1 d each. On the other hand, to describe an individual's habitual intake, multiple 1-d periods must be studied. To characterize an individual's usual intake, the study design must account for seasonal differences in food availability and varied eating patterns on different days of the week and holidays. More days of study are required to represent the individual's usual intake with the same degree of precision when intraindividual (day-to-day) variability is greater. Thus, to capture the usual intake of a particular nutrient, such as vitamin A, which is present in considerable amounts in a fairly small number of foods, more days of study would be needed than to characterize the intake of a nutrient, such as protein, which is more ubiquitous.

Quantitative assessment techniques provide data on the actual amount of individual foods acquired or consumed within a specific period of time, whereas qualitative techniques provide data on the usual types (and possibly amounts) of food consumed over some longer time frame or a description of usual feeding practices (for infants and young children). Depending on the methods employed, dietary data may reflect either food availability or food consumption. Because of the biomedical focus of this chapter, only those techniques used for the assessment of individual food consumption will be reviewed. Selected characteristics of these dietary assessment techniques and their susceptibility to different types of measurement error are summarized in Tables 1 and 2.

Individual 24-h Recall The 24-h recall history is a systematic interview conducted to identify and quantify all food consumed by an individual during a 24-h period. A trained interviewer probes for information on all meals and snacks, including drinks, condiments, and so forth, that are consumed both at home and outside the home. Consumption of individual foods must often be derived by reconstructing recipes or mixed-food preparations, unless the composition of these recipes or commercially prepared foods is already available in standard food composition tables. The accuracy of recall histories can be enhanced by using props such as food models, photos, or drawings of common food items and portion sizes. As indicated earlier, the appropriate number of days of study per individual depends on whether single individuals or population groups are being assessed.

Individual Food Record The food record is similar to the 24-h recall history, except that either the subject or an observer records the data himself or herself at the time of food preparation and consumption. The self-obtained food record may be either written or recorded on tape. Ideally, all foods that are included in recipes and all single food items or composite dishes are weighed. However, because of the burden that this imposes on the respondent and the potential bias introduced by the fact that only those individuals capable of completing the measurements can be enrolled in these studies, intakes may also be estimated from common household measures, such as cups, spoons, plates, or pre-existing data on usual portions sizes.

Food Frequency Questionnaire Food frequency questionnaires are used to provide information on the subjects' usual intakes. This data collection instrument differs from the recall history and food record because it does not capture the actual intake during a specified period of time, but, rather, the typical intake over some generally longer interval. With the food frequency questionnaire, the respondent indicates, from a pre-existing list, those foods that are usually consumed, the typical frequency of consumption, and the usual portion size. The respondent burden is minimized with this procedure, but the investigator must invest a substantial amount of time initially to develop the instrument from previously obtained recall histories or dietary records.

INTERPRETATION OF DIETARY INTAKE DATA Once the food consumption data are collected, the foods must be converted to nutrients and compared with recommended levels of intake. The conversion of food intake to nutrient intake relies on food composition tables or computerized databases, occasionally supplemented with analyses of any individual foods that are not represented in the existing tables. In some cases, nutrient content may be corrected for the amounts that are actually available for metabolism. For example, algorithms have been applied to correct for iron bioavailability, based on the form of iron (inorganic iron or heme iron) and the presence in the diet of different enhancers

Table 1
Characteristics of Selected Assessment Techniques for Measuring the Dietary Intakes of Individuals

Technique	Able to measure usual intake of group	Able to measure usual intake of individual	Requires educational component[a]	Quantitative	Relative accuracy	Relative cost
Single 24-h recall	Y	N	N	Y	++	+
Multiple 24-h recalls	(Y)[b]	Y	N	Y	++	++
Single 24-h food record (self-recorded)[c]	Y	N	Y	Y	++	+
Single 24-h food record (observed)	Y	N	N	Y	+++	+++
Multiple 24-h food records (self-recorded)[c]	(Y)[b]	Y	Y	Y	++	++
Multiple 24-h food records (observed)	(Y)[b]	Y	N	Y	+++	++++
Food frequency questionnaire	Y	Y	N	N/(Y)[d]	+	+

[a]Subject must be trained in data collection technique.
[b]Data can be used to characterize intake by group, but this is not the most efficient design.
[c]Self-collected food records may report either estimated or weighed food amounts, with expected differences in accuracy and precision.
[d]Instrument can be designed to be semiquantitative.
Note: Regarding relative accuracy and relative cost, + = less accurate, ++++ = more accurate; + = less expensive, ++++ = more expensive.

Table 2
Susceptibility of Different Dietary Assessment Techniques to Measurement Error

Source of error	24-h Recall	Estimated food record (self-recorded)	Weighed food record (self-recorded)	Observed, weighed food record	Food frequency questionnaire
Omitted foods	+	+/−	+/−	−	+
Added foods	+	−	−	−	+/−
Poorly estimated food weights	+	+	−	−	+
Poorly estimated frequency of consumption	−	−	−	−	+
Day-to-day variability	+	+	+	+	−
Intentional change of diet	−	+/−	+	+	−

Source: Adapted from *ref. 1.*
Note: + = susceptible to specific type of error, +/− = may be susceptible to specific type of error, − = not susceptible to specific type of error.

or inhibitors of inorganic iron absorption (6). It is important to recognize that the accuracy of food composition tables may be affected by many different factors, including the food sampling methods (number of foods analyzed, season obtained, production site and methods), the analytic techniques and conversion factors employed, the food storage and processing techniques used by consumer, and whether or not food wastes are considered.

After converting food intake to nutrient consumption, the nutrient intake data are compared with the recommended dietary intakes (RDI) to assess the nutrient adequacy ratio. Because the RDI for all nutrients other than energy is set at the mean requirement for particular age and physiological groups plus two standards deviations (to assure that the RDI is sufficient to meet the needs of nearly all healthy individuals, ie., approx. 98%, of the group), many individuals may consume less than the RDI, yet satisfy their own nutrient requirements. Thus, adequacy of intake is sometimes also estimated as two-thirds of the RDI, or by the "probability approach." The latter method, which is currently recommended by the US National Research Council (7), assesses the likelihood that an individual's intake of a nutrient is less than his or her requirement by assuming that the group's requirement is distributed normally and that the coefficient of variation (CV) of the requirement (for nutrients other than energy) is 15% and by assigning a probability that a particular level of intake is low considering this distribution of requirements.

VALIDITY AND PRECISION OF DIETARY ASSESSMENT METHODS It is extremely difficult to validate dietary assessment methods because of true biological variation in intake and difficulty in assuring that the validation procedures themselves do not influence intake or the accuracy of the data collection technique being evaluated (8). The best validation methods rely on either surreptitious observation or comparison of intake data with biological measures of intake, such as analysis of tissue reserves or excretion of a particular nutrient or metabolite. Studies in which reported intakes were independently observed have found that low consumers tend to exaggerate their intakes and high consumers tend to underreport, resulting in the so-called "flat-slope phenomenon" (9). However, this phenomenon does not have much influence on the mean intakes by a group of individuals. Dietary assessment methods may also be compared with each other to assess their relative precision.

ANTHROPOMETRIC ASSESSMENT

Anthropometry can be defined as the measurement of the body's mass and/or dimensions. Anthropometry is a particularly attractive method of nutritional assessment because most of the techniques are relatively simple to perform, safe, cheap, and portable. On the other hand, anthropometry is relatively insensitive to recent changes in nutritional conditions and is not specific to particular nutritional deficiencies. To assure optimal accuracy and precision of anthropometric techniques, the measurement instruments should be calibrated frequently and observers should be standardized periodically.

ANTHROPOMETRIC TECHNIQUES The aspects of the body that are most commonly measured for the purpose of nutritional assessment are described briefly in this section. Measurement of body weight indicates the amount of body tissue accrued up to a particular point in time or during some period of observation. Body weight describes the combined mass of all body compartments (fat mass, fat-free tissue mass, water, and skeleton), but does not distinguish among them. Measurement of height indicates the cumulative linear growth prior to the time of the measurement or during a period of assessment. Height is measured as supine length in children less than 2 yr of age and as stature, or standing height, in older children and adults. Mid-upper-arm circumference (MUAC) is sometimes used as a screening tool in place of weight measurements. MUAC can also be used along with the triceps skinfold thickness to calculate the arm muscle area and arm fat area, which provide an estimate of the relative size of the body fat mass and fat-free mass. Measurement of skinfold thickness at various peripheral sites (arms and legs) and central sites (back, chest, abdomen) can be used to assess the amount and distribution of body fat. Elbow breadth is measured to characterize the body "frame size," which is used in the interpretation of ideal body weight of adults. Head circumference correlates with brain size and is usually used to detect microcephaly and macrocephaly in children up to 24 mo of age, but is generally not used independently as an indicator of nutritional status.

INTERPRETATION OF ANTHROPOMETRIC TECHNIQUES

Attained Size Versus Growth Attained size (e.g., body weight or height) is the product of prior nutritional and health experience and does not necessarily reflect recent events. Growth, on the other hand, refers to the change in body size during an interval of time and reflects the nutritional and health conditions during that interval. Assessment of growth requires measurements at more than one point in time. Measurements of growth are more sensitive indicators of recent nutritional circumstances than static assessments of current size.

Anthropometric Indices and Reference Data for Assessing Children An anthropometric index is a combination of two or more measurements of body size or of a measurement of body size and age. Examples of anthropometric indices are weight-for-age, height-for-age, weight-for-height, body mass index, and arm muscle area. The height-for-age index reflects achieved linear growth in relation to that expected for children in the reference population who are of the same chronological age and sex. Low height-for-age indicates shortness (which may be normal) or "stunting" (which implies that the low height is pathological). High height-for-age indicates tallness. In rare clinical cases, this may be due to endocrine disorders, such as growth hormone-producing tumors.

Weight-for-height reflects body weight in relation to that expected for children in the reference population who are of the same height and sex. Low weight-for-height indicates thinness (which may be normal) or "wasting" (which implies recent starvation or severe disease). High weight-for-height indicates over-weight or obesity. Overweight may be due to increased fat mass or lean body mass. Thus, although there is a strong correlation between overweight and obesity, the latter can only be measured by assessing adiposity directly (e.g., by measuring skinfold thickness). Nevertheless, at the population level, most individuals with high weight-for-height are obese.

Weight-for-age is useful to describe body mass in relation to that expected for children in the reference population who are of the same chronological age and sex. This index is influenced by both the height and weight of the child, making interpretation more difficult than for the two aforementioned indices. In populations that have little wasting, weight-for-age provides similar information as height-for-age.

Growth velocity refers to the change in weight or length per unit time. For example, weight velocity = $(w_2-w_1)/(t_2-t_1)$, where w_2 is the weight at the end of the interval of observation (t_2) and w_1 is the weight at the beginning of the interval (t_1). Measures of growth velocity are the anthropometric indicators that are most sensitive to an individual's recent or current nutritional situation.

Anthropometric indices can be expressed as percentiles, percent of median, or Z-scores in relation to the distribution of values in the selected reference population. Percentiles refer to the rank position of an individual's measurement on a particular reference distribution, stated in terms of what percentage of the reference group that the individual equals or exceeds. Thus, a child of a given age whose weight falls on the tenth percentile weighs the same or more than 10% of the reference population children of the same age and sex. Percentiles are often used clinically to describe the nutritional status of individuals whose data fall within the range of the reference population. In general, percentile data are easy to interpret. However, because the same interval of percentile values corresponds to different absolute amounts of weight or height at higher or lower positions of the reference distribution, it is not possible to calculate summary statistics, such as means and standard deviations of percentiles. Percentiles are also not very useful in populations where many or most individuals fall outside the range of the reference population.

The percent of median is the ratio of a measured value of an individual to the median value of the reference data for individuals of the same age or height and sex, expressed as a percentage. This index is easy to calculate and reasonably easy to interpret. For example, if a 12-mo-old boy weighs 8.12 kg and the reference median weight-for-age is 10.15 kg, the boy's percent of expected weight-for-age = (8.12)(100)/10.15 = 80%. The percent of median is interpretable even when the individual's measurement falls outside the range of the reference data. However, there is no fixed correspondence between the percent of median and the distribution of values of the reference population across age or height. For example, 80% of the median weight-for-height may be either above or below the third percentile at different ages. Moreover, the cutoffs of percent of median that are nutritionally important vary for different anthropometric indices. To approximate a cutoff of the third percentile, for example, the usual cutoff for height-for-age is 90% of the median, whereas for low weight-for-age and weight-for-height, the usual cutoff is 80% of the median.

Z-scores express the anthropometric value as the number of standard deviations (or Z-scores) below or above the reference median. The Z-score is calculated as the difference between the subject's measurement and the reference median divided by the reference standard deviation (SD). For example, if a 69-cm-tall

Table 3
Waterlow Classification of Moderate/Severe Undernutrition

	Percent median weight-for-height	
Percent median height-for-age	>80%	<80%
>90%	Normal	Wasting
<90%	Wasting	Stunting and wasting

boy weighs 6.3 kg and reference median weight-for-height for a 69-cm-tall boy is 8.5 kg and the reference SD is 1.0 kg, then the boy's Z-score weight-for-height = $(6.3-8.5)/1.0 = -2.2\ Z$. A particular Z-score value implies a constant height or weight difference in relation to the reference population median regardless of the indicator or age. Z-scores can be subjected to summary statistics, such as means and standard deviations.

Anthropometric reference data describe the characteristics of some well-defined population and are used to provide a common basis for comparing different populations. Reference data, then, do not necessarily indicate some desirable norm or target size. The World Health Organization/Centers for Disease Control (WHO/CDC) reference population is the one that is currently used most commonly for international comparisons of children (10), and public domain software is available to convert raw weight and height data into anthropometric indices using this information (11).

Anthropometric indicators are also used to classify the degree of severity of malnutrition. The Gomez classification, for example, is based on percent of median weight-for-age, with >90% of median considered to be normal, 76–90% of median labeled as mild undernutrition, 61–75% of median as moderate undernutrition, and <61% of median as severe undernutrition. The Waterlow classification is based on a cross-tabulation of percent median height-for-age and percent median weight-for-height (Table 3).

Anthropometric Indices and Reference Data for Assessing Adults Because adults have stopped growing, indicators of linear growth no longer reflect recent or current nutritional conditions. Thus, in adults, anthropometry is used primarily to determine the presence of obesity or underweight. Several different ratios of body weight in relation to height have been used to predict the likelihood of obesity. The most common indices are the body mass index (BMI) and the ponderal index. The BMI, also known as Quetelet's index, is calculated as weight (in kg)/height^2 (in m). For example, an individual of weight of 70 kg and height of 178 cm or 1.78 m has a BMI = $70/(1.78)^2 = 70/3.17 = 22$ kg/m^2. According to WHO, a BMI <18.5 indicates chronic energy deficiency, 18.5–25 is normal, 25–30 indicates mild overweight, 30–40 indicates moderately severe overweight, and >40 indicates severe overweight (12). Other classification systems suggest that a BMI >27 may be associated with an increased risk of heart disease, hypertension, and diabetes (13). The ponderal index, which is used less frequently than the BMI, is calculated as height/(weight)$^{1/3}$.

The Metropolitan Life Insurance tables of "ideal body weight" relate the weight and height of policy holders aged 25–59 to subsequent mortality. The tables indicate the weight ranges in relation to frame size that are associated with greatest longevity. These tables can be criticized because the policyholders are not representative of the general population, pre-existing disease may

have been present, and the quality of the data is suboptimal. For example, some of the weights were reported and not measured, and the subjects' shoes and clothing were often not removed. Nevertheless, the large study sample and the fact that the anthropometric data were related to a critical functional outcome—mortality—make this a valuable resource. Reference tables of the weight and height of a representative sample of noninstitutionalized US adults 18–74 y of age is also available from the US National Center for Health Statistics (NCHS), although these data have not been related to subsequent mortality.

Measurements of skinfold thickness at various superficial anatomic sites are used to estimate total body fat. Equations that have been derived from empirical observations of different populations can be used to convert the skinfold data to body density, which is, in turn, related to the percent body fat (14,15). Total fat mass can then be calculated from body weight and percent body fat.

CLINICAL ASSESSMENT

Clinical assessment of nutritional status is comprised of the standard medical history and physical examination. Whereas dietary assessment focuses on food and nutrient intake, the clinical history elicits information on symptoms that might influence the utilization of nutrients and on other factors that might be involved in the etiology of nutritional disease. For example, symptoms of diarrhea or intestinal malabsorption would increase the likelihood of nutritional depletion, even when dietary intake appears to be sufficient, and a history of prior intestinal surgery, such as ileal resection, would heighten suspicion concerning malabsorption of specific nutrients. Likewise, consumption of drugs that are known to interfere with nutrient absorption or metabolism is an important piece of information to elicit during nutritional assessment.

The physical examination includes inspection and palpation of tissues whose integrity is affected by extreme nutritional conditions. A complete discussion of the range of physical abnormalities associated with particular nutritional diseases is beyond the scope of this chapter. Nevertheless, some of the principal physical findings associated with nutritional diseases are listed in Table 4. It is important to realize that clinical evidence of nutritional deficiency or excess is generally a fairly late indicator of nutritional disease. Thus, although clinical assessment is an important component of the general nutritional evaluation, it is less useful than other methods for detecting early or mild nutritional disease.

BIOCHEMICAL ASSESSMENT

Biochemical assessment consists of laboratory analysis of:

1. The concentrations of nutrients in body tissues, circulating fluids, or excreta;
2. Carrier or storage proteins associated with these nutrients; or
3. Enzymes whose function is directly dependent on them.

In all cases, attention must be devoted to the proper collection, handling, preparation, and analysis of specimens for the results to be interpretable. Also, the range of normal values for different biochemical indicators may vary by age group, geographic setting (e.g., altitude), racial group, and presence of infection, so caution is needed in the interpretation of laboratory results.

Space does not permit a full discussion of the entire range of available biochemical assessment techniques for all nutrients, so

Table 4
Selected Physical Signs of Nutritional Disease

Anatomic site	Clinical signs (and associated nutrients)
Hair	Depigmentation (protein); alopecia, hair loss (zinc, protein)
Eyes	Xerophthalmia, Bitot spots, corneal ulceration (vitamin A); conjunctival pallor (iron, folate, vitamin B$_{12}$)
Mouth	Angular stomatitis (riboflavin, other B vitamins); glossitis, cheilosis (B vitamins); swollen, hemorrhagic gums (vitamin C)
Neck	Goiter (iodine)
Abdomen	Hepatomegaly (protein)
Bones	Rachitic rosary, flaring of long bones (vitamin D, calcium)
Skin and nails	Capillary fragility, petechiae (vitamin C); dryness, peri-follicular hyperkeratosis (vitamin A); "flaky-paint" dermatosis (protein); erythematous macular rash of exposed skin (niacin); erythema and desquamation of intertriginous areas (zinc); subcutaneous fat (energy); palmar pallor (iron, folate, vitamin B$_{12}$); nonspecific rash, nail loss (selenium)
Nervous system	Parasthesias, depressed reflexes (vitamin B$_{12}$)
Heart	Tachycardia, congestive heart failure (thiamin); cardiomegaly, arrhythmia, congestive heart failure (selenium)
Blood	Anemia (iron, folate, B$_{12}$, vitamin A), neutropenia (copper)

assessment of just three nutrients—vitamin A, iron, and zinc—will be presented in some detail. These nutrients were chosen because they illustrate a broad range of issues concerning biochemical assessment and because each of these nutrients is believed to be involved in immune function.

BIOCHEMICAL ASSESSMENT OF VITAMIN A STATUS

In well-nourished individuals, more than 90% of the total-body vitamin A is stored in the liver, and plasma retinol concentration is homeostatically regulated within a fairly narrow range. Only at the extremes of vitamin A deficiency or toxicity does the plasma retinol concentration directly reflect total body reserves *(16)*. Thus, a number of other clinical and biochemical tests have been developed in an attempt to distinguish among the categories of deficient, marginal, adequate, excessive, and toxic vitamin A status.

Direct biopsy of the liver and measurement of tissue vitamin A concentration is considered the best quantitative indicator of vitamin status, although care must be taken because of uneven distribution of vitamin A in liver tissue *(17)*. Because of the invasiveness of this procedure, however, it is generally used only to validate other indirect measures of vitamin A status *(18,19)* or to assess population status by completing autopsies of previously healthy victims of accidental deaths *(20,21)*. Recently, isotope dilution techniques using tetra-deuterated retinol have also been applied successfully to estimate total-body vitamin A pool size quantitatively *(19,22)*. This technique is still limited by the high cost of the labeled retinol and the isotope-ratio analyses, and further validation of the technique is still required for different age groups and physiological conditions.

The plasma vitamin A concentration is the biochemical test that has been used most commonly to identify individuals and populations with a high risk of vitamin A deficiency. A plasma concentration less than 10 µg/dL (0.35 µmol/L) is considered to be indicative of deficiency, and concentrations between 10 and 20 µg/dL (0.35 and 0.70 µmol/L) are felt to be consistent with marginal vitamin A status. Plasma retinol concentrations >140 µg/dL (4.9 µmol/L) are indicative of vitamin A toxicity. At the population level, when more than 20% of individuals have a plasma retinol concentration < 20 µg/dL, the population is said to have a public health problem with regard to vitamin A status *(16)*.

In addition to its lack of direct correlation with total vitamin A reserves, as described above, the major disadvantages of the plasma retinol concentration as an indicator of vitamin A status are the need to obtain venous blood, the analytic complexities (analysis generally relies on the availability of high-performance liquid chromatography), and the confounding effects of infection and protein deficiency. Because retinol-binding protein (RBP), the vitamin A carrier protein in plasma, is an acute-phase reactant, the plasma retinol concentration is diminished in the presence of infection or systemic inflammation *(23)*. Thus, this test may be unreliable in infected individuals or in populations with a high prevalence of infectious diseases; an independent biochemical indicator of systemic inflammation, such as C-reactive protein or alpha$_1$ acid glycoprotein, should probably be measured simultaneously in individuals at high risk of infection. Likewise, the plasma RBP concentration decreases in the presence of severe protein deficiency, so the plasma retinol concentration may be unreliable under this circumstance *(24)*.

The relative dose response (RDR) test was developed to overcome the inability of plasma retinol concentration to identify individuals with marginally depleted hepatic reserves. For the RDR test, plasma retinol concentration is measured immediately before and 5 h after administering a small dose (approximately 1 mg) of retinol. In depleted individuals, there is a rapid rise in plasma retinol concentration, so that the difference between the baseline and 5-h level is at least 20% of the latter value. Although the RDR test has been validated in comparison with hepatic retinol concentrations in surgical patients *(18)*, concerns have been raised about poor intraindividual reproducibility of results from one week to the next *(25)*. Because the RDR test requires two blood samples, a modified test has also been developed using an analog of retinol (didehydro-retinol, vitamin A$_2$) for the vitamin A dose *(26)*. This analog can be distinguished from the plasma retinol in the 5-h sample and interpreted in a similar way as the standard RDR test, but without the need for a baseline blood sample.

To avoid the need for any blood sampling, breast milk retinol concentration can also be used as a measure of vitamin A status of lactating women and their infants. Although the relationship between milk retinol concentration and maternal vitamin A stores is not well understood, it does appear that women with low reserves of vitamin A also have low breast milk vitamin A concentrations. Moreover, the vitamin A content of breast milk responds to supplementation of depleted women *(27)* and vitamin A fortification of foods they consume (28). Because the concentration of retinol in milk also varies in relation to milk fat content, some investigators suggest adjusting the retinol concentration for the level of fat (24).

BIOCHEMICAL ASSESSMENT OF IRON STATUS The biochemical assessment of iron status is well developed, and techniques are available to detect deficient, adequate, and excessive iron stores, as well as functional complications of iron deficiency. In the normal individual, when dietary intake or absorption of iron is low, iron can be mobilized from the storage compounds, ferritin and hemosiderin, to permit synthesis of hemoglobin and other metabolically active iron-containing compounds. When iron reserves become depleted, hemoglobin synthesis is compromised and the concentration of free erythrocyte protoporphyrin (FEP), the iron-free precursor of heme, increases in red blood cells. At the same time, the hemogobin concentration of blood begins to fall, as does the mean corpuscular volume (MCV). Iron transport in circulating blood also decreases during iron deficiency, so the percent saturation of the iron-transport protein, transferrin, is decreased. By measuring some or all of this battery of iron-related indicators, it is possible to distinguish among different stages and severity of iron deficiency or overload.

The small quantities of ferritin that are present in serum are proportional to total-body ferritin, so, in most cases, the serum ferritin concentration provides a good estimate of total-body iron reserves. Serum ferritin is generally measured by radioimmunoassay, which requires the availability of a gamma counter, or more recently by enzyme-linked immunoassay. A concentration of less than 12 µg/L is generally accepted as evidence of iron deficiency (29), although some authors recommend a slightly higher cutoff value (30). Serum ferritin is a less reliable indicator of iron deficiency in infants (31) and shortly after initiating iron therapy (29). In both cases, serum ferritin concentrations may fall in the normal range despite the presence of other evidence of iron deficiency. The serum ferritin concentration also increases considerably in the presence of infection or systemic inflammation, and several field studies have found that the presence of infection markedly reduced the apparent prevalence of iron deficiency (32,33). Therefore, this test should not be applied in infected individuals or those with elevated acute-phase reactants.

Hemoglobin concentration can be measured spectrophotometrically, and dedicated portable instruments are now available for field use (34). Normal values for hemoglobin vary with age, sex, altitude, and, possibly, race (29). Although iron deficiency can certainly be the precursor of anemia (low hemoglobin concentration), there are many other causes as well. Thus, other nutritional deficiencies, hereditable diseases, infections, blood loss, and other reasons for anemia must be considered in the differential diagnosis. For this reason, a combination of tests is generally recommended for the diagnosis of iron-deficiency anemia.

The MCV can be measured by electronic counter or derived from the ratio of hematocrit (packed red blood cell volume) to red cell count obtained microscopically. The former technique is more precise and less subject to the sampling problems that occur with determination of hematocrit. The MCV also varies with age, so appropriate reference values must be applied. Anemia associated with a low MCV is most often due to iron deficiency, although thalassemia minor produces a similar constellation of findings.

The FEP, which is assayed fluorometrically, can be used to distinguish between iron-deficiency anemia and thalassemia minor. FEP is elevated in the former condition but not the latter. However, FEP also increases in the presence of inflammation and lead toxicity, so these conditions must be excluded for a definitive interpretation of this test result.

Because most iron in serum is bound to transferrin, the transferrin saturation is measured as the ratio of serum iron to total iron-binding capacity, expressed as a percentage. In the presence of iron deficiency, the transferrin saturation falls below 7–16%, depending on age (29). The transferrin saturation value is also affected by diurnal variation in serum iron concentration and by inflammation, so it is generally used as aid in diagnosis rather than a primary diagnostic tool. Transferrin saturation >60% is likely to indicate iron overload.

BIOCHEMICAL ASSESSMENT OF ZINC STATUS Zinc was selected as one of the nutrients reviewed in this section because it poses special problems for biochemical assessment. Unlike the situation with inadequate dietary intake of vitamin A and iron, where tissue stores can be mobilized to maintain normal physiological function until the deficiency becomes severe, there does not seem to be a large, readily exchangeable reserve of zinc (35). Instead, tissue zinc concentrations appear to be conserved by decreased fecal excretion of endogenous zinc and, in children, by a deceleration or cessation of growth. Thus, there may be no readily detectable biochemical evidence of early zinc deficiency, despite its negative impact on tissue synthesis and physical growth. Only with more severe or prolonged deficiency does plasma zinc concentration decline.

The mean plasma zinc concentration in humans is approximately 100 µg/dL (approx. 15 µmol/L), which is considerably less than its concentration in many other tissues (36,37). The total amount of zinc circulating in plasma is less than 0.2% of the total-body zinc content. Because the concentration of zinc in tissues such as muscle and liver is approximately 50 times greater than that of plasma, small variations in uptake or release of zinc from these tissues can have a profound effect on the plasma zinc concentration. For these reasons, it is not surprising that plasma zinc concentration does not portray total-body zinc stores reliably under all circumstances. For example, release of zinc from muscle tissue that is catabolized during starvation can result in transient, seemingly paradoxical, elevations in plasma zinc (38). On the other hand, meal consumption induces a considerable postprandial reduction in plasma zinc concentration, even when dietary zinc intake and tissue reserves are presumably adequate (39). Despite these apparent discrepancies, when zinc intake of adult volunteers is severely restricted, the plasma zinc concentrations do fall within a fairly short period of time (40).

Although low plasma zinc concentration may be a useful sign of zinc deficiency in many situations, there are many factors that confound the interpretation of this test. Determinants of plasma zinc concentration other than recent zinc consumption are hypoalbuminemia, which influences absorption and transport of zinc (41), infection (42,43) and other forms of stress, such as tissue injury imposed by surgery (44) and strenuous physical exercise (45), pregnancy (46), and intestinal diseases that interfere with zinc absorption (37).

The relationship between plasma zinc concentration and infection is of special importance because many of the same populations that are at greatest risk of zinc deficiency also have high rates of infections. A number of experimental studies, both in laboratory animals and adult human volunteers, have found a consistent decline in plasma zinc concentration shortly before or after the onset of febrile infections (43) or administration of bacterial endotoxin (42). These changes in circulating zinc levels are associated with elevations of selected plasma proteins, such as C-reactive protein, alpha$_1$- antitrypsin, haptoglobin, and alpha$_1$ acid glycoprotein, a predictable set of metabolic reactions to infection or tissue injury known as the acute-phase response. Researchers have found that the acute-phase response is mediated by cytokines such as interleukin-1 and tumor necrosis factor-alpha, which stimulate secretion of interleukin-6 and glucocorticoids, both of which activate, in turn, hepatic synthesis of metallothionein (MT), an intracellular metal-binding protein (47). Studies have confirmed that MT stimulates hepatic uptake of zinc and the consequent reduction in plasma zinc during inflammation (48).

Despite the fairly consistent occurrence of transient hypozincemia during acute, febrile, experimentally induced infections and following the administration of endotoxin or cytokines, several factors can modify the impact of natural infections on plasma zinc concentrations. For example, there is some evidence from clinical studies that the magnitude of change in plasma zinc concentration is related to the severity and stage of infection (49). Several studies have also shown that the cytokine response to infection is reduced in malnourished experimental animals (50) and in humans with protein-energy malnutrition (50,51). Thus, infection may exert less of a confounding effect on plasma zinc concentration in malnourished individuals.

The relationship between infection and plasma zinc has been examined in several cross-sectional, community-based studies in developing countries (32,52,53). Notably, none of these three studies detected significant relationships between the presence of infection and the children's serum or plasma zinc concentrations. The discrepancy between these results and those of the aforementioned experimental trials and clinical studies of adults may be due to methodological differences in the research protocols or to differences in the severity of the infections. For example, the studies of experimentally induced infections (42) and the clinical studies of hospitalized patients (43) were conducted in adults, whereas the community-based studies were carried out in children. Thus, it is conceivable that the distinct age ranges of the study populations contributed to the different outcomes. Also, it is likely that the children included in the community studies had less severe infections than those that were induced in the adult subjects, thereby reducing the impact of the children's infections on their plasma zinc concentrations. Whatever the explanation, the results of the small number of community studies that are currently available suggest that common, acute infections encountered in community settings may not undermine the utility mean plasma zinc concentration as an indicator of zinc status.

Several additional pieces of evidence suggest that the mean plasma zinc concentrations of groups of individuals provide useful information about their zinc status, even though the results in any particular individual may be less reliable. First, in a recently completed meta-analysis of the effects of zinc supplementation on children's growth, one of the factors that predicted whether a particular population had a significant growth response to zinc was the baseline mean plasma zinc concentration (54). Study populations with lower initial mean plasma zinc concentrations had significantly greater increments in weight and length in response to zinc supplementation. Second, in the same analysis, there were clear and sizable increases in the mean plasma zinc concentrations fol-

lowing supplementation. Thus, this assessment tool appears to be helpful both to predict whether a population is likely to have a growth response to zinc supplementation (indicating that they are zinc deficient) and to monitor intake of zinc supplements.

For plasma zinc concentrations to be useful indicators of a population's zinc status, care must be taken to avoid technical problems that may affect the results of the analyses. Many of these problems, which are related to either blood sampling or specimen processing, have been discussed previously (55,56). Briefly, plasma zinc concentration varies according to the time or day, proximity of meals, and occurrence of recent exercise or other forms of stress. Ideally, these conditions should be standardized, to the extent possible, in field settings. The sizable magnitude of the postprandial decline in plasma zinc concentration argues for particular attention to this factor. Once the blood sample is obtained, the serum or plasma should be separated as quickly as possible to prevent contamination with zinc released from cells (57). Likewise, results from hemolyzed samples should be considered unreliable because of the loss of cellular zinc to serum or plasma. Other issues, such as contamination of specimens with zinc from needles, syringes, anticoagulants, transfer pipets, rubber stoppers, dirty glassware, and impure reagents have been reviewed previously (55).

In summary, there is clear evidence that severe infections and other forms of stress, particularly when encountered in hospitalized adults or accompanied by fever or other indicators of an acute-phase response, produce a fall in plasma zinc concentrations. Nevertheless, infections do not seem to affect the mean plasma zinc concentrations of groups of children examined in community-based studies. Because the mean plasma zinc concentration has been found to be a useful predictor of children's growth response to zinc supplementation, this laboratory test should be considered a potentially useful indicator of the zinc status of populations of children, even in settings where there is a high prevalence of common childhood infections.

FUNCTIONAL ASSESSMENT

Functional assessment refers to the examination of some physiologic or behavioral competence that may be affected by nutritional deficiency or excess. Specific categories of function that are affected by nutritional status are structural integrity, host defense, transport, hemostasis, reproduction, nerve function, and work capacity/hemodynamics (58). Examples of functional assessment tests include evaluation of immune responses, psychomotor development, muscle strength, and sexual maturation. Test procedures developed to evaluate these specific categories of function have been reviewed comprehensively (58), so they will not be amplified any further in this chapter. Examination of immune responses will be described in detail in subsequent sections of this volume.

SUMMARY

Nutritional assessment is comprised of dietary, anthropometric, clinical, biochemical, and (sometimes) functional techniques to evaluate the nutritional condition of an individual or population. Dietary assessment provides information on the likelihood of low (or high) intake, and consequent risk of undernutrition (or overnutrition), but it does not characterize nutritional status *per se*. Therefore, studies of dietary intake must be combined with other measures to characterize actual nutritional conditions. Anthropometric assessment encompasses the measurement of body mass and/or physical dimensions. Anthropometry is simple to perform, safe, inexpensive, and portable, but it is relatively insensitive to recent changes in nutritional conditions and is not specific to particular nutritional deficiencies. Clinical assessment includes the medical history, which is targeted to elicit information on symptoms and signs that might influence the utilization of nutrients, and physical examination of specific issues whose integrity can be affected by extreme nutritional conditions. Biochemical assessment consists of laboratory analysis of:

1. The concentrations of nutrients in body tissues, circulating fluids, or excreta;
2. Carrier or storage proteins associated with these nutrients; and
3. Enzymes whose function is directly dependent on them.

Finally, functional assessment refers to the examination of physiologic or behavioral functions that are affected by nutritional deficiency or excess. Combinations of these tests can be applied to identify those individuals or population groups that might benefit from some form of nutritional (or other therapeutic) intervention and to evaluate the success of these interventions.

REFERENCES

1. Gibson RS. Principles of Nutritional Assessment. Oxford University Press, New York, 1990.
2. Beaton GH, Bengoa JM. Nutrition in Preventive Medicine. World Health Organization, Geneva, 1976.
3. Golden MHN. The role of individual nutrient deficiencies in growth retardation of children as exemplified by zinc and protein. In: Waterlow JC, ed, Linear Growth Retardation in Less Developed Countries, pp. 143–63. Raven, New York, 1988.
4. Beaton GH, Milner J, Corey P, McGuire V, Cousins M, Stewart E, et al. Sources of variance in 24-hour recall data: implications for nutrition study design and interpretation. Am J Clin Nutr 1979; 32:2546–59.
5. Nelson M, Black AE, Morris JA, Cole TJ. Between- and within-subject variation in nutrient intake from infancy to old age: estimating the number of days required to rank dietary intakes with desired precision. Am J Clin Nutr 1989; 50:155–67.
6. Murphy S, Beaton GH, Calloway DH. Estimated mineral intakes of toddlers: predicted prevalence of inadequacy in village populations in Egypt, Kenya, and Mexico. Am J Clin Nutr 1992; 56:565–72.
7. National Research Council. Nutrient Adequacy: Assessment Using Food Consumption Surveys. National Academy Press, Washington, DC, 1986.
8. Block G. Review of validations of dietary assessment methods. Am J Epidemiol 1982; 115:492–505.
9. Gersovitz M, Madden JP, Smiciklas-Wright H. Validity of the 24-hour dietary recall and seven-day record for group comparisons. J Am Diet Assoc 1978; 73:48–55.
10. Hamill PVV, Drizd TA, Johnson CL, Reed RB, Roche AF, Moore WM. Physical growth: National Center for Health Statistics percentiles. Am J Clin Nutr 1979; 32:607–29.
11. Dean AG, Dean JA, Burton AH, Dicker RC. Epi Info, Version 5: A Word Processing Database, and Statistical Program for Epidemiology on Microcomputers. USD, Incorporated, Stone Mountain, GA, 1990.
12. World Health Organization. Physical Status: The Use and Interpretation of Anthropometry. WHO Technical Report Series No. 854, WHO, Geneva, 1995.
13. Health and Welfare Canada. Promoting Healthy Weight: A Discussion Paper. Health Services and Promotion Branch, Health and Welfare, Ottawa, 1988.
14. Durnin JV, Wormsley J. Body fat assessed from body density and its estimation from skinfold thickness: measurements on 481 men and women aged from 16 to 72 years. Br J Nutr 1974; 32:77–97.
15. Jackson JS, Pollock ML. Generalized equations for predicting body density of men. Br J Nutr 1978; 40:497–504.
16. Underwood BA. Methods for assessment of vitamin A status. J Nutr 1990; 120:1459–63.
17. Olson JA, Gunning DB, Tilton RA. The distribution of vitamin A in human liver. Am J Clin Nutr 1979; 32:2500–7.
18. Amedee-Menasme O, Anderson D, Olson JA. Relation of the relative dose response to liver concentrations of vitamin A in generally well nourished surgical patients. Am J Clin Nutr 1984; 39:898–902.
19. Furr HC, Amedee-Menasme O, Clifford AJ, Bergen HR III, Jones AD, Anderson DP, et al. Vitamin A concentrations in liver determined by isotope dilution assay with tetradeuterated vitamin A and by biopsy in generally healthy adult humans. Am J Clin Nutr 1989; 49:713–16.
20. Hoppner K, Phillips WEJ, Murray P, Perrin DK. Survey of liver vitamin A stores in Canadians. Can Med Assoc J 1968; 99:983–6.
21. Raica NJ, Scott BS, Lowry L, Sauberlich HE. Vitamin A concentration in human tissue collected from five areas of the United States. Am J Nutr 1972; 25:291–6.
22. Haskell MJ, Handleman GJ, Peerson JM, Jones AD, Atai Rabbi M, Awal MA, et al. Assessment of vitamin A status by the deuterated-retinol-dilution technique and comparison with hepatic vitamin A concentration in Bangladeshi surgical patients. Am J Clin Nutr 1997; 66:67–74.
23. Filteau SM, Morris SS, Abbott RA, Tomkins AM, Kirkwood BR, Arthur P, et al. Influence of morbidity on serum retinol of children in a community-based study in northern Ghana. Am J Clin Nutr 1993; 58:192–7.
24. World Health Organization. Indicators for Assessing Vitamin A Deficiency and Their Application in Monitoring and Evaluating Programmes. WHO, Geneva, 1994.
25. Solomons NW, Morrow FD, Vasquez A, Bulux J, Guerrero A-M, Russell RM. Test–retest reproducibility of the relative dose response test in Guatemalan adults: issues of diagnostic sensitivity. J Nutr 1990; 120:728–44.
26. Tanumihardjo SA, Furr HC, Erdman JWJ, Olson JA. Use of the modified relative dose response (MRDR) assay in rats and its application to humans. Eur J Clin Nutr 1990; 4:219–24.
27. Stoltzfus R, Hakimi M, Miller KW, Rasmussen KM, Dawiesah S, Habicht JP, et al. High dose vitamin A supplementation of breast-feeding Indonesian mothers: effects on the vitamin A status of mother and infant. J Nutr 1993; 123:666–75.
28. Arroyave G, Aguilar JR, Flores M, Guzman MA. Evaluation of Sugar Fortification with Vitamin A at the National Level. Pan American Health Organization, Washington DC, 1979.
29. International Nutritional Anemia Consultative Group. Iron Deficiency in Infancy and Childhood. The Nutrition Foundation, Washington DC, 1979.
30. Yip R, Dallman PR. Iron. In: Ziegler EE, Filer LJ Jr, eds., Present Knowledge of Nutrition, 7th ed., ILSI, Washington DC, 1996.
31. Siimes MA, Addiego JE Jr, Dallman PR. Ferritin in serum: diagnosis of iron deficiency and overload in infants and children. Blood 1974; 43:581–90.
32. Brown KH, Lanata CL, Yuen ML, Peerson JM, Butron B, Lonnerdal B. Potential magnitude of the misclassification of a population's trace element status due to infection: example from a survey of young Peruvian children. Am J Clin Nutr 1993; 58:549–54.
33. Kuvibidila S, Mbele V, Yu L, Warrier R, Lemonnier D. Usefulness of serum ferritin in evaluation of iron status in Zairean women of the reproductive age group. Am J Clin Nutr 1991; 53:P22 (abstract).
34. PATH. Anemia Detection Methods in Low-Resource Settings: A Manual for Health Workers. PATH, Seattle, WA, 1997.
35. King JC. Assessment of zinc status. J Nutr 1990; 120:1474–9.
36. Jackson MJ. Physiology of zinc: general aspects: In: Mills CF, ed., Zinc in Human Biology, Springer-Verlag, London, 1989.
37. Cousins RJ. Systemic transport of zinc. In: Mills CF, ed, Zinc in Human Biology. Springer-Verlag, London, 1989.
38. Henry RW, Elmes ME. Plasma zinc in acute starvation. Br Med J 1975; 625–6.
39. Hambidge KM, Goodall MJ, Stall C, Pritts J. Post-prandial and daily

changes in plasma zinc. J Trace Elem Electrolytes Health Dis 1989; 3:55–7.

40. Baer MT, King JC. Tissue zinc levels and zinc excretion during experimental zinc depletion in young men. Am J Clin Nutr 1984; 39:556–70.

41. Smith KT, Failla ML, Cousins RJ. Identification of albumin as the plasma carrier for zinc absorption by perfused rat intestine. Biochem J 1978; 184:627–33.

42. Beisel WR, Pekarek RS, Wannemacher RW Jr. The impact of infectious disease on trace-element metabolism of the host. In: Hoekstra WG, Suttie J, Ganther H, Mertz W eds, Trace Element Metabolism in Animals—2, pp. 217–40. Baltimore University Park Press, Baltimore, MD, 1973.

43. Falchuk KH. Effect of acute disease and ACTH on serum zinc proteins. N Engl J Med 1977; 296:1129–34.

44. Shenkin A. Trace elements and inflammatory response: implications for nutritional support. Nutrition 1995; 11:100–5.

45. Lukaski HC, Bolonchuk WW, Klevay LM, Milne DB, Sandstead HH. Changes in plasma zinc content after exercise in men fed a low-zinc diet. Am J Physiol 1984; 247:E88–93.

46. Swanson CA, King JC. Reduced serum zinc concentration during pregnancy. Obstet Gynecol 1983; 62:313–8.

47. Schroeder JJ, Cousins RJ. Interleukin 6 regulates metallothionein gene expression and zinc metabolism in hepatocyte monolayer cultures. Proc Natl Acad Sci 1990; 87:3137–41.

48. Rofe AM, Philcox JC, Coyle P. Trace metal, acute phase and metabolic response to endotoxin in metallothionein-null mice. Biochem J 1996; 314:793–7.

49. Beisel WR. Zinc metabolism in infection. In: Brewer GJ, Prasad AS, eds., Zinc Metabolism: Current Aspects in Health and Disease. Alan R. Liss, New York, 1977.

50. Kauffman CA, Jones PG, Kluger MJ. Fever and malnutrition: endogenous pyrogen/interleukin-1 in malnourished patients. Am J Clin Nutr 1986; 44:449–52.

51. Keusch GT. Malnutrition, infection, and immune function. In: Suskind RM, Lewinter-Suskind L, eds., The Malnourished Child. Raven, New York, 1990.

52. Ruz M, Solomons NW, Mejia LA, Chew F. Alterations of circulating micronutrients with overt and occult infections in anaemic Guatemalan preschool children. J Food Sci Nutr 1995; 46:257–65.

53. Friis H, Ndhlovu P, Kaindera K, Sandstrom B, Michaelsen KF, Vennervald BJ, et al. Serum concentration of micronutrients in relation to schistosomiasis and indicators of infection: a cross-sectional study among rural Zimbabwean school children. Eur J Clin Nutr 1996; 50:386–91.

54. Brown KH, Peerson JM, Allen LH. Effect of zinc supplementation on children's growth: a meta-analysis of intervention trials. Bibliotheca Nutritio Dieta 1998; 54:76–83.

55. Smith JC, Holbrook JT, Danford DE. Analysis and evaluation of zinc and copper in human plasma and serum. J Am Coll Nutr 1985; 4:627–38.

56. Clegg MS, Keen CL, Lönnerdal B, Hurley LS. Influence of ashing techniques on the analysis of trace elements in animal tissue. Biol Trace Elements Res 1981; 3:107–15.

57. English, Hambidge KM. Plasma and serum zinc concentrations: effect of time between collection and separation. Clin Chim Acta 1988; 175:211–6.

58. Solomons NW, Allen LH. The functional assessment of nutritional status: principles, practice, and potential. Nutr Rev 1983; 41:33–50.

2 Evaluating Malnutrition

What Should the Physician Look For?

CHARLES H. HALSTED, MD

INTRODUCTION

Using a variety of defining criteria, malnutrition with increased in-hospital morbidity was described 2 decades ago in 48% of medical patients (1) and in 50% of surgical patients (2). Other historical studies showed that malnutrition leads to more frequent postoperative complications in surgical patients (3,4) and to more frequent hospital admissions in the elderly (5). A recent study from the Netherlands that used two methods of multivariate analysis to correct for concomitant disease severity found evidence of malnutrition in 45–57% of patients with gastrointestinal and other medical diseases as a predictor of increased morbidity and mortality (6). However, in spite of these compelling data, the clinical definition of malnutrition remains enigmatic and few physicians consider the nutritional state in the patient evaluation or treatment plan.

Malnutrition, or bad nutrition, occurs under many guises in clinical medicine, from the severely obese patient with multiple medical complications to the severely underweight patient who presents to the clinician with one or more of a variety of underlying disorders. As examples, the severely obese patient may exhibit hypertension, dyspnea with signs of fluid retention, epigastric pain due to esophageal reflux, and joint pain secondary to osteoarthritis. At the other end of the spectrum, clinical malnutrition may present as loss of subcutaneous fat with muscle wasting, or, less obvious, normal fat but decreased muscle mass with peripheral edema, and may be a major feature of medical and surgical patients with chronic wasting diseases such as autoimmune deficiency syndrome (AIDS) and cancer, acute pancreatitis, intestinal diseases including malabsorption syndromes, renal or hepatic failure, and prolonged surgical convalescence associated with wound or systemic infections. Given this array of clinical presentations, it is important to approach malnutrition in a systematic fashion, using the conventional approaches of the patient history, physical findings, selective laboratory tests, and specialized procedures. Because the topic of obesity is covered separately in Chapter 26, this chapter will focus on the undernourished patient.

From: *Nutrition and Immunology: Principles and Practice* (ME Gershwin et al. eds.), © Humana Press, Inc., Totowa, NJ

BODY COMPOSITION AND THE METABOLIC RESPONSE TO ILLNESS

The approach to nutritional assessment requires physician understanding of certain principles of the composition of the body compartments and the metabolic response to starvation and the stress of illness. In general, the human body is composed of about 25% fat (more in women than in men), 35% extracellular fluid, and the remaining 40% as the bony skeleton and the body cell mass, or metabolic machinery of the body, which is contributed by cells of the intestine, liver, kidneys, brain, heart, hematopoietic system, and skeletal muscle (7). Energy balance is maintained by the ingestion of dietary calories commensurate with expenditure of energy necessary to sustain life. In health, the resting, or basal, energy expenditure (BEE) is equivalent to the dietary calorie requirement and is a function of body weight (W), height (H), age (A), and gender. This value is given by the Harris–Benedict formula as

$$BEE = 66.473 + 13.751W + 5.0033H - 6.7550A \text{ kcal/d for men}$$

$$BEE = 65.50955 + 9.4634W + 1.8496H - 4.6756A \text{ kcal/day for women (8)}.$$

As an alternative to this formula, a simple rule of thumb is that basal or resting energy expenditure is roughly equal to the patient's body weight in kg times 25 kcal/d. To these calculations, one should add an additional 10% for the thermic effect of digestion and an exercise factor ranging from 10% for minimal to 40% for highly active. While the acutely ill patient is at bedrest, the stress of illness increases energy expenditure by 12.5% for every degree of fever over 37°C. Acute surgery adds 25%, sepsis 70%, and burns up to 100% to the BEE.

Simple starvation, defined functionally as failure to ingest or absorb sufficient dietary calories to sustain normal weight and function, results in body energy conservation with a decrease in the metabolic rate and BEE. Energy needs are maintained mainly by the mobilization of body fat stores at about 150 g/d, or 1350 kcal/d of stored energy, which is sufficient to sustain life for 2–3 mo, depending on body fatness. At the same time, body protein stores of about 12 kg are conserved by reducing protein catabolism (breakdown) from 75 to 20 g/d (9). Starved individuals present a clinical picture of cachexia with profound loss of body fat as

Table 1
Evaluating Patient History for Malnutrition

Cause	Clinical setting examples	Deficiencies
Impaired intake or absorption	Poverty, eating disorders, gastrointestinal obstruction, intestinal malabsorption, chronic alcoholism, AIDS	Body fat, skeletal muscle, multiple micronutrients
Abnormal nutrient metabolism	Major surgery, sepsis, cancer, AIDS, chronic liver disease	Skeletal and visceral protein, multiple micronutrients
Increased nutrient losses	Chronic diarrhea of any cause, inflammatory bowel disease	Visceral protein, phosphate, zinc, iron, magnesium, potassium

well as progressive depletion of skeletal muscle. On the other hand, metabolic stress such as occurs with acute surgery, sepsis, or other critical illness is associated with increased metabolic rate with release of glucocorticoids, epinephrine, and cytokines, all of which accelerate skeletal muscle catabolism with increased use of protein at rates up to 240 g/d in order to meet requirements of gluconeogenesis. Untreated, this rate of protein loss can result in 50% depletion of body protein stores within 2–3 wk, a condition incompatible with life. Because accelerated muscle protein catabolism is associated with increase in extracellular water, stressed individuals may not be underweight, but typically manifest clinical edema and progressive depletion of skeletal muscle (10). However, a more common clinical picture is the malnourished patient who requires surgery or develops acute or chronic illness and demonstrates a mixture of starvation and protein catabolism. Examples include patients with inflammatory bowel disease, recurrent pancreatitis, chronic infection such as AIDS and tuberculosis, and invasive cancers. These individuals are likely to present with combinations of edema together with rapid loss of body fat and skeletal muscle superimposed on an underlying body habitus of starvation.

THE PATIENT HISTORY OF MALNUTRITION

In modern society, malnutrition is typically associated with poverty, an eating disorder, chronic alcoholism or other substance abuse, a variety of gastrointestinal diseases, cancer, and chronic infectious illness such as tuberculosis and AIDS. These disorders fall under three broad etiologies of malnutrition: impaired dietary intake, inadequate absorption of nutrients, and altered metabolism with excessive nutrient losses (Table 1). Regardless of the cause, the experienced physician should focus the patient history on change in the patient's body weight and appetite, as well as on features of the underlying illness that may contribute to malnutrition. Most patients are aware of their usual body weight, which can be compared to the recorded weight; an unintentional decrease in body weight greater than 10% from the usual weight is considered significant. Concomitant with the physician's disease-oriented history, it is useful in most instances to complement the history with information from the clinic or hospital dietitian on the amount and composition of the patient's diet. For example, the physician's history of anorexia and weight loss in the absence of other clinical findings would prompt suspicion of a psychological condition such an anorexia nervosa or depression, which would be substantiated by the dietitian's quantification of reduced and inadequate food intake. A history of diarrhea and weight loss in the absence of anorexia would prompt suspicion of a malabsorption syndrome such as chronic pancreatitis, the short-bowel syndrome, or celiac disease, which would be supported by the dietitian's

history of adequate dietary intake. A history of indolent fever with weight loss would prompt consideration of AIDS or other chronic infectious diseases, whereas weight loss with diarrhea and crampy abdominal pain should lead to consideration of inflammatory bowel disease.

THE PHYSICAL EXAMINATION

The physical examination should focus initially on estimation of weight loss, then on changes in body composition and specific features of nutrient deficiencies. Body weight is considered in terms of its percentage of the patient's ideal body weight for height. Although tables are available for ideal weight for height (11), a workable formula (± 10%) is that a healthy man should weigh 106 lbs for 5 ft of height, plus another 6 lbs for every additional inch, whereas a healthy woman should weigh 100 lbs for the first 5 ft., then 5 lbs for each additional inch (12). Actual body weight less than 90% of ideal is considered significant, whereas a patient weight less than 70% of ideal body weight is consistent with severe malnutrition, and weight less than 60% is tantamount to impending death. An alternative approach is to calculate the body mass index (BMI), a measurement that accounts for body height that is given as BMI = body weight (in kg)/ body height (in m²). BMI values below 19 are consistent with malnutrition and those below 13 are incompatible with life, whereas values greater than 25 are consistent with overweight and >30 with progressive obesity, and increased risk of mortality is a J-shaped function of the BMI value (13).

ANTHROPOMETRY Anthropometry refers to measurements of subcutaneous body fat and skeletal muscle. Practically, anthropometry requires the use of skinfold calipers and a tape measure. Body fat is estimated from the thickness of the skinfold of the posterior mid-upper arm and ranges between 7.5 and 12.5 mm for men and between 10.0 and 16.5 mm for women. Muscle mass is estimated by measuring the mid-upper-arm circumference (in cm), then subtracting 3.14 (pi) times the triceps skinfold thickness (in cm). Normal mid-arm circumference values range between 20.0 and 25.5 cm for men and between 18.5 and 23.0 cm for women (14). The limitations of anthropometry include the need for an experienced observer, special calipers for measuring skinfold thickness, and the frequently obscuring variables of altered body water resulting in edema or dehydration.

SKIN TESTS AND LYMPHOCYTE COUNTS Malnutrition causes a shrinkage of lymphoid structures, a decrease in total lymphocytes, and a reduction in cell-mediated immune function, but an unchanged immunoglobulin response to infection. The total lymphocyte count, given as total white blood cells times percent as lymphocytes, correlates roughly with severity of malnutrition when the result is less than 1000/mm³. However, the total lympho-

Table 2
Physical Examination of the Malnourished Patient

Deficiency	Physical finding
Body fat	Weight loss
Essential fatty acids	Seborrheic rash
Protein	Weight loss, edema, decreased temporal and skeletal muscle mass, parotid enlargement
Vitamin A	Follicular hyperkeratosis, night blindness
Thiamine	Peripheral neuropathy, ophthalmoplegia, cerebellar gait, memory loss, confabulation
Niacin	Hyperpigmentation of sun exposed areas of skin, dementia
Riboflavin	Severe glossitis, angular stomatitis, cheilosis
Pyridoxine	Glossitis, cheilosis, angular stomatitis, peripheral neuropathy
Folic acid	Glossitis, pallor
Vitamin B_{12}	Glossitis, pallor, loss of position and vibratory sensation
Vitamin C	Perifollicular hemorrhage, swollen bleeding gums, arthropathy
Magnesium	Hyperactive reflexes
Zinc	Poor taste, delayed wound-healing, "flaky paint" rash on lower extremities
Iron	Pallor, spooning of nails
Phosphorus	Acute disorientation

cyte count is very nonspecific because it can be affected by many underlying conditions that contribute to malnutrition, such as acute or chronic infection, uremia, cancer, cirrhosis, and acute trauma. A similar caveat applies to comprehensive skin testing, where anergy is anticipated in severe malnutrition but also in the same variety of underlying diseases (15).

SPECIFIC PHYSICAL FINDINGS IN MALNUTRITION A systematic approach to the physical examination, including the general appearance, skin, mucus membranes, and neurological examination provides specific clues to specific features of malnutrition (12, Table 2). In the absence of skinfold calipers, the depletion of body fat can be estimated by the "pinch test," in which only minimal tissue is present between the examiner's thumb and first finger when compressing the posterior skin of the upper arm. Deficiency of visceral protein and skeletal muscle protein is evident by the presence of edema, easily plucked hair, transverse depigmentation of the nails, sunken temporal muscles, decreased arm circumference as evidenced by the ability to circumscribe the upper arm with one's forefinger and thumb, and muscle wasting of the thighs according to visual inspection. Specific skin rashes include perifollicular hemorrhages with corkscrew hairs in vitamin C deficiency (classical scurvy), a dry "flaky paint" rash on the lower extremities consistent with zinc deficiency, hyperpigmentation of skin-exposed areas consistent with niacin deficiency (classical pellagra), a "goose bump" rash with dry skin in vitamin A deficiency, and naso-labial seborrhea in essential fatty acid deficiency. Examination of the conjunctivae is useful for evaluating the severity of anemia. Angular stomatitis and cheilosis, or cracking of the corners of the mouth and of the lips, nonspecifically suggest deficiency of riboflavin, pyridoxine, or niacin, whereas glossitis, or a smooth red tongue, is a nonspecific manifestation of vitamin C, riboflavin, vitamin B_{12}, folate, pyridoxine, or niacin

deficiency. Hypertrophied and easily bleeding gums suggest vitamin C deficiency of scurvy, but it can also occur in dilantin toxicity. Parotid enlargement and loss of tooth enamel are indicative of recurrent vomiting with protein deficiency, prompting a potential diagnosis of anorexia/bulimia or gastric obstruction. The neurological system provides many signs of specific deficiency states. Thiamine deficiency, common in chronic alcoholic patients, is typically manifest by combinations of ophthalmoplegia, a wide-based cerebellar gait, a peripheral stocking-glove type of neuropathy (Wernicke syndrome), and, more severely, with cerebral degeneration with memory loss and confabulation (Korsakoff syndrome). Peripheral neuropathy is also consistent with pyridoxine deficiency or underlying chronic diabetes. A specific neuropathy with loss of distal position and vibratory sensation is characteristic of the subacute combined degeneration of vitamin B_{12} deficiency.

SUBJECTIVE GLOBAL ASSESSMENT

A group in Toronto developed an approach to nutritional assessment based on recognition and grading of a series of clinical parameters in the history and physical examination (16,17). According to this approach, the most significant five features of the patient evaluation include:

1. Chronic (approx 6 wk) and recent (2 wk) weight loss;
2. Anorexia with change in dietary pattern;
3. Significant gastrointestinal symptoms, including nausea, vomiting, and diarrhea;
4. Decrease in energy level and functional performance;
5. Assessment of the severity of the underlying illness.

The most significant four features of the physical examination include graded severity of:

1. Loss of subcutaneous fat tissue;
2. Skeletal deltoid and quadriceps muscle wasting;
3. Peripheral and/or sacral edema;
4. Abdominal ascites.

On the basis of these criteria, patients are rated as being well nourished, moderately malnourished, or severely malnourished. The subjective global assessment is comparable with other schemes to assess relationships between malnutrition and in-hospital morbidity and mortality. However, as in all aspects of medicine, the effectiveness of the subjective global assessment is dependent in large part on the skill and experience of the observer.

THE USE OF THE LABORATORY IN NUTRITIONAL ASSESSMENT

BLOOD MEASUREMENTS As in all aspects of cost-effective diagnosis and management, the judicious use of the laboratory is an essential part of assessing the spectrum and severity of malnutrition in any given patient. Visceral proteins can be estimated by the serum albumin, a highly sensitive but only minimally specific assay test of malnutrition (Table 3). Serum albumin represents about 40% of the total-body albumin pool, which is maintained by hepatic synthesis and which turns over at a rate of about 10% per day. Clinically, the serum albumin level is diminished in any condition that results in decreased hepatic synthesis or uncompensated accelerated turnover and by fluid shifts and/or excessive hydration that increase the intravascular fluid space (12). Common clinical conditions that lower the serum albumin level in the absence of malnutrition include acute or chronic liver disease

Table 3
Laboratory Assessment of Malnutrition

Assay	Interpretation
Serum albumin	Low value also seen in liver disease, nephrotic syndrome, and any condition expanding the vascular volume; Normal value excludes protein malnutrition
Pre-albumin, transferrin, fibronectin	Low value may be more specific for malnutrition
Vitamin and mineral assays	Generally specific, but do not always assess body stores or functional reserve
Serum homocysteine	Elevation consistent with folate or vitamin B_{12} deficiency
Serum methylmalonic acid	Elevation specific for vitamin B_{12} deficiency

which reduces liver albumin synthesis and the nephrotic syndrome or chronic inflammatory bowel disease, which accelerates albumin loss through the urine or intestine. Although simple starvation reduces albumin synthesis, the body's albumin pool may be conserved at the cost of depletion of body fat and skeletal muscle. On the other hand, the stress of surgery, infection, or other inflammatory illness contributes to the development of malnutrition while lowering the serum albumin level by dramatically decreasing albumin synthesis at the same time as expanding the extracellular fluid space. Given this multitude of variables, the best that can be said about the serum albumin assay is that a normal value in a nonstarving individual excludes malnutrition. Because the half-life of circulating albumin is about 3 wk, measurements of shorter-lived visceral proteins has been advocated as part of laboratory armamentarium for nutritional assessment. Several of these proteins with their normal half-lives include the prealbumin–retinol-binding protein complex (2–3 d), transferrin (8 d), and fibronectin (1 d). Among these, the serum prealbumin–retinol-binding complex may predict a worse prognosis in patients with gastrointestinal diseases, whereas serum transferrin appears to correlate with the nitrogen balance test in assessing recovery during nutritional support (18). However, like the serum albumin, these measurements can be affected nonspecifically by acute infection and renal and liver failure.

If the history and physical exam suggest specific micronutrient deficiencies, they can be identified by an array of commonly available measurements of vitamins and minerals in the plasma, usually by high-pressure liquid chromatography, and each with their own range of normal values established by the testing laboratory (12; Table 3). A low value of vitamin A is found in intestinal malabsorption syndromes and chronic liver disease, whereas a high level suggests excessive use and potential toxicity. The 25-OH vitamin D assay is an accurate measure of vitamin D status; low levels are seen in intestinal malabsorption syndromes and marginal levels may be found in postmenopausal women at risk for osteoporosis. Both serum folate and vitamin B_{12} can be measured accurately in the serum and are used to differentiate the cause of macrocytic anemia. However, as there may be overlap, newer complementary tests have been developed based on the metabolic cofactor functions of these vitamins. Elevation of the plasma homocysteine level is consistent with either folate or vitamin B_{12} deficiency, whereas the plasma methylmalonic acid level is only elevated in vitamin B_{12} deficiency (19).

SPECIALIZED PROCEDURES

BODY COMPOSITION BY BIOELECTRICAL IMPEDANCE ANALYSIS Bioelectrical impedance analysis (BIA) is a method for assessment of body compartments based on electrical conductivity. In practice, current-inducing electrodes are placed on the dorsal surfaces of the hands and feet, followed by passage of a weak and painless electrical current through the body. Because impedance to current flow is greatest through fat and least through water, calculations can be derived from the measured impedance of current through these two body compartments. Lean body or fat-free mass is given by subtracting fat mass from body weight, or by dividing the measurement of total body water by 0.73 (7). The practical value of BIA is a matter of debate, with a lack of clear consensus on its usefulness in the severely obese or critical or chronically ill patient (20). Conductivity measurements are compromised in the severely obese, where body fat and water are concentrated centrally away from the limbs to the intraabdominal region. On the other hand, the BIA is limited in critical or chronic illness by its inability to accurately detect differences between intracellular and extracellular water compartments. This lack of precision becomes important in estimating the body cell mass or principal metabolic machinery, which is represented by intracellular water and solids and is diminished in malnutrition. However, the extracellular fluid compartment is typically increased in malnourished and stressed patients, especially in those who have received excessive intravenous fluids or who exhibit ascites or renal or cardiac failure. Because size and changes in the body cell mass compartment are probably the most important predictors of mortality and/or response to nutritional support in the malnourished patient, the development of reliable techniques to differentiate intracellular from extracellular water is critical to the use of BIA in the acutely ill patient. At present, BIA can be considered a useful tool in comparing nutritional status among free-living population groups and in stable chronically ill patients in whom fluid retention is not a major factor (Table 4).

ENERGY EXPENDITURE Actual measurement of the patient's energy expenditure is useful in arriving at an accurate formulation of the amount and composition of dietary, enteral, or parenteral energy requirements. Although estimations of energy needs can be approximated on the basis of body weight and severity of clinical illness, mixed pictures arise in the patient with chronic inflammatory illness, in whom increased metabolic needs may be superimposed on starvation, where needs are typically reduced, and in the obese patient, whose body weight is overrepresented by stored energy as fat.

Indirect calorimetry is a procedure in which the energy cost of metabolism is calculated by respiratory gas exchange using measurements of the volumes (V) in liters of oxygen consumed and of carbohydrate produced over a given period of time. These values are entered into the modified Weir equation (21): Energy expenditure (kcal) = $3.9\ V_{O_2} + 1.1 VC_{O_2}$. Values are normalized for 24 h. The procedure is reliable in the bedridden patient receiving a constant influx of parenteral or enteral nutrition with constant body temperature during the day and is best achieved using an air-collection canopy or tracheostomy attachment via a mobile

Table 4
Specialized Procedures

Procedure	Interpretation
Bioelectrical impedance analysis (BIA)	Assessment of body fat and total body water; other compartments problematic
Indirect calorimetry	Reasonably accurate assessment of actual energy expenditure and requirements
Creatinine height index	Accurate measure of skeletal muscle protein mass; requires stable renal function and accurate 24-h urine collection
Nitrogen balance	Measures balance of net anabolism or catabolism; useful in surveillance of efficacy of nutritional support
Muscle function tests	Most sensitive measure of malnutrition, but quantitation and/or equipment can be problematic

metabolic cart. These measurements can also be used to calculate the respiratory quotient (RQ), or ratio of V_{CO_2}-produced to O_2 consumed. As an index of substrate use, the RQ is normally around 0.85 during consumption of a mixed diet or formula, but decreases to less than 0.7 when the body draws on its fat stores, as in starvation, and increases to greater than 1.0 when carbohydrate is provided in excess of needs with resultant lipogenesis. In addition to assessing total energy needs in the hospitalized patient candidate for nutrition support, indirect calorimetry is useful in monitoring the adequacy and appropriate formulation of nutrition support of the malnourished acute or chronically ill patient.

URINE MEASUREMENTS Twenty-four-hour urine collections are an excellent source of nitrogenous compounds that can be used to estimate both muscle mass and the status of anabolism, or net muscle protein accretion, versus catabolism, or net muscle protein breakdown. The success of these measurements hinges most importantly on the reliability and completeness of the urine collection as well as on optimal steady-state renal function for the individual patient, which, in turn, demands adequate constant hydration.

Creatinine Excretion Because creatinine is the metabolic product of creatine, a nearly exclusively skeletal muscle protein, measurement of the daily urinary excretion of creatinine can be used as an accurate estimation of muscle mass both at baseline and in comparisons during nutritional support. Approximately 18 kg of fat-free muscle releases 1 g creatinine daily for urinary excretion. The *creatinine coefficient* is the amount of creatinine released from muscle per kilogram of body weight. For healthy men, the creatinine coefficient is 23 mg/kg of ideal body weight, calculated as described above on the basis of body height. The creatinine coefficient for a healthy woman is 18 mg/kg ideal body weight. These values are independent of age and stable renal function, but may vary by 10% according to diet and accuracy in urine collection. The *creatinine height index* provides a close approximation of the patient's skeletal muscle mass and is calculated as the ratio of the patient's 24-h urine creatinine excretion to the predicted creatinine coefficient of a healthy person at the patient's ideal body weight. In practice, a creatinine height index

of less than 70% is indicative of severe depletion of muscle protein with estimated high likelihood of morbidity and mortality *(11,12,22)*.

Nitrogen Balance This measurement allows the physician to determine whether the patient is in a state of net anabolism or catabolism of muscle protein. As indicated, during starvation or stress, skeletal muscle and visceral protein are continuously broken down to amino acids used to meet the body's energy needs through gluconeogenesis. Muscle and visceral protein losses are balanced by the intake of protein-sparing calories and protein, which can be administered orally, by feeding tube, or by parenteral nutritional support, depending on the clinical condition of the patient. Dietary intake must be calculated carefully by a dietitian using daily calorie and protein counts, whereas intakes of protein and calories from enteral and parenteral formulas are more readily available. Calculation of nitrogen balance requires the measurement of nitrogen in all potential excretory sources. Urinary urea nitrogen measurement is available in most community hospitals, from which total nitrogen can be calculated by dividing by 0.85. However, measurement of total nitrogen excretion by the more specialized Kjeldahl technique is more precise and takes into account other sources of nitrogen such as urine ammonia that increases significantly in patients with chronic liver disease *(23)*. Measurement of total nitrogen in gastrointestinal excreta is essential in patients with protein-wasting disorders such as the inflammatory bowel diseases and in patients with pancreatic or enterocutaneous fistulas. In practice, the nitrogen balance is the net difference between protein nitrogen entering the patient and protein nitrogen exiting the patient through all routes. For this calculation, 1 g of nitrogen is equivalent to 6.25 g of protein (or 6.0 g of protein in parenteral solutions). Ideal nitrogen balance values fall between 0 and +1.0; negative values reflect the severity of the patient's metabolic response to illness and requirement for nutritional support *(12)*.

MUSCLE FUNCTION TESTS Various muscle function tests have been promoted as sensitive measures of malnutrition. These tests include measurements of hand-grip strength using a hand dynamometer or, subjectively, by squeezing the practitioner's fingers, and respiratory muscle strength by blowing against a movable paper object *(24)*, as well as the involuntary response of the adductor pollicis muscle to electrical stimulation *(25)*. The force frequency and relaxation rate of this muscle in response to a standard stimulus is more sensitive than anthropometry or serum protein measurements and can predict malnutrition before other clinical measurements of skeletal muscle deficiency *(25)*. Although sensitive, these tests are limited by the lack of quantitative standardization and by the limited availability of equipment.

Summary: Why Assess Patient Malnutrition? This chapter has provided an outline to the approach to assessing malnutrition in the clinic or hospitalized patient that follows the conventional paradigm of the patient history, physical examination, laboratory tests, and specialized procedures. Although this outline presents a reasonable clinical approach for the physician, it should, in many instances, be complemented by the dietitian's evaluation of the amount and composition of the diet. With the exception of certain of the procedures, every other method of evaluation discussed is in easy reach of the primary care physician who practices in the community setting.

Given the wide availability of methods of nutritional assessment, one must ask why only the rare practitioner considers this approach in his or her overall clinical evaluation of the sick patient. Overlooking nutritional assessment can be ascribed in part to the fact that clinical nutrition education is included in only a minority of medical schools and residency training programs and, in spite of great patient interest, a convincing argument for the role of nutrition in health and disease has not yet been made to the medical profession. There are several sides to this argument.

Clearly, malnutrition is both common and consequential in hospitalized patients, where clinical evidence continues to exist in about half of all patients with implications for prolonged hospital stay and complications of clinical illness (1,2,6). These statistics provide an *a priori* argument not only for improved awareness and techniques for evaluating nutrition but increased efforts to treat malnutrition in order to prevent costly and life-threatening complications. Furthermore, in the age of cost-conscious managed care, awareness of nutritional deficiencies in the outpatient setting and their dietary or other specialized treatment would appear to be a compelling argument for applying nutritional practices in the maintenance of health and prevention of disease. Yet, many of the tests (e.g., serum proteins, skin allergy testing, BIA, subjective global assessment) lack specificity or precision and there are very few unequivocally convincing clinical trials that prove that hospital admissions, morbidity, and mortality can be prevented or treated by proper diet and/or nutritional support. As outlined in a recent National Institutes of Health sponsored conference, the only clinical condition in which nutritional support unequivocally saves lives is the short-bowel syndrome, whereas conclusive clinical trials are lacking in common conditions such as inflammatory bowel disease, pancreatitis, and critical and postoperative care (26). Nevertheless, a compelling argument can be made for nutritional assessment as a guide to nutritional prevention or support in conditions where malnutrition has clearly been shown to present a risk of acute or prolonged illness, morbidity, and mortality, such as in severely underweight individuals and in severely catabolic patients.

REFERENCES

1. Weinsier RL, Hunker RN, Krumdieck CL, Butterworth CE Jr. Hospital malnutrition: a prospective evaluation of general medical patients during the course of hospitalization. Am J Clin Nutr 1979; 32:418–26.
2. Bistrian BR, Blackburn GL, Hallowell E, Heddle R. Protein status of general surgical patients. JAMA 1974; 239:858–60.
3. Studley HO. Percentage of weight loss. A basic indicator of surgical risk in patients with chronic peptic ulcer. JAMA 1936; 106:458–60.
4. The Veterans Affairs Total Parenteral Nutrition Cooperative Study Group. Perioperative total parenteral nutrition in surgical patients. N Engl J Med 1991; 325:525–32.
5. Sullivan DH. Protein-energy undernutrition and the risk of mortality within one year of hospital discharge: a follow-up study. J Am Geriatr Soc 1995; 43:507–12.
6. Naber THJ, Schermer T, de Bree A, Nusteling K, Eggink L, Kruimel JW, et al. Prevalence of malnutrition in nonsurgical hospitalized patients and its association with disease complications. Am J Clin Nutr 1997; 66:1232–9.
7. Shizgal HM. The effect of malnutrition on body composition. Surg Gynecol Obstet 1981; 152:22–6.
8. Harris JA, Benedict FG. Standard Basal Metabolism Constants for Physiologists and Clinicians, a Biometric Study of Basal Metabolism in Man, pp. 223–50. JB Lippincott, Philadelphia, 1919.
9. Cahill GF. Starvation in man. N Engl J Med 1970; 282:668–75.
10. Long CL, Lowry SF. Hormonal regulation of protein metabolism. J Parenter Enter Nutr 1990; 14:555–62.
11. Blackburn GL, Bistrian BR, Maini BS, Schlamm HT, Smith MF. Nutritional and metabolic assessment of the hospitalized patient. J Parenter Enter Nutr 1977; 1:11–22.
12. Halsted CH, Van Hoozen CM, Ahmed B. Preoperative nutritional assessment. In: Quigley EMM, Sorrell MF, eds., The Gastrointestinal Surgical Patient: Preoperative and Postoperative Care, pp. 27–49. Williams and Wilkins, Baltimore, MD, 1994.
13. Bray, G. Obesity. In: Ziegler EE and Filer LJ, eds., Present Knowledge of Nutrition, pp. 19–22. ILSI, Washington DC, 1996.
14. Heymsfield SB, Casper K. Anthropometric assessment of the adult hospitalized patient. J Parenter Enter Nutr 1987; 11:36S–41S.
15. Dominioni L, Dionigi R. Immunological function and nutritional assessment. J Parenter Enter Nutr 1987; 11:70S–72S.
16. Baker JP, Detsky AS, Wesson DE, Wolman SL, Stewart S, Whitewell J, et al. Nutritional assessment; a comparison of clinical judgment and objective measurements. N Engl J Med 1982; 306:969–72.
17. Detsky AS, Baker JP, Mendelson RA, Wolman SL, Wesson DE, Jeejeebhoy KN. Evaluating the accuracy of nutritional assessment techniques applied to hospitalized patients: methodology and comparisons. J Parenter Enter Nutr 1984; 8:153–9.
18. Church JM, Hill GL. Assessing the efficacy of intravenous nutrition in general surgical patients: dynamic nutritional assessment with plasma proteins. J Parenter Enter Nutr 1987; 11:135–9.
19. Savage DG, Lindenbaum J, Stabler SP, Allen RH. Sensitivity of serum methylmalonic acid and total homocysteine determinations for diagnosing cobalamin and folate deficiencies. Am J Med 1994; 96: 239–46.
20. National Institutes of Health Technology Assessment Conference. Conference Summary. Bioelectrical impedance analysis in body composition measurement. Am J Clin Nutr 1996;64:524S–32S.
21. Weir JB. New methods for calculating metabolic rate with special reference to protein metabolism. J Physiol 1949; 109:1–9.
22. Heymsfield SB, Arteaga C, McManus C, Smith J, Moffitt S. Measurement of muscle mass in humans: validity of the 24-hr urinary creatinine method. Am J Clin Nutr 1983; 37:478–94.
23. Soberon S, Pauley MP, Duplantier R, Fan A, Halsted CH. Metabolic effects of enteral formula feeding in alcoholic hepatitis. Hepatology 1987; 7:1204–09.
24. Windsor JA, Hill GL. Weight loss with physiologic impairment, a basic indicator of surgical risk. Ann Surg 1988; 207:290–6.
25. Russell D McR, Leiter LA, Whitwell J, Marliss EB, Jeejeebhoy KN. Skeletal muscle function during hypocaloric diets and fasting: a comparison with standard nutritional assessment parameters. Am J Clin Nutr 1983; 37:133–8.
26. Klein S, Kinney J, Jeejeebhoy KN, Alpers D, Hellerstein M, Murray M, et al. Nutrition support in clinical practice: review of published data and recommendation for future research directions. Am J Clin Nutr 1997; 66:683–706.

3 Evaluation of the Immune System in the Nutritionally At-Risk Host

Jonathan Powell, Andrea T. Borchers, Steven Yoshida, and M. Eric Gershwin

INTRODUCTION

Information on the influence of nutrition on immune function generally shows that suboptimal nutrition results in immunological deficiencies. Specific influences of nutrition on immunity have recently been reviewed by us *(1)* and are summarized in Tables 1–4.

As with other animal physiological systems, usable energy and the structural components required to build an immune system are derived through food intake. Without adequate nutrition, the immune system is clearly deprived of components needed to generate an effective immune response. A few of the immunological parameters that are often used as measures of the status of the immune system and its responsiveness to antigenic challenges include leukocyte number and mobility, oxidant balance, protein activity, antibody production, and interleukin (IL) release *(51)*.

The nutritional deficiencies that are of particular interest here involve those that compromise an individual's ability to resist infectious micro-organisms or cancerous growths. Decreased leukocyte proliferation and phagocytic activity could result in less clonal expansion of microbe-specific clones of lymphocytes and less vigorous microbial elimination. Shifts in oxidant balance will have repercussions on the cell cycle. In immune responses, proteins play vital roles as antibodies, cytokines, acute-phase proteins, components of the complement pathways, transcription factors, and enzymes. Alterations in proteins could, therefore, lead to immunologically important changes in enzyme-dependent antioxidant protection (e.g. selenium–glutathione peroxidase), transcription regulation (e.g. zinc-finger proteins), complement activation, antibody-mediated virus neutralization, and intercellular communication via cytokines. This, in turn, would have myriad effects on immune responsiveness and homeostasis through the disruption of cooperative leukocyte activity. Thus, the immune problems related to nutritional deficiencies could range from increased opportunistic infections and cancers to suboptimal responses to vaccinations, and perhaps other immunological disorders such as allergies. Major components of the immune system in humans and, where relevant, techniques for assessment of their function are outlined below. In particular, a tier system, which considers different local amenities, is proposed for assessment of immune parameters.

THE IMMUNE SYSTEM

PHYSICAL BARRIERS The first line of defense is the intact skin. Its impermeable nature is fortified by lactic acid and fatty acids, which decrease the pH of sweat and sebaceous secretions; this has an inhibitory effect on most bacterial growth. Similarly, the inner epithelial regions of the body are protected by mucosal layers which block the attachment of bacteria to the underlying cells. The mechanical clearing of mucus and the foreign entities trapped within it is accomplished by ciliary movement, coughing and sneezing in the lung, or peristalsis in the gut. Tears, saliva, and urine perform a washing function to protect epithelial boundaries. In addition, these mucosal and fluid layers often possess bactericidal activity due to the presence of leukocytes, antibodies, acids, metals, and enzymes.

Normal bacterial flora, typically of the skin or intestinal lumen, also protect the host from pathogenic microbes through competition for nutrients and the release of inhibitory compounds. For example, lactic acid is produced by commensal bacterial species, and colicins, antibacterial proteins produced by *Escherichia coli,* disturb the membrane of certain bacteria by forming voltage-dependent channels. When these protective microbes are disturbed through antibiotic treatment, opportunistic infections may ensue.

PHAGOCYTES Phagocytes are cells that consume other cells and particles and become important following breaches of physical barriers. Phagocytosis, an early development in the evolution of the immune system, is an activity widely used in both innate and acquired immune responses. Neutrophils (polymorphonuclear cells) and macrophages are the two main phagocytes and both are produced in the bone marrow and released into blood. Mature neutrophils are characterized by a multilobed nucleus and a large reservoir of cytoplasmic granules that are used in the degradation of phagocytosed bacteria. Myeloperoxidase, defensins, bactericidal/permeability-increasing factor, and cathepsin G are contained in the "primary azurophilic granules," whereas lactoferrin, lysozyme, alkaline phosphatase, and cytochrome b_{558} are found in the secondary granules of neutrophils.

From: *Nutrition and Immunology: Principles and Practice* (ME Gershwin et al. eds.), © Humana Press, Inc., Totowa, NJ

Table 1
Immune Consequences of Nutritional Depletion

Nutrient	Decrease in	Increase in
Food restriction (2,3)	• Immunocompetence at less than 60% of body weight • CD4+/CD8+ ratio • Plasma complement	• Circulating B cells • Circulating antibodies
Caloric restriction (mice and rats) (4–8)	• Tumor virus expression and malignancies • Proliferation of autoreactive B1 cells • Pro-inflammatory and Th1 cytokines (IL-6, TNFα and TGFβ)	• T-Cell proliferative response
Severe protein and protein-energy deficiency (9–11)	• Humoral and cell-mediated parameters	• Oxidative stress
Protein deficiency (mice)[a] (12–17)	• Delayed-type hypersensitivity • Circulating IgG • Tissue repair • Macrophage functions	• Th2 tolerance • Oxidative stress • Splenic suppressor T cells
Amino acid restriction (arginine and glutamine particularly) (18)	• Immune competence, because arginine promotes T-cell development, growth, and thymic integrity, and glutamine is an energy source for leukocytes	
Nucleic acid restriction (19,20)	• Natural-killer activity • Recovery in sepsis • Cell-mediated immune response including delayed-type hypersensitivity, graft rejection, IL-2 production, T-cell proliferation, polymorph, and natural-killer cell functions (mice)	
Fatty acid supplementation (21,22)	• Inflammation, helped by $n3$ fatty acids • Fatty acid composition and fluidity of cell membranes as influenced by diet	• Immune suppression, with saturated fats being the most immunosuppressive • Fatty acid composition and fluidity of cell membranes as influenced by diet

Note: All data from humans except where indicated in mice or rats.
[a]Mice fed an even moderately protein-deficient diet will reduce their food intake, resulting in protein-energy malnutrition.

Macrophages circulate in the blood as monocytes (52) (normally 1–6% of circulating leukocytes) and then undergo further maturation to become tissue macrophages or histiocytes. They are widely distributed in the host and, in different tissues, attain distinct morphological characteristics of separate nomenclature, such as Kupffer cells in liver or osteoclasts in bone. Macrophage granules differ from those in neutrophils in that they are cytoplasmic bodies and contain acid hydrolases such as proteases, nucleases, and lipases. Importantly, unlike the polymorphonuclear cells, macrophages can recycle degraded antigen to the cell surface for antigen presentation to lymphocytes (see the following subsection).

Phagocytes recognize bacteria in a number of ways, ranging from nonspecific attachment via hydrophobicity to specific receptor–ligand interactions. In any case, particles >100 nm in diameter activate intracellular contractile systems, which trigger phagocytosis and fusion of the cytoplasmic granules with the particle-containing phagosome. Phagocytes also generate reactive oxygen molecules for the killing of micro-organisms and this activity is called the respiratory, oxidative, or metabolic burst due to the characteristic increase in oxygen consumption (53). Cells are protected from their own toxic oxidative compounds by several antioxidant systems, including vitamins C and E, the sulfhydryl-containing tripeptide reduced glutathione, and enzymes such as catalase, which enzymatically converts H_2O_2 to water and oxygen.

The longer life-span of macrophages (months) compared to neutrophils (<48 h) is reflected by differences in their rate of degradation of engulfed materials. Phagocytosis by macrophages tends to be slower than by neutrophils and the metabolic burst is less intense. Such a strategy provides short- and long-term phagocytic function in the elimination of microbes and other particulate foreign materials.

As with all circulating leukocytes, measurement of the percentage of neutrophils and monocytes is a useful indicator of immune status in an individual. This may be assessed by microscopic analysis and counting of cells in a blood film (blood count) or by using flow cytometry, which sorts cells based on their size, granularity, or specific cell surface antigens that are detected with fluorescent monoclonal antibodies. The flow cytometer uses a hydraulic system to pass single cells, from a cell suspension, before a laser source so that leukocytes may be individually phenotyped. Prior to analysis, cells are incubated with commercially available fluorescent monoclonal antibodies, allowing identification of different leukocyte subtypes or their degree of activation. Flow cytometry is an indispensable tool for sophisticated immunological diagnostics and research. A wide range of fluorescent probes are

Table 2
Vitamins and the Immune System

Vitamin A (2,23–27)
  Deficiency reduces leukocyte numbers, lymphoid tissue weights, complement, T-cell functions, tumor resistance, NK⁻ cell numbers, antigen-specific IgG and IgE, and Th2 numbers
  Deficiency increases IFN-γ synthesis [except in one study (28)]
  Supplementation increases lymphocyte proliferation, tumor resistance, graft rejection, and cytotoxic T-cell activity
  Excess vitamin A has adjuvant effects, perhaps by inhibiting T-cell apoptosis
  Important for maintaining the integrity of epithelial and mucosal boundaries, as Th2 growth factor

Vitamin B Complex (2,29–32)
  Pyridoxine (B6) deficiency reduces lymphocyte numbers and proliferative responses to mitogen, lymphoid tissue weights, graft rejection, IL-2 production, DTH reactions, antibody responses
  Pyridoxine supplementation protects against the immunosuppressive effects of UV-B radiation
  B12 deficiency depresses phagocyte functions, DTH responses, T-cell proliferation
  Biotin deficiency reduces thymic weights, antibody responses, lymphocyte proliferation
  Pantothenic acid deficiency reduces antibody responses
  Thiamin deficiency reduces thymic weight, antibody responses, PMN mobility
  Riboflavin deficiency decreases antibody responses, thymic weight, circulating lymphocyte numbers

Vitamin C (31–33)
  Deficiency lowers phagocyte activity, tumor resistance, DTH reactions, graft rejection, wound repair
  Antioxidant function protects phagocytes from auto-oxidation

Vitamin D (34,35)
  Stimulates monocyte and macrophage development and phagocytosis
  Selectively suppresses Th1, and not Th2 or CD8⁺ T-cell activity

Vitamin E (31–33, 36–39)
  Deficiency reduces lymphocyte proliferation, phagocyte functions, tumor resistance
  Supplementation increases lymphocyte proliferation, antibody levels, DTH reactions, IL-2 and 6-keto PGF1a production, phagocytosis, Th1 activity
  Supplementation reduces PGE_2 synthesis

Table 3
Trace Elements and the Immune System

Copper (40–43)
  Deficiency reduces antibody production, phagocytic activity, IL-2 production, T cell proliferation, and neutrophil respiratory burst and candidacidal activity in mice and rats; decreases T-cell proliferation in humans
  Deficiency increases B-cell numbers
  Involved in complement function, cell membrane integrity, Cu–Zn superoxide dismutase (SOD), immunoglobulin structure

Iron (41,44)
  Deficiency reduces DTH reaction, graft rejection, and cytotoxic activity of phagocytes
  Low plasma iron selectively inhibits proliferation of Th1, and not Th2, cells
  High plasma iron interferes with IFN-γ activity
  Important in the formation of reactive oxygen and radicals during respiratory burst
  Component of metalloenzymes

Magnesium (45,46)
  Deficiency increases thymic cellularity, eosinophils, IL-1, IL-6, TNF-α, and histamine levels
  Deficiency reduces acute-phase proteins and complement activity
  Influences cytotoxicity of CTL through interactions with ATP and adhesion molecules
  A component of metalloenzymes

Selenium (47–49)
  Deficiency reduces antibody production, cytokine synthesis, cell-mediated cytotoxicity, lymphocyte proliferation
  A component of the antioxidant enzyme glutathione peroxidase

Zinc (41,50)
  Important for thymocyte development, T-cell function, and thymic integrity
  Deficiency results in reductions in T-cell development, thymic hormone release, and T-cell functions
  Component of many proteins including zinc-finger transcription factors, Cu-Zn SOD, prolactin, and MHC class I

Table 4
Antioxidants and the Immune System

Antioxidant defenses include antioxidant vitamins and trace
    element components of antioxidant enzymes.
Dietary oils oxidized by heating or frying may compromise
    antioxidant defenses.
Kwashiorkor is characterized by oxidant stress.
CD8$^+$ T cells may be more susceptible to oxidant damage than
    CD4$^+$ T cells.
Because cell-mediated immune responses produce reactive oxygen
    and radical species, the Th1 cell may be an important focus for
    feedback inhibition by products of inflammation.

available for measuring not only the presence of cell-surface markers (e.g., CD [clusters of differentiation] and adhesion molecules), but also intracellular molecules (e.g., cytoskeleton, DNA) and cellular processes (e.g., calcium release, cell cycle). The capacity to concurrently stain for more than one marker or process and the ability to quantitate the intensity of fluorescence give the user the ability to monitor the status of specific cell types *(54)*.

Functional studies of phagocytes include examining the phagocytic and chemotactic activities, lysosomal activity, metabolic burst, and the production of IL-1 by resting and stimulated macrophages and neutrophils *(55)*. The antigen-presenting capacity of macrophages can also be measured. Short-term (hours to days) cell culturing are usually sufficient to study these cellular functions. The phagocytic activity of macrophages can be assessed through the incubation of cells with phagocytic materials. Uptake of bacteria can be determined by the number of colonies recover-

able from the culture medium (and, therefore, not phagocytosed). The uptake of plastic beads is quantified by microscopic examination and counting of beads.

The ability of leukocytes to migrate toward a chemoattractant source is also a measure of immunological responsiveness. One classic method for examining this ability is the use of a Boyden chamber. In this two-compartment vial, cells are placed in one end and a chemoattractant material is added to the other. Migration is assessed by counting the number of cells that cross the boundary between the two compartments. An alternative to measuring migration is the observation of morphological changes believed to precede cell movement *(56)*.

Oxidative burst is most commonly measured through the production of reactive oxygen species (ROS), such as H_2O_2 and superoxide anion, or the generation of reactive nitrogen intermediates. Most commonly, colorimetric assays are used when color changes are detected either with a spectrophotometer or an ELISA reader *(57,58)* (enzyme-linked immunosorbent assays [ELISAs] will be described later). The measurement of IL-1 and other cytokines will be presented in the subsection on cytokines.

LYMPHOCYTES AND ANTIGEN PRESENTATION All leukocytes (Table 5) develop from a unique, self-renewing, pluripotential hematopoietic stem cell *(59),* and different developmental signals and tissue microenvironments give rise to the diversity of white blood cells. There is much interest in the identification, purification, and nature of this stem cell, as it may be ideal for bone marrow transplantation. Such a cell can potentially reconstitute the full range of leukocytes without the hazards of a graft-versus-host (GVH) reaction that may occur following the implantation of more mature effector donor cells. In GVH disease,

Table 5
The Leukocytes

Cells	Characteristics and functions
Lymphocyte	
B	Dominant B cells in the peritoneal cavity and gut-associated lymphoid tissue (GALT); produce IL-10 and autoantibodies; B1a expresses surface CD5 marker, whereas B1b does not.
B1a, B1b B2	B Cells normally found in the circulation; they produce antibodies to foreign antigens; CD5 marker not present.
T	
CD4$^+$ CD8$^-$	T Helper cells; Th1 and Th2 promote cell-mediated and antibody-mediated immune responses, respectively; Th1 produces IL-2 and IFN-γ; Th2 produces IL-4, IL-5, and IL-10
CD4$^-$CD8$^+$	T Cytotoxic cells that kill other cell types; also T suppressor cells that regulate immune responses by cytotoxicity and cytokines.
CD4$^-$CD8$^-$	T Cytotoxic cells that often express the γδ TCR and are situated at GALT.
NK	Cytotoxic for some virus-infected and tumor cells; producer of many cytokines.
Phagocyte	
Neutrophil (PMN)	First-line defense against microbes; found in circulation and GALT; producer of enzymes and reactive oxygen
Monocyte/macrophage	Monocyte found in the circulation; macrophage is the activated form of the monocyte; localized in tissues; producer of enzymes, cytokines, and reactive oxygen; important antigen-presenter to T cells.
Granulocyte	
Eosinophil	Important in antihelminth response; producer of enzymes, IL-5, reactive oxygen; involved in IgE-mediated allergies by their Fcε receptors.
Basophil/mast cell	Basophils are in the circulation, whereas mast cells are localized in tissues; producers of vasoactive molecules during the inflammatory response; involved in IgE-mediated allergies by their Fcε receptors.
Thrombocyte	
Platelet	Involved in blood coagulation; producer of vasoactive molecules and arachidonic acid metabolites.

the donor immune system recognizes the host as foreign and initiates a reaction to recipient tissues. It is still unresolved whether the implantation of donor stem cells without also manipulating the tissue microenvironments, some of which change with age (e.g., thymus), can fully reconstitute an entire immune system. Lymphocytes are key cells of the acquired immune response most commonly the subject of investigation when assessing immune function and are, therefore, discussed in some detail here.

T (THYMIC-DEPENDENT) LYMPHOCYTES T Lymphocytes develop from self-renewing progenitors which migrate from the bone marrow to the thymic gland, where maturation occurs *(60,61)*. Surface markers are commonly used in determining the developmental stage of thymocytes; progenitors are initially CD3$^-$CD4$^-$CD8$^-$, but following gene rearrangement in the thymic cortex, the T-cell receptor (TCR) is expressed (CD3$^+$). The $\gamma\delta$ T cells remain CD4$^-$CD8$^-$, whereas the $\alpha\beta$ T cells convert to a CD4$^+$CD8$^+$ phenotype and mature to either CD4$^+$CD8$^-$ (helper T) or CD4$^-$CD8$^+$ (cytotoxic T) cells. Positive clonal selection results in the restriction of T cells to recognize host major histocompatibility complex (MHC). Finally, thymocytes migrate to the thymic medulla, where clones recognizing self-antigen–MHC complexes are eliminated (negative selection) to minimize the potential for autoreactivity. Mature T cells are then released into the peripheral circulation. The mammalian thymus begins to atrophy during puberty, but T-cell development may shift to other tissues, in particular, the gastrointestinal tract *(62,63)*.

T cells normally only recognize antigen that is presented to them by an antigen-presenting cell (APC) such as a macrophage or dendritic cell. APCs process and present antigen with either MHC class I or class II. Both MHC class I and II molecules are transmembrane heterodimers which contain structural domains formed by disulfide bridging. MHC class I heterodimers are composed of a nonpolymorphic β_2-microglobulin, from chromosome 15, and a polymorphic α-chain with three disulfide-linked domains. Class II antigens are formed by polymorphic α- and β-chains, each with two immunoglobulin domains. Both MHC molecules contain clefts that bind peptide antigens through noncovalent interactions. MHC class I is usually involved in the presentation of endogenous antigen to CD4$^+$ T cells, allowing the detection of abnormal cellular proteins that may arise, for example, from tumorigenesis or viral infections. In contrast, MHC class II presents protease-degraded exogenous antigen to CD8$^+$ T cells. In both cases, interaction of the MHC–antigen complex and TCR are required for antigen recognition, although additional APC–T-cell interactions of costimulatory molecules are required to determine the magnitude and type of T-cell response.

The TCR, which is expressed with only a single antigenic specificity, is a heterodimer composed of disulfide-linked α- and β-chains *(64,65)* or γ- and δ-chains *(66)*. The two isotypes ($\alpha\beta$ and $\gamma\delta$) are encoded by separate genes and show different antigen specificity, MHC restriction, effector functions, and anatomical location. The TCR includes a complex of nonpolymorphic accessory proteins (CD3) required for TCR expression and function. The T-cell receptors bind to the MHC-presented peptide antigens via noncovalent molecular interactions such as electrostatic charges, hydrogen-bonding, and Van der Waals forces.

A major feature of the adaptive immune system is immunological memory, which reduces the probability of disease recurrence in normal individuals. Following the initial contact with an immunogen, clonal selection of lymphocytes occurs, allowing rapid expansion of antigen-specific T and B cells upon secondary antigenic exposure. Phenotypic and functional differences readily distinguish memory from naive lymphocytes. Memory T cells are more readily stimulated by succeeding contact with antigens and there are alterations in the expression of various T-cell surface markers. Adhesion molecules increase and there is a change in the isoform of the leukocyte common antigen, namely CD45, which is found in a high-molecular-weight form (CD45RA) on naive T cells and a low-molecular-weight form (CD45RO) on memory cells. The change from a CD45RA to CD45RO phenotype suggests T-cell activation, although in the absence of antigenic stimulation, CD45RO$^+$ cells may revert to the RA phenotype.

HELPER T CELLS (CD4$^+$CD8$^-$) Depending on local signaling and soluble mediators, activated CD4$^+$ T cells may differentiate into Th1- or Th2-type cells. The former favor inflammatory responses such as the activation of macrophages, whereas the latter activate humoral responses such as the production of antibodies by B cells. Potentially activated T cells are also carefully autoregulated by means of deletion, which is the elimination of certain lymphocyte clones, or anergy, which renders T cells unresponsive *(67)*. Several factors contribute to the selectivity of T cells for deletion or anergy, including maturity of the T cell, the type of APC involved in the T cell–APC interaction, and the affinity of TCR–antigen–MHC binding. In particular, costimulatory receptor–ligand interactions and cytokine signaling dictate the selectivity of T cells. In the absence of such associated signals, TCR–MHC interactions tend to result in T-cell anergy rather than activation.

The percentages of CD4$^+$ and CD8$^+$ T cells in the total lymphocyte population and their ratio to each other as well as the extent of their activation provide useful indicators of an individual's immune status and can be determined by staining cells with fluorescent antibodies and counting them on a fluorescence microscope. Such visual counts will not permit the accurate quantitation of fluorescence intensity nor the ability to segregate the fluorescence of multistained cells. However, this method can provide useful information of cells stained with a single marker. Flow cytometry (described earlier) represents a more accurate way of quantitating T-cell subsets or of distinguishing several cell types through the use of multiple markers.

The ability of lymphocytes to proliferate upon activation provides another tool for assessing lymphocyte health. In such a proliferation assay, mononuclear cells are isolated from peripheral blood and are cultured in the presence and absence of mitogens, such as phytohemagglutinin (PHA), lipopolysaccharide (LPS), or Concanavalin A (Con A), which activate the cells polyclonally (i.e., in an manner not involving the antigen-specific receptor). Following a short period of culture (approx 3 d) cells are pulsed with ^{3}H-thymidine, which is incorporated into the *de novo* synthesized DNA of proliferating cells, allowing their quantitation by scintillation counting. T-Cell proliferation may also be stimulated by the mixing of leukocytes from genetically different sources. Such allogeneic activation is induced by TCR–MHC interactions, as cells from one source will recognize the other MHC as foreign. Both cell types may proliferate simultaneously and the selective measurement of proliferating cells from one source is achieved by γ-irradiating cells from the other source prior to mixing. γ-Irradiated cells then serve solely as stimulators for the unirradiated cells and, again, proliferation is determined by ^{3}H-thymidine uptake. This test is used as one functional measure of MHC differences (histocompatibility) between individuals and is considered an in vitro counterpart to tissue mixing (e.g., tissue grafts, bone marrow transplants).

Monocyte–T cell interactions during the process of antigen presentation are important for the generation of antigen-specific immune responses. In order to measure this process, blood monocytes, T lymphocytes, and antigens are cultured together, and T-cell activation is monitored. The readouts are usually T-cell proliferation and cytokine production.

CYTOTOXIC T CELLS (CD4⁻CD8⁺) Cytotoxic T cells are required for the elimination of abnormal host cells. Mature CD4⁻CD8⁺, αβ TCR⁺ T cells are generally MHC class I restricted and traditionally fall into two major categories. Suppressor T cells inhibit the activation phase of immune responses, although reports are variable on their MHC-restricted interactions, expression of TCR, CD markers, and antigen-specificity (68–70). Cytotoxic T lymphocytes (CTLs) are important in the killing of virally infected cells and tumor cells and their origins have been outlined earlier. CTLs can themselves act as effectors, killing infected cells directly (71) through recognition of target antigens by the T-cell receptor and the polarization and release of cytoplasmic granules in the vicinity of the target cell. Cytotoxicity is accomplished by apoptosis and lysis, whereas the release of γ-interferon reduces the spread of virus to neighboring host cells.

NATURAL-KILLER (NK) CELLS Elimination of abnormal host cells is the prime function of the natural killer (NK) cell (72). NK cells constitute about 15% of circulating lymphocytes and, morphologically, appear as large granular lymphocytes with low nuclear : cytoplasmic ratios. They appear distinct from T- and B-lymphocyte lineages because certain immunodeficiency states are characterized by a lack of T and B cells but not NK cells. Nonetheless, NK cells share certain characteristics with CTLs and γδ T cells in terms of cytotoxic activities, target-cell specificities, surface markers, and cytokine production. The binding of lectinlike NK receptors to carbohydrate ligands on target cells appears important in NK-cell activity (73). Mice deficient in NK cells generally show an increased susceptibility to the metastatic spread of tumors, although NK cells do not eliminate all malignancies. Indeed, there is evidence that the expression of MHC class I molecules on target cells is inversely related to their elimination. Immediately following NK–target cell interaction, cytotoxic granules are released by NK cells at the region of contact. The best characterized granule constituent, perforin or cytolysin, is structurally and functionally similar to the complement factor C9 and forms transmembrane pores. Apoptosis (programmed cell death) of the target cell shortly follows. Natural-killer cells are protected from their own granules by the presence of chondroitin sulfate A, which is a protease-resistant, negatively charged proteoglycan that inhibits their autolysis.

Cytotoxicity assays are useful in determining the killing activity of CTLs and NK cells. A genetically compatible source of indicator or target cells is used to determine cytotoxic activity of CTLs because TCR–MHC interactions are required for this type of killing. In contrast, tumor-cell lines are commonly used to measure the NK-cell function. In either case, target cells are loaded with ⁵¹Cr, incubated with the effector lymphocytes, and release of the radiolabel is then used as a measure of target-cell killing. Fluorescent markers have also been developed that avoid the need for radioactivity. Finally, DNA fragmentation, a process characteristic of cells undergoing apoptosis, is another possible outcome measure because target-cell killing is mediated through apoptosis.

B CELLS AND IMMUNOGLOBULINS Although the mammalian fetal liver is a source of B cells early in life, most B-cell production occurs in the bone marrow. The stages of B-cell lineage are characterized by rearrangement and expression of antibody genes and cell surface markers such as CD5. It has been suggested that B2 cells (CD5⁻) and αβ TCR⁺ T cells are recently evolved, compared to B1 cells (CD5⁺) and γδ TCR⁺ cells (74). Although B cells may act as professional antigen-presenting cells, their unique role in the immune system is in the production of antigen-neutralizing antibodies.

Antibodies to every possible foreign epitope cannot be constitutively produced; therefore, antigen-specific lymphocyte clones are generated in response to antigen challenge. Each B lymphocyte synthesizes antibodies with one unique paratope and, therefore, one basic antigenic specificity (75). The host contains a large number of resting B-cell clones capable of responding to a range of immunogenic stimuli. In this way, bacteria, for example, expressing a finite quantity of antigenic epitopes will encounter a large number of B lymphocytes of differing antigenic specificities. Microbial antigens will bind to the closest complementary B-cell receptors. Upon ligation, these B-cell clones are activated and soluble antibodies with identical paratopes are released. The proliferation of activated cells ensures that the immune response is of sufficient magnitude to effectively neutralize the antigen. The B-cell antigen receptor is similar in structure to a secreted antibody (65). Indeed, the isotope and antigen specificity of the secreted and membrane-bound immunoglobulins (sIg and mIg, respectively), derived simultaneously from a B-cell clone, tend to be similar. However, important differences exist between sIg and mIg in that mIg are always monomeric and form part of a hydrophobic transmembrane receptor.

Most immunoglobulins bind to native as opposed to denatured or degraded antigens and generally, therefore, recognize conformational epitopes that are formed by protein folding. The monomeric antibody molecule is a covalently linked complex of four polypeptide subunits, two smaller "light" chains and two larger "heavy" chains. Monomeric antibodies may covalently link to form dimeric or multimeric antibodies. All antibodies contain three major functional regions, namely a pair of clonally variable antigen-binding sites, a constant "Fc" region that binds to Fc receptors (FCR) present on the surfaces of many leukocytes and, between these ends, a portion of the antibody that activates the classical complement pathway. Thus, both Fc and complement-activating regions are functions of the constant region, whereas antigen binding is a function of the variable region.

Antibodies are grouped into five isotypes (classes) according to the structure of the constant region of the heavy chain: IgM, IgG, IgA, IgE, and IgD. IgG and IgA are further divided into four and two subclasses, respectively (e.g., IgG1–4 and IgA1–2). Structural differences among heavy-chain isotypes are limited to the constant regions and these influence the non-antigen-binding characteristics of antibodies. For example, secreted antibodies are not necessarily monomeric. IgM is released as a pentamer and IgA, which is chiefly found in mucosal secretions, is secreted as a dimer. Mast cells and basophils have Fc receptors for IgE (Fcε) only, whereas neutrophils and macrophages express Fc receptors for IgG (Fcγ). Effector mechanisms also combine humoral and cellular components in what is termed "antibody-dependent cell-mediated cytotoxicity" or ADCC. Unlike opsonization, in which immune cells recognize antigen-bound antibodies via their FcRs,

ADCC denotes the "arming" of leukocytes with antibodies via Fc–FcR interactions. This facilitates leukocyte binding to antigen. Both macrophages and NK cells possess FcRs, which can presumably link with antigen-specific IgG. Cellular contact with antigens expressed on the surface of an infected cell then results in phagocytosis and/or cytotoxic killing of the target cell.

Quantification of circulating antibodies, their antigen specificity, and isotype is widely used in assessing the immune status of an individual. Immunodiffusion assays are performed on agar-coated glass microscope slides and represent a relatively inexpensive and uncomplicated means of detecting the classes, subclasses, and antigen specificity of antibodies from peripheral blood. Immunofluorescence and immunoblots are used in addition to the widely applied ELISA. ELISAs are based on the binding of plasma/serum antibodies with defined antigens onto a solid phase and using commercially available antibodies for detection. Standardized plastic plates are used for the assay and results are determined on commercially available readers.

Immunoblots are more useful for the detection of antibodies against ill-defined antigens. For example, antigens from a tissue homogenate can be separated by sodium dodecyl sulfate–polyacrylamide gel electrophoresis (SDS-PAGE), transferred to blotting strips, and incubated with patient sera. Antigen-specific antibodies can then be detected by a color reaction. The location and intensity of the color changes provide information on the relative amounts of antibody and the molecular mass of its ligand.

The ELISPOT is used to quantitate antigen-specific B cells in a fashion similar to the ELISA *(76)*. B cells are added to antigen-coated ELISA wells and nonspecifically activated to produce antibodies; B cells recognizing the antigen will then bind to the solid phase. The subsequent color reaction will be limited to those areas on the plate that captured the appropriate antibodies and produce a halo (spot) around the antigen-specific B cells. These spots, taken to represent individual B cells, are then counted visually.

CYTOKINES Cytokines are fairly small (<30 kD) proteins, often glycoproteins, produced mostly by lymphoid cells and to some extent by nonlymphoid cells *(77)*. They can be divided into four families: the interleukins (ILs), tumor necrosis factors (TNFs), interferons (IFNs), and colony-stimulating factors (CSFs). A somewhat different way of grouping cytokines is based on the cell type producing them. There are lymphocyte-derived lymphokines, monocyte-derived monokines, hematopoietic colony-stimulating factors, and connective tissue growth factors *(78)*. As the predominantly autocrine or paracrine factors controlling the proliferation and differentiation of immune cells as well as the tissue remodeling necessary for the influx of those cells into target tissues, cytokines play an important role in the interactions between cells during an immune response, thereby coordinating it *(77)*.

Cytokines are usually not constitutively expressed, but are, instead, induced by infectious challenges or other stressors. Individual cytokines may be synthesized and secreted by more than one cell type and may then act on a variety of target cells, inducing different activities in different cells. The functional activity of a cytokine is mediated by typical ligand/receptor binding. The understanding of cytokine networks is complicated by the multiple cellular sources and targets, the pleiotropic effects of most cytokines, the synergistic or antagonistic effects of cytokine mixtures, and their ability to alter the production of other cytokines and their receptors.

Distinctions between the cytokine-release profiles of type 1 and type 2 T helper (Th1, Th2) cells are important *(79)*. Although these helper-cell types cannot be distinguished phenotypically, as they are both CD4$^+$CD8$^-$ T cells, they are separable, based on the coordinated expression of distinct but overlapping sets of cytokines. Th1 cells are characterized by the release of IFN-γ, the induction of cell-mediated immune responses, and the facilitation of IgG2a production. Th2 cells, on the other hand, produce IL-4, IL-5, and IL-10, and are primarily involved in stimulating the production of antibodies (IgG, IgA, IgE). As discussed earlier, these cell types and the immune networks that they promote are antagonistic; for example, IFN-γ, released by Th1 cells, blocks the growth of Th2 cells, and IL-4, produced by Th2 cells, inhibits some functions of macrophages activated by IFN-γ. CD5$^+$ B-1 cells represent an example of the synergistic effects of cytokines: they release IL-10 and themselves are activated by IL-5, both cytokines released by Th2 cells *(80)*.

Cytokines released by cells in vitro or present in plasma are commonly measured by ELISA, whereas the levels of cytokine mRNA in cells may be measured by reverse transcription–polymerase chain reaction (RT-PCR) or Northern blot. Another method of potentially wide application is the detection of intracellular cytokines using anticytokine antibodies and flow cytometry. For this assay, the membranes of leukocytes are permeabilized with detergents, then the cells are incubated with fluorescent anticytokine antibodies. The intensity of fluorescence is measured by flow cytometry.

COMPLEMENT SYSTEM Complement is a constituent of the humoral immune response and consists of a group of plasma proteins that play a vital role in the elimination of pathogens. The early events leading to the activation of the classical pathway of complement are antibody dependent, which distinguishes it from the alternative pathway of complement activation in which the initiating events occur in the absence of antibody. In both pathways, a cascade of proteolytic cleavage steps leads to the activation of C3 convertase, an enzyme that cleaves complement component C3. Further activation steps result in the ultimate effector functions of complement, such as induction of peptide mediators of inflammation, recruitment of phagocytes, opsonization of pathogens, formation of membrane attack complex, and lysis of certain pathogens.

The activity and concentrations of complement proteins from patient sera are measurable by a variety of methods. Complement activity may be titrated by the hemolysis of sheep red blood cells (SRBC). Concentrations (but not activity) of serum complement proteins may be assayed by radial immunodiffusion or ELISA *(81)*.

HYPERSENSITIVITY SKIN TESTS Hypersensitivity to exogenous antigens or allergens is a common problem in humans. Avoiding contact with allergens, in order to minimize the frequency and intensity of allergic reactions, clearly requires identification of the environmental agents. Skin tests are often used where samples of potential allergen are injected subcutaneously and reactivity is measured by the extent of the inflammatory skin reaction. Immediate hypersensitivities (e.g., to pollen extract) are mediated by IgE and are evident in minutes.

For the determination of general immunocompetence, delayed-type hypersensitivity (DTH) reactions, which involve the recruitment of immune cells to the injection site and require 24–48 h, are widely used. The DTH reaction to tuberculin antigen is probably the most frequently determined one; however, DTH tests often employ at least three or four recall antigens. The diameter of the

Table 6
Hypothetical Tiering System

Tier	Characteristics	Methods
One	Absence of permanent public health facility	Dermatological hypersensitivity tests Hematology (hematocrit, differential)
Two	Rural medical clinic	Immunodiffusion, ELISA, and electrophoresis for immunochemical analysis Short-term cell culture for chemotaxis, phagocytosis, antibody production Immunofluorescent staining with fluorescent microscopy for cell phenotyping
Three	Medical center	Flow cytometry for cytokines analysis, cell phenotyping, cell cycle analysis *In situ* hybridization and reverse transcription–polymerase chain reaction for cytokine analysis Longer-term cell culturing for cytotoxicity, proliferation, antigen presentation

induration developing around the injection site is measured, and a size ≥ 2 mm is considered a positive reaction.

ASSESSING THE IMMUNE STATUS OF AN INDIVIDUAL OR A POPULATION

Public health management requires the constant monitoring of human populations and the resources on which they depend, especially food. Worldwide, many people are not receiving diets that allow them to reach or maintain minimal health standards. The morbidity and mortality characteristics of these underserved populations are, in part, related to underlying properties of their immune systems. Clearly, immunological monitoring should be integrated into public health management systems to understand the health problems of the undernourished more fully.

Because nutritional deficits are often associated with societal disruptions, poverty, and a lack of public services, the materials and personnel needed to obtain and interpret immunological information may be limiting. The types of immunological studies and tests that can be done on selected individuals or populations will depend on a number of factors. These factors include the ability to store and transport biological samples and test equipment, the location of test sites (a major city as opposed to an isolated village), the personnel available, and their level of expertise. The conditions in which immunological information must be obtained may vary widely.

A flexible system that can adapt to a variety of situations but still achieve the goal of obtaining useful immunological information is desired. As we have previously suggested with regard to studies of the impact of toxicological substances on the immune system, a practical testing structure for nutrition and immunity might include a tiered system *(82)*. This would apply increasingly sophisticated examinations of the study materials and subjects in moving from provincial and isolated sites to metropolitan centers. One of the authors (SY) was a Peace Corps volunteer in West Africa for 2 yr. Familiarity with conditions on the road as well as the facilities that were available at a local American Baptist missionary hospital provides a first-hand impression of the range of environments in which immunological information may be gathered.

TIER SYSTEM The following description is provided as an example of the different conditions one might confront and the studies that could be done within these circumstances (Table 6). In real situations, the feasibility and appropriateness of the methodologies will depend on the actual working environment, the particular needs of the public health personnel and the treated population, and the resources made available.

Table 7
Protocol for Cryopreservation

STEP 1.	Isolate peripheral blood mononuclear cells (PBMC)
STEP 2.	Resuspend cells with RPMI 1640 containing 20% fetal bovine serum and supplemented with 0.1% of a 50-mg/mL gentamicin solution
STEP 3.	Transfer cell suspension to 2-mL Biofreeze vials and place on ice
STEP 4.	Slowly add (dropwise) 900 mL of RPMI 1640 containing 20% dimethyl sulfoxide to cell suspension
STEP 5.	Enclose the vials in styrofoam and freeze at −80°C for 24 h
STEP 6.	Transfer samples into liquid nitrogen

When deemed necessary, biological samples could be sent to a centralized facility (e.g., from tier one or two regions to a tier-three region) in order to do tests in a more controlled environment or to gather information on additional immunological parameters. One method of preparing samples that cannot immediately be analyzed is cryopreservation (*see* Table 7 for the protocol). However, it needs to be considered that the practicality of preservation and transportation of samples would depend on a number of factors, such as distance and the condition of roads or airfields, temperature-controlled storage, and the ability to communicate and transmit information. For example, the missionary hospital mentioned earlier did have its own airfield and plane, but the expense of their use would need to be justified or compensated. The parties must also coordinate the arrival of samples with the readiness to deal with them.

However, several immunological tests are feasible, even under conditions that preclude very sophisticated analyses. The conditions likely to be encountered in tier-one, tier-two, and tier-three areas and the immunological assessments possible under these conditions are outlined here.

Tier One The first tier is embodied by a working situation in which a permanent health facility is not available. In this case, public health workers may travel into extremely rural or underdeveloped regions and may be required to perform their examinations from temporary quarters such as tents. The population being examined may reside in relatively permanent settlements (i.e., villages) or they may be potentially migratory and live in impermanent shelters. Water will come from a well or neighboring stream and electrical power should not be expected to exist. As a result, these on-site tests should not require temperature-controlled or sterile environments or a constant source of electricity (unless a portable generator is available).

Skin tests are appropriate for the first tier. These would include dermatological testing for contact hypersensitivity to various immunological stimuli, and tuberculin-type assays *(83)*. The subjects could either have a history of known contact with immunogenic materials or received past vaccinations. Subsequent skin testing could be used as an overall measure of the person's ability to generate an immunological response. Immunodeficiencies may be evidenced by lower than normal or absent responses to antigenic challenges. As above, the length of time needed for an observable skin reaction will depend on the underlying immunological mechanism in progress (i.e., antibody [IgE]-mediated "immediate hypersensitivity" will be evident in minutes, whereas cell-mediated "delayed hypersensitivity" must be followed for several days).

Blood smears may also be done in the field. Staining and microscopic analysis of blood cells for hematological counts will give general information on the numbers of different white blood cells. Concurrently, hematocrits could be obtained as a general measure of the concentration of red and white blood cells. Because hematocrit determinations require the centrifugation of capillary tubes, an electric generator would be needed.

Tier Two The tier-two scenario may be one of a clinic in a rural setting. Running water is present, although its quality may not be equal to that of a modern city in a developed country. Portable filtering devices and boiling are probably desirable. Electric power is fairly dependable but subject to occasional (maybe once-a-week) power outages.

There are other considerations that limit the feasibility of some types of research and diagnostics work. For example, depending on the location and time of year, the ambient temperature may be higher than incubator temperature. An air-conditioned workroom is an improbability (but not impossibility), but there will be no ultracold ($-70°C$) freezers for storage and no cold rooms. Sterility for cell culturing may be problematic. This type of site would not have facilities for the responsible disposal of biohazardous or radioactive wastes, thus precluding any assays generating such waste.

On the other hand, equipment such as fluorescent microscopes and ELISA readers are conceivable in such a rural setting, assuming that the number of subjects to be studied are high enough to justify such procedures. These types of material need not be permanent but could be brought into the clinic on a temporary basis when needed.

A variety of the above-described immunochemical tests are perfectly feasible in a tier-two setting. Immunodiffusion assays probably constitute the least complicated and least expensive way of determining the classes, subclasses, and antigen specificity of antibodies from peripheral blood. Enzyme-liked immunosorbent assays are more quantitative and sensitive than immunodiffusion tests and might also be appropriate for the second tier. The feasibility of these assays may be limited by the ability to obtain the necessary materials, including plasticware, ELISA reader, pipeters, and immunological reagents. However, there are no significant obstacles to their safe storage or competent use in a rural setting. The same may be said for other biochemical methods such as ELISAs for the concentrations of serum complement proteins or SDS-PAGE. The materials for these analyses are easily stored and the temperature (ambient temperature, domestic refrigerator/ freezers) and utility (electricity and water) requirements can be met by most rural clinics. Determining the activity of complement proteins from patient sera may represent somewhat of a problem because the shelf life of commercial sheep blood cells is limited.

Other assays that could be feasible in tier-two facilities include the measurement of phagocytic and chemotactic activity, the quantitation of antigen-specific B lymphocytes by the ELISPOT assay, and the staining of cells with fluorescent antibodies and counting on a fluorescent microscope to determine the relative numbers of different types of peripheral blood lymphocytes.

Tier Three The third tier envisions a modern medical center in a capital city. This facility provides the personnel, expertise, materials, storage facilities, and laboratory equipment needed for more expensive, highly specialized, and probably less frequently done tests.

In such a facility, the proliferative capacity of lymphocytes may be measured using either the mixed-leukocyte reaction or mitogen stimulation. The cytotoxic capacity of peripheral blood T lymphocytes and natural-killer cells are also more appropriate for tier three than tier two. One reason for this is that cytotoxicity must be demonstrated on live target cells. This will require facilities for the culturing of target cell lines and possibly the in vitro generation of target-specific cytotoxic T cells *(84)*. Another reason is that proliferation and cytotoxicity are both measured by using radioactive isotopes, and the cost and size of radiation counters combined with the need for safe disposal of radioactive wastes will probably preclude the use of these methods in tier-two areas.

REFERENCES

1. Yoshida SH, Keen CL, Gershwin ME. Nutrition and the immune system. In: Shields M, ed, Modern Nutrition and Health, Williams and Wilkens, New Jersey, NY, 8th ed, 1998.
2. Harbige LS. Nutrition and immunity with emphasis on infection and autoimmune disease. Nutr Health 1996; 10:285–312.
3. Kramer TR, Moore RJ, Shippee RL, Fried LKE, Martinez-Lopez L, Chan MM, Askew EW. Effects of food restriction in military training on T-lymphocyte responses. Int J Sports Med 1997; 18:S84–90.
4. Engelman RW, Day NK, Good RA. Calorie intake during mammary development influences cancer risk: lasting inhibition of C3H/HeOu mammary tumorigenesis by peripubertal calorie restriction. Cancer Res 1994; 54:5724–30.
5. Tian L, Cai Q, Bowen R, Wei H. Effects of caloric restriction on age-related oxidative modifications of macromolecules and lymphocyte proliferation in rats. Free Radical Biol Med 1995; 19:859–65.
6. Hursting SD, Perkins SN, Phang JM. Calorie restriction delays spontaneous tumorigenesis in p53-knockout transgenic mice. Proc Natl Acad Sci USA 1994; 91:7036–40.
7. Hursting SD, Perkins SN, Brown CC, Haines DC, Phang JM. Calorie restriction induces a p53-independent delay of spontaneous carcinogenesis in p53-deficient and wild-type mice. Cancer Res 1997; 57:2843–6.
8. Fernandes G, Venkatraman JT, Turturro A, Attwood VG, Hart RW. Effect of food restriction on life span and immune functions in long-lived Fischer-344 × Brown Norway F1 rats. J Clin Immunol 1997; 17:85–95.
9. Chandra RK. Protein-energy malnutrition and immunological responses. J Nutr 1992; 122:597–600.
10. Chandra RK, Kumari S. Nutrition and immunity: an overview. J Nutr 1994; 124:1433S–5S.
11. Morley JE. Nutritional modulation of behavior and immunocompetence. Nutr Rev 1994; 52:S6–8.
12. Reynolds JV, Shou JA, Sigal R, Ziegler M, Daly JM. The influence of protein malnutrition on T cell, natural killer cell, and lymphokine-activated killer cell function, and on biological responsiveness to high-dose interleukin-2. Cell Immunol 1990; 128:569–77.

13. Reynolds JV, Redmond HP, Ueno N, Steigman C, Ziegler MM, Daly JM, Johnston RG Jr. Impairment of macrophage activation and granuloma formation by protein deprivation in mice. Cell Immunol 1992; 139:493–504.

14. Nimmanwudipong T, Cheadle WG, Appel SH, Polk HC Jr. Effect of protein malnutrition and immunomodulation on immune cell populations. J Surg Res 1992; 52:233–8.

15. Redmond HP, Gallagher HJ, Shou J, Daly JM. Antigen presentation in protein-energy malnutrition. Cell Immunol 1995; 163:80–7.

16. Rana S, Sodhi CP, Mehta S, Vaipei K, Katyal R, Thakur S, Mehta SK. Protein-energy malnutrition and oxidative injury in growing rats. Hum Exp Toxicol 1996; 15:810–4.

17. Ha CL, Paulino-Racine LE, Woodward BD. Expansion of the humoral effector cell compartment of both systemic and mucosal immune systems in a weanling murine model which duplicates critical features of human protein-energy malnutrition. Br J Nutr 1996; 75:445–60.

18. Schilling J, Vranjes N, Fierz W, Joltar H, Gyurech D, Ludwig E, et al. Clinical outcome and immunology of postoperative arginine, omega-3 fatty acids, and nucleotide-enriched enteral feeding: a randomized prospective comparison with standard enteral and low calorie/low fat i.v. solutions. Nutrition 1996; 12:423–9.

19. Grimble GK. Dietary nucleotides and gut mucosal defence. Gut 1994; 35:S46–S51.

20. Adjei AA, Yamamoto S, Kulkarni A. Nucleic acids and/or their components: a possible role in immune function. J Nutr Sci Vitaminol 1995; 41:1–16.

21. Blok WL, Katan MB, Van der Meer JWM. Modulation of inflammation and cytokine production by dietary (n-3) fatty acids. J Nutr 1996; 126:1515–33.

22. Calder PC, Bond JA, Harvey DJ, Gordon S, Newsholme EA. Uptake and incorporation of saturated and unsaturated fatty acids into macrophage lipids and their effect upon macrophage adhesion and phagocytosis. Biochem J 1990; 269:807–14.

23. Zhao Z, Ross AC. Retinoic acid repletion restores the number of leukocytes and their subsets and stimulates natural cytotoxicity in vitamin A-deficient rats. J Nutr 1995; 125:2064–73.

24. Ross AC, Stephensen CB. Vitamin A and retinoids in antiviral responses. FASEB J 1996; 10:979–85.

25. Carman JA, Hayes CE. Abnormal regulation of IFN-γ secretion in vitamin A deficiency. J Immunol 1991; 147:1247–52.

26. Carman JA, Pond L, Nashold F, Wassom DL, Hayes CE. Immunity to Trichinella spiralis infection in vitamin A-deficient mice. J Exp Med 1992; 175:111–20.

27. Wiedermann U, Hanson LA, Kahu H, Dahlgren UI. Aberrant T-cell function in vitro and impaired T-cell dependent antibody response in vivo in vitamin A-deficient rats. Immunology 1993; 80:581–6.

28. Bowman TA, Goonewardene IM, Pasatiempo AM, Ross AC, Taylor CE. Vitamin A deficiency decreases natural killer cell activity and interferon production in rats. J Nutr 1990; 120:1264–73.

29. Baez-Saldana A, Diaz G, Espinoza B, Ortega E. Biotin deficiency induces changes in subpopulations of spleen lymphocytes in mice. Am J Clin Nutr 1998; 67:431–7.

30. Matthews KS, Mrowczynski E, Matthews R. Dietary deprivation of B-vitamins reflected in murine splenocyte proliferation in vitro. Biochem Biophys Res Commun 1994; 198:451–8.

31. Grimble RF. Effect of antioxidative vitamins on immune function with clinical applications. Int J Vitamin Nutr Res 1997; 67:312–20.

32. Buzina-Suboticanec K, Buzina R, Stavljenic A, et al. Ageing, nutritional status and immune response. Int J Vitamin Nutr Res 1998; 68:133–41.

33. Blumberg JB. Vitamins. In: Forse RA, ed, Diet, Nutrition, and Immunity, CRC Press, pp. 237–46. Boca Raton, FL.

34. Lemire JM. Immunomodulatory role of 1,25-dihydroxyvitamin D3. J Cell Biochem 1992; 49:26–31.

35. Benis KA, Schneider GB. The effects of vitamin D binding protein-macrophage activating factor and colony-stimulating factor-1 on hematopoietic cells in normal and osteoperotic rats. Blood 1996; 88:2898–905.

36. Tengerdy RP. The role of vitamin E in immune response and disease resistance. Ann NY Acad Sci 1990; 587:24–33.

37. Meydani SN, Barklund MP, Liu S, Meydani M, Miller RA, Conor JG, et al. Vitamin E supplementation enhances cell-mediated immunity in healthy elderly subjects. Am J Clin Nutr 1990; 52:557–63.

38. Shklar G, Schwartz JL. Vitamin E inhibits experimental carcinogenesis and tumour angiogenesis. Eur J Cancer Part B, Oral Oncol 1996; 32B:114–9.

39. Meydani SN, Meydani M, Blumberg JB, Kekal S, Siber G, Laszewski K, et al. Vitamin E supplementation and in vivo immune response in healthy elderly subjects. A randomized controlled trial. J Am Med Assoc 1997; 277:1380–6.

40. Babu U, Failla ML. Copper status and function of neutrophils are reversibly depressed in marginally and severely copper-deficient rats. J Nutr 1990; 120:1700–9.

41. Sherman AR. Zinc, copper, and iron nutriture and immunity. J Nutr 1992; 122:604–9.

42. O'Dell BL. Interleukin-2 production is altered by copper deficiency. Nutr Rev 1993; 51:307–9.

43. Kelley DS, Daudu PA, Taylor PC, Mackey BE, Turnlund JR. Effects of low-copper diets on human immune response. Am J Clin Nutr 1995; 62:412–6.

44. Johnson MA, Fischer JG, Bowman BA, Gunter EW. Iron nutriture in elderly individuals. FASEB J 1994; 8:609–21.

45. McCoy H, Kenney MA. Magnesium and immune function: recent findings. Magnesium Res 1992; 5:281–93.

46. Weglicki WB, Phillips TM. Pathobiology of magnesium deficiency: a cytokine/neurogenic inflammation hypothesis. Am J Physiol 1992; 263:R734–7.

47. Nair MPN, Schwartz SA. Immunoregulation of natural and lymphokine-activated killer cells by selenium. Immunopharmacology 1990; 19:177–83.

48. Mantero-Atienza E, Sotomayor MG, Shor-Posner G, Fletcher MA, Sauberlich HP, Beach RS. Selenium status and immune function in asymptomatic HIV-1 seropositive men. Nutr Res 1991; 11:1237–50.

49. Schrauzer GN, Sacher J. Selenium in the maintenance and therapy of HIV-infected patients. Chem–Biol Interact 1994; 91:199–205.

50. Keen CL, Gershwin ME. Zinc deficiency and immune function. Annu Rev Nutr 1990; 10:415–31.

51. Cunningham-Rundles S. Analytical methods for evaluation of immune response in nutrient intervention. Nutr Rev 1998; 56:S27–S37.

52. Gordon S, Clarke S, Greaves D, Doyle A. Molecular immunobiology of macrophages: recent progress. Curr Opin Immunol 1995; 7:24–33.

53. Rosen GM, Pou S, Ramos CL, Cohen MS, Britigan BE. Free radicals and phagocytic cells. FASEB J 1995; 9:200–9.

54. Flescher E, Dang H, Talal N. Lymphocytes, cytokines, and surface markers. In: Weir DM, ed, Weir's Handbook of Experimental Immunology, 5th ed, pp. 134.1–134.6. Blackwell Science, Cambridge, MA, 1996.

55. Lesourd BM, Mazari L, Ferry M. The role of nutrition in immunity in the aged. Nutr Rev 1998; 56:S113–25.

56. Wilkison PC. Locomotion and chemotaxis in vitro. In: Weir DM, ed, Weir's Handbook of Experimental Immunology, 5th ed. Blackwell Science, Cambridge, MA, 1996.

57. Ross GD, Cain JA, Lachmann PJ. Membrane complement receptor type three (CR3) has lectin-like properties analogous to bovine conglutinin and functions as a receptor for zymosan and rabbit erythrocytes as well as a receptor for iC3b. J Immunol 1985; 134:3307–15.

58. Stuehr DJ, Nathan CF. Nitric oxide. A macrophage product responsible for cytostasis and respiratory inhibition in tumor target cells. J Exp Med 1989; 169:1543–55.

59. Scott MA, Gordon MY. In search of the haemopoietic stem cell. Br J Haematol 1995; 90:738–743.

60. Jameson SC, Hogquist KA, Bevan MJ. Positive selection of thymocytes. Annu Rev Immunol 1995; 13:93–126.

61. Kisielow P, Von Boehmer H. Development and selection of T cells: facts and puzzles. Adv Immunol 1995; 58:87–209.

62. Abo T. Extrathymic pathways of T-cell differentiation: a primitive and fundamental immune system. Microbiol Immunol 1993; 37:247–58.

63. Franceschi C, Monti D, Sansoni P, Cossarizza A. The immunology of exceptional individuals: the lesson of centenarians. Immunol Today 1995; 13:12–6.

64. Hein WR. Structural and functional evolution of the extracellular regions of T cell receptors. Semin Immunol 1994; 6:361–72.

65. De Franco AL. Transmembrane signaling by antigen receptors of B and T lymphocytes. Curr Opin Cell Biol 1995; 7:163–75.

66. Havran WL, Boismenu R. Activation and function of gamma delta T cells. Curr Opin Immunol 1994; 6:442–6.

67. LaSalle JM, Hafler DA. T cell anergy. FASEB J 1994; 8:601–8.

68. Arnon R, Teitelbaum D. On the existence of suppressor cells. Int Arch Allergy Immunol 1993; 100:2–7.

69. Kemeny DM, Noble A, Holmes BJ, Diaz-Sanchez D. Immune regulation: a new role for the CD8+ T cell. Immunol Today 1994; 15:107–10.

70. Le Gros G, Erard F. Non-cytotoxic, IL-4, IL-5, IL-10 producing CD8+ T cells, their activation and effector functions. Curr Opin Immunol 1994; 6:453–7.

71. Podack ER. Execution and suicide: cytotoxic lymphocytes enforce Draconian laws through separate molecular pathways. Curr Opin Immunol 1995; 7:11–16.

72. Klein E, Mantovani A. Action of natural killer cells and macrophages in cancer. Curr Opin Immunol 1993; 5:714–8.

73. Gumperz JE, Parham P. The enigma of the natural killer cell. Nature 1995; 378:245–8.

74. Kantor AB, Herzenberg LA. Origin of murine B cell lineages. Annu Rev Immunol 1993; 11:501–38.

75. Klinman NR. Selection in the expression of functionally distinct B-cell subsets. Curr Opin Immunol 1994; 6:420–4.

76. Hodgkin PD, Kehry MR. Methods for polyclonal B lymphocyte activation to proliferation and Ig secretion *in vitro*. In: Weir DM, ed, Weir's Handbook of Experimental Immunology, 5th ed, pp. 89.1–89.13. Blackwell Science, Cambridge, MA, 1996.

77. Arai K, Lee F, Miyajima A, Miyatake S, Arai N, Yokota T. Cytokines: coordinators of immune and inflammatory responses. Annu Rev Biochem 1990; 59:783–836.

78. Thompson AW. The Cytokine Handbook. Academic, San Diego, CA, 1994.

79. Anderson GP, Coyle AJ. TH2 and "TH2-like" cells in allergy and asthma: pharmacological perspectives. Trends Pharmacol Sci 1994; 15:324–332.

80. O'Garra A, Howard M. Cytokines and Ly-1 (B1) B cells. Int Rev Immunol 1992; 8:219–34.

81. Dickneite G. Complement activation and inhibition. In: Weir DM, ed, Weir's Handbook of Experimental Immunology, 5th ed, pp. 218.1–218.7. Blackwell Science, Cambridge, MA.

82. Yoshida S, Golub MS, Gershwin ME. Immunological aspects of toxicology: premises not promises. Regul Toxicol Pharmacol 1989; 9:56–80.

83. Asherson GL, Zembala M. Contact and delayed hypersensitivity. In: Weir DM, ed, Weir's Handbook of Experimental Immunology, 5th ed, pp. 137.1–137.9. Blackwell Science, Cambridge, MA, 1996.

84. Stauss HJ, Sadovnikova E. Cytotoxic T lymphocytes. In: Weir DM, ed, Weir's Handbook of Experimental Immunology, 5th ed, pp. 140.1–140.12, Blackwell Science, Cambridge, MA, 1996.

SPECIFIC NUTRIENT REQUIREMENTS

II

(NORMAL POPULATIONS; POPULATIONS WITH LOW INTAKES, INCLUDING TEENS, FEMALES, ELDERLY...)

4 Caloric Intake: Sources, Deficiencies, and Excess—An Overview

DEAN A. TROYER AND GABRIEL FERNANDES

INTRODUCTION

Carbohydrates, protein, and fats are the major energy-containing constituents of food (macronutrients), and extensive animal studies indicate that decreased total caloric intake is generally a beneficial, life-extending tool. However, the proportion of calories derived from fat is also important, influencing the risks of development of cancer, obesity, and cardiovascular disease. In contrast to carbohydrates and protein, fat is an energy-dense substance that tends to be stored rather than metabolized under normal physiological conditions. Thus, not all calories are alike. Reduced consumption of fat is, therefore, a major goal for nutrition in industrialized countries. However, just as not all calories are alike, not all fats are alike. Vegetable oils, fish oils, and animal-derived fats have profoundly different effects on immune function, cancer, and atherosclerosis. Although both fish oils and vegetable oils generally ameliorate atherosclerosis, fish oils have, in addition, anti-inflammatory properties that may be of benefit for the treatment and prevention of cancer and autoimmune disease. A sedentary life-style combined with energy-dense foods rich in fat are important factors in overnutrition.

The relentless increase in the prevalence and severity of obesity over the past 30 yr *(1)* has spawned an expensive battle against fat. However, although we may all be getting more obese as average body weights increase, body weights vary widely among comparable individuals. It is these wide variations within groups that emphasize the importance of neurohormonal and genetic influences on adiposity. As a component of the economy, "nutrition" is a multimillion dollar industry and includes books, magazines, radio and television programming, numerous weight-loss programs, and the sale of nutritional supplements. The expenditures of time, effort, and money for diet books, diet foods, and other remedies have been estimated to account for 30–50 billion dollars annually *(2)*. Although obesity receives much more attention, undernutrition is also a problem. Famine is an ongoing problem in the world, and the scarcity of food can be natural or man-made. Even in the midst of abundance, there are conditions that lead to malnutrition in the United States, and the eating disorders

anorexia and bulimia nervosa may, in part, represent extreme responses to the fear of obesity. These are disorders of unknown cause, but are most common among young women who have the perception that they are overweight, even when their actual body weight is normal. A downward spiral results from a quest for thinness. Thus, there is a dark side to the war against obesity. In contrast to public campaigns promoting cessation of smoking, which has slight downside, an overly aggressive or poorly conceived campaign against obesity might promote the evolution of anorexia in those who are susceptible. A few additional issues concerning sex, age, and ethnicity will be considered. Both anorexia and obesity are more common in females than males, and obesity is more common in ethnic minority groups. Aging into middle age is associated with a steady increase of weight, but in later years of life, body weight tends to decrease. We are slowly beginning to understand the variable nutritional needs specific to age, sex, and ethnicity. Finally, there are physiological and metabolic changes that produce undernutrition in hospitalized patients and in patients with chronic diseases such as tuberculosis, cancer, and AIDS in which relentless weight loss occurs (cachexia). The causes of malnutrition and the needs of patients hospitalized for trauma, surgery, and other reasons are better understood, but much less is known about weight loss in human immunodeficiency virus (HIV) and cancer patients. The causes of anorexia, cachexia, and obesity remain elusive, but emerging scientific data suggest that eating behavior and metabolism are influenced by endocrine, physiological, and genetic factors. At the very least, we should realize that obese people do not seek obesity any more than anorexics desire starvation.

MACRONUTRIENTS

Macronutrients are the major components of food: protein, carbohydrate, and fat. Public awareness of the health risks of high-fat and high-calorie diets has increased, and the food industry has begun to introduce low-calorie, low-fat food items. Carbohydrates compose 45% of the diet in the United States and as high as 90% of dietary calories in the tropics *(3)*. Rice, cereals, and other plant-derived sources of carbohydrates are inexpensive and efficiently produced and are widely available. Proteins are typically derived from both plant and animal sources in the diet, and vegetarians must be careful to incorporate legumes, nuts, and grains with

From: *Nutrition and Immunology: Principles and Practice* (ME Gershwin et al. eds.), © Humana Press, Inc., Totowa, NJ

vegetables and fruits to assure an adequate supply of micronutrients and essential amino acids *(3)*. There are nine essential amino acids required in food for humans to produce and maintain body tissues. Fats are a potent energy source (9 cal/g versus 4 cal/g for carbohydrates and proteins) and can be derived from meats and plants (corn oil and other vegetable oils). Two fatty acids are required in the diet in humans, linoleic acid (18:2n-6) and α-linolenic acid (18:3n-3), and arachidonic acid is sometimes listed as one of the essential fatty acids *(3)*. It can be synthesized from linoleic acid by desaturation and chain elongation, but it is also available in meat products. In industrialized societies where food is widely available, overnutrition is the commonest nutritional issue. Overnutrition, in turn, is closely linked to sedentary life-styles, total caloric intake, and total fat intake. Because fat is the most calorie-dense macronutrient, reducing or substituting other macronutrients for fat presents the greatest potential for reduction of calories *(4)*. However, total caloric intake is also important, and restriction of calories is a powerful life-extending intervention.

CALORIE RESTRICTION IS BENEFICIAL   Up to one-third of all cases of human cancer are related to dietary factors, and caloric intake is a major dietary risk factor for cancer *(5)*. Restriction of calories (without malnutrition or micronutrient deficiency) slows nearly all age-sensitive biological parameters, including age-related decrements in immune function, delays tumorigenesis *(6,7)*, and increases life-span *(8,9)*. First observed in rats, the effects of calorie restriction have been observed in several other species *(8)*. In most of these studies, the animals on a calorie-restricted diet are given a diet in which the content of calories is reduced by approximately 40% that of the unrestricted controls fed *ad libitum*. All macronutrients are reduced proportionately, and it appears that this proportionate reduction of all macronutrients is as effective as the selective reduction of carbohydrates, protein, or fat *(10)*. In a typical study, the *ad libitum*-fed animals gain weight early and plateau at roughly twice the weight of the restricted animals. The result is that energy intake per kilogram body weight is very nearly the same in the two groups *(11)*. The mechanisms whereby calorie restriction ameliorates autoimmune disease, suppresses tumorigenesis, and prolongs life-span remain poorly understood. However, the free-radical theory of aging suggests that calorie restriction decreases oxidant stress and suppresses the production of reactive oxygen intermediates *(12)*. An extension of this hypothesis links the suppression of free radicals by calorie restriction to upregulation of apoptosis and suppression of free radicals *(13)*. In summary, calorie restriction is a powerful experimental tool that may be applicable to humans in understanding the general processes occurring in aging and tumorigenesis. At a practical level, 40% calorie restriction is not applicable to human dietary habits. However, overnutrition results from the interaction of excess caloric intake, decreased physical activity, and the macronutrient (especially high fat) content of food *(14)*. The importance of a sedentary life-style has been noted recently in the context of a paradoxical decline in caloric intake and fat in the diet that has paralleled a continuing rise in obesity in the United States *(15)*.

ALL CALORIES ARE NOT ALIKE   The macronutrient content of the diet influences food palatability, the amount of food and energy taken in, and the disposition of energy in the body. The increasing incidence of obesity has been accompanied by an increased intake of dietary calories derived from fat, with a parallel decrease in the total calories derived from carbohydrates *(16)*. Although not firmly established by epidemiological studies, increased fat intake is associated with increased obesity *(17)*. Fat is much more energy-dense (9 kcal/g) than either protein or carbohydrate (4 kcal/g each). After digestion by lipases into fatty acids and monoacylglycerols, fats are absorbed and stored as reserves of energy to buffer day-to-day variations in food intake *(19)*. This was probably an adaptation that allowed our ancestors to deal with periods of food scarcity. Protein and carbohydrate stores are more tightly regulated than are fats. Physical training and growth stimuli such as growth hormone and anabolic steroids lead to increased muscle mass, but protein stores do not increase following increased dietary intake of protein *(18)*. Thus, excess dietary carbohydrate or protein tend to be oxidized rather than stored and their energy liberated as heat (thermogenesis) *(20)*. Although carbohydrates are converted to storage forms such as glycogen, this is an inefficient process *(19)*. When expressed as a percentage of the energy content of the macronutrient ingested as food, storage of fat "costs" 4%, whereas the costs of converting carbohydrates into glycogen (12%) or *de novo* into lipids (23%) are substantially higher *(19)*. Storage of carbohydrates and proteins is tightly regulated within a narrow range; however, fats are stored when made available as excess calories *(21)*, particularly in individuals prone to obesity *(22,23)*. In addition to these factors governing the disposition of ingested macronutrients, total food intake contributes to energy balance. The accumulated evidence suggests that physical activity, amount and type of food, and genetic factors all contribute to body weight *(24)*. In other words, a sedentary life-style combined with a high-calorie/high-fat diet are factors that almost universally lead to obesity. However, a genetic predisposition to obesity can exacerbate the influence of these factors, leading to individual variations within a group of comparable people *(24)*.

Several mechanisms influence food intake and satiety, and macronutrients differ in their ability to satisfy hunger *(25)*. Factors such as food texture, taste, volume, and palatability influence eating behavior. Fats provide a texture and taste that most people find desirable, and fat-rich foods typically require little chewing and can be eaten quickly. In contrast, food items that contain complex carbohydrates or fiber require more chewing and must be eaten more slowly, with the effect of limiting total consumption *(19)*. There is good evidence that the weight or volume of food influences satiety. When high-fat/low-fiber diets versus low-fat/high-fiber diets are offered to people, the volume of food remains more nearly constant than energy content, with the result that high-fat diets lead to increased energy intake *(14,23)*. Once digestion has begun, the effects of digested, oxidized, and absorbed nutrients commence and these "postabsorptive" factors also influence satiety *(19)*. The rapid metabolism of carbohydrates to sugars may provide satiety by raising blood glucose and insulin levels, and fats frequently depress blood glucose *(23,26)*.

MACRONUTRIENT SUBSTITUTION   High dietary fat intake, particularly of saturated fats, has been correlated with an increased risk of heart and cardiovascular disease *(27)* and cancer *(28,29)*. The increasing evidence of the health risks of high dietary fats has led to the recommendation that dietary fat intake should be 20% of calories, with only 6% of this being saturated fats *(30)*, and the US Public Health Service has targeted a decrease in fat intake of adults to an average of 30% or less of total calories by the year 2000 *(17)*. Because food preferences are hard to change, over 6600 food products have been introduced that are familiar foods modified to have reduced energy density, reduced fat, or reduced carbohydrate content *(31)*. These products have emerged to meet the increased public awareness of the health risks of high dietary fat and the perception that total fat content in the diet should be reduced *(32)*. The following are examples of macronutrient alterations that can produce foods with decreased caloric content while preserving taste and desirability *(4)*: the introduction and promotion of artificial high-intensity sweeteners; bulking agents, including fiber; and fat replacements. Fat replacements can be absorbable and metabolizable substitutes that have a lower caloric density than fat (starch, protein, or modified low-calorie fats) or they can be noncaloric (cellulose, seaweed, gums). Alternatively, fat substitutes, such as olestra, have a texture and taste similar to fats but are not absorbed and digested (4). Olestra is a member of a family of substitutes that are composed of 8–22 carbon fatty acids esterified to sucrose. These were originally tested as cholesterol-lowering agents. Depending on the number of esterified fats, the texture can range from liquid to solid.

It is of interest to note that in a human trial of breast cancer risk in women, reduction of dietary fat to 15% of total calories led to a significant reduction in sex hormones. Estrogen, progesterone, and follicle-stimulating hormone levels were decreased by 20%, 35%, and 7%, respectively *(33)*. This confirms the influence of macronutrient composition on hormones that may be of relevance to breast cancer risk. Previous studies in animals have demonstrated the ability of calorie restriction to similarly modulate prolactin levels in breast-cancer-prone C3H mice *(34)*. Taken together, these and similar findings emphasize the importance of dietary calories and fats in tumorigenesis *(29)*.

The goals of macronutrient substitution are to reduce caloric intake and fat content in the diet. It is not certain that reduction in the fat content of foods will lead to a concomitant reduction in energy intake. This is due to a tendency for replacement of the energy lost in the low-fat/low-calorie food by other foods to maintain a constant level of energy intake *(31)*. Therefore, unless there is a conscious effort to reduce total energy intake, macronutrient substitution may reduce the fat content of the diet without decreasing energy intake and body weight.

ALL FATS ARE NOT ALIKE The association of high levels of dietary fat with increased heart and cardiovascular disease has shifted fat consumption to those of plant origin and away from animal fats in the diet. This was based on epidemiological evidence that consumption of saturated fats was correlated with the elevation of plasma cholesterol levels and an increased incidence of atherosclerotic heart and cardiovascular disease *(27)*. The substitution of vegetable-derived polyunsaturated fatty acids for saturated fats has paralleled a decrease in the incidence of cardiovascular disease. At the present time, over 90% of the fats consumed in the United States (average 170 g) are from plant sources, with very little being from fish (marine) sources *(35)*. Fats derived from fish (marine oils) taken in the diet can also decrease the incidence of heart and cardiovascular disease and favorably affect immune function *(36)*. The predominant fatty acids in marine oils have the first unsaturated (double) bond between the third and fourth carbons from the methyl carbon and are designated ω-3, whereas the plant-derived fatty acids are designated ω-6 because the first double bond is between carbons 6 and 7 from the methyl carbon.

This structural difference leads to profound differences in the effects of diets rich in ω-3 versus ω-6 fats. Diets enriched in either ω-6 or ω-3 fatty acids reduce the incidence of heart attack and atherosclerotic cardiovascular disease *(27,37,38)*. However, ω-3 lipids additionally modulate immune function *(36)* and suppress tumorigenesis *(39)*. In rodent studies, there is good evidence that ω-6 fats have a tumor-enhancing effect that is greater than even that of saturated fats, whereas ω-3 fats, in contrast, tend to be protective *(40)*. It is of interest to note that the breast-cancer-promoting effects in rats on a diet high in ω-6 fats are transmitted to the next generation when the exposure occurs *in utero (41)*. (This is of relevance to the discussion of imprinting in this chapter.) To promote these benefits of ω-3 fats, it is appropriate, therefore, to consider the recommendation that the ratio of ω-6/ω-3 fats be closer to 1 : 1 or 10 : 1 (versus the current 20 : 1) *(30)*.

A variety of biological functions are influenced by ω-6 and ω-3 fats because they become incorporated into the phospholipids of cell membranes, where they can affect membrane fluidity *(42)* and serve as substrates for the generation of inflammatory mediators (prostaglandins, leukotrienes, and thromboxanes). These compounds are pro-inflammatory, increase platelet aggregation, and can activate neutrophils *(43)*. The anti-inflammatory properties of fish oils reside in the ability of the two main ω-3 fatty acids in fish oil, eicosapentanoic acid (EPA) and docosahexanoic acid (DHA), to compete with vegetable-derived arachidonic acid both for acylation at the 2-position of membrane phospholipids and as a substrate for cyclooxygenase. The increased availability of EPA and DHA leads to increased production of 3-series prostaglandins (PG) and thromboxanes (TX). PGE_3 is less inflammatory than PGE_2 derived from arachidonic acid, and the TXA_3 generated in preference to TXA_2 is less active against platelets *(43)*. The type of fat consumed substantially alters the potency of the inflammatory mediators. Increased consumption of ω-3 (fish) oils favorably affects arthritis, cardiovascular, and kidney disease, which are diseases caused by overactivity of the immune system and/or complicated by platelet aggregation *(36)*.

Because the calories allocated to fat in the diet should be limited, it is important to carefully select those fatty acids that are most beneficial and, at the very least, do no harm. The substitution of fish-oil fatty acids for vegetable-oil fats may prove to be a beneficial step. In addition, less abundant fatty acid constituents are receiving attention with regard to their effects on serum lipids and/or their potential for influencing carcinogenesis. At least one double bond is present in most naturally occurring fatty acids, and it is usually in the cis configuration. Trans fatty acids are formed during the catalytic conversion of liquid oils to solids (e.g., for use in preparing margarine) by partial hydrogenation. Because this process destroys some naturally occurring fatty acids and generates new trans isomers that are structurally similar to saturated fats, there is concern that trans fatty acids could promote hyperlipidemia. The estimated intake of trans fatty acids ranges from 5 to 15 g/d, derived mainly from frying fats, margarines, and other spreads *(44)*. The soft-tub margarines contain much less than the solidified stick margarine. Ironically, the original reason for substitution of trans-fatty-acid-rich margarine for butter was to lower cholesterol. A recent study suggests that stick margarine is without effect on cholesterol, whereas relatively low-trans-content soft-tub margarines do lower cholesterol *(44,45)*. Therefore, trans fatty acids may not be cholesterolemic, but the presence of trans fatty acids, although not necessarily harmful, may displace other more desirable fatty acids from the diet. This emphasizes the importance of understanding the allocation of fat calories among those fats that reduce health risks. Additional individual fats are being studied for this purpose.

The isomerized forms of linoleic acid, found in red meat and dairy products, are referred to as conjugated linoleic acid. The anticarcinogenic properties of conjugated linoleic acid were originally identified in ground beef (46). Linoleic acid (18 : 2n-6) normally has two double bonds located at C_{12}–C_{13} and C_9–C_{10}, both in the cis configuration. However, conjugated linoleic acid has dienoic double bonds between carbons C_9–C_{10} and C_{11}–C_{12} or C_{10}–C_{11} and C_{12}–C_{13}, and each double bond can be cis or trans, giving rise to eight total isomers. Conjugated linoleic acid is incorporated predominantly into neutral lipids, suppresses tumorigenesis (47), and is antiatherogenic (46). In amounts as small as 1% of total fat intake, it protects against cancer in vivo and in vitro (46). The trans isomer of linoleic acid is found in dairy foods in amounts ranging up to 8 mg/g of fat (48). Recent studies indicate that the antiproliferative effects of conjugated linoleic acid are specific to estrogen-receptor positive breast cancer cells (49).

Additional examples of food constituents that significantly reduce oxidant stress and suppress cancer and/or atherosclerosis include antioxidants [vitamins C and E, quinones, selenium, and the carotenoids (50)] and estrogenlike compounds, phytoestrogens (51). Also of importance are constituents of olive oil found in the Mediterranean diet (52), where high oleic acid intake occurs at the expense of carbohydrates. In spite of this higher fat intake, consumption of this diet is associated with amelioration of both atherosclerosis and a lower incidence of breast cancer (52). Dramatically different rates of cancer are seen across the world, and these differences are attributed in part to differences in dietary fat intake and relative vitamin or trace nutrient deficiencies, particularly the antioxidants vitamin E and A (50). The emerging discipline of chemoprevention includes the study of dietary factors that can prevent or delay the onset of common age-related tumors such as colon, breast, and prostate cancers (53).

OVERNUTRITION

ATTITUDES Obesity is a term heavily laden with overtones that suggest a lack of self-control and even contempt. The common notion of obesity centers on appearance and takes little account of health risk *per se*. It is assumed that anyone who looks overweight is obese, but it is less certain that our negative perception of obesity is based on an understanding of health risks associated with obesity. A little obesity is not nearly as dangerous as a lot, and it is important that we distinguish being mildly overweight from being sufficiently overweight to endanger health. Aside from the many billions of dollars spent on weight loss, drugs used to help people slim down have the potential to cause physical harm (54,55) in addition to the fruitless expenditure of money on remedies that do not last. Thus, the benefits of treating obesity should be balanced by consideration of the risks, including those of overtreating mild obesity, for which the health risks may be nominal (56). The firmly entrenched notion that obesity is the direct result of overeating has been described as a "folk belief" (57).

CLASSIFICATION, PREVALENCE, AND DISTRIBUTION

A calculated value called the body mass index (BMI) is used to correct body weight for height and is determined by dividing body weight in kilograms by the square of the height in meters

Table 1
Classification of Obesity

Body mass index	Classification
≤25.0	Overweight
25.0–29.9	Preobesity
30.0–34.9	Class I obesity
34.9–39.9	Class II obesity
≥40.0	Class III obesity

(kg/m^2) (58). The behavioral, environmental, and genetic factors that contribute to BMI create a "set point," which is a weight toward which we return, often frustrating the best efforts of individuals to lose weight and keep it off (57). Increased BMI correlates with increases in both total body fat and percentage of fat (58), and a BMI of 19–25 is considered optimal. For a person who is 6 ft tall, the corresponding ideal weight range is from 140 to 180 lbs. Until a body mass of 27 or 28 (200–205 lbs for a 6-ft-tall individual) is reached, the risk of death increases, but modestly. When body mass increases to 29–32 (215–230 lbs for a 6-ft-tall individual), the risk of death increases 1.5-fold, and this increased risk diminishes with age (59). Table 1 shows a classification scheme for obesity, based on BMI.

The number of Americans who fall into what epidemiologists call Class III obesity (i.e., people too grossly overweight to fit into an airline seat) has risen 350% in the past 30 yr. In the mid-1960s, 17% of middle-aged Americans were clinically obese, and today the figure is 30–35% (60), and overweight in adolescence (ages 12–17 yr) increased from 15% to 21% (61). This is a worldwide trend affecting all social groups and there is no end in sight (62,63). The incidence of obesity varies greatly among racial groups and between men and women. Obesity approaches 50% among Hispanic and African-American women, nearly twice the figure among white women, particularly below the age of 55 (64,65). Native Americans, including the intensively studied Pima Indians living in present-day Arizona, have extremely high rates of obesity, particularly among younger individuals than do corresponding white populations, and the rates of obesity among the Pima have been steadily increasing throughout this century (78). This steady increase of obesity over time and among younger individuals is thought to be related to economic and cultural changes (e.g., relatively sedentary life-styles) superimposed on genetic susceptibility.

AGING AND BODY FAT Prospective studies that follow the same subjects over time show a progressive increase of weight with aging. One such study demonstrated an increase of 3.5 lbs in weight during the 2 decades from 23 to 44 yr of age and again during the 2 decades from age 45 to 65, but, thereafter, body weight decreased (65). In another study of 18- to 30-yr-old men and women initiated in 1985–86, even larger weight gains were seen during 7 yr of follow-up (66). The larger weight gains were seen in women, and weight gains were greater in African-American women. Over the 7-yr period of the study, the average weight increase ranged from 5.2 kg in white women to 8.5 kg in African-American women (66).

The distribution of fat or body shape may also affect the health risks associated with obesity. An increased waist-to-hip ratio correlates with an increased risk of adult-onset diabetes, cardiovascular disease, and overall mortality (67,68). As measured by computerized tomography, the amount of fat present within the abdominal cavity (versus subcutaneous fat) increases more dramatically than does body weight with aging (69). Women are not exempt from the accumulation of abdominal fat, demonstrating a steady increase from 91 cm^2 for women below the age of 30 to 184 cm^2 at ages 50–59 (70,71). Other studies also show a correlation between increased abdominal fat and increased risk of cardiovascular disease in both men and women (67,68). After menopause, abdominal fat accumulates 2.6 times as rapidly as it does before menopause (72), and postmenopausal women are at much greater risk of cardiovascular disease than are premenopausal women. Similarly, hormone-replacement therapy in postmenopausal women can prevent the redistribution of fat to the abdomen, which otherwise occurs with aging during the postmenopausal period (73).

CAUSES OF OVERNUTRITION Obesity is not acquired over a period of days or weeks, but typically occurs over a period of years. This slow pace implies that small metabolic changes, projected over years, could account for obesity. The size of these changes may be very difficult to measure over a period of days or weeks. It has been estimated that to achieve a weight of 150 kg at the age of 50 yr, the daily excess consumption of food would be only 50 kcal out of 2200–2500 kcal typically consumed per day (74). Generally, we do not count calories so closely as to determine an error of 50 kcal, and the real surprise may be that so many people stay lean while paying little attention to the precise caloric content of food. This ability to regulate body weight within a reasonable range implies that weight-regulating mechanisms are efficient. However, there is frequently one obese family member, with the other members weighing much less (75), and this general observation has led to the suggestion that recessive genes may play a role in obesity. In contrast, obesity in the extensively studied Pima Indians of modern-day Arizona is highly familial, and genetic factors and/or long-lasting effects of the diabetic intrauterine environment are thought to be important in the pathogenesis of obesity in this population (76). These studies suggest that rates of energy expenditure are familial, with approximately 11% of the basal metabolic rate determined by genetic factors (76). Furthermore, individuals with a low basal metabolic rate are at risk for weight gains compared to individuals with normal or elevated metabolic rates (77,78).

The following conclusions summarize the observations about the causes of obesity in the Pima Indians (78): a reduced rate of energy expenditure is a risk factor for body weight gain; at any given weight, Pima women require fewer calories for maintenance of weight than men; obesity in the Pima is unlikely to be the result of a fixed or predetermined number of adipocytes; adipocytes, although larger in obese individuals, are resistant to the action of insulin (e.g., they require more insulin to stimulate glucose transport); a relative inability of fat stores to release stored triglycerides (fats) as free fatty acids; energy expenditure is lower in obese individuals than in lean. These observations indicate that there are metabolic differences that distinguish obese and non-obese individuals.

A substantial body of evidence indicates that obese and lean people eat about the same amount of food (79–82) and caloric intake varies widely among randomly selected lean individuals (83,84). This implies the existence of autoregulatory mechanisms (a "setpoint") which maintains body weight within a fairly narrow range. It has been suggested that in the absence of any underlying differences in energy expenditure ("energy efficiency") between obese and lean people, obesity must be due to excessive intake of energy (85). This conclusion would rest on the prediction that energy requirements vary only with body size, age, and sex and can be predicted in a mathematical way that takes these variables into account. However, there is accumulating evidence that genetic factors mediate our basal rate of energy expenditure (75,86). The resting metabolic rate, which accounts for 75% of energy used each day in sedentary adults, is strongly correlated with body size (87–89). However, the variability of metabolic rates from person to person exceeds that predicted if age, sex, and body size alone are the sole determinants, leaving an estimated 20–45% of basal metabolic rate accounted for by other factors (24,90).

HEALTH CONSEQUENCES OF OVERNUTRITION Health risks of obesity begin to appear when weight is more than 20% above optimal weights using life insurance tables or when body mass index exceeds 27 (91). Individuals who are overweight are at increased risk of hypertension, diabetes, stroke, heart disease, and some forms of cancer (92). Thus, obese individuals more frequently demonstrate insulin resistance and type II diabetes, and they have other risk factors for cardiovascular disease, including hypertension, hypertriglyceridemia, and decreased high-density lipoproteins. Overweight men demonstrate high mortality rates for colorectal cancer and modestly increased death rates from prostate cancer (93). For women, obesity increases the incidence of cancers in which endocrine factors play a role, including endometrial, cervical, and ovarian cancer (94). Curiously, results for breast cancer are less clear, with some studies showing increased breast cancer in lean women (95).

INTERVENTION Although weight loss is typically regarded as the goal of treatment for obesity, it has been recently suggested that metabolic fitness be included as a measure of successful outcome (55). This notion stems, in part, from the observation that physical activity can restore insulin sensitivity and lower cholesterol levels in obese patients even in the absence of weight loss (96). Changes in eating habits and levels of physical activity come slowly and are not like the "quick fixes" we often demand.

Because successful and permanent weight loss is so frustrating and difficult to achieve, there is a huge audience for drug treatments for obesity, which fall into four general classes: those affecting satiety via effects on the brain; those that inhibit the absorption of fats and calories in the gastrointestinal tract without affecting the brain; those which increase metabolic rates and thermogenesis; those that mobilize peripheral stores of fats or that inhibit triglyceride synthesis (4). The size of the market for a quick path to thinness is demonstrated by the fact that in the year before it was removed from the market, the weight loss drug combination of fenfluramine and phentermine (fen-phen) was given to over 18 million people (54). The search for ways to fight obesity are varied and have a long history. Cigarettes were marketed as useful in weight control, particularly among young women (97). Similarly, up to half of all female cocaine users report use of cocaine as a weight-control measure (98). This is not to directly compare cocaine use to fen-phen or cigarette smoking, but merely to emphasize that pharmacological control of obesity has a powerful allure.

OVERNUTRITION, LEPTIN, AND HORMONES In 1994, the gene for a weight-regulating protein called leptin was cloned from obese mice having a mutant gene for leptin (designated ob/ob) (99). The lack of leptin in these mice causes them to eat as though they are in a perpetual state of starvation. Normally secreted by adipocytes, injection of leptin back into ob/ob mice produced weight loss, and leptin was found to be secreted in humans with a circadian nocturnal rise *(100)*. Thus, the initial data suggested that leptin was a "fat-busting" hormone that suppressed eating and hunger and that might be mutated in obese human subjects. However, mutations of the leptin gene are extremely rare, with only a few families discovered to have leptin mutations after several years of a worldwide search *(24)*. Furthermore, obese subjects have leptin levels in serum that are higher than normal-weight subjects, which closely correlate with percentage of body fat *(101)*. These results suggest that obesity may represent an insensitivity to leptin. It is possible that leptin receptors, rather than leptin itself, may be altered or malfunctioning in human obesity. Another mouse, prone to obesity and diabetes, designated db/db has been shown to have mutant-inactive leptin receptors *(102)*, but unlike the ob/ob mouse, it has normal leptin levels. As with mutants of leptin, leptin-receptor mutants are rare in humans *(24)* and do not account for the vast majority of obesity.

Leptins also stimulate production of a factor which causes death of adipocytes by apoptosis *(103)*. It is proposed that the pathway stimulated by leptin acting on the central nervous system (CNS) leads to expression of an inner mitochondrial membrane protein of adipocytes that uncouples mitochondrial respiration *(104,105)*. This uncoupled mitochondrial respiration promotes free-radical generation and eventually produces apoptosis. A patent was recently issued for a clinical assay to measure expression of one of the uncoupling proteins, and it is suggested that expression of uncoupling protein at high levels marks the ability to dispose of excess calories *(106)*. The mediator connecting the CNS and peripheral adipocytes remains unknown, but it may be the retinoic acid receptor and the peroxisome proliferator receptor *(107)*. These findings concerning leptin and its receptor prompted a search for proteins that interact with leptin to control appetite. Leptin receptors are present in the brain in the same region where another protein, neuropeptide Y (NPY), is located. NPY is markedly elevated in the leptin-deficient ob/ob mice and stimulates appetite *(108)*.

Another obese mouse strain, agouti, overproduces a protein (*agouti*) which blocks the binding of alpha melanocyte-stimulating hormone (αMSH) to a receptor designated Metabolic Clearance Rate (MCR)-1 *(109)*. Normally, αMSH causes the production of black pigment in the hair, but that is blocked by the *agouti* protein, leading to their bright yellow fur. To explain the obesity, it was proposed that a parallel system of receptor-blocking *agouti* proteins and appetite-suppressing MCR-like receptors existed in the brain. Following up on this hypothesis, a receptor called MCR-4, located in the arcuate nucleus of the brain (a region also targeted by leptin), signals suppression of feeding. Melanocortins suppressed appetite when injected into both ob/ob and normal mice, and "knock-out" of the MCR-4 receptor from normal mice leads to obesity *(110)*. Thus, the melanocortins suppress appetite in contrast to NPY, which increases appetite. The relationships among leptin, melanocortins, and NPY are shown in Fig. 1.

UNDERNUTRITION

RESPONSE TO STARVATION
There may be a connection between leptin and starvation by which starvation-induced decreases in leptin mediate some of the well-known endocrine

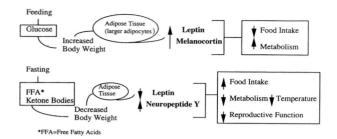

Fig. 1. Feeding/fasting, fuel sources, and body weight are shown on the left portion of the diagram. Recently discovered mediators are shown in the middle in bold with proposed physiological responses are on the right (see refs. 100–110).

and metabolic effects of starvation *(111,112)*. The endocrine consequences of starvation include decreased negative feedback of leptin and insulin on the hypothalamus and peripheral organs, decreased production of thyroid hormone and reproductive hormones with suppression of the menstrual cycle, and increased production of glucocorticoids *(111,113)*. Adults will lose approximately 25% of body weight within 6 mo of a semistarvation diet (approximately 1500 cal) *(114)*. During recovery, when caloric intake is gradually increased over a period of 3 mo to prestarvation levels, body fat stores are replenished. Subsequently, when food is made available as desired, food intake climbs well above the prestarvation levels (hyperphagia) and persists for several weeks after prestarvation body weight is reached. This period of hyperphagia correlates with restoration of muscle mass (lean body mass) *(115)*.

The metabolic responses to starvation (in the absence of other diseases) are quite predictable. In otherwise healthy individuals, glucose is the main source of fuel when food supplies are adequate. In contrast, following several days of starvation, the main fuel source shifts to gluconeogenesis primarily from fat. Although liver stores of glycogen are utilized during the early period of starvation, these last only 24–48 h. Thus, during periods of inadequate nutrition, the body generates glucose from fat stores, preserving lean (e.g., muscle) mass, as a survival mechanism *(115)*. Figure 2 illustrates the principle that production (or loss) of peptide mediators can induce weight loss in spite of normal or even increased food intake. This should serve as a reminder that the opposite problem, obesity, could reasonably be the result of mediators that alter the efficiency of utilization of calories.

Adults who survive a period of starvation are, at least physi-

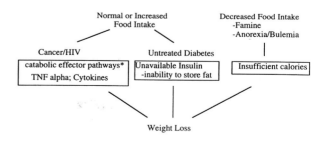

Fig. 2. Outline of the mechanisms leading to weight loss, demonstrating the principle that weight loss can occur in spite of normal or increased food intake.

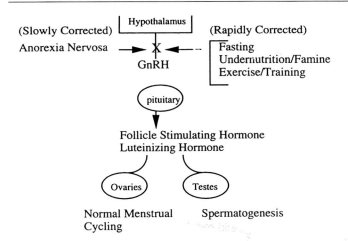

Fig. 3. Hypothalamic–pituitary axis and effects of starvation vs anorexia on menstruation and spermatogenesis.

cally, restored to their previous health status. Reproductive function, which rapidly decreases during conditions of undernutrition, is quickly restored to normal when food becomes available. The loss of normal reproductive function can occur rapidly, even following 2 d of fasting, and is accompanied by diminished secretion of gonadotropin-releasing hormone (GnRH) by the hypothalamus (see Fig. 3) (116,117). This occurs without significant loss of body weight or body fat and is accompanied by decreased secretion of luteinizing hormone and follicle-stimulating hormone by the pituitary (118). The pituitary remains responsive to exogenously administered GnRH during undernutrition, suggesting that a shift to fasting metabolism is accompanied by suppression of reproductive hormones at the level of the hypothalamus. Thus, if adults survive a famine, the evidence is that they will recover normal fertility levels (119). However, the effects of famine on children, particularly during pregnancy and the first year of life, may be more long lasting. The loss of reproductive function during periods of undernutrition may prevent conception in the first place, decreasing the likelihood that conception will occur during periods of scarcity. Nevertheless, children born after exposure to famine conditions in utero and during early life (e.g., the first year) may suffer some health consequences. The term "imprinting" has been used to describe nongenetic programming of fetal development that persists into adult life.

FETAL AND POSTNATAL IMPRINTING Epidemiological studies have led to the concept that during critical periods of growth, the fetus or newborn may be programmed in a permanent way by nongenetic conditions in utero and during early life. This hypothesis develops naturally out of observations that variations in birth weight and size are influenced much more by the maternal/uterine environment than by the fetal genome (120). Intrauterine and early postnatal life includes periods of embryological development and rapid growth, and it is reasonable to consider that undernutrition exerts effects during early life that may not be seen when adults are exposed to famine conditions.

Studies conducted in Great Britain have shown that low-birth-weight babies and babies who gain weight slowly after birth have substantially higher death rates as a result of cardiovascular disease during their adult life, and this increased risk of cardiovascular

disease is paralleled by measurable differences in cholesterol, blood pressure, and fibrinogen levels (121). The risk incurred by low birth weight (e.g., 5.5 lbs vs 8.5 lbs at birth) has been compared to the magnitude of increased risk for cardiovascular disease which is observed in cigarette smokers. Similarly, low-birth-weight babies have a higher incidence of impaired glucose tolerance and adult-onset diabetes (approximately 40% of individuals weighing 5.5 lbs or less at birth have impaired glucose tolerance or overt diabetes versus 22% of those whose birth weight was 8.5 lbs) (122). A cautious approach to these findings is warranted because other studies fail to confirm these findings directly. The hypothesis that fetal undernutrition would cause increased mortality in adults who survived as compared to an unaffected cohort has been tested in other populations. Adult survivors born during the Finnish famine years 1866–1868, when three successive crop failures caused the death of 8% of the total population of the country, did not manifest differences in mortality rates when compared to those born prior to, during, and after the famine (123).

Ongoing studies of the famine experienced in Holland during the last 6 mo of World War II (October 1944–May 1945) support the concept that extreme undernutrition during the fetal and early postpartum periods can determine effects that are observed in adult life. During this war-induced famine, rations fell to 1200 cal in November of 1945 and to between 600 and 800 cal in February of 1945. A decrease in birth weight was observed when maternal weight gain fell below a threshold of 0.5 kg/wk during the third trimester of pregnancy (119,124). Additional studies of the offspring of the Dutch famine of 1945 suggest that trimester-specific effects occur. Approximately 300,000 men whose mothers had been exposed to this famine were studied when they were inducted into the Dutch military services at age 19 (125). Exposure during the first half of pregnancy resulted in significantly higher obesity rates, whereas exposure during the last trimester of pregnancy and during the first months of life produced significantly lower rates of obesity in adult life. These data suggest that the timing of the nutritional events during pregnancy and early life can have different and even opposing effects. Finally, recently completed analyses of the offspring of mothers exposed to the Dutch famine suggest that some imprinting effects are conveyed to the next generation (126). Such studies require detailed records of prenatal care, birth weight, and postnatal feeding and weight gain. Similarly, knowledge of the characteristics of the population at large is required to enable control for potentially confounding variables.

Infant diets may also exert programming effects. Studies conducted in baboons suggest that breast vs formula feeding permanently programs the risk of atherosclerotic disease in the adult animals. Formula-fed baboons have lower rates of involvement of blood vessels by atherosclerotic plaques, and hepatic low-density lipoprotein (LDL) receptor mRNA is consistently higher in breast-fed animals (127).

CACHEXIA Weight loss is common in patients with both cancer and infection by human immunodeficiency virus (HIV). Although decreased food intake (anorexia) occurs in these conditions, the weight loss is either in spite of adequate caloric intake or it is out of proportion to the anorexia. The causes of these syndromes remain unclear, although much research has focused on circulating factors that promote weight loss, including tumor necrosis factor-alpha (TNFα) and other cytokines (128). Before insulin was widely available to treat diabetes, it was known that untreated diabetics were hyperphagic and yet they continued to lose weight. We now understand that this is due to the stimulation of lipolysis by insulin deficiency and an inability to produce the enzyme (lipoprotein lipase) that promotes uptake of fats from the blood into adipocytes *(113)*.

One of the most striking features of tuberculosis (TB) infections was the loss of body weight that occurred in patients, and TB was referred to as "consumption." Modern equivalents include the HIV wasting syndrome *(129)* and the cachexia observed in about half of all patients with cancer *(130)*. A significant number of cancer patients develop cachexia in which there is loss of both adipose tissue and skeletal muscle mass. Although cancer patients experience anorexia and therefore eat less, the loss of body mass is out of proportion to the decreased caloric intake *(130)*. In addition, unlike what one might predict, the decreased food intake of cancer patients is associated not with decreased metabolic rate, but with an increase in energy expenditure. This is accompanied by increased gluconeogenesis. It is unlikely that cancer-related cachexia is the result of competition for calories, as it occurs when tumors comprise less than 0.01% of body weight *(131)*. TNF-α is an important element in the pathogenesis of cachexia. TNF-α was isolated from rabbits with severe weight loss and hypertriglyceridemia and an associated inhibition of lipoprotein lipase, resulting in catabolic effects on fat cells *(132)*. TNF-α and other cytokines both decrease lipoprotein lipase and increase lipolysis. It is of interest to note that fish-oil supplementation of the diet of patients with pancreatic cancer, who are particularly susceptible to cancer cachexia, reverses cachexia and weight loss *(133)*. EPA derived from fish oil directly inhibits lipolysis and the breakdown of nitrogen from muscle protein in an animal model of lymphoma *(134)*. Serum from these mice promotes lipolysis in non-tumor-bearing mice, suggesting that a catabolic factor produced by tumors can induce weight loss via lipolysis. The effect occurred without increasing calorie consumption or intake of nitrogen and is specific to EPA, and EPA reverses the lipolysis and protein degradation that occurs in these mice. EPA may exert its anti-cachexia effects via altering cyclooxygenase activity or the potency of eicosanoids both at the level of target organ by inhibiting nitrogen loss and by inhibiting the generation of TNF-α by macrophages *(135)*.

Human immunodeficient virus patients also suffer weight loss in spite of adequate caloric intake. In a prospective study, in spite of counseling and maintenance of caloric intake, weight loss occurs *(136)*. This weight loss has been attributed to the hypermetabolism which occurs in HIV-infected patients *(137)*. In addition, malabsorption may account for some of the weight loss occurring in HIV-infected patients. This malabsorption occurs even in patients without diarrhea or severe weight loss *(138)*. It is of interest to note that enteral supplementation with a fish-oil-containing formula prevented the HIV-associated cachexia in human patients, whereas one lacking fish oils did not prevent it *(136)*.

Finally, it is likely that cytokines alone may not explain all of the cachexia seen in HIV-positive and cancer patients. Regions of the brain communicating with the pituitary and adrenal glands [the hypothalamic–pituitary–adrenal axis (HPA)] play a central role in regulation of body weight in response to decreased (and increased) food intake and in the wasting syndromes associated with AIDS and cancer *(139)*. It is also of interest to note that malignancy-induced cachexia is the only circumstance in which adipocytes are known to undergo death, by apoptosis *(140)*.

ANOREXIA AND BULIMIA   Fear of fatness has become a part of life among adolescent girls *(141)* and it is notable that this angst over body weight and thinness parallels the widely documented increase in the incidence of obesity over the past 20 yr among virtually all age groups. Furthermore, it is not just fear of fatness but a desire to be "ultrathin" that is found when adolescent girls are questioned about their perceptions of body weight *(142)*. It is especially troubling that dieting behavior in these adolescent girls is associated with lowered intake of micronutrients compared to girls who do not diet *(143)*.

Young women from middle school through college ages are especially susceptible to anorexia and bulimia, which are behaviors that reduce caloric intake sometimes to the point of starvation. Anorexia and bulimia are poorly understood, difficult to treat and carry staggering emotional and financial costs for patients and their families. They are presumed to be related to social pressures to lose weight and a perception of being "overweight" in spite of being of normal weight, or nearly so *(144)*. Factors that conspire to create this perception include fashion standards that promote a lean, even prepubescent, physique. The natural physical development of adolescents as they move increasingly away from this fashion standard may parallel the perception of "fatness."

Anorexia is not a newly described disease, as the essence of it was observed and characterized in the 19th century *(144)*. Anorexia and bulimia affect up to 3% of women at some point during their lives *(144,145)*. Anorexics demonstrate the following characteristics: extreme dieting, fear of eating, dangerous loss of weight, increased physical activity, depression, reduced heart rate and blood pressure, increased cortisol levels, and markedly reduced estrogen (or androgen) production with amenorrhea, which is a hallmark feature *(144,146)*. The metabolic effects of anorexia resemble semistarvation observed in marasmic children and protein malnutrition observed in hospitalized patients in affluent countries *(147)*. A recent study of albumin metabolism in anorexics has shown some of the anticipated metabolic effects of starvation: decreased body weight, decreased BMI, and decreased lean body mass *(148)*. However, in contrast to famine-induced undernutrition, serum albumin levels do not tend to fall *(148)*. Treatment of the disease is to prescribe a 2000- to 4000-cal diet combined with supervision, counseling, and monitoring at an impatient facility or a day-treatment program *(144)*. Restoration of body weight is usually achieved, but relapse is also common *(149)*. The causes of anorexia remain elusive, but normalization of these abnormalities with restoration of body weight argue against an obvious biological cause. However, the observation that serotonin metabolites and leptin levels are increased in recovered anorexics raises the possibility of an underlying biological disturbance *(144)*. Mortality from anorexia because of suicide or starvation is approximately 5% per each 10 yr of follow-up *(150)*. Problems are lifelong in at least half of all patients, including continued preoccupation with weight gain, depression, and metabolic problems such as osteoporosis, which is not prevented by estrogen-replacement therapy *(144)*.

In contrast to anorexics, who are underweight, bulimics usually have normal body weights *(144)*. Bulimia nervosa was recognized as a disorder in 1980, and bulimics share with anorexics a preoccupation with weight and body shape occurring mainly in young women *(144)*. However, in bulimics, weight loss is not as severe, and eating is in binges that are typically followed by purging behavior (self-induced vomiting, use of laxatives or diuretics, and compulsive exercise) *(151)*. Reported crude mortality rates for anorexics range from 3% to 20% during follow-up periods of 6–20 yr, and figures for bulimia nervosa are somewhat lower, around 3% *(152)*. It is increasingly recognized that bulimia and anorexia may coexist, such that up to half of all anorexics develop bulimic symptoms and severe restriction and bulimic behaviors may alternate in the same affected individual *(153)*. Treatment with either behavioral therapy or antidepressant medications is associated with resolution in up to 50% of patients *(144)*.

THE HOSPITALIZED PATIENT   Major surgery and trauma are stresses that lead to hypermetabolic states. Stored fats, glycogen, and labile protein are broken down as energy sources, and a variety of hormones, including adrenocorticotropin, catecholamines, cortisol, and glucagon, act to oppose the action of insulin and promote the generation of glucose. They also stimulate net protein catabolism with the potential for losses of as much as 20–30 g/d of nitrogen *(155)*. Up to one-third of hospitalized patients were noted by Butterworth over 20 yr ago to be severely malnourished *(146)*. Furthermore, the longer severely ill, injured, or postoperative patients stay in the hospital, the more likely they are to suffer from steadily worsening malnutrition. Parenteral and enteral nutrition have become part of the armamentarium of treating and supporting postsurgical, trauma, burn, sepsis, and other patients who have special nutritional needs *(155)*. Anticipation and prevention of nutritional stresses is now the favored approach to these patients. Catabolism accompanies major surgery and normally persists for up to 72 h when a shift to anabolic metabolism occurs. Serum albumin levels below 35 g/L and low total protein and cholesterol levels have been used as laboratory values to identify a group of patients at risk for complications associated with nutritional deficits *(156)*. There is evidence that protein-energy malnutrition is associated with increased length of hospitalizations, impaired immune and skeletal muscle function, and decreased wound healing *(157)*. However, nutritional intervention with parenteral or enteral supplemental nutrition is complicated by the potential for increased risk of infection *(158)*. At a practical level, it is suggested that if feeding cannot be resumed 5 d after surgery, nutritional support is indicated.

FAMINE   It is unlikely that you will encounter malnutrition resulting from a lack of available calories or protein in wealthy countries such as the United States. However, famine is a regular and fearsome part of human history, and a few words about the causes and consequences of famine are in order. Famine is sometimes the simple result of crop failure because of drought or plant diseases, and if populations are dependent on locally produced food, famine can result. However, famines caused by government policies have killed many millions of people during the 20th century. It is nearly impossible for us to envision famine in which starvation and associated diseases can easily carry away one-third of the population and cause entire countries to be depopulated by emigration *(159)*. The Irish potato famine and the Finnish famine of 1866–1868 were initiated by natural causes and were closely associated with diseases such as tuberculosis *(160)*. Warfare is closely associated with famine, and the 900-d siege of Leningrad, which was at its worst in November of 1941, is beyond description. During a period of 3 wk, it is estimated that 200,000 people died when the daily ration of food in Leningrad was 125 g in the form of edible grain baked into a loaf *(161)*. This is equivalent to a cup of rice or two thin slices of bread, an amount of food that sustained life for 2 wk at best, given the malnutrition

of the city's inhabitants. The Great Leap Forward, undertaken by Mao Tse-tung in China in the late 1950s, exemplifies a man-made famine caused not by war but by government policy. Astonishingly, rations of food available to residents in Pingyuan county in northeastern China during the entire period of 1959 through 1960 were similar to those available to citizens of Leningrad in November of 1941 *(161)*. The Great Leap Forward was a plan to collectivize agriculture and move more than 90 million peasants off of their lands and employ them in producing steel using primitive smelters. Peasants scoured the countryside for metal of any kind, including hoes, shovels and other farming tools, to be melted down and used for steel production. Between 30 and 50 million people died in the ensuing famine. Finally, earlier in the century, a similar plan of collectivization was developed by the Russian Communist government, led by Stalin, and directed mainly at Ukrainians. By conservative estimates, this led directly to the deaths of 11 million people from 1930 to 1937 *(162)*. Perhaps knowledge of these millions of famine-caused deaths in our own century will serve as reminders of the tenuous balance of natural and man-made forces required to maintain a reliable supply of food.

SUMMARY

This chapter introduces the concept that obesity is not a condition that is the simple result of overeating. Although populations around the world, as a whole, are becoming progressively more obese, there is an ever-increasing body of scientific evidence that genetic and neurohormonal factors drive the tendency toward obesity among individuals. In other words, although the trends toward decreasing physical activity and increased dietary fat intake may explain the ever-increasing incidence of obesity, they do not explain the wide individual variations in body weight. We are on the cusp of greater scientific understanding of the complex interactions of peripheral and central nervous system humoral and genetic factors that modulate body weight, satiety, and eating.

Obesity has been epidemiologically linked to an increased risk of death from cancer, atherosclerosis, and diabetes and with musculoskeletal morbidity resulting from bearing increased weight on joints. As with many risks, moderate obesity is less troublesome than extreme obesity and recommendations to lose weight must be tempered by a balanced view of the likely benefits. Because it is so difficult to lose weight and keep it off by following the "eat less and exercise more" prescription, drug treatment for obesity will continue to have an enormous attraction. Whether the reason for losing weight is primarily for the sake of appearances or for medical purposes, there is an intense drive to appear slim and attractive.

Although losing weight is generally a good thing for most of us, anorexia/bulimia among young girls is the tragic consequence of a poorly understood response to a "fear of fatness." This is a potentially fatal condition that presents tragedy and stress for the patients and families. Otherwise perfectly healthy girls are afflicted and essentially become starved. Other forms of undernutrition include the cachexia observed in HIV and cancer patients. Cachexia occurs in spite of adequate caloric intake, or, at least, the resulting weight loss is out of proportion to the anorexia that many cancer and HIV patients experience. Hospitalization is a risk factor for undernutrition. Patients undergoing general anesthesia and surgery are fasting, and patients who have suffered trauma, burns, and infections may be unable to take food by mouth or they may have extreme protein losses because of catabolism and/or their injuries. Although parenteral nutrition is of great value in supporting these patients, it is not without complications, particularly the risk of infection resulting from the indwelling catheters used to provide the nutrition. Famine as a cause of undernutrition is seldom merely the result of crop failure. It is almost always complicated by war, and even more tragically, it has been used as an instrument of terror and genocide. Famine, war, and pestilence will undoubtedly follow us into the next century. Finally, the chapter includes a discussion of imprinting that describes the permanent modification of genes into adult life as a result of events occurring during fetal and early postnatal life. This is a fascinating arena which offers data that contradict our usually assumed notions that "fatness" at birth is bad. In fact, most evidence suggest that there are significantly increased risks of atherosclerotic cardiovascular disease during adult life among individuals who are "skinny' at birth.

REFERENCES

1. Flegal KM, Carroll MD, Kuczmarski RJ, Johnson CL. Overweight and obesity in the United States: prevalence and trends, 1960–1994. Int J Obesity 1998; 22:39–47.
2. The painful business of losing weight. The Economist August 30, 1997; 45–47.
3. Krause MV, Mahan LK. Food Nutrition and Diet Therapy, A Textbook of Nutritional Care. WB Saunders, Philadelphia, 1984.
4. Leveille GA, Finley JW. Macronutrient substitutes. Ann NY Acad Sci 1997; 819:11–21.
5. Doll R, Pieto R. The causes of cancer: quantitative estimates of avoidable risks of cancer in the United States today. J Natl Cancer Inst 1981; 66:1191–309.
6. Fernandes G, Chandrasekar B, Troyer DA, Venkatraman JT, Good RA. Dietary lipids and calorie restriction affect mammary tumor incidence and gene expression in mouse mammary tumor virus/v-Ha-*ras* transgenic mice. Proc Natl Acad Sci USA 1995; 92:6494–8.
7. Hursting S, Perkins S, Phang J. Calorie restriction delays spontaneous tumorigenesis in p53-knockout transgenic mice. Proc Natl Acad Sci USA 1994; 91:7036–40.
8. Weindruch R, Walford RL, Fligiel S, Guthrie D. The retardation of aging in mice by dietary restriction: longevity, cancer, immunity and lifetime energy intake. J Nutr 1986; 116:641–54.
9. Fernandes G, Venkatraman JT. Dietary restriction: effect on immunological function and aging. In: Klurfeld DM, eds, Human Nutrition: A Comprehensive Treatise, pp. 91–120, Plenum, New York, 1993.
10. Masoro EJ, Yu BP. Diet and nephropathy. Lab Invest 1989; 60:165–7.
11. Troyer DA, Chandrasekar B, Thinnes T, Stone A, Loskutoff DJ, Fernandes G. Effects of energy intake on type 1 plasminogen activator inhibitor levels in glomeruli of lupus-prone B/W mice. Am J Path 1995; 146:111–20.
12. Yu BP, Lee DW, Marler CG, Choi JH. Mechanisms of food restriction: protection of cellular homeostasis. Proc Soc Exp Biol Med 1990; 193:13–5.
13. Troyer D, Fernandes G. Nutrition and apoptosis. Nutr Res 1996; 16:1959–79.
14. Rolls B, Shide D. The influence of dietary fat on food intake and body weight. Nutr Rev 1992; 50:283–90.
15. Heini AF, Weinsier RL. Divergent trends in obesity and fat intake patterns: the American paradox. Am J Med 1997; 102:259–64.
16. Danforth E. Diet and obesity. Am J Clin Nutr 1985; 41:1132–5.
17. US Public Health Service. Healthy People 2000: National Health Promotion and Disease Prevention Objectives. US Department of Health and Human Services, Washington, DC, 1991.
18. Tararanni PA, Ravussin E. Effect of fat intake on energy balance. Ann NY Acad Sci 1997; 819:37–43.
19. Golay A, Bobbioni E. The role of dietary fat in obesity. Int J Obesity 1997; 21:S2–S11.
20. Schutz Y, Acheson KJ, Jequier E. Twenty-four-hour energy expenditure and thermogenesis: response to progressive carbohydrate overfeeding in man. Int J Obesity 1985; 9:S111–S1114.
21. Abbott WGH, Howard BV, Christin L, Freymond D, Lillioja S, Boyce VL, et al. Short-term energy balance: relationship with protein, carbohydrate, and fat balances. Am J Physiol 1988; 255:E332–7.
22. Astrup A, Buemann B, Christensen NJ, Toubro S. Failure to increase lipid oxidation in response to increasing dietary fat content in formerly obese women. Am J Physiol 1994; 266:E592–9.
23. Duncan K, Bacon J, Weinsier R. The effects of high and low energy diets on satiety, energy intake, and eating time of obese and nonobese subjects. Am J Clin Nutr 1983; 37:763–7.
24. Pi-Sunyer FX. Energy balance: role of genetics and activity. Ann NY Acad Sci 1997; 819:29–35.
25. McHugh P, Moran T, Barton G. Satiety: a graded behavioral phenomenon regulating caloric intake. Science 1975; 190:167–9.
26. van Amerlsvoort J, van Stratum P, Kraal J, Lussenburg R, Houtsmuller U. Effects of varying the carbohydrate : fat ratio in a hot lunch on postprandial variables in male volunteers. Br J Nutr 1989; 61:267–83.
27. Ascherio A, Willett WC. New directions in dietary studies of coronary heart disease. J Nutr 1995; 125:647S–55S.
28. Fernandes G, Venkatraman J. Micronutrient and lipid interactions in cancer. Ann NY Acad Sci 1993; 587:78–91.
29. Kritchevsky D. Overview of fat and calories in tumorigenesis. Adv Exp Med Biol 1996; 399:1–12.
30. Connor WE, Connor SL. Diet, atherosclerosis, and fish oil. Adv Intern Med 1990; 35:139–71.
31. Anderson GH. Nutritional and health aspects of macronutrient substitution. Ann NY Acad Sci 1997; 819:1–9.
32. Nabors LO. Consumer attitudes and practices. Ann NY Acad Sci 1997; 819:115–20.
33. Boyd NF, Lockwood GA, Greenberg CV, Martin LJ, Tritchler DL. Effects of a low-fat high-carbohydrate diet on plasma sex hormones in premenopausal women: results from a randomized controlled trial. Br J Cancer 1997; 76:127–35.
34. Sarkar NH, Fernandes G, Telang NT, Kourides IA, Good RA. Low-calorie diet prevents the development of mammary tumors in C3H mice and reduces circulating prolactin level, murine mammary tumor virus expression, and proliferation of mammary alveolar cells. Proc Natl Acad Sci USA 1982; 79:7758–62.
35. Chung OK, Pomeranz Y. Recent trends in usage of fats and oils as functional ingredients in the baking industry. JAOCS 1983; 60: 1848–1851.
36. Fernandes G, Jolly CA. Nutrition and autoimmune disease. Nutr Rev 1998; 56:91–9.
37. Zhu BQ, Parmley WW. Modification of experimental and clinical atherosclerosis by dietary fish oil. Am Heart J 1990; 119:168–78.
38. Fernandes G, Venkatraman JT. Role of omega-3 fatty acids in health and disease. Nutr Res 1993; 13:S19–S45.
39. Galli C, Butrum C. Dietary ω-3 fatty acids and cancer. World Rev Nutr Dietet 1991; 66:446–61.
40. Fay MP, Freedman LS, Clifford CK, Midthune DN. Effect of different types and amounts of fat on the development of mammary tumors in rodents: a review. Cancer Res 1997; 57:3979–88.
41. Hilakivi-Clarke L, Clarke R, Onojafe I, Raygada M, Cho E, Lippman M. A maternal diet high in n-6 polyunsaturated fats alters mammary gland development, puberty onset, and breast cancer risk among female rat offspring. Proc Natl Acad Sci USA 1997; 94:9372–77.
42. Fernandes G, Flescher E, Venkatraman JT. Modulation of cellular immunity, fatty acid composition, fluidity and Ca²⁺ influx by food restriction in aging rats. AGING: Immunol Infect Dis 1990; 2:117–25.
43. Simopoulos AP. Omega-3 fatty acids in health and disease and in growth and development. Am J Clin Nutr 1991; 54:438–463.
44. Zock PL, Katan MB. Butter, margarine and serum lipoproteins. Atherosclerosis 1997; 131:7–16.
45. Zock PL, Katan MB. Trans fatty acids, lipoproteins, and coronary risk. Can J Phys Pharm 1997; 75:211–16.

46. Ip C. Review of the effects of trans fatty acids, oleic acid, n-3 poly-unsaturated fatty acids, and conjugated linoleic acid on mammary carcinogenesis in animals. Am J Clin Nutr 1997; 66:1523S–9S.

47. Schultz T, Chew B, Seaman W. Differential stimulatory and inhibitory responses of human MCF-7 breast cancer cells to linoleic acid and conjugated linoleic acid in culture. Anticancer Res 1992; 12:21–43.

48. Lin H, Boylston TD, Chang MJ, Luedecke LO, Shultz TD. Survey of the conjugated linoleic acid content of dairy products. J Dairy Sci 1995; 78:2358–65.

49. Durgam VR, Fernandes G. The growth inhibitory effect of conjugated linoleic acid on MCF-7 cells is related to estrogen response system. Cancer Lett 1997; 116:121–30.

50. van Poppel G, van den Berg H. Vitamins and cancer. Cancer Lett 1997; 114:195–202.

51. Kurzer MS, Xu X. Dietary phytoestrogens. Ann Rev Nutr 1997; 17:353–81.

52. Trichopoulou A, Lagiou P. Healthy traditional Mediterranean diet: an expression of culture, history, and lifestyle. Nutr Rev 1997; 55:383–9.

53. Prasad KN, Cole W, Hovland P. Cancer prevention studies: past, present, and future directions. Nutrition 1998; 14:197–210.

54. Kolata G. Companies recall 2 top diet drugs at FDA's urging. New York Times September 16, 1997:A1.

55. Campfield, LA. In: Dalton S, ed. Overweight and Weight Management, pp. 466–85. Aspen, Gaithersburg, MD, 1997.

56. Stevens J, Cai J, Pamuk ER, Williamson DF, Thun MJ, Wood JL. The effect of age on the association between body-mass index and mortality. N Engl J Med 1998; 338:1–7.

57. Bennett WI. Beyond overeating. N Engl J Med 1995; 332:673–4.

58. Kuczmarski RJ, Carroll MD, Flegal KM, Troiano RP. Varying body mass index cutoff points to describe overweight prevalence among U.S. adults: NHANES III (1988 to 1994). Obesity Res 1997; 5:542.

59. Rosenbaum M, Leibel RL, Hirsch J. Obesity. N Engl J Med 1997; 337:396–407.

60. Kuczmarski RJ, Flegal KM, Campbell SM, Johnson CL. Increasing prevalence of overweight among US adults: The National Health and Nutrition Examination Surveys 1960–1991. JAMA 1994; 272:205–11.

61. Troiano RP, Flegal KM, Kuczmarski RJ, Campbell SM, Johnson CL. Overweight prevalence and trends for children and adolescents: the National Health and Nutrition Examination Surveys, 1963–1991. Arch Pediatr Adolesc Med 1995; 149:1085.

62. Seidell JC. Obesity in Europe: scaling an epidemic. Int J Obesity 1995; 19(suppl 1):1.

63. World Health Organization (WHO) Consultation on Obesity. Obesity: Preventing and Managing the Global Epidemic of Obesity. Report of the WHO Consultation on Obesity (Geneva, June 3–5, 1997). WHO, Geneva, 1998; xvii, 276:111.

64. Kumanyika S. Obesity in black women. Epidemiol Rev 1987; 9:31–50.

65. Hazuda HP, Mitchell BD, Haffner SM, Stern MP. Obesity in Mexican American subgroups: findings from the San Antonio Heart Study. Am J Clin Nutr 1991; 53:1529S–34S.

66. Shimokata H, Andres R, Coon PJ, Elahi D, Muller DC, Tobin JD. Studies in the distribution of body fat. II. Longitudinal effects of losing weight. Int J Obesity 1988; 13:455–64.

67. Lewis CE, Smith DE, Wallace DD, Williams OD, Bild DE, Jacobs DR. Seven-year trends in body weight and associations and lifestyle and behavioral characteristics in black and white young adults: the CARDIA study. Am J Public Health 1997; 87:635–42.

68. Kissebah AH, Krakower GR. Regional adiposity and morbidity. Physiol Rev 1994; 74:761–811.

69. Zamboni M, Armellini F, Sheibban I, De Marchi M, Todesco T, Bergamo-Andreis IA, Cominacini L, Bosello O. Relation of body fat distribution in men and degree of coronary narrowings in coronary artery disease. Am J Cardiol 1992; 70:1135–8.

70. Depress JP, Moorjani S, Ferland M, Tremblay A, Lupien PJ, Nadeau A, Pinault S, Theriault G, Bouchard C. Adipose tissue distribution and plasma lipoprotein levels in obese women: importance of intra-abdominal fat. Arteriosclerosis 1989; 9:203–10.

71. Zamboni M, Armellini F, Harris T, Turcator E, Micciolo R, Bergamo-Andreis IA, et al. Effects of age on body fat distribution and cardiovascular risk factors in women. Am J Clin Nutr 1997; 66:111–5.

72. Kotani K, Tokunaga K, Fujiooka S, Kobatake T, Keno Y, Yoshida S, Shimomura I, Tarui S, Matsuzawa Y. Sexual dimorphism of age-related changes in whole-body fat distribution in the obese. Int J Obesity 1994; 18:207–12.

73. Haarbo J, Marslew U, Gotfredsen A, Christiansen C. Postmenopausal hormone replacement therapy prevents central distribution of body fat after menopause. Metabolism 1991; 40:1323–30.

74. Bjorntorp P. Body fat distribution, insulin resistance, and metabolic diseases. Nutrition 1997; 13:795–803.

75. Bouchard C. Genetics of obesity: overview and research directions. In: Bouchard C, ed, The Genetics of Obesity, p. 223. CRC, Boca Raton, FL, 1994.

76. Bogardus C, Lillioja S, Ravussin E, Abbott W, Zawadzki JK, Young A, Knowles WC, et al. Familial dependence of the resting metabolic rate. N Engl J Med 1986; 315:96–100.

77. Ravussin E, Lillioja S, Knowler WC, Christin L, Freymond D, Abbott, et al. Reduced rate of energy expenditure as a risk factor for body-weight gain. N Engl J Med 1988; 318:467–72.

78. Howard BV, Bogardus C, Ravussin E, Foley JE, Lillioja S, Mott DM, Bennett PH, Knowles WC. Studies of the etiology of obesity in Pima Indians. Am J Clin Nutr 1991; 53:1577S–85S.

79. Stefanik PA, Heald FP Jr, Mayer J. Caloric intake in relation to energy output of obese and non-obese adolescent boys. Am J Clin Nutr 1959; 7:55–62.

80. McCarthy MC. Dietary and activity patterns of obese women in Trinidad. J Am Diet Assoc 1966; 48:33–37.

81. Maxfield E, Konishi F. Patterns of food intake and physical activity in obesity. J Am Diet Assoc 1966; 49:406–8.

82. Kromhout D. Energy and macronutrient intake in lean and obese middle-aged men (the Zutphen Study). Am J Clin Nutr 1983; 37:295–9.

83. Widdowson EM. A study of English diets by the individual method, I. Men. J Hyg (Camb) 1936; 36:269–92.

84. Widdowson EM. A study of English diets by the individual method, II. Women. J Hyg (Camb) 1936; 36:293–309.

85. Garrow JS. Energy balance in man, an overview. Am J Clin Nutr 1987; 45(suppl 5):1114–9.

86. Comuzzie AG, Allison DB. The search for human obesity genes. Science 1988; 280:1374–7.

87. Roza AM, Shizgal HM. The Harris–Benedict equation reevaluated: resting energy requirements and the body cell mass. Am J Clin Nutr 1984; 40:168–82.

88. Bernstein RS, Thornton JC, Yang MU, Wang J, Redmond AM, Pierson RN Jr., et al. Prediction of the resting metabolic rate in obese patients. Am J Clin Nutr 1983; 37:595–602.

89. Ravussin E, Burnand B, Schutz Y, Jequier E. Twenty-four-hour energy expenditure and resting metabolic rate in obese, moderately obese and control subjects. Am J Clin Nutr 1981; 35:566–73.

90. Seidell CS, Muller DC, Sorkin JD, Andres R. Fasting respiratory exchange ratio and resting metabolic rate as predictors of overweight gain: The Baltimore Longitudinal Study on Aging. Int J Obesity 1992; 16:667–674.

91. Pi-Sunyer FX. Health implications of obesity. Am J Clin Nutr 1991; 53:1595S–1603S.

92. Centers for Disease Control. Prevalence of overweight—Behavioral Risk Factor Surveillance System 1987. MMWR 1989; 38:421–3.

93. Nomura A, Heilbrun LK, Stermmermann GN. Body mass index as a predictor of cancer in men. J Natl Cancer Inst 1985; 74:319–23.

94. Garfinkel L. Overweight and cancer. Ann Intern Med 1985; 103:1034–6.

95. Willet WC, Browne ML, Bain C, Lipnik RJ, Stampfer MJ. Relative weight and risk of breast cancer among premenopausal women. Am J Epidemiol 1985; 122:731–40.

96. Hill JO, Peters JC. Environmental contributions to the obesity epidemic. Science 1998; 280:1371–3.

97. French SA, Perry CL, Leon GR, Fulkerson JA. Weight concerns, dieting behavior and smoking initiation among adolescents: a prospective study. Am J Public Health 1994; 84:1818–20.

98. Cochrane CE, Malcolm R, Brewerton T. The role of weight control as a motivation for cocaine abuse. Addict Behav 1998; 23:201–7.

99. Zhang Y, Proenca R, Maffei M, Barone M, Leopold L, Friedman JM. Positional cloning of the mouse obese gene and its human homologue. Nature 1994; 372:425–31.

100. Sinha MK, Ohannesian JP, Heiman ML, Kriauciunas A, Stephens TW, Magosin S, Marco C, Caro JF. Nocturnal rise of leptin in lean, obese, and non-insulin-dependent diabetes mellitus subjects. J Clin Invest 1996; 97:1344–7.

101. Considine RB, Sinha MK, Heiman ML, Kriauciunas A, Stephens TW, Nyce MR, et al. Serum immunoreactive-leptin concentrations in normal-weight and obese humans. N Engl J Med 1996; 334:292–5.

102. Tartaglia LA. The leptin receptor. J Biol Chem 1997; 272:6093–6.

103. Qian H, Azain MJ, Compton MM, Hartzell DL, Hausman GJ, Baile CA. Brain administration of Leptin causes deletion of adipocytes by apoptosis. Endocrinology 1998; 139:791–4.

104. Negre-Salvayre A, Hirtz C, Carrera G, Cazenave R, Troly M, Salvayre R, et al. A role for uncoupling protein-2 as a regulator of mitochondrial hydrogen peroxide generation. FASEB J 1997; 11:809–15.

105. Gura, T. Uncoupling proteins provide new clue to obesity's causes. Science 1998; 280:1369–70.

106. Bonn D. Diagnosing weight disorders by measuring uncoupling proteins. Mol Med Today 1998; 4:185.

107. Chawla A, Lazar MA. Peroxisome proliferator and retinoid signaling pathways co-regulate preadipocyte phenotype and survival. Proc Natl Acad Sci USA 1994; 91:1786–90.

108. Stephens TW, Basinski M, Bristow PK, Bue-Valleskey JM, Burgett SG, Craft L, et al. The role of neuropeptide Y in the antiobesity action of the obese gene product. Nature 1995; 377:530–2.

109. Lu D, Willard D, Patel IR, Kadwell S, Overton L, Kost T, et al. Agouti protein is an antagonist of the melanocyte-stimulating-hormone receptor. Nature 1994; 371:799–802.

110. Huszar D, Lynch CA, Fairchild-Huntress V, Dunmore JH, Fang Q, Berkmeier LR, et al. Targeted disruption of the melanocortin-4 receptor results in obesity in mice. Cell 1997; 88:131–41.

111. Flier JS, Maratos-Flier E. Obesity and the hypothalamus: novel peptides for new pathways. Cell 1998; 92:696.

112. Ahima RS, Prabakaran D, Mantzoros C, Qu D, Lowell B, Maratos-Flier E, Flier JS. Role of leptin in the neuroendocrine response to fasting. Nature 1996; 382:250–2.

113. Schwartz MW, Seeley RJ. Neuroendocrine responses to starvation and weight loss. N Engl J Med 1997; 336:1802–11.

114. Keys A, Brozek JJ, Henschel A, Mickelsen O, Taylor HL. The Biology of Human Starvation. Minneapolis University of Minnesota Press, 1950.

115. Dulloo AG. Human pattern of food intake and fuel-partitioning during weight recovery after starvation: a theory of autoregulation of body composition. Proc Nutr Soc 1997; 56:25–40.

116. Cameron JL, Wiltzin T, McConaha C, Helmreich DL, Kaye WH. Suppression of reproductive axis activity in men undergoing a 48 hour fast. J Clin Endocrinol Metab 1991; 73:35–41.

117. Cameron JL. Nutritional determinants of puberty. Nutr Rev 1996; 54:S17–S22.

118. Bronson FH, Manning JM. The energetic regulation of ovulation: a realistic role for body fat. Biol Reprod 1991; 44:945–50.

119. Lumey LH, Stein AD. In utero exposure to famine and subsequent fertility: the Dutch famine birth cohort study. Am J Public Heallth 1997; 87:1962–6.

120. McCance RA, Widdowson EM. The determinants of growth and form. Proc Roy Soc Lond (Biol) 1974; 185:1–17.

121. Barker DJP. Growth in utero and coronary artery disease. Nutr Rev 1996; 54:S1–7.

122. Valdez R, Athens MA, Thompson GH, Bradshaw BS, Stern MP.
Birthweight and adult health outcomes in a biethnic population in the USA. Diabetologia 1994; 37:624–31.

123. Kannisto V, Christensen K, Vaupel JW. No increased mortality in later life for cohorts born during famine. Am J Epidem 1997; 145:987–94.

124. Lumey LH, Stein AD. Offspring birth weights after maternal intrauterine undernutrition: a comparison within sibships. Am J Epidem 1997; 46:810–9.

125. Ravelli G-P, Stein ZA, Susser MW. Obesity in young men after famine exposure in utero and early infancy. N Engl J Med 1976; 295:349–53.

126. Lumey LH, Stein AD. Offspring birth weights after maternal intrauterine undernutrition: A comparison within sibships. Am J Epidem 1997; 146:810–9.

127. Mott GE. Early feeding and atherosclerosis, In: Boulton J, et al., eds. Long-term Consequences of Early Feeding. Nestle Nutrition Workshop Series 1996; 36:113–22.

128. Matthys P, Billiau A. Cytokines and cachexia. Nutrition 1997; 13:763–70.

129. Coodley GO, Loveless MO, Merrill TM. The HIV wasting syndrome: a review. J Acquired Immune Deficiency Synd 1994; 7:681.

130. Tisdale MJ. Biology of cachexia. J Natl Cancer Inst 1997; 89:1763–73.

131. Fearon KCH, Carter DC. Cancer cachexia. Ann Surg 1988; 208:1–5.

132. Rouzer CA, Cerami A. Hypertriglyceridemia associated with *Trypanosoma brucei* infection in rabbits. Role of defective triglyceride removal. Mol Biochem Parasitol 1980; 2:31.

133. Wigmore SJ, Ross JA, Falconer JS, Plester CE, Tisdale MJ, Carter DC, Fearon KC. The effect of polyunsaturated fatty acids on the progress of cachexia in patients with pancreatic cancer. Nutrition 1996; 12:S27–30.

134. Tisdale MJ. Inhibition of lipolysis and muscle protein degradation by EPA in cancer cachexia. Nutrition 1996; 12:S31–33.

135. Erickson KL, Hubbard NE. Dietary fish oil modulation of macrophage tumoricidal activity. Nutrition 1996; 12:S34–S38.

136. Chlebowski RT, Beall G, Lillington L, Richards EW, Abbruzzese BC, McCamish MA, Cope FO. Nutritional intervention in the course of HIV disease. Nutrition 1995; 11:S250–S254.

137. Grunfeld C, Feingold DR. Metabolic disturbance and wasting in AIDS. N Engl J Med 1992; 327–329.

138. Jao DV, Tai VW, Beall GN, Chlebowski RT. Malabsorption as measured by D-xylose testing in HIV-infected patients without diarrhea of severe weight loss. Oncology (Live Sci Adv). 1994; 13:135.

139. Meguid MM, Yang ZJ, Gleason JR. The gut-brain brain-gut axis in anorexia: toward an understanding of food intake regulation. Nutrition 1996; 12:S57–62.

140. Prins JB, Walker NI, Winterford CM, Cameron DP. Apoptosis of human adipocytes in vitro. Biochem Biophys Res Commun 1994; 201:500–7.

141. Walthon MA. MMWR 1991; 40:747.

142. Ryan YM, Gibney MJ, Flynn MAT. The pursuit of thinness: a study of Dublin schoolgirls aged 15 y. Int J Obesity 1998; 22:485–7.

143. Crawley HF, Shergill-Bonner R. The nutrient and food intakes of 16–17 year old female dieters in the UK. J Hum Nutr Dietet 1995; 8:25–34.

144. Walsh BT, Devlin MJ. Eating disorders: progress and problems. Science 1998; 280:1387–90.

145. Woodside DB. The review of anorexia nervosa and bulimia nervosa. Curr Prob Pediatr 1995; 25:67–89.

146. Butterworth Revised diagnostic subgroupings for anorexia nervosa. Nutr Rev 1994; 52:213–5.

147. Waterlow JC. On serum albumin in anorexia nervosa. Nutrition 1996; 12:720–1.

148. Smith G, Robinson PH, Fleck A. Serum albumin distribution in early treated anorexia nervosa. Nutrition 1996; 12:677–84.

149. Walsh BT. Eating Disorders In: Tasman A, Kay J, Lieberman JA, eds, Psychiatry, pp. 1202–16. W. B. Saunders, Philadelphia, 1997.

150. Sullivan PF. Mortality in anorexia nervosa. Am J Psychiatry 1995; 152:1073–4.

151. Anonymous. Revised diagnostic subgroupings for anorexia nervosa. Nutr Rev 1994; 52:213–5.

152. Eckert ED, Halmi KA, Marchi P, Grove W, Crosby R. Ten-year follow-up of anorexia nervosa: clinical course and outcome. Psychol Med 1995; 25:143–56.

153. Lucas AR, Beard CM, O'Fallon WM, Kurlan LT. 50-year trends in the incidence of anorexia nervosa in Rochester, Minn.: a population-based study. Am J Psychiatry 1991; 148:917–22.

154. Smith G, Robinson PH, Feck A. Serum albumin distribution in early treated anorexia nervosa. Nutrition 1996; 12:677–84.

155. Meguid MM, Muscaritoli M. Current use of total parenteral nutrition in clinical practice. Am Family Phys 1993; 47:383.

156. Blackburn GL, Ahmad A. Skeleton in the hospital closet—then and now. Nutrition 1995; 11:S193–5.

157. Moore FA, Feliciano DV, Andreassy RJ, McArdle AH, Booth FV, Morgenstein-Wagner TB, Kellum JM Jr., et al. Early enteral feeding compared with parenteral reduces postoperative septic complications. The results of a meta-analysis. Ann Surg 1992; 216:172.

158. Anonymous. The Veterans' affairs total parenteral nutrition cooperative study group. Perioperative nutrition in surgical patients. N Engl J Med 1991; 325:525.

159. Moberg W. The Emigrants. Simon and Schuster, New York, 1951.

160. Kannisto V, Christensen K, Vaupel JW. No increased mortality in later life for cohorts born during famine. Am J Epidemiol 1997; 145:987–94.

161. Salisbury HE. The New Emperors: China in the era of Mao and Deng. Little Brown and Co., Boston, 1992.

162. Conquest R. The Harvest of Sorrow. Oxford University Press, New York, 1986.

5 Protein and Amino Acids

Vernon R. Young

INTRODUCTION

The usual source of amino acids the body cannot make (the nutritionally indispensable, or essential, amino acids) and of the nitrogen required for the synthesis of other amino acids (the nutritionally dispensable or nonessential amino acids) and numerous physiologically important nitrogen-containing compounds is from the protein-containing component of the diet. In the case of special nutritional therapies, the required amino acids and nitrogen can be supplied by formulations that are given via enteral or parenteral administration. Inadequate protein or amino acid intakes cause diminished content of protein in cells and organs and deterioration in the capacity of cells to carry out their normal function. This then results in growth faltering in the young and, in all individuals, increased morbidity and eventually death if the poor diet continues. Furthermore, intakes in considerable excess of physiologic needs also might be disadvantageous. Thus, an adequate diet, whether consisting of normal foods or specially formulated medical/nutritional products, must contain an appropriate level of protein (nitrogen) and balance of amino acids one to another, so that adequate growth, development, and/or long-term health can be achieved and sustained.

Before focusing on the quantitative needs for dietary protein (nitrogen) and for specific amino acids, it might be worthwhile to begin with a short survey of the functions of amino acids and proteins. This will then be followed by a brief overview of some general features of amino acids and proteins. This will then be followed by a brief overview of some general features of protein metabolism, at the whole-body level, and particularly those that serve to determine the nutritional needs of the host. This is intended to provide a better understanding for the basis of the approaches taken to estimate human and amino acid needs. The currently accepted values for these requirements and host factors that affect them will then be reviewed and critiqued.

AMINO ACID AND PROTEIN FUNCTIONS

Amino acids serve as the currency of the nitrogen and protein economy of the host. Although there are hundreds of amino acids in nature, only 20 of these commonly appear in proteins, via charging by their cognate tRNAs and subsequent recognition of

From: *Nutrition and Immunology: Principles and Practice* (ME Gershwin et al. eds.), © Humana Press, Inc., Totowa, NJ

a codon on the mRNA. In the special case of selenoproteins, such as glutathione peroxidase and type 1 iodothyronine 5′ deiodinase, the formation and incorporation of selenocysteine into these proteins involves a complex process, including conversion of a seryl-tRNA to selenocysteinyl-tRNA, which is then recognized by a UGA codon (1). Other amino acids, such as hydroxyproline or N^τ-methylhistidine, as examples, are also present in proteins. These arise via a posttranslational modification of specific amino acids residues, which endows particular structural and functional properties to proteins; for example, there is a vitamin K-dependent carboxylation of glutamic acid residues in a number of proteins, such as those involved in blood coagulation and bone matrix deposition (2). It is, however, the common 20 amino acids, together with a selected few others that are not in peptide-bound form, such as ornithine, citrulline, and taurine, that are of major quantitative importance in the maintenance of nitrogen economy and protein nutritional status of the human subject.

Whereas all plants can synthesize the 18 amino acids and 2 amides (asparagine and glutamine) commonly found in proteins, the animal kingdom, from protozoa up to mammals, is dependent on at least 9 of the amino acids being supplied from exogenous sources; these amino acids are referred to as the essential or indispensable amino acids (3) and we will return to these later.

The nutritionally relevant amino acids serve multiple and diverse physiologic functions; examples of these are listed in Table 1, as well as an indication of those functions played by the proteins elaborated from their individual amino acids via peptide bond formation. In the course of carrying out their physiologic and functional roles, the proteins and amino acids turn over and part of their nitrogen and carbon is irretrievably lost via the excretory pathways, including CO_2 in expired air, and urea and ammonia in urine. Hence, to maintain an adequate body protein and amino acid nutritional status, these losses must be balanced by an appropriate exogenous, or dietary, supply of (1) a utilizable source of nitrogen for synthesis of physiologically important nitrogen-containing compounds to support cell and organ function and (2) the indispensable amino acids, together with certain so-called "conditionally indispensable" amino acids under specific pathophysiological states. These dietary components are used to replace those lost during the course of daily metabolic transactions and/ or that are needed for deposition of new tissues during growth or for repair and protein repletion following disease or other unfavorable nutritional conditions.

Table 1
Some Functions of Amino Acids and Proteins

Function	Example
Amino acids	
Substrates for protein synthesis	Those for which there is a codon
Regulators of protein turnover	Leucine, arginine
Regulators of enzyme activity (allosteric)	Arginine and NAG synthetase; Phe and PAH activation
Precursor of signal transducer	Arginine and nitric oxide
Methylation reactions	Methionine
Neurotransmitter	Tryptophan (serotonin); glutamate
Ion fluxes	Taurine; glutamate
Precursor of "physiologic" molecules	Arg (creatinine); glycine (purines)
Transport of nitrogen	Alanine; glutamine
Oxidation-reduction properties	Cyst(e)ine; glutathione
Precursor of conditionally indispensable amino acids	Methionine (cys); phe (tyr)
Gluconeogenic substrate and fuel	Alanine; serine; glut (NH_2)
Proteins	
Enzymatic catalysis	BCKADH
Transport	B-12 binding proteins; ceruloplasmin; apolipoproteins
Messenger/signals	Insulin; growth hormone
Movement	Kinesin; actin
Structure	Collagens; elastin
Storage/sequestration	Ferritin; metallothionein
Immunity	Antibodies; TNF; interleukins
Growth; differentiation; gene expression	EGF; IGFs; transcription factors

Note: PAH: phenylalanine hydroxylase; BCKADH: branched-chain ketoacid dehydrogenase; TNF: tumor necrosis factor; NAG: *N*-acetyl-glutamate.

THE MAJOR SYSTEMS INVOLVED IN BODY PROTEIN AND AMINO ACID METABOLISM

The principal metabolic systems responsible for the maintenance of body protein and amino acid homeostasis are shown in Fig. 1. They are:

1. Protein synthesis;
2. Protein breakdown or degradation;
3. Amino acid oxidation, with elimination of carbon dioxide and urea production; and
4. Amino acid synthesis, in the case of the nutritionally dispensable or conditionally indispensable amino acids.

Dietary and nutritional factors determine the dynamic status of these systems; such factors include the intake levels relative to the host's protein and amino acid requirements, the form and route of delivery of nutrients (i.e., parenteral and enteral nutritional support) and timing of intake during the day, especially in relation to the intake of the major energy yielding substrates. Changes in the rates of these systems lead to an adjustment in whole-body nitrogen (protein) balance and retention, with the net direction and the extent of the balance depending upon the sum of the interactions occurring among the prevailing factor(s).

Protein synthesis rates are high in the newborn and per unit of body weight, these rates decline with progressive growth and development (Table 2) *(4)*. Three points that are relevant to nutritional requirements might be drawn from the data summarized here. First, the higher rate of protein synthesis in the very young, as compared to that in the adult, is related to the fact that a net protein deposition occurs during growth and also a high rate of protein turnover (synthesis and breakdown), which is associated with tissue remodeling. Hence, protein *synthesis* in the premature

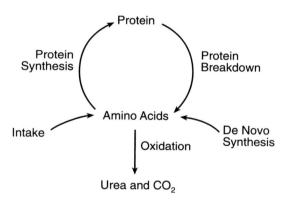

Fig. 1. The principal biochemical systems responsible for homeostasis of protein and amino acid metabolism in vivo. Changes in the rates of these systems account for the adaptation to alterations in dietary protein/amino acid intakes.

infant *(5)* is about twice as high as in the preschool child and approximately three or four times as high as in the adult. Second, at all ages in healthy subjects, the rates of whole-body protein synthesis and breakdown are considerably greater than usual intakes or levels of dietary protein thought to be necessary to meet the needs for maintenance or for the support of adequate growth *(2)*. It follows, therefore, that there is an extensive reutilization within the body of the endogenous amino acids liberated during the course of protein breakdown. Third, a general relationship can be seen here between the age-related differences in protein turnover and in the dietary protein needs for each specific age group. This suggests that when rates of synthesis and breakdown of body proteins change in response to various stimuli, such as

Table 2
Comparison of Whole-Body Protein Synthesis Rates
with Dietary Protein Allowances at Different Ages[1]

Age group	Protein synthesis[a] (A)	Protein allowance[b] (B)	Ratio A/B
Infant (premature)	11.3, 14	~3	4.3
Newborn	6.7	1.85	3.6
Child (15 mo)	6.3	1.3	4.8
Child (2–8 yr)	3.9	1.1	3.5
Adolescent (~13 yr)	~5	1.0	~5
Young adult (~20 yr)	~4.0	0.75	~5.3
Elderly (~70 yr)	~3.5	0.75	4.7

[a]Extended slightly from Young et al. *(4)*.
[b]In units of g protein/kg/d.

Table 3
Whole-Body Protein Turnover in Relation
to Resting Metabolic Rate (MR) in Adult
of Mammalian and Avian Species

Species	Weight (kg)	Protein turnover (A) (g/kg/d)	MR (B) (k/kg/d)	Ratio B/A
Mouse	0.04	43.5	760	11
Rat	0.35	22.0	364	17
Rabbit	3.6	9.2	192	20
Wallaby (Parma)	4.2	7.5	163	21
Sheep	63	5.6	96	17
Man	70	4.6	107	23
Cow	575	3.0	60	20
Birds (chickens)	1.4	27	439	16

Note: From a summary of literature by Young et al. *(8)*, where original references are given.

in sepsis and trauma, the dietary requirement for nitrogen and specific amino acids intakes will change. This supposition is consistent with the increased total nitrogen needs of injured patients *(6,7)*.

An additional metabolic relationship, of nutritional interest, is that there is also a general relationship between the basal or resting metabolic rate of the organism and the rate of whole-body protein turnover; from an interspecies survey (Table 3), it can be estimated that about 15–20 kJ (4–5 kcal) of basal energy expenditure are expended in association with each gram of whole-body protein synthesis *(8)*. It then follows from this relationship that amino acid transport and peptide synthesis alone might account for at least 20% of total basal metabolism. This being so, it could be concluded that major changes in body protein turnover resulting from, for example, severe infection or major trauma would not only affect the protein and amino acid requirements but also the status of body energy expenditure and requirements. In turn, changes in energy status will affect protein turnover *(9)* and thus, influence the requirement for protein.

Because the basal metabolic rate accounts for a significant proportion of total daily energy expenditure, where ATP is the currency *(10)* and because of the relationship with protein turnover noted in the previous paragraph, a point might be raised here about the contributions made by the major different ATP-consuming reactions to the metabolic rate, including that for protein synthesis.

Table 4
Some Energy-Dependent Processes Associated with Protein
Turnover and Amino Acid Homeostasis

Protein turnover
  Formation of initiation complex
  Peptide bond synthesis
  Protein degradation
    Ubiquitin dependent
    Ubiquitin independent
    Autophagic degradation (sequestration, lysosomal, proton pump)
RNA turnover
  rRNA; tRNA
  Pre-mRNA splicing (spliceosome) and mRNA
Amino acid transport
Regulation and integrity
  Reversible phosphorylation, enzymes, factors
  GTP–GDP exchange proteins (signal transduction)
  Second messengers (phosphatidyl inositol system)
  Ion pumps and channels
  ATP-dependent heat-shock proteins (folding)
  Protein translocation
Nitrogen metabolism
  Glutamate–glutamine cycle
  Glucose–alanine cycle
  Urea synthesis

Table 4 lists a number of energy-dependent processes that are associated with protein and amino acid function and homeostasis, and in this context, Rolfe and Brown *(11)* have estimated that the sodium–potassium ATPase pump, protein turnover, and urea synthesis, combined, account for about 40–50% of whole-body oxygen use. Using a similar set of assumptions, Yu and co-workers *(12)* estimated that 25% of the increase in energy expenditure in burn patients was due to the increased rate of protein synthesis and urea production. The point of emphasis is that there are significant quantitative interrelationships between energy and protein metabolism and their nutritional requirements.

Clearly, then, it should not be difficult to appreciate that both the level of protein as well as level of energy intake can affect body N balance; the available data reveal that the effects of these two nutritional factors are interdependent and their interactions can be complex. It was pointed out more than 40 yr ago by Calloway and Spector *(13)* that the level of caloric intake, whether above or below requirements, determines the degree of change in the N balance that is prompted by a change in N intake. Furthermore, the level of N-intake determines the quantitative effect of energy intake on N balance. Munro *(14)* captured this complexity in schematic form, as shown in Fig. 2.

In quantitative terms, for human subjects, an excess energy intake at adequate levels of N intake causes a retention of approximately 1–2 mg N/kcal *(15)*, but at limiting or low N intakes, this relationship is markedly attenuated *(14)*. However, at lower energy intakes, within the submaintenance range, there is a greater impact of changes in energy intake on N balance. Hence, in normal men, for each kilocalorie change in energy intake, it appears that at low energy, the N balance is altered by as much as 8 mg, with the relationship "breaking" at a total energy intake of about 1400 kcal daily *(15)*. This energy-level effect also applies for depleted, hospitalized patients for whom a value of approximately 7.5 mg

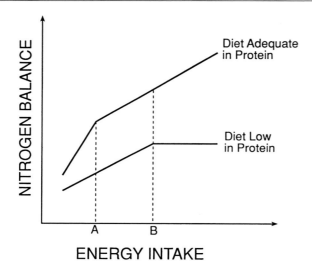

Fig. 2. Relationship of nitrogen balance and energy intake with diets of differing protein content. Between energy intakes A (low) and B (higher), the two lines are parallel. (From ref. *14.*)

N/kcal has been established, with energy intakes up to about the equivalent of 15 kcal/kg body weight/d *(16)* (Fig. 3).

The foregoing energy–nitrogen relationships have been emphasized because of their profound consequences for the design and interpretation of N-balance experiments, especially those intended to aid in the determination of protein and amino acid requirements. Thus, Garza et al. *(17)* and Inoue et al. *(18)* showed how relatively small changes in the level of energy intake can affect N balance and, therefore, the estimated protein requirements in healthy adult men. Indeed, the excess energy intakes given to subjects in the balance studies by Rose *(19)* were a concern to the investigator and this is a problem that has undoubtedly contributed to a underestimation of the quantitative needs for the indispensable amino acids in healthy adults *(8,20).*

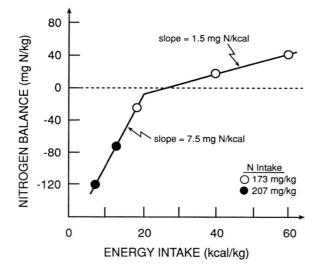

Fig. 3. Relationship between N balance and energy intake in postabsorptive and depleted patients. (From ref. *16.*)

GENERAL NUTRITIONAL ASPECTS OF AMINO ACIDS

AMINO ACIDS CLASSIFIED The nutritional requirement for dietary protein consist of two components: They are (i) a utilizable source of nitrogen (often called nonspecific nitrogen or NSN) that may be supplied as a specific amino acid or a nitrogen compound such as urea or diammonium citrate or as a mixture of dispensable (nonessential) amino acids and (ii) the indispensable amino acids (essential) amino acids. Under certain conditions, there are the "conditionally essential" or "conditionally indispensable" amino acids. These various classes of amino acids are listed in Table 5 *(4,21).*

It will be noted from Table 5 that the conceptual organization of the present classification differs from that proposed by Rose et al. *(21),* following their classical N-balance studies carried out about 45 yr ago. Thus, it is now accepted that the human being requires at least nine indispensable amino acids under all conditions. Furthermore, from research carried out subsequent to the classic studies in Illinois *(19,21),* an assessment of the dietary significance of the various amino acids is more elaborate than the earlier classification suggested. Several developments have contributed to this expanded understanding of the role of dietary (exogenous) amino acids in human metabolism and function: These include (a) the successful clinical application of parenteral and enteral feeding techniques, requiring specific, chemically defined formulations, (b) the potential benefit of perioperative artificial nutrition, whether by the enteral or parenteral routes *(22),* and the possibility of maintaining patients on highly regulated and well-defined feeding regimens for prolonged periods, and (c) an increased understanding of the metabolism and function of the amino acids *(see refs. 23* and *24* for review). In consequence, research in the area of amino acid nutrition has shifted away from the earlier and rather narrow focus on nitrogen balance, as the dominant paradigm for establishing the qualitative and quantitative aspects of nutritional needs, toward a more comprehensive evaluation of the consequences of altered amino acid levels and balance of intake on the metabolic and functional status of individuals. A paradigm shift has been enabled, to a major extent, by the application and further development of tracer techniques, especially the use of stable nuclides, in metabolic/nutritional research *(25).* It has also been promoted by the availability and study of new and novel amino-acid-based substrates, which include glutamine-enriched total parenteral nutrition solutions *(26),* short-chain peptides containing glutamate, tyrosine, or cysteine, and taurine conjugated *(4).* Hence, an additional class of amino acids has emerged in human amino acid nutrition and these are the so-called conditionally indispensable amino acids *(28).* Depending on the physiological and metabolic condition of the host, these may include arginine *(29,30),* proline *(30,31),* glutamine *(26,32),* cysteine *(33),* and, possibly, glycine *(34).*

The metabolic regulation of the conditionally indispensable amino acids and their roles in nutrition are a current focus of research in human protein and amino acid metabolism. Studies in healthy human adults *(35)* have led to the conclusion that the endogenous synthesis of arginine is relatively constant, whereas the degradation of arginine varies with dietary change. Thus, it seems as though the status of arginine degradation determines the arginine status of the body, and if this is so, then this would seem to explain the apparent increase in the need for arginine in catabolic

Table 5
The Changing View of the Role of Amino Acids in Human Nutrition

Indispensable (essential)		Conditionally indispensable	Dispensable	
1954[a]	Present[b]	Present	1954[a]	Present[b]
Valine	Valine	Glycine	Glycine	
Isoleucine	Isoleucine	Cystine	Cystine	
Leucine	Leucine	Glutamine	Glutamic acid	Glutamic acid?
Lysine	Lysine	Tyrosine	Tyrosine	
Methionine	Methionine	Proline	Proline	
Phenylalanine	Phenylalanine	Arginine	Arginine	
Threonine	Threonine	Taurine	Alanine	Alanine
Tryptophan	Tryptophan	Glutamic acid?	Serine	Serine
	Histidine		Aspartic acid	Aspartic acid
			Histidine	Asparagine
			Hydroxyproline	
			Citrulline	

[a]Based on "final classification" by Rose et al. (21).
[b]A current interpretation.

states (36,37). On the other hand, it appears that the endogenous synthesis of arginine plays an important role in regulating arginine homeostasis in neonatal (38) and in postweaning pigs (39). Hence, it will be important to know whether this also applies to the status of arginine metabolism in human infants and young children. Similarly, proline synthesis appears to be limited in the newborn pig (40) and laying hen (41) and the state of proline synthesis balance in the human neonate (42) and in burn patients (31) also suggests a dietary requirement for this amino acid in these cases.

A likelihood that there is a limiting availability of endogenously synthesized glycine under conditions of high metabolic demand, as in the rapid recovery state from malnutrition, has been hypothesized (34). Measurements of urinary L-5-oxoproline excretion, used as an index of glycine status, have indicated a number of possible physiological conditions (43,44) under which an enriched intake of glycine might be beneficial. There are no data, however, on which to base an estimate of what this actual intake of glycine should be.

In this chapter, we are principally concerned with the quantitative needs for protection and amino acids and so it must be stated that little can be said yet about the amounts of the individual, conditionally indispensable amino acids needed to optimally support the nitrogen economy of the host, under any specific condition. There is even doubt now about the quantitative nutritional interrelationships between the two sulfur amino acids methionine and cyst(e)ine, for which a close metabolic association has long been recognized. For example, earlier nitrogen-balance investigations in adults suggest that dietary cystine could spare the requirement for methionine by approximately 16% to as much as 90% (45). This nutritional problem has been explored in a series of investigations using labeled methionine as a tracer. From studies with both healthy young adults (46,47) and elderly men and women (48), there does not appear to be a profound methionine-sparing effect of dietary cyst(e)ine. Therefore, it has been proposed (47,48) that approximately two-thirds of the requirement for the total sulfur amino acids (SAAs) should be supplied as methionine, together with a generous addition of cysteine. However, the optimum ratio of methionine-to-cyst(e)ine and the desirable total SAA intake cannot yet be stated with any substantial degree of confidence.

In view of the role played by cyst(e)ine in the regulation of glutathione (L-γ-glutamyl-L-cysteinylglycine) synthesis and homeostasis (49–51), the quantitative determination of the nutritional relationships between cystine and methionine deserve to be more completely established.

NONSPECIFIC NITROGEN Although the required intake levels of the conditionally indispensable amino acids for specific situations are not known, it is clear, as reviewed elsewhere (28), that studies in the growing rat, chick, human infant, and adult have revealed the importance of an adequate level and appropriate dietary source of "nonspecific nitrogen" (NSN) for maintenance of an adequate state of body protein balance and nutriture. Indispensable amino acids alone, even when supplied in excess of their physiological requirements, do not maintain either adequate growth or maintenance in the rat (52). Furthermore, in human studies, the nutritional value of diets that supply a low amount of total nitrogen or diets containing predominantly the indispensable amino acids may be improved when NSN is added (53).

To summarize, in addition to the nitrogen obtained from the indispensable amino acids, there is a requirement for a sufficient intake of "nonspecific nitrogen." This can be met effectively from the dispensable amino acids or from utilizable nitrogen sources but not from an excessive intake of indispensable amino acids alone. The extent to which a single specific chemical source(s) of the nonspecific nitrogen component might be sufficient to meet total "protein" (nitrogen) and amino acids needs is not entirely clear. Thus, a 1965 FAO/WHO (54) Expert Group on protein requirements concluded that the healthy human body is able to utilize most "nonessential" nitrogen compounds with equal efficiency. However, recent work describing the metabolism of the amino acids within the lumen of the intestine and the metabolic fate of dietary glutamate, in particular, might soon lead to a possible reassessment of the nutritional significance of specific amino acids (55,56). Dietary glutamate, for example, appears to be an important source for glutathione synthesis and for energy metabolism in the intestinal mucosa and little of the dietary glutamate reaches the portal circulation. Finally, an additional reason why it is important to better establish the nutritional requirement relationships between the "nonspecific nitrogen" and the indis-

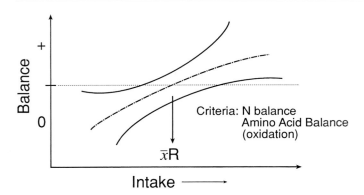

Fig. 4. Nitrogen balance in relation to N intake and estimation of the nitrogen (protein) requirement. Similarly, amino acid balance can be determined by measurement of amino acid loss via oxidation. $\bar{x}R =$ mean requirement.

pensable amino acid component of the total protein requirement is because it has been hypothesized that high levels of nonspecific nitrogen in the diet can diminish the oxidative losses of the indispensable amino acids (57) and that this accounts for the relatively low requirement values for the indispensable amino acids as have been recommended by the FAO/WHO/UNU (58). However, stable isotope tracer studies (59) in young adults failed to demonstrate any significant sparing effect of dietary specific nitrogen on leucine oxidation or phenylalanine hydroxylation, which were used as indices of indispensable amino acid losses or of the sparing by nonspecific nitrogen.

PROTEIN REQUIREMENTS

The foregoing has concentrated on the qualitative nature of the amino acids in human nutrition and so we now turn to the question of the quantitative needs for dietary protein and the individual indispensable amino acids. The protein requirement will be considered first, beginning with a short account of the ways by which the quantitative needs are established. Emphasis is given here to the approaches used by the United Nations (58) because the publications arising from these bilateral agencies have served to establish global nutrition policy and programs. They have also frequently been used as a major basis for establishing dietary recommendations by various national and/or professional groups.

COMMENTS ON APPROACHES AND METHODS The requirement for protein (nitrogen) is defined as the lowest level of intake that will balance the losses of nitrogen and amino acids (via oxidative catabolism) from the body in persons maintaining energy balance and a modest level of physical activity (58). In the case of children and pregnant and lactating women, the requirement also includes the needs associated with the deposition of protein in tissues or the secretion of milk at rates consistent with good health.

Hence, the starting point for estimating total protein needs is the direct measurement of nitrogen needed for achieving zero balance in adults during short-term and long-term studies (58) (Fig. 4). Most estimates of protein requirements, therefore, are obtained directly or indirectly from measurements of the N balance. Although this approach has been discussed in detail in the 1985 FAO/WHO/UNU (58) report on energy and protein requirements, some points might be made here before summarizing the estimates of protein requirements for the various age groups.

Table 6
Criteria for Valid Nitrogen-Balance
Measurement of Protein Requirements

Design and technical criteria
  Sufficient period of stabilization to new test protein level
  Periods sufficiently long for a stable response
  Urine collections complete and precisely timed
  Fecal collections complete and suitably aliquoted
  Correction for integumenal and miscellaneous N losses
  Overall design must be appropriate for intended purpose
Dietary criteria
  Energy intake to match energy expenditure
  Fluid intake controlled
  Protein intake precisely controlled and monitored
  Multiple test levels encompassing near requirement level
Host Factors
  Subjects should be fully replete
  Subjects free of mild infections
  Daily physical activity regular and not excessive

Source: Based on *ref. 60.*

First, the nitrogen-balance technique involves the determination of the difference between the intake of nitrogen and the amount excreted in urine, feces, and sweat, together with minor losses via other routes. There are (i) a number of inherent sources of error in nitrogen-balance measurements and (ii) a number of experimental requirements must be met if reliable N balance data are to be obtained. These have been summarized by Scrimshaw (60) (Table 6) and they include:

1. The need to closely match energy intake with energy need, for the various reasons discussed earlier,
2. An appropriate stabilization period to the experimental diet and periods long enough to reliably establish the full response to a dietary change,
3. Timing and completeness of urine collections, and
4. The absence of even mild infections and of other sources of stress.

A detailed review of the concepts behind and techniques involved in reference to nitrogen-balance measurements and their application has been made by Manatt and Garcia (61), which should be consulted for further details.

In most previous N-balance experiments, only the nitrogen content of the diet, urine, and feces has been measured. Therefore, losses by other routes must be assumed and these are based on a rather limited body of published data (62). However, for this purpose, the UN group (58) accepted a value of 8 mg N/kg/d as a suitable correction, or allowance, for these unmeasured losses. Although Millward and Roberts (63) propose a value of 5 mg N/kg/d based on their assessment of the literature, it would seem prudent to accept the higher value at this time, especially because it has been used to set current international recommendations for protein intakes.

Second, the minimum physiological requirement is estimated by extrapolating or interpolating the N-balance data to the zero balance point (N equilibrium) for adults or for the achievement of adequate growth (positive N balance) in children. Some of the early balance studies involved a diet period without protein and, often, the levels of protein intake tested were far below the requirement. However, from studies in experimental animals and in man, it is known that the N-balance response is not linear throughout the entire submaintenance range: The slope decreases as the intakes approach and slightly exceed zero balance *(64)*. Therefore, it is now preferred that studies assessing requirements should include several levels of intake test protein and that these encompass but not greatly exceed the expected range of requirements. Therefore, the multicenter studies on adult protein requirements sponsored by the United Nations University applied a standardized N-balance protocol, in accordance with these principles that have been described elsewhere *(65)*.

Where direct N-balance determinations of the protein requirement data are lacking, as is the case for a number of age groups, an interpolation of requirements between two age groups might be made. In addition, a factorial approach may also be applied, as was done previously by the 1973 FAO/WHO Expert Group *(66)* on energy and protein requirements. In this approach the so-called obligatory urine and fecal nitrogen losses are determined, following a change to a protein-free diet, and these are summated with other obligatory losses. For children, estimates of N deposition or retention are also included. The estimates of average requirements, as obtained by the 1973 FAO/WHO group, were the summated factorial losses that were then corrected by a factor of 1.3 to account for the fact that even high-quality dietary proteins are not used with 100% efficiency; in this case, the efficiency was taken to be close to 70%. This factorial approach was discarded largely by the 1985 FAO/WHO/UNU Expert Group *(58)*, although this group used a modification of it to arrive at the protein requirements of children from 6 mo onward. In this latter case, the maintenance requirement for this age group was derived from results of several short-term N-balance studies and it was judged to be 120 mg N/kg/d at 1 yr falling to 100 mg N/kg/d at 20 yr *(58)*. Then, the requirement for growth was estimated, using (a) published values for N accretion, which were increased by 50% to account for intra-individual variation in the day-to-day deposition of protein and (b) then, again, the figure was adjusted assuming a 70% efficiency of dietary N retention. Finally, an assessment of interindividual variability in maintenance and growth requirements was then made in order to arrive at a safe level of protein intake, which would cover the needs of virtually all healthy children.

For infants 0–6 mo, the 1985 UN report *(58)* derived their protein requirements from estimated intakes by fully breast-fed infants. This required adoption of values for the protein content of human milk, the breast milk intake, and an assumed utilization of the nonprotein nitrogen fraction in human milk, a major proportion of which is urea *(67)*. These points will be addressed further later.

Protein requirements for young adult men and women have been based on both short- and long-term studies *(58)* (Table 7). This also applies to the healthy elderly, whose protein requirements were judged *(58)* not to be different from those of younger adults, although some have even speculated on the possibility that they may be even lower for the old as compared to the young *(63)*. In the case of pregnant women, the FAO/WHO/UNU group *(58)* estimated their additional requirements based on (i) an assumed average protein gain during pregnancy of 925 g plus 30% to account for variation (2 standard deviations [SD]) of birth weight and (ii) an assumed efficiency factor for dietary N utilization. The extra protein requirements for lactation were arrived at from

Table 7
Summary of Approaches for Arriving at Protein Requirements of Adults

1. Short-term N-balance studies
   Intakes expected to promote N equilibrium
   Mean 0.63 g/kg highly digestible, good quality protein
   For variability in requirements, a coefficient of 12.5% assumed;
   ∴ Mean + 2 SD (25%) = safe protein intake
2. Longer-term N-balance studies (24–89 d)
   Six investigations: proposed that the data suggested a mean requirement of 0.5 g/kg/d
3. Safe level of protein intake: 0.75 g/kg/d
4. Young women; older adults and elderly: same recommendations

Source: ref. 58.

estimates of breast milk output, protein content, and an allowance for variation in breast milk volume.

PROTEIN REQUIREMENTS, AS PROPOSED IN 1985 BY FAO/WHO/UNU *(58)* Because the 1985 report of the FAO/WHO/UNU Expert Consultation *(58)* includes an extensive discussion of the approaches taken to arrive at estimates of the mean requirements for protein in various age and physiological groups, a summary of the safe protein intakes for infants and young children, together with those for adults and lactating, and pregnant women, as proposed by this Expert Consultation group is presented in Table 8.

It should be emphasized that the recommendations for safe protein intakes shown in Table 8 include a factor for variation in protein requirements among apparently similar individuals. For adults, FAO/WHO/UNU *(58)* estimated that the biological variability in protein requirements amounted to a coefficient of variation of 12.5. Therefore, the Consultation group accepted that a value of 25% (2 SD) above the *mean* physiological requirement (0.6 g/kg/d) would be expected to meet the needs of all but 2.5% of individuals within the population. Hence, the mean requirement was increased to a level of 0.75 g/kg/d to give the *safe protein intake* for the healthy adult. Of course, most individuals would

Table 8
1985 FAO/WHO/UNU Safe Protein Intakes for Selected Age Groups and Physiological States

Group	Age (yr)	Safe protein level (g/kg/d)
Infants	0.3–0.5	1.47
	0.75–1.0	1.15
Children	3–4	1.09
	9–10	0.99
Adolescent	13–14 (girls)	0.94
	13–14 (boys)	0.97
Young adults	19 +	0.75
Elderly		0.75
Women:		
Pregnant	2nd trimester	+6 g daily
	3rd trimester	+11 g daily
Lactating	0–6 mo	~+16 g daily
	6–12 mo	~+11 g daily

Note: Data summarized from FAO/WHO/UNU *(58)*. Values are for proteins such as those of quality equal to hen's egg, cow's milk, meat, or fish.

require less than this intake to maintain protein nutrition al status with some subjects requiring as little as 0.45 g high-quality/kg/ d. Because it is impossible to identify those subjects whose requirements fall at the lower end of the range of requirements in a given population without directly determining their individual needs, it would not be prudent to generally accept a level lower than about 0.6 g/kg/d of good quality protein (68) where protein restriction was advisable on clinical grounds, such as in renal disease.

Another point worth underscoring is that the recommendations shown in Table 8 apply to healthy individuals. However, it is highly likely, as alluded to earlier, that the needs of sick or less healthy patients would differ from and presumably usually exceed those of healthy subjects. In this case, the values given in this table can only be regarded as a basis from which to begin an evaluation of how disease and stress, including surgery, affect the needs for dietary protein. Unfortunately, the quantitative needs for protein (total nitrogen) in sick, hospitalized patients can only be very crudely approximated. In fact, very little headway seems to have been made on this aspect of protein requirements since Munro and Young (69) made some tentative recommendations in 1980; these are reproduced with slight modification in Table 9 (70).

Increased interest has also been given recently to the metabolism (71,72) and needs for protein in older individuals. Based on their data and a review of the literature, Campbell and Evans (73) have concluded that the safe level of protein intake for older adults may be higher than currently recommended. This contrasts with the conclusion drawn by Millward and Roberts (63) that the available studies on the protein requirements of older individuals do not indicate a change with advancing age or a mean requirement value that exceeds that defined by FAO/WHO/UNU (58). Because older individuals are generally less healthy than young adults and stress increases requirements, Young et al. (70) propose a modestly higher protein intake recommendation for this age group, which they set at not less than 12–14% of energy intake for protein of quality similar to that of a balanced, mixed-protein diet.

INTERNATIONAL DIETARY ENERGY CONSULTANCY GROUP The UN protein recommendations presented above serve, as already noted, as a major basis for various national recommendations worldwide. In 1994, the International Dietary Energy Consultancy Group (IDECG) conducted a workshop to assess (a) whether the 1985 FAO/WHO/UNU (74) recommendations needed to be revised and (b) if so, on what basis and what any new recommendations might be (74). This more recent expert group reassessed the protein requirements of infants and children (75).

The IDECG determination of intakes by breast-fed infants included new assumptions about values for the protein content and volume of breast milk and efficiency of utilization of the nonprotein nitrogen component. Thus, the revised estimate of "adjusted" protein intake was arrived at from (i) a new analysis of breast milk volume from two studies (76,77) and (ii) an assess-

Table 9
Some Tentative Estimates of Protein Needs in Specific Diseases

I. Normal adult:
  (a) for N equilibrium: 0.75 g/kg, raised to 0.83 g/kg for dietary protein digestibility of 90%
  (b) Customary intake: 1–2 g/kg
II. Metabolic response to severe burn injury and trauma:
  (a) acute phase: 2–4 g/kg plus energy
  (b) convalescence: 2+ g/kg
III. Malabsorption and GI diseases:
  (a) malabsorption syndrome: 1 g/kg
  (b) ulcerative colitis: 1–1.4 g/kg[a]
  (c) ileocecostomy: 1–1.4 mg/kg[a]
IV. Liver disease:
  (a) acute hepatic encephalopathy; very low[b]
  (b) recovered encephalopathy: 1–1.5 g/kg
  (c) chronic encephalopathy: 0.5 g/kg
V. Renal disease:
  (a) uremia: 0.6 g/kg[b] (including ketoanalogs)
  (b) nephrosis: 1–1.4 g/kg[a]
VI. Malignant disease: increased protein energy needs

[a]Intake restricted on clinical grounds.
[b]In each condition, losses of protein and double minimal requirement.
Source: ref. 70.

Table 10
Revised Estimates by IDECG (75) of the 1985 FAO/WHO/UNU (58) Intakes of "Protein" by Breast-Fed Infants

Age (mo)	N	Breast milk intake (g/d)[a]	Weight (kg)	Total nitrogen intake[b] mg/d	mg/kg/d	Crude "protein" intake g/d	g/kg/d	Adjusted protein intake[c] g/d	g/kg/d
1[d]	37	794	4.76	1723	362	10.8	2.26	9.3–9.7	1.95–2.04
2[d]	40	766	5.62	1486	264	9.3	1.65	7.9–8.3	1.41–1.48
3[d]	37	764	6.30	1406	233	8.8	1.46	7.5–7.9	1.19–1.25
3[e]	61	812	6.24	1472	236	9.2	1.48	7.9–8.3	1.27–1.33
4[d]	41	782	6.78	1408	208	8.8	1.30	7.5–7.8	1.11–1.16
6[e]	12	881	7.54	1486	197	9.3	1.23	8.0–8.4	1.05–1.11

[a]Exclusively breast-fed infants; data for milk intake from Butte et al. (77) and Heinig et al. (76) were corrected for insensible water loss [+5.7%, Heinig et al. (76)].
[b]Including nonprotein nitrogen.
[c]Based on milk protein concentration plus 46–61% of the NPN (protein=6.25 × nitrogen).
[d]From *ref. 77*.
[e]From *ref. 76*.
Source: ref. 75.

Table 11
IDECG (75) Revised Estimates for the Average Requirements and Safe Level of Protein Intakes for Infants

Age (mo)	Average protein requirement[a]		IDECG safe protein[a,b] intake
	IDECG (75)	1985 FAO/WHO/UNU (58)	
0–1	1.99	—	2.69
1–2	1.54	2.25	2.04
2–3	1.19	1.82	1.53
3–4	1.06	1.47	1.37
4–5	0.98	1.34	1.25
5–6	0.92	1.30	1.19
6–9	0.85	1.25	1.09
9–12	0.78	1.15	1.02

[a]In units of g protein/kg/d.
[b]Includes separate variations for maintenance (12.5% Coefficient of Variation) and growth, as described in Table 5 of IDECG (75).

Table 12
IDECG (75) Revised Estimates of the 1985 FAO/WHO/UNU (58) Requirements for Protein for Selected Age Groups in Children and Adolescents

Age (yr)	Average requirement (g protein/kg/d)	Safe intake (g protein/kg/d)
2–3	0.74	0.93
5–6	0.69	0.86
7–8	0.69	0.86
9–10	0.69	0.86
Girls		
12–13	0.69	0.85
14–15	0.66	0.82
17–18	0.63	0.78
Boys		
12–13	0.71	0.88
14–15	0.69	0.86
17–18	0.66	0.81

Data taken and calculated from Tables 19 and 20 in ref. 75.

ment of the utilization of the nonprotein nitrogen fraction of breast milk. Here, it was assumed that all of the α-amino nitrogen and glucosamines are used and that 17–40% of the remaining nonprotein nitrogen can be utilized. Thus, the new values summarized in Table 10 are given for a range representing 46–61% utilization of nonprotein nitrogen in human milk. When expressed per kilogram of body weight, the intakes are about 0.20–0.46 g/kg/d less than the values listed in Table 29 of the 1985 report (58), or a difference of about 10–26%, depending on the age used for comparison. This is largely the result of the proportion of nonprotein nitrogen fraction utilized, but it is also the result of differences in the value used for milk protein concentration and means for birth weight of infants.

For infants and children over 6 mo, the IDECG group (75) also examined the assumptions involved in the modified factorial method used in the 1985 FAO/WHO/UNU report (58), as described earlier. Thus, (i) a maintenance requirement value of 90 mg N/kg/d was chosen (rather than the FAO/WHO/UNU value of 120 mg N/kg/d), (ii) values for body protein gain for infants after 6 mo were taken to be lower than those used by the UN group, and (iii) no additional augmentation was made for day-to-day (intraindividual) variability in growth. Instead, this latter factor was considered to be covered adequately by the interindividual variation in growth. These changes gave rise to requirement estimates for infants between 6 and 12 mo that were about 27–35% lower than the 1985 values (Table 11). Nevertheless, the IDECG group concluded that there was strong epidemiological support based, in part, on an analysis by Beaton and Chery (78) for the lower recommendations that it made for infants, as compared to those made in 1985 by FAO/WHO/UNU (58).

Similarly, the average protein requirements and estimates for a safe level of protein intake for children and adolescents were reassessed by IDECG (75), using a maintenance requirement of 100 mg N/kg/d and without the 50% augmentation for intraindividual variation in growth used in the 1985 report (58). This new assessment gave estimates for preschool children that were about 17–20% lower than the 1985 values, whereas for older children and adolescents, the IDECG group concluded that the available data suggests that the 1985 values were probably appropriate

(Table 12). The IDECG group did not review the protein needs of adults in any detail. Hence, the 1985 FAO/WHO/UNU (58) values remain, as far as official, international recommendations are concerned.

INDISPENSABLE AMINO ACID REQUIREMENTS

With respect to the amino acids, it is possible to slightly modify the earlier definition for the requirements for protein (nitrogen) such that the dietary need for a specific indispensable amino acid can be stated to be as follows: "the lowest level of intake that achieves nitrogen balance or that balances the irreversible oxidative loss of the amino acid, without requiring major changes in normal protein turnover and where there is energy balance with a modest level of physical activity." Again, in infants, children, and pregnant and lactating women, the requirements for the amino acid will also include that amount of the amino acid needed additionally for net protein deposition and for the synthesis and secretion of milk proteins. The foregoing is an operational definition of requirement, as in the case of protein. Ideally, a functional definition and determination of these requirements inherently would seem to be preferable but the choice and nature of the functional index or (indices) and its quantitative definition remains a challenge for future research.

COMMENT ON APPROACHES AND METHODS In general, the approaches and methods that have been used to determine specific indispensable amino acid requirements are similar to those that have been applied for the estimation of total protein needs. Thus, amino acid requirements have been assessed by nitrogen balance in male adults, starting with the classical work of Rose (19) and through similar studies in women by other investigators (45): by determining the amounts needed for normal growth and N balance in infants, preschool children (79–82), and school children (82,83) by assessment of the intakes provided by breast milk (58,75) or those supplied from intakes of good quality proteins (84). In addition, factorial predictions of the amino acid requirements of infants (75) and adults (85,86) have been made.

For adults, Millward and Rivers (57) proposed that minimum rates of oxidation or losses of the indispensable amino acids might be estimated from obligatory nitrogen losses *(66)* and Young et al. *(85–87)* extended this estimation as a basis for predicting the average minimum physiological intakes (requirement) necessary to maintain body amino acid balance in a healthy, well-nourished individual. The approach used by these investigators involves three major assumptions:

1. The total obligatory nitrogen losses are taken to be approximate 54 mg/kg nitrogen/d in the adult *(58)*.
2. The average amino acid composition of body proteins can be used to estimate the contribution made by each amino acid to this obligatory nitrogen output (equivalent, therefore, to the obligatory amino acid losses) *(85)*.
3. At requirement intake levels, an absorbed amino acid is used to balance its obligatory oxidative loss with an efficiency of approximately 70%. This value is derived from published nitrogen-balance data in adults *(58)*.

This predictive approach is analogous to the factorial method used by the 1973 FAO/WHO/UNU Expert Committee *(66)* for estimating the total-nitrogen (protein) requirement of individuals at various ages. Although, as already stated, the factorial approach was abandoned for this purpose by the 1985 FAO/WHO/UNU Expert Committee *(58)*, the MIT group *(86,87)* considered it to be a useful procedure for an initial reassessment of the indispensable amino acid requirements in healthy adults. This approach has been criticized by some *(88,89)*, but Young and El-Khoury *(85)* concluded that there is reasonable justification and validity for the approach, as an *initial* basis for establishing the requirement value in the absence of more direct studies.

Finally, in relation to establishing adult amino acid requirements, which also are a current focus of active research and vigorous debate *(88–92)*, tracer techniques are now being applied in the further assessment of the quantitative needs for the indispensable amino acids. Two major tracer paradigms have been applied and they are (1) the indicator amino acid oxidation method and (2) the direct tracer balance technique.

First, in the indicator amino acid oxidation approach, the oxidation of a ^{13}C-labeled "indicator" amino acid at different levels of the test amino acids is used as a means of establishing a requirement value *(93)*. When the test amino acid intake reaches a requirement level, the oxidation of the indicator amino acid reaches its lowest rate (Fig. 5). The biochemical rationale that underlies this methodology is that the body requires a pattern of amino acids, and for protein synthesis to proceed at an adequate rate, all of the necessary amino acids must be present in sufficient amounts at the active site of polypeptide chain initiation and elongation. If the intake of the test amino acid is too low, or limiting, then the other amino acids (including the indicator amino acid) would be present in relative excess and would be oxidized rather than being used efficiently for protein anabolic purposes. This indicator amino acid oxidation approach has been used successfully by Zello and co-workers in Toronto to estimate the lysine *(94,95)* and tryptophan *(96)* requirement in human adults. In those studies, measurements of the oxidation of ^{13}C-phenylalanine as an indicator were made at different dietary levels of lysine and tryptophan intake. The oxidation rate was measured in subjects during the fed state and while receiving the test diet only on the day during which the oxidation measurements are made. The Toronto investigations have been criticized *(97)* because of a lack of dietary adaptation period for the test amino acid levels examined, prior to the conduct

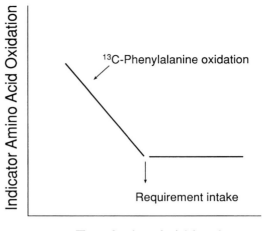

Fig. 5. A schematic presentation of the indicator amino acid oxidation approach for estimating the requirements for specific indispensable amino acids. Here, the indicator used is ^{13}C-phenylalanine.

of the tracer studies. However, a counterargument could be made that the lack of an adaptation period at more limiting lysine intakes would, in fact, tend to result in a lower rather than a higher requirement value with this experimental design *(98)*. Fereday et al. *(99)*, in their assessment of the protein requirements of the elderly, also did not include a period of dietary adaptation before conducting their ^{13}C-leucine-balance studies.

A modification of the original indicator amino acid oxidation technique was recently introduced by Kurpad and co-workers *(100)* to estimate leucine balance, in which ^{13}C-leucine was used as an indicator while coupled to a 24-hr tracer infusion protocol. The purpose of that study, carried out for healthy Indian adults, was to assess the appropriateness of the MIT-derived estimates of the lysine requirements of healthy adults (see below) for healthy, Third World populations, whose habitual intakes of IAAs are likely to be much lower than those characteristic of US individuals.

The second technique is the direct tracer balance method, which is analogous to the classical nitrogen-balance approach because it involves a direct estimate of the amount of the amino acid needed in the diet to replace its losses from the body; the amino acid loss is estimated directly by the loss (oxidation) of carbon from a labeled amino acid. Here, a ^{13}C-carboxyl-labeled amino acid is given as the tracer, either by mouth or by vein, and the amount of the amino acid oxidized is determined by measuring the $^{13}CO_2$ exhalation in the breath and the isotopic ^{13}C abundance of the test amino acid in the plasma (taken to be an index of the isotopic level in the pool undergoing oxidation). Tracer protocols have been conducted for either 8 h (tracer given for 3 h during the fast state followed by tracer infusion during ingestion of small meals over 5 h) *(86,87)* or for 24 h (12 h fast followed by ingestion of small meals over the remaining 10–12 h) *(100–103)*. Using this tracer balance approach, the group at MIT has determined new requirement estimates for the IAAs leucine, lysine, valine, threonine, methionine, tryptophan, and phenylalanine, which will be presented later.

There are a number of difficult technical problems associated with the 24 h tracer balance approach; these include:

Table 13
1985 FAO/WHO/UNU[1] Estimates of Amino Acid Requirements (mg/kg/d) at Different Ages

Amino acid	Infants (3–4 mo)	Children (2 yr)	School boys (10–12 yr)	Adults
Histidine	28	?	?	[8–12]
Isoleucine	70	31	28	10
Leucine	161	73	44	14
Lysine	103	64	44	12
Methionine and cystine	58	27	22	13
Phenylalanine and tyrosine	125	69	22	14
Threonine	87	37	28	7
Tryptophan	17	12.5	3.3	3.5
Valine	93	38	25	10
Total	714	352	216	84
Total per gram of protein[a]	434	320	222	111

[a]Total mg/g crude protein. Taken from Table 38 in *ref. 58* and based on all amino acids minus histidine.
Source: ref. 58.

Table 14
IDECG (75) Factorial Estimate of the Amino Acid Needs of the Infant and Amino Acid Supply from Breast Milk: age 3–6 mo; Median Body Weight 6.3 kg

Amino acid	Requirement Growth (mg/d)	Requirement Total (mg/kg/d)	Requirement Total (mg/d)	Intake from 800 mL milk (mg/d)
Lysine	134	63	347	482
Aromatic	132	60	378	564
Sulfur	68	27	170	244
Valine	89	38	239	346
Leucine	142	54	340	707
Isoleucine	65	32	202	360
Threonine	78	34	214	299
Tryptophan	34	11	69	170
Glycine	307			150
Arginine	237			244
Alanine	225			238
Total	1890			6800
Essential	742	320	2016	3196
Nonessential	1148			3604

Source: Data extracted and calculated from Table 18 in *ref. 75.*

1. The substantial amount of ^{13}C-labeled that is given over the 24-h period in those studies.
2. The difficulties of estimating the true rates of oxidation because the isotopic enrichment of the free amino acid pools that serve as the site for oxidative losses cannot be directly probed.
3. The possible overestimation of the net loss of amino acids as determined using the ^{13}C tracer approach, because of a hypothesized substantial inflow of IAAs into the body that is caused by and arises from the metabolic activity of the intestinal flora.

These potential problems have been discussed elsewhere *(104)* and are not repeated here, except to say that point 3. does not appear to be a problem.

INDISPENSABLE AMINO ACID REQUIREMENTS There are principally three major sets of proposed amino acid requirements for healthy subjects that should be mentioned and are summarized here. First, there are the requirements proposed by FAO/WHO/UNU *(58)* for the various age groups, which are presented in Table 13. As noted earlier, IDECG *(75)* also has assessed the amino acid needs of infants by using a factorial method; these are summarized in Table 14. It should be noted that the latter would approximate the average requirements, whereas the intakes supplied by the breast milk (shown in Table 14 for comparison) are well above the mean requirement in order to meet the needs of virtually all infants (e.g., *ref. 78*).

It should be noted that the requirement values given in Tables 13 and 14 are based on limited data; the values for the preschool child age group are derived from a single set of investigations carried out at the Institute for Central America and Panama *(80,81)*, whereas those for the school-age child come from studies conducted by a single group of investigators in Japan *(82)*. Those for the adult (Table 13) are based on the studies in men by Rose *(19)* and in women by various investigators (summarized in *ref. 45*).

There are multiple reasons for questioning the nutritional sig-

nificance of the adult FAO/WHO/UNU *(58)* values (Table 13) and the arguments have been presented by the MIT investigators in a number of reviews *(92,98,104,105)*. The major concerns for the international adult amino acid requirement values are related to the inappropriate experimental design of the studies by Rose *(19)*, as discussed by Young and Marchini *(106)* and the inadequacy of the nitrogen-balance technique and the criterion of nitrogen balance used to judge the nutritional adequacy of the levels of amino acid intake tested. However, not all N-balance studies suffer from the design flaws that characterize so many of the earlier N-balance investigations of adult amino acid requirements. One acceptable investigation was that by Jones et al. *(107)* on the lysine requirements of adult women. Nevertheless, with a re-evaluation of the nitrogen-balance data as reported by Jones et al. *(107)* using standard statistical techniques and after adjusting their published nitrogen-balance data for an assumed 8-mg/kg N/d loss via unmeasured miscellaneous routes *(58)*, it seems apparent that the lysine requirement in these young adult women was considerably higher than the value (<10 mg/kg/day) proposed by the original authors; this unpublished analysis (108) suggests the medium requirement to approx 28 mg/kg/d, with a wide variation among the 14 women studied.

Therefore, the MIT group has proposed new, tentative amino acid requirement values for the adult and these are shown in Table 15 together with a comparison with the 1985 FAO/WHO/UNU *(58)* adult values. It might also be noted that when these adult amino acid requirements are expressed as a pattern, or concentration, of the individual amino acids in relation to the protein requirement, it is not profoundly different from that for the preschool child or that is even not much lower than the factorially derived amino acid requirement pattern for the 6-mo-old infant, according to the IDECG *(75)* (Table 16).

In summary and in contrast to the reasonable consensus regarding the requirements for total protein in the nutrition of healthy

Table 15
Newly Revised MIT Estimates of Amino Acid Requirements in Adults
and a Proposed New MIT Amino Acid Scoring Pattern for This Age Group

	1985 FAO/WHO/UNU		New revised MIT estimates[b]	
Amino acid	Requirement[a] (mg/kg/d)	Pattern[a] (mg/g protein)	Requirement (mg/kg/d)	Pattern (mg/g protein)
Isoleucine	10	13	23	38
Leucine	14	19	39	65
Lysine	12	16	30	50
Met + Cys (SAA)	13	17	15	25
Phe + Tyr	14	19	39	65
Threonine	7	9	15	25
Tryptophan	3.5	5	6	10
Valine	10	13	20	35
Total	83.5	111	187	313

[a]Estimates from *ref. 58.*
[b]Data from *ref. 86.*

Table 16
Comparison of Various Amino Acid Requirement (Scoring)
Patterns for Infants, Preschool Children and Adults

	Amino acid pattern			
			Adult	
Amino acid	Infant, 3–6 mo (IDECG)[a]	Preschool child (FAO/WHO/UNU)[b]	FAO/WHO/UNU[b]	MIT[c]
Isoleucine	32	28	13	38
Leucine	54	66	19	65
Lysine	63	58	16	50
Met + Cys (SAA)	27	25	17	25
Phe + Tyr	60	63	19	65
Threonine	34	34	9	25
Tryptophan	11	11	6	10
Valine	38	35	13	35
Total	319	320	111	313

[a]Data calculated from *ref. 76.*
[b]Data from Table 38 in *ref. 56.*
[c]Based on data from *ref. 86.*

human adults, the requirements for the individual indispensable amino acids and, under certain pathophysiological conditions, for the conditionally indispensable amino acids are far less securely established. Tentative estimates based on the use of tracer techniques are generally much higher than earlier determinations based on the nitrogen-balance approach.

DIETARY PROTEIN QUALITY Knowledge of the requirements for the specific indispensable amino acids provides the basis for evaluating the relative capacity (or quality) of individual protein foods or mixture of food protein sources to meet human amino acid requirements. Therefore, brief consideration might be given here to the application of amino acid requirement values or, specifically, amino acid scoring patterns for the evaluation of dietary protein quality. This topic has been reviewed extensively *(109–111)* and so some of the key features and issues only need to be covered here.

Briefly, the use of amino acid scoring systems has progressed over the years since the earlier expectation that not only should an amino acid score be able to predict the potential protein nutritional value of a food or diet for humans but that it also should (with or without a protein digestibility consideration) correlate directly with the results of animal assays, such as net protein utilization (NPU) *(109).* However, it is now generally agreed that scoring systems developed to predict the nutritional value of protein sources for humans need not necessarily be expected to agree with values obtained with growing rats. Thus, it is now contended that the appropriate standard for dietary assessment should be via direct experimental study in human subjects or predicated from the human amino acid requirement or scoring pattern. Furthermore, for animal bioassays to be useful, they should be designed to give predictions in line with those based on human amino acid requirements rather than the reverse.

Thus, accepting the validity and usefulness of the amino acid scoring approach, the various estimates made of the amino acid requirements in humans at all ages would serve as the reference amino acid scoring pattern. In 1991 a Joint FAO/WHO Expert

Table 17
Predicted Quality (Amino Acid Score) of Wheat Proteins in Relation
to Use of Various Amino Acid Requirement (Scoring) Patterns

| Protein | Lysine content (mg/g protein) | Amino acid score (%) based on | | |
| | | 1985 FAO/WHO/UNU | | MIT pattern |
		Adult pattern	Preschool	
Whole wheat flour	24	>100 (L)	41 (L)	48 (L)
Wheat flour	20	>100 (L)	34 (L)	40 (L)
Wheat bran	16	100 (L)	28 (L)	32 (L)
"Animal proteins"	85±9	>100		>100
Legumes	65±7	>100		>100

Note: Data combined from Tables 6 and 7 in *ref. 105.*
(L) = Lysine is the linking amino acid.

Consultation *(110)* reviewed the appropriate methods for measuring quality of food proteins for the nutrition of human populations. This consultation concluded that the most appropriate method available was the protein digestibility-corrected amino acid score method (PDCAAS method) and it was recommended for international use. This amino acid scoring procedure, including a correction corrected for digestibility, uses the amino acid requirement pattern for the 2- to 5-yr-old child as proposed in 1985 by FAO/WHO/UNU *(58)* (Table 16, column 2) as the reference pattern for this purpose *(110)*.

The PDCAAS is estimated from the following equation:

$$\text{PDCAAS} = \frac{\begin{array}{c}\text{Concentration of most limiting digestibility-}\\\text{corrected amino acid in a test protein}\end{array}}{\begin{array}{c}\text{Concentration of that amino acid in the 1991}\\\text{FAO/WHO amino acid scoring pattern}\end{array}}$$

In addition to establishing the amino acid reference pattern for use in the PDCAAS method, the FAO/WHO Consultation *(110)* also considered the procedures for measuring and estimating amino acids and digestibility. This approach offers considerable benefits over that of animal bioassays, which traditionally have been used to assess protein quality of food protein in human diets. An important benefit is that the PDCAAS approach uses human amino acid requirements as the basis of evaluation, which ensures that appropriate levels of indispensable amino acids will be provided in the diet. Also, use of the proposed amino acid scoring procedure facilitates an evaluation of blending of foods to optimize nitrogen utilization and meeting protein and amino acid needs.

The development of an internationally derived procedure for evaluating protein quality using the amino acid scoring concept is a step that had long been required. This PDCAAS procedure can be modified as new knowledge about specific amino acid requirements emerges and as the determination of availability of dietary amino acids is improved and the factors affecting digestibility and availability are better understood. For the present, the PDCAAS proposed by FAO/WHO *(110)* would appear to be very useful for evaluating the nutritional quality of human food protein sources.

Two additional points in reference to adult amino acid nutrition might be emphasized. First, comparisons can be made of the prediction of the protein quality of whole wheat protein based on the 1991 FAO/WHO scoring pattern, on the one hand, and the

Table 18
Biological Assessment of the Nutritional Quality of
Whole Wheat Proteins in Young Adults

| Measure of quality | Experimental value | Predicted from amino acid values | |
		1985 FAO/WHO/UNU	MIT pattern
RPV[a]	54[b]	>100	48
RNR[c]	56[b]	>100	48

[a]RPV = relative protein value *(see ref. 109).*
[b]Expressed in comparison with beef protein as reference protein *(112).*
[c]RNR = relative nitrogen requirement.

1985 FAO/WHO/UNU adult amino acid requirement pattern, on the other. Thus, as shown in Table 17, the nutritional value of wheat is predicted to be quite different from that based on the 1985 adult amino acid scoring pattern showing a predicted value that is comparable to those for high-quality animal protein source. Clearly, the appropriate choice of the reference amino acid scoring pattern is obviously very important.

Second, when the nutritional quality of wheat protein is evaluated by use of the MIT adult amino acid requirement pattern (see Table 16, column 4), the comparative nutritional value of whole wheat is estimated to be about half of that for high-quality animal proteins, or slightly higher than that value predicted by use of the 1991 FAO/WHO *(110)* amino acid scoring pattern. In contrast, as already noted, the nutritional value of whole wheat proteins is similar to that for high-quality proteins when the 1985 FAO/WHO/UNU *(58)* adult requirement pattern is used for reference purposes. However, the lower estimate of the nutritional quality of whole wheat protein when based on use of the MIT pattern is entirely consistent with the results of nitrogen-balance experiments in healthy adults carried out at MIT approximately 25 yr ago *(112)*. Thus, the nitrogen-balance response to graded intakes of test dietary protein in healthy adults, expressed as relative protein value (RPV=[N-balance slope with wheat ÷ *N*-balance slope with reference protein] × 100), was 54 for whole wheat protein, using beef protein as a reference *(112)*. Expressed as relative nitrogen requirement (RNR = 1/[amount of wheat protein to achieve nitrogen balance is 97.5% of population ÷ amount of beef protein] × 100), the response was about 56 (Table 18). The MIT amino acid requirement pattern predicted a value of 48. Hence, it is apparent that there is good agreement between the experimentally derived (nitrogen balance) and predicted (from amino acid score) estimates of the nutritional quality of whole wheat proteins. In contrast, use of the 1985 FAO/WHO/UNU adult amino acid pattern gives a contradictory estimate of the nutritional value of wheat protein. Notwithstanding the problems that occur in attempts to aggregate nitrogen-balance data across separate studies carried out in different laboratories or within the same laboratory on different occasions *(89)*, the above supports the conclusion that the 1985 FAO/WHO/UNU lysine requirement value of 12 mg/kg/d for the adult should be discarded *(113)*. Furthermore, they provide additional justification for the MIT tentative working value of 30 mg/kg/d (or 50 mg lysine/g protein), and they support the recommendation that this figure be used until additional data become available that may make any further change in the amino acid requirement pattern both necessary and desirable. It is important that these uncertainties be resolved, in view of the importance of reliable amino acid requirement data for the appropriate planning of future world food and protein needs *(114)*. Use of either the 1991 FAO/WHO *(110)* amino acid scoring pattern, or possibly, preferably, the MIT amino acid scoring pattern (Table 16, column 4), with its modestly lower concentration of lysine, would be prudent in considerations of dietary protein quality and human protein nutrition.

SUMMARY

The functions of amino acids and the metabolic basis for their requirements, including energy–protein relationships, and for a utilizable source of nitrogen were reviewed briefly. Also, the methods and approaches used to arrive at estimates of the total protein and specific amino acid requirements of individuals from infancy to the later years of adult life have been reviewed. The current international assessments of protein requirements and recommendations for safe protein intakes were then summarized, together with an account of some of the more recent revisions proposed by IDECG for infants and children *(75)*. The protein requirements in elderly people remain somewhat elusive, but the current international recommendations for this age group provide a reasonable benchmark for planning diets for individuals, recognizing that the elderly may need a somewhat higher protein intake because of the effects of stress and disease in increasing nutrient needs. Current knowledge about the requirements of specific indispensable amino acids was outlined, with the conclusion that there is a great deal of uncertainty and imprecision attached to the amino acid requirement values for all age groups. Results from tracer studies of the amino acid requirements in adults suggest that the international figures are far too low. Thus, for the evaluation of protein quality and planning of diets, it is considered prudent to use the 1991 FAO/WHO amino acid scoring (requirement) pattern *(110)* or a proposed modification of it based on data obtained from tracer studies *(86)*.

REFERENCES

1. Burke RF, Hill KE. Regulation of selenoproteins. Annu Rev Nutr 1993; 13:65–81.
2. Ferland G. The vitamin K-dependent proteins: an update. Nutr Rev 1998; 56:223–30.
3. Munro HN. Evolution of protein metabolism in mammals. In: HN Munro, ed, Mammalian Protein Metabolism, Vol. 3, Chap. 25. Academic, New York, 1969.
4. Young VR, El-Khoury AE, Sanchez M, Castillo L. The biochemistry and physiology of protein and amino acid metabolism, with reference to protein nutrition. In: Raiha NCR, ed, Protein Metabolism During Infancy, pp. 1–27, Raven, New York, 1994.
5. Van Goudoever JB, Sulkers EJ, Halliday D, Degenhart HJ, Carnielli VP, Wattimena JL, et al. Whole body protein turnover in premature appropriate for gestational age and small for gestational age infants: comparison of [^{15}N]glycine and [$1-^{13}$C]leucine administered simultaneously. Pediatr Res 1995; 37:381–8.
6. Kinney JM, Elwyn DH. Protein metabolism and injury. Annu Rev Nutr 1983; 3:433–66.
7. Young VR, Yu Y-M. Protein and amino acid metabolism. In: Fischer JE, ed, Nutrition and Metabolism in the Surgical Patient, 2nd ed, pp. 159–201. Little, Brown & Co., Boston, 1996.
8. Young VR, Yu Y-M, Fukagawa NK. Energy and protein turnover. In: Kinney JM, Tucker HN, eds, Energy Metabolism: Tissue Determinants and Cellular Corollaries, pp. 439–66, Raven, New York, 1992.
9. Garlick PJ, Clugston GA, Waterlow JC. Influence of low-energy diets on whole-body protein turnover in obese subjects. Am J Physiol 1980; 238:E235–E244.
10. Elia M. Energy expenditure in the whole body. In: Kinney JM and Tucker HN, eds, Energy Metabolism: Tissue Determinants and Cellular Corollaries, pp. 19–59, Raven, New York, 1992.
11. Rolfe DFA, Brown GC. Cellular energy utilization and molecular origin of standard metabolic rate in mammals. Physiol Rev 1997; 77:731–58.
12. Yu YM, Tompkins RG, Ryan C, Young VR. The metabolic basis of the rise in energy expenditure in severely burned patients. J Parent Enteral Nutr 1999; (in press).
13. Calloway DH, Spector H. Nitrogen balance as related to caloric and protein intake in active young men. Am J Clin Nutr 1954; 2:405–12.
14. Munro HN. General aspects of the regulation of protein metabolism by diet and hormones. In: Munro HN, Allison JB, eds, Vol. 1, pp. 381–481. Academic, New York, 1964.
15. Young VR, Yu Y-M, Fukagawa NK. Whole body energy and nitrogen (protein) relationships. In: Kinney JM, Tucker HN, eds, Energy Metabolism: Tissue Determinants and Cellular Corollaries, pp. 139–60, Raven, New York, 1992.
16. Elwyn DH. Nutritional requirements of adult surgical patients. Crit Care Med 1980; 8:9–20.
17. Gaza CG, Scrimshaw NS, Young VR. Human protein requirements: the effect of variations in energy intake within the maintenance range. Am J Clin Nutr 1976; 29:280–7.
18. Inoue G, Fujita Y, Nijyama Y. Studies on protein requirements of young men fed egg protein and rice protein with excess and maintenance energy intakes. J Nutr 1973; 103:1673–87.
19. Rose WC. The amino acid requirements of adult man. Nutr Abst Rev 1957; 27:631–67.
20. Young VR. Protein and amino acid requirements in humans: metabolic basis and current recommendations. Scand J Nutr (Näringsforskning) 1992; 30:47–56.
21. Rose WC, Haines WJ, Warner DJ. The amino acid requirements of man. V. The role of lysine, arginine, and tryptophan. J Biol Chem 1954; 206:421–30.
22. Silk DBA, Green CJ. Perioperative nutrition: parenteral versus enteral. Curr Opin Clin Nutr Metab Care 1998; 1:21–7.
23. Schauder P, Wahren J, Paoletti R, Bernardini R, Rinetti M. eds. Branched-Chain Amino Acids: Biochemistry, Physiopathology, and Clinical Science. New York, 1992.
24. Cynober LA, ed. Amino Acid Metabolism and Therapy in Health and Nutritional Disease. CRC, Boca Raton, FL, 1995.
25. Young VR, Ajami AM. The Rudolf Schoenheimer Centenary Lecture: isotopes in nutrition research. Proc Nutr Soc (Engl) 1999; 58:1–18.
26. Souba WW. Nutritional support. N Engl J Med 1997; 336:41–8.
27. Furst P. Old and new substrates in clinical nutrition. J Nutr 1998; 128:789–96.
28. Young VR, El-Khoury AE. The nature of the nutrition essentiality of amino acids, revisited, with a note on the indispensable amino acid requirements in adults. In: Cynober L, ed, Amino Acid Metabo-

lism and Therapy in Health and Nutritional Disease. CRC, Boca Raton, FL, 1995.

29. Visek WJ. Arginine and disease states. J Nutr 1985; 115:532–41.

30. Hurson M, Regan MC, Kirk SJ, Wasserkrug HL, Barbul A. Metabolic effects of arginine in a healthy elderly population. J Parent Enteral Nutr 1995; 19:227–30.

31. Jaksic T, Wagner DA, Burke JF, Young VR. Proline metabolism in adult male burned patients and healthy control subjects. Am J Clin Nutr 1991; 54:408–13.

32. Fürst P, Stehle P. Glutamine and glutamine-containing peptides. In: Cynober L. ed, Amino Acid Metabolism and Therapy in Health and Nutritional Disease, pp. 373–83. CRC, Boca Raton, FL, 1995.

33. Fomon SJ. Nutrition of Normal Infants, p. 122. Mosby, St. Louis, MO, 1993.

34. Jackson AA. The glycine story. Eur J Clin Nutr 1991; 45:59–65.

35. Castillo L, Chapman TE, Sanchez M, Yu Y-M, Burke JF, Ajami AM, et al. Plasma arginine and citrulline kinetics in adults given adequate and arginine-free diets. Proc Natl Acad Sci USA 1993; 90:7749–53.

36. Yu Y-M, Ryan CM, Burke JF, Tompkins RG, Young VR. Relations among arginine, citrulline, and ornithine and leucine kinetics in adult burn patients. Am J Clin Nutr 1995; 62:960–8.

37. Yu YM, Sheridan RL, Burke JF, Chapman TE, Tompkins RG, Young VR. The kinetics of plasma arginine and leucine in pediatric burn patients. Am J Clin Nutr 1996; 61:60–6.

38. Flynn NE, Wu G. An important role for endogenous synthesis of arginine in maintaining arginine homeostasis in neonatal pigs. Am J Physiol 1996; 271:R1149–R1155.

39. Wu G, Davis PK, Flynn NE, Krabe DA, Davidson JT. Endogenous synthesis of arginine plays an important role in maintaining arginine homeostasis in postweaning growing pigs. J Nutr 1997; 127:2342–9.

40. Ball RO, Atkinson JL, Bayley HS. Proline as an essential amino acid for the young pig. Br J Nutr 1986; 55:659–68.

41. Berthold HK, Hachey DL, Reeds PJ, Thomas OP, Hoeksema S, Klein PD. Uniformly ^{13}C-labeled algae protein used to determine amino acid essentiality in vivo. Proc Natl Acad Sci USA 1991; 88:8091–5.

42. Miller RG, Jahoor F, Reeds PJ, Heird WC, Jaksic T. A new stable isotope tracer technique to assess human neonatal amino acid synthesis. J Pediatr Surg 1995; 30:1325–9.

43. Jackson AA, Badaloo AV, Forrester T, Hibbert JM, Persaud C. Urinary excretion of 5-oxoproline (pyroglutamic aciduria) as an index of glycine insufficiency in normal man. Br J Nutr 1987; 58:207–14.

44. Jackson AA, Persaud C, Werkmesiter G, McClelland SM, Bodaloo A, Forrester T. Comparison of urinary 5-L-oxoproline (L-pyroglutamate) during normal pregnancy in women in England and Jamaica. Br J Nutr 1997; 77:183–96.

45. Irwin MI, Hegsted DM. A conspectus of research in amino acid requirements of man. J Nutr 1971; 101:539–66.

46. Hiramatsu T, Fukagawa NK, Marchini JS, Cortiella J, Yu Y-M, Chapman TE, et al. Methionine and cysteine kinetics at different intakes of cysteine in healthy adult men. Am J Clin Nutr 1994; 60:525–33.

47. Raguso CA, Ajami AM, Gleason R, Young VR. Effect of cysteine intake on methionine intake and oxidation, determined with oral tracers of methionine and cysteine in healthy adults. Am J Clin Nutr 1997; 66:283–92.

48. Fukagawa NK, Yu Y-M, Young VR. Methionine and cysteine kinetics at different intakes of methionine and cysteine in elderly men and women. Am J Clin Nutr 1998; 68:380–8.

49. Beutler E. Nutritional and metabolic aspects of glutathione. Annu Rev Nutr 1989; 9:287–302.

50. Meister A. Glutathione metabolism and its selective modification. J Biol Chem 1998; 263:17,205–8.

51. Taniguchi M, Hirayama K, Tagaguchi K, Tateishi N, Suzuki M. Nutritional aspects of glutathione metabolism and function. In: Dolphin D, Poulson R, Avramovic C, eds, Part B, pp. 645–727. Wiley, New York, 1989.

52. Young VR, Zamora J. Effects of altering the proportions of essential to nonessential amino acids on growth and plasma amino acid levels in the rat. J Nutr 1958; 96:21–7.

53. Kies C. Comparative value of various sources of non-specific nitrogen for the human. J Agric Food Chem 1974; 22:190.

54. FAO/WHO. Protein Requirements. Report of a Joint FAO/WHO Expert Group. In: FAO Nutrition Meetings Report, Series No. 37. Food & Agriculture Organization of the United Nations, Rome, 1965.

55. Reeds PJ, Burrin DG, Jahoor F, Wykes L, Henry J, Frazer EM. Enteral glutamate is almost completely metabolized in first pass by the gastrointestinal tract of infant pigs. Am J Physiol 1996; 270:E413–8.

56. Reeds PD, Burrin DG, Stoll B, Jahoor F, Wykes L, Henry J, et al. Enteral glutamate is the preferential source for mucosal glutathione synthesis in fed piglets. Am J Physiol 1997; 273:E408–15.

57. Millward DJ, Rivers JP. The nutritional role of indispensable amino acids and the metabolic basis for their requirements. Eur J Clin Nutr 1988; 42:367–93.

58. FAO/WHO/UNU. Energy and Protein Requirements, Technical Report series No. 724. WHO, Geneva, 1985.

59. Hiramatsu T, Cortiella J, Marchini JS, Chapman TE, Young VR. Source and amount of dietary nonspecific nitrogen in relation to whole-body leucine, phenylalanine and tyrosine kinetics in young men. Am J Clin Nutr 1994; 59:1347–55.

60. Scrimshaw NS. Criteria for valid nitrogen balance measurement of protein requirements. Eur J Clin Nutr 1996; 50(suppl 1):S196–7.

61. Manatt MW, Garcia PA. Nitrogen balance: Concepts and techniques. In: S. Nissen, ed, Modern Methods in Protein Nutrition and Metabolism, pp. 9–66. Academic, San Diego, 1992.

62. Calloway DH, Odell ACF, Margen S. Sweat and miscellaneous nitrogen losses in human balance studies. J Nutr 1971; 101:775–86.

63. Millward DJ, Roberts SB. Protein requirements of older individuals. Nutr Res Rev 1996; 9:67–87.

64. Young VR, Taylor YSM, Rand WM, Scrimshaw NS. Protein requirements of man: efficiency of egg protein utilization at maintenance and submaintenance levels in young men. J Nutr 1973; 103:1164–74.

65. Rand WM, Uauy R, Scrimshaw NS, ed, Protein-Energy-Requirement Studies in Developing Countries: Results of International Research. The United National University, Tokyo, 1984.

66. FAO/WHO. Energy and protein requirements. Report of a joint FAO/WHO Ad Hoc Expert Committee. Technical Report Series No. 522. WHO, Geneva, 1973.

67. Donovan SM, Lonnerdal B. Isolation of the non-protein nitrogen fraction from human milk by gel-filtration chromatography and its separation by fast protein liquid chromatography. Am J Clin Nutr 1989; 50:53–7.

68. Young VR. Some metabolic and nutritional considerations of dietary protein restriction. In: WE Mitch, ed, Contemporary Issues in Nephrology, pp. 263–83. Churchill Livingstone, Edingburgh, 1984.

69. Munro HN, Young VR. Protein and amino acid requirements. In: AN Exton-Smith, FI Caird, eds, Metabolic and Nutritional Disorders of the Elderly, p. 13. Wright, Bristol, UK, 1980.

70. Young VR, Munro HN, Fukagawa NK. Protein and functional consequences of deficiency. In: A Horwitz, DM Macfadyen, H Munro, NS Scrimshaw, B Steen, TF Williams, eds, Nutrition in the Elderly, pp. 65–84. Oxford University Press, Oxford, 1989.

71. Millward DJ, Fereday A, Gibson N, Pacy PJ. Aging, protein requirements, and protein turnover. Am J Clin Nutr 1997; 66:774–86.

72. Pannemans D. Energy and protein metabolism in the elderly. Thesis. CIP Gegevens Koninkljke Bibliotheck, Den Haag, Netherlands, 1994.

73. Campbell WW, Evans WJ. Protein requirements of elderly people. Eur J Clin Nutr 1996; 50(suppl 2):S180–5.

74. Scrimshaw NS, Waterlow JC, Schürch B, eds, Energy and protein requirements. Eur J Clin Nutr 1996; 50(suppl 1):S1–S197.

75. Dewey KG, Beaton G, Fjeld C, Lonnerdal B, Reeds P. Protein requirements of infants and children. Eur J Clin Nutr 1996; 50(suppl 1):S119–50.

76. Heinig MJ, Nommsen LA, Peerson JM, Lonnerdal B, Dewey KG. Energy and protein intakes of breast-fed and formula-fed infants during the first year of life and their association with growth velocity: the DARLING study. Am J Clin Nutr 1993; 58:152–61.

77. Butte NF, Garza C, O'Brien-Smith E, Nichols BL. Human milk intake and growth in exclusively breast-fed infants. J Pediatr 1984; 104:187–95.

78. Beaton GH, Chery A. Protein requirements of infants: a re-examination of concepts and approaches. Am J Clin Nutr 1998; 48:1403–12.

79. Holt LE Jr, Snyderman SE. Protein and amino acid requirements of infants and children. Nutr Abstr Rev 1965; 35:1–13.

80. Pineda O, Torun B, Viteri FE, Arroyave G. Protein quality in relation to estimates of essential amino acid requirements. In: Bodwell LE, JS Adkins, DT Hopkins, eds, Protein Quality in Humans: Assessment and In Vitro Estimation, pp. 29–42. AVI, Westport, CT, 1981.

81. Torun B, Pineda O, Viteri FE, Arroyave G. Use of amino acid composition data to predict protein nutritive value for children with specific reference to new estimates of their essential amino acid requirements. In: CE Bodwell, JS Adkins, DT Hopkins, eds, Protein Quality in Humans: Assessment and In Vitro Estimation, pp. 374–89. AVI, Westport, CT, 1981.

82. Nakagawa I, Takahashi T, Suzuki T, Koboyashi K. Amino acid requirements of children: nitrogen balance at the minimal level of essential amino acids. J Nutr 1964; 83:115–8.

83. Williams HH, Harper AE, Hegsted DM, Arroyave G, Holt LE Jr. Nitrogen and Amino Acids, Food and Nutrition Board, National Research Council. Improvement of Protein Nutriture, pp. 23–63. National Academy of Sciences, Washington, DC, 1974.

84. Fomon SJ, Thomas LN, Filer LJ Jr, Anderson TA, Bergmann KE. Requirements for protein and essential amino acids in early infancy. Studies with soy-isolate formula. Acta Paediatr Scand 1973; 62:33–45.

85. Young VR, El-Khoury AE. Can amino acid requirements for nutritional maintenance in adults be approximated from the amino acid composition of body mixed proteins? Proc Natl Acad Sci USA 1995; 92:300–4.

86. Young VR, Bier DM, Pellett PL. A theoretical basis for increasing current estimates of the amino acid requirements in adult man, with experimental support. Am J Clin Nutr 1989; 50:80–92.

87. Young VR. Adult amino acid requirements: The case for a major revision. J Nutr 1994; 124:1517S–23S.

88. Fuller MF, Garlick PJ. Human amino acid requirements: can the controversy be solved? Annu Rev Nutr 1994; 14:217–41.

89. Millward DJ, Jackson AA, Price G, Rivers JPW. Human amino acid requirements: current dilemmas and uncertainties. Nutr Res Rev 1989; 2:109–32.

90. Young VR, El-Khoury AE. Human amino acid requirements. A re-evaluation. Food Nutr Bull 1996; 17:191–203.

91. Waterlow JC. The requirement of adult man for indispensable amino acids. Eur J Clin Nutr 1996; 50:151–79.

92. Young VR, Pellett PL. Current concepts concerning indispensable amino acid needs in adults and their implications for international nutritional planning. Food Nutr Bull 1990; 12:289–300.

93. Zello GA, Wykes LJ, Ball RO, Pencharz PB. Recent advances in methods of assessing dietary amino acid requirements for adult humans. J Nutr 1995; 125:2907–15.

94. Zello GA, Pencharz PB, Ball RO. Dietary lysine requirements of young adult males determined by oxidation of L-[1-13C]phenylalanine. Am J Physiol 1993; 264:E677–85.

95. Duncan AM, Ball RO, Pencharz PB. Lysine requirement of adult males is not affected by decreasing dietary protein. Am J Clin Nutr 1996; 64:718–25.

96. Lazaris-Brunner G, Rafii M, Ball RO, Pencharz PB. Tryptophan requirement in young adult women as determined by indicator amino

acid oxidation with L-[1-13C]phenylalanine. Am J Clin Nutr 1998; 68:303–10.

97. Millward DJ. Human amino acid requirements. J Nutr 1997; 127:1842–6.

98. Young VR. Human amino acid requirements: counterpoint to Millward and the importance of tentative revised estimates. J Nutr 1998; 128:1570–3.

99. Fereday A, Gibson NR, Cox M, Pacy PJ, Millward DJ. Protein requirements and aging: metabolic demand and efficiency of utilization. Br J Nutr 1997; 77:685–702.

100. Kurpad AV, El-Khoury AE, Beaumier L, Srivatsa A, Kuriyan R, Raj R, et al. An initial assessment, using 24h [13C]leucine kinetics, of the lysine requirement of healthy adult Indian subjects. Am J Clin Nutr 1998; 67:58–86.

101. El-Khoury AE, Fukagawa NK, Sanchez M, Tsay RH, Gleason RE, Chapman TE, et al. Validation of the tracer balance concept with reference to leucine intravenous tracer studies with L-[1-13C]leucine and [15N-15N]urea. Am J Clin Nutr 1994; 59:1000–11.

102. El-Khoury AE, Fukagawa NK, Sanchez M, Tsay RH, Gleason RH, Chapman TE, et al. The 24h pattern and rate of leucine oxidation, with particular reference to tracer estimates of leucine requirements in healthy adults. Am J Clin Nutr 1994; 59:1012–20.

103. Basile A, Beaumier L, El-Khoury AE, Kenneway M, Gleason RE, Young VR. Twenty-four hour L-[1-13C]tyrosine and L-[3,3²H₂] phenylalanine oral tracer studies at generous, intermediate and low phenylalanine intakes to estimate aromatic amino acid requirements in adults. Am J Clin Nutr 1998; 67:640–50.

104. Young VR, Borgonha S. Adult human amino acid requirements. Curr Opin Clin Nutr Metab Care 1999; 2:39–45.

105. Young VR, El-Khoury AE. Human amino acid requirements. A re-evaluation. Food Nutr Bull 1996; 17:191–203.

106. Young VR, Marchini JS. Mechanisms and nutritional significance of metabolic response to altered intakes of protein and amino acids, with references to nutritional adaptation in humans. Am J Clin Nutr 1990; 51:270–89.

107. Jones EM, Baumann CA, Reynolds MS. Nitrogen balances of women maintained on various levels of lysine. J Nutr 1956; 60:549–59.

108. Rand WM, Young VR. Statistical Analysis of N Balance Data with Reference To The Lysine Requirement in Adults. J Nutr (Submitted) 1999.

109. Pellett PL, Young VR. Nutritional Value of Protein Foods. United Nations University World Hunger Programme. Food and Nutrition Bull, Supplement 4, The United Nations University, Tokyo, 1980.

110. FAO/WHO. Protein quality evaluation. Report of Joint FAO/WHO Expert Consultation. FAO Food and Nutrition Paper No. 51. Food and Agriculture Organization of the United Nations, Rome, 1991.

111. Bodwell CE, Adkins JS, Hopkins DT, eds, Protein Quality in Humans: Assessment and In Vitro Estimation. AVI, Westport, CT, 1981.

112. Young VR, Fjardo L, Murray E, Rand WM, Scrimshaw NS. Protein requirements of man: comparative nitrogen balance response within the submaintenance-to-maintenance range of intakes of wheat and beef proteins. J Nutr 1975; 105:534–42.

113. Clugston G, Dewey KG, Fjeld C, Millward J, Reeds P, Scrimshaw NS, et al. Report of the working group on protein and amino acid requirements. Eur J Clin Nutr 1996; 50(suppl 1):S193–5.

114. Young VR, Scrimshaw NS, Pellett PL. Significance of dietary protein source in human nutrition: animal or plant proteins? In: JC Waterlow, DG Armstrong, L Fowden, R Riley, eds, Feeding a World Population of More Than Eight Billion People: A Challenge to Science, pp. 205–12. Oxford University Press, New York, in association with the Rank Prize Funds, 1998.

6 Specific Nutrient Requirements

Trace Elements

Janet C. King

INTRODUCTION

Trace elements, like vitamins, are needed for vital cellular functions. Often they function as cofactors for enzymes. The quantity of trace elements required in the diet to maintain those functions is very small. Dietary intakes range from as little as 20 μg/d to about 20 mg/d. The requirements for macrominerals, such as calcium, phosphorus, magnesium, and potassium, are 20-fold to 1000-fold higher. Furthermore, the sum weight of the essential trace elements in an adult is less than 10 g; they constitute less than 1% of the weight of all of the minerals in the body.

Fifteen trace elements are considered to be important for health (iron, zinc, copper, selenium, chromium, iodine, fluoride, manganese, molybdenum, boron, nickel, silicon, vanadium, arsenic, and cobalt), but questions currently exist about the essentiality of four of these trace elements (chromium, boron, fluoride, and vanadium). Their essentiality is questioned because they fail to meet all of the following criteria for essentiality:

1. It is present in all healthy tissue of living things;
2. Its tissue concentration from one animal to the next is fairly constant;
3. Its withdrawal from the body induces the same physiological and structural changes reproducibly, regardless of the species;
4. Its addition either reduces or prevents the functional abnormalities;
5. The functional abnormalities induced by deficiencies are always accompanied by specific biochemical changes;
6. The biochemical changes are prevented or cured when the deficiency is prevented or cured; and
7. Excessive intakes also induce functional abnormalities that are accompanied by specific biochemical changes.

Trace elements generally are required as components or cofactors for enzymes (Table 1). Some of the elements have additional unique functions: Iron is required for the normal synthesis of heme, iodine for the synthesis of thyroid hormones, and fluoride for increasing the resistance of teeth enamel to acid erosion. Severe deficiencies cause multiple biochemical and physiological changes that lead to clinical signs and symptoms that are easy to recognize (i.e., skin rashes, hair loss, reduced immunity, growth retardation). For example, deficiencies of iron, zinc, iodine, copper, and manganese cause a failure to grow normally. Impaired immune function occurs when the intakes of iron, zinc, copper, and selenium are inadequate. Marginal or subclinical deficiencies are more difficult to recognize. This is particularly true in humans because a deficiency of one trace element often coexists with deficiencies of other nutrients.

Deficiencies of trace elements often stem from one or more of the following conditions:

1. *Low intakes* of the trace element resulting from poor food selection or consumption of foods grown in trace element poor soil;
2. *Low bioavailability* of the trace element resulting from the presence of factors in the diet that inhibit absorption; and
3. *Presence of underlying disease or use of drugs* that increases trace element loss or reduces whole-body utilization.

A deficiency resulting from poor intakes and/or poor bioavailability of the element for the food source is called a primary deficiency; a deficiency resulting from the presence of underlying disease is termed a secondary deficiency. In developed countries such as the United States or the European Union, trace element deficiencies are generally secondary to underlying disease or use of drugs. In developing countries where cereal products are the dietary staple, primary trace element deficiencies generally occur as a result of low bioavailability of the trace element.

Because more than one trace element may share binding sites for intestinal absorption or membrane transport or because trace elements may substitute for each other as cofactors for enzymes, interactions between them is not uncommon. An excess of one trace element may cause a deficiency of another. For example, a slight manganese overload aggravates an iron deficiency, and iron supplementation reduces zinc absorption. Conversely, a deficiency of one trace element may increase susceptibility to a toxic reaction from another. Iron deficiency, for example, makes the body more susceptible to lead toxicity. Some of the common trace element interactions are summarized in Table 2.

From: *Nutrition and Immunology: Principles and Practice* (ME Gershwin et al. eds.), © Humana Press, Inc., Totowa, NJ

Table 1
Functions of Some of the Trace Elements

Mineral	Function	Deficiency symptoms
Iron	Part of hemoglobin, myoglobin, and cytochrome enzymes	Microcytic anemia, fatigue, reduced work performance
Zinc	Catalytic, structural, and regulatory functions in over 50 different enzymes	Growth retardation, reduced immunity, loss of appetite, skin rashes, failure in wound healing
Copper	Cofactor or component of enzymes that often catalyze reactions involving molecular oxygen; required for normal iron metabolism	Microcytic anemia, neutropenia, poor growth, impaired immunity, abnormal bone growth
Selenium	Cofactor for enzymes involved in peroxide metabolism and thyroid hormone metabolism	Cardiomyopathy, muscle pain, and weakness
Iodine	Component of thyroid hormones	Goiter, poor growth and development, cretinism
Manganese	Component of enzymes (i.e., arginase, pyruvate carboxylase, and MnSOD)	None in humans
Molybdenum	Component of enzymes (i.e., xanthine dehydrogenase)	None in humans
Fluoride	Increases resistance to acid erosion of teeth	Increased risk of dental caries
Chromium	May increase insulin action	None in healthy humans; may improve glucose tolerance in diabetics

Table 2
Trace Element Interactions

Interaction	Proposed mechanism	Physiologic effect
Iron–zinc	High iron intakes may compete with zinc absorption.	Secondary zinc deficiency; supplemental zinc recommended if >60 mg supplemental iron is taken.
Zinc–copper	Excess zinc intakes (>150 mg/d) may interfere with copper absorption.	Symptoms of copper deficiency with chronic zinc supplementation.
Selenium–iodine	Selenium is required for iodothyronine deiodinase.	Serious thyroid failure has occurred in endemic cretins undergoing selenium repletion.
Iron–manganese	Supplemental manganese may interfere with iron absorption	Chronic manganese supplementation is not common in humans; potentially could cause a secondary iron deficiency in individuals with marginal iron status.

Whenever the concentration of trace elements in tissues is too high, function is also impaired and clinical signs of trace element toxicity may become evident. For some trace elements, such as selenium, toxicities occur at levels that are only several-fold higher than the amounts required for normal function. Others have a broader range of tolerance. To avoid the risk of trace element toxicity, the total intake from the diet and supplements should remain within the range associated with normal function and health. Keeping total intake to less than two times the recommended intake is a good rule of thumb.

Immune function and resistance to disease is influenced by trace element nutrition. Infections, particularly of the gastrointestinal tract, can lead to increased losses and a secondary deficiency. These relationships between trace elements and immune function and disease are discussed elsewhere in this volume. Because the roles of iron, zinc, copper, and selenium in immune function are best known, the specific functions and requirements for these elements are discussed in this chapter. Emphasis is placed on those populations of increased risk because of growth, such as in infants, adolescents, and pregnant women, or because of reduced utilization, such as in the elderly.

IRON

Total-body iron averages about 3.8 g in men and 2.3 g in women. Iron-containing compounds in the body can be grouped into two

categories: functional compounds that serve a metabolic or enzymatic role and storage compounds that represent transport or storage iron. Approximately two-thirds of the total-body iron exists in a functional form, and most of this is as hemoglobin. Men tend to have much higher amounts of storage iron; about one-third of the total body iron is storage iron in men and one-eighth is in women. The two principal forms of storage iron are ferritin and hemosiderin.

IRON METABOLISM The iron status, or health, of an individual is determined by three factors: amount absorbed, stored, and excreted. Dietary iron intakes and the capacity to absorb that iron dictates the amount absorbed. Iron balance is regulated primarily by the gastrointestinal tract. The amount of iron absorbed can range from <1% to >50% of the food iron. The amount absorbed is determined by the interaction between the food supply and the regulatory mechanisms reflecting total-body iron need. Heme and nonheme iron are absorbed by different mechanisms. Heme iron comes primarily from hemoglobin and myoglobin in animal flesh, and it accounts for less than 20% of the total iron intake. It is absorbed two to three times more efficiently than nonheme iron, however. Nonheme iron absorption is dependent on its solubility in the upper part of the small intestine. A number of dietary factors enhance or inhibit iron absorption. Enhancers include vitamin C and the presence of meat in the meal. Inhibitors include phytic acid from unprocessed whole grain cereals, bran, calcium phosphate, and polyphenols (in tea and some vegetables). Iron entry into the body from the mucosal cells is regulated in some manner by total-body stores. Nonheme iron absorption is regulated to a greater extent than heme iron absorption. Iron is transported in circulation bound to transferrin. The delivery of iron to cells is accomplished by the binding of transferrin to cell-membrane-specific receptors for transferrin (1). The number of receptors is highly regulated (2). When the iron supply to the cell is inadequate, the number of transferrin receptors increases. Serum transferrin receptors are proportional to the number of cell surfaces and serve as a biochemical indicator of iron status (3).

Iron is stored in the liver, reticuloendothelial cells, and bone marrow as ferritin and hemosiderin (4). On average, ferritin contains about 25% iron by weight. Iron is stored in ferritin as a hydrated ferric phosphate surrounded by 24 polypeptide units. Hemosiderin contains iron as a large iron–salt–protein aggregate. Ferritin iron is mobilized more readily than hemosiderin iron. The amount of iron stores can vary widely without any apparent impairment to body function. Storage iron is almost completely depleted before the signs of iron deficiency are apparent; a >20-fold increase over normal may occur before any tissue damage is evident.

Daily iron losses average about 1.0 mg/d in men and about 1.3 mg/d in menstruating women. Most of the loss (approx 0.6 mg/d) is via the feces from bile, desquamated mucosal cells, and the loss of minute amounts of blood (5). Another 0.2–0.3 mg/d is lost via desquamated skin cells and sweat, and a minor amount is lost in the urine (approx 0.1 mg/d). The most common cause of a negative iron balance is excessive blood loss. Hookworm infection causes gastrointestinal blood loss and is a major cause of iron deficiency in tropical countries (6). In the United States a sensitivity to cow's milk in children, the use of aspirin, bleeding ulcers, or tumors may cause gastrointestinal blood loss and iron depletion.

IRON FUNCTION   Functional forms of iron can be divided into heme and nonheme compounds. The heme-containing compounds include hemoglobin for oxygen transport, myoglobin for muscle storage of oxygen, and cytochromes for oxidative production of cellular energy in the form of adenosine triphosphate. Hemoglobin possesses the unique ability to become almost fully oxygenated in lung tissue and to then become largely deoxygenated during its transit through tissue capillaries. Anemia, or a reduced oxygen-carrying capacity in the blood, is frequently the result of an iron deficiency, although many other pathological conditions can affect hemoglobin or erythrocyte synthesis. In moderate anemia, biochemical changes occur in the tissues to compensate for reduced oxygen-carrying capacity. In severe anemia, reduced oxygen delivery causes a chronic tissue hypoxia.

Whereas hemoglobin is only present in erythrocytes, myoglobin is only present in muscles. Myoglobin transports and stores oxygen in the muscle so it can be released quickly when needed for muscle contractions. Iron-deficient rats tend to have reduced amounts of myoglobin in their skeletal muscles (7).

Cytochromes a, b, and c are essential for the production of energy by oxidative phosphorylation; they serve as electron carriers in transforming adenosine dephosphate (ADP) to adenosine triphosphate (ATP). Animals with severe iron deficiency have lower levels of cytochromes b and c and reduced rates of oxidation by the electron-transport chain (7). Cytochrome P450 is located in the microsomal membranes of the liver and intestine. This enzyme degrades endogenous compounds or environmental toxins by oxidative degradation.

Nonheme-iron-containing enzymes include the iron–sulfur complexes of NADH dehydrogenase and succinate dehydrogenase. These enzymes are required for the first reaction in the electron-transport chain. Hydrogen peroxidases, such as catalase and peroxidase, are another group of iron-dependent enzymes that protect against the accumulation of highly reactive hydrogen peroxide (H_2O_2). Rat and human erythrocytes show increased lipid peroxidative damage with iron deficiency (8). Other nonheme-iron-containing enzymes include aconitase, phosphoenolpyruvate carboxykinase, and ribonucleotide reductase.

IRON DEFICIENCY AND EXCESS   Iron deficiency is the most common nutritional problem in the United States and worldwide affecting primarily older infants, young children, and women of childbearing age (9). The primary causes of iron deficiency are reduced absorption because of the presence of inhibitors of iron uptake in the diet, excessive iron loss due to chronic blood loss, and repeated pregnancies in women with marginal iron intakes.

Unless the anemia is severe, the clinical symptoms of iron deficiency are subtle and difficult to detect (10). Anemia is the best known consequence of iron deficiency. Mild anemia has little effect on function because compensatory mechanisms maintain the tissue oxygen supply. Those compensatory mechanisms include an improved extraction of oxygen from hemoglobin by the tissues, redistribution of blood flow to vital organs, and increased cardiac output (11). With severe anemia (hemoglobin <70 g/l), compensation is no longer possible and acidosis develops. The risk for maternal and infant mortality rises as hemoglobin concentrations drop below 70 g/L (12). Reduced resistance to infection is observed in experimental iron deficiency in rats and humans (13). Iron-deficient children tend to have impaired lymphocyte and neutrophil functions, but an increased number of infections resulting from iron deficiency *per se* has not been demonstrated. Although iron deficiency and infections often coexist in children in the developing countries, a cause and effect has not been established.

Other functional consequences of iron deficiency include a reduced work capacity, impaired intellectual performance and behavioral changes, a decreased capacity to maintain body temperature, and adverse pregnancy outcome. The impaired work capacity may be the result, in part, of poor tissue oxygenation associated with anemia, but studies in experimental animals suggest that a marked oxidative capacity in skeletal muscles may contribute to the problem (14). Cognitive changes in association with iron deficiency have been demonstrated primarily in iron-deficient infants. The effects include a decreased responsiveness and activity with a greater tendency toward fatigue (15). The longer the presence of iron deficiency, the greater the severity of the symptoms. Most studies show that the developmental deficits are corrected with iron treatment, but others do not (16,17). The decreased ability to maintain body temperature appears to be related to a reduction in thyroid-stimulating hormone and thyroid hormones; a blood transfusion corrects the abnormality (18). Adverse pregnancy outcomes because of iron deficiency include preterm delivery, low birth weight, and fetal death (19,20).

Recently, there has been growing concern that iron overload may increase the risk of certain chronic diseases. This concern stems from the fact that iron may serve as a catalyst for redox reactions by donating or accepting electrons. When redox reactions are not modulated by iron-binding proteins or antioxidants, cellular components such as fatty acids, proteins, or nucleic acids may be damaged. Epidemiological studies suggest that elevated levels of serum ferritin or transferrin saturation are associated with cancer and coronary heart disease *(21,22)*. The potential impact of iron overload on health disorders needs to be investigated. In the interim, active programs to identify and prevent iron overload, especially hereditary hemochromatosis, will reduce any potential morbidity related to iron.

POPULATIONS AT RISK The populations at greatest risk for iron deficiency include older infants and children, adolescents, menstruating women, and pregnant women. The prevalence of iron deficiency is higher among the poor. Factors increasing the risk of iron deficiency in children include birth from an iron-deficient mother, preterm birth, or low birth weight because those infants are often born with lower iron stores and the more rapid growth rates during infancy will deplete their marginal iron stores. During the rapid growth phases of adolescence the need for iron is high due to expansion of the red blood cell mass and the deposition of iron as myoglobin in the muscle. Heavy menstrual losses place women at risk, particularly if they also are of high parity. The demand for iron during gestation is high due to the expansion of the blood volume of the mother and the demands for fetal and placental tissue synthesis.

For the U.S. population as a whole, approximately 9% of children between 1–2 years of age have iron deficiency. During the later childhood years the incidence falls to about 6%, but it rises again during adolescence to as much as 12% in males and 6% in females. The incidence in males is higher due to the more rapid growth rates and the greater gain of muscle tissue. Five to 14% of menstruating or pregnant females are iron deficient *(23)*. The incidence of iron deficiency in women living in developing countries is much higher, possibly as much as 35–50%.

DIAGNOSIS OF IRON DEFICIENCY The clinical symptoms of iron deficiency are too subtle to prompt concern. Therefore, evidence of increased risk based on the dietary and medical history along with measurement of a low hemoglobin or hematocrit can prompt physicians to evaluate individuals at risk. A low mean corpuscular volume (MCV) is strong supportive evidence of iron deficiency. If the history and blood count suggest a risk for iron depletion, a hemoglobin analysis of venous blood is indicated. Additional tests that may be conducted include an erythrocyte protoporphyrin, serum ferritin, and transferrin saturation. A simplified erythrocyte protoporphyrin test has been developed for the measurement of lead poisoning in children; this test can also be used to assess individuals for iron deficiency *(7)*. A screening cutoff for erythrocyte protoporphyrin is 0.35 mg/L of whole blood or 3.0 µg/g of hemoglobin.

IRON REQUIREMENTS AND DIETARY SOURCES The estimated need for absorbed iron is based on the amount of iron loss. Additional needs for growth is added to that value for infants and children. To estimate the dietary requirement, an assumption must be made about the proportion of dietary iron available for absorption. A value of 5% is used for cereal-based diets; 15% is proposed for more varied diets that are rich in meat and ascorbic acid. In the United States, a working value of 12.5% for availability is reasonable. Thus, the iron requirement for replacement and growth needs is multiplied by 8 to derive the dietary requirement *(7)*.

The current Recommended Dietary Allowances (RDAs) *(24)* are summarized in Table 3. A factor of 1.25 is added to the

Table 3
Recommended Dietary Allowances
for Iron, Zinc, Selenium and Copper

Age group	Iron (mg/d)	Zinc (mg/d)	Selenium (µg/d)	Copper (mg/d)
0–6 mo	6	5	10	0.4–0.6
7–12 mo	10	5	15	0.6–0.7
1–10 yr	10	10	20–30	0.7–2.0
11–14 yr	M: 12	M: 15	M: 40	1.5–2.5
	F: 15	F: 12	F: 45	
15–18 yr	M: 12	M: 15	50	1.5–2.5
	F: 15	F: 12		
19–24 yr	M: 10	M: 15	M: 70	1.5–3.0
	F: 15	F: 12	F: 55	
25–50 yr	M: 10	M: 15	M: 70	1.5–3.0
	F: 15	F: 12	F: 55	
50+ yr	10	M: 15	M: 70	1.5–3.0
		F: 12	F: 55	

Source: ref. 24.

estimated requirement for absorbed iron to cover individual variability. The RDA for pregnancy, 30 mg/d, cannot be met from food iron alone and supplementation is recommended. Although selected foods in the bread, legume, or fruit and vegetable groups are good sources of iron, meat iron is more available because much of it is in the heme form that is absorbed two to three times more readily than nonheme iron in the other foods. Nonheme iron absorption can be enhanced by ascorbic acid if it is ingested with the meal.

ZINC

The adult total-body content of zinc ranges from about 1.5 g in women to 2.5 g in men. Zinc is present in all tissues and fluids in the body. It is primarily an intracellular ion with over 95% found within the cells; 60–80% of the cellular zinc is located in the cytosol. Approximately 85% of the whole-body zinc is found in the skeletal muscle and bone *(25)*.

ZINC METABOLISM The zinc status, or health, of an individual is determined largely by the regulation of zinc absorption and endogenous excretion in the small intestine. Zinc is absorbed all along the small intestine, but most seems to be taken up in the jejunum *(26)*. Various exogenous and endogenous ligands in the lumin can either enhance or inhibit zinc uptake. Histidine and cysteine enhance zinc absorption; zinc in animal proteins rich in these amino acids tends to be higher than absorption from vegetable proteins. Phytic acid, the storage form of phosphorus in cereals, inhibits zinc absorption. The presence of large amounts of other divalent cations, such as iron and calcium, may compete with zinc for mucosal-cell-binding sites.

As intraluminal concentrations of zinc rise, the efficiency or fractional absorption of zinc declines, but the total amount of zinc absorbed increases. This is because transcellular uptake of zinc increases as the luminal concentrations rise. Thus, regulation of the intestinal absorption of zinc only provides "coarse control" over total-body zinc. Endogenous fecal zinc losses are thought to provide the "fine control." However, the mechanisms regulating endogenous gastrointestinal excretion are not known. Fractional absorption of zinc from a typical diet varies widely from about 20% to 40%. This variation may reflect differences in zinc status of the individual as well as differences in the availability of zinc from the foods in the diet.

Albumin is the primary portal carrier for newly absorbed zinc. Changes in the systemic level of albumin may alter zinc absorption *(27)*. In the general circulation, plasma zinc comprises only 0.1% of the whole-body zinc with approximately 70% bound to albumin and 20% bound to alpha-2-macroglobulin. Plasma zinc fluctuates markedly in response to specific physiological stimuli and dietary intakes; zinc circulating in the plasma turns over about 100 times or more in a day.

There is no specific store for zinc, although cytosolic zinc may serve as a cellular reserve.

In addition to endogenous fecal zinc, small amounts of zinc are also lost in the urine (about 0.5 mg/d). Reductions in urinary zinc excretion only occur if the dietary supply is very low; however, increased zinc intake from highly available sources, such as zinc supplements, can lead to an increase in urinary zinc. Surface zinc losses through desquamation of skin cells, out growth of hair, and sweat contribute another milligram of zinc lost daily. Semen is high in zinc, and approximately 1 mg is lost per ejaculate.

ZINC FUNCTION   The ubiquitous distribution of zinc among cells coupled with zinc being the most abundant intracellular trace element points to it having very basic functions *(28)*. Its functions can be grouped into three general areas: catalytic, structural, and regulatory. Catalytic roles are found in all six classes of enzymes. Over 50 different enzymes require zinc for normal activity. There are numerous examples of zinc depletion and changes in the activity or concentration of zinc metalloenzymes in the literature. It is difficult, however, to show a clear relationship between zinc intake and enzymatic function in humans. The physiological consequence of a change in enzyme activity may not be evident unless the zinc-requiring enzyme was acting at a rate-limiting step *(28)*.

The role of zinc in metalloenzymes is often structural. The zinc-finger motif is an example of an important structural function for zinc. Zinc fingers tend to have the following general structure: $-C-X_2-C-X_n-C-X_2-C-$, where C designates cysteine and X designates other amino acids *(28)*. This structure allows zinc to be bound as a tetrahedral complex with four cysteines. Zinc fingers are associated with multiple functions. They are located in the nucleus and in the transcription factors for retinoic acid and 1,25-dihydroxycholecalciferol receptors *(29)*. Zinc-finger motifs are also associated with protein–protein interactions affecting cellular differentiation, signal transduction, and cellular adhesion. The influence of zinc nutrition on the zinc fingers is unknown, but three observations are clear: (1) Considering their abundance, zinc fingers contribute to the overall zinc requirements, (2) they explain the tight homeostatic control for zinc, and (3) they may explain the basic functions of zinc in membrane integrity, receptor actions, and cellular proliferation and differentiation *(28)*.

Regulation of gene expression is the third biochemical function of zinc. A role for zinc in the expression of metallothionein has been demonstrated *(30)*. A metal-binding transcription factor and a metal-responsive element in the promotor region of the regulated gene are required. The metal-binding transcription factor in the cell cytosol acquires zinc and then binds with the metal responsive element to stimulate transcription.

It is difficult to reconcile these basic biochemical functions of zinc with physiological functional changes during zinc depletion. Changes in immune function, apoptosis, membrane integrity, lipid peroxidation, and reproduction have been observed in zinc deficiency. Immune defects associated with zinc deficiency include reduced thymic hormone production and activity, impaired functions of lymphocytes, natural-killer cells and neutrophils, impaired antibody-dependent cell-mediated cytotoxicity, altered immunologic ontogeny, and defective lymphokine production *(31)*. Zinc deficiency reduces the mass of lymphoid tissues more than any other tissue. A reduction in cell-division rates may explain some of these changes in immune function. Also, zinc may be needed for structure and activity of thymulin, a nine-amino-acid peptide found in plasma that stimulates T-cell development *(32)*. There is also evidence that intracellular zinc concentrations alter the cell selection process through apoptosis. Increased apoptosis appears to signal cellular zinc deficiency, whereas high concentrations inhibit cellular death *(33)*.

ZINC DEFICIENCY AND TOXICITY   The classical symptoms of zinc deficiency in experimental animals include retarded growth, depressed immune function, skin lesions, depressed appetite, skeletal abnormalities, and impaired reproduction. In humans, zinc deficiency causes severe growth retardation and sexual immaturity *(34)*. The characteristic rapid reduction in growth in zinc deficiency occurs without a reduction in tissue concentrations *(35)*. Anorexia and cyclic food intake is a classical response to zinc deficiency in experimental animals *(36)*. Poor appetite is also a sign of zinc deficiency in children *(35,37)*. The reduction in food intake may be adaptive because tissue concentrations are conserved by limiting growth. Also, cyclical food intake leads to an intermittent breakdown of muscle tissue and release of zinc for essential functions *(38)*.

A deficiency of zinc during early development is highly teratogenic. Typical malformations include brain and eye defects, spina bifida, cleft lip and palate, and numerous malformations of the heart, lung, skeleton, and urogenital system *(39)*. Zinc deficiency during gestation can also cause parturition difficulties, with delayed deliveries and excessive bleeding. Male reproductive function is also altered by zinc deficiency. The testes are reduced in size with atrophy of the seminiferous epithelium and impaired spermatogenesis and testosterone secretion *(40)*.

Marginal or mild zinc depletion is more typical in humans, but it is difficult to detect because impaired growth velocity is an early response. Furthermore, the marked reduction in endogenous zinc losses with reduced intakes conserves tissue zinc and prevents the onset of specific features of zinc deficiency *(41)*.

Acute zinc toxicity with intakes in the range of 1–2 g causes gastric distress, dizziness, and nausea. High chronic intakes from supplements (150–300 mg/d) may impair immune function and reduce concentrations of high-density lipoprotein cholesterol *(28)*. Also, hypocupremia occurred when sickle cell anemia patients were treated with 150 mg Zn/d *(42)*. Subsequently, high intakes of zinc have been used to treat Wilson's disease, a copper-accumulation disorder. It is thought that zinc induces the synthesis of metallothionein in the intestinal mucosal cells, which preferentially bind copper and leads to copper loss via desquamation of the cells. On balance, zinc is relatively nontoxic, but chronic use of zinc supplements may induce nutrient imbalances and physiological effects not encountered when zinc is supplied by food.

DIAGNOSIS OF ZINC DEFICIENCY   Despite our knowledge of zinc function and metabolism, the diagnosis of zinc deficiency has proven to be difficult because of the lack of a sensitive, specific indicator of zinc status *(43)*. Plasma/serum zinc concentrations do not fall with low zinc intakes, unless the dietary levels are so low that homeostasis cannot be re-established. Also, a number of other metabolic states influence plasma zinc concentrations. Stress, infection, food intake, short-term fasting, and the hormonal state of the individual all influence plasma zinc. Other static measures also hold little promise. Erythrocyte zinc responds very slowly to changes in dietary zinc. Leukocyte zinc is difficult to measure and the response to poor zinc intake is not consistent among various laboratories. Hair zinc levels seem to be depressed in mild zinc depletion, but they are unchanged in severe states where hair growth is arrested. Urinary zinc excretion falls in severe depletion, but this measurement is not sensitive to less severe states and is confounded by many clinical conditions that increase urinary zinc losses.

Currently, zinc deficiency is best diagnosed by using a combination of dietary, static, and functional signs of depletion. There should be evidence that the dietary supply is low and/or poorly available or that the individual has a clinical disorder known to impair zinc nutrition. Second, a low plasma or hair zinc concentration is a static indicator of poor status. Finally, a functional marker provides definitive evidence of zinc depletion. This might be a low erythrocyte metallothionein concentration, a decline in lymphocyte messenger RNA for metallothionein, an increase in the fragility of erythrocyte membranes, or a decrease in the activity of a zinc-dependent enzyme, such as 5′ nucleotidase.

ZINC REQUIREMENTS AND DIETARY SOURCES Dietary zinc requirements have been estimated from a variety of methods: balance studies, measures of total endogenous losses, and radioactive and stable isotope studies of zinc turnover. The Recommended Dietary Allowances are based on the amount required in the diet to maintain balance. Because the absorption of zinc varies with endogenous need and food sources, a standard fractional absorption of 20% was assumed (24). Using this approach, the zinc RDA is 5 mg/d for infants, 10 mg/d for children under 10 yr of age, 15 mg/d for males over age 10, 12 mg/d for females over age 10, 15 mg/d for pregnancy, and 19 and 16 mg/d for lactation during the first and second 6 mo, respectively. (Table 3).

Foods vary greatly in their inherent zinc content, with red meat and shellfish constituting the best sources. Foods of vegetable origin tend to be low, except for the germ of grains and seeds, such as nuts and legumes. Although the amount of zinc provided by a vegetarian diet may reach recommended intakes, the availability of the zinc from those foods is reduced by the presence of phytic acid, and fractional absorption is likely to fall below 20%.

COPPER

The total amount of copper in adults is approximately 110 mg (44). Kidneys have the highest concentrations, followed by liver and brain and then heart and whole bone. Whole blood and plasma contain about 1 μg of copper/g.

COPPER METABOLISM Copper absorption occurs primarily in the duodenum. The efficiency of copper absorption tends to be higher than that of other essential cations, about 40–70%. The efficiency of absorption declines, however, with high intakes and increases with low intakes (45). Copper absorption is affected by the presence of other trace elements in the diet. As explained earlier, high intakes of zinc decrease copper absorption. It is thought that this is due to the induction of metallothionein by zinc, which then traps the copper and makes it unavailable for

absorption. The presence of certain amino acids and citrate appears to enhance copper absorption, possibly by acting as copper ligands.

After being absorbed, copper enters the bloodstream bound to albumin and is quickly deposited in the liver. In rats, virtually all of the absorbed copper is cleared from after circulating 2 h and can be found almost exclusively in the liver, kidney, and liver-derived products, such as the bile (46). After this initial uptake of copper by the liver, it reappears in circulation as ceruloplasmin. This copper in ceruloplasmin is available for uptake by most tissues of the body.

Copper is not stored in tissues. There is some deposition in the liver, as metallothionein-bound copper, but this is not a store *per se*. Deposition of hepatic copper occurs *in utero*, possibly to serve as a reserve of copper for rapid postnatal growth because milk is not rich in copper (47,48).

Although there is some regulation of absorption with more being absorbed in deficiency and less in the face of copper adequacy, copper homeostasis is maintained primarily via excretion. The bile is the major excretory route for copper, but copper is also lost in gastric, pancreatic, and intestinal secretions. The total amount of copper secreted into the gastrointestinal tract is about three times the amount consumed in the diet. Most of this copper is reabsorbed, although there is some evidence that biliary copper is not readily absorbed (44). Very little copper is lost in the urine, hair, or desquamated skin cells.

COPPER FUNCTION Copper functions primarily as a cofactor or component of enzymes. Almost without exception, copper-dependent enzymes catalyze reactions that involve molecular oxygen. At least three copper enzymes have a role in antioxidant defense. These are the intracellular and extracellular superoxide dismutases (SODs), extracellular ceruloplasmin, and the intracellular copper thioneins. All SODs catalyze the conversion of superoxide anions to peroxides, which are then converted to H_2O by catalase or glutathione peroxidase. Several other copper enzymes are involved in molecular oxygen-requiring reactions that lead to cross-linking or polymerization of amino acids or other substituents. Examples include lysyl oxidase of connective tissue, which is needed for maturation of collagen and elastin. The copper-containing enzyme tyrosinase is involved in the synthesis of the melanin polymer that determines the pigment in our skin, hair, and eyes. Copper-containing enzymes are also involved in the formation and inactivation of hormones. For example, dopamine-β-monoxygenase catalyzes the synthesis of epinephrine and norepinephrine (44).

Copper appears to be essential for the normal utilization of iron. Ceruloplasmin and ferroxidase II (a copper-containing enzyme) oxidize iron to Fe^{3+} so that it can bind to transferrin in the plasma and facilitate the transport of iron to the bone marrow for hematopoiesis (44).

COPPER DEFICIENCY AND TOXICITY The symptoms of copper deficiency in both experimental animals and humans include hypochromic anemia, neutropenia, hypopigmentation of the hair and skin, abnormal bone formation with skeletal fragility and osteoporosis, vascular abnormalities, and uncrimped or steely hair (49). In addition, alterations in lipid and glucose metabolism have been observed in copper-deficient animals. The symptoms include hypercholesterolemia, hypertriglyceridemia, glucose intolerance, and enhanced sorbitol production. The exact role of copper in the development of these symptoms is unknown (44). Fertility and immunity also appear to be dependent on copper sufficiency. Pups born to copper-deficient dams have impaired hematopoiesis and abnormally developed bone and vasculature. Sperm motility is also reduced in copper deficiency (50). With respect to immunity, copper-deficient animals are much more susceptible to infection. Specific defects observed in the immune function include hyporesponsiveness of lymphoid cells to mitogens, decreased antibody production, decreased thymus weight, decreased activity of natural killer cells, and decreased antimicrobial activity of phagocytes (51–53).

Copper is relatively nontoxic. A few cases of liver cirrhosis have been reported, however, as a result of ingesting a chronic excess of copper. With very high intakes (i.e., 2000 µg/g), the gastrointestinal tract is damaged. Epigastric pain, nausea, vomiting, and diarrhea occur. Most of the toxic effects of copper are thought to be due to the production of oxygen radicals by Cu^+ chelates; ascorbic acid may be involved in producing those Cu^+ chelates (45). Those oxygen radicals scar liver tissue, leading to changes in liver function.

POPULATIONS AT RISK FOR COPPER DEFICIENCY

Although primary copper deficiency due to poor intakes is rare in humans, deficiencies have been observed in several special circumstances. Infants recovering from malnutrition, preterm and low-birth-weight infants fed milk-based diets, and patients supported on total parenteral nutrition have developed copper deficiency. The deficiency probably was a result of increased tissue need for tissue synthesis along with a marginal dietary supply. Chronic use of zinc supplements providing at least 150 mg zinc/d may induce a secondary copper deficiency. The prevalence of subclinical copper deficiency is unknown. Many diets provide less than 2 mg copper/d. Until the symptoms of mild copper depletion are known, the presence of subclinical copper deficiencies in the population should not be dismissed.

ASSESSMENT OF COPPER STATUS

Serum copper and ceruloplasmin concentrations fall rapidly with severe copper depletion and are reliable biomarkers of copper status (54). However, they may not be sensitive to mild deficiency, and ceruloplasmin, as an acute-phase protein, may be elevated in a variety of conditions masking a copper deficiency. Other potential indicators of copper status include erythrocyte superoxide dismutase, erythrocyte cytochrome oxidase, or possibly hair or urinary copper concentrations.

COPPER REQUIREMENTS AND DIETARY SOURCES

The estimated safe and adequate daily dietary intake of copper recommendation by the Institute of Medicine, Food and Nutrition Board, is 1.5–3.0 mg copper/d (24). The World Health Organization (49) recently published standards for copper intake. They estimate that the requirement for absorbed copper is between 0.7 and 0.8 mg/d. The minimum intake of a population of adults to provide the estimated need for absorbed copper is 1.2 mg/d for women and 1.3 mg/d for men.

Copper is widely distributed in plants and animals. Good dietary sources of copper (> 2 µg/g) include seafood, organ meats, legumes and nuts. Refined cereals and dairy products tend to be low.

SELENIUM

Most selenium in animal tissues is present in two forms: selenomethionine and selenocysteine. Selenomethionine must be derived from the diet because it cannot be synthesized in tissues. Selenocysteine is the form of selenium in its various biological roles (55).

SELENIUM METABOLISM

Seleno-amino acids are the dietary forms of selenium, whereas inorganic selenium is often the form used in experimental diets and some supplements. Inorganic selenium absorption is not regulated; it tends to be high (approx 70–80%) and is not influenced by selenium status (56,57). The absorption of selenomethionine is like that of methionine. The uptake of selenocysteine is not known. The metabolism of absorbed selenium is regulated to maintain an available supply of selenocysteine and to achieve tissue selenium homeostasis. Selenide is the common form of selenium found in the cells. Selenocysteine derived from selenomethionine, the diet, or selenoprotein catabolism is converted to selenide via selenocysteine β-lyase (58). Selenide is metabolized to selenophosphate, which is used for the synthesis of selenoproteins and seleno-tRNA (55). Selenide is also methylated to form the typical excretory products of selenium found in the urine and breath.

Selenium homeostasis is maintained through urinary excretion. As dietary intakes of selenium rise, urinary losses also increase. A small percentage of urinary selenium is trimethylated (59); the remaining forms have not been characterized.

SELENIUM FUNCTION

As is the case for other trace elements, selenium also functions as a cofactor for several enzymes. Approximately 10 different selenoproteins have been identified in rats (55). Four selenium-dependent glutathione peroxidases have been characterized. GSHPx-1 is the most abundant and is found in all cells. It reduces H_2O_2 and free hydroperoxides. GSHPx-2 is located in the gastrointestinal tract and GSHPx-3 is the plasma form. GSHPx-4 is high in the testis but is present in most cells. It is the only form of GSHPx that can reduce fatty acid hydroperoxides present in phospholipids (60).

Recent evidence shows that type I iodothyronine deiodinase is a selenoprotein (61). Selenium deficiency causes the activity of this enzyme to decline, but if iodine status and thyroid function are good, a compensatory rise in plasma T_4 prevents hypothyroidism. Type II and type III iodothyronine deiodinases were also recently shown to be selenoproteins. Type II regulates T_3 production in brain, pituitary, brown fat and placental tissue and controls thyroid-stimulating hormone secretion (62). Type III also degrades T_3 and other thyroid hormones.

Selenoprotein P is an extracellular protein rich in selenocysteine residues (55). Its function is not known, but it may be an extracellular antioxidant. Selenoprotein W is found in the muscle. It may be involved in the muscle degeneration seen with selenium deficiency.

SELENIUM DEFICIENCY AND TOXICITY

Selenium deficiency has been seen among women and children in certain regions of China. They develop a characteristic disorder, Keshan Disease, which includes myocardial necrosis. The coronary arteries are not affected, but the membranous organelles, such as mitochondria, show early necrotic changes (63). Kashin-Beck disease is another disorder linked with low selenium status. It is an endemic osteoarthropathy that affects children in certain parts of China and the Soviet Union. Degeneration and necrosis of the hyaline cartilage tissue seems to be the primary defect. Although these disorders are considered to be primarily due to a selenium deficiency, marginal vitamin E deficiency may also be involved, and a role for infection-induced oxidative stress has also been suggested (63). Beck and co-workers (64) have shown that selenium-deficient mice are more susceptible to heart damage because of coxsackievirus B than selenium-sufficient mice. In addition, inoculation of a benign strain of coxsackievirus B$_3$ into selenium-deficient mice cause a mild degree of heart damage. Isolation of the virus from the selenium-deficient mice and reinoculation into normal mice also caused heart damage (65). This suggests that the benign virus had undergone a genotypic change in the selenium-deficient animals that increased its virulence. A change in the RNA at six of seven sites confirmed the genotypic change (66). Similar viral changes were also observed when the virus was passed through vitamin E-deficient mice.

High intakes of selenium have been protective against tumorigenesis in experimental animals. A double-blind selenium-supplementation cancer prevention trial was just completed in 1312 individuals living in the southeastern United States. Individuals receiving 200 μg selenium/d for about 4.5 yr had a significant reduction in total cancer mortality, total cancer incidence, and incidences of lung, colorectal, and prostate cancers. Primarily because of the apparent reductions in total cancer mortality and total cancer incidence in the selenium group, the blinded phase of the trial was stopped early (67). A follow-up study in seven countries is planned.

The risk of selenium toxicity is higher than that of most other trace elements. Selenium poisoning occurred in China where individuals were ingesting nearly 5 mg selenium/d in a vegetable diet (68). The clinical signs of selenosis include hair and nail loss, skin lesions, and abnormalities of the nervous system. It is thought that the symptoms of selenosis stem from interference with sulfur metabolism and inhibition of protein synthesis (69). The Environmental Protection Agency has established a reference dose (RfD) of 350 μg/d, or 5 μg/kg/d (70).

POPULATIONS AT RISK FOR SELENIUM DEFICIENCY

Selenium deficiency in humans seems to be limited to individuals in selected regions where the soil content is low and, therefore, the food supply of selenium is also low. Although the soil in certain parts of the United States is low in selenium (i.e., Oregon), the population does not seem to be at risk because food is supplied from all over the country. Furthermore, concomitant vitamin E deficiencies or infections may be necessary for the expression of selenium deficiency.

ASSESSMENT OF SELENIUM STATUS Blood selenium concentrations appear to reflect dietary intakes (71). Plasma selenium concentrations respond rapidly to changes in the diet and are a measure of short-term selenium status (72). Plasma selenium concentrations tend to be low among people living in areas with selenium-poor soil, such as New Zealand. Supplementation with selenomethionine raises blood levels markedly because this form of selenium is not subject to homeostatic regulation. Hair selenium concentrations have been used to evaluate selenium status in China, but it may not be valid in the United States because many hair products contain selenium. Blood glutathione peroxidase activity is correlated with blood selenium concentrations up to 1.27 μmol/L (73). Above that value, the activity of glutathione peroxidase plateaus; however, it is a useful functional indicator of selenium status within the range of usual dietary selenium intakes.

SELENIUM REQUIREMENTS AND DIETARY SOURCES The RDA for selenium is 55 μg/d for women and 70 μg/d for men (24) (Table 3). This standard is based on the amount needed in the diet to maximize plasma glutathione peroxidase activity. The WHO (63) recently estimated that the requirement for absorbed selenium is about 0.4 μg/kg/d in adult men and women. Based on the normal variation in selenium intakes, 30 μg/d are needed

in the diet of women to meet this need and 40 μg/d are needed by men.

The selenium content of foods varies widely depending on the amount of selenium available in the soil for uptake by plants. Thus, the values for selenium in foods given in food composition tables are of marginal use in estimating the amount of selenium consumed. The selenium content of cereal products tends to vary the most, based on the amount of selenium in the soil. Concentrations of selenium in cereals ranges from <0.1 to >0.8 mg/kg wet weight (63). If the soil is rich in selenium, cereals may comprise about 75% of the total selenium intake; if the soil is poor, cereals may provide less than 10% of the intake. Liver, kidney, and seafood tend to have the highest amounts of selenium (0.4–1.5 mg/kg wet weight). Dairy products provide <0.1 to 0.3 mg/kg, and fruits and vegetables are low, with <0.1 mg/kg.

SUMMARY

At least 15 trace elements are required in the diet for normal cellular functions. The tissue concentrations and the total dietary need for these nutrients are very small (ppm concentrations). Analysis of minute quantities of trace elements in tissues and foods became routine with the widespread availability of atomic absorption spectroscopy in the early 1960s. Furthermore, the use of isotopic tracers, both stable and radioactive, extended the scope of studies from mere measurements of the quantity consumed and lost to measurements of tissue distribution, turnover, and metabolism. Like vitamins, trace elements primarily function as cofactors for enzymes. Some have additional unique functions; for example, the requirement for iron to facilitate oxygen transport or the need for iodine to synthesize thyroid hormones. The metabolism, function, deficiency symptoms, methods for assessment, and dietary requirements and food sources for four trace elements (iron, zinc, copper, and selenium) are discussed in this chapter. All four of these elements have been shown to affect immune function or the risk for infectious disease. Iron and zinc deficiencies are common in populations of growing infants and children and pregnant women who are subsisting on cereal-based diets with poor iron/zinc bioavailability. Selenium deficiency is a problem in some regions of the world (e.g., China), where the soil is low in selenium and the population is consuming a vegetable diet. Because copper is widely distributed in foods and is readily absorbed, copper deficiency among healthy humans is unusual. Human deficiencies have been reported, however, in preterm or low-birth-weight infants, in patients supported on total parenteral nutrition, and in individuals chronically taking supplemental zinc. Because trace elements are cofactors for enzymes, organ meats, and animal flesh are good sources.

REFERENCES

1. Huebers HA, Finch CA. The physiology of transferrin and transferrin receptors. Physiol Rev 1987; 67:520–81.
2. Casey JL, DiJeso B, Rao K, Rouault TA, Klausner RD, Harford JB. The promoter region of the human transferrin receptor gene. Ann NY Acad Sci 1988; 526:54–64.
3. Skikne BS, Flowers CH, Cook JD. Serum transferrin receptor: a quantitative measure of tissue iron deficiency. Blood 1990; 75:1870–6.
4. Halliday JW, Ramm GA, Powell LW. The cellular iron processing and storage. In: Brock JH, Halliday JW, Pippard MJ, Powell LW, eds, Iron Metabolism in Health and Disease, pp. 97–121. WB Saunders, London, 1994.
5. Green R, Charlton RW, Seffel H, Bothwell T, Mayet F, Adams B,

et al. Body iron excretion in man: a collaborative study. Am J Med 1968; 45:336–53.

6. Ziegler EE, Fomon SJ, Nelson SE, Rebouche CJ, Edwards BB, Rogers RR, et al. Cow milk feeding in infancy: further observations on blood loss from the gastrointestinal tract. J Pediatr 1990; 116:11–8.

7. Yip R, Dallman PR. Iron. In: Ziegler EE and Filer LJ Jr, eds, Present Knowledge in Nutrition, pp. 277–92. ILSI, Washington, DC, 1996.

8. Jain SK, Yip R, Dallman PR, Shohet SB. Evidence of peroxidative damage to the erythrocyte membrane in iron deficiency. Am J Clin Nutr 1983; 37:26–30.

9. Dallman PR, Yip R, Johnson C. Prevalence and causes of anemia in the United States, 1976–1980. Am J Clin Nutr 1984; 39:437–45.

10. Dallman PR. Manifestations of iron deficiency. Semin Hematol 1982; 19:19–30.

11. Varat MA, Adolph RJ, Fowler NO. Cardiovascular effects of anemia. Am Heart J 1972; 83:416–26.

12. Van den Broeck J, Eeckels R, Vuylsteke J. Influence of nutritional status on child mortality in rural Zaire. Lancet 1993; 341:1491–5.

13. Dallman PR. Iron deficiency and the immune response. Am J Clin Nutr 1987; 46:329–34.

14. Davies KJA, Donovan CM, Refino CA, Brooks GA, Packer L, Dallman PR. Distinguishing effects of anemia and muscle iron deficiency on exercise bioenergetics in the rat. Am J Physiol 1984; 246:E535–43.

15. Lozoff B, Brittenham GM, Viteri FE, Wolf AW, Urrutia JJ. The effects of short-term oral iron therapy on developmental deficient anemic infants. J Pediatr 1982; 100:351–7.

16. Lozoff B. Behavioral alterations in iron deficiency. Adv Pediatr 1988; 35:331–59.

17. Oski FA, Honig AS, Helu B, Howanitz P. Effect of iron therapy on behavior performance in nonanemic, iron-deficient infants. Pediatrics 1983; 71:877–80.

18. Beard J, Green W, Miller L, Finch CA. Effect of iron-deficiency anemia on hormone levels and thermoregulation during cold exposure. Am J Physiol 1984; 247:R114–9.

19. Garn SM, Ridella SA, Petzold AS, Falkner F. Maternal hematologic levels and pregnancy outcomes. Semin Perinatol 1981; 5:155–62.

20. Scholl TO, Hediger ML, Fischer RL, Shearer JW. Anemia vs iron deficiency, increased risk of preterm delivery in a prospective study. Am J Clin Nutr 1992; 55:985–8.

21. Steves RG, Jones DY, Micozzi MS, Taylor PR. Body iron stores and the risk of cancer. N Engl J Med 1988; 319:1047–52.

22. Salonen JT, Nyyssonen K, Korpela H, Tuomilehto J, Seppanen R, Salonen R. High stored iron levels are associated with excess risk of myocardial infarction in Western Finnish men. Circulation 1992; 86:803–11.

23. Life Sciences Research Office. Summary of a report on assessment of the iron nutritional status of the United States population. Am J Clin Nutr 1985; 42:1318–30.

24. Subcommittee on the Tenth Edition of the RDAs, Food and Nutrition Board, Commission on Life Sciences, National Research Council. Recommended Dietary Allowances, 10th ed. National Academy Press, Washington DC, 1989.

25. Jackson MJ. Physiology of zinc: general aspects. In: Mills CF, ed, Zinc in Human Biology, pp. 1–14. Springer-Verlag, New York, 1989.

26. Lönnerdal B. Intestinal absorption of zinc. In: Mills CF, ed, Zinc in Human Biology, pp. 33–56. Springer-Verlag, New York, 1989.

27. Smith KT, Failla M, Cousins RJ. Identification of albumin as the plasma carrier for zinc absorption by perfused rat intestine. Biochem J 1979; 184:627–33.

28. Cousins RJ. Zinc. In: Ziegler EE, Filer LJ Jr, eds, Present Knowledge in Nutrition, pp. 293–306. ILSI, Washington, DC, 1996.

29. Klug A, Schwabe JWR. Zinc Fingers FASEBJ (1995) 9:597–604.

30. Cousins RJ. Metal elements and gene expression. Annu Rev Nutr (1994) 14:449–69.

31. Keen CL, Gershwin ME. Zinc deficiency and immune function. Annu Rev Nutr 1990; 10:415–31.

32. Dardenne M, Pleau JM, Nabarra B, Lefrancier P, Derrien M, Choay J, Bach JF. Contribution of zinc and other metals to the biological

activity of the serum thymic factor. Proc Natl Acad Sci USA 1982; 79:5370–3.

33. McCabe MJ, Jiang SA, Orrenius S. Chelation of intracellular zinc triggers apoptosis in mature thymocytes. Lab Invest 1993; 69:101–10.

34. Prasad AS. Zinc in human nutrition. CRC, Boca Raton, FL 1979.

35. Golden MNH. The diagnosis of zinc deficiency. In: Mills CF (ed), Zinc in human biology, pp. 323–33. Springer-Verlag, New York, 1989.

36. O'Dell BL, Reeves PG. Zinc status and food intake. In: Mills CF (ed), Zinc in human biology, pp. 173–81. Springer-Verlag, New York, 1989.

37. Hambidge KM, Casey CE, Krebs NF. Zinc. In: Mertz W (ed), Trace elements in human and animal nutrition Vol. II, pp. 1–37. Academic, Orlando, FL.

38. Masters DG, Lönnerdal B, Hurley LS. Release of zinc from maternal tissues during zinc deficiency or simultaneous zinc and calcium deficiency in the pregnant rat. J Nutr 1986; 116:2148–54.

39. Keen CL, Hurley LS. Zinc and reproduction: effects of deficiency on fetal and postnatal development. In: Mills CF (ed), Zinc in human biology, pp. 183–220. Springer-Verlag, New York 1989.

40. McClain CJ, Gavaler JS, Van Thiel DH. Hypogonadism in the zinc-deficient rat: localization of the functional abnormalities. J Lab Clin Med 1984; 104:1007–15.

41. Baer MT, King JC. Tissue zinc levels and zinc excretion during experimental zinc depletion in young men. Am J Clin Nutr 1984; 39:556–70.

42. Prasad AS, Brewer GJ, Shoomaker EB, Rabbani P. Hypocupremia induced by zinc therapy in adults. JAMA 1978; 240:2166–8.

43. King JC. Assessment of zinc status. J Nutr 1990; 120:1474–9.

44. Linder MC. Copper. In: Ziegler EE, Filer LJ Jr, eds, Present Knowledge in Nutrition, pp. 307–19. ILSI, Washington, DC, 1996.

45. Turnlund JR, Scott KC, Peiffer GL, Jang AM, Keyes WR, Keen CL, et al. Copper status of young men consuming a low-copper diet. Am J Clin Nutr 1997; 65:72–8.

46. Weiss KC, Linder MC, Los Alamos Radiological Medicine Group. Copper transport in rats involving a new plasma protein. Am J Physiol 1985; 249:E77–88.

47. Linder MC. The Biochemistry of Copper. Plenum, New York, 1991.

48. Linder MC, Munro HN. Iron and copper metabolism in development. Enzyme 1973; 15:111–38.

49. World Health Organization. Trace Elements in Human Nutrition and Health, pp. 123–43. WHO, Geneva, 1996.

50. Morisawa M, Mohri H. Heavy metals and spermatozoan motility. I. Distribution of iron, zinc and copper in sea urchin spermatozoa. Exp Cell Res 1972; 70:311–5.

51. Lukasewyycz OA, Prohaska JR. The immune response in copper deficiency. Ann NY Acad Sci 1990; 587:147–59.

52. Mulhern SA, Koller LM. Severe or marginal copper deficiency results in a graded reduction in immune system status of mice. J Nutr 1988; 118:1041–7.

53. Vyas D, Chandra RK. Thymic factor activity, lymphocyte stimulation response and antibody producing cells in copper deficiency. Nutr Res 1983; 3:343–9.

54. Turnlund JR. Copper. In: Shils ME, Olson JA, Shike M, eds, Modern Nutrition in Health and Disease I, 8th ed, pp. 231–41. Lea & Febiger, Philadelphia, 1994.

55. Levander OA, Burk RF. Selenium. In: Ziegler EE, Filer LJ Jr, eds, Present Knowledge in Nutrition, pp. 320–8. ILSI, Washington, DC, 1996.

56. Whanger PD, Pedersen ND, Hatfield J, Weswig PH. Absorption of selenite and selenomethionine from ligated digestive tract segments in rats. Proc Soc Exp Bio Med 1976; 153:295–7.

57. Brown DG, Burk RF, Seely RJ, Kiker KW. Effect of dietary selenium on the gastrointestinal absorption of $^{75}SeO_3^{-2}$. Int J Vitam Nutr Res 1972; 42:588–91.

58. Esaki N, Nakamura T, Tanaka H, Soda K. Selenocysteine lyase, a novel enzyme that specifically acts on selenocysteine: mammalian distribution and purification and properties of pig liver enzyme. J Biol Chem 1982; 257:4386–91.

59. Burk RF. Selenium in man. In: Prasad A, ed, Trace Elements in Human Health and Disease, Vol II, pp. 105–33. Academic, New York, 1976.

60. Roveri A, Maiorino M, Nisii C, Ursini F. Purification and characterization of phospholipid hydroperoxide glutathione peroxidase from rat testis mitochondrial membranes. Biochim Biophys Acta 1994; 1208:211–21.

61. Berry MJ, Larsen PR. The role of selenium in thyroid hormone action. Endocrin Rev 1992; 13:207–19.

62. Davey JC, Becker KB, Schneider MJ, St Germain DL, Galton VA. Cloning of a cDNA for the type II iodothyronine deiodinase. J Biol Chem 1995; 270:26,786–9.

63. World Health Organization. Trace Elements in Human Nutrition and Health, pp. 105–22. WHO, Geneva, 1996.

64. Beck MA, Kolbeck PC, Shi Q, Rohr LH, Morris VC, Levander OA. Increased virulence of a human enterovirus (coxsackievirus B3) in selenium-deficient mice. J Infect Dis 1994; 170:351–7.

65. Beck MA, Kolbeck PC, Rohr LH, Shi Q, Morris VC, Levander OA. Benign human enterovirus becomes virulent in selenium-deficient mice. J Med Virol 1994; 43:166–70.

66. Beck MA, Shi Q, Morris VC, Levander OA. Rapid genomic evolution of a non-virulent coxackievirus B3 in selenium-deficient mice results in selection of identical virulent isolates. Nature Med 1995; 1:433–6.

67. Clark LC, Combs GF Jr, Turnbull BW, Slate EH, Chalker DK, Chow J, et al. Effects of selenium supplementation for cancer prevention in patients with carcinoma of the skin. A randomized controlled trial. Nutritional Prevention of Cancer Study Group. JAMA 1996; 276: 1957–63.

68. Yang GQ, Wang S, Zhou R, Sun S. Endemic selenium intoxication of humans in China. Am J Clin Nutr 1983; 37:872–81.

69. Levander OA. Selenium: biochemical actions, interactions, and some human health implications. In: Prasad AS, ed, Clinical, Biochemical, and Nutritional Aspects of Trace Elements, pp. 345–68. Alan R. Liss, New York, 1983.

70. Levander OA. Human selenium nutrition and toxicity. In: Mertz W, Abernathy CO, Olin SS, eds, Risk Assessment of Essential Elements, pp. 147–55. ILSI, Washington, DC, 1994.

71. World Health Organization. International Programme on Chemical Safety: Environmental Health Criteria 58. Selenium. WHO, Geneva, 1987.

72. Thomson CD, Robinson MF. Selenium in human health and disease with emphasis on those aspects peculiar to New Zealand. Am J Clin Nutr 1980; 33:303–23.

73. Thomson CD, Rea HM, Doesburg VM, Robinson MF. Selenium concentrations and glutathione peroxidase activities in whole blood of New Zealand residents. Br J Nutr 1977; 37:457–60.

7 Vitamins

Overview and Metabolic Functions

ROBERT RUCKER

INTRODUCTION

The concept that specific food components play important roles in tissue growth and repair has been evident since the writings of early Egyptian, Greek, and Asian philosophers. For example, nutrition is a topic in the Hippocratic collection; the *Papyrusebers* (written about 1580–1570 B.C.) prescribes beef liver for eye diseases. The concept that vitamins are essential dietary compounds, however, did not evolve with any clarity until the early 1900s. Up to the early 1900s, it was widely held that only the major constituents in the diet (i.e., carbohydrates, protein, fat, and some minerals) were needed for nourishment (1). Nevertheless, the view that small amounts of certain factors seemed necessary for optimal growth and development eventually became apparent. It is now appreciated that vitamin status influences a number of relationships important to metabolic regulation. Consequently, a goal in this chapter is to provide a summary of the functions for each of the compounds now conventionally classified as vitamins or vitamin-like. A perceptive on vitamin requirements will also be developed. To the extent that vitamin status influences the ability to deal with foreign antigens and infections, another goal is to amplify those aspects of vitamin function important to the discussion of acquired, adaptive, and innate immunity that are developed elsewhere throughout this volume.

NOMENCLATURE

As a group of compounds, vitamins have been defined as organic substances present in minute amounts in natural foodstuffs that are essential to normal metabolism, the lack of which causes deficiency diseases. This definition, however, is not specific and could apply to a number of compounds derived from the secondary metabolism of amino acids, simple sugars, and fatty acids. Vitamins may also be classified according to their chemical and physical properties (i.e., whether they are soluble in aqueous solutions or lipid solvents). The varied functions of vitamins, however, complicate the development of a simple system for nomenclature. The chemical structures for many of the vitamins were also poorly understood initially; thus, a system of letter designations was

developed as a method of simple categorization based on physiologic function (2). This system became less useful when it was discovered that some of the functions originally ascribed to vitamins were due to other substances, such as the essential amino acids. The lack of chemical composition data also resulted in a complex system of expressing dosages as arbitrarily defined units, in which a unit was defined in relationship to a biological phenomenon or response in a given animal model. Table 1 summarizes some of the common designations for the vitamins.

GENERAL FEATURES OF VITAMIN METABOLISM AND UTILIZATION

The vitamins that are soluble in lipid solvents are absorbed and transported by conventional lipid-transport processes (3; Fig. 1). For water-soluble vitamins, their respective aqueous solubility coefficients, in part, dictate relative absorption. Within normal, physiological ranges of intakes, active transport and receptor-mediated processes are utilized for water-soluble vitamin absorption (4,5). At higher concentrations (5–10 times the physiological need) passive and pericellular processes may also be involved. Most vitamins are absorbed in the upper intestine. Notable exceptions are folic acid and vitamin B_{12}. Folacin or folate (the family of folic acid derivatives) is absorbed through the mid-intestine; vitamin B_{12} is absorbed primarily in the ileum (6).

A general appreciation for the diversity and complexity of vitamin metabolism and processing is important. Vitamins in foods are often present as cofactors or chemically complex forms. Pancreatic and intestinal cell-derived enzymes are required to initiate normal uptake and absorption. Nucleosidases, phosphatases, and peptidases are key factors in processing cofactors to vitamins (Fig. 2). Once absorbed, most vitamins are processed and modified chemically in the liver for eventual delivery to given target cells and tissues. Table 2 indicates specific proteins known to be involved in vitamin transport. Such proteins serve a number of important functions; for example, delivery to specific cellular sites, protection from unwanted interactions and side reactions, and refinements in overall regulation.

FAT-SOLUBLE VITAMINS

VITAMIN A Descriptions of vitamin A-related deficiency occur throughout written history (2). From a modern perspective, the

From: *Nutrition and Immunology: Principles and Practice* (ME Gershwin et al. eds.), © Humana Press, Inc., Totowa, NJ

Table 1
The Vitamins

Vitamin	Trivial and IUPAC Designations[a]	Adult daily need (per 1000 kcal or 4180 kJ) or RDA[b]	Sources
Vitamin A	Antixerophthalmic factor, retinol, metinol, axerophthol	0.3–0.4 mg as retinol; 300–400 as retinol equivalents (RE), where one RE = 1 μg of retinol; 1000–1300 international units (IU), where 1 IU = 0.3 μg of retinol; current RDA: 1000 μg/d (males) or 800 μg/d (females) as RE	Plant carotinoids; palm oil, many germ oils, tubers, legumes, maize, pigmented fruits, peppers, vegetables; most organ meats, particularly liver, and marine fish
Vitamin D	Ergocalciferol or D_2 derived from plant sources; cholecalciferol or D_3 derived from 7-dehydro-cholesterol; rachitic factor, calciol (D_3)[4], ercalciol (D_2)	Adults 1 μg to infants/children 2–4 μg as vitamin D_3; 400–1600 IU where 1 IU = 0.025 μg as vitamin D_2 or D_3	Animal products, edible skins (poultry), fish oils
Vitamin E	Various isomers of tocopherols, the most potent of which is R,R,R-α-tocopherol (formally d-α-tocopherol) or all-rac-α-tocopherol	2–4 mg as R,R,R-α-tocopherol, 1 international unit = 1 mg of R,R,R-α-tocopherol acetate; current RDA: 10 mg/d (males) or 8 mg/d (females)	Various plant oils
Vitamin K	K_2 from micro-organisms: menaquinone (MK), phylloquinones (from plants); antihemorrhagic factor, K_3 is menadione, a synthetic precursor of vitamin K	50–150 μg as MK[c]; current RDA: 80 μg/d (males) or 65 μg/d (females)	Green leafy vegetables, certain plant oils (grape seed, olive, soybean)
Ascorbic acid	Vitamin C, antisorbutic or scurvy factor	30–60 mg, current RDA: 60 mg/d	Fruit and vegetable juices, many berries, peppers
Niacin	Antipellagra factor, vitamin B_5	6–12 mg; current RDA: 15 mg/d (males) or 12 mg/d (females)	Organ meats, fish, white grains
Riboflavin	Vitamin B_2, vitamin G	0.5–1.0 mg; current RDA: 1.7 mg/d (males) or 1.3 mg/d (females)	Milk, cheese, organ meats, green vegetables tryptophan-rich protein sources
Thiamin	Vitamin B_2, anti-beri-beri factor	0.3–0.6 mg; current RDA: 1.5 mg/d (males) or 1.1 mg/d (females)	Seeds, nuts, meat, yeast
Vitamin B_6	Now used as the designation for the vitamins: pyridoxine ($-CH_2NH_2$ form), pyridoxylamine ($-CH_2NH_2$ form), and pyridoxal (–CHO).	0.6–1.8 mg; current RDA: 2.0 mg/d (males) or 1.6 mg/d (females)	Organ meats, muscle, eggs, cereals
Pantothenic acid	Antidermatitis factor	2–4 mg	Meats, cereals, and most vegetables, yeast
Biotin	Vitamin H	75–250 μg	Dairy products, egg yolk, grains, oil seed meals, molasses
Folate (pteroylglutamate) and folic acid/ pteroylglutamic acid)	Folacin, folate polymers; pteroates (PteGlu, $PteGlu_2$, $PteGlu_3$, etc.)	Current RDA: 200 μg/d (males) or 180 μg/d (females)	Green vegetables, organ meats, eggs cheese, yeast
Vitamin B_{12}	Designation for various forms of the cobalamines	300–1000 ng; current RDA: 2000 ng/d	Animal products, milk, eggs, fish and seafood (clams and oysters)

[a]International Union of Pure and Applied Chemistry.
[b]Recommended Daily Allowances, if established.
[c]Based on the amount that optimizes osteocalcin carboxylation based on the most recent information from balance studies.

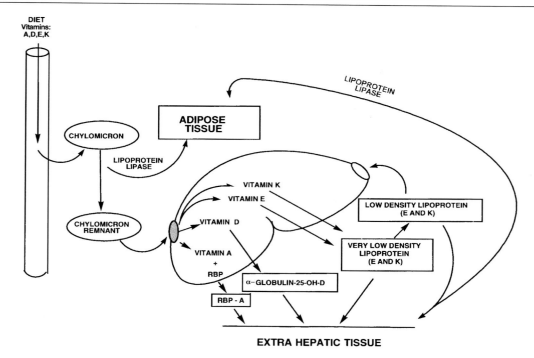

Fig. 1. Fat-soluble-vitamin absorption. Fat-soluble vitamins (A, E, K, and D) are absorbed into and transported from intestinal cells by processes important to the absorption and transport of lipids in general. For vitamin A, the oxidation of β-carotene to retinal (*see* Fig. 4) and the esterification and re-esterification of retinol (*see* Fig. 4) are specific features. From the liver, vitamin A is transported to extrahepatic tissues bound to retinal-binding protein (RBP). Vitamins E and K are transported by low-density and very-low-density lipoprotein particles. The levels of vitamins E and K are influenced by factors that also influence the assembly and metabolism of low-density and very-low-density lipoprotein particles. Vitamin D and its metabolites are transported by proteins designed for secosteroid transport. Receptors for the chylomicron remnant is depicted by the shaded oval and the low-density lipoprotein receptor is depicted by the open circle.

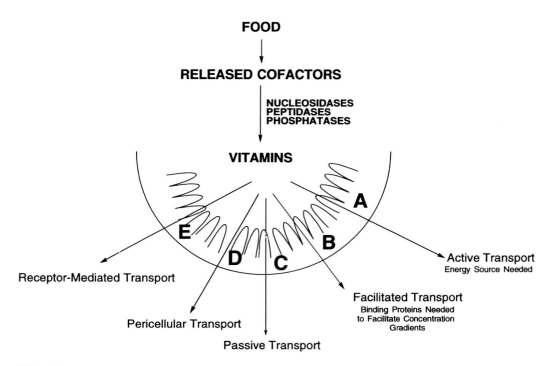

Fig. 2. Water-soluble-vitamin absorption. The processing of water-soluble vitamins as cofactors in food requires, first, the action of pancreatic and intestinal enzymes (e.g., nucleosidases, phosphatases, and specific peptidases) and active or facilitative processes (**A** or **B**). At high concentrations, the absorption of many vitamins is passive (**C**) or can occur by pericellular diffusion (**D**). The uptake of vitamins from the luminal surface may be facilitative, whereas active transport is often involved in delivery of given vitamins into circulation from the serosal membrane. The liver is the next major step in water-soluble vitamin processing. In the liver, given vitamins are modified (e.g., converted into cofactors), directed to a specific liver-derived transport protein for eventual delivery to a target cell or tissue, degraded, or shunted into bile.

Table 2
Vitamins for Which Plasma Transport Proteins Have Been Characterized

Vitamin	Transport proteins in plasma
Vitamin A	Retinol-binding protein
Retinyl esters	Very low-density lipoprotein
Vitamin D	Vitamin D-binding protein (member of the globulin family of proteins)
Vitamin E	Low-density lipoprotein
Vitamin K	Very low-density lipoprotein
Riboflavin	Riboflavin-binding protein
Vitamin B_6	Albumin
Folate	Folate-binding protein
Vitamin B_{12}	A family of transcobalmins (I, II, and III); transcobalmin II predominates

observations by Hopkins, Stepp, and others that a growth-stimulating factor could be extracted from milk into lipid solvents eventually led to the identification of vitamin A *(7)*. Vitamin A was next identified as being present in egg yolk, butter, and cod liver oil. In nature, compounds with vitamin A are largely present as retinyl esters in animal tissues and as carotenoids, the provitamin form vitamin A in plants (Fig. 3).

Over 600 carotenoids have been isolated; however, only about 50 appear to have some degree of provitamin A activity *(8)*. In plants and prokaryotes, carotenoids serve as mediators of photoenergy-related processes. Carotenoids can also quench singlet oxygen and act as weak antioxidants. In plants, carotenoids occur in association with chloroplasts, complexed with protein and other lipids which can decrease their availability *(9)*. General features of vitamin A metabolism are given in Fig. 4. Once inside targeted cells, vitamin A, as retinol, interacts with cellular binding proteins that function to control its subsequent metabolism (e.g., oxidation to retinal or to retinoic acid). Some cellular binding proteins are also a part of the superfamily of glucocorticoid–retinoid–thyroxine transcriptional factors. It is the role of such proteins in the transcription and regulation of specific genes that makes vitamin A and retinoic acid important to many facets of cellular regulation *(8)*.

Metabolism of retinoids in liver cells proceeds by two pathways. The principal pathway is cystolic and involves one or more of the alcohol dehydrogenase isozymes. The other pathway involves microsomal (smooth endoplasmic reticulum) enzymes that are inducible by dietary excesses (e.g., chronic and acute alcohol consumption or drugs); for example, high doses of phenobarbital or ethanol can cause depletion of liver retinol by the induction of microsomal enzymes *(10)*.

The major functions of vitamin A are in vision, cell differentiation, and tissue growth *(8,11)*. With respect to vision, only a small

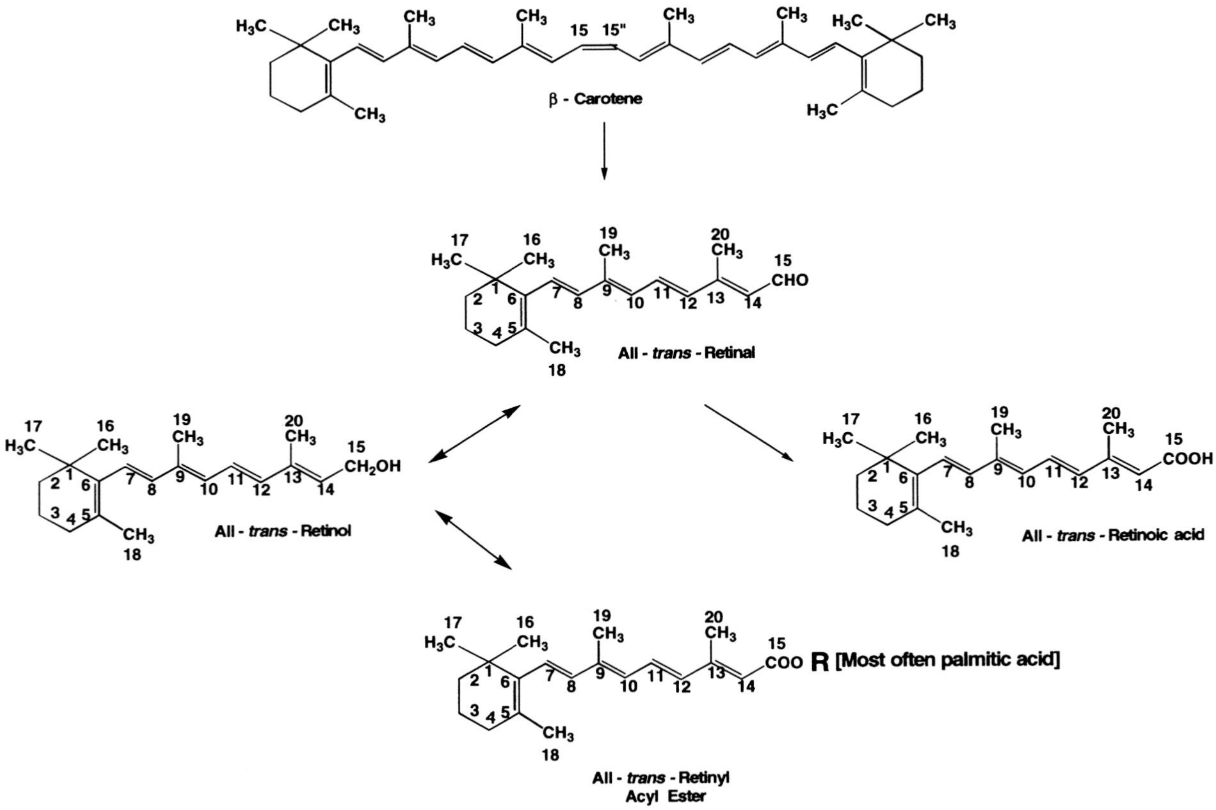

Fig. 3. Vitamin A derivatives and β-carotene. The structures for all-*trans*-retinol, retinal, retinyl acyl ester, and retinoic acid are shown. The interconversions occur in all cells. Oxidation of retinal to retinoic acids is not reversible. β-Carotene is the most potent vitamin A precursor. For vitamin A activity, the presence of the β-ionone ring structure is essential. For structures similar to β-carotene oxidation at the 15, 15′ position is a requirement to eventually generate a molecule of vitamin A. Retinyl esters are found in animal products. The carotinoids are common plant pigments.

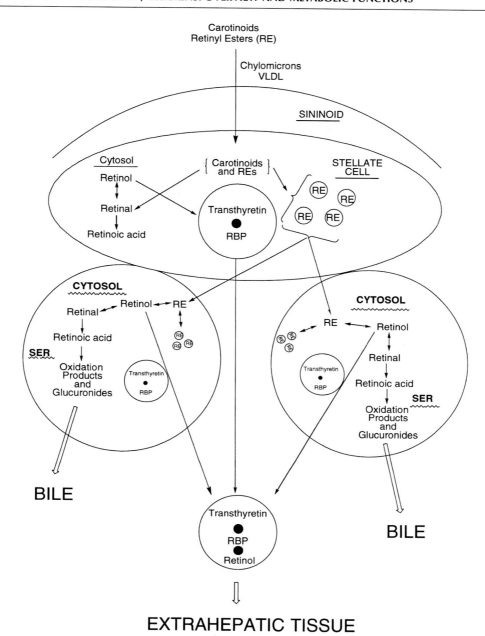

Fig. 4. Major steps in vitamin A metabolism. Carotenoids, retinoids, and retinyl esters associated with chylomicra and intestinal very low-density lipoprotein particles are transported to the liver sininoids via the lymphatic system. These compounds are transported first into liver stellate cells. Liver stellate cells communicate with adjacent liver parenchymal cells. Each of these cells produces retinol-binding protein (RBP), which facilitates the transport of retinol into secretory pathways that allow the delivery of retinol into blood and to extrahepatic tissue. Excess retinol in cells is stored as retinyl ester (RE). Excess retinol is also oxidized by dehydrogenases in the cytosol as well as by microsomal oxidases associated with the smooth endoplasmic reticulum (SER). The SER oxidase system results in a variety of oxidation products as well as retinyl glucuronides. Some of these products are delivered via bile into the intestine. In given target cells, specific retinoids act as important signaling and regulatory agents in the transcription of specific genes.

fraction of the total vitamin A requirement is involved in this process. In vision, vitamin A, as a component of rhodopsin, facilitates the efficient transfer of energy from photons of light to electrochemical signals (Fig. 5).

Regarding vitamin A's importance to growth, a key feature is the role of the vitamin A metabolites, retinoic acid, in the maintenance and differentiation of epithelial cells. Vitamin A deficiency causes abnormal differentiation of epithelial cells to squamous,

keratin-enriched cells *(12)*. In response to very low doses of retinoids, epithelial cells undergo "terminal differentiation." Retinoids and associated transcription factors control the expression of various proteins important to mucus formation and cytoskeletal integrity (e.g., keratin and transglutaminase) and the rate of cell cycling. In response to reduced levels of retinoids, vitamin A, and retinoic acids, epithelial cells lose their normal columnar shape, become flattened or squamous, and increase their cytosolic content of

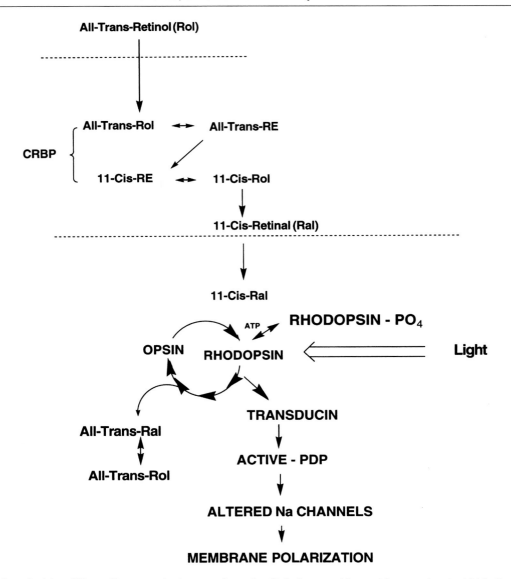

Fig. 5. Vitamin A and vision. When all-*trans*-retinol enters the rod cell, it first combines with cytosol retinoid-binding protein (CRBP). Retinol and the all-*trans*-retinyl ester are capable of isomerization. Reactions involving all-*trans*-retinol and retinyl esters occur by pathways that utilize CRBP–retinoid complexes as substrates. Retinol is oxidized to retinal. *Cis*-retinal reacts with opsin to form rhodopsin. The multiple arrows from rhodopsin back to opsin are meant to represent conformational changes in rhodopsin that occur upon light stimulation. Activated rhodopsin interacts with transducin, which, in turn, activates phosphodiesterase, which eventually causes a decrease in cGMP levels. This sequence of reactions causes an alteration in sodium channels and alters membrane polarization to activate optic-nerve signal propagation. With incremental decreases in active rhodopsin, there is the need for an increasing intensity of light to activate nerve signal propagation.

keratin (stabilized by transglutaminase catalyzed cross-links). In the dermis, this process can normally result in a protective outer layer. However, in locations in which the primary function of the epithelial cell is to provide a moist surface or to function in the process of absorption, squamization and overkeratinization leads to loss of functional integrity. The normal expression of phagocytic cells associated with the immune response (e.g., the production of normal differentiation of the B cells and T cells) is also responsive to changes in vitamin A status *(13)*.

The requirement for vitamin A depends on age, sex, rate of growth, and reproductive status. The current Recommended Dietary Allowance for vitamin A is given in Table 1. Pathological conditions that influence vitamin A status include malabsorption, pancreatic insufficiency, cholestatic disease, cystic fibrosis, liver disease, and kidney disease. Many forms of liver disease also interfere with the production or release of retinal-binding protein, which results in a lower plasma level of vitamin A. Renal failure can result in the loss of retinal-binding protein in urine. Vitamin A toxicity is also a concern *(14)*. In high concentrations, vitamin A and its pharmacological analogs are teratogenic.

VITAMIN D   The D vitamins are 9,10 secosteroids. Their various designations are given in Table 1. Under most instances, humans can synthesize sufficient quantities of vitamin D_3 if they receive adequate exposure to ultraviolet light (280–320 nm). As vitamin D_3 is produced at one site (skin) and acts at other sites, including bone and intestine, it fulfills the definition of a prohormone *(15)*.

Initially, it was assumed that vitamin D was a cofactor for

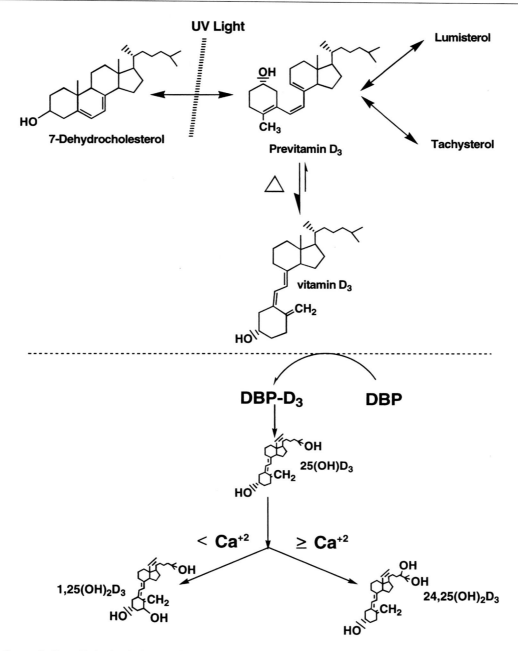

Fig. 6. Vitamin D metabolism. Dehydrocholesterol in skin can be converted to pre-vitamin D by the action of ultraviolet light. At body temperature, pre-vitamin D is spontaneously converted to vitamin D_3 (also known as cholecalciferol or calcitriol). Related derivatives (e.g., lumisterol and tachysterol) are also formed. Vitamin D-binding protein (DBP) aids in the transport of vitamin D from skin to the liver, where vitamin D is converted to 25-hydroxy-vitamin D_3. Next, calcitriol or 1,25-dihydroxycholecalciferol production occurs primarily in the kidney, although recent evidence suggests calcitriol production can also occur in macrophages, placenta, and intestine. In an eucalcemic or hypercalcemic state, 24,25-dihydroxycholecalciferol (24R-hydroxycalcidiol) production is the primary product. The primary function of 1,25-dihydroxychole-calciferol (calcitriol) is in regulation of intestinal calcium absorption, although newer evidence also suggests a broader range of functions. Calcitriol receptors are present in most cells involved in optimal immune function.

reactions that served to maintain calcium and phosphorus (a phosphate). When isotopes of calcium became available, it was soon appreciated that there was a time lag between the administration of vitamin D and its effect on calcium-related metabolism. This lag was shown to result from the conversion of vitamin D_3 to active forms of the vitamin *(16)*. The sequence of events is outlined in Fig. 6 *(17)*. The kidney is the major site of 1,25 dihydroxychole-calciferol (calcitriol, 1,25-$(OH)_2$-D_3 production. Other organs, such

the placenta, bone, and macrophages are also capable of synthesis in vitamin D_3 small quantities. This discovery together with the finding that 1,25-$(OH)_2$-D_3 is found in the nuclei of intestinal cells suggested that vitamin D_3 functions mechanistically analogous to steroid hormones *(18)*. The production of 1,25-dihydroxychole-calciferol is normally regulated through feedback control by the action of 1,25-dihydroxycholecalciferol and/or parathyroid hormone [PTH *(18,19)*]. A fall in plasma calcium also triggers the release of PTH from the parathyroid gland. These events reduce plasma calcium (specifically ionizable calcium) and/or PTH stimulates the production and activation the 1 α-hydroxylase that catalyzes formation of 1,25-(OH)$_2$-D$_3$. A separate hydroxylase, 25-hydroxyvitamin D$_3$-24-hydroxylase, which catalyzes 24,25-(OH)$_2$-D$_3$ formation, is activated under eucalcemic and hypercalcemic states. Whether 24,25-(OH)$_2$-D$_3$ has unique hormonal activity is controversial. There is evidence that 24,25-(OH)$_2$-D$_3$ is required for some of the biological responses attributed to vitamin D *(19)*.

Vitamin D receptors have been found in a large number of cell types, ranging from skeletal muscle cells to cells important to immune and phagocytic functions (e.g., macrophages) *(20)*. In pancreatic beta calls, 1,25-(OH)$_2$-D$_3$ has also been observed to be important to normal insulin secretion. Vitamin D increases insulin release from isolated perfused pancreatic cells. Moreover, vitamin D metabolites can suppress immunoglobulin production by activated lymphocytes. T Cells are also affected by vitamin D metabolites. 1,25-(OH)$_2$-D$_3$ exhibits permissive or enhancing effects on T-cell suppressor activity *(19)*.

Humans require 5 μg or less of vitamin D$_3$ per 1000 kcal of diet. When intake exceeds 5–10 times this amount, there is a risk of toxicity, characterized by hypercalcemia and eventual calcification of soft tissues—in particular, blood vessels of the lung, kidney, and heart. Acute doses of vitamin D (20 times the requirements) can eventually result in a negative calcium balance, because bone resorption is accelerated *(19)*.

VITAMIN E   Vitamin E plays an important role in defending cell membranes from oxidants. In the diet, vitamin E comes primarily from plant seed oils. The most active form of vitamin E is RRR-α-tocopherol. In cell membranes, vitamin E functions to block free-radical-mediated chain reactions and peroxide radical formation (Fig. 7).

The identification of vitamin E as an essential dietary factor evolved from studies that were carried out in the early 1920s, when rats fed diets composed of rancid lard failed to reproduce. When whole wheat was added to diets containing rancid fat, reproduction was improved. Thus, a bioassay was conceived that allowed testing for a unique factor not previously ascribed to the known nutritional factors. Once the connection to compounds with the properties of tocopherols was made, progress regarding the role of vitamin E was rapid. Vitamin E deprivation can cause degeneration of tissues rich in unsaturated lipids. It is now generally accepted that the primary role of vitamin E in such processes is related to its ability to act as an antioxidant *(21)*.

Vitamin E is used as the generic term for all of the forms that exhibit functional activity in biological or chemical tests of antioxidation. RRR-α-tocopherol is possibly the most biologically active of the tocopherols. This form of vitamin E is found in plant oils, particularly in germ seeds. Synthetic vitamin E is obtained as a mixture of isomeric forms and is designated all-rac-α-tocopherol. Tocopherols are stable to heat and dilute alkali in the absence of oxygen. They are also unaffected by acids at temperatures up to 100°C. Vitamin E is prepared commercially as an ester, which, in part, protects from vitamin E oxidation during storage. Oxidized end products of vitamin E include tocopheryl quinone and various tocopherol polymers.

It is important to underscore that the antioxidant functions of vitamin E can be linked directly to the signs and symptoms associated with vitamin E deficiency. For example, myopathies, signs of muscular dystrophy, defects in capillary permeability, and reproductive failure in experimental animals appear to be associated with peroxidative damage. The signs of peripheral neuropathy in humans is also associated with vitamin E deficiency, particularly in those individuals who suffer from genetic defects that involve defects in low-density lipoprotein (LDL) expression or who suffer from long-term fat malabsorption. Polymorphism in a hepatic protein that is involved in the transfer of the D-form of tocopherol to LDL may also influence vitamin E status *(22)*. Patients who receive their nutrition from a parenteral (intravenous) route may also be susceptible to signs of vitamin E deficiency *(21–22)*.

Tocopherols are transported in plasma in LDL particles. Tocopherols are not easily transported across the placenta into the fetus. As a consequence, infants are often born with relatively low levels of tocopherols, which can cause accelerated cell-membrane damage if the infant is subjected to abnormally high levels of oxidants. One well-characterized sign of such damage is red blood cell fragility. Fragility of red cells can result in hemolytic anemia. The anemia occurs because red cells damaged by oxidation become fragile and lyse upon mechanical stress (e.g., as they are forced through vessels and capillaries). Such lysis causes a release of hemoglobin into circulation, which may result in further tissue damage, because of the subsequent accumulation of iron in given tissues. Other disorders associated with low vitamin E status are retinopathy, bronchopulmonary dysplasia, thromocytosis, and abnormal platelet aggregation. In severe cases of vitamin E deficiency in infants, hypoflexia and ataxia may occur.

The nutritional status of vitamin E is often difficult to assess. Enzymes such as superoxide dismutases, catalase, glutathione peroxidase, and related systems for oxidant defense can moderate the absolute need for vitamin E. Further high dietary intakes of polyunsaturated dietary fats increase the vitamin E requirement, because of their eventual deposition in cell membranes and higher susceptibility to oxidation. In adult humans, signs of vitamin E deficiency are difficult to demonstrate. In part, this relates to the elaborate and redundant system in well-differentiated cells for dealing excesses of oxidants and adult organs. However, data from numerous prospective studies and intervention trials provide compelling arguments that vitamin E supplementation in the 200- to 400-mg/d range may be protective against cardiovascular disease *(23)*.

VITAMIN K   In the 1940s, it became clear that substances synthesized by bacteria and leafy plants possessed what is now recognized as K activity. As this work progressed, information also became available regarding compounds in spoiled clover and certain grasses that caused hemorrhagic disorders in cattle and served as antagonists to vitamin K. With the isolation and identification of vitamin K, an understanding of mechanism of its action evolved, although not without controversy. A number of questions were also raised regarding the structural requirements for vitamin K activity.

The mechanism of action for vitamin K became clear after it was demonstrated that the formation of γ-carboxyglutamic acid (GLA) residues in prothrombin and other proteinases/precursors associated with the blood-clotting cascade was vitamin K dependent *(24)*. The GLA residues serve as calcium-binding sites in the proforms of proteinases associated with blood coagulation. Calcium binding is a requisite for their eventual activation. In this regard, vitamin K serves as cofactor for microsomal carboxylases, which are responsible for GLA formation. The vitamin K-dependent carboxylase utilizes oxygen and bicarbonate as substrates (Fig. 8).

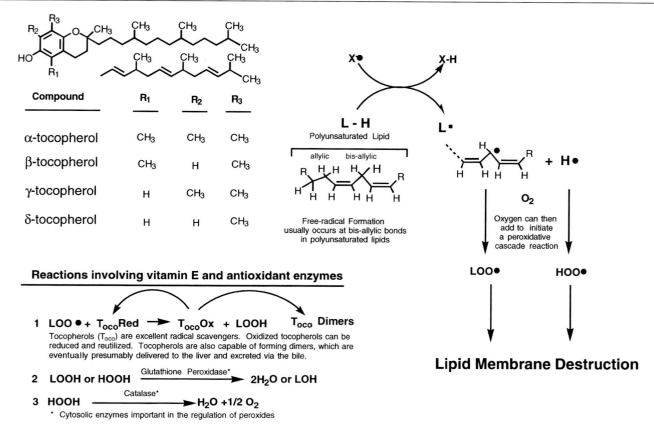

Compound	R_1	R_2	R_3
α-tocopherol	CH_3	CH_3	CH_3
β-tocopherol	CH_3	H	CH_3
γ-tocopherol	H	CH_3	CH_3
δ-tocopherol	H	H	CH_3

Reactions involving vitamin E and antioxidant enzymes

1 LOO• + T_{oco}Red ⟶ T_{oco}Ox + LOOH T_{oco} Dimers

Tocopherols (T_{oco}) are excellent radical scavengers. Oxidized tocopherols can be reduced and reutilized. Tocopherols are also capable of forming dimers, which are eventually presumably delivered to the liver and excreted via the bile.

2 LOOH or HOOH $\xrightarrow{\text{Glutathione Peroxidase*}}$ $2H_2O$ or LOH

3 HOOH $\xrightarrow{\text{Catalase*}}$ $H_2O + 1/2 O_2$

* Cytosolic enzymes important in the regulation of peroxides

Fig. 7. Structure and function of vitamin E. The principle forms of vitamin E, tocopherol and tocotrienol, are depicted. The tocopherols are the most potent antioxidants in biological systems. Vitamin E is particularly important in quenching free radicals that generate from the allelic and bis-allelic unconjugated bonds found in membrane polyunsaturated lipids. Other enzymes important to regulation of oxidants are also depicted.

In addition to prothrombin and proteins associated with blood coagulation. GLA residues are also found in proteins that are involved in the regulation of new bone formation and calcification (e.g., osteocalcins) *(25)*. The presence of GLA-containing proteins in bone helps to explain why administration of vitamin K antagonists at levels that cause hemorrhagic disease also can result in bone defects, particularly in neonates. The mineralization disorders are characterized by complete fusion of the proximal tibia growth plate and cessation of longitudinal bone growth. GLA-containing proteins are also present in lymphocytes.

The establishment of the dietary requirement for vitamin K has been difficult, in part due to its short half-life and the synthesis of vitamin K isomers by intestinal bacteria. Recent assessment of nutritional requirements suggest that small animals should obtain approximately 500–1000 μg as phyllo- or menaquinone/kg diet. Oxidized squalene and high intakes of vitamin E may act as vitamin K antagonists. The human requirement is currently set at approximately 50 μg per day, but recent data based on optimal GLA formation in osteocalcin suggest the daily need may be 300 μg per day or more (i.e., similar on a dry-food basis to the requirement for most animals).

WATER-SOLUBLE VITAMINS

Water-soluble vitamins serve primarily as enzymatic cofactors and cosubstrates (Figs. 9 and 10). For example, niacin, riboflavin, and ascorbic acid serve to facilitate redox reactions *(26)*. The roles of thiamin, pyridoxine (vitamin B₆), and pantothenic acid (as a component of coenzyme A) are distinguished because of their unique roles in carbohydrate metabolism, protein and amino acid metabolism, and acyl and acetyl transport, respectively. Biotin, folic acid, and vitamin B₁₂ (cobalamin) have roles in single-carbon metabolism.

Other vitaminlike compounds include inositol, choline, and carnitine, compounds that are derived from carbohydrate, amino acid, or fatty acid metabolic pathways and perform mainly specialized transport functions or are involved in signal transduction and cell signaling. However, there are "conditional" requirements for such compounds (e.g., during developmental periods where utilization exceeds the synthesis).

ASCORBIC ACID   Ascorbic acid functions primarily as a cofactor for microsomal mono-oxygenases (hydroxylases) and oxidases. In most animals, ascorbic acid is synthesized from glucose in the liver or kidney *(27,28)*. In humans, a deficiency of gulonolactone oxidase, the last step in ascorbic acid synthesis, results in the need for a dietary source. Because of its importance in humans, vitamin C deficiency (scurvy) has often determined the course of history (e.g., outbreaks of scurvy have influenced the outcome of military campaigns and territorial explorations).

Ascorbic acid, a 2,3-enediol-L-gluonic acid, is the most powerful reducing agent available to cells and is of general importance

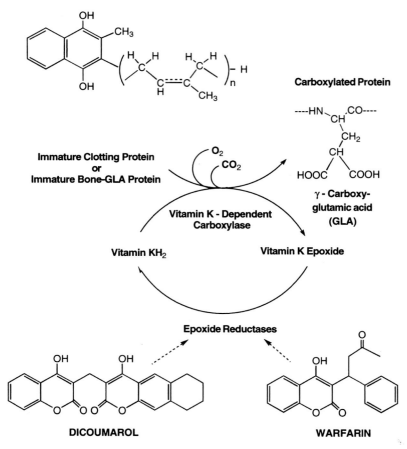

Fig. 8. Structure and function of vitamin K. Vitamin K functions as a cofactor for microsomal carboxylases that act on immature clotting proteins in the liver or immature proteins in metabolically active bone to cause the formation of peptidyl-γ-carboxyglutamyl residues (e.g., prothrombin [important in blood coagulation] and osteocalcin [important in bone mineralization]). During the course of this unusual carboxylation reaction, vitamin K is converted to vitamin K epoxide. The epoxides may be converted back to vitamin K. The site of action of vitamin K antagonists, such as dicoumarol and warfarin, is the reductase regeneration system, which is important to vitamin K regeneration.

as an antioxidant because of its high reducing potential. Both of the hydrogens of the enediol group can dissociate, which results in the strong acidity of ascorbic acid (pK =4.2). Enediols are also excellent reducing agents; the reaction usually occurs in a stepwise fashion with monodehydroascorbic acid, as a semiquinone intermediate *(29)*. This intermediate then disproportionates to ascorbic acid and dehydroascorbic acid. Dehydroascorbic acid is not as hydrophilic as ascorbic acid, as it exists in a deproteinated form. As such, this form of ascorbic acid can move easily across cell membranes. The dehydro form, however, is easily cleaved by alkali (e.g., to oxalic acid and threonic acid) and oxidized *(29)*.

Dietary ascorbic acid is absorbed from the duodenum and proximal jejunum. Measurable amounts can also cross the membranes of the mouth and gastric mucosa. Studies indicate that within the normal ranges of intake (50–200 mg/d), 80–90% of the vitamin may be absorbed.

In tissues, the highest concentration of ascorbic acid is found in the adrenal and pituitary glands, followed by the liver, thymus, brain, and pancreas. Cellular uptake of ascorbic acid occurs by both active and simple diffusion processes. In diabetes, the ascorbic acid content of tissue is often depressed, which suggests elevated glucose, and factors responding to hyperglycemic states can compromise ascorbic acid uptake and status *(30)*.

Ascorbic acid is maintained in cells by several mechanisms.

Ascorbate reductases maintain L-ascorbic acid in the reduced form, which prevents leakage from the cells as dehydroascorbic acid. Ascorbic acid may also be converted to the 2-sulfate derivative. In rats, about 5% of a labeled dose of ascorbic acid is recovered in urine as 2-0-methyl ascorbic acid. The ability to modify ascorbic acid as the 2-sulfate or 2-0-methyl derivative as well as to easily degrade an excess of ascorbic acid is a way for cells to compartmentalize or modulate functional ascorbic acid levels. In the neonate, maintenance of relatively high gluthathione levels is also important for ascorbate recycling and regeneration.

Ascorbic acid also been suggested to play a number of regulatory roles. Ascorbic acid influences histamine metabolism in some animals, particularly humans. There is an inverse correlation between ascorbic acid levels and serum histamine levels *(31)*.

As a cellular reducing agent, ascorbic acid serves as a cofactor for mixed-function oxidations that result in the incorporation of molecular oxygen into various substrates *(32)*. Most of the enzymes involved in these processes are metal-requiring enzymes, in which the role of ascorbic acid is to maintain the metal (usually Cu or Fe) in a reduced state. Examples include prolyl hydroxylase, lysyl hydroxylase, dopamine hydroxylase, and various steroid hydroxylases.

Furthermore, steps in the transcriptional regulation of certain proteins, such as the fibrillar collagens, also appear to be influenced

Water Soluble Vitamins and Cofactors

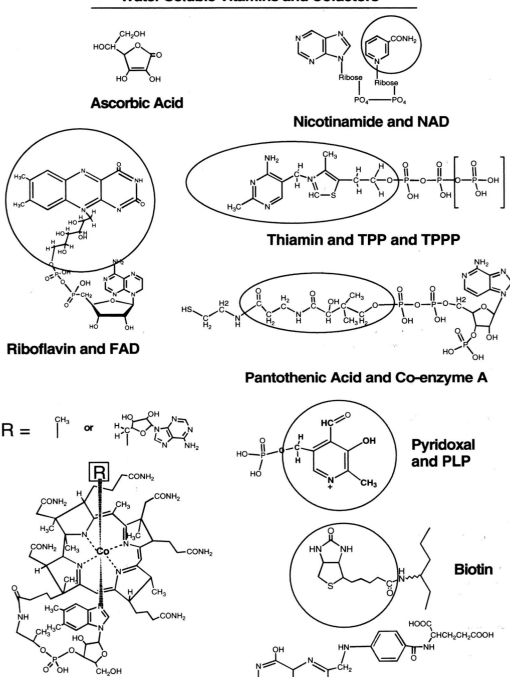

Fig. 9. The water-soluble vitamins and selected corresponding cofactors. The structure of the vitamin moiety is shown within the circle. NAD = nicotinamide adenine dinucleotide; TPP = thiamin pyrophosphate; TPPP = thiamin triphosphate; FAD = flavin adenine dinucleotide; PLP = pyridoxal-5'-phosphate.

by the presence or absence of strong reducing agents, such as ascorbic acid *(32)*.

In humans, impaired collagen synthesis is a principle feature of ascorbate deficiency; signs include capillary fragility, bleeding gums, delayed wound healing, and impaired bone formation. Connective tissue lesions are primarily a result of underhydroxylated collagen (at specific prolyl and lysyl residues) being abnormally susceptible to degradation. In addition, the inability to deal with metabolic stress requiring normal adrenal gland function and the reduced ability to metabolize fatty acids, possibly the result of impaired carnitine synthesis, contribute to signs of scurvy. Ascorbic acid is also essential to phagocytic cell oxidative burst

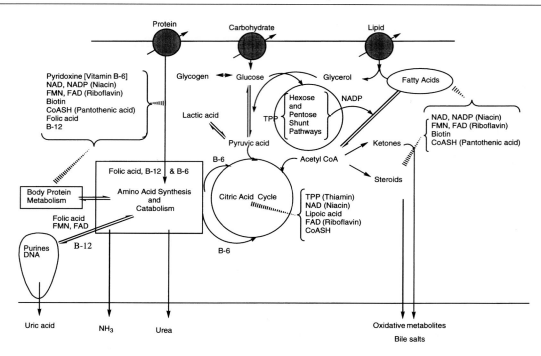

Fig. 10. Vitamins in cellular metabolism. The products of protein, carbohydrate, and lipid metabolism enter cellular compartments in a highly regulated fashion (●). Note that pyridoxine and vitamins involved in single carbon metabolism and transfers are particularly important to amino acid metabolism. Carbohydrate metabolism has specific requirements for thiamin, pantothenic acid, niacin, and riboflavin. Similarly, lipid metabolism has specific requirements for thiamin, pantothenic acid, niacin, and riboflavin, as well as biotin. Also note that NADP is generated from the hexose monophosphate shunt pathway. NADP in its reduced form is required for synthetic pathways (e.g., fatty acid synthesis).

activity and to lymphocyte B- and T-cell functions (13). Ascorbic acid acts as a primary reductant to maintain iron in a reduced state to facilitate Fenton reactions, $H_2O_2 \rightarrow OH + OH$, important to the eventual generation of hypochlorite (OCl) and hydroxyl free-radical formation important to phagocytic and chemical destruction of foreign material.

Animals that generate their own ascorbic acid make from 20 to 60 mg of ascorbic acid per 1000 kcal utilized during the course of normal metabolism. As might be expected, the ascorbic acid requirement for humans also ranges from 20 to 60 mg/1000 kcal of energy utilized (see the section Perspectives on Vitamin Assessment and Related Needs).

When consumed in gram amounts per day, ascorbic acid can result in gastrointestinal distress and bleeding. Also, tissue levels of ascorbic acid are homeostatically maintained. Homeostasis occurs by the induction of ascorbic acid decarboxylases and cleavage enzymes that catalyze the degradation of ascorbic acid to CO_2 plus ribulose, or oxalic acid plus threonic acid. These conversions protect cells against ascorbic excesses and nonspecific or unwanted Fenton-type reactions.

THE B VITAMINS: NIACIN, RIBOFLAVIN, VITAMIN B6, THIAMIN, PANTOTHENIC ACID, BIOTIN, FOLACIN, AND COBALAMIN

The B vitamins provide a diverse set of cofactor functions. Figure 10 provides an overview of those functions key to energy regulation. A description of pyruvate decarboxylation and acetyl-CoA's entry into the citric acid cycle is described in Fig. 11 as a way of highlighting attributes that are important to given cofactor functions.

NIACIN Niacin is the vitamin moiety of the nicotinamide adenine dinucleotide cofactors: NAD and NADP. Through the

elegant work Goldberger and others, the nutritional deficiency disease pellagra was linked to a dietary deficiency of niacin and decreased NAD formation. Throughout the 18th and 19th centuries, pellagra was prevalent in Western Europe and the southern region of the United States. Pellagra is associated with the consumption of corn (maize). Niacin deficiency occurs when available niacin and the amino acid, tryptophan, are limiting. Tryptophan is important to niacin status, because niacin is generated upon tryptophan degradation (Fig. 12). NAD and NADP both contain an unsubstituted pyridine 3-carboxamide that is essential to redox reactions with a chemical potential near −0.32 V. Virtually all cells are capable of converting niacin to NAD. Most enzymes that require NAD are oxidoreductases (dehydrogenases) that aid in the catalysis of a diverse array of reactions, such as the conversion of alcohols and polyols to aldehydes or ketones. The most common mechanism involves the stereospecific abstraction of a hydride ion (H:) from the substrate with its subsequent transfer. It is of interest that cells generally delegate NAD to enzymes in catabolic pathways, whereas NADP is utilized in synthetic pathways (33–34).

An additional and equally important function of NAD is its role as a substrate in monoribosylation and polyribosylation reactions (35) and in the generation of cyclic ADP. Cyclic ADP, similar to inositol 1,4,5-triphosphate is an important secondary messenger in intracellular calcium mobilization (36). Monoribosylation and polyribosylation are important to a broad array of cellular regulatory functions. Enzymes that undergo monoribosylation can become activated or deactivated upon addition of ADP-ribose. Somewhat analogous to phosphorylation, ribosylation represents another example of covalent modification as a regulatory control. In the nuclei of cells, polyribosylation of histones precedes the normal process of DNA repair. This later phenomenon may be important

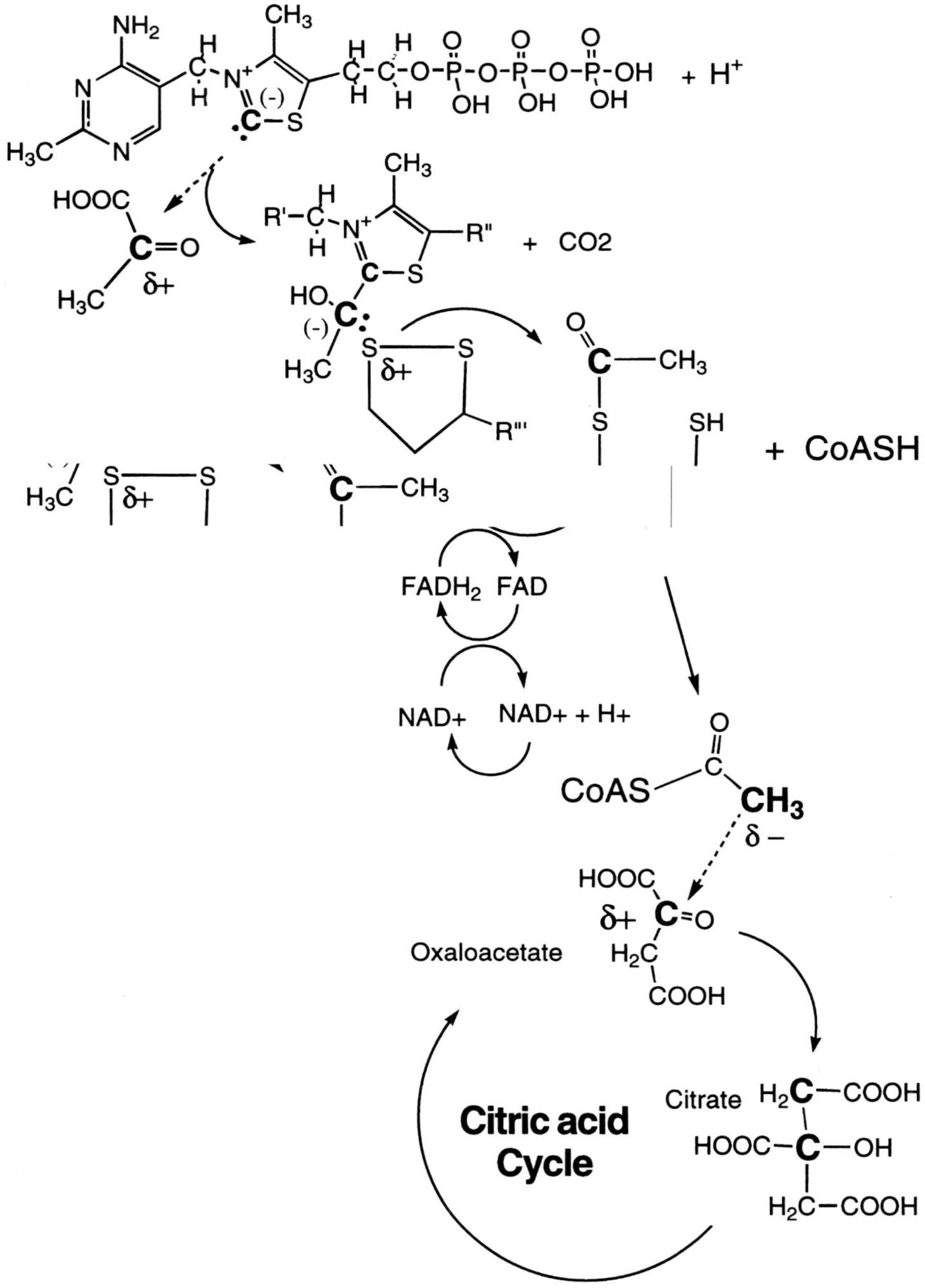

Fig. 11. Mechanistic features of vitamin action: Selected example—Thiamin and pyruvic acid decarboxylation. The first step in the citric acid cycle (the decarboxylation of pyruvate and generation of acetyl CoA) illustrates a major strategy that is important to biochemical transformations involving vitamin-derived cofactors. Focus on the carbon atoms in bold. To facilitate decarboxylation, the carbon adjacent to the carboxyl group must acquire carbanion character, which can be catalyzed by the interaction of pyruvate with thiamin pyrophosphate (TPP) as a part of pyruvate decarboxylase. A principle function of TPP is stabilization of carbanion intermediates. The thiazole ring of thiamin maintains negative ion character. The arrangement of atoms, N^+=CH–S, known as a ylid, causes the carbon in bold to take on a considerable anion (negative ion) character. Carbanions have a negative character and are prime targets for electrophilic substitutions. In this regard, oxidized lipoic acid is designed to engage in an electrophilic substitutions. The resulting thiol ester is not stabilized by resonance; accordingly, it may be viewed as a "high-energy" intermediate. Thus, the transfer of acetate from coenzyme A can be accomplished without an energy source, such as ATP. Riboflavin- and niacin-derived cofactors are also important. Electrons to and from lipoic acid go from NADH + H^+ through FADH. Flavin cofactors are well suited chemically to carry out oxidations and reductions, one electron and one proton at a time. Oxidation of electronegative atoms with the chemical characteristics of sulfur or oxygen prefer to undergo redox in a stepwise manner, where one-electron transfers are a principle feature. In the second step of the sequence, the reaction is again staged because the α-carbon of oxaloacetate has positive or carbonion ion character. The β-carbon of acetyl CoA takes on a negative ion character because of the lack of resonance stabilization of thiol esters. This facilitates an addition that results in citrate formation. At each step the character of cofactors and the active sites of associated enzymes elicit catalytic reactions by providing properties that optimize given electrophilic and nucleophilic substitutions reactions.

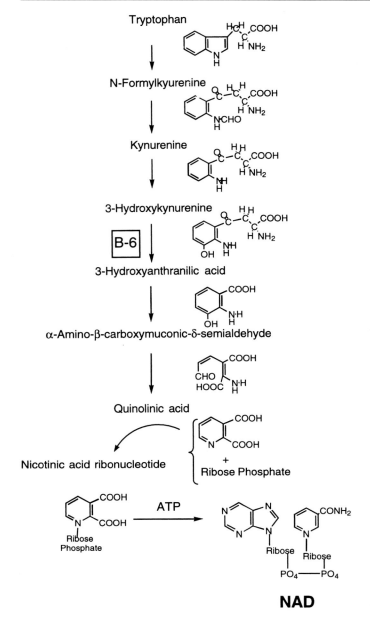

Fig. 12. The niacin and tryptophan relationship. NAD can be derived from tryptophan through the quinolinate pathway. A diet containing 250–500 mg of tryptophan (easily derived from consuming 50–80 g of high-quality protein) produces the equivalent of 3–8 mg of niacin.

to pellagra-related lesions of skin following exposure to ultraviolet (UV) light. UV exposure results in the dark pigmented lesions associated with pellagra when there is a lack of niacin and, therefore, NAD *(35)*. It is this nonredox function of NAD that accounts for the rapid turnover of NAD in cells. Some estimates suggest that as much as 40–60% of the NAD in cells is involved in monoribosylation or polyribosylation reactions *(37)*.

Niacin is needed in amounts corresponding to 3–6 mg/1000 kcal of diet. The conversion of tryptophan to niacin is about 1 mg of niacin for very 50–70 mg of tryptophan degraded. Niacin (nicotinamide) is relatively nontoxic, although nicotinic acid can cause vasodilatation when consumed in excess of 100 mg. Conse-

quently, there are a number of therapeutic uses for pharmacological doses of niacin-derived compounds when increased blood flow is desirable.

RIBOFLAVIN Riboflavin was one of the first of the B vitamins identified (*see* Fig. 9). Originally, it was thought to be the heat-stable factor responsible for the prevention of pellagra. Riboflavin is present in tissue and cells as FAD (flavin adenine dinucleotide) and FMN (flavin mononucleotide). FAD and FMN are cofactors in aerobic processes, usually as cofactors for oxidases, although FAD also can function in anaerobic environments as a dehydrogenase cofactor *(26)*. Many flavin-containing proteins are found in the smooth endoplasmic reticulum of cells (i.e., as microsomal enzymes).

Riboflavin deficiency is uncommon, but it can occur when high doses of certain antibiotics are prescribed. For example, imipramine, chlorpromazine, and amitriptyline interfere with riboflavin processing and binding to transport proteins. Glossitis and cheilosis are signs of B-vitamin deficiency, which occur when a poor diet and antibiotics are factors *(38)*.

THIAMIN Thiamin in cells occurs either as the pyrophosphate (TPP) or the triphosphate (TPPP). There are two general types of reactions, wherein TPP functions as a magnesium-coordinated coenzyme for active aldehyde transfer reactions *(39)*. One example is the decarboxylation of α-keto acids (Figs. 9 and 10). Decarboxylation of α-keto acids occurs twice in the TCA cycle (Figure 10); the conversion of pyruvate to acetyl-CoA and α-ketoglutarate to succinyl CoA. The other reaction of TPP is the transformation of "ketols" (ketose phosphates) in the pentose phosphate pathway, designated as a transketolase reaction. In this pathway, NADP is reduced to NADPH. As noted in the section Niacin, NADPH is an essential reducing agent for synthetic reactions.

Thiamin triphosphate predominates in neural tissue and in brain *(40)*. In the brain, TPPP is proposed to be involved in sodium regulation (i.e. the flux of sodium ions across neuronal cell membranes).

Thiamin status should be routinely considered in disease assessment, because a number of factors influence thiamin availability and may induce a deficiency. Thiamin is heat and alkali labile. Extensive destruction of thiamin can occur in the various steps of food processing and preservation. Tannins in tea and other brewed beverages can cause thiamin to polymerize, which results in decreased thiamin absorption. Alcohol also interferes with thiamin utilization. Thiamin can be destroyed enzymatically by thiaminases, whose levels are measurable in raw fish and certain fermented sauces.

Thiamin deficiency is characterized by cardiac myopathies, neurologic deficits, wasting, and mental distortions (e.g., confabulations). Thiamin-deficiency disease is known as beri-beri. This disease still occurs in "rice-eating" cultures (rice is low in thiamin), wherein tea, raw fish, and fermented sauces are also consumed. The mental disturbances associated with alcohol-induced thiamin deficiency are often classified under the heading of a collection of physiological and psychological syndromes [e.g., Wernicke and Korsakoff *(40)*].

PYRIDOXINE Vitamin B$_6$ is a collective term for pyridoxine, pyridoxal, and pyridoxamine (Fig. 9). Pyridoxine is most abundant in plants, and pyridoxal and pyridoxamine are most abundant in animals tissues *(41)*. Each of these compounds can be interconverted. The active form of pyridoxal is phosphorylated at the 5′

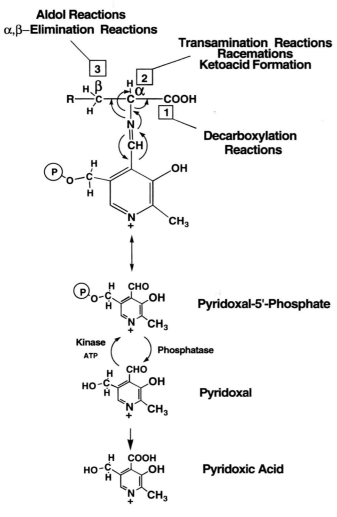

Aldol Reactions
α,β–Elimination Reactions

Transamination Reactions
Racemations
Ketoacid Formation

Decarboxylation Reactions

Pyridoxal-5'-Phosphate

Kinase / Phosphatase
ATP

Pyridoxal

Pyridoxic Acid

Fig. 13. Vitamin B$_6$. Vitamin B$_6$ is a collective term for pyridoxal and its amidated and reduced derivatives, pyridoxamine and pyridoxine. The active form of pyridoxial is phosphorylated and carries out decarboxylation reactions, transamination reactions (including racemations and keto acid formation and aldol reactions (including α–β elimination reactions). The phosphate group of pyridoxal-5'-phosphate is utilized in glycogen phosphorylase, an enzyme that catalyzes the hydrolysis of ether bonds in glycogen to form glucose-6-phosphate.

position. When pyridoxal-5'-phosphate is in cellular excess, it is converted to pyridoxic acid, which is transported into plasma and eventually excreted.

The reactions carried out by vitamin B$_6$ fall into four general categories; three related to the metabolism and interconversion of amino acids (Fig. 13) and the fourth, the hydrolysis of ether bonds in glycogen in the formation of glucose-t-phosphate, which is catalyzed by glycogen phosphorylase *(42)*. It is the association of vitamin B$_6$ with glycogen phosphorylase that accounts for the high concentration of vitamin B$_6$ in muscle *(43)*.

The requirement of vitamin B$_6$ in animals is positively related to the intake of protein and amino acids *(41)*. Although vitamin B$_6$ deficiency is rarely seen in nature, drug-induced vitamin B$_6$ deficiency can occur following administration of the tuberculo-

static drug isoniazid (isonicotinic acid hydrazide). This drug forms a hydrazone derivative with pyridoxal or pyridoxal phosphate which inhibits the pyridoxal-requiring enzymes. Penicillamine, β-dimethylcysteine, used in the treatment of Wilson's disease can also induce a vitamin B$_6$ deficiency resulting from the formation of thioazole derivatives. Moreover, there are naturally occurring antagonists to vitamin B$_6$, (e.g., linatine [1-amino-D-proline]), which is present in flax seed. To iterate, vitamin B$_6$ deficiency is uncommon, although the recent focus on homocysteine and its relationship to atherosclerosis has renewed interest in this vitamin. Pyridoxal-5'-phosphate is a cofactor for cystathiamin synthetase, which is importance to homocysteine clearance *(44)*.

PANTOTHENIC ACID The functional importance of pantothenic acid was put into perspective in the 1950s when Lippman and his associate demonstrated that pantothenic acid was a component of coenzyme A. Pantothenic acid is essential to all forms of life and is found in nature in amounts ranging from 20 to 50 µg/g of typical animal and plant edible tissues. Thus, it is possible to meet the currently recommended ranges of intakes for adults with a mixed diet containing as little as 100–200 g of solid food (i.e., equivalent to a mixed diet corresponding to 600–1200 kcal). In this regard, the typical American daily diet contains approximately 6 mg of pantothenic acid *(45)*.

Once pantothenic acid is absorbed, the rate of tissue uptake or diffusion do not appear to be rate limiting with respect to utilization (*see* Fig. 14). For example, the pantothenic acid content of red blood cells (RBCs) can be calculated with reasonable precision knowing only the daily intake of pantothenic acid and the daily net pantothenic acid excretion. Most of the pantothenic acid in blood is found in erythrocytes and the available data suggest uptake, and the content of pantothenic acid at equilibrium in RBCs is closely related to relative dietary intake. Likewise, the transport of pantothenic acid from the mammary into milk also appears to be a function of intake minus excretion. Human milk delivers about 5–6 mg of pantothenic acid/1000 kcal. Furthermore, for every milligram of pantothenic acid consumed, about 0.4 mg can be transported into milk when lactation is active.

Because of the widespread occurrence of the vitamin in foods, deficiencies are extremely rare. Urinary output of pantothenic acid is directly proportional to dietary input and has been used as an index of adequacy. For humans, the mean excretion of pantothenic acid is 4 mg/d.

B VITAMINS INVOLVED IN SINGLE-CARBON METABOLISM: BIOTIN, FOLIC ACID, AND VITAMIN B$_{12}$

BIOTIN In food, biotin is present in relatively high concentrations in cereals including soybeans, rice, barley, oats, corn, and wheat *(46)*. Biotin is covalently bound to the enzymes it serves as a cofactor; the chemical linkage is a peptide bond between the carboxylic acid moiety on biotin and the ε-amino function of peptidyl lysine in the enzyme (Fig. 9). When biotin-containing carboxylases are degraded, biotin is released as biocytin. Biocytinase is an important liver enzyme that catalyzes the cleavage of the peptide linkage between biotin and lysine to release free biotin for reutilization. In the absence of the enzyme, biotin deficiency can occur in the newborn.

Biotin is found in highest concentrations in the liver. Biotin-containing enzymes include acetyl-CoA carboxylase (important

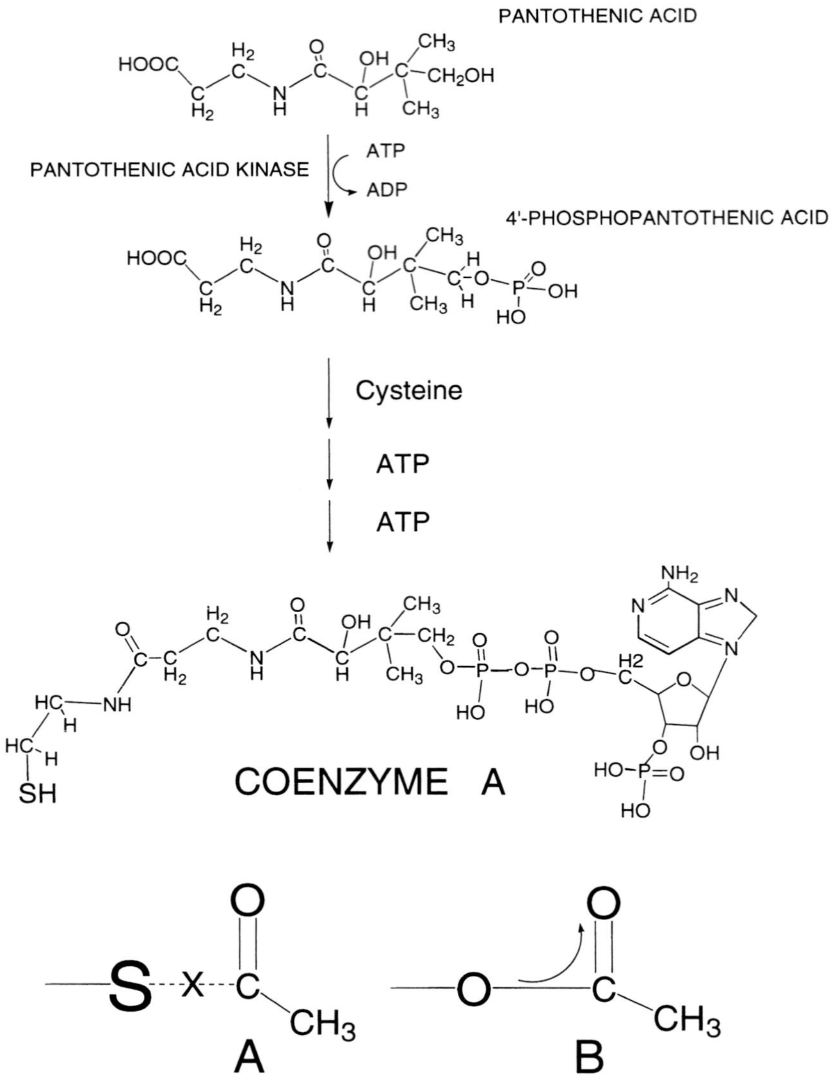

Fig. 14.   Pantothenic acid and coenzyme A. Pantothenic acid is a component of coenzyme A. The choice of coenzyme A, a thiol ester, rather than an oxygen ester for acyl transfers is very pragmatic. Thiol esters are more reactive than oxygen esters (*A*). Oxygen esters are kinetically more stable than thiol esters in reactions at the acyl carbon atom as a result of greater stabilization of the ground state by resonance interactions (*B*). Such interactions are largely absent in thiol esters (*A*).

to malonyl-CoA formation), pyruvate carboxylase, a key enzyme in gluconeogenesis, and malonyl-CoA carboxylase (important to succinyl CoA production).

Biotin and biocytin also have high affinities for certain proteins, particularly avidin in egg white. The consumption of raw egg albumin can induce biotin deficiency, because of the strong association of biotin with avidin, which can render dietary biotin unavailable. Biotin deficiency leads to impairment of gluconeogenesis and fat metabolism. Biotin deficiencies can also induce severe metabolic acidosis. The inability to carry out fat metabolism also markedly affects the dermis with biotin deficiency. Alopecia and dermatitis are characteristics of biotin deficiency in most animals. Biotin deficiency in humans is rare. Congenital deficiency of the enzyme, biocytinase or biotinidase, causes the inability to release biotin from carboxylases *(47)*.

FOLIC ACID AND VITAMIN B$_{12}$ Knowledge regarding folic acid and vitamin B$_{12}$ evolved from efforts to better understand macrocytic anemias and a certain degenerative neurologic disorders *(48,49)*. The Scottish physician Combe recognized in the early 1800s that certain form of macrocytic anemia appears related to a disorder of the digestive organs. In classic studies by Minot and Murphy, Castle, and others, it became a clearer that the disorder was associated with gastric secretions and, in some cases, could be reversed by consuming raw or lightly cooked liver *(2)*. Through careful clinical investigations and inferences, Castle postulated the existence of an intrinsic factor in gastric juice, which appeared to combine with a dietary extrinsic factor to modulate the severity of the anemia. In parallel studies, folic acid was associated with macrocytic anemia *(49,50)*. The key to understanding the essential role of folic acid and vitamin B$_{12}$ is an appreciation

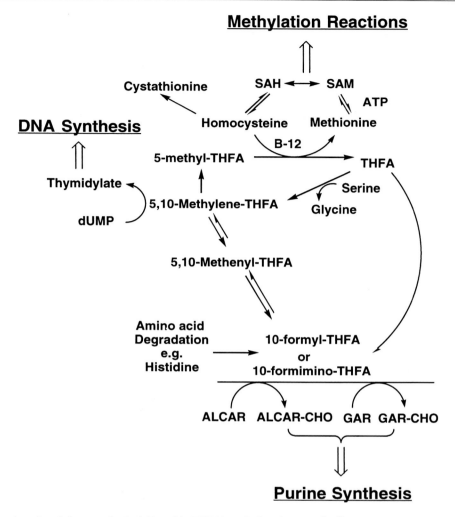

Fig. 15. Interactive reactions involving tetrahydrofolic acid (THFA) and vitamin B_{12}. N^5,N^{10}-methylene THFA is important for thymidylic acid formation from deoxyuridylic acid. The single carbon unit of other forms of THFA, such as the formyl and N^5,N^{10}-methenyl derivatives are important for purine synthesis. The single carbon, when reduced, can be ultimately transferred through vitamin B_{12} to form methionine from homocysteine. The reaction of ATP with methionine to produce S-adenosylmethionine (SAM) results in an activated form of methionine for methylation reactions. This intermediate is important to the methylation of phospholipids, DNA, and the production of methylated forms of various amino acids and carbohydrates. GAR = glycinamide ribonucleotide; AIGAR = aminoimidazolecarboxamide ribonucleotide, which are precursors in the purine synthesis pathway.

of their roles in purine, DNA synthesis, and methyl transfer reactions (Fig. 15). The source of single carbons is primarily from amino acid degradation. End products, such as formaldehyde and formimino groups, are transferred to folate acid. For these conversions to occur, folic acid must be in its completely reduced state as 5, 6, 7, and 8 tetrahydrofolic acid (THFA). Reduction brings the nitrogen at positions 5 and 10 closer together and changes electrochemical properties of both nitrogens, which facilitate the formation of the various THFA single-carbon derivatives.

Two vitamin B_{12} coenzymes participate in mammalian metabolism. Vitamin B_{12} in its methylated form is the cofactor in the THFA–homocysteine transmethylase system in which the methyl group is transferred from methyl THFA to homocysteine. In its adenosylated form as 5-deoxyadenosylcobalamin, vitamin B_{12} serves as a coenzyme of methylmalonyl-CoA mutase (Fig. 9). In the latter reaction, methylmalonyl-CoA is converted to succinyl CoA for ultimate use

as a metabolic fuel. In the absence of vitamin B_{12}, methylmalonic acid accumulates in blood and is excreted in urine.

The requirements for folic acid range from 1 to 3 mg/kg of diet for most animals. There are some conditions in which the folic acid requirements are conditionally high (e.g., when either natural or pharmacological folic acid antagonists are present in the diet or administered). The requirement for vitamin B_{12} for most animals is in the range of 2–6 g/kg of typical diet. Deficiencies of both vitamin B_{12} and folic acid produce clinical signs of macrocytic anemia and dissynchronies in growth and development owing to the importance of folic acid to purine and DNA synthesis. Chronic deficiencies of either folic acid or vitamin B_{12} can also promote fatty liver disease and indirectly influence extracellular matrix maturation stability by causing abnormal elevations in homocysteine. Such signs and symptoms are attributable to both THFA and vitamin B_{12} deficiencies, because of the integral relationship of

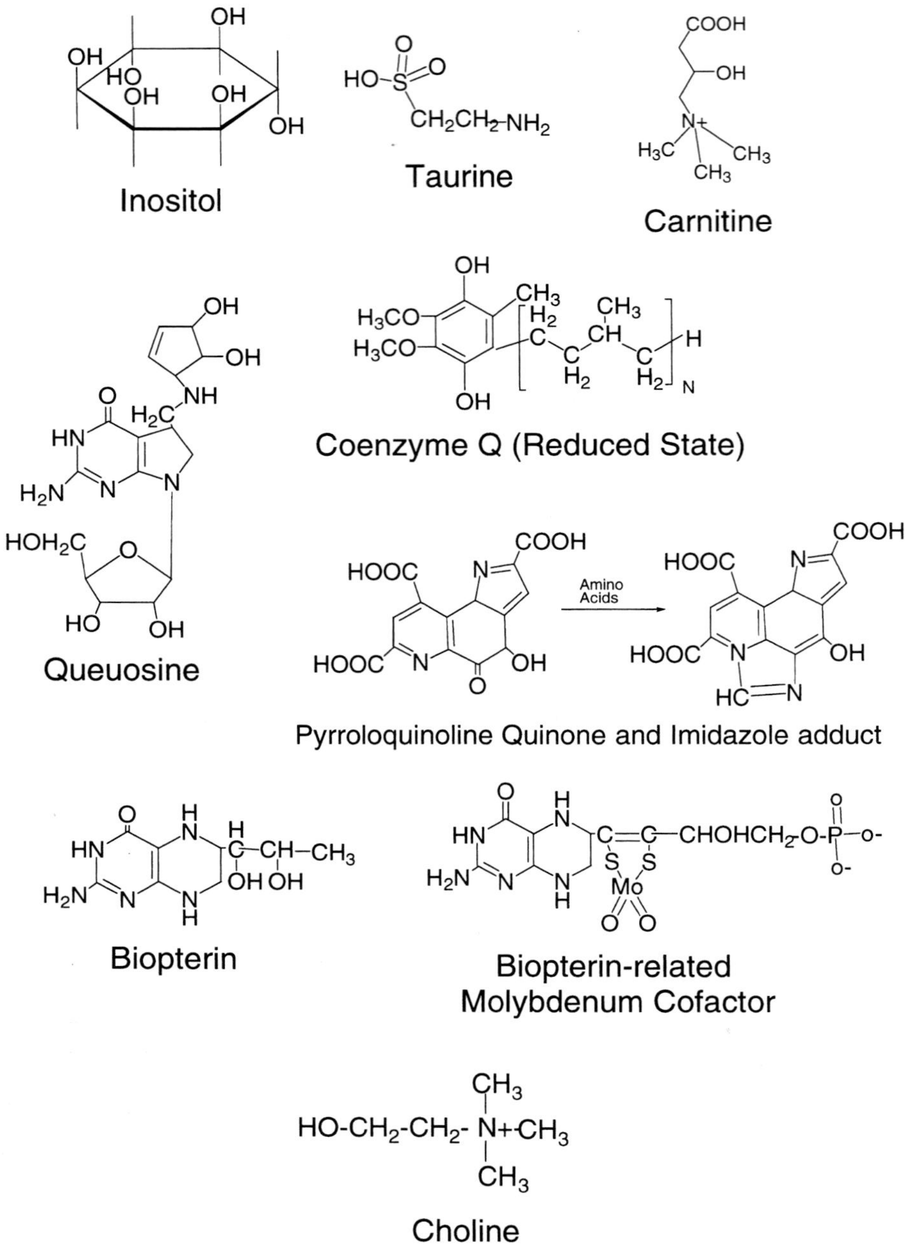

Fig. 16. Structures of compounds that are sometimes defined as "vitaminlike."

vitamin B_{12} to reduced folic acid regeneration. Dietary intakes of folic acid, sufficient to maintain functional levels, can mask the initial signs of vitamin B_{12} deficiency (e.g., macrocytic and megaloblastic anemia). Prolonged vitamin B_{12} deficiency results in serious neurologic disorders (e.g., degeneration of the myelin sheath).

VITAMINLIKE COMPOUNDS

LIPOTROPIC FACTORS Nutritional requirements exist for a number of compounds at specific periods in development, particularly neonatal development, and periods of rapid growth. These compounds typically perform specialized transport function, particularly in relation to fatty acids. Apart from specific amino acids, such as methionine, examples include choline, inositol, and carnitine (Fig. 16).

Choline plays a key role in methyl group metabolism, carcinogenesis, and lipid transport (51). Choline is generally the major source of methyl groups in the diet, but it can also be synthesized *de novo* from ethanolamine when methionine, dimethylcysteine, or betaine are in adequate supply. The most abundant source of choline in the diet is lecithin. The primary sign of a choline deficiency is fatty liver. In monkeys, dogs, and rats, it has also been shown that prolonged choline deficiency results in hepatocellular cancer, a unique example of nutrition deficiency resulting in neoplasm. The choline requirement is 100–200 mg/100 kcal of diet or about 0.5–1.0 g/kg of dry food.

Another lipotropic factor is carnitine (52,53). Carnitine plays a major role in the lipid-transport process by accepting activated fatty acids and facilitating their transport. Carnitine comes both

Table 3
Vitamin Assessment

Vitamin	Analytical methods	Clinical and chemical methods
Vitamin A	High-performance liquid chromatography[a] (HPLC) separation and extraction into lipids solvents, UV absorption, HPLC and mass spectrophotometry of isolated retinoids	Impaired vision
Vitamin D	Extraction into lipid solvents, HPLC separation, and UV absorption or mass spectrophotometry	Signs of rickets or osteomalacia
Vitamin E	Extraction into lipid solvents, HPLC separation, and UV absorption	Malonaldehyde detection, diene conjugation, lipid peroxidation, hexane and pentane expiration, tissue fluorescence
Vitamin K	Extraction into lipid solvents, HPLC separation, and UV absorption	GLA[b] content in osteocalcin or prothrombin
Vitamin C (ascorbic acid)	Plasma assays based on oxidation to dehydroascorbic acid coupled to a chromaphoric substance with a high extinction coefficient, HPLC separation, and UV detection	Signs of scurvy
Riboflavin	HPLC separation and fluorescent detection of urinary or plasma riboflavin	Erythrocyte glutathione reductase activity; stimulation without or with added riboflavin, fatigue, cheilosis, angular stomatitis
Niacin	HPLC separation and UV detection of NAD and NADP or detection by redox enzyme activity	Signs of pellagra
Thiamin	Urinary thiamin excretion and plasma thiamin determined following HPLC separation and fluorescent detection of thiochrome (produced by alkali treatment).	Erythrocyte transketolase activity; stimulation without and with thiamin added
Vitamin B_6	Plasma pyridoxal-5′-phosphate (PLP) estimation using assays based on activation of PLP-requiring enzymes.	Anemia, increased urinary xanthurenic acid after a tryptophan load
Biotin	HPLC separation and fluorescence detection, avidin-binding bacterial growth assays	Signs of macrocytic anemia formimino glutamic acid excretion following a histidine load
Vitamin B_{12}	Competition assays based on binding to cobalamin-binding proteins	Measurement of holo-*trans*-cobalamin II levels. Signs of macrocytic anemia: positive Schilling test (indirectly measures B-12 absorption), deoxyuridine suppression test (indirectly measures methylation potential and DNA synthesis)

[a]High-performance liquid chromatography employing straight-phase, reverse-phase, isocratic, or gradient chromatography.
[b]γ-Carboxyglutamic acid.

from the diet and a complex synthesis pathway in which trimethyl lysine serves as a key substrate. Ascorbic-acid-dependent hydroxylation and novel cleavage steps result in carnitine. Given the importance of carnitine to the β-oxidation of long-chain fatty acids, carnitine deficiency can have a profound effect on lipid utilization. The inability to synthesis carnitine is rare. More important are inherited deficiencies of carnitine acyl transferase. Meats and dairy products, in contrast to plant foods, are good sources of carnitine. Cereal grains are low in carnitine.

Inositol is also a component of phospholipid, and similar to choline, a dietary deficiency results in a fatty liver *(54)*. Inositol is synthesized from glucose-6-phosphate. For most adults, the estimated daily intakes ranges from 250 to 1000 mg/d. Inositol is particularly important in signal transduction and phospholipid assembly. A number of excellent sources are available on this topic. Plasma levels of inositol are increased during renal disease and nephrectomy. Otherwise, there is constant turnover resulting from the incorporation and release from phospholipids.

OTHER COFACTORS AND POTENTIAL VITAMINS Figure 16 contains structures of other compounds that are also occasionally defined as "vitaminlike." Each are highlighted because of their known role as coenzymes in prokaryotes and eukaryotes

or roles as a probiotic (growth-promoting substances) in higher animals (*see* Table 4). These compounds include taurine, queuosine, coenzyme Q, pteridines (other than folic acid), such as biopterin and the molybdenum-containing pteridine cofactor (utilized as cofactors in several mono-oxygenases, phenylalanine hydroxylase and xanthine oxidase), lipoic acid, and pyrroloquinoline quinone (PQQ).

PERSPECTIVE ON VITAMIN ASSESSMENT AND RELATIVE NEED

Nutritional deficiencies of vitamins usually occur when monotonous diets are fed for therapeutic or other reasons. Other contributory factors include interference with normal food intake, loss of appetite (anorexia), impaired absorption and/or utilization, increased excretion, or the interaction with antagonists. Certain physiological states (e.g., lactation) may influence vitamin status.

The problem of assessing the dietary adequacy for various vitamins, however, has presented problems for nutritionists. Merely measuring the concentrations of vitamins in the diet does not account for their availability from food. Measures of status are often arbitrary and imprecise. Approaches include:

Table 4
Vitaminlike Compounds

Compound	A Major Function	Ref.
Taurine	Formation of taurocholic acid; antioxidant	60
Quesuosine	Can substitute for guanine in tRNA, when available for the diet	61
Coenzyme Q	Mitochondrial redox cofactor	62
Pteridines	Several redox cofactors are pteridines, e.g., molybdopterin in xanthine oxidase, tetrahydropterin in phenylalanine hydroxylase.	63
Lipoic acid	Acetyl and acyl transfer reactions, antioxidant	64
Pyrroloquinoline quinone	Potent growth factor for neonatal mice and rodents	65

1. Vitamin concentrations in biological fluids, such as blood plasmas.
2. Administering the vitamin and measuring urinary excretion of corresponding metabolites as an index of the saturation of body stores.
3. "Loading" tests in which a compound that requires the vitamin for its metabolism is administered and the urinary excretion of a product is measured.
4. Enzyme-stimulation tests in which the rate of a reaction is measured before and after the addition of the vitamin.

With regard to human vitamin requirements, it is important to appreciate that on a comparative basis, the relative vitamin requirements are often of the same order across animal species. Differences in requirements between species are usually the result of the presence or absence of pathways important to the production of a given vitamin, vitamin cofactor, or its degradation or disposal. Ascorbic acid and niacin are examples of vitamins that cannot be synthesized by some animals, therefore becoming "true" vitamins (e.g., ascorbate in humans and niacin in cats). As noted, vitamin deficiencies are often the result of consuming monotonous diets (i.e., diets based on a limited number of food sources). Furthermore, young and growing animals may have a relatively higher nutritional need for some nutrients. The processing of foods can result in substantial losses of natural and added vitamins. While single-vitamin deficiencies of the fat-soluble vitamins occur naturally, frequently multiple-vitamin deficiencies of the B complex are encountered. Foods that are poor sources of one of the B vitamins tend to be poor sources of the several B vitamins.

Vitamin requirements are also influenced by many of these same factors that influence macronutrient requirements. A case can easily be made that in homeotherms, there is a positive correlation between the metabolic rate and the requirement for those vitamins utilized directly in energy-driven processes. This perspective comes largely from the work of Kleiber (55).

Water-soluble vitamin requirements may be described and comparisons between homeothermic species, "warm-blooded" animals, can be made as proportions to weight (in kilograms) expressed exponentially (e.g., often to the three-fourths power). For homeotherms, the estimation of relative "metabolic body size" ($kg^{3/4}$) correlates with direct estimates of the metabolic rate for animal species whose body weights vary by several orders of magnitude. It can be shown that for the water-soluble vitamins, their relative needs are often in direct relationship to the energy need to sustain normal basal metabolism. For sedentary to moderately active humans, the implication is that 60–80% of most water-soluble-vitamin requirements is directly related to the energy costs for basal metabolism.

To further make the case that vitamin requirements are a function of basal metabolism, there should be an excellent correspondence between requirements between species of homeotherms when expressed on a basal-energy need basis. The requirements for growing animals and animal at maintenance are established for a number of species. These values correlate with those for adult humans derived primarily from data based on nutrient-balance techniques when expressed as a function of metabolic body size ($wt_{kg}^{3/4}$).

As an illustrative example, ascorbic acid synthesis in homeotherms will be considered. It is well established that most homeotherms are capable of ascorbic acid synthesis. In humans, the absence of gulonolactone oxidase dictates that ascorbic acid be consumed as a dietary essential. One can ask, do the amounts of ascorbic acid synthesized per day in differing species correspond to the amounts needed in the human diet. For such calculations, data originally offered by Grollman and Lehninger (56), Chatterjee (28), Chaudhuri and Chatterjee (57) [also cf. Rucker et al. (58) and Ginter (59)] can be used. These data describe, in general, the potential synthesis of ascorbic acid from D-glucuronic acid or gulonic acid, for which glucose and galactose serve as precursors. When expressed relative to the metabolic body size or basal metabolic needs of the species used, extrapolation to humans give values that are in keeping with the requirement (see Table 5). For example, Grollman and Lehninger (56) used liver homogenates and gulonic acid as a substrate to measure ascorbic acid synthesis. They found that the amounts varied from 0.01 g of ascorbic acid synthesized per day per kg body weight for the pig to 0.2 g/kg body weight for the rat. Such values have been used to infer that the ascorbic acid needs in humans are in the gram/day range. However, what is ignored is that ascorbic acid production can be no more than the amount of glucose or galactose shunted through the direct oxidative pathway. In a 70-kg person, this value ranges from 5 to 15 g/d. In the article by Grollman and Lehninger (56), in addition to the data on ascorbic acid synthesis, they also provided data on the ratio of ascorbic acid production to gulonic acid oxidation. For a 70-kg animal, the ratio is between 0.008 and 0.011; that is, only about 1% of the gulonic acid flux is in the direction of ascorbate synthesis. Given that 5–15 g of glucose and galactose are shunted through the glucuronic and gulonic acid pathways in humans, this amounts to about 50–150 mg of ascorbate today.

Chatterjee (28) provided data on the synthesis of L-ascorbic acid by crude liver microsomes using gulonolactone as a substrate. By using simple "rules of thumb" drawn from pharmokinetic estimates and transformations based on metabolic body size and extrapolation to 70 kg, it may also be concluded that the amount needed is in the range of 100–200 mg of ascorbic acid/d (58). Furthermore, additional support comes from observations on the turnover of ascorbic acid in vivo. Ginter (59) has provided excellent data on the rates of ascorbate metabolism in the rat, mouse, guinea pig, rabbit, hamster, and human. The transfer rate of a substance into and out of the body (i.e., turnover) is a function of $Wt_{kg}^{1/4}$, that is, $([Wt_{kg}] \div [Wt_{kg}^{3/4}])$. This is derived by assuming

Table 5
Ascorbic Acid Synthesis

I. Based on extrapolation from the data provided by Grollman and Lehniger (56)

Specie	Body weight (kg)	Ascorbic acid production (mg/liver/d)	Relative Synthesis L-Gulonic acid to ascorbic acid (molar ratio)
Mouse	0.033	3.0	0.39
Rat	0.350	70	0.117
Rabbit	2	264	0.053
Dog	10	816	0.013
Pig	125	1014	0.008
Cow	488	8921	0.004

II. Based on extrapolated from data by Chatterjee (28)

Species	Ascorbic acid production (μg/mg of microsomal protein/h)[a]	Theoretical net synthesis (mg/liver/d)[b]	Amount (g) per day per (70 kg)$^{3/4}$
Goat	68	646	0.8
Cow	50	3042	0.7
Sheep	43	495	0.6
Rat	38	5.4	0.3
Mouse	35	0.3	0.1
Squirrel	30	5.7	0.2
Gerbil	26	2.0	0.2
Rabbit	23	17.3	0.3
Cat	5	7.6	0.1
Dog	5	20	0.1

III. Ascorbate turnover in guinea pig and humans based on extrapolation from data provided by Ginter[c]

Animal	$(Wt_{kg})^{1/4}$	Guinea pig (d)	Man (d)
Mouse	0.414	3.4	9.8
Hamster	0.569	4.7	13.7
Rat	0.669–0.775	3.6–3.7	10.4–10.8
Rabbit	1.41	2.8	8.0
Average		3.6	10.5

[a]Represent the micrograms of ascorbic acid synthesized per milligram of liver microsomal protein per hour using L-gulonolactone as a substrate.
[b]The theoretical net synthesis in vivo of ascorbic acid per whole liver per day was calculated in the following manner. Michaelis–Menten kinetics were applied with the assumption that the values expressed as rates were close to the estimates for V_{max}. The K_m for the gulonolactone oxidase was taken as 5 mM in each case. The tissue concentration of L-gulonolactone was assumed to be no greater than 0.05 mM. Subsequently, a theoretical observed rate was obtained by substituting into the equation $V_0 = V_{max}S/K_m + S$. The values were then multiplied by 40 (1 g of liver contains approx 40 mg of microsomal protein), times 24 (to convert to 1 d), and then times the total grams of liver. The body and liver weights used in the calculations were respectively goat (50 kg, 1 kg), cow (488 kg, 6.4 kg), sheep (50 kg, 1.2 kg), rat (0.35 kg, 0.015 kg), mouse (0.025 kg, 0.001 kg), and squirrel (0.5 kg, 0.02 kg).
[c]Values under columns labeled guinea pig and man were computed by dividing the $(wt_{kg})^{1/4}$ for the guinea pig (body weight taken to be 1 kg) or man (body weight taken to be 70 kg) by the values in the column labeled $(wt_{kg})^{1/4}$ and then multiplying by the appropriate values for the ascorbate half-life as determined by Ginter (59).

that the body pool size of the substance (total content) is directly proportional to weight. The ascorbic acid turnover rate in humans can be predicted by knowing the ascorbic acid turnover in the rat, mouse, rabbit, or hamster. This observation provides additional validation of the connection between vitamin need and energy utilization.

CONCLUSIONS

In this chapter, selected functions of vitamins have been highlighted. It should be clear that vitamins represent a diverse array of molecules, which have equally diverse functional roles. Nevertheless, when expressed on an energy basis, most vitamin requirements are often of the same order when interspecies comparisons are made. Vitamin deficiencies are most often the result of consuming monotonous diets (i.e., diets based on a limited number of food sources).

The requirements for vitamins are usually greatest during the neonatal period. There are also numerous possibilities for interactions that can have deleterious physiological consequences. The processing of foods can result in losses of natural and added vitamins. As noted, whereas single-vitamin deficiencies of the fat-soluble vitamins occur naturally, frequently multiple-vitamin deficiencies of the B complex are encountered. Foods that are poor sources of one of the B vitamins tend to be poor sources of the several B vitamins. The vitamins evolved to serve unique and complex roles as cofactors, as signaling agents in cells, as regulators of gene expression, and as redox and free-radical quenching agents. As is the case of any substance that is essential to a given function, all vitamins at some point in development can be viewed as limiting nutrients, the absence of which results in specific deficiency signs and symptoms.

REFERENCES

1. Darby WJ, Jukes TH, eds. Founders of Nutrition Science, Volumes 1 and 2 American Institute of Nutrition, Bethesda, MD, 1992.
2. Guggenheim YK. Nutrition and Nutritional Disease: The Evolution of Concepts. Collamore, New York, 1981.
3. Sokol RJ. Fat-soluble vitamins and their importance in patients with cholestatic liver diseases. Gastroenterol Clinics North Am 1994; 23:673–705.
4. McCormick DB, Zhang Z. Cellular assimilation of water-soluble vitamins in the mammal: riboflavin, vitamin B-6, biotin, and vitamin C. Proc Soc Exp Biol Med 1993; 202:265–70.
5. Rose RC. Intestinal absorption of water-soluble vitamins. Proc Soc Exp Biol Med 1996; 212:191–8.
6. Pruthi RK, Tefferi A. pernicious anemia revisited. Mayo Clinic Proc 1994; 69:144–50.
7. Diplock, AT, ed. Fat Soluble Vitamins. William Heinemann Medical Books, London, 1985.
8. Sporn MB, Roberts AB, Goodman DS, eds. The Retinoids: Biology, Chemistry, and Medicine, 2nd ed. Raven, New York, 1994.
9. de Pee S, West CE. Dietary carotenoids and their role in combating vitamin A deficiency: a review of the literature. Eur J Clin Nutr 1996; 50(suppl 3):S38–53.
10. Lieber, C.S. Mechanisms of ethanol-drug-nutrition interactions. J Tox Clin Tox 1994; 32:631–681.
11. Hinds TS, West WL, Knight EM. Carotenoids and retinoids: a review of research, clinical and public health applications. J Clin Pharmacol 1997; 37:551–8.
12. Sucov HM, Evans RM. Retinoic acid and retinoic acid receptors in development. Mol Neurobiol 1995; 10:169–84.
13. Bendich A. Physiological role of antioxidants in the immune system. J Dairy Sci 1993; 76:2789–94.

14. Morriss-Kay G, ed. Retinoids and Teratogenesis, Oxford University Press, Oxford, New York, 1992.

15. Collins ED, Norman AW. In: Machlin LJ, ed, Vitamin D. Handbook of Vitamins: Nutritional, Biochemical and Clinical Aspects. Marcel Dekker, New York, 1991.

16. Balmain N, Calbindin A. Vitamin-D-dependent, calcium-binding protein in mineralized tissues. Clin Orthopaed Related Res 1991; 25: 265–76.

17. Wasserman RH, Fullmer CS. Vitamin D and intestinal calcium transport: facts, speculations and hypotheses. J Nutr 1995; 25:1971S–9S.

18. Kumar MV, Tindall DJ. Transcriptional regulation of the steroid receptor genes. Prog Nucleic Acid Res Mol Biol 1998; 59:289–3.

19. Norman AW. Pleiotropic actions of 1 alpha, 25-dihydroxyvitamin D3: an overview. J Nutr 1995; 125(suppl 6):1687S–9S.

20. Strugnell SA, Deluca HF. The vitamin D receptor—structure and transcriptional activation. Proc Soc Exp Biol Med 1997; 215:223–8.

21. Traber MG, Packer L. Vitamin E: beyond antioxidant function. Am J Clin Nutr 1995; 62(suppl 6):1501S–9S.

22. Kayden HJ, Traber MG. Absorption, lipoprotein transport, and regulation of plasma concentration of vitamin E in humans. J Lipid Res 1995; 34:343–58.

23. Gey KF. Vitamins E plus C and interacting conutrients required for optimal health. A critical and constructive review of epidemiology and supplementation data regarding cardiovascular disease and cancer. Biofactors 1998; 7:113–74.

24. Suttie JW. The importance of menaquinones in human nutrition. Annu Rev Nutr 1998; 15:399–417.

25. Binkley NC, Suttie JW. Vitamin K nutrition and osteoporosis. J Nutr 1995; 125:1812–21.

26. Bender DA. Nutritional Biochemistry of the Vitamins. Cambridge University Press, Cambridge, 1992.

27. Banhegyi G, Braun L, Csala M, Puskas F, Mandl J. Ascorbate metabolism and its regulation in animals. Free Radical Biol Med 1997; 23:793–803.

28. Chatterjee I. Evolution and biosynthesis of ascorbic acid. Science 1973; 182:1271–4.

29. Packer L, Fuchs J, eds. Vitamin C in Health and Disease. Marcel Dekker, New York, 1997.

30. Bode AM. Metabolism of vitamin C in health and disease. Sies, H. (Eds.), Adv Pharmacol 1997; 38:21–47.

31. Johnston CS, Solomon RE, Corte C. Vitamin C depletion is associated with alterations in blood histamine and plasma free carnitine in adults. J Am Coll Nutr 1996; 15:586–91.

32. England S, Seifer S. The biochemical functions of ascorbic acid. Annu Rev Nutr 1986; 6:365–406.

33. Lanska DJ. Stages in the recognition of epidemic pellagra in the United States: 1865–1960. Neurology 1996; 47:829–34.

34. Henderson LM. Niacin. Annu Rev Nutr 1983; 3:289–97.

35. Rawling JM, Jackson TM, Driscoll ER, Kirkland JB. Dietary niacin deficiency lowers tissue poly(ADP-ribose) and NAD+ concentrations in Fischer-344 rats. J Nutr 1994; 124(9):1597–603.

36. Takasawa S, Akiyama T, Nata K, Kuroki M, Tohgo A, Noguchi N, et al. Cyclic ADP-ribose and inositol 1,4,5-triphosphate as alternate second messengers for intracellular Ca2+ mobilization in normal and diabetic beta-cells. J Biol Chem 1998; 273(5):2497–500.

37. Poirier GG, Moreau P, eds. ADP-Ribosylation Reactions. Springer-Verlag, New York, 1992.

38. D'Arcy PF. Nutrient-drug interactions. Adverse Drug React Toxicol Rev 1995; 14:233–54.

39. Sable HZ, Gubler CJ, eds. Thiamin. New York Academy of Science, New York, 1982, vol. 378:1–470.

40. Bettendorff L, Mastrogiacomo F, Kish SJ, Grisar T. Thiamine, thiamin phosphates, and their metabolizing enzymes in human brain. J Neurochem 1998; 66:250–8.

41. Coburn SP. A critical review of minimal vitamin B6 requirements for growth in various species with a proposed method of calculation. Vitamin Horm 1994; 48:259–300.

42. Dakshinamurti K, ed. Vitamin B-6. New York Academy of Science, New York, 1990, vol. 585.

43. Palm D, Klein HW, Schinzel R, Buehner M, Helmreich EJ. The role of pyridoxal 5'-phosphate in glycogen phosphorylase catalysis. Biochemistry 1990; 29:1099–107.

44. Mayer EL, Jacobsen DW, Robinson K. Homocysteine and coronary atherosclerosis. J Am Coll Cardiol 1996; 27:517–27.

45. Fox HM. Pantothenic Acid. In: Macklin LJ, ed, Handbook of Vitamins: Nutritional, Biochemical and Clinical Aspects. Marcel Dekker, New York, 1991.

46. Mock DM. Determinations of biotin in biological fluids. Methods Enzymol 1997; 279:265–75.

47. Oizumi J, Hayakawa K. Biocytin-specific 110kDa biotinidase from human serum. Clin Chim Acta 1993; 215(1):63–71.

48. Ellenbogen L, Cooper BA. Vitamin B-12. In: Macklin LJ, ed. Handbook of Vitamins: Nutritional, Biochemical and Clinical Aspects. Marcel Dekker, New York, 1991.

49. Aving JF, Nair NG, Baugh CM, eds. Chemistry and Biology of Pteridines and Folates. Plenum, New York, 1991.

50. Kamaeo B. Folate and antifolate pharmacology. Semin Oncol, 1997; 24(suppl 18):S18-30–39.

51. Zeisel SH. Choline. A nutrient that is involved in the regulation of cell proliferation, cell death, and cell transformation. Adv Exp Med Biol 1996; 399:131–41.

52. Borum PR. The Clinical Aspects of Human Carnitine Deficiency, Pergamon, New York, 1986.

53. McGarry JD, Brown NF. The mitochondrial carnitine palmitoyltransferase system. From concept to molecular analysis. Eur J Biochem 1997; 244:1–14.

54. Holub BJ. The cellular form sand functions of inositol phospholipids and their metabolic derivatives. Nutr Rev 1987; 45:65–71.

55. Klieber M. The Fire of Life. Wiley, New York, 1961.

56. Grollman AP, Lehniger A. Enzymatic synthesis of L-ascorbic acid in different species. Arch Biochem Biophys 1957; 69:458–64.

57. Chaudhuri CR, Chatterjee I. Ascorbic acid synthesis in birds: phylogenic trends. Science 1969; 164:435.

58. Rucker RB, Dubick MA, Mouritsen J. Hypothetical calculations of ascorbic acid synthesis based on estimates in vitro. Am J Clin Nutr 1980; 33:961–4.

59. Ginter E. Endogenous ascorbic acid synthesis and recommended dietary allowances for vitamin C. Am J Clin Nutr 1981; 34:1448–51 (letter).

60. O'Flaherty L, Stapleton PP, Redmond HP, Bouchier-Hayes DJ. Intestinal taurine transport: a review. Eur J Clin Invest 1997; 27:873–80.

61. Farkas WR. Effect of diet on the queuosine family of tRNAs of germfree mice. J Biol Chem 1980; 255:6832–5.

62. Ernster L, Dallner G. Biochemical, physiological and medical aspects of ubiquinone function. Biochim Biophys Acta 1995; 1271:195–204.

63. Kaufman S. New tetrahydrobiopterin-dependent systems. Annu Rev Nutr 1993; 13:261–86.

64. Packer L, Witt EH, Tritschler HJ. Alpha-lipoic acid as a biological antioxidant. Free Radical Biol Med 1995; 19:227–50.

65. Steinberg FM, Gershwin ME, Rucker RB. Dietary pyrroloquinoline quinone: growth and immune response in BALB/c mice. J Nutr 1994; 124(5):744–53.

8 α-Lipoic Acid
The Metabolic Antioxidant

JOHN K. LODGE AND LESTER PACKER

INTRODUCTION

There is increasing evidence that thiols play a role in various biological processes. This arises from their ability to undergo redox reactions; thus, they can act as efficient electron donors or acceptors. α-Lipoic acid is a dithiol-containing compound that plays an essential role in mitochondrial dehydrogenase reactions, but it has recently gained considerable interest as an antioxidant. Further investigations have shown lipoate to be an effective redox modulator of cell signaling and gene transcription. The various effects of α-lipoic acid at a cellular level are discussed here, highlighting the remarkable therapeutic potential for lipoate in a variety of disorders where oxidative stress is a factor.

LIPOIC ACID PLAYS AN INTEGRAL ROLE IN OXIDATIVE METABOLISM Lipoic acid (thioctic acid, 1,2-dithiolane-3-pentanoic acid) was first purified in 1951 by Reed and co-workers *(1)* after being recognized that this compound was responsible for a number of compounds displaying the same activity *(2)*. Such compounds were found to be required for normal growth of bacteria *(3)* and were found to be able to replace acetate *(4)* and to allow the oxidation of pyruvate *(5)*. Lipoic acid was tentatively described as a vitamin after isolation, but it was later discovered to be synthesized by both plants and animals *(6)*. The complete biosynthetic pathway is still widely unknown; however, the immediate precursor is thought to be octanoic acid *(7)*. The thiolation may arise from cysteine residues. Lipoic acid is an eight-carbon chain, dithiol-containing compound (Fig. 1). It has a chiral center; therefore, two optical isomers exist; the *R* form being the naturally occurring variety and a racemic mixture exists in synthetic preparations.

In vivo lipoic acid is found bound to the ε-amino group of a lysine residue of five distinct mitochondrial proteins *(8)*. As lipoamide, it functions as a cofactor in multienzyme complexes that catalyze the oxidative decarboxylation of pyruvate, α-ketoglutarate, and branched-chain α-keto acids (Fig. 2). The complexes that catalyze these reactions share structural similarities. They are all composed of multiple copies of three enzymes, E_1, E_2, and E_3.

The E_2 subunit, called dihydrolipoyl acyltransferase, contains the lipoyl domains, which, depending on the species, can vary between 1 and 3.

The lipoyl group of the E_2 subunit receives the acetylated thiamine pyrophosphate group from E_1 (pyruvate dehydrogenase) and transfers the acetyl group to coenzyme A, forming acetyl CoA. In this process, lipoamide is reduced to the dihydrolipoamide form. E_3, dihydrolipoamide dehydrogenase, is the enzyme that reoxidizes this back to lipoamide, using NAD^+, which is converted to NADH. The E_2 and E_3 subunits are held together by protein X, which also contains a lipoyl group. This protein is believed to have only a structural role *(9)*; however, it has recently been thought to be involved in the reoxidation of dihydrolipoamide to lipoamide *(10)*.

The fifth lipoyl-containing protein is found in the glycine cleavage system *(11)*, which catalyzes the oxidation of glycine to CO_2 and ammonia, forming NADH and 5,10-methylenetetrahydrofolate. The lipoyl moiety is present on the H-protein (one of four labeled P-, H-, T-, and L-) and is involved in the transfer of the methylene moiety from the decarboxylated glycine. Dihydrolipoamide dehydrogenase is also present here to reform the lipoamide moeity.

Dihydrolipoamide dehydrogenase is able to reduce lipoamide in a reverse reaction at the expense of NADH. This enzyme may also act independently of the above complexes and, thus, may have alternative roles. It is found associated with the plasma membrane in rat adipocytes *(12)*, E. coli and various strains of Archaebacteria *(13)*, which lack the keto acid dehydrogenase complexes. In addition, eukaryotic cells contain dihydrolipoamide not associated with these multienzyme complexes.

CELLULAR UPTAKE AND REDUCTION OF LIPOIC ACID Current interest in lipoic acid arises from its potential as a drug to combat a variety of disorders. Therefore, it is of interest to understand the cellular fate of exogenously supplied free lipoic acid. When α-lipoic acid is orally administered, it is absorbed, transported into tissues, taken up by cells, and reduced to dihydrolipoic acid (DHLA). DHLA is then released outside the cells. The uptake of exogenously supplied α-lipoic acid has been studied in the perfused rat liver and isolated hepatocytes *(14)*. Two different transport mechanisms were reported: carrier-mediated uptake, which is prominent below 75 μ*M,* and passive diffusion, which

From: *Nutrition and Immunology: Principles and Practice* (ME Gershwin et al. eds.), © Humana Press, Inc., Totowa, NJ

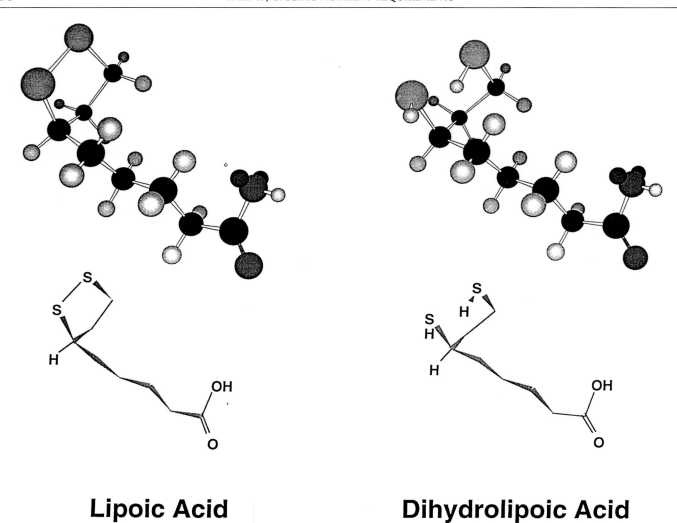

Lipoic Acid   **Dihydrolipoic Acid**

Fig. 1. Structures of α-lipoic and dihydrolipoic acid.

is prominent at higher concentrations. This study also showed that the carrier-mediated uptake can be blocked by medium-chain fatty acids, suggesting that the same translocator was in use *(14)*. However the exact mechanism is still in doubt. The cellular reduction of α-lipoic acid was proposed by Peinado et al. *(14);* however, this was not shown directly until a study by Handelman et al. with T lymphocytes *(15)*, using high-performance liquid chromatography (HPLC) with electrochemical detection.

This reduction to DHLA has now been observed in several cell lines, including hepatocytes *(16)*, erythrocytes *(17)*, keratinocytes *(18)*, and lymphocytes *(15)*. Further work on the mechanisms of reduction have shown both cytosolic and mitochondrial activity, with varying specificities *(16)*. The mitochondrial enzyme E_3 (dihydrolipoamide dehydrogenase) is capable of reducing α-lipoic acid, in a reverse reaction, which is at the expense of NADH. This enzyme shows a marked preference for the naturally occurring *R*-enantiomer of lipoic acid *(19)*. Alternatively, the cytosolic enzyme glutathione reductase (E.C. 1.6.4.2) can also catalyze the reduction using NADPH as a cofactor; however, the preference of this enzyme is for the unnatural *S*-enantiomer *(19)*. Recently, it has been found that thioredoxin reductase, a cytosolic enzyme that catalyzes the NADH-dependent reduction of oxidized thioredoxin,

efficiently reduces both lipoic acid and lipoamide *(20)*. This may not be so surprising, as thioredoxin reductase, glutathione reductase, and dihydrolipoamide dehydrogenase belong to the same family of proteins.

Thus, α-lipoic acid can be reduced by different enzymatic systems from various cellular compartments (Fig. 3). The reduction has also been found to be tissue-specific, and the relative reduction pathways in terms of mitochondrial and cytosolic enzymes are different in each case *(16)*. For example, the liver appears to reduce lipoate to an equal extent by both glutathione reductase and dihydrolipamide reductase *(16)*. In contrast, the heart reduces lipoate almost completely (90%) by dihydrolipo-amide reductase *(16)*. It appears that the reducing activity will correlate with the relative amounts and activities of the enzymes involved, and this is also related to the mitochondrial content, which differs markedly from tissue to tissue *(16)*. Because the stereospecificities of the enzymes are markedly different, this has implications for the form in which exogenously supplied α-lipoate is provided and could even provide a means for tissue-specific targeting *(16)*. Recently, the content of the naturally occurring protein-bound form of lipoic acid (lipoyllysine) has been deter-mined in various bovine and murine tissues *(22)*. The content was

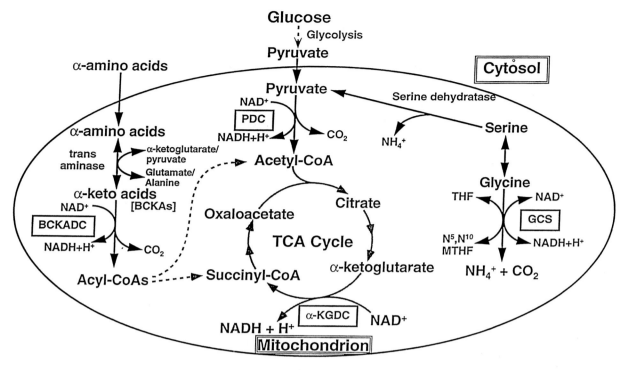

Fig. 2. The role of lipoic-acid-containing enzymes in energy metabolism. PDC = pyruvate dehydrogenase complex; BCKADC = branched-chain keto acid dehydrogenase complex; α-KGDC = α-ketoglutarate dehydrogenase complex; GCS = glycine cleavage system. (Courtesy of Dr. Mulchand S. Patel and Dr. Lester Packer.)

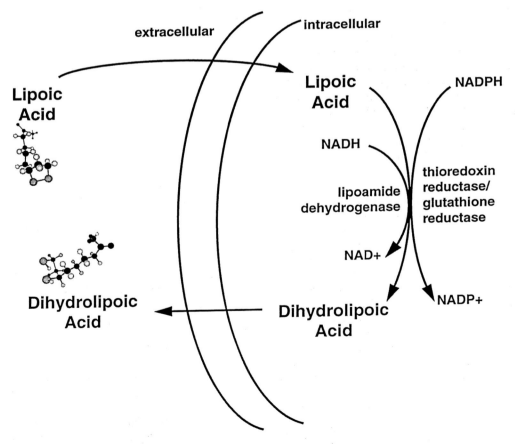

Fig. 3. Cellular pathways of α-lipoic acid reduction. (Adapted from ref. 21.)

found to be tissue-specific with values ranging from 2.6–0.1 µg/ g dry weight. The highest content was found in the kidney, heart, liver, and muscle. Interestingly, these values correlate exactly with the amount of NADH-dependent lipoate reduction in these tissues found by Haramaki et al. *(16)*. This is no surprise because dihydro-lipoamide dehydrogenase (E_3) is a component of the mitochondrial enzyme complexes which contain lipoyl groups. Therefore, the content of lipoic acid in tissues will correlate with the metabolic activity *(22)*.

Reduction contributes one way to lipoate metabolism. Other routes have been demonstrated using radiolabeled lipoic acid, administered either orally *(23)* or via injection *(24)* into the rat. Several components were identified, including the short-chain homologs bisnorlipoic and tetranorlipoic acids *(24)*. Interestingly, no evidence for the oxidation of the dithioline ring was observed. Following the radioactivity after administration of [1,6-^{14}C]lipoic acid indicates that lipoic acid is rapidly absorbed in the gut and passed to various tissues for catabolism *(23)*. The localization of administered lipoate was greatest in the liver, other intestinal organs, and the skeletal muscle *(23)*. Another study confirmed that α-lipoic acid supplementation results in lipoic acid and DHLA accumulation in tissues of vitamin E-deficient mice *(25)*; however, these researchers found the greatest localization to be in the heart. Nevertheless, these studies confirm that exogenously administered lipoic acid is distributed to tissues where it can be taken up by cells and reduced.

LIPOIC ACID AS AN ANTIOXIDANT

Recently, there has been a great deal of interest in the antioxidant properties of α-lipoic acid and especially its reduced form, dihydrolipoic acid. These studies originated from the observations of Rosenberg and Culik in 1959 *(26)*, who noticed that administration of α-lipoic acid prevented the symptoms of both vitamin C and vitamin E deficiency in rats. Over the last decade, a number of reports have shown the effectiveness of lipoic acid and DHLA in scavenging a number of reactive oxygen species. α-Lipoic acid can scavenge hydroxyl radicals *(27)*, hypochlorous acid *(28,29)*, singlet oxygen *(30,31)*, and hydrogen peroxide (J. Lodge, unpublished results). In addition, it is thought to be able to chelate a number of metal ions *(32–34)*. DHLA can also scavenge the above radicals and superoxide *(35,36)* and peroxyl radicals *(36,37)*, which α-lipoic acid cannot. Again, it is also thought to be able to chelate metal ions. These actions are summarized in Table 1.

Hydroxyl radicals are extremely reactive radicals potentially formed in vivo wherever transition metal complexes come into contact with hydrogen peroxide. Hydroxyl radical scavenging has been demonstrated in a metal catalysis system *(35)* and by ultraviolet A (UVA) irradiation of NPIII [*N,N'-bis*(2-hydroperoxy-2-methoxyethyl)-1,4,5,8-napthalenetetracarboxylic diimide] *(27)*. This latter system confirms actual hydroxyl radical scavenging and not simply the result of metal chelation properties of lipoic acid. DHLA appears to be a more effective hydroxyl radical scavenger, as concentrations of 0.5 mM completely eliminated the dimethyl pyrroline oxide DMPO–hydroxyl radical electron spin resonance radical (ESR) signal *(38)*, whereas concentrations up to 1 mM of lipoic acid were required.

The respiratory burst of neutrophils in response to stimuli produces highly reactive oxygen species. Superoxide ($O_2^{\cdot-}$) is formed, which forms H_2O_2 in the presence of superoxide dismutase

Table 1
Antioxidant Activity of α-Lipoic Acid and DHLA

Oxidant	Scavenged by α-lipoic acid	Scavenged by DHLA
Hydroxyl radical	Yes *(28)*	Yes *(33,39)*
Singlet oxygen	Yes *(31,32)*	No *(32)*
Superoxide	No *(33,36)*	Yes *(36,37)*
Peroxyl radical	No *(38)*	Yes *(38)*
Hypochlorite	Yes *(29,30)*	Yes *(29,30,33)*
Hydrogen peroxide	Yes[a]	Yes[a]
Nitric oxide radical	Yes[a]	Yes[a]
Peroxynitrite	Yes[a]	Yes[a]
Metal chelation	Possibly *(33–35)*	Possibly *(33,40,41)*

[a]Unpublished data

(SOD). This can then be converted to hypochlorous acid (HOCl) by the action of myeloperoxidase. Various groups have demonstrated the HOCl scavenging ability of lipoic acid via α_1-antiproteinase inactivation *(29,32)* and by prevention of protein carbonyl formation *(28)*. This latter report evaluated a number of antioxidants and showed DHLA to be the most effective in scavenging hypochlorite. DHLA was twice as effective as reduced glutathione and *N*-acetyl cysteine, and five time more effective than lipoic acid *(28)*. DHLA appears to be able to scavenge superoxide, whereas lipoic acid cannot. Using xantine–xanthine oxidase to generate superoxide, DHLA was found to abolish the superoxide–DMPO ESR adduct in two separate reports *(35,36)*. The reactions were confirmed by assaying sulfhydryl content, and the formation of hydrogen peroxide as a product. DHLA is an effective peroxyl radical scavenger. Peroxyl radicals are present during the formation of lipid hydroperoxides, and this measurement is often used as an indicator of oxidative damage to membranes and low-density lipoproteins. Both lipophilic and hydrophilic peroxyl radicals, generated from AAPH and AMVN, respectively, were scavenged by DHLA *(37)*.

The presence of transition metal ions in biological systems may catalyze Fenton-type reactions, which lead to the production of hydroxyl radicals. Metal ions have also been shown to be toxic in their own right, especially in overload conditions and poisoning episodes. The metal-chelating abilities of lipoate are still rather indecisive. Direct studies on the bivalent-ion-binding capacity revealed that lipoate forms stable complexes with Mn^{2+}, Cu^{2+}, and Zn^{2+} *(34)* and that the complexes were mediated via the carboxylate group. Two different studies have indicated that lipoic acid may chelate iron. Scott et al. *(32)* showed that α-lipoic acid inhibited site-specific degradation of deoxyribose by a $FeCl_3$–H_2O_2–ascorbate system and attributed this effect to the removal of deoxyribose-bound iron by lipoate. Devasagayam et al. *(30)* found that the protective effect of lipoate against singlet-oxygen-induced DNA strand breaks was lowered in the presence of EDTA, indicating that the protective effect was somewhat dependent on metal-ion chelation. In terms of oxidative systems, lipoic acid was found to prevent Cu^{2+}-induced ascorbic acid oxidation; liposomal peroxidation *(33)*, however, was found to be ineffective against Cu^{2+}-induced low-density lipoprotein (LDL) peroxidation *(39)*, whereas DHLA was *(39)*. It has also been found that lipoate decreased Cd^{2+}-induced toxicity in isolated hepatocytes, although the authors speculate that the true chelating agent was DHLA formed via cellular reduction. DHLA is able to chelate iron in both oxidation states and is also able to remove iron from ferritin *(42)*. However, DHLA may actually act as a pro-oxidant under certain conditions, especially because it can reduce Fe^{3+}. Indeed, DHLA was found to act as a pro-oxidant in the peroxidation of rat liver microsomes *(40)*, and DHLA has also been shown to induce single-strand DNA breaks in the presence of Cu^{2+}, but not Fe^{3+} or Fe^{2+}. This in contrast to recent research showing the ability of DHLA to prevent Cu^{2+}-mediated LDL peroxidation via chelation *(39)*. Such inconsistent data in this area warrant further work for clarification.

LIPOATE INTERACTS WITH OTHER ANTIOXIDANTS

During the interaction between an antioxidant and a reactive oxygen species, the antioxidant is generally converted to a form that is no longer able to function and is thus said to be consumed. This oxidized product needs to be recycled to its native form in order to function again. The DHLA–lipoate redox couple is a very potent reductant (potential −0.32 V) and is thus able to regenerate oxidized antioxidants.

α-Lipoate protection of antioxidants was first suggested and shown by Rosenberg and Culik in 1959 *(26)*, when supplementation of α-lipoic acid prevented symptoms of both vitamin E and vitamin C deficiency. They stated that lipoate might act as an antioxidant for ascorbic acid and tocopherols. These early observations have been confirmed in a study by Podda et al. *(25)* in tocopherol-deficient hairless mice. Vitamin E, being a potent peroxyl radical scavenger, is the major chain-breaking antioxidant protecting biological membranes from lipid peroxidation *(41)*. This is not an easy task because, on average, the ratio of phospholipid molecules to vitamin E is 1000–2000 : 1. However, oxidation of membranes does not readily occur nor is vitamin E rapidly depleted. This paradox can be explained by the fact that vitamin E is constantly recycled by circulating antioxidants. A number of antioxidants can regenerate vitamin E, including vitamin C, ubiquinols, and thiols *(43,44)*. DHLA only has a weak direct interaction with the tocopheroxyl radical *(45)* and so the major recycling of vitamin E by DHLA occurs via the intermediary recycling of other antioxidants. The ascorbate-dependent recycling of vitamin E by DHLA has been demonstrated in DOPC liposomes *(37)*, erythrocyte membranes *(46)*, and human low-density lipoproteins *(47)*. In these electron spin resonance studies, the ascorbyl radical generated from oxidation by a chromanoxyl radical was recycled by DHLA, thereby allowing more ascorbate to be made available for direct recycling of vitamin E. It was also demonstrated by Kagan et al. *(37)* that DHLA interacts with NADH and NADPH-dependent electron-transport chains to recycle vitamin E.

Other studies have suggested that DHLA may also recycle vitamin E by reducing oxidized glutathione (GSSG) directly, the reduced glutathione (GSH) can then recycle vitamin E *(48)*. DHLA can reduce GSSG to GSH, but GSH is incapable of reducing α-lipoate to DHLA *(49)*. This role of GSH was based on the observation that a combination of DHLA and GSSG prevented lipid peroxidation induced by iron/ascorbate, whereas DHLA alone had no effect *(40)*. DHLA can also reduce thioredoxin *(50)*, an important cytosolic protein that functions to transfer electrons in various biochemical processes. Another lipophilic antioxidant is ubiquinol. There is now evidence that lipoate supplementation increases tissue ubiquinol content even in a oxidative stress situation *(51)*, and ubiquinol is also known to recycle vitamin E *(52)*.

Therefore, α-lipoate can directly interact with ascorbate, glutathione, NADH, and ubiquinol, recycling these antioxidants and indirectly replenishing the pool of vitamin E, which will enhance both lipid and aqueous-phase antioxidant defenses (Fig. 4).

METABOLIC EFFECTS OF EXOGENOUSLY SUPPLIED α-LIPOATE

Normal metabolic processes in cells require free energy, in the form of ATP, and an efficient electron acceptor. This role is undertaken partly by nicotinamide adenine dinucleotide (NAD^+), and its reduced form, NADH, can also donate electrons where required. Because most cell processes involve NAD^+/NADH, any compound that can modulate these ratios can affect numerous aspects of cell metabolism. α-Lipoate can affect this balance because the intracellular reducing power arises from NADH and NADPH. When lipoic acid is supplied to cells, there is a decrease in the cellular NADH/NAD^+ ratio *(53)*. In Wurzburg T cells exposed to 0.5 m*M* α-lipoate, NADH depletion was evident after 30 min, and after 24 h, lipoate decreased by 30%. This treatment also decreased cellular NADPH levels *(53)*, but relatively less and slower, consistent with the major pathway of lipoate reduction being the NADH-dependent mitochondrial E_3 enzyme and not the cytosolic NADPH-dependent glutathione reductase pathway. In these studies, it was also found that this treatment increased the pyruvate/lactate ratio by 35% *(53)*. This may also be a consequence of the altered NAD^+/NADH ratio; however, the reduced form of lipoate (DHLA) has been found to decrease respiration of NADH-dependent substrates in intact rat liver mitochondria (N. Haramaki, unpublished data). High cellular levels of NADH inhibits metabolic pathways such as glycolysis. Supplementation of lipoic acid to cells increased glucose uptake in a concentration-dependent manner *(53)*, which is consistent of another report in which α-lipoate enhanced glucose disposal in patients with Type II diabetes *(54)*. These events are summarized in Fig. 5.

α-Lipoate has been shown to cause an increase in intracellular glutathione in vitro *(55)* and in vivo *(54)*. Glutathione is the major extracellular oxidant that acts as a sulfhydryl buffer, protecting cysteine residues in proteins from oxidation. The modulation of GSH has been discussed as a potential therapeutic strategy *(57)*. Han et al. showed that α-lipoic acid increases intracellular glutathione in human Jurkat T lymphocytes *(55)*. More recently, it was hypothesized that this increase is a consequence of increased glutathione synthesis by the improvement of cystine utilization *(58)*. This effect has now been shown in a number of cell lines, including Jurkat T cells, erythrocytes, glial cells, and neuroblastoma cells. The rate-limiting step in the synthesis of glutathione is the availability of cysteine. Lipoic acid enters the cells, is reduced to DHLA, and is then released into the medium. DHLA subsequently reduced cystine to cysteine, and this is taken up by the ascorbate ASC transporter. This system is at least 10 times more efficient than the glutamate-sensitive cystine transporter. Thus, there is an influx of cysteine resulting in an elevation of cellular GSH levels *(58)* (Fig. 6).

Another important intracellular component is calcium. Ca^{2+} plays an important role as a second messenger that regulates a variety of metabolic processes, and it is a known requirement for protein phosphorylation reactions. Oxidants have been shown to stimulate Ca^{2+} signaling, which has led to suggestions that oxidants may play a physiological role in Ca^{2+} regulation and signaling.

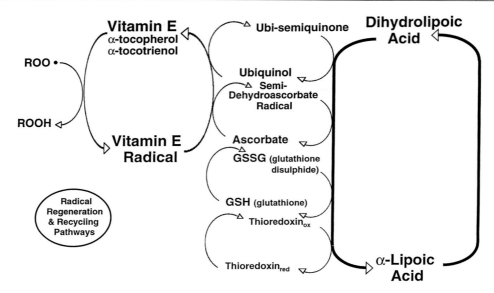

Fig. 4. The vitamin E cycle, and the recycling of antioxidants by α-lipoate.

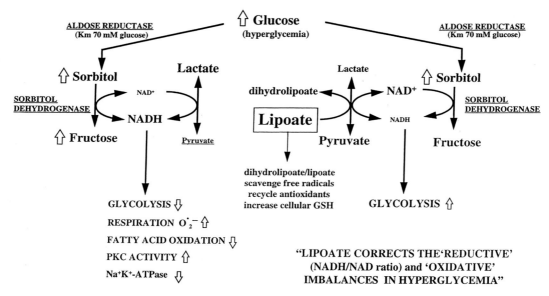

Fig. 5. Representation of the influence of α-lipoate supplementation on metabolic pathways that result in the alteration of NADH/NAD⁺ ratios. (Adapted from ref. 53.)

When cells are challenged with oxidants, there is a rapid perturbation of intracellular calcium homeostasis resulting in elevated intracellular calcium concentration *(54)*. Possible sites of oxidants may include enhancement of Ca^{2+} channels, the inhibition of Ca^{2+} pumps *(60)* or the mobilization of intracellular calcium pools in the sarco-endoplasmic reticulum and mitochondria *(61)*; however, the exact mechanisms remain unknown. It has been reported that most of the oxidant-induced intracellular calcium originated from intracellular stores *(62)*. This oxidant-induced transient increase in cytosolic Ca^{2+} is stabilized in cells pretreated with α-lipoate *(63)*. In this flow cytometric study with Jurkat T cells, treatment of 0.25 mM hydrogen peroxide resulted in a multifold increase in intracellular Ca^{2+} within 10–30 s. This was not observed in cells pretreated with α-lipoic acid for 18 h, and the effect was dose dependent. Consistent with these results is a recent report showing that α-lipoate also affects mitochondrial calcium transport *(64)*. The authors suggest that the α-lipoate stimulated Ca^{2+}-release pathway from mitochondria was the result of the oxidation of vicinal thiols, which stimulates the hydrolysis of pyridine nucleotides *(64)*. Thus, by affecting various aspects of calcium mobilization, lipoate will affect various signaling pathways. Such pathways are involved in signal transduction.

LIPOIC ACID AS A MODULATOR OF SIGNAL TRANSDUCTION

The process that relays an extracellular message across the plasma membrane and into the cytosol, which will eventually lead to the induction of a biological response, is termed signal transduction.

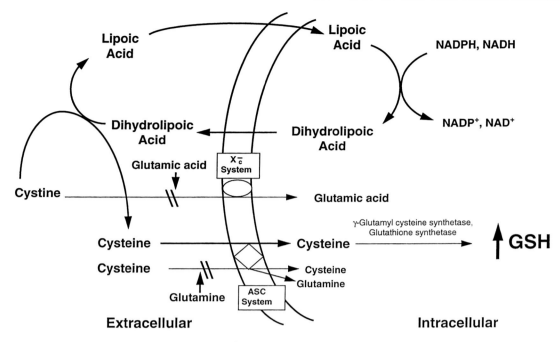

Fig. 6. Mechanism for the α-lipoate-induced increase in intracellular glutathione. (From ref. 58.)

Recently, vast attention has been focused on the role of oxidants *(60)* and antioxidants *(63)* in the regulation of these processes. Redox changes in cells trigger molecular responses. Nuclear Factor kappa B NF-κB is a well-characterized redox-sensitive transcription factor. The activation of NF-κB is involved in the expression of a wide variety of genes involved in oxidative stress and cellular response mechanisms. Most agents activating NF-κB tend to trigger the formation of reactive oxygen species or are oxidants by themselves (e.g., $O_2^{.-}$, H_2O_2, or lipoxygenase products) *(65);* therefore, it is not surprising that a number of antioxidants and reducing agents have the ability to inhibit NF-κB activation. These include various thiol-containing compounds (2-mercaptoethanol, glutathione, *N*-acetylcysteine, cysteine), phenolic and catecholic compounds (tocopherol derivatives), and chelators (desferrioxamine). α-Lipoate was also found to inhibit NF-κB activation induced by phorbol ester or tumor necrosis factor α (TNFα) in Jurkat T-cells in a dose-dependent fashion *(66)*. Both enantiomers of lipoate were found to be effective *(67)*, as was DHLA added directly to the medium; however, at higher concentrations of DHLA, there was an effect on cell viability not observed with α-lipoate *(67)*. It has recently been shown that the ability of α-lipoate to inhibit NF-κB was not dependent on increased intracellular glutathione levels *(63)*. In these experiments, Wurzburg T cells were preincubated with buthionine sulfoxamine (BSO), an inhibitor of glutathione synthesis. Lipoate treatment could not increase GSH levels in these cells but was able to inhibit NF-κB activation induced by phorbol ester, TNFα or H_2O_2 *(63)*. Following the activation of NF-κB, there is translocation into the nucleus and binding to specific areas of DNA, which elicits the response. α-Lipoate has been shown to inhibit the DNA binding of NF-κB *(68);* however, DHLA was found to enhance binding. Also, the inhibition of DNA binding by diamide can be overcome by the addition of DHLA. These observations suggest that two modes of redox regulation exist in cell signaling for NF-κB *(69)*: the first, a requirement of oxidative processes in activating NF-κB, and, the second, a requirement for reductive processes in DNA binding. A scheme summarizing redox regulation in gene transcription is shown in Fig. 7.

LIPOIC ACID IN HEALTH AND DISEASE

The properties of α-lipoate lead to the possibility that administration may influence intracellular function via antioxidant actions and through affecting the redox status of thiol-containing proteins *(45)*. Indeed, α-lipoic acid administration has been shown to be effective in various pathologies in which reactive oxygen species have been implicated (reviewed in refs. 21, 45, and 69). α-Lipoic acid can be thought of as a metabolic antioxidant, as it is a naturally occurring substance and is acted on by cellular enzymatic systems as a substrate. Beneficial effects of lipoic acid administration have been reported in diabetic complications *(54,70)*, ischemia-repurfusion injury *(71,72)* and liver disease *(73)*. Also, lipoic acid may be a good candidate for treatment in AIDS *(74)*, neurodegenerative diseases *(21)*, and heavy metal poisoning *(45)*.

One well-documented example of the therapeutic effectiveness of α-lipoic acid is in diabetes. α-Lipoic acid appears to act in a number of ways that maybe protective in diabetes. In an animal model, supplementation of lipoate prevented β-cell destruction, which leads to Type I diabetes *(75)*. In a separate study, α-lipoic acid supplementation enhanced glucose uptake in rats *(76)* and in humans with Type II diabetes *(54)*. Both studies demonstrated enhanced insulin-stimulated whole-body glucose by 50%. In vitro studies have shown α-lipoate to prevent glycation of various proteins *(77)*. A nuclear magnetic resonance (NMR) study revealed that α-lipoic acid can bind to human serum albumin *(78)*, and this may be the means by which lipoate protects against glycation *(79)*. A common complication of diabetes is neuropathy. Various studies have shown α-lipoate supplementation to be effective in the alleviation of some symptoms of this condition *(80,81)*, and

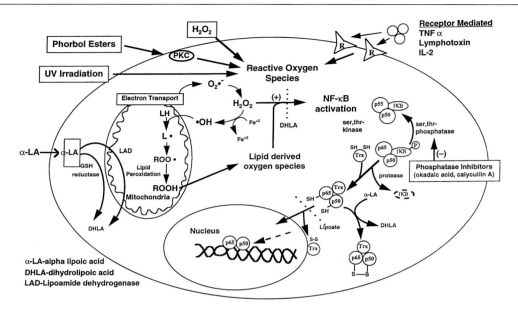

Fig. 7. Various steps in redox regulation of gene transcription, including possible sites of action for α-lipoate. (Adapted from ref. 69.)

now α-lipoate is approved in Germany for this treatment. Another common complication is cataracts. In vitro cataractogenesis in rat lenses exposed to high glucose levels was prevented by α-lipoate supplementation in the medium *(82)* and when cataractogenesis in newborn rats was induced by BSO treatment, α-lipoic acid treatment resulted in a 60% decrease in cataract formation *(83)*. It was also observed in these studies that other antioxidants such as ascorbate, tocopherol, and glutathione were spared. Therefore, one further role of lipoate in this disease is to replenish ascorbate, whose transport is affected in diabetes *(84)*. Also, because lipoate can inhibit NF-κB activation, this has implications in diabetic-associated atherosclerosis. Advanced glycosolation end products (AGE) can induce the expression of vascular-cell-adhesion molecules (VCAM-1), which is an early feature in the pathogenesis of atherosclerosis *(85)*. Therefore, the attenuating effect on NF-κB activation may dampen the acceleration of atherosclerosis associated with diabetes.

SUMMARY

The lipoic acid–dihydrolipoic acid couple has been described as a universal antioxidant *(37)*. Both are able to scavenge a wide variety of reactive oxygen species, as well as possessing metal-chelating properties. Because of the high reducing potential, DHLA can interact and recycle other antioxidants, forming an antioxidant network that can protect vitamin E. Such sparing effects have been demonstrated in vitro and in vivo. When supplemented, α-lipoic acid is rapidly absorbed, distributed to tissues, and taken up by cells. There, it is reduced to DHLA, and this process can increase the ratio of NAD^+ to NADH, thus having the potential of stabilizing conditions where NADH levels are increased. Intracellular glutathione levels are also increased markedly after lipoic acid supplementation; thus, lipoic acid can affect cellular redox status. Increasing evidence has now also shown lipoic acid to modulate certain signal transduction pathways; thus, it has the potential to work at different cellular levels. These wide-ranging effects have paved the way for the potential usefulness

of α-lipoic acid as a therapeutic agent for the treatment of energy-impaired and redox-unbalanced conditions.

REFERENCES

1. Reed LJ, DeBusk BG, Gunsalus IC, Hornberger J. Crystalline α-lipoic acid: a catalytic agent associated with pyruvate dehydrogenase. Science 1951; 114:93–4.
2. Snell EE, Broquist HP. On the probability of several growth factors. Arch Biochem Biophys 1949; 23:326–8.
3. Snell EE, Strong FM, Peterson WH. Growth factors for bacteria. VI. Fractionation and properties of an accessory factor for lactic acid bacteria. Biochem J 1937; 31:1789–99.
4. Guirard BM, Snell EE, Williams RJ. The nutritional role of acetate for lactic acid bacteria. I. The response to substances related to acetate. Arch Biochem Biophys 1946; 9:361–79.
5. O'Kane DJ, Gunsalus IC. Accessory factor requirement for pyruvate oxidation. J Bacteriol 1947; 54:20–1.
6. Carreau JP. Biosynthesis of lipoic acid via unsaturated fatty acids. Methods Enzymol 1979; 62:152–8.
7. Dupre S, Spoto G, Matarese RM, Orlando M, Cavallini D. Biosynthesis of lipoic acid in the rat: incorporation of 35S- and 14C-labeled precursors. Arch Biochem Biophys 1980; 202:361–5.
8. Reed LJ. Multienzyme complexes. Acc Chem Res 1974; 7:40–6.
9. Lawson JE, Behal RH, Reed LJ. Disruption and mutagenesis of the *Saccharomyces cervisiae* PDX1 gene encoding the protein X component of the pyruvate dehydrogenase complex. Biochemistry 1991; 30:2834–9.
10. Patel MS, Roche TE. Molecular biology and biochemistry of pyruvate dehydrogenase complexes. FASEB J 1990; 4:3224–33.
11. Patel MS, Smith RL. Biochemistry of lipoic acid containing proteins: past and present. In: Schmidt K, Diplock AT, Ulrich H, eds, The Evolution of Antioxidants in Modern Medicine, pp. 65–77. Hippocrates Verlag, Stuttgart, 1994.
12. Danson MJ. Dihydrolipoamide dehydrogenase: a "new" function for an old enzyme? Biochem Soc Trans 1987; 16:87–9.
13. Danson MJ, Eisenthal R, Hall S, Kessell SR, Williams DL. Dihydrolipoamide dehydrogenase from halophilic archaebacteria. Biochem J 1984; 218:811–8.
14. Peinado J, Sies H, Akerboom TPM. Hepatic lipoate uptake. Arch Biochem Biophys 1989; 273:389–95.
15. Handelman GJ, Han D, Trischler H, Packer L. α-lipoic acid reduction

by mammalian cells to the ditiol form, and released into the culture medium. Biochem Pharmacol 1994; 47:1725–30.

16. Haramaki N, Han D, Handelman GJ, Tritschler HJ, Packer L. Cytosolic and mitochondrial systems for NADH–NADPH-dependent reduction of α-lipoic acid. Free Radicals Biol Med 1997; 22:535–42.

17. Constantinescu A, Pick U, Handelman GJ, Haramaki N, Han D, Podda M, Tritschler HJ, Packer L. Reduction and transport of lipoic acid by human erythrocytes. Biochem Pharmacol 1995; 50:253–61.

18. Podda M, Han D, Koh B, Fuchs J, Packer L. Conversion of lipoic acid to dihydrolipoic acid in human keratinocytes. Clin Res 1994; 42:41a.

19. Pick U, Haramaki N, Constantinescu A, Handelman GJ, Tritschler HJ, Packer L. Glutathione reductase and lipoamide dehydrogenase have opposite stereospecificities for α-lipoic acid enantiomers. Biochem Biophys Res Commun 1995; 206:724–30.

20. Arner ESJ, Nordberg J, Holmgren A. Efficient reduction of lipoamide and lipoic acid by mammalian thioredoxin reductase. Biochem Biophys Res Commun 1996; 225:268–74.

21. Packer L, Tritschler HJ, Wessel K. Neuroprotection by the metabolic antioxidant α-lipoic acid. 1997; 22:359–78.

22. Lodge JK, Youn H-D, Handelman GJ, Konishi T, Matsugo S, Mathur W, Packer L. Natural sources of lipoic acid: determination of lipolyllysine released from protease-digested tissues by high performance liquid chromatography incorporating electrochemical detection. J Appl Nutr 1997; 49:3–11.

23. Harrison EH, McCormick DB. The metabolism of *dl*-(1.6-14C) lipoic acid in the rat. Arch Biochem Biophys 1974; 160:514–22.

24. Spence JT, McCormick DB. Lipoic acid metabolism in the rat. Arch Biochem Biophys 1976; 174:13–9.

25. Podda M, Tritschler HJ, Ulrich H, Packer L. α-Lipoic acid supplementation prevents symptoms of vitamin E deficiency. Biochem Biophys Res Commun 1994; 204:98–104.

26. Rosenberg HR, Culik R. Effect of α-lipoic acid on vitamin C and vitamin E deficiencies. Arch Biochem Biophys 1959; 80:86–93.

27. Matsugo S, Yan L-J, Han D, Tritschler HJ, Packer L. Elucidation of antioxidant activity of alpha-lipoic acid toward hydroxyl radical. Biochem Biophys Res Commun 1995; 208:161–7.

28. Yan L-J, Traber MG, Kobuchi H, Matsugo S, Tritschler HJ, Packer L. Efficacy of hypochlorous scavengers in the prevention of protein carbonyl formation. Arch Biochem Biophys 1996; 327:330–34.

29. Haenen GR, Bast A. Scavenging of hypochlorous acid by lipoic acid. Biochem Pharmacology 1991; 42:2244–6.

30. Devasagayam TP, Subramanian M, Pradhan DS. Prevention of singlet oxygen-induced DNA damage by lipoate. Chem–Biol Interact 1993; 86:79–92.

31. Kaiser S, Di Mascio P, Sies H. Lipoat und Singulettsauerstoff. In: Borbe HO, Ulrich H, eds, Thioctsäure, pp. 69–76. pmi Verlag GmbH, Frankfurt, 1989.

32. Scott BC, Aruoma OI, Evans PJ, O'Neill C, Vander Vliet A, Cross AE, Tritschler H, Halliwell B. Lipoic and dihydrolipoic acids as antioxidants. A critical evaluation. Free Radical Res 1994; 20:119–33.

33. Ou P, Tritschler HJ, Wolff SP. Thioctic (lipoic) acid: a therapeutic metal-chelating antioxidant? Biochem Pharmacol 1995; 50:123–6.

34. Sigel H, Prijs B, McCormick DB, Shih JCH. Stability of binary and ternary complexes of a-lipoate and lipoate derivatives with Mn^{2+}, Cu^{2+}, and Zn^{2+} in solution. Arch Biochem Biophys 1978; 187:208–14.

35. Suzuki YJ, Tsuchiya M, Packer L. Thioctic acid and dehydrolipoic acid are novel antioxidants which interact with reactive oxygen species. Free Radical Res. Commun 1991; 15:255–63.

36. Suzuki YJ, Tsuchiya M, Packer L. Antioxidant activities of dihydrolipoic acid and its structural homologues. Free Radical Res. Commun 1993; 18:115–22.

37. Kagan VE, Shvedova A, Serbinova E, Khan S, Swanson C, Powell R, Packer L. Dihydrolipoic acid—a universal antioxidant both in the membrane and in the aqueous phase. Reduction of peroxyl, ascorbyl and chromanoxyl radicals. Biochem Pharmacol 1992; 44:1637–49.

38. Matsugo S, Yan L-J, Han D, Tritschler HJ, Packer L. Elucidation of antioxidant activity of dihydrolipoic acid toward hydroxyl radical using a novel hydroxyl radical generator NP-III. Biochem Mol Biol Int 1995; 37:375–83.

39. Lodge JK, Traber MG, Packer L. Thiol chelation of Cu^{2+} by dihydrolipoic acid prevents human low density lipoprotein peroxidation. Free Radical Biol Med 1998; 25:287–97.

40. Bast A, Haenen GRMM. Interplay between lipoic acid and glutathione in the protection against microsomal lipid peroxidation. Biochim Biophys Acta 1988; 963:558–61.

41. Burton GW, Ingold KU. Autoxidation of biological molecules. 1. The antioxidant activity of vitamin E and related chain-breaking phenolic antioxidant in vitro. J Am Chem Soc 1981; 103:6472–7.

42. Bonomi F, Pagani S. Removal of ferritin-bound iron by *dl*-dihydrolipoate and *dl*-dihydrolipoamide. Eur J Biochem 1986; 155:295–300.

43. Sies H. Strategies of antioxidant defense. Eur J Biochem 1993; 215: 213–9.

44. Packer L. New horizons in vitamin E research—the vitamin E cycle, biochemistry and clinical applications. In: Ong ASH, Packer L, eds, Lipid-Soluble Antioxidants: Biochemistry and Clinical Applications, pp. 1–16. Birkhauser Verlag, Boston, 1992.

45. Packer L, Witt EH, Tritschler HJ. Alpha-lipoic acid as a biological antioxidant. Free Radical Biol Med 1995; 19:227–50.

46. Constantinescu A, Han D, Packer L. Vitamin E recycling in human erythrocyte membranes. J Biol Chem 1993; 268:10,906–13.

47. Kagan VE, Serbinova EA, Forte T, Scita G, Packer L. Recycling of vitamin E in human low density lipoproteins. J Lipid Res 1992; 33: 385–97.

48. Bast A, Haenen GRMM. Regulation of lipid peroxidation of glutathione and lipoic acid: involvement of liver microsomal vitamin E free radical reductase. In: Emerit I, Packer L, Auclair C, eds, Antioxidants in Therapy and Preventive Medicine, pp. 111–6. Plenum, New York, 1990.

49. Jocelyn PC. The standard redox potential of cysteine–cystine from the thiol–disulphide exchange reaction with glutathione and lipoic acid. Eur J Biochem 1967; 2:327–31.

50. Gleason FK, Holmgren A. Thioredoxin and related protein in procaryotes. FEMS Microbiol Rev 1988; 54:271–97.

51. Gotz ME, Dirr A, Burger R, Janetzky B, Weinmuller M, Chan WW, Chen SC, Reichman H, Rausch WD, Riedcer P. Effect of lipoic acid on redox state of coenzyme Q in mice treated with 1-methyl-4-phenyl-1,2,3,6-tetrahydropyridine and diethyldithiocarbamate. Eur J Pharmacol 1994; 266:291–300.

52. Kagan V, Serbinova E, Packer L. Antioxidant effects of ubiquinones in microsomes and mitochondria are mediated by tocopherol recycling. Biochem Biophys Res Commun 1990; 169:851–7.

53. Roy S, Sen CK, Tritschler H, Packer L. Modulation of cellular reducing equivalent homeostasis by alpha lipoic acid: mechanisms and implication for diabetes and ischemic injury. Biochem Pharmacol 1997; 53:393–9.

54. Jacob S, Henriksen EJ, Schiemann AL, Simon I, Clancy DE, Tritschler HJ, Jung WI, Augustin HJ, Dietze GJ. Enhancement of glucose disposal in patients with type 2 diabetes by alpha lipoic acid. Arzneimittel-Forschung 1995; 45:872–4.

55. Han D, Tritschler HJ, Packer L. Alpha-lipoic acid increases intracellular glutathione in a human T-lymphocyte Jurkat cell line. Biochem Biophys Res 1995; 207:258–64.

56. Busse E, Zimmer G, Schopohl B, Kornhuber B. Influence of α-lipoic acid on intracellular glutathione in vitro and in vivo. Arzneimittel-Forschung/Drug Res 1992; 43:829–31.

57. Meister A. In: Dolphin D, Poulson R, Avramovic O, eds, Glutathione: Chemical, Biochemical, and Medical Aspects, pp. 367–73. Wiley, New York, 1989.

58. Han D, Handelman G, Marcocci L, Sen CK, Roy S, Kobuchi H, Tritschler HJ, Flohe L, Packer L. Lipoic acid increases de novo synthesis of cellular glutathione by improving cystine utilization. Biofactors 1997; 9:1–18.

59. Trump BF, Berezesky IK. The role of cytosolic Ca^{2+} in cell injury, necrosis and apoptosis. Curr Opin Cell Biol 1992; 4:227–32.

60. Suzuki YJ, Forman HJ, Sevanian A. Oxidants as stimulators of signal transduction. Free Radical Biol Med 1997; 22:269–85.

61. Bootman MD, Berridge MJ. The elemental principles of calcium signaling. Cell 1995; 83:675–8.

62. Sen CK, Roy S, Packer L. Involvement of intracellular Ca^{2+} in oxidant-induced NF-κB activation. FEBS Lett 1996; 385:58–62.

63. Sen CK, Packer L. Antioxidant and redox regulation of gene transcription. FASEB J 1996; 10:709–20.

64. Schweizer M, Richter C. Stimulation of Ca^{+2} release from rat liver mitochondria by the dithiol reagent a-lipoic acid. 1996; 52:1815–20.

65. Baeuerle PA, Henkel T. Function and activation of NF-κB in the immune system. Annu Rev Immunol 1994; 12:141–79.

66. Suzuki YJ, Aggarwal BB, Packer L. Alpha-lipoic acid is a potent inhibitor of NF-κB activation in human T cells. Biochem Biophys Res Commun 1992; 189:1709–15.

67. Suzuki YJ, Packer L. Alpha-lipoic acid is a potent inhibitor of NF-κB activation in human T cells: does the mechanism involve antioxidant activities. In: Packer L, Cadenas E, eds, Biological Oxidants and Antioxidants. Hippokrates Verlag, Stuttgart, 1994.

68. Suzuki YJ, Mizuno M, Tritschler HJ, Packer L. Redox regulation of NF-κB DNA binding activity by dihydrolipoate. Biochem Mol Biol Int 1995; 36:241–6.

69. Packer L, Roy S, Sen CK. α-Lipoic acid: a metabolic antioxidant and potential redox modulator of transcription. Adv Pharmacol 1996; 38:79–101.

70. Ziegler D, Hanefeld M, Ruhnau KJ, Meissner HP, Lobish M, Schutte K, Gries FA. Treatment of symptomatic diabetic peripheral neuropathy with the anti-oxidant a-lipoic acid. A 3-Week Multicentre Randomized Control Trial (ALADIN Study). Diabetologia 1995; 38: 1425–33.

71. Cao X, Phillis JW. The free radical scavenger, α-lipoic acid, protects against cerebral ischemia-reperfusion injury in gerbils. Free Radical Res 1995; 23:365–70.

72. Panigrahi M, Sadguna Y, Shivakumar BR, Kolluri SV, Roy S, Packer L, Ravindranath V. Alpha lipoic acid protects against reperfusion injury following cerebral ischemia in rats. Brain Res 1996; 717:184–8.

73. Bustamante J, Lodge JK, Marcocci L, Tritschler HJ, Packer L, Rihn B. a-Lipoic acid in liver metabolism and disease. Free Radical Biol Med 1998; 24:1023–39.

74. Baur A, Harrer T, Peukert M, Jahn G, Kalden JR, Fleckenstein B. Alpha-lipoic acid is an effective inhibitor of human immuno-deficiency virus (HIV-1) replication. Klin Wochenschr 1991; 69:722–4.

75. Faust A, Burkart V, Ulrich H, Weischer CH, Kolb H. Effect of lipoic acid on cyclophophoamide-induced diabetes and insulitis in nonobese diabetic mice. Int J Immunopharmacol 1994; 16:61–6.

76. Henriksen EJ, Jacob S, Tritschler H, Wellel K, Augustin HJ, Dietze GJ. Chronic thioctic acid treatment increases insulin-stimulated glucose transport activity in skeletal muscle of obese Zucker rats. Diabetes 1994; 1 (suppl) 122A.

77. Suzuki JY, Tsuchiya M, Packer L. Lipoate prevents glucose-induced protein modifications. Free Radical Res Commun 1992; 17:211–7.

78. Schepkin V, Kawabata T, Packer L. NMR study of liopoic acid binding to bovine serum albumin. Biochem Mol Biol Int 1994; 33:879–86.

79. Kawabata T, Packer L. Alpha-lipoate can protect against glycation of serum albumin, but not low density lipoprotein. Biochem Biophys Res Commun 1994; 203:99–104.

80. Sachse G, Willms B. Efficacy of thioctic acid in the therapy of peripheral diabetic neuropathy. In: Gries FA, Freund HJ, Rabe F, Berger H, eds, Aspects of Autonomic Neuropathy in diabetes, pp. 105–8, 1980.

81. Ziegler D, Mayer P, Muhlen H, Gries FA. Effeckte einer Therapie mit α-Liponsaure gegenüber Vitamin B1 bei der diabetischen Neuropathie. Diab Stoffw 1993; 2:443–8.

82. Kilic F, Handelman G, Serbinova E, Packer L, Trevithick JR. Modelling cortical cataractogenesis. 17: In vitro effect of a-lipoic acid on glucose-induced lens membrane damage, a model of diabetic cataractogenesis. Biochem Mol Biol Int 1995; 37:361–70.

83. Maitra I, Serbinova E, Tritschler H, Packer L. Alpha-lipoic acid prevents buthionine sulfoximine-induced cataract formation in newborn rats. Free Radical Biol Med 1995; 18:823–9.

84. Packer L. The role of anti-oxidative treatment of diabetes mellitus. Diabetologia 1993; 36:1212–13.

85. Marui N, Offermann MK, Swerlick R, Kunsch C, Rosen CA, Ahmad M, Alexander RW, Medford W. Vascular cell adhesion molecule-1 (VCAM-1) gene transcription and expression are regulated through an antioxidant-sensitive mechanism in human vascular endothelial cells. J Clin Invest 1993; 92:1866–74.

9 Defining the Role of Dietary Phytochemicals in Modulating Human Immune Function

HAROLD SCHMITZ AND KATI CHEVAUX

As this volume clearly demonstrates, the interaction between nutrition and immune function is multidimensional, highly integrated, and extremely complex. A growing number of reports in the literature suggest that this interaction is true for both "nonessential" components of the diet as well as the classically defined essential micronutrients and macronutrients, with "nonessential" components comprising plant-derived compounds (phytochemicals), certain bacteria and their metabolites, certain fatty acids and peptides, and so forth. Indeed, epidemiological data strongly suggest that intake of foods rich in certain phytochemicals, such as fruits, vegetables, and nuts, is protective against chronic diseases such as cancer *(1–3)* and cardiovascular disease *(4,5)*. Given the critical role of immune cells and signaling molecules in these health conditions, these data imply a potential interaction of phytochemicals with immune function. This hypothesis is supported by a large amount of data demonstrating the ability of some phytochemicals to modulate immune cells and signaling molecules in vitro and in certain animal models. However, it must be recognized that current knowledge of the interaction between these "nonessential" components, including phytochemicals, and immune function generally lags behind that available in the literature on essential nutrients, especially with respect to human clinical data.

INTRODUCTION

Research on phytochemicals and their impact on immune function has increased significantly during the past two decades as a result of encouraging epidemiological associations, such as those cited above. Our understanding of the immunological impact of a *few* of these dietary constituents has increased concomitantly. Indeed, in vitro data strongly suggest that some nonessential components of human diets, including several phytochemicals, have a significant immunomodulating potential *(6)*. With respect to these phytochemicals, the carotenoids and flavonoids are two classes of compounds that represent our current state-of-the-art understanding of

how "nonessential" plant constituents may impact human immune function and, possibly, be useful for both the maintenance of optimal health and/or treatment of certain immunological disorders. Accordingly, these two classes of compounds will be used as working examples where appropriate to emphasize the following key points of this chapter.

- The fundamental role that phytochemicals can potentially play in modulating immune function.
- The importance of utilizing appropriate animal and in vitro experiments to elucidate the potential mechanisms by which phytochemicals may modulate immune function.
- The need for well-designed clinical trials to assess the impact of phytochemicals on human immune function.

Underlying each of these points is a recurring theme of why a fundamental understanding of the chemical and biological properties of phytochemicals should be aggressively pursued and integrated into the design of experiments if meaningful data are to be obtained regarding their impact on human immune function.

Upon examination of this chapter, the reader should appreciate the potential of certain phytochemicals to impact human immune function. More importantly, it is hoped that the reader will recognize the need for research teams to integrate expertise capable of understanding the fundamental chemistry of phytochemicals, the complex biochemistry of phytochemicals, and the ability to properly evaluate the actions of these phytochemicals in human clinical trials if we can ever hope to fully understand and leverage these dietary components to enhance human health and well-being.

HISTORICAL PERSPECTIVES

The influence of phytochemicals on immune function has been studied for thousands of years. Although the tools of modern science could obviously not be employed throughout most of this time, many effects now termed as "clinically relevant" were observed using animal models and human subjects *(7)*. During this century, a tremendous amount of research during this century using a variety of analytical techniques (especially liquid chromatography) has identified a plethora of compounds, or phytochemicals, in plants *(8)*. Although a thorough review of these compounds

From: *Nutrition and Immunology: Principles and Practice* (ME Gershwin et al. eds.), © Humana Press, Inc., Totowa, NJ

and their chemical families is beyond the scope of this chapter, a brief review of select aspects of carotenoid and flavonoid research as it relates to their respective immunomodulatory properties will provide insight into both the discovery process often associated with phytochemicals as well as how a foundation is developed for subsequent research efforts.

Members from both the carotenoid and flavonoid families have a rich history as objects of scientific investigation, and evidence suggesting that compounds from each class could influence the general nutrition, health, and well-being of humans began to arise in the late 1920s and early 1930s. In the case of carotenoids, carotenes and xanthophylls were first isolated in the 19th century by Wackenroder and Berzelius (8). It is significant to note that carotenoids were one of the fractions separated by Tswett in the early part of this century, when he employed his pioneering liquid-chromatographic technique to separate components from a plant extract (9). The impact of carotenoids on human health began to crystallize when it was demonstrated by Moore in 1929 that certain carotenoids can be precursors to vitamin A-active retinoids and Karrer determined the chemical structures of beta-carotene (BC) and vitamin A (10). An immense body of research then followed, which demonstrated that these retinoids, derived from provitamin A carotenoids, are essential to several biological functions in humans, including satisfactory immune function (11). During the early part of the 1980s, largely in response to the hypothesis paper by Peto et al. (1) postulating a potential effect of BC on the incidence of cancer in humans, researchers began to investigate whether *intact* carotenoids might play critical roles in prevention of chronic disease. Previously, research in this area was focused on vitamin A-active retinoid metabolites of select carotenoids, as well as available synthetic retinoid analogs. Thus, the epidemiological association with cancer preventative properties was the catalytic agent, which stimulated aggressive investigation into the influence of carotenoids on the immune function, with the operative hypothesis being that modulation of the immune response was a key factor in cancer prevention (12).

Like the carotenoids, the flavonoids have been recognized as having biological activity relevant to human health for several decades. Indeed, certain members were once thought to have vitaminlike attributes, and a mixture of citrus flavonoids were, in fact, assigned the name vitamin P in the late 1930s because of their putative activity in stabilizing the biological activity of ascorbic acid (13). Over the next few decades, it became clear that these compounds did not possess classically defined vitamin activity, and the designation was dropped. However, research demonstrating the ability of select flavonoids to modulate biological systems relevant to human health has continued to appear in the literature (14), and the evidence supporting the value of consuming these compounds in the diet is, in some cases, quite compelling (4,15–17). Similar to the carotenoids, recognition of the hypothesis that immune function is a critical component of chronic disease prevention/treatment coupled with epidemiological data associating high flavonoid intake with decreased risk of certain chronic diseases (14) has stimulated research examining the influence of these compounds on the immune system. In contrast to the carotenoids, substantial evidence exists suggesting that some flavonoids can be deleterious to normal biological function and, indeed, toxic to some species when consumed in acute doses (18).

The thoughtful reader will appreciate the influence of 20th-century nutrition research philosophy and the way in which phyto-chemicals have been studied in this context; that is, emphasis has been given to studying the properties of individual compounds (e.g., BC and quercetin) within these often large and diverse chemical families rather than the mixtures which typically occur in foodstuffs and the diet. Only recently have deliberate efforts by a few investigators been made to begin researching the biological effects of *mixtures* of these compounds using state-of-the-art techniques. Unfortunately, this shortcoming is coupled with an historical paucity of good clinical data regarding the ability of dietary phytochemicals, including carotenoids and flavonoids, to modulate human immune function.

CHEMISTRY AND OCCURRENCE

Basic structural information and general occurrence in nature is available for many phytochemicals of interest (6). With respect to carotenoids and flavonoids, a complete review of their chemistry and occurrence is beyond the scope of this chapter and the reader is therefore directed to other references available in the literature (8,13). However, it is important to appreciate the usefulness of understanding the chemistry of these and other phytochemicals and the implication this chemistry has in defining their ability to modulate immune function. Hence, a brief description of key chemical characteristics to consider is given here to provide a foundation for meaningful experimentation in biological systems and clinical application, with the hope that the reader will pursue more thorough reviews on the chemistry of phytochemicals of interest to obtain a deeper knowledge of their biological potential.

Both carotenoids and flavonoids occur widely in the plant kingdom and impart distinctive color and flavor characteristics to many foods. However, their presence and availability in the diet differs dramatically in both quantity and type, depending on the individual foodstuff and the techniques used to harvest, process, and/or cook the food (19,20). The biosynthesis of both classes of compounds is reasonably well understood and has been reviewed elsewhere (13,21). A critical point that must be appreciated and will therefore be emphasized throughout the rest of this chapter is that individual compounds within these families can have, and often do have, significantly different chemical and biological properties. Thus, it is incorrect to assume that the relevant properties/bioactivities of a given carotenoid or flavonoid can be *a priori* extrapolated to other members of their respective families, even when they are seemingly closely related in structure.

CAROTENOIDS In general, carotenoids are a class of compounds composed of eight isoprene units such that the linking of the isoprene units in the middle of the molecule is reversed (Fig. 1). The numbering of the carbon atoms proceeds from one end to the center of the molecule as 1–15, and from the other end to the center as 1′–15′. The additional numbering of the methyl groups present are 16–20 and 16′–20′, respectively. The Greek letters beta, epsilon, kappa, phi, chi, and psi indicate the configurations of the end groups. Beta and epsilon are used to indicate six-carbon-atom ring end groups, kappa indicates five-carbon-atom ring groups, phi and chi indicate aromatic end groups, and psi indicates no ring or aromatic structures at the specified end of the carotenoid. Complete rules for carotenoid nomenclature may be found in Isler's monograph (22).

Straub listed 563 characterized individual carotenoids in 1987, with several more having been characterized since, putting the actual number at something greater than 600 (8). The actual number of naturally occurring carotenoids is significantly larger

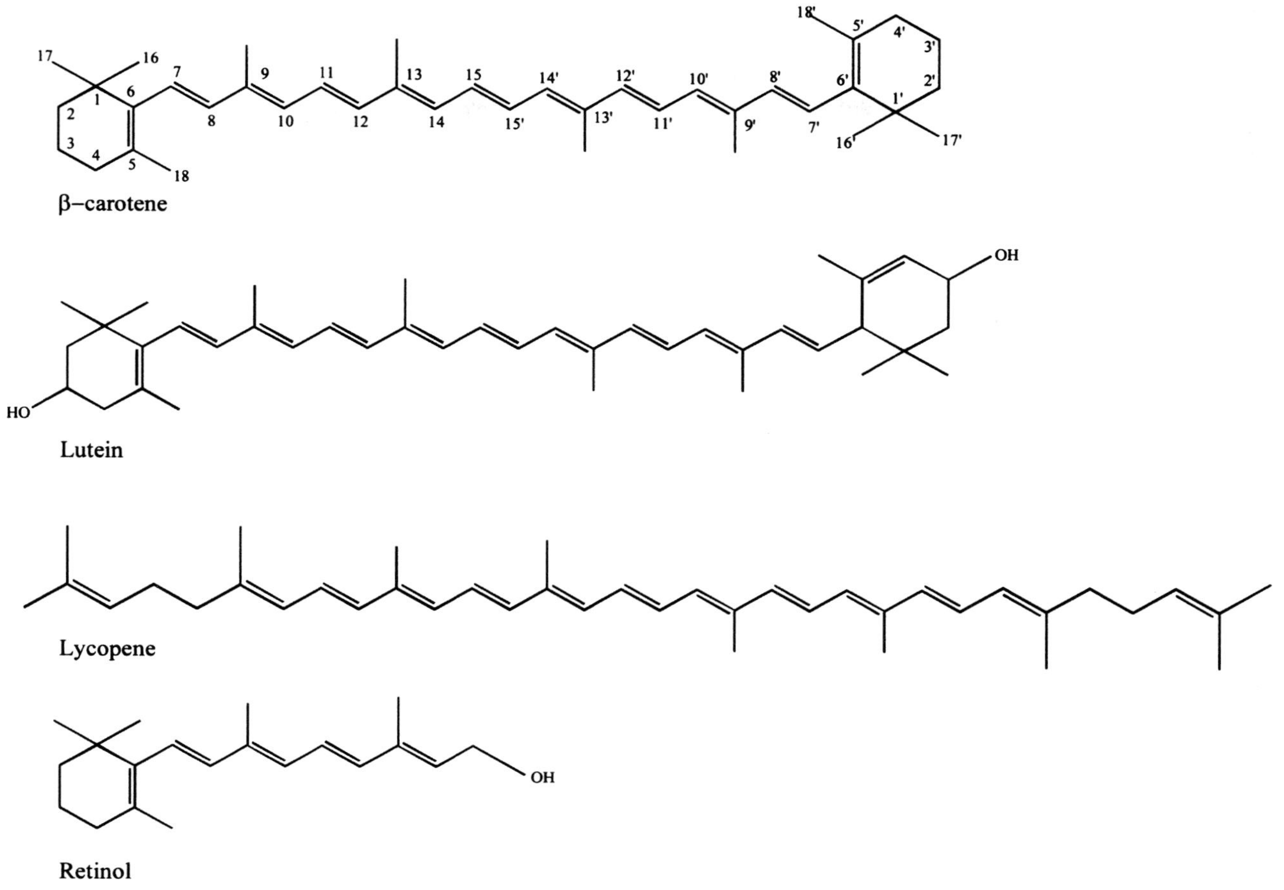

β−carotene

Lutein

Lycopene

Retinol

Fig. 1. Structures of beta-carotene, lutein, lycopene, and retinol.

because of the number of optical and/or geometric isomers of individual carotenoids not listed separately in the aforementioned texts and are known to exist in the diet as a result of food processing practices *(23)*. Most of the carotenoids are oxygenated (xanthophylls), and relatively few are exclusively hydrocarbon in nature (carotenes), with the entire class being systematically arranged into four major groups:

1. C40 hydrocarbons, which consist of acyclic, alicyclic, and aromatic carotenoids.
2. C40 xanthophylls, which consist of mono-, di-, and poly-hydroxy compounds, ethers, aldehydes, ketones, and acids, which may be arranged in a number of ways, including acyclic, alicyclic, aromatic, epoxide, and other arrangements.
3. Carotenoids with more than 40 carbon atoms.
4. Apo-carotenoids with less than 40 carbon atoms.

Most carotenoids are brightly colored pigments that can be detected by the human eye, an analytically useful property that is the result of a chromophore consisting of multiple conjugated double bonds present in most carotenoids. However, the high degree of conjugation present in most carotenoids may lead to facile isomerization and/or degradation of the original compound. Indeed, the stability of carotenoids is dependent on a number of factors, including the matrix in which a given carotenoid is delivered, as well as the exposure to heat, light, and oxygen over time

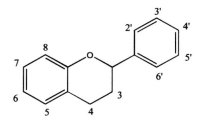

Fig. 2. Basic structure of flavonoids.

to which the compound is exposed *(24,25)*. Control experiments to define the stability within a given matrix and administration protocol of the carotenoid(s) in question should *always* be done to ensure interpretable results. Finally, it should be noted that a relatively wide range of solubilities exists within the carotenoid family because of the variety of structures and their respective isomers. The impact this may have on delivery of select carotenoids to either in vitro systems or as part of experimental diets must always be considered.

FLAVONOIDS Flavonoids are phenolic compounds composed of a C15 flavane nucleus made up of two benzene rings connected by a pyrane ring (Fig. 2). The over 4000 individual flavonoid compounds can be subdivided into a few basic structures: flavonols, flavones, catechins, flavonones, anthocyanidins, and isoflavones (Fig. 3). With the exception of catechins, most

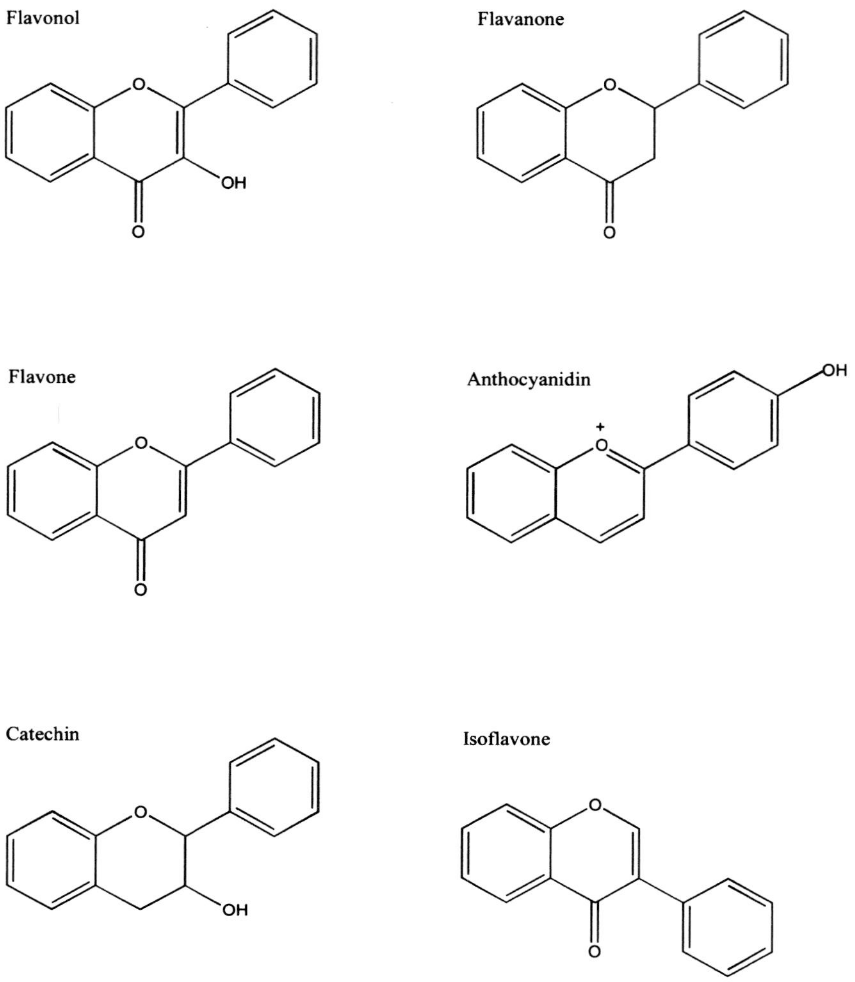

Fig. 3. Classes of flavonoids.

flavonoids occur in nature as a glycoside (i.e., having a sugar moiety attached to a hydroxyl group). In addition, individual flavonoids can be further characterized by hydroxylation, methoxylation, and acylation at various positions, as well as naturally occurring polymerization, which results from the linking of individual flavonoid monomers. The procyanidin series found in tea and cocoa are examples of foods in which these polymers may be found *(19,26)*. As with carotenoids, this polymeric class of flavonoids has an enormous number of potential isomeric variations. Taken together, these structural variations have important implications for the physiological functions discussed in this chapter; for example, the well-established antioxidant activity of flavonoids has been related to specific structural characteristics *(27)*.

Because of the probable dependence of most flavonoid functions on chemical structure and stereochemistry, alterations resulting from storage, handling, and processing must be considered when drawing conclusions about the physiological relevance of flavonoid intake from foods. For example, a range of structurally diverse products and molecular weights can develop during the processing and fermentation of green to black tea, such as oxidation products, theaflavins, and condensed flavonoids *(19)*. Another important consideration when studying the chemistry and functionality of flavonoids is the extent to which they may have other

chemical moieties attached. For example, there are many examples of glycated compounds that have distinctly different chemical and biological properties when compared to their respective aglycones *(28,29)*. Beyond structure, chemical properties that are of importance to the investigator include solubility, stability, and redox activity of different flavonoids. As might be guessed given the large number of flavonoid compounds naturally present in foods, these properties are wide ranging and, thus, must be considered carefully on a case-by-case basis when designing experiments.

As with the carotenoids and many other classes of phytochemicals, the complexity of chemical characteristics briefly described earlier places a premium on structural identification of flavonoids and understanding their unique chemical properties in order to accurately assess their ability, through dietary intake, to modulate immune function.

DIETARY INTAKE, ABSORPTION AND METABOLISM

Key considerations for understanding the influence of phytochemicals on immune function include the quantity and type of compound of interest consumed in the diet, their bioavailability or lack thereof, and what metabolic transformations take place either in the gastrointestinal (GI) tract or subsequent to absorption. In the context of immunomodulation, it is important to note that dietary components *not* absorbed into portal or lymphatic circulation can still impact immune function through interaction with the GI tract, which is rich in cells either directly or indirectly related to immune function *(30)*.

INTAKE Historically, the ability to accurately assess dietary intake of individual phytochemicals has been difficult because of the lack of appropriate databases. Recently, however, the tools for better assessing carotenoid intake have become available as a result of the database compiled and published by the United States Department of Agriculture *(31)*. Use of this and similar databases has yielded results suggesting that intakes of several milligrams per day is common in the United States, with the majority of this intake comprised of BC, lutein, and lycopene *(32)*. A similar database is not yet available for flavonoids or for most other phytochemical families. However, a review of the data currently used for flavonoids demonstrates how a rough estimate of intake can be obtained and that sufficient quantities of these compounds can be consumed to potentially impact immune function, assuming at least some of their in vitro bioactivity is relevant in vivo to humans. It should be noted that this is likely true for other classes of dietary phytochemicals.

Five flavonoids have been quantified in various beverages and certain fruits and vegetables, as has the isoflavonoid content of soybean products *(33,34)*. Onions emerge as a rich source of quercetin, with kale, broccoli, endive, French beans, turnip tops, apples and apple juice, wine, and tea having measurable quantities of various flavonoids. This data set provides the basis for flavonoid food composition data, but caution must be used when drawing conclusions based on these values because of the early stages of analytical method development and the limited number of flavonoids quantified. Flavonoids excluded from such analyses may have potential health benefits based on in vitro data. For example, a relatively substantial body of in vitro data and animal experiments indicates that components of tea may have health benefits, however, intake data using the above database of flavonols and flavones would not represent the main flavonoid component of tea, namely the catechins.

An early estimate of daily flavonoid intake was 1 g/d *(13)* of the glycone, with the major sources in the United States being beverages (cocoa, cola, coffee, tea, beer), fruits, and juices *(35)*. More recent estimates of flavonol and flavone intake were proposed in the Seven Countries Study in which intake ranged from 2.6 to 68.2 mg/d *(15)*. Other studies using the same food composition data placed mean intake in the 4- to 40-mg/d range *(4,16,17,36,37)*. Because of the limited number of flavonoids quantified in the diet, total flavonoid intake calculated in these studies is probably an underestimate of total flavonoid intake.

Although considerable work remains to be done before the intake, absorption, transport, and metabolism of phytochemicals is well defined, many phytochemicals, including members from both the carotenoid *(24,38)* and flavonoid *(28,39)* families, can be absorbed and, in some cases, excreted as metabolites in the urine. Although tissue uptake and distribution of carotenoids has been studied *(24)*, little is known on this subject for the flavonoids. A brief review of some of the work done to elucidate aspects of flavonoid and carotenoid absorption and metabolism will illustrate the complicated nature of this process. It is important to understand the fate of phytochemicals after ingestion when designing appropriate in vitro, in vivo, and clinical experiments that define if and

how select phytochemicals can impact immune function. A recent article by Novotny et al. *(40)* describing the use of deuterium-labeled BC in combination with mathematical modeling techniques demonstrates a method by which the absorption and metabolism of phytochemicals may be better understood in the future.

The absorption, metabolism, and bioavailability of flavonoids have been reviewed recently *(39)*, with tea being one of the most studied food sources *(41)*. Although the absorption of flavonoids has been shown in some animal models, definitive data on the absorption of a wide range of flavonoid compounds in humans are not available. In general, catechins were better absorbed than quercetin *(39)*. With the exception of catechins, most flavonoids present in foods are bound to sugar moieties as glycosides. Unfortunately, it is unknown whether humans can liberate free flavonoid from glycosides, although enzymes capable of liberating free flavonoid have not been found in the small intestine. Based on the difference between intake and excretion in ileostomy patients, the intake of onions containing quercetin glycosides resulted in the absorption of quercetin to a greater extent than absorption of the pure aglycone, but plasma quercetin was not measured in these subjects *(28)*. Catechins have been identified in the blood of rats after oral administration and in human plasma after consumption of tea or catechin-containing beverage *(41)*. Preliminary evidence exists, based on the absorption of radioactive catechin dimer in mice and the increase in plasma polyphenol levels after consumption of tea, that catechin condensation products are absorbed *(41)*. Whether the condensation products are absorbed intact is not known. Beyond this limited amount of information, very little is known about tissue distribution and accumulation of the flavonoids.

Flavonoid metabolites can be produced by colonic bacteria and liver enzymes and should also be considered as potential regulators of immune function. Flavonoids, which escape absorption in the small intestine, can potentially undergo hydrolysis and ring fission to phenolic acids *(13)*. After absorption, flavonoid hydroxy groups can be conjugated with glucuronic acid or sulfate in the liver and methylation may occur. Metabolism after absorption also includes the addition or exposure of hydroxyl groups, conjugation with glucuronic acid, sulfate, or glycine, resulting in a molecule that can be excreted in the urine. *O*-Methylation can occur, resulting in the inactivation of the catechol. The fate of flavonoids unabsorbed in the small intestine or those reabsorbed from circulation with bile includes hydrolysis of any sugar or conjugate and ring cleavage by colonic bacteria, with the susceptibility of flavonoids to ring cleavage being dependent on structure *(39)*. These metabolic transformations of flavonoids are only beginning to be defined, and it is important to remember that they are specific to the flavonoid under study.

Other important factors to consider regarding absorption of flavonoids from food include protein content, especially proline-rich proteins such as those found in milk, as they are known to bind and reduce the bioavailability of polyphenols *(42)*. Conversely, the effects of polyphenols on the absorption of these proteins as well as minerals such as nonheme iron in the diet must also be considered *(41)*.

In contrast to the flavonoids, the carotenoids are an example of a phytochemical whose absorption and metabolism has been studied more extensively. Indeed, the absorption of carotenoids has been studied for decades, especially with regard to the fate of BC and other provitamin A carotenoids. In general, absorption

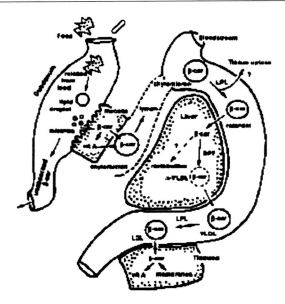

Fig. 4. Pathways and processes involved in the absorption plasma transport and tissue uptake of carotenoids such as beta-carotene. (Adapted from Parker RS. Absorption, metabolism, and transport of carotenoids. FASEB J 1996; 10:542–51.)

of carotenoids is dependent on mechanisms common to fat-soluble micronutrients, with the presence of conjugated bile salts being a requirement for uptake of BC into epithelial cells (10,38). In addition, some carotenoids, specifically the xanthophylls, can exist as esters or as part of a protein complex and can be absorbed in their free form after exposure to digestive actions. Of great importance to clinical investigators is the observation that carotenoids fed in oil or detergent are better absorbed than those from foods. It is also important to note that, unlike vitamin A, as the dose of carotenoids given increases, the percentage absorbed decreases (10). The amount of various carotenoids absorbed is not specifically known with estimates reported in the literature ranging from 10% to 60% of a given dose, depending on the type of carotenoid, fat content of the meal, fiber, presence of other fat-soluble nutrients, food or pill matrix, and other factors (10,11,38).

The transport of carotenoids after absorption is dependent on incorporation into chylomicra and secretion into the lymphatic system (10,38). Subsequently, more hydrophobic carotenoids such as BC are partitioned into very low-density lipoprotein (VLDL) and low-density lipoprotein (LDL) fractions, whereas the more polar xanthophylls tend to accumulate in the high-density lipoprotein (HDL) fraction. Both polar and nonpolar carotenoids are distributed to many tissues within the body (10,24), including liver, lung, muscle, kidney, adipose, testes, and adrenal. Present knowledge regarding the absorption and transport of BC in vivo is summarized in Fig. 4.

Following absorption and transport to specific tissues, it is important to recognize the potential for metabolite formation from intact phytochemicals and the role these metabolites can play in modulating immune function. A classic example is the conversion of provitamin A carotenoids such as BC to vitamin A, which plays a key role in maintaining a healthy immune system (11). The susceptibility of the highly unsaturated carotenoids to oxidative attack, either chemically or enzymatically, suggests that

metabolites having no vitamin A activity may also be formed in vivo (10), and their potential to modulate aspects of immune function should also be considered.

Taken together, it can be concluded from our current understanding of carotenoids and flavonoids that members of these phytochemical families and their in vivo metabolites are available for potential immunomodulating activities in vivo in humans, whether within the GI tract or other tissues following absorption and transport. Regarding phytochemicals in general, it is apparent from the preceding discussion that classes of compounds, and specific compounds within these classes in many cases, must be considered on an individual basis to truly understand their potential to reach target tissues important for immunomodulation. In addition, the potential for formation of bioactive metabolites from phytochemical compounds must also be considered. Use of synthetically or biosynthetically labeled compounds will undoubtedly play an important part in helping to provide more definitive information in these areas.

USE OF PHYTOCHEMICALS IN IN VITRO, IN VIVO, AND CLINICAL EXPERIMENTS

The labile and reactive natures of carotenoids and flavonoids have been referred to in previous sections. Although not always facile, the propensity for alteration or degradation of the chemical structure of any phytochemical should always be considered. This is true not only when isolating or synthesizing the compound but also when assessing the biological activity of the given phytochemical(s). Thus, the quantitative and qualitative aspects of the compound(s) being tested must be understood as clearly as possible from an analytical chemistry perspective. For example, carotenoids generally exist in foodstuffs as complex mixtures, unless specifically fortified with a synthetically derived compound (Fig. 5). When a foodstuff appears to contain reasonable phytochemical candidate components vis à vis their/its potential impact on the immune system, an effort should be made to extract this portion of the foodstuff for further evaluation by model systems. Already at this very early stage, a number of considerations must be made to ensure the reproducibility of future experiments based on the results of this initial work. Using carotenoids as a working example, these considerations include the following:

1. Does the extract contain one carotenoid (very unlikely), such as BC, or is it a mixture of several (very likely) carotenoids? Further, does it contain geometric and/or optical isomers? As represented in Fig. 6, the carotenoid profile in biological samples, such as human serum, can be quite complex. This is a critical point given that different carotenoids, even those that are structural (i.e., alpha-carotene, beta-carotene, and lycopene) or geometric isomers (i.e., all-*trans*-beta-carotene and 9-*cis*-beta-carotene), can have very different biological activities. Two examples germane to the interaction between nutrition and immune function clearly illustrate the importance of this point. The former is the well-known fact that each of the candidate carotenoids listed above have significantly different provitamin A activity, with alpha-carotene and 9-*cis*-beta-carotene (43) having much less than that of all-trans BC and others having no activity at all (11). Thus, if the immunomodulating ability of the extract is based on the ability of the model system to convert provitamin A carotenoids into

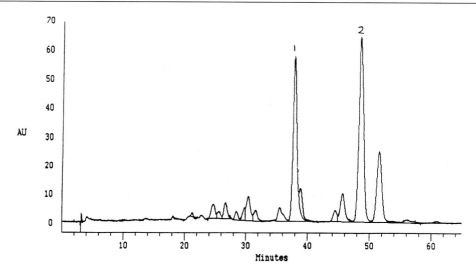

Fig. 5. High-performance liquid chromatographic (HPLC) separation of carotenoids in palm oil using a YMC C$_{30}$ stationary phase in combination with a mobile phase consisting of 11% Methyl Tert Butyl Ether (MTBE) in MeOH at 2.0 mL/min. Peak 1 is all-*trans*-alpha-carotene and peak 2 is all-*trans*-beta-carotene. The other peaks are additional carotenoids and geometric carotenoid isomers present in palm oil.

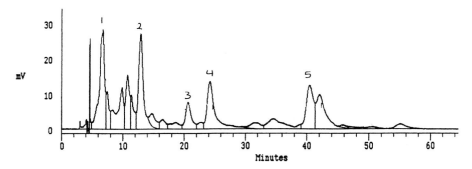

Fig. 6. HPLC separation of carotenoids in human serum using a 25-cm Vydac 201 C$_{18}$ stationary phase in combination with a mobile phase consisting of 1% THF in MeOH (+0.05% Triethylamine (TEA) at 0.7 mL/min. Peak 1 is lutein + zeaxanthin, peak 2 is beta-cryptoxanthin, peak 3 is alpha-carotene, peak 4 is beta-carotene, and peak 5 is lycopene. The other peaks are additional carotenoids and geometric isomers present in human serum.

vitamin A active retinoids, standardization of the extract for use in human trials should focus on the most active provitamin A component, or BC in this case. If, on the other hand, the immunomodulating ability of the extract is based on the ability to quench singlet oxygen in the model system, standardization should focus on the best antioxidant present with this activity, or lycopene in this case *(44)*. Therefore, the researcher must understand the type and amount of carotenoids present in the extract so that this can be matched against future extracts that, although obtained from the same type of foodstuff, may have been taken from a different cultivar, undergone significant exposure to light, oxygen and/or heat during storage and processing, and so forth, and thus contain a significantly different mixture of carotenoids with significantly different biological potential.

2. Has the extract been prepared and stored in such a manner that no alteration/degradation of the carotenoids has occurred as compared to those originally contained in the foodstuff? As noted previously, carotenoids are generally sensitive to light, heat, oxygen, and extreme pH's, especially when removed from the food matrix they are within naturally. Thus, isomerization and degradation products are often generated during the extraction and storage of carotenoids from biological samples, unless proper procedures are followed *(24,25)*. This consideration is of great concern to the investigator because of two possible outcomes, both of which can result incorrect conclusions by the researcher and, thus, inappropriate future research direction. The first is that immunomodulating activity in the extract may be lost because of the conversion from active carotenoid components to inactive isomers or degradation products. The second is the inverse of the first; that is, the extract will demonstrate significant immunomodulating activity because of the formation of active isomers or degradation products.

3. What is the chemical nature of the extract and of each of the carotenoids contained in the extract? This has tremendous potential impact on experimental design in that solvent systems must be developed and validated that ensure

proper and nontoxic delivery of the carotenoids to target cells or tissues. This is often accomplished using hydrophobic systems owing to the lipophilicity of many carotenoids. However, some extracts may contain carotenoids with a wide range of solubilities (i.e., lutein vs beta-carotene), requiring a solvent system with appropriate physicochemical characteristics to deliver these carotenoids to the cell culture system. Its worth noting that geometric isomers can have different solubilities, as demonstrated by the significantly different chromatographic retention times of all-*trans*- and 9-Z-beta-carotene on a calcium hydroxide stationary phase *(23)* and potentially different antioxidant activities *(45)*.

From a biological perspective, species differences must be considered with respect to both absorption and metabolism of the immunomodulating candidate phytochemical. For example, it is well known that there are differences in qualitative and quantitative absorption of carotenoids among species *(46,47)*. Given the well-known ability of vitamin A nutriture to profoundly influence immune function, this is not a subtle difference to contemplate with regard to the potential bioactivity of provitamin A carotenoids.

Thus, knowledge of a few key chemical and biological characteristics of candidate phytochemicals is essential to begin understanding how a given phytochemical may impact immune function in humans, including the following:

1. Understanding the type and amount of chemicals in a given extract, especially when focusing on large and diverse families such as carotenoids and flavonoids
2. Understanding the chemistry of candidate phytochemicals in order to ensure stability during extraction and storage and to ensure appropriate delivery to in vitro or in vivo experimental models and during clinical trials
3. Understanding the absorption and metabolism of candidate phytochemicals to assess the true structure–function relationships responsible for immunomodulation and appreciating the potential species differences when using animal models

HUMAN CLINICAL EXPERIMENTS

Appropriately designed and well-controlled clinical experiments will ultimately define the role of phytochemicals in modulating immune function. In this context, carotenoids are among a small group of compounds that have been tested in at least a few reasonably good clinical trials. However, it is important to note that this research has focused exclusively on BC, and thus nothing is really known about how mixtures of carotenoids, such as those typically found in the diet, may modulate immune function. The reasons for this focus include the documented safety of BC *(48)*, the availability of large quantities of synthetic BC, and epidemiological literature that indicate associations between dietary intake of BC and/or its presence in the serum of populations and health benefits such as decreased cancer risk. This emphasis on BC has also been amplified by promising in vitro and animal model data suggesting immunoenhancing properties of this carotenoid (a brief review of which follows this section). The choice of BC was a sensible one, given these considerations; however, the provitamin A nature of this carotenoid presents a significant confounding factor because of the immunomodulating properties of vitamin A.

A number of trials have been reported in the literature; however, the findings from this research are equivocal. Although a number of researchers have found an immunoenhancing effect when subjects were given BC supplements, some investigators have found no effect. In addition, some trials indicated immunoenhancing effects that peaked at an intermediate time point during the study and then declined for the remaining portion of the study, suggesting the promise as an immunoenhancing agent only in the context of short-term use applications. A brief review of some of the key papers in the field will illustrate the current confusion in the area and serve to underscore the need for more well-designed clinical trials.

Watson et al. have investigated the effects of BC supplementation in older adults (mean age >55 yr) and found indications of an immunostimulatory effect *(49,50)*. This interpretation was suggested by significant increases observed in surface markers for T-helper and natural-killer (NK) cells on lymphoid cells, as well as for PBMCs having interleukin-2 receptors (IL-2R) when BC was given orally for at least 2 mo in doses of 30 mg or greater. In addition, one of the trials suggested a dose-response relationship between BC and markers of immunostimulation, including IL-2R and NK cells *(50)*. Doses administered in this trial were 0, 15, 30, 45, and 60 mg/d for 3 mo. Interestingly, values for these markers had returned to pretrial levels 2 mo after cessation of treatment. Others have reported positive associations with immunostimulation as a result of BC supplementation, although the results have not always agreed with respect to which aspect of the immune system was being stimulated *(51)*.

In contrast to the above-cited reports, there are also data from other clinical trials suggesting that BC has no effect on immune function in humans. Daudu et al. observed no effect of BC depletion, repletion, or moderate supplementation on markers of immune function in adult women over a time period of several months *(52)*. These markers included IL-2R and lymphocyte subsets. It is important to note that this trial was designed to investigate BC *depletion* from the diet rather than supplementation with large doses (e.g., >30 mg/d). Another trial investigated the effects of ingesting 0, 15, 45, 180, or 300 mg of BC for 1 mo in adults (mean age of 34 yr). As with the work of Daudu et al., these investigators observed no effects on immunological indexes, including NK cells, IL-2R, and lymphocyte subsets *(53)*.

The contrasting results reviewed above do not appear to present conclusive evidence of an immunomodulatory role for BC (or other carotenoids) in humans; however, a closer examination of the data suggests that further research is warranted. This is especially true for subpopulations that may be immunocompromised or are undergoing immunosenescence, such as the elderly. Indeed, in the above-reviewed studies, positive results were seen in the trials using elderly subjects, whereas the two trials reporting no effect were completed using younger subjects. Recent work by Meydani's group supports this observation, as it was observed that the BC supplementation protocol in the Physician's Health Trial (50 mg BC given on alternating days for 10–12 yr) eliminated differences in NK cell activity between elderly subjects and middle-aged subjects. BC supplementation had no effect on immune function in middle-aged subjects *(51)*.

Factors other than age also have to be considered when assessing the potential immunomodulatory effects of carotenoids, including vitamin A status, overall nutrient status, purity of carotenoid supplements, and environmental factors. An excellent example of influence of environment is the work of Roe et al., who demonstrated a protective effect of carotenoid supplementation against ultraviolet (UV)-induced immunosuppression *(54)*. This work was stimulated by earlier work done by Mathews-Roth demonstrating a protective effect of BC supplementation in individuals suffering from erythropoietic protoporphyria *(55)*. This is an especially intriguing piece of work given the well-established role of carotenoids in providing photoprotection for plants and the exceptional ability of carotenoids to quench singlet oxygen *(56)*. Thus, it is possible that carotenoids can protect immune function against damage by UV radiation *(57)*. In this context, it is interesting to note that other investigators have shown that lycopene concentrations in skin is reduced to a greater extent than BC *(58)* and, thus, may be participating in photobiological-catalyzed reactions relevant to immunomodulation.

Finally, although the epidemiological work supporting an immunomodulatory role for carotenoids was, by definition, an association with complex mixtures of carotenoids found in the diet, no clinical work has been reported using these types of mixtures. This type of work is desperately needed and will require fundamental understanding of the differences in chemistry and biological activity of different carotenoids commonly found in the diet. Clearly, these needs extend across all of the phytochemical classes thought to have immunomodulatory activities.

IN VITRO AND IN VIVO ANIMAL EXPERIMENTS

Although clinical trials provide final proof of bioactivity, well-designed in vitro and in vivo animal model experiments can be quite useful in elucidating structure–function and mechanistic relationships between phytochemicals and immune function. A considerable amount of work has been done examining the effect of select carotenoids and flavonoids on immune function in in vitro and in vivo models. With regard to BC, this work has been used to provide the foundation for assays performed on samples taken from subjects in clinical trials. A brief review of the in vitro and in vivo work done to explore the immunomodulating potential of carotenoids and flavonoids will give perspective on the scope of information that can be obtained about phytochemicals and their biological activities prior to initiation of clinical experiments.

A large proportion of the work done to understand the mechanism and role of carotenoids in immune function has focused on their effect on the production of select cytokines (the key immunomodulating roles of this class of compounds is discussed in other chapters of this volume). This work has demonstrated the ability of select carotenoids, primarily BC, to influence the production of certain cytokines in a number of cell culture models. Because of the evidence for how immune function might influence cancer prevention, initial focus was placed on the cytokines most thought to possess anticancer activity, namely tumor necrosis factor alpha (TNF-α) and interleukin-1 (IL-1) as well as the ability of beta-carotene to stimulate T-lymphocyte proliferation *(51–59–61)*. Research using animal models has provided supporting evidence for much of this work, with Shapiro and Bendich demonstrating significant increases in T- and B-lymphocyte responses upon mitogen stimulation after feeding rats a diet containing 0.2% by weight of either BC or canthaxanthin *(62)*. This report was especially important because it described an immunomodulating potential for a non-provitamin A carotenoid (canthaxanthin), thus leading to the conclusion that carotenoids may possess significant immunomodulating activities independent of vitamin A activity.

Although most of the focus on carotenoids and immunomodula-

tion have centered on the above-cited areas, a small amount of data has been reported in the literature regarding the potential of carotenoids to impact arachidonic acid metabolism as well as the humoural immune response *(51,63,64)*. Although a large body of evidence is not yet available to support these types of actions, it is important to recognize the usefulness of investigating immuno-modulating pathways complementary to the work examining the relationship between BC and cytokine expression.

As with carotenoids, certain flavonoids have been shown to affect many aspects of the immune response in vitro and using in vivo models, including inflammation, cytokine production, lymphocyte production, and granulocyte function. Although it is difficult to isolate aspects of immune function that may be effected by flavonoids, we will discuss the state of knowledge as it applies to inflammation, phagocytosis and extracellular killing and, finally, acquired immunity, including lymphocyte and cytokine production. Much of this research has focused on the following possible mechanisms of action: (1) protection from free-radical damage, (2) regulation of nitric oxide production, and (3) regulation of arachidonic acid metabolism.

Inflammation is an important component to the immunological defense. At the same time, prevention of excess or chronic inflammation is necessary for recovery of the subject. Proper regulation of the negative aspects of inflammation may help prevent the development of certain chronic diseases potentially propagated through inflammation, such as cardiovascular disease *(65,66)*. Modern science has begun to attribute the effects of several botanicals traditionally used to treat inflammation to specific components of the botanical, which demonstrate anti-inflammatory abilities when used as isolated components in in vitro and in vivo studies. The flavonoids include several such components with potential anti-inflammatory activity *(67)*.

A proposed mechanism for the anti-inflammatory action of flavonoids is the inhibition of arachidonic acid metabolism. Arachidonic acid is released from mast cells and can mediate the inflammatory response. Subsequent to its release, arachidonic acid is metabolized by either lipoxygenase to produce leukotrienes or by the cyclooxygenases to produce thromboxanes and prostaglandins. Oral ingestion of several flavonoids isolated from medicinal plants inhibited mouse paw edema induced by carrageenin injection *(68)*. Interestingly, the flavonoid glycosides exhibited a greater inhibition of paw edema than their aglycones. In this same study, prostaglandin E2 and leukotriene B4 levels were reduced. Several flavonoids have also been shown to inhibit the formation of thromboxane B2 by human platelets stimulated by either bovine thrombin or arachodonic acid in vitro *(69)*. Quercetin and flavone were the most potent with IC50 values at 44–80 μM, and rutin, phloridzin, and naringen had no effect. In addition, the flavonoids differed in the reversibility of their effect on arachidonic acid metabolism. For example, both quercetin and catechin inhibited cyclooxygenase and lipoxygenase pathways, but quercetin was an irreversible inhibitor of C12 lipoxygenase and catechin was an irreversible inhibitor of cyclooxygenase.

Histamine release is also a component of the immune response leading to inflammation. Histamine release by human basophils *(70)* and rat mast cells (71) was diminished in the presence of some but not all flavonoids. Of structure–function significance is that flavonoids with saturation and of the C2–C3 bond, those lacking the C4 carbonyl group (catechins) and flavonoid glycosides had little activity in reducing histamine release *(70)*. Also, the apigenin dimer amentoflavone exhibited greater inhibitory activity than the apigenin monomer as well as other flavonoids tested [71].

Regarding the effect of flavonoids on cytokines potentially involved in cancer etiology, epigallocatechin gallate (EGCG) isolated from green tea significantly stimulated the production of IL-1 beta and TNF by human peripheral blood mononuclear cells in vitro [72]. EGCG also stimulated the production of both IL-1α production by mononuclear cells and stimulated the adherence of mononuclear cells. In addition, EGCG-enhanced IL-1α mRNA synthesis but not that of IL-1β.

Flavonoids have also been shown to influence acquired immunity. Using human peripheral blood mononuclear cells (PBMC), spontaneous and mitogen-stimulated lymphocyte proliferations were enhanced after the flavonoid cianidanol was added to the culture medium [73]. Cianidanol also enhanced the synthesis of IgG by human PBMC.

Seven of 34 flavonoids tested showed significant inhibition of Concanavilin A (Con A)-induced T-cell lymphocyte proliferation of mouse splenocytes: apigenin, luteoline, flavonol, chrysin, fisetin, keampferol, quercetin, and myricetin [74]. Only myricetin was shown to suppress Lipopolysaccharide LPS-induced B-cell lymphocyte proliferation. Also, none of the glycosides tested were found to suppress either Con A- or LPS-induced lymphocyte proliferation, indicating the structure–function relationship of the aglycone. Apigenin, luteolin, fisetin, keampferol, and quercetin suppressed lymphocyte proliferation in a mixed-lymphocyte culture.

Several biflavonoids tested also suppressed Con A- and LPS-induced lymphocyte proliferation [75]. Ochnaflavone and isocryptomerin (apigenin dimers) irreversibly inhibited Con A-induced lymphocyte proliferation because the inhibition remained even after lymphocytes were washed. In contrast, the inhibition of proliferation brought about by quercetin and apigenin was restored after washing. In addition, the biflavonoids suppressed activity for up to 48 h during which time apigenin lost its suppressive effect. These results indicate that dimeric flavonoids can have significantly different effects on immune function parameters than the monomeric flavonoids.

The role of reactive nitrogen and oxygen species has been identified as key modulators of inflammation and, thus, immune function during the past decade [51,76]. Several phytochemicals, including the flavonoid EGCG from tea, were shown to reduce nitrite production by stimulated mouse peritoneal cells [79]. EGCG was also shown to reduce the inducible nitric oxide synthase gene expression and inhibit enzyme activity [78].

After stimulation of a neutrophil by an agonist, oxygen uptake increases and subsequent release of microbicidal products such as superoxide, hydrogen peroxide, nitric oxide, and hydroxy radical occurs. This respiratory burst, although effective in the killing of foreign particles, may also play a detrimental role through inflammation and oxidative damage to tissues. Flavonoids may be involved in net oxygen consumption of the cell and this effect appears to correlate with flavonoid structure [81]. Formation of reactive oxygen species, as measured by chemiluminescence (CL), was inhibited by quercetin in Polymorphonuclear leukocyte PMN cells at a $10^{-5}M$ concentration of quercetin. Quercetin, at concentrations of $1 \times 10^{-6}M$ to 1×10^{-5}M, also reduced the production of superoxide as well as reduced neutrophil oxygen consumption at concentrations of $10^{-4}M$. All nine flavonoids tested reduced the neutrophil CL response to opsonized zymosan [80]. These results indicate that the role of flavonoids in protection against oxidative damage is supported by the significant in vitro evidence that flavonoids possess strong antioxidant activity [27,82].

In addition to the above-mentioned immune functions, flavonoids have been screened for potential inhibition of human immunodeficiency virus infection and replication [82,83]. Regarding flavonoid monomers, the flavans showed selective inhibition against HIV infection with epicatcchin-3-O-gallate showing the greatest activity [82]. When investigating higher oligomers and tannins, it was found that for hydrolyzable tannins, a higher number of units corresponded with greater anti-HIV activity; condensed tannins and lower-molecular-weight polyphenols had little anti-HIV activity [83].

The fundamental mechanisms by which some phytochemicals are able to impart immunomodulatory activities in vitro and in vivo are largely speculative at this time. The use of well-designed experiments at the molecular biological level should reveal some of these mechanisms with respect to modulation of levels of cytokines and other important signaling molecules. Many of the phytochemicals showing potential activity have also demonstrated antioxidant activities, with carotenoids and flavonoids being part of this group. In fact, a brief review of the antioxidant potential of carotenoids, coupled with the corresponding information for flavonoids discussed earlier, is useful for demonstrating the complexity of antioxidant chemistry and how it may or may not be biologically relevant and, thus, important for immunomodulation [84].

Carotenoids are known to be essential for protection of plant photosynthetic centers against the destructive actions of oxidation catalyzed by UV light [56]. This knowledge led to the rationale extrapolation that intact carotenoids may also play an analogous protective role in humans [55] and that this activity may be related to their ability to modulate immune function [51]. Although a good possibility, it is important to recognize the chemistry of carotenoids and what this means with respect to their potential activity as antioxidants. Of great significance is the extensive conjugation present in the backbone of most carotenoids and the ability of this conjugation to dissipate the energy associated with singlet oxygen [44]. Indeed, this is exactly why carotenoids play such a critical role in the protection of plants from photooxidation. However, this same structural characteristic makes these carotenoids outstanding targets for oxidative abstraction of a hydrogen atom, with subsequent modification and degradation seen for other unsaturated lipids that are easily oxidized and participate in auto-oxidative processes [85]. Thus, in instances where singlet oxygen is a critical oxidant, carotenoids may be important in defending biological tissues against oxidative damage; however, the presence of singlet oxygen in vivo in humans is unclear at present. Conversely, carotenoids may be of little value in preventing or attenuating other forms of oxidative stress and may, in fact, promote oxidation of certain substrates due to their highly unsaturated structure. Understanding this is further complicated by the potential for carotenoids to have different antioxidant potential under different oxygen pressures [86].

The antioxidant potential of flavonoids and certain other phytochemicals in biological systems is equally complex to that described above for the carotenoids [87]. Thus, although the potential for phytochemicals to modulate immune function via their ability to act as antioxidants is enormous, there is still a large amount of research left to be done to understand the mechanisms by which they can function to do this. Additional work to achieve this goal includes a better understanding of the chemistry of individual phytochemicals as well as the biological environment in which they may function.

CONCLUSION

The human immune system is extremely complex, and a multitude of dietary factors play key roles in its regulation. Based on a large amount of in vitro data, it appears that certain dietary phytochemicals, most of which are commonly deemed "nonessential," possess the potential to modulate at least some aspects of immune function in humans. Although promising, defining the role that phytochemicals may play in immunomodulation will be challenging. To understand this role, a concordance of epidemiological, mechanistic, and clinical data will have to be achieved for phytochemicals of interest. In many cases, this will require not only isolation and testing of individual compounds but also mixtures of closely related compounds such as those that typically occur in plant foods.

In this chapter, we have used research on carotenoids and flavonoids in the field of immunomodulation as a working example to illustrate the potential that certain classes of phytochemicals have for bioactivity in this area. In addition, these examples illustrate the complex chemical, biochemical, and biological issues that face scientists who endeavor to define the role of phytochemicals in modulating human immune function. Indeed, it is sobering to consider that although these two classes of phytochemicals have been intensely studied in a nutrition and health context for decades, there is still a tremendous amount of work to accomplish before we can draw conclusions about their immunomodulating potential. And yet, we do not want to lose perspective on the valuable insights gained from this research. For example, it is clear that at least a few members from each of these phytochemical classes demonstrate immunomodulating activity in vitro and in vivo models. In addition, preliminary clinical evidence suggests that beta-carotene may have immunoenhancing effects in elderly populations and applications to other populations that are environmentally or otherwise stressed. Most importantly, the research on carotenoids and flavonoids has demonstrated the essentiality of understanding the fundamental chemical and biological aspects of phytochemicals in order to design the appropriate in vivo model and clinical experiments necessary for defining the role of dietary phytochemicals in human immune function.

REFERENCES

1. Peto R, Doll R, Buckley JD, and Sporn MB. Can dietary beta-carotene materially reduce human cancer rates? Nature 1981; 290:201–8.
2. Beyers T, Perry G. Dietary carotenes, vitamin C and vitamin E as protective antioxidants in human cancers. Annu Rev Nutr 1992; 12:139–59.
3. Steinmetz KA, Potter JD. Vegetables, fruits, and cancer prevention: A review. J Am Diet Assoc 1996; 96:1027–39.
4. Hertog MGL, Feskens EJM, Hollman PCH, Katan MB, Kromhout D. Dietary antioxidant flavonoids and risk of coronary heart disease: the Zutphen Elderly Study. Lancet 1993; 342:1007–11.
5. Fraser GE, Sabate J, Beeson WL, Strahan M. A possible protective effect of nut consumption of risk of coronary heart disease. Arch Intern Med 1992; 152:1416–24.
6. Bruneton J, ed. Parmacognosy Phytochemistry Medicinal Plants. Lavoisier Publishing, Paris, 1995.
7. Borchers AT, Hackman RM, Keen CL, Stern JS, Gershwin E. Complementary medicine: a review of immunomodulatory effects of Chinese herbal medicines. Am J Clin Nutr 1997; 66:1303–12.
8. Pfander H. Carotenoids: An overview. Methods Enzymol 1992; 213:3–13.
9. Tswett M. Physikalisch-chemische studien uber das chlorophyll. Die adsorptionen. Ber Deut Botan Ges 1906; 24:316–23.
10. Olson JA. Formation and function of vitamin A. In: JW Porter and SL Spurgeon, eds., Biosynthesis of Isoprenoid Compounds. Wiley, New York, 1983.
11. Olson JA. Vitamin A, retinoids and carotenoids. In: Modern Nutrition in Health and Disease (Shil ME, Olson JA, and Shike M, eds), 8th ed. Lea and Febiger, Philadelphia, 1994.
12. Malter M, Schriever G, Eilber U. Natural killer cells, vitamins, and other blood components of vegetarian and omnivorous men. Nutr Cancer 1989; 12:271–8.
13. Kuhnau J. The flavonoids: a class of semi-essential food components; their role in human nutrition. World Rev Nutr Diet 1976; 24:117–91.
14. Rice-Evans CA, Packer L, eds. Flavonoids in Health and Disease. Marcel Dekker, New York, 1997.
15. Hertog GL, Kromhout D, Aravanis C. Flavonoid intake and long-term risk of coronary heart disease and cancer in the seven countries study. Arch Intern Med 1995; 155:381–6.
16. Hertog MGL, Sweetnam PM, Fehily AM, Elwood PC, Kromhout D. Antioxidant flavonols and ischemic heart disease in a Welsh population of men: the Caerphilly Study. Am J Clin Nutr 1997; 65:1489–94.
17. Knekt P, Jarvinen R, Seppanen R, Heliovaara M, Teppo L, Pukkala E, et al. Dietary flavonoids and the risk of cancer and other malignant neoplasms. Am J Epidemiol 1997; 146:223–30.
18. Reed JD. Nutritional toxicology of tannins and related polyphenols in forage legumes. Anim Sci 1995; 73(5):1516–2.
19. Balentine DA, Wiseman SA, Bouwens CM. The chemistry of tea flavonoids. Crit Rev Food Sci Nutr 1997; 38(8):693–704.
20. Khachik F, Beecher GR, Goli MB. Separation, identification, and quantification of carotenoids in fruits, vegetables and human plasma by high performance liquid chromatography. Pure Appl Chem 1991; 63:71–80.
21. Goodwin TW. Biosynthesis of carotenoids: an overview. Methods Enzymol 1993; 214:330–40.
22. Isler O. Tentative rules for the nomenclature of carotenoids. In: Isler O, ed. Carotenoids. Birkhauser Verlag, Basel, 1971.
23. O'Neil CA, Schwartz SJ. Chromatographic analysis of cis/trans carotenoid isomers. J Chromatogr 1992; 624:235–52.
24. Schmitz HH, Poor CL, Gugger ET, Erdman JW. Analysis of carotenoids in human and animal tissues. Meth Enzymol 1993; 214:102–16.
25. Scita G. Stability of beta-carotene under different laboratory conditions. Methods Enzymol 1992; 213:175–85.
26. Hammerstone JF, Lazarus SA, Mitchell AE, Rucker R, Schmitz HH. Identification of procyanidins in cocoa (theobroma cacao) or chocolate using high-performance liquid chromatography/mass spectometry. J Agric Food Chem 1999; 47:490–6.
27. Rice-Evans CA, Miller NJ, Paganga G. Structure–antioxidant activity relationships of flavonoids and phenolic acids. Free Radical Biol Med 1996; 20(7):933–56.
28. Hollman PCH, de Vries JHM, van Leeuwen SD, Mengelers MJB, Katan M. Absorption of dietary quercetin glycosides and quercetin in healthy ileostomy volunteers. Am J Clin Nutr 1995; 62:1276–82.
29. Leung KH, Ip MM. Regulation of rat natural killing II. Inhibition of cytolysis and activation by inhibitors of lipoxygenase: possible role of leukotrienes. Cell Immunol 1986; 100:474–84.
30. Brantzaeg P. Development and basic mechanisms of human gut immunity. Nutr Rev 1998; 56(1):S5–S18.
31. US Department of Agriculture, Agriculture Research Service. 1997. USDA-NCI Carotenoid Food Composition Database. Nutrient Data Laboratory Home Page, http://www.nal.usda.gov/fnic/foodcomp.
32. VandenLangenberg GM, Brady WE, Nebeling LC, Block G, Forman M, Bowen PE, et al. Influence of using different sources of carotenoid data in epidemiological studies. J Am Diet Assoc 1996; 96(12): 1271–5.
33. Hertog MGL, Hollman PGH, Katan MB. Content of potentially anti-

carcinogenic flavonoids of 28 vegetables and 9 fruits commonly consumed in The Netherlands. J Agric Food Chem 1992; 40:2379–83.

34. Hertog MGL, Hollman PGH, van de Putte B. Content of potentially anticarcinogenic flavonoids of tea infusions, wines, and fruit juices. J Agric Food Chem 1993; 41:1242–6.

35. Pierpoint WS. Flavonoids in the human diet. In: Plant Flavonoids in Biology and Medicine: Biochemical, Pharmacological, and Structure–Activity Relationships, pp. 125–40. Alan R. Liss, New York, 1986.

36. Rimm EB, Katan MB, Ascherio A, Stampfer MJ, Willett W. Relation between intake of flavonoids and risk for coronary heart disease in male health professionals. Ann Intern Med 1996; 125(5):384–9.

37. Hertog MGL, Hollman PCH, Katan MB, Kromhout. Intake of potentially anticarcinogenic flavonoids and their determinants in adults in the Netherlands. Nutr Cancer 1993; 20(1):21–9.

38. Erdman JW. The physiologic chemistry of carotenes in man. Clin Nutr 1988; 7:101–6.

39. Hollman PCH, Katan MB. Absorption, metabolism, and bioavailability of flavonoids. In: Rice-Evans, Packer L, eds, Flavonoids in Health and Disease, pp. 483–522. Marcel Dekker, New York, 1997.

40. Novotny JA, Dueker SB, Zech LA, Clifford AJ. Compartmental analysis of the dynamics of beta-carotene metabolism in an adult volunteer. J Lipid Res 1995; 36:182–38.

41. Hollman PCH, Tijburg LBM, Yang CS. Bioavailability of flavonoids from tea. Crit Rev Food Sci Nutr 1997; 37(8):719–38.

42. Spencer CM, Cai Y, Martin R, et al. Polyphenol-complexation—some thoughts and observations. Phytochemistry 1988; 27:2397–409.

43. Sweeney JP, Marsh AC. Liver storage of vitamin A in rats fed carotene stereoisomers. J Nutr 1973; 103:20–5.

44. Di Mascio P, Sundquist AR, Devasagayam TPA, Sies H. Assay of lycopene and other carotenoids as singlet oxygen quenchers. Methods Enzymol 1992; 213:429–38.

45. Levin G, Mokady S. Antioxidant activity of 9-*cis* compared to all-*trans* beta-carotene in vitro. Free Radical Biol Med 1994; 17:77–82.

47. Yang A, Larsen TW, Tume RK. Carotneoid and retinol concentrations in serum, adipose tissue and liver and carotenoid transport in sheep, goats and cattle. Aust J Agric Res 1992; 43:1809–17.

48. Hathcock JN, Hattan DG, Jenkins MY, McDonald JT, Ramnathan Sundaresan P, Wilkening VL. Evaluation of vitamin A toxicity. Am J Clin Nutr 1990; 52:183–202.

49. Prabhala RH, Garewal HS, Hicks MJ, Sampliner RE, Watson RR. The effects of 13-cis-retinoic acid and beta-carotene on cellular immunity in humans. Cancer 1991; 67:1556–60.

50. Watson RR, Prabhala RH, Plezia PM, Alberts DS. Effects of beta-carotene on lymphocyte subpopulations in elderly humans: evidence for a dose-response relationship. Am J Clin Nutr 1991; 53:90–4.

51. Meydani SN, Wu D, Santos MS, Hayek MG. Antioxidants and immune response in aged persons: overview of present evidence. Am J Clin Nutr 1995; 62(suppl):1462S–76S.

52. Daudu PA, Kelley DS, Taylor PC, Burri BJ, Wu MM. Effect of a low beta-carotene diet on the immune functions of adult women. Am J Clin Nutr 1994; 60:969–72.

53. Ringer TV, DeLoof MJ, Winterrowd GE, Francom SF, Gaylor SK, Ryan JA. Beta-carotene's effects on serum lipoproteins and immunologic indices in humans. Am J Clin Nutr 1991; 53:668–94.

54. Fuller CJ, Faulkner H, Bendich A, Parker RS, Roe DA. Effect of beta-carotene supplementation on photosuppression of delayed-type hypersensitivity in normal young men. Am J Clin Nutr 1992; 56:684–90.

55. Mathews-Roth MM. Photoprotection by carotenoids. Fed Proc 1987; 461:890–3.

56. Krinsky NI. Antioxidant functions of carotenoids. Free Radical Biol Med 1989; 7:617–35.

57. Schoen DJ, Watson RR. Prevention of UV irradiation induced suppression of monocyte functions by retinoids and carotenoids *in vitro*. Photochem Photobiol 1988; 48:659–3.

58. Ribaya-Mercado JD, Garmyn M, Gilchrest BA, Russell RM. Skin lycopene is destroyed preferentially over beta-carotene during ultraviolet irradiation in humans. J Nutr 1995; 125:1854–9.

59. Abdel-Fatth G, Watzl B, Huang D, Watson RR. Beta-carotene in vitro stimulates tumor necrosis factor alpha and interleukin-1 alpha secretion by human prepheral blood mononuclear cells. Nutr Res 1993; 13:863–71.

60. Prabhala RH, Garewal HS, Meyskens FL, Watson RR. Immunomodulation in humans caused by beta-carotene and vitamin A. Nutr Res 1990; 10:1473–86.

61. Schwartz JL. In vitro biological methods for determination of carotenoid activity. Methods Enzymol 1993; 214:226–56.

62. Bendich A and Shapiro SS. Effect of beta-carotene and canthaxanthin on the immune responses of the rat. J Nutr 1986; 116:2254–62.

63. Halevy O, Sklan D. Inhibition of arachidonic acid oxidation by beta-carotene, retinol and alpha-tocopherol. Biochim Biophys Acta 1987; 918:304–7.

64. Jyonouchi H, Zhang L, Tomita Y. Studies of immunomodulating actions of carotenoids. II. Astaxanthin enhances in vitro antibody production to T-dependent antigens without facilitating polyclonal B-cell activation. Nutr Cancer 1993; 19:269–80.

65. Seifert PS, Kazatchkine MD. The complement system in atherosclerosis. Atherosclerosis 1988; 73:91–104.

66. Meydani M. Nutrition, immune cells, and atherosclerosis. Nutr Rev 1998; 56(1):5177–82.

67. Pietta P. Flavonoids in medicinal plants. In: Flavonoids in Health and Disease (Rice-Evans CA, Packer L, eds). Mercel Dekker, New York, 1998.

68. Ferrandiz ML, Alcaraz MJ. Anti-inflammatory activity and inhibition of arachidonic acid metabolism by flavonoids. Agents Actions 1991; 32(3/4):283–8.

69. Corvasier E, Maclouf J. Interference of some flavonoids and non-steroidal anti-inflammatory drugs with oxidative metabolism of arachidonic acid by human platelets and neutrophils. Biochim Biophys Acta 1985; 85:315–21.

70. Middleton E, Drzewiecki G. Flavonoid inhibition of human basophil histamine release stimulated by various agents. Biochem Pharmacol 1984; 33(21):3333–8.

71. Amella M, Bronner C, Briancon F, Haag M, Anton R, Landry Y. Inhibition of mast cell histamine release by flavonoids and biflavonoids. Planta Med 1985; 1:16–20.

72. Sakagami H, Takeda M, Sugaya K, Omata T, Takahashi M, Yamamoto M. Stimulation by epigallocatechin gallate of interleukin-1 production by human peripheral blood mononuclear cells. Anticancer Res 1995; 15:971–4.

73. Brattig NW, Diao G-J, Berg PA. Immunoenhancing effect of flavonoid compounds on lymphocyte proliferation and immunoglubulin synthesis. Int J Immunopharmacol 1984; 6(3):205–15.

74. Namgoong SY, Son KH, Chang HW, Kang SS, Kim HP. Effects of naturally occurring flavonoids on mitogen-induced lymphocyte proliferation and mixed lymphocyte culture. Life Sci 1993; 54:313–20.

75. Lee SJ, Choi JH, Son KH, Chang HW, Kang SS, Kim HP. Suppression of mouse lymphocyte proliferation in vitro by naturally-occurring biflavonoids. Life Sci 1995; 57(6):551–8.

76. Beck MA. The influence of antioxidant nutrients on viral infection. Nutr Rev 1998; 56(1):S140–6.

77. Chan MM-Y, Ho C-T, Huang H-I. Effects of three dietary phyochemicals from tea rosemary and turmeric on inflammation-induced nitrite production. Cancer Lett 1995; 96:23–9.

78. Chan MM, Fong D, Ho CT, Huang HI. Inhibition of inducible nitric oxide synthase gene expression and enzyme activity by epigallocatechin gallate, a natural product from green tea. Biochem Pharmacol 1997; 54(12):1281–6.

79. Pagonis C, Tauber AI, Pavotsky N, and Simons E. Flavonoid impairment of neutrophil response. Biochem Pharmacol 1986; 35:237–45.

80. Busse WW, Kopp DE, Middleton E. Flavonoid modulation of human neutrophil function. J Allergy Clin Immunol 1984; 73:801–9.

81. Rice-Evans CA, Miller NJ. Antioxidant activities of flavonoids as bioactive components of food. Biochem Soc Trans 1996; 24:790–4.

82. Mahmood N, Pizza C, Aquino R. Inhibition of HIV infection by flavonoids. Antivir Res 1993; 22:189–99.

83. Nakashima H, Murakami T, Yamamoto N. Inhibition of human immu-

nodeficiency viral replication by tannins and related compounds. Antivir Res 1992; 18:91–103.

84. Krinsky NI. Antioxidant functions of carotenoids. Free Radical Biol Med 1989; 7:617–35.

85. Frankel EN. Lipid oxidation: mechanisms, products and biological significance. JAOCS 1984; 61:1908–17.

86. Vile GF, Winterbourn CC. Inhibition of adriamycin-promoted microsomal lipid peroxidation by beta-carotene, alpha-tocopherol and reti-

nol at high and low oxygen partial pressures. FEBS Lett 1988; 238: 353–6.

87. Decker EA. Phenolics: prooxidants or antioxidants? Nutr Rev 1997; 55(11):396–407.

88. Ganguly J, Krischnamurthy S, Mahadevan S. The transort of carotenoids, vitamin A and cholesterol across the intestines of rats and chicks. Biochem J 1959; 71:756–62.

10 Dietary n-3 Polyunsaturated Fatty Acids Modulate T-Lymphocyte Activation

Clinical Relevance in Treating Diseases of Chronic Inflammation

Robert S. Chapkin, David N. McMurray, and Christopher A. Jolly

DIETARY FISH OIL THERAPY IN INFLAMMATORY DISEASES

Approximately 40 million Americans (1 in 7) are afflicted with arthritis. Arthritis costs the economy an estimated $54.6 billion annually in medical care and indirect costs (i.e., lost wages) and is the number one cause of disability in the United States. The Centers for Disease Control and Prevention project that by the year 2020, the number of cases of arthritis will increase to 59.4 million Americans *(1)*. Current therapy includes the use of nonsteroidal anti-inflammatory drugs (NSAIDs) and slow-acting antirheumatic drugs, but because of side effects, these drugs are usually not administered for more than 2 yr *(2,3)*. The development of safer therapeutic strategies are required to improve patient quality of life in the long term. One such therapeutic approach has been the use of fish oil supplementation. Epidemiological data collected in the 1970s indicate that Greenland Eskimos have a decreased incidence of inflammatory disease despite their high-fat diet. Similar observations were made in the Japanese population, which led to the correlation between a lower incidence of inflammatory disease and high consumption, relative to Americans, of cold-water marine fish *(4)*. Scientists have tested the effects of dietary fish oil supplementation on rheumatoid arthritis (RA) in human clinical trials *(3,5)*.

Rheumatoid arthritis is a chronic inflammatory disease and the most severe and disabling type of arthritis, afflicting approximately 2.1 million Americans *(1)*. Double-blind, placebo-controlled clinical trials showed that supplementation with fish oil containing 2.7–5.6 g/d of eicosapentaenoic acid (EPA) and docosahexaenoic acid (DHA), the two n-3 polyunsaturated fatty acids enriched in fish oil, over a 12-wk period led to significant improvement in the number of tender and swollen joints, grip strength, and global

disease activity *(3,5)*. The average American normally consumes approximately 100 mg/d of EPA and DHA (in the form of fish) compared to 8000 mg/d in clinical trials and 6000–12,000 mg/d by Greenland Eskimos *(6–10)*; (Table 1). Taken together, these clinical trials indicate that, similar to drug therapy, dietary fish oil does not cure rheumatoid arthritis but does significantly alleviate symptoms. Most recently, research has focused on the use of fish oil supplementation as an adjunct to drug therapy. A 4-mo double-blind placebo-controlled study in which patients were given 5.8 g/d of EPA and DHA in conjunction with naproxen indicated an added benefit of including the fish oil supplements *(10)*. Furthermore, supplementation for 6 mo with 3.0 g/d of EPA and DHA resulted in a significant decrease in NSAID usage *(11)*. Similar results were obtained in two other double-blind, placebo-controlled clinical trials in which patients were supplemented with approximately 2.8 g/d EPA and DHA for 12 mo *(12,13)*, which represents the longest clinical trials to date. Increasing supplementation to 6.2 g/d EPA and DHA for 22 wk allowed some patients to discontinue NSAID therapy *(14)*. Although dietary fish oil has been shown to be beneficial in managing rheumatoid arthritis, fish oil does not appear to influence inflammatory skin disorders such as atopic dermatitis and psoriasis *(15)*. Therefore, fish oil cannot be used as a general anti-inflammatory agent. One drawback to these studies is that the fish oil protocol required the consumption of at least 10 capsules/d (depending on the source of fish oil), which could lead to compliance problems and significant cost to patients. Future investigations need to determine whether the same beneficial effects come from the substitution of fish and fish products in the diet.

Studies have also been conducted in rodent models of inflammatory disease in order to elucidate the biological mechanism(s) of dietary fish oil's anti-inflammatory properties. In the 1970s, it was shown that feeding low-fat (1.2% wt/wt) diets increased the life-span in autoimmune-prone mice compared to a high-fat (9–18%) diet *(16)*. In the 1980s, it was revealed that not only the amount of fat but the type of fat was an important variable in the

From: *Nutrition and Immunology: Principles and Practice* (ME Gershwin et al. eds.), © Humana Press, Inc., Totowa, NJ

Table 1
Comparison of the Fatty Acid Consumption Among Epidemiological, Clinical, and Experimental Studies

Fatty acid	Greenland Eskimo	Japanese	Canadian[a]	Mouse	United States[a]	Clinical trials
% Energy as fat	39[b]	30	39	7	38	40
Fat[c]	130[b]	70	80–110	0.150	80	88
18:2n-6[c]	2–3[d]	2–5[d]	14–19	0.080[e]	14.7	14.7
18:3n-3[c]	13.7[b]	0.4[d]	1.4–2.8	0	1.6	1.6
20:4n-6[c]	1.3	2.6	0.25	0	0.1	0.1
20:5n-3+						
22:6n-3[c]	6–12[d]	1–3[d]	0.15	0.048[e]	0.1	8[f]

[a]From Ref. 9.
[b]From Ref. 6.
[c]Values represent grams per day.
[d]From ref. 7.
[e]From ref. 8.
[f]From ref. 3.

modulation of inflammatory disease. The first study to show a beneficial effect of dietary fish oil on rodent inflammatory disease was in 1983. This study showed that feeding 25% (wt/wt) fish oil increased the survival of NZB×NZW/F1 mice, which are prone to developing autoimmune nephritis. Control mice fed a lard-based diet died from renal failure (17). This mouse strain serves as a model for the human inflammatory disease systemic lupus erythematosus (SLE). Using the same mouse model, similar results were obtained by feeding 20% fish oil compared to corn oil controls (18,19). Mrl lpr/lpr (Mrl/l) mice, a model for human SLE and RA, exhibited decreased severity of renal pathology when fed a 25% (wt/wt) fish oil diet (20).

The effects of fish oil supplementation in murine inflammatory disease models are more dramatic when compared to human clinical trials. This could be explained, in part, by the fact that fish oil feeding in rodent disease models begins prior to disease onset, whereas human clinical trials initiate fish oil supplementation after disease onset. Initiating fish oil supplementation prior to the development of clinical signs of RA might have a greater impact on disease incidence and/or severity. One would predict that early supplementation would enhance the beneficial effects of fish oil because of the overwhelming epidemiological evidence in Greenland Eskimos and the Japanese (4). One study has addressed this issue and showed that feeding 5% (wt/wt) fish oil starting after disease onset in NZB×NZW mice did increase survival rate (21), but the effect was not as dramatic as initiating the feeding regimen prior to clinical disease (20). As with human inflammatory disease, high-dose fish oil feeding (25% wt/wt) is not effective in all rodent models of inflammatory disease (e.g., collagen-induced arthritis in rats) (22). In contrast, a lower-dose (5%) fish oil feeding suppressed the susceptibility of mice to collagen-induced arthritis (23). One possible explanation for this discrepancy is that too much fish oil could be deleterious in some inflammatory diseases. These observations underscore the need to carefully determine optimal doses of fish oil that should be used clinically for treating different inflammatory diseases.

REGULATION OF T-CELL FUNCTION BY DIETARY FISH OIL

The etiology of RA is currently unknown; however, the pathogenesis is understood, although not fully. RA is an autoimmune disease, meaning that the immune system has become deregulated and is responding actively to self-antigen(s). Several immune cells, including T and B lymphocytes and macrophages are involved in this chronic, destructive joint inflammation (24). In an attempt to elucidate the mechanisms of the anti-inflammatory action of fish oil, research has focused primarily on the T cell and, to a lesser extent, on the macrophage.

The T cell is a key player in propagating an immune response by responding to antigen. Antigen presentation to the T cell in the context of the major histocompatibility complex (MHC) is mediated via interaction with the antigen specific T-cell receptor/CD3 complex (TCR/CD3). This signal is necessary but not sufficient to induce a functional response (i.e., proliferation). A second, or costimulatory, signal is required, which is derived via accessory cells such as macrophages (25). The costimulatory signal can come from soluble mediators such as interleukin-1 (IL-1) and/or tumor necrosis factor (TNF) (26) interacting with the T-cell IL-1 receptor (IL-1R) and/or TNF receptor (TNFR). Alternatively, the costimulatory signal could be derived from macrophage-expressed plasma membrane receptors, of which B7-1 and B7-2 provide the strongest T-cell costimulation. The B7-1 and B7-2 receptors interact with the T-cell ligands CD28 and CTLA-4, respectively. The net result of the two stimulatory or activating signals is secretion of interleukin-2 (IL-2), a potent autocrine and paracrine T-cell growth factor, and expression of the IL-2 receptor α-chain (IL-2R α). The IL-2R α-chain interacts with the constitutively expressed β- and γ-chains to yield a high-affinity IL-2R complex. The secreted IL-2 binds to the high-affinity IL-2R, which drives the T cell through the cell cycle. The proliferating T cells increase in number and differentiate into effector cells, secreting a plethora of lymphokines (hormonelike glycoproteins). These include IL-2, IL-4, IL-5, and IL-6, which enhance immunoglobulin production (humoral immunity), and interferon-γ (IFN-γ) as well as IL-2, which enhance cell-mediated immunity (25). Therefore, T cells play important regulatory roles in both major arms (humoral and cell mediated) of the immune system.

Generally, dietary fish oil suppresses T-cell proliferation (27–31). Supplementing healthy human volunteers with 18 g/d of fish oil for 6 wk diminished T-cell proliferation associated with reductions in IL-2 secretion in peripheral blood lymphocytes stimulated in vitro with phytohemagglutinin (PHA), a polyclonal T-cell mitogen (32). Supplementation with a lower dose of fish oil (3 g/d) for 12 wk resulted in suppressed PHA-induced T-cell proliferation and impaired IL-2 secretion in the cultured peripheral blood mononuclear cells of healthy female volunteers *(33)*. Recently, the effect of fish in the diet (instead of fish oil capsule supplementation) on human T-cell function was determined. Consumption of 180 g fish/d for 24 wk resulted in suppressed concanavalin A (Con A; a polyconal T-cell mitogen)-induced proliferation, which was associated with reductions in the T-cell-dependent delayed-type hypersensitivity response in vivo *(34)*. Similar results were found in rodent studies. Rats fed a diet containing 20% (wt/wt) fish oil for 10 wk exhibited suppressed Con A-induced T-cell proliferation in splenic lymphocytes *(35)* and whole blood *(36)*. Feeding mice half the amount of fish oil (10% wt/wt) for 8 wk also reduced PHA-induced T-cell proliferation in murine splenic lymphocytes *(37)*. In contrast to all these reports, a recent study demonstrated that feeding monkeys 3.3% of energy as EPA and DHA for 14 wk increased Con A- and PHA-induced T-cell proliferation and IL-2 secretion in peripheral blood mononuclear cells *(38)*. The reason for this discrepancy is currently unknown. A human study showed that ingestion of 4 g/d EPA ethyl esters for 8 wk enhanced T-cell PHA-mediated proliferative responses *(39)*. However, these patients were asthmatic and the effects of the pathology of asthma on T-cell function and responses was not determined.

Taken together, the majority of these data suggest that the anti-inflammatory effects of fish oil are mediated, in part, via downregulation of T-cell proliferation. Impaired proliferation and IL-2 secretion in response to fish oil supplementation has been well documented; however, the mechanism(s) by which these phenomena occur is not known.

MECHANISMS BY WHICH FISH OIL MODULATES T-CELL FUNCTION

There are several possible mechanisms for the suppressed T-cell proliferation observed in the vast majority of fish oil supplementation studies. These include

1. Alterations in the relative distribution of T-cell subsets.
2. Modifications of T-cell membrane structure.
3. Changes in accessory cell (primarily the macrophage) ability to costimulate the T cell.
4. Modified T-cell intracellular signals.

In general, the suppressive effects of fish oil are attributed to EPA [20:5n-3] and DHA [22:6n-3]. Dietary fish oil mediates its biological effects via incorporation of these polyunsaturated fatty acids into the membrane lipids of a variety of cells, including T cells *(8)* and macrophages *(40,41)*.

One potential explanation for fish oil supplementation suppressing T-cell proliferation is reduced numbers of T cells or alterations of T-cell subsets. There are two major T-cell subsets that can be distinguished phenotypically based on the plasma membrane expression of either the CD4+ or CD8+ molecules. These subsets also differ functionally. The CD4+ T cells are helper/inducers of the immune response and produce high levels of IL-2, whereas the CD8+ T cells are cytotoxic/suppressors of immunity and utilize IL-2 *(25)*. Therefore, relative increases in CD8+ T cells could result in reduced T-cell proliferation because of the reduced availability of IL-2 or putative suppressor activity. Alternatively, reductions in the proportion of CD4+ T cells could yield a lower proliferative response. The effect of dietary fish oil on T-cell subsets varies depending on the experimental system used.

Consumption of 180 g/d of fish by human volunteers for 24 wk yielded decreased CD4+ and CD8+ T cells in the peripheral blood *(34)*. Similar results were obtained in the spleens from mice fed a diet containing 10% (wt/wt) fish oil for 8 wk *(37)*. In contrast, there was no effect of feeding a 20% (wt/wt) fish oil diet to rats on T-cell populations in whole blood *(36)*, spleen, lymph node, or thymus *(35)* or in mice fed highly purified EPA or DHA ethyl esters *(42)*. These contradictory results justify the continued examination of the effects of fish oil on T-cell phenotype distribution.

Alternatively, EPA and DHA could alter the membrane structure of T cells, resulting in a suppressed proliferative response. Incorporation of EPA and DHA into membrane phospholipids could alter membrane fluidity (ability of proteins to move in the lipid bilayer), thereby influencing the ability of T cells to be triggered by environmental signals (e.g., antigen–MHC, costimulatory molecules) *(43)*. However, T cells appear to possess compensatory mechanisms, which allow them to maintain a homeostatic fluidity *(44,45)*. Although bulk or overall membrane structure may remain intact, annular domains (area immediately surrounding membrane proteins) could be modified, ultimately affecting cellular responses *(46)*. To date, this mechanism has not been evaluated in T cells.

T-cell activation (i.e., proliferation) could be indirectly inhibited by fish oil feeding by modifications of accessory cells, primarily macrophages. The macrophage provides an obligatory costimulatory signal, without which the T cell cannot proliferate. By far, the most extensively studied mechanism by which dietary fish oil could modulate macrophage-derived T-cell costimulation is eicosanoid metabolism. Feeding fish oil leads to an increase in EPA and DHA in some membrane phospholipids with a concomitant decrease in arachidonic acid (AA) *(20;* 4n-6) content *(40,47,48)*. The cyclooxygenase enzymes metabolize AA, yielding prostaglandin E_2 (PGE_2) which directly suppresses T-cell proliferation. A decrease in PGE_2 production is observed in response to fish oil feeding because of reduced levels of AA *(47,49)*. The increased EPA in cellular phospholipids yields more PGE_3, which is less biologically active than PGE_2. DHA does not yield PGs, but it can suppress PGE_2 formation by inhibiting the cyclooxygenase enzyme *(50)*. Therefore, decreased PGE_2 production would result in enhanced T-cell proliferation. However, the T-cell proliferative response is suppressed, not enhanced, in fish oil feeding studies, suggesting the involvement of additional mechanisms *(51–55)*. Alternative mechanisms by which fish oil supplementation might influence macrophage function, leading to suppression of the T-cell proliferative response, have been investigated. Feeding fish oil to mice decreased the antigen-presenting function of spleen cells (the macrophage is the major antigen-presenting cell in the spleen) suggesting downregulation of macrophage MHC expression *(56)*. Studies in humans show that fish oil supplementation (3 g/d) was accompanied by downregulation of macrophage MHC as well as adhesion molecule expression *(57)*. The diminished expression of adhesion molecules could reduce the interaction between the T cell and the macrophage resulting in suppression of T-cell proliferation. Dietary fish oil may also influence the production of macrophage-derived costimulatory molecules. A 10% (wt/wt) fish oil diet was shown to suppress the costimulatory molecule IL-1 mRNA in murine macrophages *(58)*. Interestingly, fish oil feeding enhanced murine macrophage TNF secretion *(59,60)*. The mechanism most likely involves the downregulation of PGE_2 because PGE_2 suppresses macrophage-derived TNF production *(60)*. In this scenario, the extracellular concentration of TNF could increase to the point that it inhibits T-cell proliferation. Taken together, dietary fish oil can indirectly suppress T-cell proliferation via modifications of macrophage prostaglandin production, cell-surface receptor expression, and secretion of costimulatory proteins.

Finally, dietary fish oil could modulate T-cell function directly. Research, to date, has focused primarily on the expression of membrane receptors that play integral roles in T-cell function. Fish oil feeding (10% wt/wt) in mice has been shown to suppress CD8+ cell-surface expression in splenic T cells *(61)*. CD8+ is a receptor that interacts with the MHC in conjunction with the TCR/CD3 complex and generates intracellular signals important for T-cell function. Humans fed 6 g/d of EPA and DHA ethyl esters for 4 mo showed suppressed IL-2R α-chain expression at the cell surface in response to PHA activation *(62)*. Decreased IL-2R α expression would suppress the number of high-affinity IL-2Rs, which could blunt the T-cell proliferative response. We have recently demonstrated that both EPA and DHA significantly suppress T-cell proliferation *(42)*. To further elucidate the mechanism(s) of action of EPA and DHA on T-cell function, we determined the production of IL-2, a potent polyclonal autocrine T-cell growth factor, in Con A-stimulated splenic lymphocytes. Con A-induced IL-2 production was significantly reduced in both the EPA- and DHA-fed mice *(42)*, which paralleled the suppressed proliferative response. Flow cytometric analysis revealed that the suppressed IL-2 production and proliferative response was not the result of major alterations in the primary splenic T-cell subpopulations (CD4+ and CD8+). Although dietary EPA and DHA have been shown to alter the expression of select cell-surface receptors, the intracellular events influenced are largely unknown. Clearly, the effects of dietary fish oil on the T-cell processes leading to proliferation is an area of research that needs serious examination in the future.

In summary, dietary fish oil can potentially modulate T-cell function directly and/or indirectly via alterations in accessory cell function. Alterations in prostaglandin metabolism has been the focus of a majority of studies to date. However, changes in the types of prostaglandins produced cannot completely explain the suppressed T-cell proliferation. Shifts in T-cell CD4+ and CD8+ subsets cannot explain the suppressed proliferative response in all the studies. Although changes in annular membrane lipid domains could play a role in fish oil's effects, current methodologies are not yet available to allow scientists to decisively answer this question. The effect of dietary fish oil on relevant intracellular signal transduction and gene expression leading to T-cell proliferation has received the least attention to date.

T-CELL SIGNAL TRANSDUCTION

Optimal T-cell proliferation requires perturbation of the TCR/CD3 complex and additional costimulatory receptors *(63–65)*. Stimulation by these receptors generates intracellular signaling pathways, which activate transcription factors that induce the coordinate transcription of the IL-2 and IL-2R α genes *(66)*. Transcription of the IL-2 gene is mediated by transcription-factor-binding sites located in the promoter region. These include nuclear factor of activated T cells (NF-AT), Oct-1, nuclear factor κB (NF-κB), and activating protein-1 (AP-1, a heterodimer composed of fos and jun) *(67,68)*. Currently, the only known transcription factor regulating IL-2R α-gene expression is NF-κB *(69–72)*; however, the presence of other potential DNA-binding sites has recently

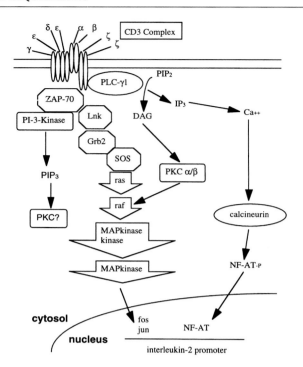

Fig. 1. *T-cell receptor intracellular signal transduction.* Stimulation of the T-cell receptor leads to the activation of the MAP kinase, PKC, PI-3-kinase and calcineurin signal transduction pathways. NF-AT = nuclear factor of activated T-cells; PKC = protein kinase C; PLC-γ1 = phospholipase C-γ1; PIP_3 = phosphatidylinositol-3,4,5-triphosphate; PIP_2 = phosphatidylinositol-4,5-bisphosphate; IP_3 = inositol-1,4,5-triphosphate; Grb2 = growth factor bound protein-2; SOS = son of sevenless; DAG = diacylglycerol; MAP kinase = mitogen activated protein kinase.

been investigated *(73–75)*. The net result of these transcriptional events is the secretion of IL-2 and expression of the IL-2R α-chain at the plasma membrane. Binding of IL-2 with the IL-2R initiates a second set of intracellular signals, driving the T cell to proliferate *(76)*. In terms of the cell cycle, the TCR/CD3 complex plus costimulatory receptor perturbation drives the G_0 to G_1 transition and the IL-2/IL-2R signaling system controls G_1 to S-phase transition, ultimately leading to T-cell mitosis *(77)*.

Intracellular signaling via stimulation of the TCR/CD3 complex has been extensively studied (Fig. 1). The TCR/CD3 complex is composed of the α and β transmembrane peptides (TCR), forming the antigen-specific part of the complex. The CD3 portion is comprised of the γ, δ, two ε, and two covalently bound ζ transmembrane peptides. The α- and β-chains have short (approximately 5–10 amino acids) cytoplasmic tails; therefore, the longer cytoplasmic tails of the CD3 complex are thought to possess the signal transduction potential. Stimulation of the TCR/CD3 complex by monoclonal antibodies to the CD3 portion or mitogenic lectins (Con A) induces the tyrosine phosphorylation of the ζ-chains on two tyrosine residues by the nonreceptor tyrosine kinase, fyn. Zeta-chain phosphorylation induces recruitment and subsequent association of the nonreceptor tyrosine kinase, ZAP-70. ZAP-70 is then activated via tyrosine phosphorylation, presumably by fyn or lck (another nonreceptor tyrosine kinase) *(78)*. Once activated, Zap-70 tyrosine phosphorylates phospholipase C-γ1 (PLC-γ1), leading to its activation. PLC-γ1 hydrolyzes phosphatidylinositol-4,5-bisphosphate (PIP_2), yielding inositol-1,4,5-triphosphate (IP_3) and diacylgycerol (DAG) (79). The IP_3 generated causes an increase in cytoplasmic calcium concentrations, which activates calcineurin, a serine/threonine phosphatase. Calcineurin dephosphorylates the cytoplasmic NF-AT, allowing it to translocate to the nucleus, where it binds to the IL-2 gene promoter and contributes to the upregulation of IL-2 gene transcription. Increased levels of DAG activate the serine/threonine kinase protein kinase C (PKC) (80,81). PKC α and/or β then phosphorylate, hence activating raf-1 kinase (82). The raf-1 kinase activates mitogen-activated protein kinase, which phosphorylates and activates mitogen-activated protein (MAP) kinase. MAP kinase ultimately enhances transcription of the *fos* and *jun* genes by a currently unknown mechanism. The fos and jun proteins form AP-1, which binds to the IL-2 promoter, enhancing IL-2 gene transcription (80). Interestingly, the TCR/CD3 complex possesses an alternative mechanism for raf-1 kinase activation. The phosphotyrosine residues of the CD3 chains recruits a 36-kDa adaptor protein (83), recently termed Lnk in CD4+ T cells (48), allowing it to be phosphorylated by ZAP-70. The 36-kDa protein then associates with Grb2 (growth factor receptor bound protein 2), another adaptor protein. The Grb2, in turn, binds the son of sevenless (SOS) protein, which is a guanine nucleotide-exchange protein. By facilitating the exchange of bound GTP for GDP, the serine/threonine kinase ras is activated. The ras enzyme can then activate raf-1 kinase, initiating the MAP kinase pathway described earlier (83). Finally, Lnk has been shown to recruit phosphatidylinositol-3-kinase (PI-3-Kinase) to the TCR/CD3 complex (48). The tyrosine phosphorylation and subsequent activation of PI-3-Kinase generates the 3-phosphorylated series of phosphoinositides (84), of which TCR stimulation has been shown to produce PIP_3. PIP_3 has been shown to activate PKC β1, ε, η, and ζ in vitro (85).

Interleukin-2 receptor activates a novel signaling cascade referred to as the JAK/STAT pathway (janus kinase/signal transducers and activators of transcription) (Fig. 1). IL-2 binding induces recruitment of the nonreceptor tyrosine kinase JAK3 to the cytoplasmic tails of the IL-2R, where they are activated by transphosphorylation (86,87). The JAK3 then tyrosine phosphorylates cytoplasmic STAT5 (88–90) and STAT3 (91,92) proteins, allowing them to translocate to the nucleus and bind DNA, inducing gene transcription (86). The nonreceptor tyrosine kinase lck is also associated with the IL-2R, which phosphorylates the adaptor protein Shc, which plays an identical role as the 36-kDa protein in TCR/CD3 signal transduction. The Shc binds Grb2, which, in turn, interacts with and stimulates SOS. SOS stimulates ras activity, leading to the activation of raf-1 kinase, thus stimulating the MAP kinase cascade (83).

The TCR/CD3 signaling cascades are crucial to T-cell proliferation, but additional receptor-mediated events are necessary to induce IL-2 secretion, leading to the equally important IL-2R-generated intracellular signals. The signaling cascades activated by the T-cell costimulatory receptors [CD28, TNF (26), and IL-1] are not well established. However, what is known about these receptors will be discussed in conjunction with the TCR/CD3 and IL-2R signaling systems in relation to PKC activation.

ROLE OF PROTEIN KINASE C IN T-CELL FUNCTION

It is well accepted that PKC plays an important role in upregulating T-cell proliferation (93,94). T-Cell activation with phorbol esters induces IL-2 and IL-2R α expression both at the protein (95–98) and mRNA (93,99) levels in normal and transformed T cells. This effect is suppressed by the addition of PKC pseudosubstrates (100). The addition of staurosporine, a PKC inhibitor, to mitogen-activated human T cells suppresses IL-2 secretion by reducing IL-2 gene levels as well as disrupting the intracellular transport of the IL-2 protein (101). The influence of pharmacologic agents on IL-2 gene expression is thought to be mediated by the PKC-dependent activation of ras. Recent evidence indicates that ras can be activated by both PKC-dependent and PKC-independent mechanisms (82,102,103), suggesting a redundancy of intracellular signals resulting in ras activation in T cells. However, inhibition of PKC with pharmacologic agents suppresses IL-2 gene levels; therefore, PKC may influence signaling cascades in addition to the ras pathway. Unfortunately, many pharmacological agents are nonspecific activators relative to PKC isoforms and can potentially stimulate other intracellular events. In order to obtain a clear understanding of PKC's role in T-cell activation, the development of tools necessary for the elucidation of individual functions for PKC isozymes is required.

Protein kinase C is a family of serine/threonine kinases currently consisting of 12 isoforms divided into 3 classes. The classical PKCs (cPKC) are α, β1, β2, and γ and require phosphatidylserine (PS), calcium, and DAG. The novel PKCs (nPKC) include δ, ε, η, θ, and μ and differ from the cPKCs by their independence from calcium. The atypical PKCs are ζ and ι/λ and are calcium and DAG independent (81); however, ζ can be activated by ceramide (104). The T cell expresses α, β1, δ, ε, η, θ, μ, and ζ (λ has not been determined) (12,81). It is accepted that PKC plays an important, although currently unknown, role(s) in upregulating T-cell proliferation (82). The lack of understanding of PKC in T-cell function is, in part, the result of the multiple and differential expression of the PKC isoforms in T-cell lineages. Human peripheral blood T cells from elderly individuals have less PKC α protein relative to their young counterparts (105). PKC α has also been shown to be absent from CD4+/CD8+ double positive thymocytes, which are functionally immature T cells (106). CD45RA+ cells, T cells that have not been stimulated or are naive, express higher protein levels of PKC α, β, and δ compared to CD45RO+ cells (memory T cells that have previously been activated) (107). In normal human CD4+ T cells, there is more β than α protein, whereas in CD8+ T cells, the relative levels of α and β are equal (108). Differences also exist between normal and transformed T cells. Mature T lymphocytes express higher PKC β relative to α, whereas in Jurkat cells, a T-cell line, more α is expressed compared to β (106,109). There are even differences between T-cell clones, with some not expressing PKC α, whereas others lack PKC β (110). Because malignant transformed cell lines are routinely used for the elucidation of T-cell signal transduction pathways (e.g., Jurkat cells), caution should be used when extrapolating these data to normal cells.

Functionally, the α and β PKC isoforms are the most extensively studied in the T cell. Stimulation of T cells with Con A or the phorbol ester PMA results in the translocation of PKC α and β from the cytosol to the membrane fraction in Jurkat cells (111). Similar observations have been in anti-CD3 stimulated human T cells (112). This is important because translocation allows PKC to interact with cofactors (DAG and PS) in the membrane which activate the classical and novel isozymes. Transgenic mice overexpressing PKC α exhibited enhanced IL-2 secretion and proliferation in anti-CD3-stimulated thymocytes; however, the effects on mature T cells were not investigated *(113)*. Transfection resulting in overexpression of PKC α in Jurkat cells enhanced AP-1 and NF-AT but not NF-κB DNA-binding activity; however, no functional responses were determined *(114)*. Overexpression of a constitutively active PKC β mutant in Jurkat cells induced the activity of an IL-2 gene reporter plasmid *(115)*. In a similar cell model, PKC β-induced IL-2 promoter activity was associated with the activation of AP-1 *(116)*. Inhibition of PKC β1 with a β1-specific agonist reduced the expression of IL-2 and IL-2R α protein levels *(117)*. Direct comparison of PKC α and β function in human T cells has shown that anti-CD3 monoclonal antibody stimulation induced a transient activation of PKC α at 10 min, followed by a prolonged increase in PKC β activity from 30 to 240 min. Suppression of PKC β activity by a monoclonal antibody resulted in suppressed IL-2 secretion and subsequent proliferation *(118)*. Furthermore, specific downregulation of PKC β by ouabain reduced IL-2 gene levels without affecting IL-2R α expression, suggesting the influence on differential signaling pathways involving distinct PKC isoforms *(93)*. Despite this evidence, controversy still exists regarding the importance of PKC β in T-cell proliferation. Three T-cell lines do not express PKC β but still proliferate and produce IL-2 in response to phorbol ester *(119–121)*. However, these cell lines may not accurately represent the intracellular events in normal cells. In addition to studies examining translocation and enzymatic activity, some evidence has been gathered showing upregulation of PKC α and β mRNA expression in response to stimulation. The addition of phorbol ester and calcium ionophore enhances PKC α and β protein and mRNA, which was positively associated with enhanced IL-2 production and IL-2R α expression in human T cells *(122)*. Mitogenic stimulation of thymocytes induces multiphasic expression of PKC β mRNA over time *(123)*. Mature, human T-cell stimulation with PHA transiently increased the time-dependent expression of PKC α and β *(124)*.

Studies examining the role of PKC isoforms other than α and β are somewhat limiting. PMA induces the translocation of PKC ε in Jurkat cells *(125)*. In normal human T cells stimulated with anti-CD3 monoclonal antibody, PKC δ and ε translocated to the membrane *(112)*. PMA stimulation does not affect PKC ζ translocation or redistribution to other intracellular compartments. However, stimulation with anti-CD3 led to a redistribution of PKC ζ to a possible cytoskeletal compartment *(126)*. This study underlines the potential differences in PKC isozyme function when using different stimuli. Mitogenic stimulation of thymocytes induces multiphasic expression of PKC ε, ζ, and δ mRNA over time *(123)*. A recent study showed that PKC ε activated AP-1 and NF-AT but not NF-κB, whereas PKC ζ did not affect any of the three transcription factors *(114)*. Unfortunately, these observations were not made in the context of a functional response.

Another area of controversy in T-cell PKC biology is whether PKC plays a role in IL-2-mediated signaling. Downregulation of PKC by PMA did not affect IL-2-mediated proliferation in Ar-5 cells, a T-cell clone, whereas Con A-induced, TCR/CD3-mediated, proliferation was suppressed *(127)*. IL-2 also induced proliferation in a murine T-cell clone that lacks the expression of the DAG and phospholipid-dependent PKC isoforms *(128)*. In contrast, a selective PKC inhibitor suppressed IL-2-mediated proliferation in TS1 cells, a T-cell line *(129)*. Using two other murine T-cell clones, this same group showed that the addition of antisense oligonucleotides to PKC β, ε or ζ reduced IL-2-mediated prolifera-

tion *(130)*. In CT6 cells, an IL-2-dependent murine T-cell clone, IL-2 induces the translocation and subsequent activation of PKC *(131)*. Clarification of these contradictory data requires studies examining the role of PKC in normal T cells. Clearly, the majority of the work examining the role of PKC isoforms in T cells has focused on translocation and subsequent activity. However, one study showed that IL-2 transiently induced the activity of an inactive membrane-associated pool of PKC *(132)*, suggesting that the lack of PKC translocation does not indicate that PKC is not activated. Activation-mediated mRNA expression and induction of protein levels, as well as functions of individual PKC isoforms, are areas that need to be examined in the future in order to elucidate the role of PKC in T-cell activation.

One of the many important events in T-cell activation is the production of the intracellular lipid second messenger, DAG, which activates protein kinase C α, β, γ, δ, ε, η, θ, and μ. It is well accepted that stimulation of the TCR/CD3 complex transiently generates DAG *(79,82)* through activation of PLC-γ1, hydrolyzing PIP_2 to DAG and IP_3. DAG has also been shown to be produced via the hydrolysis of phosphatidylcholine (PC) in Jurkat cells stimulated with PHA or anti-CD3 monoclonal antibody *(133–135)*. PC is hydrolyzed by phospholipase D (PLD), yielding phosphatidic acid (PA), which is then converted to DAG by phosphatidyl phosphohydrolase *(136)*. The duration of DAG production is also important. For example, a single transient increase in DAG is not sufficient to induce T-cell proliferation, as suggested by the requirement for multiple additions of exogenous DAG *(137,138)* or stimulation of the CD3/TCR complex *(139)* over a 2- to 4-h time period to induce T-cell proliferation. Interestingly, the PLD activity in stimulated Jurkat cells occurs at 10–30 min poststimulation *(135)*, whereas PLC-γ1 activity transiently peaks at 5 min poststimulation, suggesting that DAG can be produced for prolonged periods by PLD activation *(135)*. These observations are in agreement with the generally accepted model that DAG is biphasically produced, with the initial increase resulting from PIP_2 hydrolysis and a more sustained increase generated by the hydrolysis of PC *(140)*. Additional contributors to the intracellular pool of DAG are the costimulatory receptors (e.g., IL-1 *[141,142]* and CD28 *[143]*.) Equally important to the duration of DAG production is the molecular species of DAG produced. It has been shown that T-cell activation by either PHA or anti-CD3 generates DAGs with different fatty acid compositions *(144)*. The relevance of this observation in regard to PKC activation remains unknown. Alternatively, DAG has been shown to be generated by the IL-2R *(145)* that does not stimulate PIP_2 hydrolysis *(146)*. The IL-2R-mediated DAG appears to come from a novel source, the hydrolysis of glycosylphosphatidylinositol molecules *(147)*. The physiologic relevance of these observations remains to be determined. In conclusion, DAG is produced from multiple sources over distinct time periods and acts coordinately to induce T-cell proliferation. The key questions are as follows: What are the kinetics of DAG formation and degradation in normal T cells and how does this precisely relate to T-cell proliferation? What are the lipid sources of DAG?

Recently, ceramide has emerged as a positive effector molecule in T-cell proliferation *(148)*. This is quite surprising because ceramide is generally thought to be a molecule that induces growth suppression and/or cell death *(149)*. Ceramide can be generated by the hydrolysis of sphingomyelin (SM) via sphingomyelinase (SMase) or *de novo* by the condensation of palmitoyl CoA and serine, yielding sphingosine. A fatty acid is then added to sphingosine by ceramide synthase, yielding ceramide *(150)*. Most reports to date indicate that the hydrolysis of SM is the pathway used for intracellular signaling. There are currently two major isoforms of SMase. The neutral SMase (N-SMase) is located at the plasma membrane, whereas the acidic SMase (A-SMase) is thought to be located in lysosomes. These two isoforms have pH optimas of 7.4 and 5.0, respectively *(151)*. The T-cell costimulatory molecules TNF and IL-1 stimulate the generation of ceramide by a N-SMase *(152,153)*. However, both TNF and IL-1 T-cell receptors produce DAG *(131)*, which, at this point, is thought to have antagonistic effects on ceramide *(149)*. A series of experiments in Jurkat cells show that ceramide is produced by both N-SMase and A-SMase in response to TNF stimulation. The N-SMase is transiently activated at 1.5 min, whereas the A-SMase is transiently activated at 4 min post-TNF addition *(153)*. It has also been shown that DAG, derived from a PC-specific PLC, activates A-SMase *(154,155)*, thereby linking the DAG and ceramide signal transduction pathways. Activation of this TNF-mediated pathway is associated with the activation of NF-κB, allowing the cytosolic transcription factor to translocate to the nucleus in both Jurkat *(156)* and murine spleen T cells *(157)*. These observations have been associated with cell death; however, at lower concentrations, TNF is costimulatory with respect to T-cell proliferation *(26)*. Further evidence for the positive role of ceramide in T-cell function came from EL-4 cells, a thymocyte cell line, in which IL-1-induced ceramide formation and IL-2 secretion *(158)*. Additionally, CD28 stimulates ceramide production by A-SMase in Jurkat and freshly isolated murine spleen T cells *(159)*. In the same cell system, it was shown that ceramide mediated its costimulatory effects by enhancing IL-2 mRNA levels via inducing gene transcription and stabilizing IL-2 mRNA *(160)*. Interestingly, ceramide levels are suppressed in IL-2 stimulated human T cells *(161)*. This study indicates the possibility that ceramide may play a positive role at distinct times in the cell cycle. The mechanism by which ceramide modulates T-cell proliferation remains unclear. However, ceramide can activate several cellular enzymes, including ceramide-activated protein kinase (CAPK), ceramide-activated protein phosphatase *(162)*, and PKC ζ *(104)*. The enhancement of IL-2 production in EL-4 cells by ceramide was associated with enhanced CAPK activity *(158)*. Recently, CAPK has been shown to phosphorylate, hence activate, raf-1 kinase *(163)*, which has been attributed to the N-SMase and not the A-SMase *(164)*. This could explain the mechanism by which exogenous ceramide enhances MAP kinase activity and proliferation in fibroblasts *(165)*. An additional mechanism is via the ceramide-dependent activation of PKC ζ, which has been shown to activate NF-κB *(104)*. Alternatively, ceramide has been shown to stimulate AP-1 DNA-binding activity via activation of the Jun nuclear kinase *(166)*. However, some of the biological effects of ceramide could be attributed to sphingosine, which is generated by the hydrolysis of ceramide by ceramidase. Recently, sphingosine has been shown to inhibit apoptosis in the IL-2-dependent T-cell line CTLL-2. In this study, inhibition of sphingosine formation resulted in apoptosis. Specifically, at 2 μ*M* sphingosine, apoptosis was inhibited, but the addition of 5 μ*M* sphingosine induced apoptosis *(167)*. When 20 μ*M* sphingosine is added to Jurkat cells, DAG kinase, which phosphorylates DAG to PA, is activated *(168,169)*. Similar observations were made in porcine thymus cytosolic extracts *(170)*. Sphingosine also induces the activity of several, to date uncharacterized, protein kinases in

Jurkat cell lysates *(171)*. These results implicate the importance of the intracellular levels of sphingolipids in T-cell function.

In summary, it is clear that the lipid intracellular second messengers DAG and ceramide play important roles in enhancing T-cell proliferation. Although DAG and ceramide could mediate their effects independently, there, clearly, are several points where the two lipid second messengers interact. This is complicated by the fact that DAG and ceramide are continuously produced by activated T cells in a multiphasic fashion *(172)*.

DIETARY FISH OIL MODULATION OF T-CELL SIGNALING EVENTS

Fatty acids play an important role in T-cell function. Stimulation of T cells with mitogen results in an enrichment of polyunsaturated fatty acids and a moderate decrease in saturated fatty acids in the cellular membranes *(173,174)*. This effect is most noticeable in PC fatty acid composition *(173,175)*, which appears to be mediated by the activation of lysophosphatide acyltransferase activity following T-cell activation *(82)*. This observation is important because PC in T cells contains predominantly saturated fatty acids, which, when hydrolyzed to DAG, are relatively poor activators of PKC. However, following stimulation, there is an increase in the amount of polyunsaturated fatty acids in PC, making the hydrolized DAG a better physiologic PKC activator. These observations suggest the importance of polyunsaturated fatty acids versus saturated fatty acids, but the question still remains as to whether or not the type of polyunsaturated fatty acid is important. EPA and DHA, when fed in highly purified form, are significantly incorporated into murine splenic T-cell phospholipids with a concomitant decrease in AA content *(8)*. Feeding cod liver oil, enriched in EPA, leads to an increase in the fatty acid 24:ln-9 in SM and concomitant decreases in 22:0 and 20:0 *(176)*. Because dietary n-3 polyunsaturated fatty acids can modulate the composition (structure) of phospholipids, we speculated that it might also affect the composition, metabolism, and/or effector function of DAG and/or ceramide. To further investigate the possibility, we determined the mass and molecular species composition of DAG in murine splenic lymphocytes following short-term EPA and DHA feeding *(177)*. Generally, there was a higher n-3 fatty acid content (i.e., an increase in DAG 18:1-22:5n-3 and 16:1-20:5n-3 species) following EPA and DHA feeding. Long-chain 22:5n-3 was derived from elongation of EPA and the retroconversion of DHA. A reduction of arachidonoyl-containing species (i.e., 18:1-20:4n-6, 16:0-20:4n-6, and 18:0-20:4n-6) was also noted. Taken together, these alterations could potentially influence signal transduction pathways regulating lymphocyte function. Additional data have been gathered to support this hypothesis. For example, feeding 14.4 g/d EPA and DHA for 3 wk to humans resulted in a decrease in IP_3 formation in stimulated neutrophils *(178)*. These data imply that the production of DAG might be suppressed. This implication is supported by a recent study where a 10% (wt/wt) fat diet enriched in EPA and DHA ethyl esters resulted in suppressed DAG formation in thioglycollate-elicited peritoneal macrophages in response to ionomycin stimulation *(179)*. Furthermore, feeding highly purified EPA and DHA to mice for 10 d significantly increased the n-3 fatty acid composition of DAG from murine splenic T cells *(177)*. It is important to note that, to date, only one published study has determined the ability of dietary n-3 polyunsaturated fatty acids to modulate ceramide formation or structure *(42)*. In this study, Con A-induced DAG and ceramide

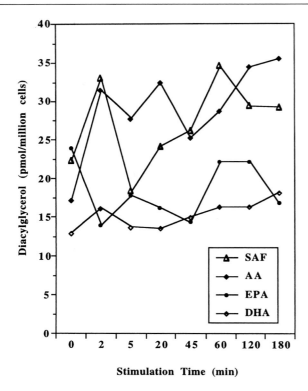

Fig. 2. *Blunted DAG kinetics in activated lymphocytes in response to dietary EPA and DHA.* Murine splenic lymphocytes were isolated and incubated with 10 μg/ml Con A. At 0, 2, 5, 20, 45, 60, 120 and 180 min, cell aliquots were obtained. Cellular lipids were extracted and DAG mass determined using the DAG kinase phosphorylation assay. △ = SAF (safflower oil ethyl esters, contains no n-3 polyunsaturated fatty acids); ● = AA (arachidonic acid triglyceride, contains no n-3 polyunsaturated fatty acids); ○ = EPA; ■ = DHA. Values represent means ± SEM, n = 4-5. All time points from 2-180 min were significantly ($p < 0.05$) lower, EPA = DHA < AA = SAF. Adapted from reference *42*.

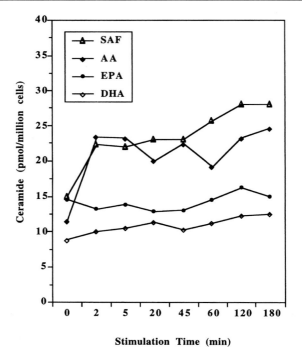

Fig. 3. *Dietary EPA and DHA suppress ceramide kinetics in activated lymphocytes.* Murine splenic lymphocytes were isolated and incubated with 10 μg/ml Con A. At 0, 2, 5, 20, 45, 60, 120 and 180 min, cell aliquots were obtained. Cellular lipids were extracted and ceramide mass quantitated using the DAG kinase phosphorylation assay. Refer to Figure 2 for details. △ = SAF; ◆ = AA; ● = EPA; ◇ = DHA. Values represent means ± SEM, n = 5-6. All time points from 2-180 min were significantly ($p < 0.05$) lower, EPA = DHA < AA = SAF. Adapted from reference *42*.

kinetic responses in splenic lymphocytes from EPA- and DHA-fed mice were determined *(42)*. Interestingly, both EPA and DHA significantly blunted DAG (Fig. 2) and ceramide (Fig. 3) production at most time points in response to Con A. However, n-3 PUFA feeding did not influence basal (time 0) DAG and ceramide levels, indicating that basic homeostatic mechanisms were not altered. Collectively, these data demonstrate that highly purified dietary EPA and DHA suppress the production of early/immediate second messengers, DAG and ceramide, in activated T cells.

The blunted activation signals (reduced DAG and ceramide production at 0–3 h) and reduced secretion of IL-2 (48 h) *(42)* suggest that dietary EPA and DHA influence T-cell proliferation by either a pretranscriptional or posttranscriptional mechanism involving the IL-2 and/or IL-2R α gene. Therefore, we also determined the effects of dietary EPA and DHA on Con A-induced IL-2 and IL-2R α-gene expression in murine splenocytes *(174)*. Dietary EPA and DHA moderately suppressed IL-2 gene expression at 3 h after mitogen addition; however, maximal expression did not differ between diet groups (Fig. 4). The differences observed in IL-2 gene expression can only partly explain the drastic reduction in IL-2 secretion. The expression of IL-2R α was suppressed 3 h after Con A addition by dietary EPA and DHA, and maximal expression was moderately reduced in EPA-

fed mice, and to a greater extent in the DHA-fed mice (Fig. 5). Interestingly, DHA feeding resulted in higher IL-2R α expression at 9 h, which may indicate a compensatory mechanism for suppressed IL-2 secretion. These data show, for the first time, that EPA and DHA do not affect IL-2 mRNA expression but suppress IL-2R α mRNA levels.

It is well established that PKC plays an important positive role in T-lymphocyte activation *(81)* via regulation of IL-2 *(92)* and IL-2R α-gene expression. We have demonstrated that dietary EPA and DHA enhance mitogen-induced PKC α, PKC β1, and PKC ζ mRNA expression relative to the SAF and AA groups (Jolly, McMurray, and Chapkin, unpublished data). Interestingly, PKC α and β1 basal (time 0) mRNA levels were elevated in DHA-fed mice relative to the SAF, AA, and EPA groups. These results are surprising because both EPA and DHA suppress IL-2 secretion and impair proliferation *(42)*. It is possible that the basal changes reflect a compensatory mechanism whereby EPA and DHA feeding suppress DAG and ceramide formation *(42)*, which could result in reduced PKC activity. The cells might respond to the suppressed PKC activity and upregulate PKC transcription to generate additional PKC protein. However, this compensatory mechanism would be ineffective because the PKC activators, DAG and ceramide, are reduced by either EPA or DHA feeding *(42)*. The assumption that increased mRNA levels result in more protein yielding higher enzyme activity is not always valid because PKC can be modulated by multiple posttranscriptional mechanisms

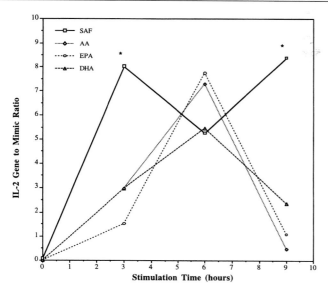

Fig. 4. *Effects of dietary EPA and DHA on IL-2 gene expression.* Mice were fed SAF, AA, EPA or DHA diets for 10 days. Splenic lymphocytes were isolated and incubated with 5 µg/ml Con A. At 0, 3, 6, or 9 h, cell aliquots were obtained and RNA isolated. The mRNA was reverse-transcribed and samples were analyzed by relative competitive-polymerase chain reaction (RC-PCR) using IL-2 specific primers. The integrated density represents the ratio of IL-2 gene product to internal standard (mimic). Values represent n = 3. Note: At time 0, IL-2 message was virtually undetectable in all groups. (*) Indicates significant ($p < 0.05$) differences between diets within a time point. Adapted from reference 180.

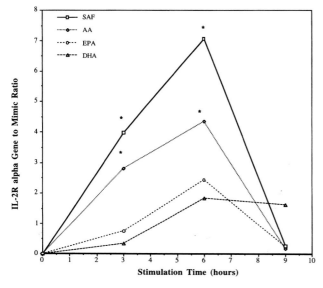

Fig. 5. *Effects of dietary EPA and DHA on IL-2Rα gene expression.* Mice were fed the experimental diets and splenic lymphocytes were isolated and stimulated as described in Figure 4. Samples were analyzed by relative competitive-PCR using IL-2Rα specific primers. The integrated density represents the ratio of IL-2Rα gene product to internal standard (mimic). Values represent n = 3. (*) Indicates significant ($p < 0.05$) differences between diets within a time point. Adapted from reference 180.

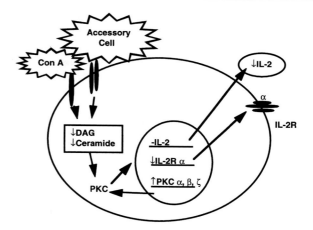

Fig. 6. *Model of dietary n-3 fatty acid effects on T-lymphocyte interleukin-2 secretion, signal transduction and gene expression.* Arrows pointing down represent events suppressed by dietary EPA and DHA, while arrows pointing up indicate events that are up-regulated by dietary EPA and DHA. A dash represents no effect by EPA and DHA. PKC = protein kinase C; Con A = concanavalin A; DAG = diacyglycerol; IL-2 = interleukin-2; IL-2R = interleukin-2 receptor.

(180,181). Therefore, a clear interpretation of the enhanced PKC α, β1, and ζ mRNA levels in this system will have to await determination of PKC α, β1, and ζ protein levels.

In summary, our results show that highly purified dietary EPA and DHA, which are constituents of fish oil, do not affect mitogen-induced splenic lymphocyte IL-2 gene expression but suppress IL-2R α mRNA levels. In addition, EPA and DHA feeding enhances PKC α, β1, and ζ mRNA levels. These results indicate that the suppressed IL-2 secretion and impaired proliferative response we previously reported *(42)* are not due to reductions in IL-2 mRNA levels. However, reduced IL-2R α-gene transcription may play a role in blunting the T-lymphocyte proliferative response previously reported *(42).* These data are the first to demonstrate that highly purified dietary EPA and DHA influences T-lymphocyte intracellular signal transduction. Future studies will address the specific mechanism(s) by which dietary EPA and DHA selectively modulate T-lymphocyte gene expression.

SUMMARY

Human and rodent inflammatory disease studies have shown that dietary fish oil, enriched in eicosapentaenoic acid (20:5n-3 [EPA]) and docosahexaenoic acid (22:6n-3 [DHA]), is therapeutic with respect to inflammatory diseases such as rheumatoid arthritis. The anti-inflammatory properties of fish oil are correlated with impaired T-cell IL-2 production and proliferative response. This is important because the T cell plays an obligatory role in propagating the immune response and IL-2 is a potent autocrine and paracrine T-cell growth factor. To date, few studies have examined the mechanism(s) by which fish oil alters intracellular signal transduction and/or gene expression in activated T cells.

Growing evidence indicates that the anti-inflammatory effects of dietary fish oil are mediated by both EPA and DHA. Furthermore, both EPA and DHA exert similar effects on T cells, indicating, at this point, no clear divergence with respect to mechanism of action. The suppressive effect of highly purified dietary EPA and DHA on activated T-cell gene expression implies that the reduced IL-2 secretion and impaired proliferative response are not due to nonspecific epiphenomena.

Future studies will need to focus on the potential role of accessory cells (macrophage) in the EPA- and DHA-mediated modulation of T-cell function. Additionally, experiments need to be conducted to elucidate the mechanism(s) by which EPA and DHA selectively modulate T-cell IL-2R α and PKC isozyme gene expression.

ACKNOWLEDGMENTS

This work was supported in part by USDA Hatch Funds (H-6983), Texas Agricultural Experiment Station and the Interdisciplinary Research Initiatives Program Grant, Texas A&M University.

REFERENCES

1. Adapted from the Arthritis Foundation. World Wide Web address: http://www.arthritis.org/facts/index.html.
2. Pincus T, Callahan LF. What is the natural history of rheumatoid arthritis? Rheum Dis Clin North Am 1993; 19:123–51.
3. Kremer JM. Clinical studies of omega-3 fatty acid supplementation in patients who have rheumatoid arthritis. Rheum Dis Clin North Am 1991; 17:391–402.
4. Simopoulos AP. Omega-3 fatty acids in health and disease and in growth and development. Am J Clin Nutr 1991; 54:438–63.
5. Nielsen GL, Farrvang KL, Thomsen BS, Teglbjerg KL, Jensen LT, Hansen TM, et al. The effects of dietary supplementation with n-3 polyunsaturated fatty acids in patients with rheumatoid arthritis: a randomized, double blind trial. Eur J Clin Invest 1992; 22:687–91.
6. Bang HO, Dyerberg J, Sinclair HM. The composition of the Eskimo food in north western Greenland. Am J Clin Nutr 1980; 33:2657–61.
7. Kinsella JE. Dietary fats and cardiovascular disease. In: Kinsella JE, ed, Seafoods and Fish Oils in Human Health and Disease, pp. 14–260. Marcell Dekker, New York, 1987.
8. Hosack-Fowler K, Chapkin RS, McMurray DN. Effects of purified dietary n-3 ethyl esters on murine T lymphocyte function. J Immunol 1993; 151:5186–97.
9. Jonnalagadda SS, Egan SK, Heimbach JT, Harris SS, Kris-Etherton PM. Fatty acid consumption pattern of Americans: 1987–1988 USDA nationwide food consumption survey. Nutr Res 1995; 15: 1767–81.
10. Kjeldsen-Kragh J, Lund JA, Riise T, Finnanger B, Haaland K, Finstad R, et al. Dietary omega-3 fatty acid supplementation and naproxen treatment in patients with rheumatoid arthritis. J Rheumatol 1992; 19:1531–6.
11. Skoldstam L, Borjesson O, Kjallman A, Seiving B, Akesson B. Effect of six months of fish oil supplementation in stable rheumatoid arthritis. A double-blind, controlled study. Scand J Rheumatol 1992; 21:178–85.
12. Lau CS, Morley KD, Belch JJ. Effects of fish oil supplementation on non-steroidal anti-inflammatory drug requirement in patients with mild rheumatoid arthritis—a double-blind placebo controlled study. Br J Rheumatol 1993; 32:982–89.
13. Geusens P, Wouters C, Nijs J, Jiang Y, Dequeker J. Long-term effect of omega-3 fatty acid supplementation in active rheumatoid arthritis. Arthritis Rheum 1994; 37:824–29.
14. Kremer JM, Lawrence DA, Petrillo GF, Litts LL, Mullaly PM, Rynes RL, et al. Effects of high-dose fish oil on rheumatoid arthritis after stopping nonsteroidal antiinflammatory drugs. Arthritis Rheum 1995; 38:1107–14.
15. Endres S, De Caterina R, Schmidt EB, Kristensen SD. n-3 polyunsaturated fatty acids: update 1995. Eur J Clin Invest 1995; 25:629–38.
16. Morrow WJW, Homsy J, Levy JA. The influence of nutrition on experimental autoimmune disease. In: Cunningham-Rundles S, ed,

17. Prickett JD, Robinson DR, Steinberg AD. Effects of dietary enrichment with eicosapentaenoic acid upon autoimmune nephritis in female NZB×NZW/F1 mice. Arthritis Rheum 1983; 26:133–9.
18. Venkatraman JT, Fernandes G. Mechanisms of delayed autoimmune disease in B/W mice by omega-3 lipids and food restriction. In: Chandra RK, ed, Nutrition and Immunology, pp. 309–23. ARTS Biomedical Publishers and Distributors, St. John's, Newfoundland, Canada, 1992.
19. Alexander NJ, Smythe NL, Jokinen MP. The type of dietary fat affects the severity of autoimmune disease in NZB/NZW mice. Am J Pathol 1987; 127:106–21.
20. Westberg G, Tarkowski A, Svalander C. Effect of eicosapentaenoic acid rich menhaden oil and MaxEPA on the autoimmune disease of Mrl/l mice. Int Arch Allergy Appl Immunol 1989; 88:454–61.
21. Watson J, Godfrey D, Stimson WH, Belch JJF, Sturrock RD. The therapeutic effects of dietary fatty acid supplementation in the autoimmune disease of the MRL-mp-lpr/1pr mouse. Int J Immunopharmacol 1988; 10:467–71.
22. Prickett JD, Trentham DE, Robinson DR. Dietary fish oil augments the induction of arthritis in rats immunized with type II collagen. J Immunol 1984; 132:725–9.
23. Leslie CA, Gonnerman WA, Ullman MD, Hayes KC, Franzblau C, Cathcart ES. Dietary fish oil modulates macrophage fatty acids and decreases arthritis susceptibility in mice. J Exp Med 1985; 162: 1336–49.
24. Panayi GS. The pathogenesis of rheumatoid arthritis: from molecules to the whole patient. Br J Rheumatol 1993; 32:533–6.
25. Abbas AK, Lichtman AH, Pober JS. Lymphocyte specificity and activation. In Wonsiewicz MJ, ed, Cellular and Molecular Immunology, pp. 35–68, WB Saunders Company, Philadelphia, 1991.
26. Munoz-Fernandez MA, Pimentel-Muinos FX, Alonso MA, Campanero M, Sanchez-Madrid F, Silva A, et al. Synergy of tumor necrosis factor with protein kinase C activators on T cell activation. Eur J Immunol 1990; 20:605–10.
27. Calder PC. Fatty acids, dietary lipids and lymphocyte functions. Biochem Soc Trans 1995; 23:302–9.
28. VanMeter AR, Ehringer WD, Stillwell W, Blumenthal EJ, Jenski LJ. Aged lymphocyte proliferation following incorporation and retention of dietary omega-3 fatty acids. Mech Age Dev 1994; 75:95–114.
29. Vallette L, Croset M, Prigent AF, Meskini N, LaGarde M. Dietary polyunsaturated fatty acids modulate fatty acid composition and early activation steps of concanavalin A-stimulated rat thymocytes. J Nutr 1991; 121:1844–59.
30. Hwang D. Essential fatty acids and immune response. FASEB J 1989; 3:2052–61.
31. Fritsche KL, Johnston PV. Effect of dietary omega-3 fatty acids on cell-mediated cytotoxic activity in BALB/C mice. Nutr Res 1990; 10:577–88.
32. Endres S, Meydani SN, Ghorbani R, Schindler R, Dinarello CA. Dietary supplementation with n-3 fatty acids suppresses interleukin-2 production and mononuclear cell proliferation. J Leuk Biol 1993; 54:599–603.
33. Meydani SN, Endres S, Woods MM, Goldin BR, Soo C, Morrill-Labrode A, et al. Oral (n-3) fatty acid supplementation suppresses cytokine production and lymphocyte proliferation: comparison between young and older women. J Nutr 1991; 121:547–55.
34. Meydani SN, Lichtenstein AH, Cornwall S, Meydani M, Goldin BR, Rasmussen H, et al. Immunologic effects of National Cholesterol Education Panel Step-2 diets with and without fish-derived n-3 fatty acid enrichment. J Clin Invest 1993; 92:105–13.
35. Yaqoob P, Newsholme EA, Calder PC. The effect of dietary lipid manipulation on rat lymphocyte subsets and proliferation. Immunology 1994; 82:603–10.
36. Yaqoob P, Newsholme EA, Calder PC. The effect of fatty acids on leucocyte subsets and proliferation in rat whole blood. Nutr Res 1995; 15:279–87.
37. Shapiro AC, Wu D, Hayek MG, Meydani M, Meydani SN. Role

of eicosanoids and vitamin E in fish oil-induced changes of spleno-cyte proliferation to T cell mitogens in mice. Nutr Res 1994; 14:1339–54.

38. Wu D, Meydani SN, Meydani M, Hayek MG, Huth P, Nicolosi RJ. Immunologic effects of marine- and plant-derived n-3 polyunsaturated fatty acids in nonhuman primates. Am J Clin Nutr 1996; 63:273–80.

39. Payan DG, Wong MYS, Chernov-Rogan T, Valone FH, Pickett WC, Blake VA, et al. Alterations in human leukocyte function induced by ingestion of eicosapentaenoic acid. J Clin Immunol 1986; 6:402–10.

40. Surette MEJ, Whelan J, Lu G, Hardard'ottir I, Kinsella JE. Dietary n-3 polyunsaturated fatty acids modify Syrian hamster platelet and macrophage phospholipid fatty acyl composition and eicosanoid synthesis: a controlled study. Biochim Biophys Acta 1995; 1255: 185–91.

41. Chapkin RS, Coble KJ. Remodeling of mouse kidney phospholipid classes and subclasses by diet. J Nutr Biochem 1991; 2:158–64.

42. Jolly CA, Jiang YH, Chapkin RS, McMurray DN. Dietary n-3 polyunsaturated fatty acid modulation of murine lymphoproliferation and interleukin-2 secretion: correlation with alterations in diacyl-glycerol and ceramide mass. J Nutr 1997; 127:37–43.

43. Brenner RR. Effect of unsaturated acids on membrane structure and enzyme kinetics. Prog Lipid Res 1984; 23:69–96.

44. Hagve TA. Effects of unsaturated fatty acids on cell membrane functions. Scand J Clin Lab Invest 1988; 48:381–8.

45. Conroy DM, Stubbs CD, Belin J, Pryor CL, Smith AD. The effects of dietary (n-3) fatty acid supplementation on lipid dynamics and composition in rat lymphocytes and liver microsomes. Biochim Biophys Acta 1986; 861:457–62.

46. Housley MD, Stanley KK. Lipid–protein interactions. In: Houslay MD, Stanley KK, eds, Dynamics of Biological Membranes, pp. 92–151, Wiley, New York, 1982.

47. Brouard C, Pascaud M. Effects of moderate dietary supplementations with n-3 fatty acids on macrophage and lymphocyte phospholipid and macrophage eicosanoid synthesis in the rat. Biochim Biophys Acta 1990; 1047:19–28.

48. Huang X, Li Y, Tanaka K, Moores KG, Hayashi JI. Cloning and characterization of Lnk, a signal transduction protein that links T-cell receptor activation signal to phospholipase Cγ1, Grb2, and phosphatidylinositol 3-kinase. Proc Natl Acad Sci 1995; 92:11,618–22.

49. Chapkin RS, Akoh CC, Miller CC. Influence of dietary n-3 fatty acids on macrophage glycerophospholipid molecular species and peptido leukotriene synthesis. J Lipid Res 1991; 32:1205–13.

50. Zurier RB. Prostaglandins, fatty acids, and arthritis. In: Cunningham-Rundles, S, ed, Nutrient Modulation of the Immune Response, pp. 201–21. Marcel Dekker, New York, 1993.

51. Raclot T, Groscolas R, Langin D, Ferre P. Site-specific regulation of gene expression by n-3 polyunsaturated fatty acids in rat white adipose tissues. J Lipid Res 1997; 38:1963–72.

52. Wander RC, Hall JA, Gradin JL, Du SH, Jewell DE. The ratio of dietary (n-6) to (n-3) fatty acids influences immune system function, eicosanoid metabolism, lipid peroxidation and vitamin E status in aged dogs. J Nutr 1997; 127:1198–205.

53. Scherer JM, Stillwell W, Jenski LJ. Spleen survival and proliferation are differentially altered by docosahexaenoic acid. Cell Immunol 1997; 180:153–61.

54. Rossetti RG, Seiler CM, DeLuca P, Laposata M, Zurier RB. Oral administration of unsaturated fatty acids: effects on human peripheral blood T lymphocyte proliferation. J Leuk Biol 1997; 62:438–43.

55. Masters C. Omega-3 fatty acids and the peroxisome. Mol Cell Biochem 1996; 165:83–93.

56. Fujikawa M, Yamashita N, Yamazaki K, Sugiyama E, Suzuki H, Hamazaki T. Eicosapentaenoic acid inhibits antigen-presenting cell function of murine splenocytes. Immunology 1992; 75:330–35.

57. Hughes DA, Pinder AC, Piper Z, Johnson IT, Lund EK. Fish oil supplementation inhibits the expression of major histocompatibility complex class II molecules and adhesion molecules on human mono-cytes. Am J Clin Nutr 1996; 63:267–72.

58. Renier G, Skamene E, DeSanctis J, Radzioch D. Dietary n-3 polyunsaturated fatty acids prevent the development of atherosclerotic lesions in mice. Arterioscler Thromb 1993; 13:1515–24.

59. Somers SD, Erickson KL. Alteration of tumor necrosis factor-α production by macrophages from mice fed diets high in eicosapentaenoic and docosahexaenoic fatty acids. Cell Immunol 1994; 153: 287–97.

60. Hardard'Ottir I, Whelan J, Kinsella JE. Kinetics of tumour necrosis factor and prostaglandin production by murine resident peritoneal macrophages as affected by dietary n-3 polyunsaturated fatty acids. Immunology 1992; 76:572–7.

61. Jenski LJ, Bowker GM, Johnson MA, Ehringer WD, Fetterhoff T, Stillwell W. Docosahexaenoic acid-induced alteration of Thy-1 and CD8 expression on murine splenocytes. Biochim Biophys Acta 1995; 1236:39–50.

62. Soyland E, Lea T, Sandstad B, Drevon A. Dietary supplementation with very long-chain n-3 fatty acids in man decreases expression of the interleukin-2 receptor (CD25) on mitogen-stimulated lympho-cytes from patients with inflammatory skin diseases. Eur J Clin Invest 1994; 24:236–42.

63. Fraser JD, Straus D, Weiss A. Signal transduction events leading to T-cell lymphokine gene expression. Immunol Today 1993; 14: 357–62.

64. Liu Y. Molecular basis of T cell costimulation. In: Liu Y, ed, The Costimulatory Pathways for T Cell Responses, pp. 30–67. R. G. Landes Company, Austin, TX, 1994.

65. Weiss A, Imboden J, Hardy K, Manger B, Terhorst C, Stobo J. The role of the T3/antigen receptor complex in T-cell activation. Annu Rev Immunol 1986; 4:593–619.

66. Ullman KS, Northrop JP, Verweij CL, Crabtree GR. Transmission of signals from the T lymphocyte antigen receptor to the genes responsible for cell proliferation and immune function. Annu Rev Immunol 1990; 8:421–52.

67. Serfling E, Avots A, Neumann M. The architecture of the interleukin-2 promoter: a reflection of T lymphocyte activation. Biochim Biophys Acta 1995; 1263:181–200.

68. Pahlavani MA, Harris MD, Richardson A. The increase in the induction of IL-2 expression with caloric restriction is correlated to changes in the transcription factor NFAT. Cell Immunol 1997; 180:10–9.

69. Nabholz M, Soldaini E, Sperisen P, Pla M, Wang SM, MacDonald HR, et al. The cis-acting elements controlling mouse IL-2Rα transcription. Immunobiology 1995; 193:259–62.

70. Sperisen P, Wang SM, Soldaini E, Pla M, Rusterholz C, Bucher P, et al. Mouse interleukin-2 receptor α gene expression. J Biol Chem 1995; 270:10,743–53.

71. Pimentel-Muinos FX, Mazana J, Fresno M. Regulation of interleukin-2 receptor α chain expression and nuclear factor-kB activation by protein kinase C in T lymphocytes. J Biol Chem 1994; 269: 24,424–9.

72. Soldaini E, Pla M, Beermann F, Espel E, Corthesy P, Barange S, Waanders GA, et al. Mouse interleukin-2 receptor α gene expression. J Biol Chem 1995; 270:10,733–42.

73. Ng J, Cantrell D. STAT3 is a serine kinase target in T lymphocytes. J Biol Chem 1997; 272:24,542–9.

74. Meyer WKH, Reichenbach P, Schindler U, Soldaini E, Nabholz M. Interaction of STAT5 dimers on two low affinity binding sites mediates interleukin 2 (IL-2) stimulation of IL-2 receptor α gene transcription. J Biol Chem 1997; 272:31,821–8.

75. Ascherman DP, Migone TS, Friedmann MC, Leonard WJ. Interleukin-2 (IL-2)-mediated induction of the IL-2 receptor α chain gene. J Biol Chem 1997; 272:8704–9.

76. Mills GB, Schmandt R, Gibson S, Leung B, Hill M, May C, et al. Transmembrane signaling by the interleukin-2 receptor: progress and conundrums. Semin Immunol 1993; 5:345–64.

77. Downward J, Graves J, Cantrell D. The regulation and function of p21ras in T cells. Immunol Today 1992; 13:89–92.

78. Howe LR, Weiss A. Multiple kinases mediate T-cell-receptor signaling. TIBS 1995; 20:59–64.

79. Park DJ, Rho HW, Rhee SG. CD3 stimulation causes phosphorylation of phospholipase C-γ1 on serine and tyrosine residues in a human T-cell line. Proc Natl Acad Sci USA 1991; 88:5453–6.

80. Weiss A, Littman DR. Signal transduction by lymphocyte antigen receptors. Cell 1994; 76:263–74.

81. Hug H, Sarre TF. Protein kinase C isoenzymes: divergence in signal transduction. Biochem J 1993; 291:329–43.

82. Szamel M, Leufgen H, Kurrle R, Resch K. Differential signal transduction pathways regulating interleukin-2 synthesis and interleukin-2 receptor expression in stimulated human lymphocytes. Biochim Biophys Acta 1995; 1235:33–42.

83. Izquierdo M, Leevers SJ, Williams DH, Marshall CJ, Weiss A, Cantrell D. The role of protein kinase C in the regulation of extracellular signal-regulated kinase by the T cell antigen receptor. Eur J Immunol 1994; 24:2462–8.

84. Rudd CE, Janssen O, Cai Y, da Silva AJ, Raab M, Prasad KVS. Two-step TCRζ/CD3-CD4 and CD28 signaling in T cells: SH2/SH3 domains, protein-tyrosine and lipid kinases. Immunol Today 1994; 21:123–32.

85. Palmer RH, Dekker LV, Woscholski R, Le Good JA, Gigg R, Parker PJ. Activation of PRK1 by phosphatidylinositol 4,5-bisphosphate and phosphatidylinositol 3,4,5-triphosphate. J Biol Chem 1995; 270:22,412–6.

86. Ihle JN, Witthuhn BA, Quelle FW, Yamamoto K, Thierfelder WE, Kreider B, et al. Signaling by the cyokine receptor superfamily: JAKs and STATS. TIBS 1994; 19:222–7.

87. Kawahara A, Minami Y, Miyazaki T, Ihle JN, Taniguchi T. Critical role of the interleukin-2 (IL-2) receptor γ-chain-associated JAK3 in the IL-2-induced c-fos and c-myc but not bcl-2, gene induction. Proc Natl Acad Sci 1995; 92:8724–8.

88. Kirken RA, Rui H, Malabarba MG, Howard OMZ, Kawamura M, O'Shea JJ, et al. Activation of JAK3, but not JAK1, is critical for IL-2-induced proliferation and STAT5 recruitment by a COOH-terminal region of the IL-2 receptor β-chain. Cytokine 1995; 7:689–700.

89. Gilmour KC, Pine R, Reich NC. Interleukin 2 activates STAT5 transcription factor (mammary gland factor) and specific gene expression in T lymphocytes. Proc Natl Acad Sci 1995; 92:10,772–6.

90. Gaffen SL, Lai SV, Xu W, Gouilleux F, Groner B, Goldsmith MA, et al. Signaling through the interleukin 2 receptor β chain activates a STAT-5-like DNA-binding activity. Proc Natl Acad Sci 1995; 92:7192–6.

91. Nielsen M, Svejgaard A, Skov S, Odum N. Interleukin-2 induces tyrosine phosphorylation and nuclear translocation of STAT3 in human T lymphocytes. Eur J Immunol 1994; 24:3082–6.

92. Brunn GJ, Falls EL, Nilson AE, Abraham RT. Protein–tyrosine kinase-dependent activation of STAT transcription factors in interleukin-2- or interleukin-4-stimulated T lymphocytes. J Biol Chem 1995; 270:11,628–35.

93. Szamel M, Resch K. T-cell antigen receptor-induced signal-transduction pathways: activation and function of protein kinases C in T lymphocytes. Eur J Biochem 1995; 228:1–15.

94. Keenan C, Long A, Kelleher D. Protein kinase C and T cell function. Biochim Biophys Acta 1997; 1358:111–26.

95. Depper JM, Leonard MJ, Kronke M, Noguchi PD, Cunningham RE, Waldmann TA, et al. Regulation of interleukin 2 receptor expression: effects of phorbol diester, phospholipase C, and reexposure to lectin or antigen. J Immunol 1984; 84:3054–61.

96. Farrar WL, Ruscetti FW. Association of protein kinase C activation with IL 2 receptor expression. J Immunol 1986; 136:1266–73.

97. Hengel H, Allig B, Wagner H, Heeg K. Dissection of signals controlling T cell function and activation: H7, an inhibitor of protein kinase C, blocks induction of primary T cell proliferation by suppressing interleukin (IL) 2 receptor expression without affecting IL 2 production. Eur J Immunol 1991; 21:1575–82.

98. Isakov N, Altman A. Human T lymphocyte activation by tumor promoters: role of protein kinase C. J Immunol 1987; 138:3100–7.

99. Kumagai N, Benedict SH, Mills GB, Gelfand EW. Requirements for the simultaneous presence of phorbol esters and calcium ionophores in the expression of human T lymphocyte proliferation-related genes. J Immunol 1987; 139:1393–9.

100. Barja P, Alavi-Nasab A, Turck CW, Freire-Moar J. Inhibition of T cell activation by protein kinase C pseudosubstrates. Cell Immunol 1994; 153:28–38.

101. Modiano JF, Kolp R, Lamb RJ, Nowell PC. Protein kinase C regulates both production and secretion of interleukin 2. J Biol Chem 1991; 266:10,552–61.

102. Izquierdo M, Downward J, Graves JD, Cantrell DA. Role of protein kinase C in T-cell antigen receptor regulation of p21ras: evidence that two p21ras regulatory pathways coexist in T cells. Mol Cell Biol 1992; 12:3305–12.

103. William DH, Woodrow M, Cantrell DA, Murray EJ. Protein kinase C is not a downstream effector of p21ras in activated T cells. Eur J Immunol 1995; 25:42–7.

104. Lozano J, Berra E, Municio MM, Diaz-Meco MT, Dominguez I, Sanz L, et al. Protein kinase C ζ isoform is critical for kB-dependent promoter activation by sphingomyelinase. J Biol Chem 1994; 269:19,200–2.

105. Whisler RL, Newhouse YG, Grants IS, Hackshaw KV. Differential expression of the α- and β-isoforms of protein kinase C in peripheral blood T and B cells from young and elderly adults. Mech Age Dev 1995; 77:197–211.

106. Tarantino N, Debre P, Korner M. Differential expression of PKCα and PKCβ isozymes in CD4+, CD8+ and CD4+/CD8+ double positive human T cells. FEBS Lett 1994; 338:339–42.

107. Corrigan E, Kelleher D, Feighery C, Long A. Protein kinase C isoform expression in CD45RA+ and CD45RO+ T lymphocytes. Immunology 1995; 85:299–303.

108. Gupta S, Harris W. Phorbol myristate acetate-induced changes in protein kinase C isozymes (α, β, γ and ζ) in human T cell subsets. In: Gupta VS, ed, Mechanisms of Lymphocyte Activation and Immune Regulation, pp. 143–448. Plenum, New York, 1994.

109. Lucas S, Marais R, Graves JD, Alexander D, Parker P, Cantrell, DA. Heterogeneity of protein kinase C expression and regulation in T lymphocytes. FEBS Lett 1990; 260:53–6.

110. Terajima J, Tsutsumi A, Freire-Moar J, Cherwinski HM, Ransom JT. Evidence for clonal heterogeneity of the expression of six protein kinase C isoforms in murine B and T lymphocytes. Cell Immunol 1992; 142:197–206.

111. Kvanta A, Jondal M, Fredholm BB. Translocation of the α- and β-isoforms of protein kinase C following activation of human T-lymphocytes. FEBS Lett 1991; 283:321–4.

112. Fulop T Jr, Leblanc C, Lacombe G, Dupuis G. Cellular distribution of protein kinase C isozymes in CD3-mediated stimulation of human T lymphocytes with aging. FEBS Lett 1995; 375:69–74.

113. Iwamoto T, Hagiwara M, Hidaka H, Isomura T, Kioussis D, Nakashima I. Accelerated proliferation and interleukin-2 production of thymocytes by stimulation of soluble anti-CD3 monoclonal antibody in transgenic mice carrying a rabbit protein kinase Cα. J Biol Chem 1992; 267:18,644–8.

114. Genot EM, Parker PJ, Cantrell DA. Analysis of the role of protein kinase C-α, -ε, and -ζ in T cell activation. J Biol Chem 1995; 270:9833–9.

115. Muramatsu MA, Kaibuchi K, Arai KI. A protein kinase C cDNA without the regulatory domain is active after transfection in vivo in the absence of phorbol ester. Mol Cell Biol 1989; 9:831–6.

116. Hama N, Paliogianni F, Fessler BJ, Boumpas DT. Calcium/calmodulin-dependent protein kinase II downregulates both calcineurin and protein kinase C-mediated pathways for cytokine gene transcription in human T cells. J Exp Med 1995; 181:1217–22.

117. Aggarwal S, Lee S, Marthur A, Gollapudi S, Gupta S. 12-Deoxyphorbol-13-O-phenylacetate 20 acetate [an agonist of protein kinase Cβ1 (PKCβ1)] induces DNA synthesis, interleukin-2 (IL-2) production, IL-2 receptor α-chain (CD25) and β-chain (CD122) expression, and translocation of PKCβ isozyme in human peripheral blood lymphocytes: evidence for a role of PKCβ1 in human T cell activation. J Clin Immunol 1994; 14:248–56.

118. Szamel M, Bartels F, Resch K. Cyclosporin A inhibits T cell receptor-induced interleukin-2 synthesis of human T lymphocytes by selectively preventing a transmembrane signal transduction pathway leading to sustained activation of a protein kinase C isoenzyme, protein kinase C-β. Eur J Immunol 1993; 23:3072–81.

119. Koretzky GA, Wahi M, Newton ME, Weiss A. Heterogeneity of protein kinase C isoenzyme gene expression in human T cell lines. J Immunol 1989; 143:1692–5.

120. Kelleher D, Long A. Development and characterization of a protein kinase C β-isozyme-deficient T-cell line. FEBS Lett 1992; 301:310–4.

121. Long A, Kelleher D. Conventional protein kinase C isoforms are not essential for cellular proliferation of a T cell lymphoma line. FEBS Lett 1993; 333:243–7.

122. Altman A, Mally MI, Isakov N. Phorbol ester synergized with Ca²⁺ ionophore in activation of protein kinase C (PKC)α and PKCβ isoenzymes in human T cells and in induction of related cellular functions. Immunology 1992; 76:465–71.

123. Freire-Moar J, Cherwinski H, Hwang F, Ransom J, Webb D. Expression of protein kinase C isoenzymes in thymocyte subpopulations and their differential regulation. J Immunol 1991; 147:405–9.

124. Isakov N, Mally MI, Altman A. Mitogen-induced human T cell proliferation is associated with increased expression of selected PKC genes. Mol Immunol 1992; 29:927–33.

125. Tsutsumi A, Kubo M, Fujii H, Freire-Moar J, Turck CW, Ransom JT. Regulation of protein kinase C isoform proteins in phorbol ester-stimulated Jurkat T lymphoma cells. J Immunol 1993; 150:1746–54.

126. Keenan C, Kelleher D, Long A. Regulation of non-classical protein kinase C isoenzymes in a human T cell line. Eur J Immunol 1995; 25:13–7.

127. Valge VE, Wong JGP, Datlof BM, Sinskey AJ, Rao A. Protein kinase C is required for responses to T cell receptor ligands but not to interleukin-2 in T cells. Cell 1988; 55:101–12.

128. Mills GB, Girard P, Grinstein S, Gelfand EW. Interleukin-2 induces proliferation of T lymphocyte mutants lacking protein kinase C. Cell 1988; 55:91–100.

129. Gomez J, De La Hera A, Silva A, Pitton C, Garcia A, Rebollo A. Implication of protein kinase C in IL-2 mediated proliferation and apoptosis in a murine T cell clone. Exp Cell Res 1994; 213:178–82.

130. Gomez J, Pitton C, Garcia A, De Aragon AM, Silva A, Rebollo A. The ζ isoform of protein kinase C controls interleukin-2 mediated proliferation in a murine T cell line: Evidence for an additional role of protein kinase C ε and β. Exp Cell Res 1995; 218:105–13.

131. Farrar WL, Anderson WB. Interleukin-2 stimulates association of protein kinase C with plasma membrane. Nature 1985; 315:233–5.

132. Lu Y, Tramblay R, Jouishomme H, Chakravarthy B, Durkin JP. Evidence that the activation of an inactive pool of membrane-associated protein kinase C is linked to the IL-2-dependent survival of T lymphocytes. J Immunol 1994; 153:1495–504.

133. Mollinedo F, Gajate C, Flores I. Involvement of phospholipase D in the activation of transcription factor AP-1 in human T lymphoid Jurkat cells. J Immunol 1994; 153:2457–69.

134. Aussel C, Pelassy C, Rossi B. Breakdown of a phosphatidylcholine pool arising from the metabolic conversion of phosphatidylethanolamine as a novel source of diacylglycerol in activated T cells. J Lipid Med 1990; 2:103–16.

135. Stewart SJ, Cunningham GR, Strupp JA, House FS, Kelley LL, Henderson GS, et al. Activation of phospholipase D: a signaling system set in motion by perturbation of the T lymphocyte antigen receptor/CD3 complex. Cell Regul 1991; 2:841–50.

136. Exton JH. Phosphatidylcholine breakdown and signal transduction. Biochim Biophys Acta 1994; 1212:26–42.

137. Berry NK, Ase K, Kishimoto A, Nishizuka Y. Activation of resting human T cells requires prolonged stimulation of protein kinase C. Proc Natl Acad Sci 1990; 87:2294–8.

138. Asaoka Y, Oka M, Yoshida K, Nishizuka Y. Metabolic rate of membrane-permeant diacylglycerol and its relation to human resting T-lymphocyte activation. Proc Natl Acad Sci 1991; 88:8681–5.

139. Davis LS, Lipsky PE. T cell activation induced by anti-CD3 antibodies requires prolonged stimulation of protein kinase C. Cell Immunol 1989; 118:208–21.

140. Nishizuka Y. Intracellular signaling by hydrolysis of phospholipids and activation of protein kinase C. Science 1992; 258:607–14.

141. Rosoff PM, Savage N, Dinarello CA. Interleukin-1 stimulates diacylglycerol production in T lymphocytes by a novel mechanism. Cell 1988; 54:73–81.

142. Dobson PRM, Plested CP, Jones DR, Barks T, Brown BL. Interleukin-1 induces a pertussis toxin-sensitive increase in diacylglycerol accumulation in mouse thymoma cells. J Endocrinol 1989; 2:R5–R8.

143. Nunes J, Klasen S, Franco MD, Lipcey C, Mawas C, Bagnasco M, et al. Signalling through CD28 T-cell activation pathway involves an inositol phospholipid-specific phospholipase C activity. Biochem J 1993; 293:835–42.

144. Pelassy C, Mary D, Aussel C. Diacylglycerol production in Jurkat T-cells: differences between CD3, CD2 and PHA activation pathways. Cell Signal 1991; 3:35–40.

145. Eardley DD, Koshland ME. Glycosylphosphatidylinositol: a candidate system for interleukin-2 signal transduction. Science 1991; 251:78–81.

146. Mills GB, Stewart DJ, Mellors A, Gelfand EW. Interleukin 2 does not induce phosphatidylinositol hydrolysis in activated T cells. J Immunol 1986; 136:3019–24.

147. Merida I, Pratt JC, Gaulton GN. Regulation of interleukin 2-dependent growth responses by glycosylphosphatidylinositol molecules. Proc Natl Acad Sci USA 1990; 87:9421–25.

148. Kolesnick R, Fuks Z. Ceramide: a signal for apoptosis or mitogenesis? J Exp Med 1995; 181:1949–52.

149. Hannun YA, Obeid LM. Ceramide: an intracellular signal for apoptosis. TIBS 1995; 20:73–7.

150. Blusztajn JK, Hudson PL, Slack BE. Sphingoid-base-containing modulators of biological signalling. In: Liscovitch M, ed, Signal-Activated Phospholipases, pp. 212–30, R. G. Landes Company, Austin, TX, 1994.

151. Heller RA, Kronke M. Tumor necrosis factor receptor-mediated signaling pathways. J Cell Biol 1994; 126:5–9.

152. Schutze S, Machleidt T, Kronke M. The role of diacylglycerol and ceramide in tumor necrosis factor and interleukin-1 signal transduction. J Leuk Biol 1994; 56:533–41.

153. Wiegmann K, Schutze S, Machleidt T, Witte D, Kronke M. Functional dichotomy of neutral and acidic sphingomyelinases in tumor necrosis factor signaling. Cell 1994; 78:1005–15.

154. Schutze S, Potthoff K, Machleidt T, Berkovic D, Wiegmann K, Kronke M. TNF activates NF-kB by phosphatidylcholine-specific phospholipase C-induced "acidic" sphingomyelin breakdown. Cell 1992; 71:765–76.

155. Kolesnick RN. 1,2-diacylglycerols but not phorbol esters stimulate sphingomyelin hydrolysis in GH₃ pituitary cells. J Biol Chem 1987; 262:16,759–62.

156. Dbaibo GS, Obeid LM, Hannun YA. Tumor necrosis factor-α (TNF-α) signal transduction through ceramide. J Biol Chem 1993; 268:17,762–6.

157. Machleidt T, Wiegmann K, Henkel T, Schutze S, Baeuerle P, Kronke M. Sphingomyelinase activates proteolytic IκB-α degradation in a cell-free system. J Biol Chem 1994; 269:13,760–5.

158. Mathias S, Younes A, Kan CC, Orlow I, Joseph C, Kolesnick RN. Activation of the sphinomyelin signaling pathway in intact EL4 cells and in a cell-free system by IL-1β. Science 1993; 259:519–22.

159. Boucher LM, Wiegmann K, Futterer A, Pfeffer K, Machleidt T, Schutze S et al. CD28 signals through acidic sphingomyelinase. J Exp Med 1995; 181:2059–68.

160. Chan G, Ochi A. Sphingomyelin-ceramide turnover in CD28 co-stimulatory signaling. Eur J Immunol 1995; 25:1999–2004.

161. Borchardt RA, Lee WT, Kalen A, Buckley RH, Peters C, Schiff S, et al. Growth-dependent regulation of cellular ceramides in human T-cells. Biochim Biophys Acta 1994; 1212:327–36.

162. Dobrowsky RT, Hannun YA. The sphingomyelin cycle and ceramide second messengers. In: Liscovitch M, ed, Signal-Activated Phospholipases, pp. 85–99. R. G. Landes Company, Austin, TX, 1994.

163. Yao B, Zhang Y, Delikat S, Mathias S, Basu S, Kolesnick R. Phosphorylation of raf by ceramide-activated protein kinase. Nature 1995; 378:307–10.

164. Belka C, Wiegmann K, Adam D, Holland R, Neuloh M, Herrmann F, et al. Tumor necrosis factor (TNF)-α activates c-raf-1 kinase via the p55 TNF receptor engaging neutral sphingomyelinase. EMBO J 1995; 14:1156–65.

165. Sasaki T, Hazeki K, Hazeki O, Ui M, Katada T. Permissive effect of ceramide on growth factor-induced cell proliferation. Biochem J 1995; 311:829–34.

166. Westwick JK, Bielawska AE, Dbaibo G, Hannun YA, Brenner DA. Ceramide activates the stress-activated protein kinases. J Biol Chem 1995; 270:22,689–92.

167. Nakamura S, Kozutsumi Y, Sun Y, Miyake Y, Fujita T, Kawasaki T. Dual roles of sphingolipids in signaling of the escape from and onset of apoptosis in a mouse cytotoxic T-cell line, CTLL-2. J Biol Chem 1996; 271:1255–57.

168. Yamada K, Sakane F, Imai S, Takemura H. Sphingosine activates cellular diacylglycerol kinase in intact Jurkat cells, a human T-cell line. Biochim Biophys Acta 1993; 1169:217–24.

169. Yamada K, Sakane F. The different effects of sphingosine on diacylglycerol kinase isozymes in Jurkat cells, a human T-cell line. Biochim Biophys Acta 1993; 1169:211–16.

170. Sakane F, Yamada K, Kanoh H. Different effects of sphingosine, R59022 and anionic amphiphiles on two diacylglycerol kinase isozymes purified from porcine thymus cytosol. FEBS Lett 1989; 255:409–13.

171. Pushkareva MY, Khan WA, Alessenko AV, Sahyoun N, Hannun YA. Sphingosine activation of protein kinases in Jurkat T cells. J Biol Chem 1992; 267:15,246–51.

172. Jolly CA, Laurenz JC, McMurray DN, Chapkin RS. Diacylglycerol and ceramide kinetics in primary cultures of activated T-lymphocytes. Immunol Lett 1996; 49:43–8.

173. Goppelt-Strube M, Resch K. Polyunsaturated fatty acids are enriched in the plasma membranes of mitogen-stimulated T-lymphocytes. Biochim Biophys Acta 1987; 904:22–8.

174. Anel A, Naval J, Gonzalez B, Torres JM, Mishal Z, Uriel J, et al. Fatty acid metabolism in human lymphocytes. I. Time-course changes in fatty acid composition and membrane fluidity during blastic transformation of peripheral blood lymphocytes. Biochim Biophys Acta 1990; 1044:323–31.

175. Szamel M, Rehermann B, Krebs B, Kurrle R, Resch K. Incorporation of polyunsaturated fatty acids into plasma membrane phospholipid regulates IL-2 synthesis via sustained activation of protein kinase C. J Immunol 1989; 143:2806–13.

176. Ahmed AA, Holub BJ. Alteration and recovery of bleeding times, platelet aggregation and fatty acid composition of individual phospholipids in platelets of human subjects receiving a supplement of cod-liver oil. Lipids 1984; 19:617–24.

177. Hosack-Fowler K, McMurray DN, Fan YY, Aukema HM, Chapkin RS. Purified dietary n-3 polyunsaturated fatty acids alter diacylglycerol mass and molecular species composition in concanavalin A-stimulated murine splenocytes. Biochim Biophys Acta 1993; 1210: 89–96.

178. Sperling RI, Benincaso AI, Knoell CT, Larkin JK, Austen KF, Robinson DR. Dietary ω-3 polyunsaturated fatty acids inhibit phosphoinositide formation and chemotaxis in neutrophils. J Clin Invest 1993; 91:651–60.

179. Marignani PA, Sebaldt RJ. Formation of second messenger diradylglycerol in murine peritoneal macrophages is altered after in vivo (n-3) polyunsaturated fatty acid supplementation. J Nutr 1995; 125:3030–40.

180. Jolly CA, McMurray DN, Chapkin RS. Effect of dietary n-3 fatty acids on interleukin-2 and interleukin-2 receptor α expression in activated murine lymphocytes. Prost Leuk Essen Fatty Acids 1998; 58:287–97.

181. Jiang YH, Lupton JR, Chapkin RS. Dietary fish oil blocks carcinogen-induced down-regulation of colonic protein kinase C isozymes. Carcinogenesis 1997; 18:351–7.

11 Nucleotides

GEORGE K. GRIMBLE AND OLWYN M. R. WESTWOOD

INTRODUCTION TO THE DIETARY NUCLEOTIDE PARADOX

There is no overriding biochemical reason why dietary nucleotides should be considered as essential nutrients. Pathways for their synthesis or salvage are (with one exception) present in every tissue and interorgan traffic should provide sufficient substrate for any tissue with increased requirements for DNA and RNA turnover. Indeed, dietary nucleotides have had a rather negative implication because of their role in the etiology of gout. Nevertheless, this model of metabolic complacency has been punctured by successive research publications which suggest that dietary nucleotide deficiency may impair liver, heart, intestine, and immune function.

The paradox is that dietary nucleotide intake is quite modest and may be extremely modest in relation to whole-body rates of RNA and DNA synthesis. This is summarized in Fig. 1, which will be referred to extensively. If a comparison were made with amino acid and protein metabolism, dietary nucleotides are akin to nonessential amino acids because of the large component of *de novo* synthesis within the system. Except in one important case, omission of individual nonessential amino acids from the diet has no deleterious consequences for whole-body amino acid and protein homeostasis *(1)*. The one exception is arginine, whose omission is fatal for cats and dogs *(2)* and was known to provoke hyperammonemia in infants parenterally fed with the early crystalline L-amino acid-based solutions *(3)*. However, adult humans can tolerate arginine-free diets *(4)*. Even for an amino acid such as glutamine, which is considered conditionally essential, its omission from the diet has been shown to have no adverse effect on growth *(5)*. This is because the rate of glutamine synthesis *de novo* (from glucose) or by salvage (from glutamate) is extremely high. Because it could be argued that nucleotide metabolism is subject to the same type of homeostatic control, dietary intake should not have marked effects on cellular metabolism. However, recent data suggest that this analysis is flawed and this chapter will, therefore, attempt to provide a metabolic rationale for the

exciting observations that have been made about the ability of dietary nucleotides to modulate the immune function.

CLINICAL AND EXPERIMENTAL STUDIES OF NUCLEOTIDE SUPPLEMENTATION

Evidence for the effectiveness of nucleotides on the immune function has come from several sources. Body growth in neonates provides the most direct evidence for a genuine requirement for any nutrient. One prospective double-blind trial, in small-for-gestational age babies who were fed formula supplemented with nucleotides, showed that compared to controls, weight gain was enhanced by 12.2% and 11.6% over the first 2 and 6 months of life, respectively ($p < 0.02$). Longitudinal growth was increased by 10.6% and 8%, respectively, and head circumference growth increased by 9.2% at 6 mo *(6)*. This effect was clearly not a result of an extra nitrogenous substrate because of the small amount of nucleotides added to the diets [approx. 0.1–0.15% of milk protein nitrogen *(7)*] and because children absorb dietary nucleotides modestly and utilize them inefficiently *(8)*. Second, evidence for a positive effect on development of the immune system in children has come from a study of children from a low socioeconomic background in Santiago in Chile *(9)*. Nucleotide supplementation of cow's milk formula significantly reduced the incidence of diarrheal disease. Finally, supplementation has been shown to increase IgG titer against beta-lactoglobulin *(10)* in premature infants and was shown to nearly double the responsiveness to *Haemophilus influenzae* type b polysaccharide in infants receiving Hib vaccine, and diphtheria, tetanus toxoids, and oral polio virus immunization *(11)*.

Breast milk confers passive immune protection to the infant in the form of maternal-derived immunoglobulins and immune cells that enter the infant's gut and fulfill an antibacterial function *(11a)*. The nonprotein nitrogen sources of breast milk have also been implicated in neonatal physiology. Although the composition of human milk varies during the course of lactation, it contains high levels of nucleotides. However, this nonprotein source of nitrogen is generally undetectable in cow's milk-based formulas. It has also been suggested that dietary nucleotides have a role in the metabolism of linoleic acid in infants *(12)*. Although these data are generally positive, the decision to supplement human milk given to premature infants should be considered with caution, for

From: *Nutrition and Immunology: Principles and Practice* (ME Gershwin et al. eds.), © Humana Press, Inc., Totowa, NJ

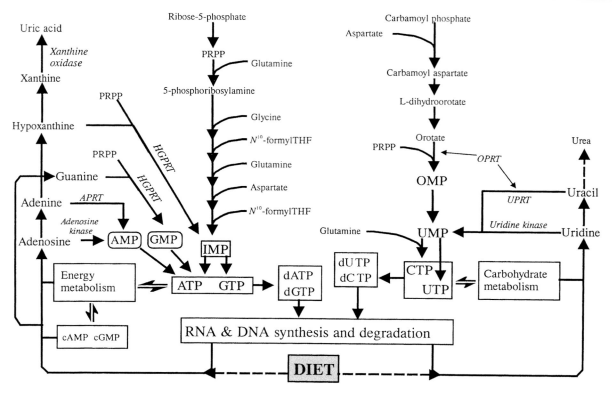

Fig. 1. Outline of purine and pyrimidine salvage and *de novo* pathways. PRPP = phosphoribosylpyrophosphate; N^{10}–formylTHF = N^{10}–formyl-tetrahydrofolic acid, APRT = adenine phosphoribosyltransferase; OPRT = orotidine phosphoribosyltransferase; HGPRT = hypoxanthine–guanine phosphoribosyltransferase.

others have suggested that nutritional additives could impair its anti-infective properties *(13)*.

BACKGROUND BIOCHEMICAL CONSIDERATIONS

Figure 1 summarizes the pathways of nucleotide metabolism in mammals. Purines and pyrimidines are synthesized *de novo* (at considerable energy cost) from simple molecules such as CO_2, ammonia and ribose (pyrimidines) or glycine, aspartate, and formyl and amine groups from folic acid and glutamine, respectively, in the case of purines. Although nucleotide triphosphates can be formed directly by *de novo* synthesis, they may also be salvaged from the degradative pathway that occurs below the level of the nucleotide monophosphates. Thus, for a nucleotide monophosphate (e.g., AMP), successive loss of the phosphate and ribose groups (to form the purine base adenine) increases the likelihood of rapid degradation to uric acid. Efficient salvage of adenine relies on direct addition of a ribose–phosphate moiety to form AMP, a nucleotide monophosphate that can be rephosphorylated back to ATP. There are four important concepts in this process. The first is that the ratio of salvage and *de novo* pathways may vary markedly between tissues. Those with a heavy reliance on salvage are likely to be most affected by dietary nucleotide supply or by interorgan transfer. Second, the ratio of salvage to *de novo* synthesis may change in individual organs according to metabolic needs or to organ or tissue function. Salvage or *de novo* enzymes may be expressed at different points in the cell cycle. Third, humans do not make large amounts of purines or pyrimidines *de*

novo. If it were true, then urinary uric acid excretion would be much higher than it is. This does not negate the fourth concept: that within the constraints of a salvage-adapted economy, some tissues may exert a strong homeostatic role in maintaining interorgan flows of purines and pyrimidines (e.g., liver).

Before considering the effects of nucleotide supplementation on immune function in detail, it is important to establish the quantitative significance of nucleotide turnover in man and, in particular, the relative amounts of nucleic acids synthesized in different tissues. This type of analysis gives several clues as to why modest supplementation may have clinically significant effects.

NUCLEOTIDE AND NUCLEIC ACID TURNOVER IN DIFFERENT TISSUES

SKELETAL MUSCLE Synthesis of rRNA occurs at approximately the same rate as that of skeletal muscle protein *(14–16)*. It is depressed by protein deprivation *(16)* and by diabetes *(17)*. Little is known about the effect of trauma on control of the muscle ribosome pool (i.e., at the level of synthesis or degradation), but the amount of tissue ribosomes and polyribosomes engaged in protein synthesis is acutely reduced by stress hormone infusion *(18)* and by elective surgery *(19)*. Loss of muscle ribosomes following an inflammatory stimulus will reduce requirements for *de novo*/salvage pathways and will require increased salvage uptake during recovery in order to maintain adequate rates of RNA synthesis (see Table 1).

HEART Cardiac rRNA synthesis occurs at approximately 15%/d *(56)* and is markedly increased during work-induced hyper-

Table 1
Summary of the Distribution of *De Novo* and Salvage Pathways in Mammalian Tissues and Organs

Tissue or organ	Purines	Refs.	Pyrimidines	Refs.
Liver	*De novo* and salvage	20,21	*De novo* = salvage	21,46
Kidney	Salvage >> *de novo* synthesis	22	Salvage from exogenous uridine << exogenous orotic acid (*de novo*)	42,47
Intestine				
Small intestines	Adenine salvage upregulated (HGPRT) by dietary purines; slow *de novo* pathway induced by nucleotide deficiency	23–25	Salvage of uridine from liver sources; depends on stage of maturation (see text)	48
Colon	*De novo*	24	*De novo*	46
Skeletal muscle	*De novo* and salvage; *de novo* synthesis stimulated by severe exercise	26–29	Salvage >> *de novo*?	49,50
Heart	Salvage > *de novo* in restoring low postischemia nucleotide pools	30–32	Salvage	51,52
Brain	Salvage predominates over *de novo*	33	Salvage, *de novo* synthesis low but upregulated in tumors	53,54
Mammary gand	*De novo*? Probably	34,35	*De novo*	34
Adrenal gland	Salvage >> *de novo*	36	Not known	
Lymphocytes	Salvage >> *de novo*, but latter strongly inducible PHA stimulation	37,38	Salvage >> *de novo*, but latter strongly inducible PHA stimulation	38
Lymphocytes from AIDS patients	*De novo* and salvage	39	Salvage only	39
Erythrocytes	Salvage	40	Salvage	55
Fetus	*De novo*	41	*De novo*	41
Implanted tumors	*De novo* synthesis commonly thought to predominate but salvage pathway is inducible	42–45	*De novo* : salvage (5 : 1)	46

Data for this table is derived from many sources and, where possible, has been from whole animal studies rather than from cell culture.

trophy, being one of the earliest changes to occur some time before increases in myofibrillar protein synthesis *(57)*. It is likely that the increase in nucleotide requirements is met from salvage pathways *(58)*, as suggested in Table 1.

LIVER The rRNA synthesis occurs at 12–25%/d *(15,49,59)*, and is slow in comparison to liver protein synthesis *(60)*. It is profoundly depressed by starvation *(61)*, which results in loss of about half of the ribosomal mass. In contrast, stimuli such as partial hepatectomy *(62,63)* or induction acute-phase response *(64)* strongly stimulate ribosome production and accumulation rates while suppressing ribosome degradation (Fig. 2). The liver is uniquely adapted to rapid induction of supply of nucleotides for RNA and DNA synthesis. Thus, in growing cultured hepatocytes, the log phase was associated with a marked increase in *de novo* purine and pyrimidine synthesis and increased pyrimidine salvage (Fig. 3). Surprisingly, purine salvage remained unaltered *(65)*. The liver may be quite dependent on adequate salvage rates of pyrimidines, as shown by one recent murine study of the fate of dietary ^{13}C-labeled nucleic acids *(21)*.

INTESTINE Little is known about the quantitative importance of rRNA synthesis in the small intestine. Along the crypt to tip axis of the villus, synthesis rates fall *(66)* while the amounts of cellular rRNA remain constant *(67,68)*. The distribution of synthesis is probably similar in colonic mucosal cells *(69)*. Detailed analysis of *de novo* and salvage pathways from ^{3}H-orotic acid and ^{3}H-uridine labeling, respectively, led Uddin and colleagues *(70)* to conclude that rRNA synthesis (i.e., nucleolar labeling) in jejunal crypts was supported mainly from pyrimidine salvage pathways and that this declined with longitudinal cellular maturation. In contrast, incorporation of pyrimidines synthesized

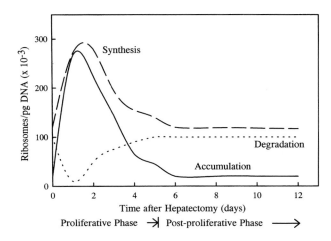

Fig. 2. Ribosome metabolism following partial hepatectomy in the rat. (Data recalculated from ref. *62*.)

by the *de novo* pathway into rRNA was low at all levels, but it made an increasingly important contribution to mRNA synthesis. It would be reasonable to assume that the quantitative synthesis rates of total mucosal RNA are high, in line with protein synthesis rates [i.e., > 100%/d *(71)*]. Intestinal disease markedly increases rRNA synthesis rates (and purine and pyrimidine salvage requirements), as suggested by an elegant histochemical study of the number of nucleolar organizer regions in colonic mucosal cells *(72)*. Thus, ulcerative colitis probably increased rRNA transcription approximately twofold, whereas the rate is probably threefold higher in adenomatous

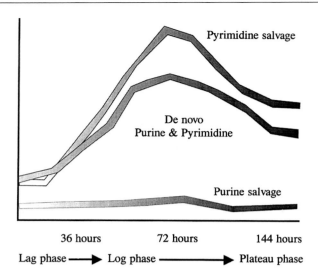

Fig. 3. Purine and pyrimidine metabolism during growth of hepatocytes. (Based on data from ref. *65*.)

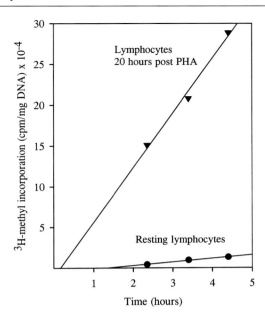

Fig. 4. Magnitude of rRNA synthesis after lymphocyte stimulation. (Redrawn from ref. *73*.)

polyps. We would suggest that intestinal RNA turnover and nucleotide requirements are of great significance in the whole-body nucleic acid economy.

LYMPHOCYTES As will be described later, lymphocyte activation is accompanied by greatly increased nucleic acid synthesis. The scale of this can be judged by an old, but still elegant quantitative study by Cooper *(73),* which suggests a 15-fold increase in synthesis rates, which would require a similar increase in precursor supply by *de novo* or salvage pathways (Fig. 4). In reality, the process of activation is managed by the lymphocyte in such a way that increases in *de novo* synthesis are minimized as a result of adaptive increases in salvage, efficiency of ribosome synthesis [i.e., less "wastage" *(74)*], and storage [i.e., utilization of inactive ribosomes *(75)*]. Figure 5 summarizes the processes and their magnitude *(37,38,76)* and should be compared to Figs. 2 and 3 (liver). It is clear that, unlike liver, the lymphocyte strongly upregulates purine salvage and that *de novo* synthesis does not become a major source of precursors for nucleic acid synthesis *(76a).* Therefore, the efficiency of lymphocyte activation will be sensitive to blood purines and pyrimidines, which depend partly on dietary intake. Nucleosides are more efficient than bases in this process because in the lectin-stimulated lymphocyte *(77),* they were better able to relieve the effects of glutamine deprivation (Fig. 6).

Thus, having established the different strategies by which tissues maintain an adequate precursor supply for nucleic acid synthesis, it may be possible to explain why dietary nucleotides have such an important effect on immune function.

NUCLEOTIDES AND LIVER FUNCTION

Intravenous nucleotide supplementation has been shown to improve the rate of liver regeneration following hepatectomy *(78,79).* This mode of delivery is also effective in minimizing hepatic damage arising from galactosamine-induced liver failure *(80).* More recently, Gil and colleagues have confirmed that hepatocellular damage and cirrhosis arising from thioacetamide treatment can be partially reversed by oral nucleotide supplementation *(81–83).* Their conclusions were based on data [i.e., reduction in

area and number of fibrous septa *(81)*] and histochemical analysis [i.e., reduced tissue collagen *(83)*]. The nucleolar area was increased threefold. It is, therefore, likely that the protective effect was partly mediated through restoration of ribosome production and, thus, protein synthesis. Indeed, the liver has a significant role in immune function of the mononuclear phagocytic system. In response to stressors (e.g., infection), the liver rapidly produces acute-phase proteins and complement that are used as opsonins to promote phagocytosis. Such is the level of immune cell activity within the liver that around 3% of liver transplant patients suffer graft-versus-host disease, a disorder caused by donor leukocytes emerging from the transplanted organ and proliferating in response to the new host *(11a).*

NUCLEOTIDES AND GUT FUNCTION

In vivo and ex vivo intestinal perfusion studies in the rat demonstrated that luminal AMP was converted to uric acid on the serosal side, thus suggesting that the intestine was an organ of active purine metabolism *(23,84).* Indeed, in mice and rats fed radiolabeled RNA, >80% of ^{14}C was promptly excreted in the urine, but of the small amount retained, most was found in the intestines and liver *(85,86).* The first suggestion that the intestine may be unique in having a poor capacity for *de novo* synthesis, was made by Munro's group *(24)* when they demonstrated low incorporation of ^{14}C–glycine into mucosal RNA together with much lower mucosal levels of the key enzyme of purine *de novo* synthesis (glutamine–amidophosphoribosyltransferase) than in the colonic mucosa or liver. Furthermore, the activity of this enzyme (and ^{14}C–glycine incorporation) was only slightly increased by dietary purine deficiency. It was, therefore, not surprising that Leleiko and colleagues *(87)* subsequently showed that the mRNA for the salvage pathway enzymes hypoxanthine–guanine phosphoribosyl transferase and adenine phosphoribosyl transferase were upregulated or downregulated by the presence or absence of purines in the diet, whereas total enterocyte cellular RNA content was

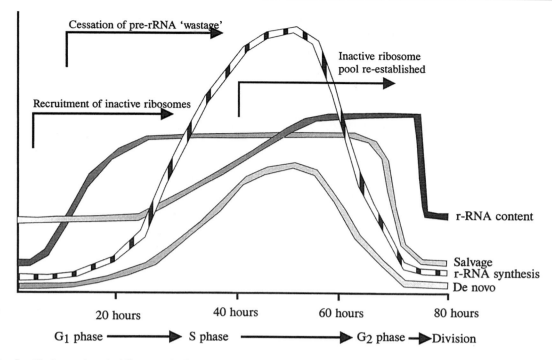

Fig. 5. Purine and pyrimidine metabolism after lymphocyte stimulation. (Based on data from refs. *37, 38,* and *76.*)

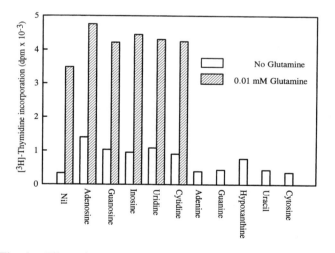

Fig. 6. Effect of exogenous nucleosides and bases on proliferation of PHA-treated lymphocytes. (Based on data from ref. *77.*)

correlated to purine intake *(87,88)*. It can be strongly argued that this indicates that the small intestine is an organ of purine homeostatis that controls portal purine intake by metabolizing excess adenosine/adenine to uric acid, thus preventing excess reliance on renal excretion. It should be noted that excess circulating adenosine and adenine can be converted to 2,8-dihydroxyadenine, which is both immunosuppressive *(89)* and nephrotoxic, being deposited as microcrystalline kidney stones *(90,91)*. It is also possible that the phenomenon of an inducible salvage pathway is a reflection of two specific small intestinal adaptations. The first is the ability to upregulate transport of glucose *(92)* and other substrates in response to increased luminal concentrations *(93)*. The second is the metabolic "channeling," which occurs in response to a relatively steady arterial nutrient supply with periods of wildly fluctuating "feast and famine," as a result of luminal absorption of nutrients [e.g., in the case of glucose *(94)*]. Metabolic requirements for "housekeeping" purposes (such as macromolecular synthesis) are more likely to be met from the arterial supply, as seems to be the case for amino acids *(95)*. In contrast to this analysis, it has been possible to argue that the small intestine is uniquely dependent on a luminal supply of nucleotides in order to maintain its function *(96)*. Purine-free diets result in loss of a significant portion of total mucosal RNA *(87)*, whereas nucleotide-free diets have been shown to result in significant depression of mucosal DNA, RNA, and protein content, as well as brush-border membrane hydrolases *(97)*. Similarly, the intestinal mucosal atrophy that accompanies total parenteral nutrition in the rat can be partially reversed by nucleotide/nucleoside supplementation *(98,99)*. Finally, two studies suggest that dietary nucleotide supplementation partially reverses mucosal damage arising from chronic lactose administration and diarrhea *(100)* and will reduce both the rate of translocation of luminal bacteria to mesenteric lymph nodes and impaired intestinal morphometry arising from endotoxin administration *(101,102)*. This argument has been strengthened by the large amount of research on the significance of the nucleotide content of human milk (see above) and its possible effects on intestinal maturation in the young *(103)*.

NUCLEOTIDES AND HEART FUNCTION

As can be seen from Table 1, the heart is primarily adapted to maintenance of adequate intracellular concentrations of the high-energy intermediate, ATP in the right ratio to ADP and AMP. To date, most interest in nucleotide supplementation has arisen from the transplant program because it was recognized early that storage and rinsing solutions for the donor organ should contain sufficient precursors to allow prompt restoration of intracellular ATP levels upon connection of the heart *(104)*. This concept has been applied to intravenous nucleoside/nucleotide solutions for use after myocardial infarction. The normal postischemia pattern of reduced ATP fructose 1,6-diphosphate and increased AMP, glucose-6-phosphate, fructose-6-phosphate, and lactate was partially reversed by prompt infusion *(105–107)*.

NUCLEOTIDES AND THE IMMUNE SYSTEM

The tissues and cells of the immune system are extremely dynamic in their aggressive elimination of dangerous antigen and are coordinated and regulated, at least in part, by the cytokine network. The areas of significant activity are the bone marrow, thymus, spleen, and lymph nodes that accommodate the proliferating immune cells. T lymphocytes arising from the bone marrow migrate and mature in the thymus, where a large proportion (up to 90%) of reactive T lymphocytes are deleted, never entering into the circulation. The signal transduction within a mature and functional T or B lymphocyte that follows the recognition and binding to its specific antigen results in intense activity. Protein synthesis is required for the production of cytokines and antigen receptors; in the case of B lymphocytes, it includes the production and secretion of immunoglobulins. Moreover, these cells also respond with rapid cell division to produce many identical clones. Therefore, in normal lymphocytes, there is a massive turnover of nucleic acids to service the rapid mititic division that occurs in response to antigen stimulation *(11a)*.

INHERITED IMMUNODEFICIENCY There is a heterogeneous group of primary immune disorders referred to as severe combined immunodeficiency (SCID). They may have either X-linked or autosomal inheritance and are characterized by marked depletion in B- and T-lymphocytes numbers. Hence, patients with SCID have an increased susceptibility to infection and failure to thrive. Over 50% of cases are the result of a defective gene on the X-chromosome that encodes for the γ-chain of number of cytokine receptors (e.g., interleukin-2 [IL-2], IL-4, IL-7). Of importance is the IL-7 receptor, for as a result of γ-chain deficiency, there are inadequate signals available to promote T-lymphocyte growth and maturation. Two autosomal recessive forms of SCID are the result of inherited deficiencies of enzymes involved in the purine degradation pathway (i.e., adenosine deaminase [ADA] or purine nucleoside phosphorylase [PNP]). As a result of these enzyme deficiencies, dATP and dGTP accumulate, which are toxic to the lymphoid stem cells because they inhibit the enzyme ribonucleotide reductase required for DNA synthesis and mitosis (Fig. 7). The reason suggested for the susceptibility of lymphocytes is their relative deficiency of 5′-nucleotidase. Deficiency in ADA or PNP activity is compensated for in other cell types by preventing accumulation of dATP and dGTP *(108)*. The only cure for SCID at present is bone marrow transplantation. There is no evidence to date of nutritional regimes using nucleotide supplementation as palliative care prior to transplantation.

ACQUIRED IMMUNODEFICIENCY The control of nucleotide synthesis has attracted great interest because it is clear that proliferative failure in T lymphocytes from HIV patients may reside at the level of precursor supply. Simmonds and colleagues have shown that even in asymptomatic patients *(39)*, lectin-stimulated lymphocytes were unable to activate the *de novo* purine synthesis pathway *(see* Fig. 5). The salvage pathway was sufficient for housekeeping purposes in resting lymphocytes, but during

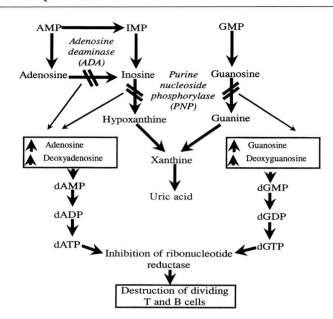

Fig. 7. Metabolic defects in severe combined immunodeficiency (SCID). (Based on ref. *108*.)

activation, infected cells underwent metabolic cell death. These data are consistent with apoptosis seen in activated infected lymphocytes; they do not seem to provide much scope for nutritional treatment with dietary nucleotides. This may be because of the action of ADA in controlling levels of adenosine or 2′-deoxyadenosine, both of which are toxic to lymphocytes *(see* Figs. 1 and 7). The extracellular form of the enzyme (which is different) normally interacts with CD26 to provide a costimulatory signal for T cells. HIV infection blocks this and is, therefore, more likely to potentiate the toxicity of adenosine *(109)*.

NUCLEOTIDE SUPPLEMENTS AND THE IMMUNE RESPONSE

Clearly, activated lymphocytes have an increased requirement of energy, proteins, and nucleotides to service the rapid cell cycle. Nucleotide omission from experimental diets can have a significant immunosuppressive effect, as shown by T-lymphocyte function following heart allografting *(110)* and reduced severity of trinitrobenzensulfonic acid-induced colitis in rats *(111,112)*. Conversely, T-lymphocyte-dependent immune responses can be augmented by supplementing a nucleotide-free diet fed to mice, with mononucleotides *(113,114)*.

THE IMMUNE RESPONSE AND ENTERAL AND PARENTERAL NUCLEOTIDES

One of the key problems of parenteral nutrition is that it does not stimulate intestinal function and can lead to marked villus atrophy. Animal studies have shown that nucleotide supplementation can attenuate the atrophic response and improve crypt cell turnover following massive bowel resection *(115,116)*. In both studies, however, nucleotides were supplied in an oral diet, and in order to consider a more stressed situation, Kishibuchi and colleagues examined the relationship between oral and parenteral feeding (with and without added nucleotides) and gut barrier function

(117). Total Parenteral Nutrition (TPN) increased intestinal permeation of sugar probes and the dimensions of the tight junction between enterocytes (10.7 ± 0.9 nm vs 15.5 ± 1.8 nm, *p*<0.05). Similarly, cathepsins G, H, and L were increased, suggesting that TPN had induced local protein catabolism. All of these changes were partially reversed by nucleotide/nucleoside supplementation *(117)*. Although no studies have shown whether nucleotides can reduce the effectiveness of mucosal-associated lymphatic tissue (MALT) in preventing the ingress of bacteria [compared to oral studies *(101,102)*], we would suggest that it is likely to do so. The gut is part of the MALT and is both a physiological and immunological barrier. In effect, the internal lymphatic circulation of immune cells and immunoglobulins (mainly IgA) between other areas of the MALT (e.g., respiratory and genitourinary tracts) are a guard at the interface between the internal and external environments. Enteral feeding assists in maintaining the active immune barrier mechanism of the gut. Regardless of the route of administration, purine nucleotides alter intestinal gene transcription *(87)*. Because many of the effects of nucleotides on gut function in TPN-fed animals are similar to those triggered by luminal nutrition, there may be a common set of signals for maintenance of the mucosal cell and MALT populations. Unfortunately, there are little data from clinical studies that shed light on this central question. The most recent study in critically ill patients showed that early enteral feeding stabilized posttrauma immunosuppression *(118)*. This was a very small study and was unable to demonstrate any advantage of a special nucleotide-containing enteral diet.

NUCLEOTIDES AND IMMUNONUTRITION

"Immunonutrition" is a term which has been adopted to describe diets that contain several additives in the form of glutamine, arginine, fish oils, and nucleotides alone or in combination. The most studied of these diets contains additions of all of these components except for glutamine and is marketed under the tradename Impact. In two recent reviews of clinical results obtained with this diet *(119,120)*, the outcome was generally positive in that most studies have shown some reduction in sepsis or hospital stay. However, the exact mechanism is elusive because of the presence of three added dietary components, each of which have marked effects on immune function.

CONCLUSIONS AND SUMMARY

We have attempted to present all of the relevant evidence on the possible benefits which might arise from dietary nucleotide supplementation. As initially stated, the data relating to children are fairly unambiguous and suggest that nucleotide supplementation will improve growth and reduce susceptibility to infection. The argument is fairly clear because the attempt has been made to model formula feed more closely to mother's milk. However, when these simple concepts have been applied to the situation of the critically ill adult or the patient with inflammatory bowel disease, the conclusions are more difficult to derive. The answer depends on the context in which the question is asked. Thus, dietary supplementation with nucleotides and arginine have been shown to promote healing and repair of small-bowel ulcers in indomethacin-induced ulcerative ileitis in rats *(121)* but to exacerbate chemically induced colitis *(112)*. This suggests that nucleotides promote healing in the presence of a nonsteroidal anti-inflammatory drug, even though they are clearly pro-inflammatory, as highlighted by Yamamoto et al. *(122)*. Oral administration appeared to lead to local increased levels of cytokines, such as tumor necrosis factor-alpha (TNF-α) and interleukin-8, in the inflamed colon *(122)*. The significance of augmenting an inflammatory response rather than the natural immune suppression that follows surgery is an immunological finding which remains contentious. For instance, Senkal et al. found that enteral nutritional support supplemented with arginine, RNA, and omega-3 fatty acids had modulated the acute-phase response, as indicated by a *reduction* in levels of TNF-α and IL-6 *(123)*. However, they also claimed an accelerated recovery of levels of the IL-1β and IL-2 receptor that was considered to assist in the recovery of patients with gastrointestinal cancer. Again, the nature of the pathology being treated demands consideration, because by definition, a tumor arose because an abnormal cell escaped immune surveillance.

Preventing infection, weight loss, and other symptoms of cachexia can prolong the survival of patients with advanced stages of neoplastic disease. Administration of dietary nucleotides were shown to improve animal survival to a challenge with *Candida albicans (120,124)*. Critically ill patients who suffer bacterial infections could develop septic shock as a consequence of acutely high levels of the cytokines, in particular TNF-α, released in response to the infection. Yet, in patients in intensive care units given enteral feeds where the supplements included nucleotides (pro-inflammatory), infectious complication were less frequent *(125)*, although this has not been observed in all studies *(126)*. It has also been proposed that the catecholamine-induced downregulation of the immune response following injury or trauma is beneficial. Although this can lead to an increased risk of infection, an augmented immune response in conjunction with the posttraumatic catabolic activity could have a deleterious effect on survival. Indeed, a return to normal immune activity has been suggested as a clinical gauge of recovery *(127)*.

Finally, prostaglandin inhibitors and morphine are prescribed for pain and inflammatory processes. Dietary nucleotides appear to modulate polyunsaturated fatty acid conversion and eicosanoid synthesis. Interestingly, studies in mice have shown that a nucleotide-free diet can attenuate morphine withdrawal symptoms. Thus, there is the suggestion that the immune status can impact also on the central nervous system—opioid-related pathways and that certain nucleotides such as uracil may have a possible immune-brain signaling role *(128)*.

REFERENCES

1. Grimble GK. Essential and conditionally-essential nutrients in clinical nutrition. Nutr Res Rev 1993; 6:97–119.
2. Morris JG, Rogers QR. Ammonia intoxication in the near-adult cat as a result of a dietary arginine deficiency. Science 1978; 199:431–2.
3. Chan JCM, Asch MJ, Lin S, Hays DM. Hyperalimentation with amino acid and casein hydrolysate solutions: mechanism of acidosis. JAMA 1972; 220:1700–5.
4. Carey GP, Kime Z, Rogers QR, et al. An arginine-deficient diet in humans does not evoke hyperammonemia or orotic aciduria. J Nutr 1987; 117:1734–9.
5. Itoh H, Kishi T, Chibata I. Comparative effects of casein and amino acid mixture simulating casein on growth and food intake in rats. J Nutr 1973; 103:1709–15.
6. Cosgrove M, Davies DP, Jenkins HR. Nucleotide supplementation and the growth of term small for gestational age infants. Arch Dis Childh 1996; 74:F122–5.

7. Janas L, Picciano M. The nucleotide profile of human milk. Pediatr Res 1982; 16:659–62.

8. Golden MHN, Waterlow JC, Picou D. Metabolism in ^{15}N nucleic acids in children. In: Waterlow JC, Stephen JML, eds. Nitrogen Metabolism in Man, pp. 269–273. Applied Science Publishers, London, 1981.

9. Brunser O, Espinoza J, Araya M, Cruchet S, Gil A. Effect of dietary nucleotide supplementation on diarrhoeal disease in infants. Acta Paediatr 1994; 83:188–91.

10. Martinez-Augustin O, Boza JJ, Del Pino JI, Lucena J, Martinez-Valverde A, Gil A. Dietary nucleotides might influence the humoral immune response against cow's milk proteins in preterm neonates. Biol Neonate 1997; 71:215–23.

11. Pickering LK, Granoff DM. Erickson JR, et al. Modulation of the immune system by human milk and infant formula containing nucleotides. Pediatrics 1998; 101:242–9.

11a Westwood OMR. The Scientific Basis for Health Care. Times Mirror International Publishers, London, 1999.

12. Gil A, Pita M, Martinez A, Molina JA, Sánchez Medina F. Effect of dietary nucleotides on the plasma fatty acids in at-term neonates. Hum Nutr Clin Nutr 1986; 40:185–95.

13. Quan R, Yang C, Rubinstein S, Lewiston NJ, Stevenson DK, Kerner JA Jr. The effect of nutritional additives on anti-infective factors in human milk. Clin Pediatr (Phila) 1994; 33:325–8.

14. Goodlad GAJ, Onyezili FN. Glucocorticoids and muscle RNA: the effect of daily administration of prednisolone to rats on the turnover of gastrocnemius ribosomal RNA. Biochem Med 1981; 25:34–47.

15. Grimble GK, Millward DJ. The measurement of ribosomal ribonucleic acid synthesis in rat liver and skeletal muscle in vivo. Biochem Soc Trans 1977; 5:913–16.

16. Hájek I, Buresóvá M. The synthesis of RNA species in the skeletal muscle of the mouse. Physiol Bohemoslov 1973; 22:623–31.

17. Ashford AJ, Pain VM. Effect of diabetes on the rates of synthesis and degradation of ribosomes in rat muscle and liver in vivo. J Biol Chem 1986; 261:4059–65.

18. Hammarqvist F, von der Decken A, Vinnars E, Wernerman J. Stress hormone and amino acid infusion in healthy volunteers: short-term effects on protein synthesis and amino acid metabolism in skeletal muscle. Metabolism 1994; 43:1158–63.

19. Petersson B, Wernerman J, Waller S, von der Decken A, Vinnars E. Elective abdominal surgery depresses muscle protein synthesis and increases subjective fatigue: effects lasting more than 30 days. Br J Surg 1990; 77:796–800.

20. Clifford AJ, Riumallo JA, Baliga BS, Munro HN, Brown PR. Liver nucleotide metabolism in relation to amino acid supply. Biochim Biophys Acta 1972; 277:443–58.

21. Berthold HK, Crain PF, Gouni I, Reeds PJ, Klein PD. Evidence for incorporation of intact dietary pyrimidine (but not purine) nucleosides into hepatic RNA. Proc Nat Acad Sci USA 1995; 92:10,123–7.

22. Natsumeda Y, Prajda N, Donohue JP, Glover JL, Weber G. Enzymic capacities of purine de novo and salvage pathways for nucleotide synthesis in normal and neoplastic tissues. Cancer Res 1984; 44:2475–9.

23. Salati LM, Gross CJ, Henderson LM, Savaiano DA. Absorption and metabolism of adenine, adenosine-5′-monophosphate, adenosine and hypoxanthine by the isolated vascularity perfused rat small intestine. J Nutr 1984; 114:753–60.

24. Leleiko NS, Bronstein AD, Baliga BS, Munro HN. De novo purine nucleotide synthesis in the rat small and large intestine: effect of dietary protein and purines. J Pediatr Gastroenterol Nutr 1983; 2:313–9.

25. Walsh MJ, Sánchez-Pozo A, Leleiko NS. A regulatory element is characterized by purine-mediated and cell-type-specific gene transcription. Mol Cell Biol 1990; 10:4356–64; erratum 1990; 10:5600.

26. Tully ER, Sheehan TG. Purine metabolism in rat skeletal muscle. Adv Exp Med Biol 1979; 122B:13-7.

27. Tullson PC, Terjung RL. Adenine nucleotide synthesis in exercising and endurance-trained skeletal muscle. Am J Physiol 1991; 261:C342–7.

28. Arabadjis PG, Tullson PC, Terjung RL. Purine nucleoside formation in rat skeletal muscle fiber types. Am J Physiol 1993; 264:C1246–51.

29. Tullson PC, Terjung RL. Adenine nucleotide metabolism in contracting skeletal muscle. Exerc Sport Sci Rev 1991; 19:507–37.

30. Gerlach E, Nees S, Becker BF. The vascular endothelium: a survey of some newly evolving biochemical and physiological features. Basic Res Cardiol 1985; 80:459–74.

31. Finelli C, Guarnieri C, Muscari C, Ventura C, Caldarera CM. Incorporation of [14C]hypoxanthine into cardiac adenine nucleotides: effect of aging and post-ischemic reperfusion. Biochim Biophys Acta 1993; 1180:262–6.

32. Smolenski RT, Simmonds HA, Garlick PB, Venn GE, Chambers DJ. Depressed adenosine and total purine catabolite production in the postischemic rat heart. Cardioscience 1993; 4:235–40.

33. Watts RW. Some regulatory and integrative aspects of purine nucleotide biosynthesis and its control: an overview. Adv Enzyme Regul 1983; 21:33–51.

34. Kunjara S, Sochor M, Bennett M, Greenbaum AL, McLean P. Pyrimidine nucleotide synthesis in the rat mammary gland: changes in the lactation cycle and the effects of diabetes. Biochem Med Metab Biol 1992; 48:263–74.

35. Thorell L, Sjoberg LB, Hernell O. Nucleotides in human milk: sources and metabolism by the newborn infant. Pediatr Res 1996; 40:845–52.

36. Rotllan P, Miras Portugal MT. Purine nucleotide synthesis in adrenal chromaffin cells. J Neurochem 1985; 44:1029–36.

37. Barankiewicz J, Cohen A. Purine nucleotide metabolism in phytohemagglutinin-induced human T lymphocytes. Arch Bichem Biophys 1987; 258:167–75.

38. Fairbanks LD, Bofill M, Ruckemann K, Simmonds HA. Importance of ribonucleotide availability to proliferating T-lymphocytes from healthy humans. Disproportionate expansion of pyrimidine pools and contrasting effects of de novo synthesis inhibitors. J Biol Chem 1995; 270:29,682–9.

39. Bofil M, Fairbanks LD, Ruckemann K, Lipman M, Simmonds HA. T-lymphocytes from AIDS patients are unable to synthesize ribonucleotides de novo in response to mitogenic stimulation. Impaired pyrimidine responses are already evident at early stages of HIV-1 infection. J Biol Chem 1995; 270:29,690–7.

40. Shenoy TS, Clifford AJ. Adenine nucleotide metabolism in relation to purine enzymes in liver, erythrocytes and cultured fibroblasts. Biochim Biophys Acta 1975; 411:133–43.

41. Boza JJ, Jahoor F, Reeds PJ. Ribonucleic acid nucleotides in maternal and fetal tissues derive amost exclusively from synthesis de novo in pregnant mice. J Nutr 1996; 126:1749–58.

42. Stet EH, De Abreu RA, Bokkerink JP, et al. Inhibition of IMP dehydrogenase by mycophenolic acid in Molt F4 human malignant lymphoblasts. Ann Clin Biochem 1994; 31:174–80.

43. Johnson DL, Mullin RJ, Duch DS, Benkovic SJ. Direct demonstration of the active salvage of performed purines by murine tumors. Biochem Biophys Res Commun 1990; 170:1164–9.

44. Natsumeda Y, Ikegami T, Olah E, Weber G. Significance of purine salvage in circumventing the action of antimetabolites in rat hepatoma cells. Cancer Res 1989; 49:88–92.

45. Ahmed N, Weidemann MJ. Purine metabolism in promyelocytic HL60 and dimethylsulphoxide-differentiated HL60 cells. Leuk Res 1994; 18:441–51.

46. Zaharevitz DW, Anderson LW, Malinowski NM, Hyman R, Strong JM, Cysyk RL. Contribution of de-novo and salvage synthesis to the uracil nucleotide pool in mouse tissues and tumors in vivo. Eur J Biochem 1992; 210:293–6.

47. Cortes P, Dumler F, Levin NW. Glomerular uracil nucleotide synthesis. Am J Physiol 1988; 255:F635–46.

48. Zaharevitz DW, Napier EA, Anderson LW, Strong JM, Cysyk RL. Stimulation of uracil nucleotide synthesis in mouse liver, intestine

and kidney by ammonium chloride infusion. Eur J Biochem 1988; 175:193–8.

49. Grimble GK. RNA metabolism in skeletal muscle. PhD thesis. University of London, 1981.

50. Jacobs AE, Oosterhof A, Veerkamp JH. Purine and pyrimidine metabolism in human muscle and cultured muscle cells. Biochim Biophys Acta 1988; 970:130–6.

51. Lortet S, Aussedat J, Rossi A. Synthesis of pyrimidine nucleotides in the heart: uridine and cytidine kinase activity. Arch Int Physiol Biochim 1987; 95:289–98.

52. Olivares J, Rossi A. [Incorporation of orotic acid in myocardial uridine nucleotides: effect of isoproterenol and ribose] Incorporation de l'acide orotique dans les nucleotides uridyliques du tissu myocardique: effet de l'isoprenaline et du ribose. J Physiol (Paris) 1982; 78:175–8.

53. Bardot V, Dutrillaux AM, Delattre JY, et al. Purine and pyrimidine metabolism in human gliomas: relation to chromosomal aberrations. Br J Cancer 1994; 70:212–8.

54. Madani S, Baillon J, Fries J, et al. Pyrimidine pathways enzymes in human tumors of brain and associated tissues: potentialities for the therapeutic use of N-(phosphonacetyl-L-aspartate and 1-β-D-arabinofuranosylcytosine. Eur J Cancer Clin Oncol 1987; 23:1485–90.

55. Simmonds HA, Fairbanks LD, Duley JA, Micheli V. Importance of the human erythrocyte in the diagnosis of inherited purine and pyrimidine disorders. Biomed Biochim Acta 1990; 49:S259–64.

56. Ray A, Mandel P, Dessaux G. Distribution des acides ribonucléiques dans le myocarde du rat. Cinétique de marquage par le ^{32}P *in vivo* [Distribution of ribonucleic acids in the myocardium of the rat. Kinetics of labeling of ^{32}P *in vivo*]. Arch Int Physiol Biochem 1973; 81:249–72.

57. Watson PA, Haneda T, Morgan HE. Effect of higher aortic pressure on ribosome formation and cAMP content in rat heart. Am J Physiol 1989; 256:C1257–61.

58. Zimmer HG. Regulation of and intervention into the oxidative pentose phosphate pathway and adenine nucleotide metabolism in the heart. Mol Cel Biochem 1996; 160–161:101–9.

59. Eliceiri GL. Turnover of ribosomal RNA in liver. Biochim Biophys Acta 1976; 447:391–4.

60. Garlick PJ, Waterlow JC, Swick RW. Measurement of protein turnover in rat liver: analysis of the complex curve for decay of a mixture of proteins. Biochem J 1976; 156:657–63.

61. Conde RD, Franze-Fernández MT. Increased transcription and decreased degradation control and recovery of liver ribosomes after a period of protein starvation. Biochem J 1980; 192:935–40.

62. Nikolov EN, Dabeva MD, Nikolov TK. Turnover of ribosomes in regenerating rat liver. Int J Biochem 1983; 15:1255–60.

63. Loeb JN, Yeung LL. Synthesis and degradation of ribosomal RNA in regenerating liver. J Exp Med 1975; 142:575–87.

64. Piccoletti R, Aletti MG, Bernelli-Zazzera A. Inflammation associated events in liver nuclei during acute-phase reaction. Inflammation 1986; 10:109–17.

65. Mayer D, Natsumeda Y, Ikegami T, et al. Expression of key enzymes of purine and pyrimidine metabolism in a hepatocyte-derived cell line at different phases of the growth cycle. J Cancer Res Clin Oncol 1990; 116:251–8.

66. Morrison A, Porteous JW. Changes in the synthesis of ribosomal ribonucleic acid and of poly(A)-containing ribonucleic acid during the differentiation of intestinal epithelial cells in the rat and in the chick. Biochem J 1980; 188:609–18.

67. Maheshwari Y, Rao M, Sykes DE, Tyner AL, Weiser MM. Changes in ribosomal protein and ribosomal RNA synthesis during rat intestinal differentiation. Cell Growth Differ 1993; 4:745–52.

68. Altmann GG, Leblond CP. Changes in the size and structure of the nucleolus of columnar cells during their migration from crypt base to villus top in rat jejunum. J Cell Sci 1982; 56:83–99.

69. Morais M, Dockery P, White FH. A quantitative study of silver-stained NORs in different segments of the normal human colorectal crypt. J Anat 1996; 188:521–7.

70. Uddin M, Altmann GG, Leblond CP. Radioautographic visualization of differences in the pattern of [^{3}H]uridine and [3H]orotic acid incorporation into the RNA of migrating columnar cells in the rat small intestine. J Cell Biol 1984; 98:1619–29.

71. McNurlan MA, Tomkins AM, Garlick PJ. The effect of starvation on the rate of protein synthesis in rat liver and small intestine. Biochem J 1979; 178:373–9.

72. Jain R, Malhotra V, Gondal R, Tatke M, Vij JC. Nucleolar organiser regions in different colonic epithelia. Trop Gastroenterol 1997; 18:27–29.

73. Cooper HL. Studies on RNA metabolism during lymphocyte activation. Transplant Rev 1972; 11:3–38.

74. Cooper HL. Degradation of 28S RNA late in ribosomal RNA maturation in nongrowing lymphocytes and its reversal after growth stimulation. J Cell Biol 1973; 59:250–4.

75. Harms-Ringdahl M, Cooper HL. Sequential changes in ribosomal activity during the activation and cessation of growth in lymphocytes stimulated with concanavalin A. J Cell Physiol 1978; 97:253–63.

76. Schobitz B, Wolf S, Christopherson RI, Brand K. Nucleotide and nucleic acid metabolism in rat thymocytes during cell cycle progression. Biochim Biophys Acta 1991; 1095:95–102.

76a Cohen A, Barankiewicz J, Lederman HM, Gelfand EW. Purine metabolism in human T lymphocytes: role of the purine nucleoside cycle. Can J Biochem Cell Biol 1984; 62:577–83.

77. Szondy Z, Newsholme EA. The effect of various concentrations of nucleobases, nucleosides or glutamine on the incorporation of [^{3}H]thymidine into DNA in rat mesenteric-lymph-node lymphocytes stimulated by phytohaemagglutinin. Biochem J 1990; 270:437–40.

78. Ogoshi S, Iwasa M, Tonegarua T, Tamiya T. Effect of nucleotide and nucleoside mixture on rats given total parenteral nutrition after 70% hepatectomy. J Parent Ent Nutr 1985; 9:339–42.

79. Ogoshi S, Mizobuchi S, Iwasa M, Tamiya T. Effect of a nucleoside–nucleotide mixture on protein metabolism in rats after seventy percent hepatectomy. Nutrition 1989; 5:173–8.

80. Ogoshi S, Iwasa M, Kitagawa S, et al. Effects of total parenteral nutrition with nucleoside and nucleotide mixture on D-galactosamine-induced liver injury in rats. J Parent Ent Nutr 1988; 12:53–7.

81. Torres MI, Fernàndez MI, Gil A, Rios A. Effect of dietary nucleotides on degree of fibrosis and steatosis induced by oral intake of thioacetamide. Dig Dis Sci 1997; 42:1322–8.

82. Torres MI, Fernàndez MI, Foutana L, Gil A, Rios A. Influence of dietary nucleotides on liver structural recovery and hepatocyte binucleoarity in cirrhosis induced by thioacetamide. Gut 1996; 38:260–4.

83. Torres MI, Fernàndez MI, Gil A, Rios A. Dietary nucleotides have cytoprotective properties in rat liver damaged by thioacetamide. Life Sci 1998; 62:13–22.

84. Wilson DW, Wilson HC. Studies in vitro of digestion and absorption of purine ribonucleotides by the intestine. J Biol Chem 1962; 237:1643–7.

85. Sonoda T, Tatibana M. Metabolic fate of pyrimidines and purines in dietary nucleic acids ingested by mice. Biochim Biophys Acta 1978; 521:55–66.

86. Greife HA, Molnar S. ^{14}C-tracerstudien zum nukleinsauren-stoffwechsel von jungratten, kuken und ferkeln. 1: Mitteilung. Untersuchungen zum purinestoffwechsel der jungratte. Z Tierphysiol Tierernahr Futtermittelkd 1983; 50:79–91.

87. Leleiko NS, Martin BA, Walsh M, Kazlow P, Rabinowitz S, Sterling K. Tissue-specific gene expression results from a purine- and pyrimidine-free diet and 6-mercaptopurine in the rat small intestine and colon. Gastroenterology 1987; 93:1014–20.

88. Leleiko NS, Walsh MJ, Abraham S. Gene expression in the intestine: the effect of dietary nucleotides. Adv Pediatr 1995; 42:145-69-145-169.

89. Chalmers AH, Rotstein T, Mohan Rao M, Marshall VR, Coleman M. Studies on the mechanism of immunosuppression with adenine. Int J Immunopharmacol 1985; 7:433–2.

90. Brule D, Sarwar G, Savoie L, Campbell J, van Zeggelaar M. Differences in uricogenic effects of dietary purine bases, nucleosides and nucleotides in rats. J Nutr 1988; 118:780–6.

91. Engle SJ, Stockelman MG, Chen J, et al. Adenine phosphoribosyl-transferase-deficient mice develop 2,8-dihydroxyadenine nephrolithiasis. Proc Natl Acad Sci USA 1996; 93:5307–12.

92. Debnam ES, Denholm EE, Grimble GK. Acute and chronic exposure of rat intestinal mucosa to dextran promotes SGLT1-mediated glucose transport. Eur J Clin Invest 1998; 28:651–8.

93. Ferraris RP, Diamond JM. Specific regulation of intestinal nutrient transporters by their dietary substrates. Annu Rev Physiol 1989; 51:125–41.

94. Fernandez Lopez JA, Casado J, Argiles JM, Alemany M. In the rat, intestinal lymph carries a significant amount of ingested glucose into the bloodstream. Arch Int Physiol Biochim Biophys 1992; 100:231–6.

95. Egan CJ, Rennie MJ. Relative importance of luminal and vascular amino acids for protein synthesis in rat jejunum. J Physiol 1986; 378:49P (abstract).

96. Grimble GK. Dietary nucleotides and gut mucosal defence. Gut 1994; 35(suppl):S46–51.

97. Uauy R, Stringel G, Thomas R, Quan R. Effect of dietary nucleosides on growth and maturation of the developing gut in the rat. J Pediatr Gastroenterol Nutr 1990; 10:497–503.

98. Iijima S, Tsujinaka T, Kido Y, et al. Intravenous administration of nucleosides and a nucleotide mixture diminishes intestinal mucosal atrophy induced by total parenteral nutrition. J Parent Ent Nutr 1993; 17:265–70.

99. Tsujinaka T, Iijima S, Kido Y, et al. Role of nucleosides and nucleotide mixture in intestinal mucosal growth under total parenteral nutrition. Nutrition 1993; 9:532–5.

100. Nuñez MC, Ayudarte MV, Morales D, Suarez MD, Gil A. Effect of dietary nucleotides on intestinal repair in rats with experimental chronic diarrhea. J Parent Ent Nutr 1990; 14:598–604.

101. Adjei AA, Yamamoto S. A dietary nucleoside-nucleotide mixture inhibits endotoxin-induced bacterial translocation in mice fed protein-free diet. J Nutr 1995; 125:42–8.

102. Adjei AA, Ohshiro Y, Yamauchi K, et al. Intraperitoneal administration of nucleoside–nucleotide mixture inhibits endotoxin-induced bacterial translocation in protein-deficient mice. Tohoku J Exp Med 1994; 174:1–10.

103. Uauy R, Quan R, Gil A. Role of nucleotides in intestinal development and repair: implications for infant nutrition. J Nutr 1994; 124:1436S–41S.

104. Swanson DK, Pasaoglu I, Berkoff HA, Southard JA, Hegge JO. Improved heart preservation with UW preservation solution. J Heart Transplant 1988; 7:456–67.

105. Kano S, Nakai T, Kohri H, Ichihara K. Effects of OG-VI, a nucleoside/nucleotide mixture, and its constituents on myocardial stunning in dogs. Coron Artery Dis 1995; 6:811–8.

106. Okazaki Y, Kano S, Ogoshi S, Ichihara K. Effects of OG-VI, a nucleoside–nucleotide mixture, on ischemic myocardial metabolism in dogs. Coron Artery Dis 1997; 8:39–43.

107. Yoshiyama M, Ishikawa M, Miura I, Takeuchi K, Takeda T. Time course of the recovery of adenosine triphosphate content with adenosine in post-ischemic hearts—a ^{31}P magnetic resonance spectroscopy study. Jpn Circ J 1994; 58:662–70.

108. Rosen F. Primary immunodeficiencies. In: Roitt I, Brostoff J, Male D, eds, Immunology, 5th ed, pp. 285–292. Times Mirror International Publishers, London, 1997.

109. Franco R, Valenzuela A, Lluis C, Blanco J. Enzymatic and extraenzymatic role of ecto-adenosine deaminase in lymphocytes. Immunol Rev 1998; 161:27–42.

110. Rudolph FB, Kulkarni AD, Schandle VB, van Buren CT. Involvement of dietary nucleotides in T lymphocyte function. Adv Exp Med Biol 1984; 165:175–8.

111. Adjei AA, Ameho CK, Harrison EK, et al. Nucleoside–nucleotide-free diet suppresses cytokine production and contact sensitivity responses in rats with trinitrobenzene sulphonic acid-induced colitis. Am J Med Sci 1997; 314:89–96.

112. Adjei AA, Morioka T, Ameho CK, et al. Nucleoside–nucleotide free diet protects rat colonic mucosa from damage induced by trinitrobenzene sulphonic acid. Gut 1996; 39:428–33.

113. Navarro J, Ruiz-Bravo A, Jimenez-Valera M, Gil A. Modulation of antibody-forming cell and mitogen-driven lymphoproliferative responses by dietary nucleotides in mice. Immunol Lett 1996; 53:141–5.

114. Yamauchi K, Adjei AA, Ameho CK, et al. A nucleoside–nucleotide mixture and its components increase lymphoproliferative and delayed hypersensitivity responses in mice. J Nutr 1996; 126: 1571–7.

115. Iijima S, Tsujinaka T, Kishibuchi M, et al. A total parenteral nutrition solution supplemented with a nucleoside and nucleotide mixture sustains intestinal integrity, but does not stimulate intestinal function after massive bowel resection in rats. J Nutr 1996; 126:589–95.

116. Tsujinaka T, Kishibuchi M, Iijima S, Yano M, Monden M. Role of supplementation of a nucleic acid solution on the intestinal mucosa under total parenteral nutrition. Nutrition 1997; 13:369–71.

117. Kishibuchi M, Tsujinaka T, Yano M, et al. Effects of nucleosides and a nucleotide mixture on gut mucosal barrier function on parenteral nutrition in rats. J Parent Ent Nutr 1997; 21:104–11.

118. Engel JM, Menges T, Neuhauser C, Schaefer B, Hempelmann G. Effects of various feeding regimens in multiple trauma patients on septic complications and immune parameters. Anasthesiol Intensivmed Notfallmed Schmerzther 1997; 32:234–9.

119. Zaloga GP. Immune-enhancing enteral diets: where's the beef? Crit Care Med 1998; 26:1143–6.

120. Imoberdorf R. Immuno-nutrition: designer diets in cancer. Support Care Cancer 1997; 5:381–6.

121. Sukumar P, Loo A, Magur E, Nandi J, Oler A, Levine RA. Dietary supplementation of nucleotides and arginine promotes healing of small bowel ulcers in experimental ulcerative ileitis. Dig Dis Sci 1997; 42:1530–6.

122. Yamamoto S, Wang MF, Adjei AA, Ameho CK. Role of nucleosides and nucleotides in the immune system, gut reparation after injury, and brain function. Nutrition 1997; 13:372–4.

123. Senkal M, Kemen M, Homann H, Eickoff U, Baier J, Zumtobel V. Modulation of postoperative immune response by enteral nutrition with a diet enriched with arginine, RNA, and omega-3 fatty acids in patients with upper gastrointestinal cancer. Eur J Surg 1995; 161:115–22.

124. Fanslow WC, Kulkarni AD, van Buren CT, Rudolph FB. Effect of nucleotide restriction and supplementation on resistance to experimental murine candidiasis. J Parent Ent Nutr 1988; 12:49–52.

125. Schilling J, Vranjes N, Fierz W, et al. Clinical outcome and immunology of postoperative arginine, omega-3 fatty acids, and nucleotide-enriched enteral feeding: a randomized prospective comparison with standard enteral and low calorie/low fat i.v. solutions. Nutrition 1996; 12:423–9.

126. Saffle JR, Wiebke G, Jennings K, Morris SE, Barton RG. Randomized trial of immune-enhancing enteral nutrition in burn patients. J Trauma 1997; 42:793–800.

127. Salo M. Effects of anaesthesia and surgery on the immune response. Acta Anaesthesiol Scand 1992; 36:201–20.

128. Kulkarni A, McVaugh W, Lawrence B, et al. Nutritional supplementation of nucleotides restores opioid CNS-mediated phenomena in mice. Life Sci 1997; 61:1691–6.

NUTRIENT-IMMUNE INTERACTIONS

III

12 Impact of Nutritional Status on Immune Integrity

Pam Fraker

THE HIGH CORRELATION BETWEEN IMMUNE STATUS AND NUTRITIONAL STATUS

Nutritional immunology remains an area ripe for further investigation. Many important relationships between specific nutrients and immune function remain to be identified. In some cases, these studies will reveal new biological roles for the nutrient or new modes of regulation of the immune system, thereby making important contributions to basic as well as clinical sciences. Although many nutritionists have a keen interest in the interrelationships between nutrients and the immune function, this area has not been widely embraced by the immunological community. Thus, nutritional immunology was left for many years in the hands of those investigators brave enough to try to master two separate and complex disciplines. As a result, only a few areas of nutritional immunology have received extensive investigation. Although some like to point out that hundreds of articles can be found describing the impact of diet on the immune function, the bulk of the early literature was a patchwork of studies. Interesting data often of limited scope received little follow-up investigation. There were, however, some persistent and wonderful pioneering efforts put forth by Chandra, Beisel, Scrimshaw, and Newberne to name a few *(1–3)*. Joined by other labs, these investigators have provided extensive detail regarding the effects of deficiencies in zinc, copper, and protein calories on a number of facets of immune defense in both humans and animal models. These early studies, along with more recent investigations to be discussed, provide compelling evidence that nutritional status and immune status are tightly linked and that immune integrity can be rapidly altered by changes in nutritional status.

This review will survey some of the areas where it is already evident that nutrients impact on specific aspects of immune function and will also attempt to address a series of important questions regarding the benefits of nutritional–immunological studies. What have the extensive investigations of deficiencies in zinc, copper, and protein calories taught us about their effects on immune status?

Have mechanisms been found to explain their rapid and profound effects on host defense mechanisms? Have they led to the identification of any new biological roles for nutrients? We know that many Western diseases such as alcoholism, sickle cell anemia, renal disease, chronic gastrointestinal disorders, AIDS, cancer, and others listed in Table 1 lead to marginal deficiencies in many nutrients that, in turn, create immunodeficiencies in the patient *(1,4,5)*. Once a chronic disease has been diagnosed, can more be done to enhance immune defense via management of diet? Should nutritional supplementation be the same for all types of chronic disease or do some seem to demand a unique nutritional focus? Do immunodeficiency diseases such as AIDS, autoimmune disease, and so forth, in turn, create unique nutritional needs?

In vitro studies can also provide important insights into the roles of nutrients in specific immune phenomena. They may not directly portend to health issues, but they may provide clues to important links between the immune function and nutrients. As will be discussed, general deprivation of nutrients as manifested by serum deprivation and fluxes in levels of calcium or zinc within the cell can cause thymocytes, precursor B cells, T cells, B cells, and so forth to readily undergo apoptosis *(6,7)*. In addition, zinc has been shown to both induce and inhibit apoptosis in a variety of kinds of cells, including thymocytes, appearing to be able to modulate cell death *(7)*. These in vitro studies, like the in vivo studies, also suggest there is a tight link between cells of the immune system and nutrients right up to and including death.

ZINC DEFICIENCY: WHAT WE HAVE LEARNED FROM A WELL-DEVELOPED NUTRITIONAL-IMMUNOLOGICAL MODEL

Extensive animal model research using rodents and primates along with human data makes the impact of zinc deficiency on immune function one of the best characterized nutritional–immunological models *(5,8)*. The literature is extensive, so the focus here will be on what we have learned about specific roles for zinc in the immune function and/or the underlying mechanisms whereby suboptimal zinc so profoundly affects immune status.

Early investigations by clinicians indicated that a suboptimal intake of zinc led to lymphopenia and thymic atrophy *(4)*. Height-

From: *Nutrition and Immunology: Principles and Practice* (ME Gershwin et al. eds.), © Humana Press, Inc., Totowa, NJ

Table 1
Some of the Diseases and Disease States
Accompanied by Nutritional Deficiencies
That Alter Immune Status and Increase
the Incidence of Infection

Diseases	Disease states
Autoimmune diseases	Aging
AIDS	Anorexia
Chronic gastrointestinal disorders	Alcoholism
Crohn's disease	Burns
Infections	Malnutrition
Renal disease	Trauma
Cirrhosis of the liver	
Sickle cell anemia	

ened numbers of infections were also observed in deficient subjects *(4,5)*. Our laboratory and several others followed these observations with extensive studies of zinc-deficient mice that showed that they had reduced ability to generate cell- and antibody-mediated responses that generally correlated with the degree of zinc deficiency *(5,8–11)*. Moreover, the loss in absolute response capacity declined sharply as zinc depletion advanced *(11)*. The immune system appeared to degenerate much faster than the function of liver, kidney, and so forth. However, the decline in immune response capacity also correlated with the degree of lymphopenia and thymic atrophy, leaving one to wonder if we had really added very much to our understanding of how suboptimal zinc affected the immune function *(11)*.

With regard to specific biochemical effects of suboptimal zinc, the thymic hormone thymulin not only declined significantly during zinc deficiency but was shown to be dependent on zinc as a cofactor for its function *(12)*. Thus, at least one new function for zinc emerged from these studies, although one would have hoped for more revelations. If one examined the ability of lymphocytes from zinc-deficient mice to produce antibody, cytokines, and so forth on a per cell basis, one found that they appeared normal when tested either in vivo or in vitro, even in autologous sera *(11,13)*. Our laboratory could find no overt evidence of defects among lymphocytes from zinc-deficient mice that might be directly related to a zinc-dependent function. However, this was not the case for macrophages. Macrophages from zinc-deficient mice had reduced capacity to take up and kill the parasite *Trypanosoma cruzi* *(14)*. It appeared to be zinc related because a 1-h preincubation in 10 µg Zn/mL of exogenous zinc restored the ability of these cells to both carry out phagocytosis and generate an oxygen burst via measurement of peroxide production *(14)*. Superoxide dismutase, phospholipase c, and the regulation of other phospholipases were some of the enzymes that are partially or overtly dependent on zinc and play key roles in the oxygen burst *(15)*. Thus, some of these studies were reinforcing and/or revealed new roles for zinc in cell function. Because phagocytosis was altered in macrophages from the zinc-deficient mice, it led us to wonder if there were not general defects in the membrane substructure of the macrophages from the zinc-deficient mouse that would alter both phagocytosis and the oxygen burst *(14,15)*. This might be an affirmation of the work of O'Dell's laboratory where zinc had been shown to stabilize membranes *(16)*. More

importantly, this difference in the functional status of lymphocytes versus phagocytic cells would not be the first dichotomy in the effects of suboptimal zinc on the myeloid versus the lymphoid compartment of the immune system.

IMPORTANT ENDOCRINE CHANGES BROUGHT ABOUT BY NUTRITIONAL DEFICIENCIES THAT IMPACT ON IMMUNE STATUS

The lymphopenia and thymic atrophy and adrenal hypertrophy noted by early investigators for both zinc deficiency and protein-calorie deficiency made us wonder whether glucocorticoids were chronically elevated during malnutrition as it was known to be during other stresses. We found that zinc deficiency in mice did, indeed, cause chronic elevation of glucocorticoids and that removal of the steroid from the equation via adrenalectomy afforded the thymus great protection from the deficiency in zinc *(17)*. Similar findings were made in protein-calorie-deficient children and rodents *(18)*. Although an important finding, some nutritionists were not pleased to learn that something other than zinc itself was creating havoc with the immune system. However, recognition that endocrine status can also be altered by changes in nutritional status has won more converts and become important to our understanding of the secondary changes that suboptimal nutriture may create. Moreover, it is also evident that glucocorticoids readily induce apoptosis in precursor cells of the immune system of both mice and humans *(19,20)*. Using highly sensitive flow cytometric methods for measuring apoptosis in heterogenous populations of cells, it has been shown that the moderate, but chronically produced endogenous glucocorticoids analogous to that found in zinc deficiency can readily induce apoptosis in thymocytes and precursor B cells of the marrow both in vivo and in vitro *(19,20)*. Moreover, in vitro serum deprivation and chelation of zinc also act to induce apoptosis, especially in cells of the immune system *(6,21)*. Thus, one would assume that there might be some synergy between the combination of suboptimal zinc and chronic production of glucocorticoids that might accelerate apoptosis. As will be discussed, these events appear to account, at least in part, for reduced lymphopoiesis and resultant lymphopenia.

The loss of early progenitor lymphoid cells during zinc deficiency followed a defined pattern in both the marrow and thymus. As zinc deficiency advanced in the mouse, a rapid, almost devastating depletion of 60–90% of the B-cell compartment of the marrow and the T cells in the thymus was observed *(22)*. If one looked at specific subsets, one saw high losses in the precursor B-cell population that are actively rearranging their Ig genes *(22)*. The same was observed in the thymus among CD4+CD8+ cells that are engaged in the rearrangement of the T-cell receptor *(36)*. Interesting, both groups of cells are highly programmed to die as a result of the generation of nonsense and anti-self-clones that must be eliminated. There were moderate losses of immature or IgM-bearing B cells. Not surprisingly, the mature IgM+IgD+ B cells are fairly resistant to zinc deficiency. Somewhat surprisingly, very early pro-B and pro-T cells (CD4−CD8−) showed substantial resistance to both zinc deficiency and glucocorticoids *(23)*. These earliest of progenitor cells may not be highly programmed to die, as they are not yet a threat and have not formed an anti-self-clone or nonsense clone, as would be the case for the precursor cells. Moreover, it was recently shown that not unlike the more mature T and B cells, these earliest of B and T cells contain high levels of the proto-oncogene Bcl-2, which provides resistance to apoptosis (24).

REGULATION OF THE CHANGES IN IMMUNE STATUS AS A NUTRITIONAL DEFICIENCY ADVANCES

We are familiar with the metabolic changes that occur as the body moves from the well-fed to the starved state. We are even aware that as a nutrient like zinc becomes limiting, it is redistributed from the serum to vital tissues, especially the liver (4). It was less obvious why the immune system, which is so vital to our survival, appears to be rapidly dismantled, leaving the subject highly vulnerable to the next pathogen or tumor. The immune system did not appear to be a protected function. Recent studies of changes in marrow function as zinc deficiency advances have shed some light on this subject.

As zinc or protein calories become limiting, it appears that choices regarding immune function must be made. Why does lymphopenia, thymic atrophy, and rapid depletion of the marrow of early T and B progenitors quickly follow? Perhaps, because lymphocytes are our second line of defense. The vast majority (>90%) live only a few weeks and never actively engage in an immune response. Yet, the marrow is obliged to produce billions of new lymphocytes each day, some 90% of which must be eliminated due to faulty rearrangement of the Ig or T-cell receptor genes (6). Taken together, lymphopoiesis is a very expensive process to maintain as a nutrient or nutrients become limiting. Although important, lymphocytes are not as vital as the heart, brain, liver, and so forth, and may be put on the "not to be maintained" list as deficiencies advance to reserve nutrients.

Recent data, however, provide reassurance, because part of the immune system appears to be protected during zinc deficiency. There is a dichotomy in the effect of zinc deficiency on myeloid versus lymphoid cells that may be of considerable importance in our understanding of the regulation of the immune system during a dietary deficiency (25). These data suggest that as zinc deficiency advances there are concerted and defined changes put into place rather than a general disassembly of the entire immune system. Use of a phenotypic marker system for mapping out six compartments of the bone marrow (26) has made evident that while there is rapid depletion of the lymphoid compartment in the zinc-deficient mouse, the myeloid compartment remains intact (25). Indeed, the myeloid compartment gradually becomes a greater portion of the marrow, increasing 30–50% because of its greater survival. The difference between the myeloid and lymphoid compartments over time is striking. It seems evident that the neutrophils and macrophages that are our first line of defense are spared as zinc becomes limiting in the body.

The above finding provides an important new understanding, namely that a key segment of our immune system is protected during zinc deficiency. Is this protection happenstance or is it the outcome of a defined regulatory process? Our hypothesis is that as zinc becomes limiting, choices have to be made regarding the immune system because it is large and in a high rate of turnover. The suboptimal zinc induces the stress axis that results in the chronic production of glucocorticoids, which has now been shown to be sufficient to readily induce apoptosis in precursor lymphoid cells, reducing their production and sparing nutrients for vital tissues (5,19,20,22). Conversely, implantation and delivery of glu-

Table 2
Nutrients That Can Initiate or Block Apoptosis in Precursor Cells of the Immune System of Humans and Rodents

Chelation of copper	Serum deprivation
Chelation of zinc	Protein-calorie deficiencies
High zinc	Zinc deficiency
Iron	Vitamin D_3
Calcium fluxes	
Selenite	

cocorticoids analogous to that found in zinc deficiency have been shown to have little effect on myeloid cells (25). Moreover, several investigators have noted that a brief incubation of human neutrophils in glucocorticoids does not induce apoptosis, as it does in lymphocytes; instead, it substantially extends their half-life (27). Interestingly, immunologists have long known that addition of small amounts of glucocorticoids to long-term bone marrow cultures promotes the development of myeloid cells to the exclusion of lymphoid cells (28). Thus, there is precedence in the literature for this dichotomy of effects of glucocorticoids on the development of lymphoid versus myeloid cells in the marrow. Taken together, these studies add additional importance to the role of hormone-mediated changes created by suboptimal nutriture to immune status. However, the most important outcome of these studies is the revelation that during zinc deficiency, there is regulation in how the immune system is altered.

ABILITY OF NUTRIENTS TO MODULATE APOPTOSIS IN CELLS OF THE IMMUNE SYSTEM

During the last decade, a terrific effort has been put forth to better understand cell death, especially apoptosis. It is hard to underestimate the importance of this phenomenon to biology and immunology in particular. Clearly, apoptosis plays a critical role in the removal of nonsense clones generated during Ig gene and T-cell receptor rearrangements, as well as removal of anti-self-clones (6). Irradiation and glucocorticoids known to have devastating effects on developing cells of the immune system have been shown to be able to readily initiate apoptosis in these cells (20). Even nutritional deprivation as represented by serum deprivation initiates apoptosis in many kinds of cells (6). The cytolytic removal of virally infected and cancerous cells is via apoptotic mechanisms (6). Some of the more efficacious chemotherapy agents are effective because they can induce apoptosis. Thus, chemicals that enhance or block apoptosis are readily sought because of their potential to regulate so many facets of health and disease. Zinc is one such regulator and there is growing evidence that other nutrients can modulate cell death as well (see Table 2).

Glucocorticoid-induced apoptosis of murine thymocytes became an early model frequently used to better understand the biochemistry of cell death (6). It was subsequently shown that the precursor and immature B cells of the marrow were also very susceptible to glucocorticoid-induced apoptosis, as already discussed (19,20). Indeed, the low but chronic levels of steroids known to be present in zinc deficiency and protein-calorie deficiencies was sufficient to reduce 40–90% of the early B cells both in vitro and in vivo (22). However, for over a decade, it was also known that zinc, in turn, could block cell death in a variety of systems, which included blocking glucocorticoid-induced death of precursor B cells and thymocytes *(6,7,29)*. Thus began a complex role for zinc in cell death.

Perhaps the earliest evidence that zinc could block apoptosis was the 1984 data provided by Cohen and Duke, where high zinc inhibited apoptosis in murine thymocyte nuclei *(29)*. Hence, it was thought that zinc inhibited the endonuclease that digests DNA at the linker regions of the nucleosomes and yields the 180-bp (basepairs) DNA fragments characteristic of apoptosis. What followed was a raft of apoptotic cues that zinc was shown to be able to block *(7,30–32)*. However, the problem for those in the trace element field was the fact that 500–1000 μM of zinc was required to bring about this inhibition. This high amount of zinc set off alarms among those who knew zinc to be a trace element that often had deleterious effects at the high concentrations used by those investigators.

Curious about this phenomenon, we wondered if zinc could block the death signal itself, as there seemed to be multiple sites in a cell where zinc might have inhibiting effects beyond the endonuclease. For example, another metal, molybdate, was associated with the docked glucocorticoid receptor *(33)*. Furthermore, it had been shown that cadmium would bind to the receptor, preventing binding of the steroid *(34)*. Thus, it seemed probable that zinc might alter glucocorticoid-mediated signaling in cell death. Indeed, cells that were incubated simultaneously with zinc and ^{3}H-dexamethasone failed to initiate apoptosis. As suspected, zinc had blocked binding of the ^{3}H-dexamethasone to the receptor, and Western analysis showed the receptor remained intact and docked *(35)*. Yet, zinc was not a strong inhibitor because it was unable to reverse the binding or block cell death if added after steroid had bound to the glucocorticoid receptor. Moreover, the reducing agent dithiothreitol (DTT) could overcome the inhibitory effects of zinc. This suggested that zinc was binding to the vicinal cysteines at sites 656 and 660, which are critical to the ligand-binding region of the glucocorticoid receptor *(35)*. Thus, zinc, albeit at high levels, can inhibit the glucocorticoid-mediated death signal.

As we sought to determine whether lower or higher physiological concentrations of zinc would protect thymocytes, we made a surprising discovery. At about 80 μM, zinc became a good inducer of apoptosis, killing 25–45% of all thymocytes in a few hours *(36)*. This suggested that zinc could modulate cell death. Other trace metals such as nickel, copper, and cadmium failed to either initiate or block apoptosis.

However, there was a cloud over these findings. Follow-up studies showed that few of the cells presumed to be protected from undergoing glucocorticoid-induced apoptosis via the addition of high zinc survived more than a few hours before dying. Repeated washing to remove steroid and zinc also failed to generate any long-term survivors *(7)*. The high nonphysiological concentrations of zinc left in the cell eventually took a toll and probably induced cell death in the cells that had temporarily managed to survive glucocorticoid-induced death. This could be chalked up to test-tube chemistry with a disappointing ending. However, the dramatic effect that the combination of suboptimal dietary zinc and the accompanying glucocorticoids have on the thymus and B-cell compartment of the marrow makes one also wonder if there is not some synergy between the two. It is very possible that in the microenvironment of the cells of the immune system that fluxes in cellular zinc might enhance or inhibit death signals.

The literature is also replete with many examples that changes in calcium status within a cell definitely modulate apoptosis *(6,29)*. It is thought that intracellular release of calcium is a critical event in many, although perhaps not all, death pathways. The calcium ionophore A23187 is able to induce apoptosis in a variety of types of cells, especially thymocytes and other cells of the immune system *(6,37)*. Investigators struggle to identify the function Bcl-2, a protooncogene, that protects cells from apoptosis. Some hypothesize that Bcl-2 regulates the movement of calcium ions. Some of the proteases such as the calpains that are activated during apoptosis are calcium dependent. Calcium is also needed for endonuclease activity *(29)*.

Other minerals and metals can also promote apoptotic cell death, especially among cells of the immune system. In the case of mouse leukemic cells L1210, the addition of selenite caused concentration-dependent DNA strand breaks that were characteristic of apoptotic death *(38)*. When thymocytes were exposed to metal chelators, apoptosis was induced, supposedly by the eight-fold elevation in copper. Copper was presumably the sole metal transported into the cell by pyrrolidine dithiozine carbamate *(39)*. Chelation of either iron or zinc created deficits in the metals, which induced apoptosis as well *(21,40)*. Of particular interest was the ability of vitamin D_3 to arrest the growth of MCF-7 breast cancer cells. A 48-h time-course of treatment followed by *in situ* labeling of DNA strand breaks indicated that D3 had gradually increased apoptosis in the cancer cells *(41)*.

The above literature is just a small sampling of the many studies that suggest that intracellular fluxes in a variety of nutrients can promote or inhibit apoptosis, especially among leukocytes. Clearly, so-called death signals can be intensified or neutralized by a variety of metals and other nutrients. These seem to further evidence of the tight link between nutritional status and immune status that would seem to include influences on life and death decisions within a cell. Moreover, it is yet another argument for the need to give greater consideration to the role of nutritional supplements in chronic diseases.

THE POTENTIAL VALUE OF APPROPRIATE NUTRITIONAL SUPPLEMENTATION TO CHRONIC DISEASES

There are numerous examples of the positive impact of zinc supplementation, especially on growth and the immune function. The pioneering studies of Prasad that established that zinc was an essential trace element for humankind *(4,42)* also showed that zinc supplementation rapidly restored growth, sexual development, lymphocyte counts, and so forth, of zinc-deficient children in the Middle East *(42)*. Immune parameters were also improved by zinc supplementation of a child with *Acrodermatitis enteropathica,* a genetic disorder that creates malabsorption of zinc *(43)*. Although the zinc status of the elderly presents a complex picture, several investigators have shown that zinc supplementation will improve some immune functions in the aged *(44,45)*. More recently, zinc supplementation of malnourished children provided enhanced growth with reductions in the incidence of infection *(46)*. In the case of rodent studies, zinc-deficient mice that had experienced greater than 30% body weight loss and a 70% reduction in thymus weight were provided 50 ppm zinc in their diet *(47)*. Recovery of the immune function was amazing. Within 2 weeks, the thymus was restored, as were antibody-mediated responses. Amazingly, this immune repair preceded restoration of body weight. Moreover, at a certain point in the repair process, a significant number of thymuses were 25–40% larger than normal. Spleens containing 130–150% the normal number of lymphocytes were also noted in a substantial proportion of the repairing mice only 10 d after supplementation. This was reminiscent of an overshoot in the immune repair process that had been noted many years before by those studying immune repair in irradiated animals. Although repair studies are tedious and expensive to carry out, there is evidence that repair of zinc deficiency is also a regulated process that may have its own unique regulating events.

As will also be discussed, a subset of AIDS patients has been shown by several investigators to have low serum zinc levels (48). The provision of zinc to a number of AIDS patients at a midpoint in the etiology of the disease reduced infection by nearly half (48). Even though zinc has been shown to be suboptimal in a variety of disease states, it is odd that patient care and management does not routinely include supplementation with this inexpensive nutrient. However, suggestions that holding a zinc lozenger in one's mouth will reduce the duration of colds has led to inclusion of zinc in a variety of pharmaceutical products in the hopes of increasing sales in spite of other studies which suggest zinc has no discernible effect on colds (49,50). It takes fairly substantial amounts of zinc supplementation to create a deficiency in copper because they share common metal-binding ligands for absorption in the gut (51). It appears to take rather extraordinary zinc dosage to create toxicity (51). Thus, it remains puzzling that this essential trace element so readily available is an inexpensive supplement but is not an integral part of the care of patients with chronic diseases, especially where appetite reduction, malabsorption, and wasting are known to be part of the disease state that will clearly compromise immune defense. Although the focus here was on zinc, there are many other studies in which a specific nutrient or group of nutrients are altered by disease or infection (1–5).

SIMILARITIES AND VARIANCES IN THE IMPACT OF NUTRITIONAL DEFICIENCIES ON THE IMMUNE FUNCTION

Zinc deficiency and protein-calorie deficiencies (PCM) are observed among peoples of the Third World and among patients with chronic disease states such as cancer, AIDS, renal disease, gastrointestinal disorders, and so on (4,5,18). These two nutritional–immunological models have been extensively studied. Because the immunological changes noted in humans or animals that are either zinc deficient or PCM are similar, it gives a sense that there is a lot of common ground in how nutritional deficits impact on the immune system. It is well documented that PCM and zinc deficiency causes thymic atrophy, lymphopenia, and reductions in cell- and antibody-mediated responses (1–18). Increased infections and reduced potential to defend against pathogenic challenges have been noted in PCM and zinc-deficient subjects (1,4,5,18). Moreover, glucocorticoids are also chronically elevated in both humans and mice with PCM (52–54). As was the case for zinc deficiency, adrenalectomy of PCM mice prior to the induction of PCM protected the thymus from atrophy (55).

The similarities between zinc deficiency and PCM probably provide too much assurance that nutritional deficiencies may have similar effects on the immune function. For example, it is well known that PCM accompanies zinc deficiency, because appetite suppression and reduced calorie intake ensue as the deficiency advances (4,5). More often than not, low serum zinc is noted in

PCM (56). This, along with the fact that the two deficiencies alter endocrine function in similar ways, may account for the many parallels between PCM and zinc deficiency.

The careful work of Prohaska and Failla provide comparison and contrast for the effects of copper deficiency on immune function to the above models (57). Although not frequently seen in the human population, increased infections have been noted in copper-deficient children. Copper-deficient mice have a smaller thymuses, with impaired cell-mediated immunity. They generate poor protective immunity when challenged with bacteria or parasites. It is not clear whether a thorough enough examination has been made of whether or not copper deficiency induces the production of glucocorticoids, although it is thought not to do so (57). However, testosterone and estradiol levels were lower in the plasma of copper-deficient male mice. Copper-deficient rats also showed reductions in the proportion of the T cells not altered in zinc-deficient mice (58). The spleen also contained blastoidlike cells, and in addition to having lower copper content, it had lower iron content as well. Failla's laboratory found that interleukin-2 (IL-2) production was diminished in copper-deficient rats and mitogenic responses were reduced (59). This is also of significance because IL-2 production mitogenically was thought to be normal for T cells from zinc-deficient mice (11,13). Moreover, healthy males fed low-copper diets exhibited reduced response to T cell mitogens with reduced production of IL-2, providing good correlation to the rodent studies (60). Surprisingly, 3 wk of copper supplementation did not bring about full immune repair. It is hoped that a longer period of supplementation would give full repair. More recently, human Jurkat T cells cultured in copper-chelated media also exhibited decreased production of IL-2 (61). Thus, there are some common effects of zinc, copper, and PCM on the branches of the immune system, but important differences appear at the cellular and biochemical level.

If we turn our attention to the comprehensive review provided by Kuvibidila, one finds that iron deficiency also impairs cell- and antibody-mediated responses and causes lymphopenia (18). Vitamin A deficiencies in rats create reductions in the thymus and reduce antibody-mediated responses, and so forth while increasing the susceptibility of humans to infection (18). Space does not permit the examination of all nutrients of potential interest; however, the above data suggest that some nutritional deficiencies have common effects on immune status. They often cause thymic atrophy, lymphopenia, and reduced cell and antibody response. As a consequence, nutritionally deficient hosts often have greater chances of infections and reduced capacity to withstand pathogenic challenges. Not surprisingly, we still have patients dying of sepsis, pneumonia, and a variety of infections rather than their primary disease such as cancer, renal disease, gastrointestinal disorders, and so on, which create a variety of nutritional deficiencies that compromise immune status. Better nutritional management of a host of chronic diseases would undoubtedly extend the life of the patient and reduce the chance of death from an infection. As we become concerned about the cost of health care, we may finally begin to give greater attention to the efficacy of nutritional supplements, which cost very little.

AIDS: AN IMMUNE DEFICIENCY CREATES NUTRITIONAL DEFICIENCIES

The devastating effects of AIDS generated an intense effort to identify its cause. More recently, the focus has been on drugs and drug cocktails to slow the advance of the disease while a vaccine is sought. Only in the last few years have studies been launched in the hopes of enhancing the quality of life of the AIDS patient by including better nutritional management. A number of studies were initiated in the nineties to look at the nutritional status of the AIDS patient, although such studies are fraught with a plethora of problems. Obviously, one would expect to see more changes in nutritional status as AIDS advances and wasting sets in. Because it is indeed an immunodeficiency disease, many of the subjects have opportunistic infections. Whether the infection is *Pneumocystis carinii* or more routine viral, fungal, or bacterial infections, they each could contribute unique and potentially different changes in the subject's nutritional status. There are a number of past studies that provide evidence that pathogens can cause their own unique changes in the body's nutritional status *(2)*. No doubt that the various drugs given in an effort to arrest HIV virus will also alter the nutrient balance to some extent. Thus, each AIDS patient comes to a study with many variables that are very difficult to control. In a 1996 study of 228 patients with AIDS, Koch et al. attempted to control some of the many variables among subjects by taking care to subdivide them by degree of malnutrition, CD4 count, type of infection, and so forth *(62)*. They began by examining the serum zinc levels of the patients. Almost 30% of the subjects exhibited rather low serum zinc levels. The remaining subjects had borderline or normal levels of zinc. Surprisingly, a low serum zinc did not seem to correlate with the subject's degree of malnutrition, CD4 count, and so on. In a related study of this same group of patients, the investigators tried to determine if there was a correlation between zinc status and albumin levels, as both are often low in advanced states of malnutrition *(63)*. There was no correlation there either. A smaller study by Lambl et al. noted significantly lower serum zinc levels in those HIV⁺ patients with chronic diarrhea and *Microsporidia* infection *(64)*. This might be an important but secondary outcome of HIV⁺ because gastrointestinal disturbances accompanied by diarrhea are known to alter zinc absorption *(4)*. The most recent study, which included 125 HIV⁺ patients studied for 3.5 yr, continues to show that mineral status is altered in AIDS patients *(65)*. However, in this study, selenium emerged as being suboptimal. Although zinc was also suboptimal in some of these subjects, only selenium had a strong correlation to CD4 counts and mortality *(65)*.

The above studies leave one in a quandary. However, an Italian group headed by Mocchegiani provides a very valuable addition to these studies *(48)*. This group found that stage IV AIDS patients had substantial reductions in serum zinc and the zinc-dependent hormone thymulin, whereas mid-stage subjects manifested more moderate reductions in these entities. Subsequently, zinc sulfate was provided to a group of mid-stage HIV⁺ patients, with encouraging results that suggest additional studies are warranted. Over the course of 24 mo, the zinc-supplemented patients gained weight, exhibited increased numbers of CD4⁺ cells, and had active thymulin levels. Most importantly, zinc supplementation reduced opportunistic infections to half the number of unsupplemented subjects!

Although the potential immune alteration created by suboptimal zinc is well documented, the role of selenium in the immune function has not been adequately described. Thus, points of focus for potential beneficial effects of selenium supplementation in the etiology of AIDS are not clear. Once again, a disease state with nutritional deficits that may need to be managed collide with lack of sufficient information. Clearly, selenium is important to glutathione peroxide function. It protects all cells, especially phagocytic cells, from oxidative damage created by peroxides *(66)*. Clearly, selenium deficiencies depressed the oxygen burst in cattle; however, its effect on the same function in the rat was inconsistent *(66)*. Earlier work by Spallholz showed that selenium deficiencies depressed antibody-mediated responses, but supplementation with modest levels of selenium greatly enhanced these responses in mice *(67)*. More recently, selenium deficiency not only increased the virulence but also the viral phenotype of Coxsackie virus in mice *(68)*. Perhaps of greatest importance is the finding that selenium deficiency in mice substantially reduced the cytolytic T-cell function in selenium-deficient mice, whereas modest supplementation of a regular diet with selenium provided enhanced cytolytic responses *(69)*. The latter are, of course, critical to AIDS patients, given their high incidence of viral infection and cancer such as Kaposi's sarcoma.

Together, these studies suggest that zinc and/or selenium supplementation of AIDS patients may be a low-cost means of improving immune defense in these individuals, especially in the later stages of the disease. Reduced appetite, wasting, infection, drugs, and so forth, could all create a low level of zinc or selenium deficiency that could be difficult to detect via analysis of serum *(4)*. The profound impact that zinc deficiency has on the immune system, especially if combined with deficits in other nutrients and protein-calorie deficiency, could, indeed, hasten the demise of the already handicapped immune system of the AIDS patient. It also seems clear that if modest deficiencies in some nutrients can have substantial effects on host defense, AIDS also provides evidence that an immunodeficiency state can create nutritional deficiencies.

EVIDENCE OF THE POTENTIAL OF NUTRITIONAL SUPPLEMENTS TO IMPROVE AN AUTOIMMUNE DISEASE

Most autoimmune diseases remain an enigma, being difficult to diagnose. Moreover, the original cause of these diseases is often unknown. Crohn's disease is a chronic inflammation of the gut, which creates abdominal pain and diarrhea in its more benign form but can lead to fistulas and diseased areas that require surgical removal. The gut area is often infiltrated with large numbers of lymphocytes, with some evidence that faulty T-cell function exacerbates the disease. Various deficiencies develop, especially in iron and zinc resulting from altered absorption *(70)*. In its more severe form, appetite induction and weight loss are factors suggestive of protein-calorie deficiency. Thus, dietary management quickly became part of the treatment program for these patients. It is another, albeit unique, example of nutritional status affecting immune status.

If Crohn's is bad, multiple sclerosis, myasthenia gravis, muscular dystrophy, and lupus are worse. They are more debilitating and invariably shorten the victim's life. However, the laboratory of Hayes has come upon a potentially important nutritional answer for experimental autoimmune in encephalomyelitis (EAE), a murine model of multiple sclerosis (MS) *(71)*. EAE was induced in BIO.PL mice by injecting them with myelin basic protein. When symptoms of autoimmunity began to appear, the mice were given 1,25-dihydroxy vitamin D_3 (D3), which was able to prevent the progression of disease. Withdrawal of D3 resulted in the resumption of autoimmunity *(71)*.

To their credit, the investigators are advancing the above study beyond the phenomenological realm, toward one with a scientific basis. They hypothesize that D3 acts as a selective immune regulator that may inhibit the undesired immune reactions that probably initiate this autoimmune disease (72). Under low-sunlight conditions, they point out that less D3 will be produced, thereby increasing the risk of MS. In support of their theory, they point out that geographics greatly impact on the prevalence of MS in a population. Indeed, MS is apparently nearly zero in equatorial regions around the world. If their hypothesis is correct, supplementation of individuals with MS with vitamin D_3 may have great therapeutic potential and, perhaps, some preventative capacity for those with a clear genetic predisposition for MS. This is another important example of investigators linking nutrition to an immune dysfunction.

DIETARY RESTRICTION: WHEN LESS MAY BE MORE FOR THE IMMUNE SYSTEM

Over the years, a compelling body of literature has accumulated, showing that modest restriction in calorie intake over an extended period of time will substantially lengthen the life-span of mice (73). From a more immunological point of view, calorie restriction also prolonged the onset of autoimmunity in NZB and MRL/lpr mice, while also reducing spontaneous tumor development in a variety of strains of mice (74). As might be expected, a number of age-related changes in the immune function were significantly offset by dietary restriction (75–77).

These are fascinating findings that indicate dietary restriction has a plethora of positive health effects, some of which have an impact on the immune system. Although the data generated were tantalizing, it had been generated over a period of 20 yr without provision of an underlying mechanism(s) that would explain the observed extension of life. Clearly, attempting to identify a single unifying mechanism(s) is a daunting task. However, without it, these potentially important studies could remain on the clinical shelf. There is, however, some recent progress in this area. As a result of the recent interest in the role of reactive oxygen species (ROS) in aging, Tian et al. compared the levels of lipid peroxidation and oxidation of plasma proteins in *ad libitum*-fed and calorie-restricted Fischer rats over a period of 31 mo (76). Although one would like to have seen a more extensive evaluation of immune parameters, especially in vivo, the primary immunological assessment was the in vitro response of T cells to mitogens. Nevertheless, these investigators found that the decline in T-cell response with age correlated with the levels of lipid and protein peroxidation. Caloric restriction partially offset both peroxidation and the age-associated decline in T cell function. Indeed, the reduction in ROS production appears to be a promising explanation for the many protective effects noted for dietary restriction.

The problem with ROS in understanding how diverse types of dietary restriction ranging from withholding calories to reducing zinc intake would reduce ROS production. Moreover, how would reduced ROS production offset the onset of autoimmunity in calorie-restricted NZB mice? An interesting new angle is provided by Spaulding et al. (77) that adds new dimension to the picture. They propose that the well-documented reduction in aging among T cells is the result of malfunction of a subset of T cells within the population rather than a decline in function among all T cells. They further note that in calorie-restricted mice, there is some

lymphopenia that would otherwise seem to have a negative impact on immunity until one looks at rates of cell death. They noted reduced rates of apoptosis among T cells from aged mice that was normalized in calorie-restricted mice. These findings may mean that calorie restriction enhances or normalizes the removal of faulty cells as rodents age, including ROS damaged cells, via maintaining or perhaps even heightening the rate of apoptosis. As discussed, it is well established that serum or nutrient deprivation and deprivation of zinc apoptosis in vitro not just among cells of the immune system but also many other types of cell (6,7,21). Thus, modest dietary restriction could well be a cue that promotes apoptosis. However, one wonders if dietary restriction like protein-calorie and zinc restriction might also alter the circadian rhythm of glucocorticoids. Small but chronic elevations in glucocorticoid production that might be difficult to measure might also be sufficient to elevate apoptosis just a few percent. This, in turn, might be more than sufficient to facilitate removal of faulty cells that accumulate with aging, spontaneous tumor cells, or the anti-self-lymphocytes that are the underpinning of autoimmunity. Regardless, these investigators are much closer to being able to explain why a variety of kinds of dietary restriction can have a positive impact on such diverse phenomena as aging, autoimmunity, and malignancy. This could well have a significant impact in the United States, where the overfed continue to be one of the greatest health problems.

THE COMPLEX INTERACTIONS AMONG INFECTION, NUTRITION, AND THE IMMUNE SYSTEM

Each infection has its own unique pathogenesis, which makes it difficult to generalize about their effects on nutritional status (2). However, more often than not, infections cause significant losses from nutritional reserves of the body. This is particularly true for infections that initiate an acute-phase response, where loss of appetite and wasting are key components of the response. One assumes that the many deleterious effects for PCM on immune status would be potential problems for these patients as well. Therefore, there is a high probability that the nutritional deficiencies created by the infection will lead to immune system derangement as a secondary consequence, thereby exacerbating recovery. Suboptimal intake of zinc, PCM, and copper have already been shown to increase the incidence of infection and morbidity in human and animals (1–3,18,57). This, of course, has the obvious potential of creating a vicious and life-threatening circle, where the infection impairs the immune system, creating a higher level of infection with a concomitant heightened level of impairment of immune defense. Thus, death becomes a possible outcome of sepsis, toxic shock syndrome, and other serious infections that compromise the immune system and for which no nutritional management is provided.

Viral infections as well as some other intracellular infections may be cleared early by natural-killer cells or by more sustained responses on the part of cytolytic T cells. Defense against bacterial infections is somewhat better understood; however, they are multi-faceted. Moreover, bacterial infection can elicit an innate response from phagocytic cells that readily adhere to a protein or carbohydrate on the surface of the microbe, making for rapid clearance. Others initiate the alternate complement pathway that can lead to removal by lysis and/or phagocytosis. Still others gradually generate an antibody-mediated response, with antibody-mediated agglutination of the pathogens leading to an arrest in their growth. A potent antibody-mediated response will also provide memory that results in the generation of rapid protective responses upon the next encounter.

Failure of these responses can lead to toxic shock syndrome in the case of *Streptococcus, Staphylococcus, Clostridium tetani,* and *Vibrio cholerae.* Gram-negative bacteria, especially *Escherichia coli* and *Salmonella typhi,* that currently represent a significant food safety problem can also overtake the immune system, becoming a catastrophic condition known as sepsis. As these responses advance, there is further activation of monocytes and macrophages. A variety of cytokines are produced, including Interleukin I and tumor necrosis factor that reduce appetite and initiate fever. Continuance of this process can lead to an intense acute-phase response. A marked change in metabolism is then noted with decreases in blood nitrogen observed, followed by enhanced gluconeogenesis as reductions in food intake increase and body wasting sets in *(2)*. In addition, early investigators noted marked depletion in serum of iron and zinc status associated with some of these infections *(1,2)*. Clearly, the nutritional costs mount as these infections advance.

Although infections, in general, and sepsis and toxic shock syndrome, in particular, are of considerable current concern and interest, the development of nutritional strategies to manage these infections seems to be limited. Moreover, there are a host of parasite, fungal diseases, and so forth, some of which continue to cause significant health problems and mortality in underdeveloped countries, that are receiving little or no attention as far as identifying the sort of nutritional changes that they might create. As in many other areas, the early literature is replete with preliminary evidence that the relationships among infection, nutrition, and immune status are definitely linked *(1,2)*. This is another important area ripe for more thorough investigation. Future nutritional strategies for providing specific or optimized nutrition for a specific infection also remain open for study. Beyond protein-calorie deficiencies created by infection, there are probably any number of infections for which the addition of the right array of trace elements, iron, vitamins, and so forth would provide beneficial support that might make the difference between a prolonged and a short-term illness, or even life versus death.

SUMMARY

It is evident from the examples provided in this chapter and throughout the book that nutritional status and immune status are tightly linked. Indeed, recent evidence suggests that at the cellular level, fluxes in nutrients can even modulate apoptotic death pathways, especially in cells of the immune system. In spite of these interesting revelations, there are many nutrients whose impact on immune status remain to be explored. As also discussed, there are a number of chronic diseases, some of which were listed in Table 1, that create nutritional deficiencies that compromise the immune system. Clearly, this increases the chances of infections and mortality in the patient. Interestingly, immune deficiencies and defects (e.g., some autoimmune diseases and AIDS) appear to also alter nutritional status. This undoubtedly exacerbates the disease process further. A plethora of studies indicate that infections alter nutritional status, thereby compromising immune defense systems in a way that helps the pathogens gain the upper hand. In spite of the overwhelming evidence that there is a glaring

need for incorporating more nutritional supplementation into our management and care of chronic diseases, disease states, and infections, we are doing so at a surprisingly slow rate. There is a clear and growing need for additional studies, especially of human subjects, to explore the efficacy of nutritional supplementation to optimize immune defense systems where suboptimal nutriture and wasting are a component of the disease process.

REFERENCES

1. Chandra R, Newberne P. Nutrition Immunity and Infection. Plenum, New York, 1977.
2. Beisel W. Impact of infectious disease in the interaction between nutrition and immunity. In: Cunningham-Rundles S, ed, Nutritional Modulation of the Immune Response, pp. 475–80. New York, 1993.
3. Scrimshaw N, Taylor C, Gordon J. Interaction of nutrition and infection. Am J Med Sci 1959; 237:367–72.
4. Endre L, Beck F, Prasad A. The role of zinc in human health. J Trace Element Exp Med 1990; 3:337–75.
5. Fraker PJ, King L, Garvy B, Medina C. Immunopathology of zinc deficiency: a role for apoptosis. In: Klurfeld D, ed, Human Nutrition—A Comprehensive Treatise, Vol. 8, pp. 267–83. Plenum, New York, 1993.
6. Cohen J, Duke R. Apoptosis and programmed cell death in immunity. Annu Rev Immunol 1992; 10:267–93.
7. Fraker P, Telford W. Reappraisal of the role of zinc in life and death decisions of cells. Proc Soc Exp Biol Med 1997; 215:229–36.
8. Keen CL, Gershwin ME. Zinc deficiency and immune function. Annu Rev Nutr 1990; 10:415–31.
9. Fraker PJ, Haas SM, Luecke RW. Effect of zinc deficiency on the immune response of the young adult A/J mouse. J Nutr 1977; 107:1889–95.
10. Fernandes G, Nair M, Onoe K, Tanaka T, Floyd R, Good R. Impairment of cell mediated immunity function by dietary zinc deficiency in mice. Proc Natl Acad Sci USA 1979; 76:457–61.
11. Cook-Mills J, Fraker PJ. Functional capacity of residual lymphocytes from zinc deficient adult mice. Br J Nutr 1993; 69:835–48.
12. Dardenne M, Pleau J, Nabarra B, LeFrancier P, Derrien M, Choay J, et al. Contribution of zinc and other metals to the biological activity of the serum thymic factor. Proc Natl Acad Sci USA 1982; 79:370–6.
13. Dowd P, Kelleher J, Guillou P. T lymphocyte subsets and interleukin-2 production in zinc deficient rats. Br J Nutr 1986; 55:59–69.
14. Wirth JJ, Fraker PJ, Kierszenbaum F. Zinc requirement for macrophage function: effect of zinc deficiency on uptake and killing of a protozoan parasite. Immunology 1989; 68:114–9.
15. Cook-Mills J, Wirth J, Fraker PJ. Possible roles for zinc in destruction of *Trypanosoma cruzi* by toxic oxygen metabolites produced by mononuclear phagocytes. In: Phillips M, ed, Antioxidant Nutrients and Immune Function, pp. 111–21. Plenum, New York, 1990.
16. Bettger W, O'Dell B. A critical physiological role for zinc in the structure and function of biomembranes. Life Sci 1981; 28:1425–36.
17. DePasquale-Jardieu P, Fraker PJ. Further characterization of the role of corticosterone in the loss of humoral immunity in zinc-deficient A/J mice as determined by adrenalectomy. J Immunol 1980; 124:2650–5.
18. Kuvibidila S, Yu L, Ode D, Warrier RP. The immune response in protein-energy malnutrition and single nutrient deficiencies. In: Klurfeld DM, ed, Human Nutrition—A Comprehensive Treatise, Vol. 8, pp. 121–57. Plenum, New York, 1993.
19. Garvy B, King L, Telford W, Morford L, Fraker PJ. Chronic levels of corticosterone reduces the number of cycling cells of the B-lineage in murine bone marrow and induces apoptosis. Immunology 1993; 80:587–92.
20. Garvy B, Telford W, King L, Fraker PJ. Glucocorticoids and irradiation induced apoptosis in normal murine bone marrow B-lineage lymphocytes as determined by flow cytometry. Immunology 1993; 79:270–7.

21. McCabe M, Jiang S, Orrenuis S. Chelator of intracellular zinc triggers apoptosis in mature thymocytes. Lab Invest 1993; 69:101–10.

22. King LE, Osati-Ashtiani F, Fraker P. Depletion of cells of the B-lineage in the bone marrow of zinc deficient mouse. Immunology 1995; 85:69–73.

23. Osati F, King L, Fraker P. Survival of pro B-cells in zinc deficient mice. Immunology, 1998; 94:94–100.

24. Merino R, Ding L, Veis D, Korsmeyer S, Nunez G. Development regulation of the Bcl-2 protein and susceptibility to death in B-lymphocytes. EMBO 1994; 13:683–9.

25. Fraker P, King L. Changes in regulation of lymphopoiesis and myelopoiesis in the zinc deficient mouse. Nutr Rev 1998; 56:565–9.

26. de Bruijn M, Slieker W, van der Loo J, Voerman J, van Ewijk W, Leenen P. Distinct mouse bone marrow macrophage precursors identified by differential expression of ER-MP12 and ER-MP20 antigens. Eur J Immunol 1994; 24:2279–84.

27. Liles W, Dale D, Klebanoff S. Glucocorticoids inhibit apoptosis of human neutrophils. Blood 1995; 86:3181–8.

28. Dexter T, Allen T, Lajtha L. Conditions controlling the proliferation of hemopoietic stem cells in vitro. J Cell Physiol 1977; 91:335–44.

29. Cohen J, Duke R. Glucocorticoid activation of calcium dependent endonuclease in thymocyte nuclei leads to cell death. J Immunol 1984; 132:38–43.

30. Waring P, Egan M, Braithwaite A, Mullbacher N, Siarda A. Apoptosis induced in macrophages and T blasts by the mycotoxin sporodismin and protection by Zn^{+2} salts. Int J Pharmacol 1990; 12:445–57.

31. Flieger D, Riethmuller G, Ziegler-Hutbrock H. Zn^{++} inhibits both tumor necrosis factor mediated DNA fragmentation and cytolysis. Int J Cancer 1989; 44:315–9.

32. Shimuzu T, Kubota M, Tanizawa A, Sano H, Kasai Y, Hashimoto H, Akiyama Y, Mikawa H. Inhibition of both etoposide-induced DNA fragmentation and activation of poly (ADP)-ribose synthesis by zinc ion. Biochem Biophys Res Commun 1990; 169:1172–7.

33. Carson-Jurica M, Shrader W, O'Malley B. Steroid receptor family: structure and function. Endocr Rev 1990; 11:201–20.

34. Simmons S, Chakraborti P, Cavanaugh A. Arsenite and cadmium as probes of glucocorticoid receptor structure and function. J Biol Chem 1990; 265:1938–45.

35. Telford W, Fraker P. Zinc reversibility inhibits steroid binding to the glucocorticoid receptor. Biochem Biophys Rev Commun 1998; 283:86–91.

36. Telford W, Fraker P. Preferential induction of apoptosis in mouse $CD4^+CD8^+\alpha\beta TCR^{lo}CD3\epsilon^{lo}$ thymocytes by zinc. J Cel Physiol 1995; 164:259–70.

37. Wyllie A, Morris R, Smith A, Dunlop D. Chromatin cleavage in apoptosis: association with condensed chromatin morphology and dependence on macromolecular synthesis. J Pathol 1984; 142:67–77.

38. Lu J, Kaeck M, Jiang C, Wilson A, Thompson H. Selenite induction of DNA strand breaks and apoptosis in mouse leukemic L1210 cells. Biochem Pharmacol 1994; 47:1531–5.

39. Nobel C, Kimland M, Lind B, Orrenius, Slater A. Dithiocarbamates induce apoptosis in thymocytes in raising the intracellular level of redox active copper. J Biol Chem 1995; 270:26,202–8.

40. Kovar J, Stunz L, Stewart B, Kriegerbeckova K, Ashman R, Kemp J. Direct evidence that iron deprivation induces apoptosis in murine lymphoma 38C13. Pathobiology 1977; 65:61–8.

41. Simboli-Campbell M, Narvaez C, Tenniswood M, Welsh J. 1,25-Dihydroxyvitamin D3 induces morphological and biochemical markers of apoptosis in MCF-7 breast cancer cells. J Steroid Biochem Mol Biol 1996; 58:367–76.

42. Prasad A. Discovery and importance of zinc in human nutrition. Fed Proc 1984; 43:2829–35.

43. Oleske J, Westphal ML, Shore S, Gordon D, Bogden J, Nahmias A. Zinc therapy of depressed cellular immunity in Acrodermatitis Enteropathica. Am J Dis Childh 1979; 133:915–18.

44. Duchateau J, Delepesse G, Vrijins R, Collet H. Beneficial effects of oral zinc supplementation on the immune response of old people. Am J Med 1981; 70:1001–4.

45. Bogden JD, Oleske JM, Lavenhar MA, Muhves IM, Kemp FW, Bruening KS, Holding KJ, et al. Zinc supplementation in elderly people: effects of zinc supplementation for 3 months. Am J Clin Nutr 1988; 48:655–63.

46. Castillo-Duran C, Heresi G, Fisberg M, Uaury R. Controlled trial of zinc supplementation during recovery from malnutrition: effects on growth and immune function. Am J Clin Nutr 1987; 45:602–8.

47. Fraker PJ, De Pasquale-Jardieu P, Zwickl CM, Luecke RW. Regeneration of T-cell helper function in zinc-deficient adult mice. Proc Natl Acad Sci USA 1978; 75:5660–5.

48. Mocchegiani E, Veccia S, Ancarani F, Scalise G, Fabris N. Benefit of oral zinc supplementation as an adjunct to zidovudine (AZT) therapy against opportunistic infections in AIDS. Int J Immunopharmacol 1995; 17:719–27.

49. Jackson J, Peterson C, Lesko E. A meta-analysis of zinc salt lozenges and the common cold. Arch Intern Med 1997; 157:2373–6.

50. Eby G, Davis D, Halcomb W. Reduction in derivative of common colds by zinc gluconate lozenges in a double blind study. Antimicrob Agents Chemother 1984; 25:20–4.

51. Walsh C, Sandstead H, Prasad A, Newberne P, Fraker P. Zinc: health effects and research priorities for the 1990s. Environ Health Perspect 1994; 102:5–46.

52. Smith HF, Latham MC, Azaburke JA, Butler W, Phillips L, Pend W, et al. Blood plasma levels of cortisol, insulin, growth hormone, and somatomedin in children with marasmus, kwashiorkor and intermediate forms of protein-energy malnutrition. Proc Soc Exp Biol Med 1981; 167:607–11.

53. Alleyne GA, Young VH. Adrenocortical function in children with severe protein-calorie malnutrition. Clin Sci 1967; 33:189–200.

54. Becker DJ. The endocrine response to protein calorie malnutrition. Annu Rev Nutr 1983; 3:187–212.

55. Wing EG, Magee DM, Barczynski LK. Acute starvation in mice reduces number of T cells and suppresses the development of T-cell mediated immunity. Immunology 1988; 63:677–82.

56. Golden M, Golden B, Harland P, Jackson A. Zinc and immune competence in protein-energy malnutrition. Lancet 1978; 1:1226–8.

57. Prohaska J, Failla M. Copper and immunity. In: Klurfeld D, ed, Human Nutrition: A Comprehensive Treatise, Vol. 8, pp. 309–22. Plenum, New York, 1993.

58. King L, Fraker P. Flow cytometric analysis of the phenotypic distribution of splenic lymphocytes in zinc-deficient adult mice. J Nutr 1991; 121:1433–8.

59. Failla M, Hopkins R. Is low copper status immunosuppressive? Nutr Rev 1998; 56:559–64.

60. Kelley D, Daud P, Taylor P. Effects of low copper diets on human immune response. Am J Clin Nutr 1995; 62:412–6.

61. Hopkins R, Failla M. Copper deficiency reduced interleukin 2 production and IL-2 mRNA in human T lymphocytes. J Nutr 1997; 127:257–62.

62. Koch J, Neal EA, Schlott MJ, Garcia-Shelton YL, Chan MF, Weaver KE, Cello JP. Zinc levels and infections in hospitalized patients with AIDS. Nutrition 1996; 12:515–8.

63. Koch J, Neal EA, Schlott MJ, Garcia-Shelton YL, Chen MF, Weaver KE, Cello JP. Serum zinc and protein levels: lack of a correlation in hospitalized patients with AIDS. Nutrition 1996; 12:511–4.

64. Lambl BB, Federman M, Pleskow D, Wanke CA. Malabsorption and wasting in AIDS patients with microsporidia and pathogen-negative diarrhea. AIDS 1996; 10:739–44.

65. Baum MK, Shor-Posner G, Lu Y, Rosner B, Sauberlich HE, Fletcher MA, et al. Micronutrients and HIV-1 disease progression. AIDS 1995; 9:1051–6.

66. Stabel J, Spears J. Role of selenium in immune responsiveness and disease resistance. In: Klurfeld D, ed, Human Nutrition—A Comprehensive Treatise, Vol. 8, pp. 333–56. Plenum, New York, 1993.

67. Spallholz E. Selenium: what role in immunity and immune cytotoxicity? In: Selenium in Biology and Medicine. Spallholz J, Morton L, Gunther H, eds, pp. 103–17. AVI Publishing, Westport, CT, 1981.

68. Beck M. Increased virulence of Coxsackievirus B3 in mice due to vitamin E or selenium deficiency. J Nutr 1997; 127:9665–705.

69. Roy M, Kiremidjian-Schumacher L, Wishe H, Cohen M, Stotzky G. Selenium and immune cell function II effect on lymphocyte mediated cytotoxicity. Proc Soc Exp Biol Med 1990; 193:143–8.

70. Stroker W, James S. The immunological basis of inflammatory bowel disease. J Clin Immunol 1986; 6:415–26.

71. Cantorna MT, Hayes CE, DeLuca HF. 1,25-Dihydroxyvitamin D3 reversibly blocks the progression of relapsing encephalomyelitis, a model of multiple sclerosis. Proc Natl Acad Sci USA 1996; 93:7861–4.

72. Hayes CE, Cantorna MT, DeLuca HF. Vitamin D and multiple sclerosis. Proc Soc Exp Biol Med 1997; 216:21–7.

73. Fernandes G. Dietary restriction: effects on immunological function and aging. In: Klurfeld D, ed, Human Nutrition—A Comprehensive Treatise, Vol. 8, pp. 91–120. Plenum, New York, 1993.

74. Beach R, Gershwin M, Hurley L. Nutritional factors and autoimmunity I. Immunopathology of zinc deprivation in New Zealand mice. Immunology 1981; 126:1999–2006.

75. Good RA, Lorenz E. Nutritional indications for cancer prevention-calorie restriction. In: Cunningham-Rundles S, ed, Nutrient Modulation of the Immune Response, pp. 481–90. Marcel Dekker, New York, 1993.

76. Tian L, Cai Q, Bowen R, Wei H. Effects of caloric restriction on age-related oxidative modifications of macromolecules and lymphocyte proliferation in rats. Free Radical Biol Med 1995; 19:859–65.

77. Spaulding CC, Walford RL, Effros RB. The accumulation of non-replicative, non-functional, senescent T cells with age is avoided in calorically restricted mice by an enhancement of T cell apoptosis. Mech Ageing Dev 1997; 93:25–33.

13 Nutritional Modulation of Inflammation by Polyunsaturated Fatty Acids/Eicosanoids

Vincent A. Ziboh

INTRODUCTION AND HISTORICAL PERSPECTIVES

The first indication that dietary fat may be essential for healthy growing animals was presented in 1918 by Aron, who proposed that butter has a nutrient value that cannot be provided by other dietary components *(1)*. This report suggested that there was a special nutritive value inherent in fat apart from its caloric contribution and that this possibly was related to the presence of certain lipids. In 1929, Burr and Burr *(2)* presented the first in a series of articles outlining a "new deficiency disease produced by the rigid exclusion of fat from the diet." In the series of conclusions put forth, they developed the hypothesis that warm-blooded animals, in general, cannot synthesize appreciable quantities of certain fatty acids. In 1930, both investigators significantly added to their earlier work by presenting evidence that the dietary inclusion of linoleic acid alone could reverse all deficiency symptoms resulting from a fat-free diet and thus linoleic acid (LA or 18:2n-6)[1] was heralded as an *essential fatty acid* (EFA) *(3)*. The recognition that some unsaturated fatty acids could not be synthesized from endogenous precursors by mammals and were *essential* dietary elements led to the designation of essential and nonessential fatty acids. It was originally thought that there are only two essential fatty acids, linoleic acid (9,12-octadecadienoic acid, LA, 18:2n-6) and α-linolenic acid (9,12,15-octadecatrienoic acid [ALA], 18:3n-3), but continued nutritional studies revealed positive essential growth responses not only for linoleic acid and α-linolenic acid, but also for arachidonic acid as well as the long-chain highly unsaturated fatty acids in fish oil (eicosapentaenoic acid, 20:5n-3) and docosahexaenoic acid, 22:n-3) *(4–6)*. More recent reports on the biologi-

cal significance of the longer-chain n-3 PUFAs do qualify these long-chain fatty acids as *essential* PUFAs.

BIOLOGICAL SIGNIFICANCE OF ESSENTIAL FATTY ACIDS

STRUCTURAL FORMS The two major families of polyunsaturated fatty acids (PUFAs) characteristic of the mammalian species (the n-6, and the n-3 PUFAs) are shown in Fig. 1. The n-6 and n-3 PUFAs are defined by the position of the double bond closest to the terminal methyl group of the fatty acid molecule. In the n-6 family, the first double bond occurs between the sixth and seventh carbons from the methyl group end of the molecule, whereas in the n-3 family, the first double bond occurs between the third and fourth carbons. PUFAs with these basic structures cannot be biosynthesized *de novo* in appreciable amounts by vertebrate animals nor are the n-3 and n-6 families of PUFAs interconvertible. Thus, these *essential* PUFAs must be supplied from dietary sources.

DIETARY SOURCES The 18-carbon n-6 and n-3 polyunsaturated fatty acids (PUFAs) are synthesized on land by many plants and, therefore, are dietarily obtained from vegetable oils. The longer-chain members of each family are either biosynthesized in vivo after dietary ingestion of the shorter 18-carbon precursors or they are obtained directly from animal or marine sources. For example, the longer-chain n-3 PUFAs, especially eicosapentaenoic acid (5,8,11,14,17,EPA,20:5n-3) and docosahexaenoic acid (4,7,10,13,16,19,DHA,22:6n-3) are found in fish and shellfish. They can be ingested directly from these sources. The longer-chain n-6 PUFA, arachidonic acid (AA, 20:4n-6), is found in the liver, brain, and meat, which are rich dietary sources of this PUFA.

DIETARY REQUIREMENTS Attempts have been made to estimate the human EFA requirement, but these have been met with a plethora of problems regarding what criteria to use for physiological normality. For instance, human infants and children are generally thought to require 1–2% of total calories as LA in order to avoid EFA deficiency *(7)*. It is generally believed that children require more LA as a percentage of total daily calorie intake than adults, because growth increases the demand of this fatty acid for cell membrane components *(8)*. Comparative studies

---

[1]Fatty acids and acyl groups are denoted 18:2n-6, 18:3n-3 and so on, with the first number representing the number of carbons in a straight chain and the number following the colon indicating the number of methylene interrupted cis double bonds. The number after *n* indicates the number of carbon atoms from the methyl end of the acyl chain to the nearest double bond.

From: *Nutrition and Immunology: Principles and Practice* (ME Gershwin et al. eds.), © Humana Press, Inc., Totowa, NJ

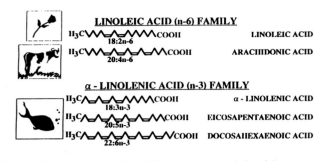

Fig. 1. Two major families of PUFAs characteristic of the mammalian species.

on the metabolic equivalence of LA and AA demonstrate that AA has three times the potency of LA (7).

ASSESSMENT OF ESSENTIAL FATTY ACID STATUS The classical biochemical method of establishing EFA deficiency (EFAD) is to calculate the ratio of triene (5,8,11-eicosatrienic acid, 20:3n-9) to tetraene (AA, 20:4n-6) fatty acids (9). A competitive interaction between the n-6 and n-3 acids results in the suppression of long-chain n-9 acid biosynthesis. Furthermore, n-3 fatty acids have been shown to moderately suppress the metabolism of n-6 acids. Thus, when the tissue level of 18:2n-6 acid is normal, relatively little oleic acid (18:1n-9, OA) acid is desaturated and elongated into 20:3n-9, resulting in a low triene/tetraene ratio. On the other hand, when LA acid is very low or inadequate, as is the case in EFAD, OA acid (derived from *de novo* glucose metabolism) undergoes desaturation/elongation reactions resulting in the elevation of 20:3n-9 in tissue lipids. Correspondingly, the triene/tetraene ratio is elevated. The triene/tetraene ratios above 0.2 and 0.4 are considered the upper limits of normalcy in human plasma and tissue lipids.

DEFICIENCY SYMPTOMS The various deficiency symptoms apparent in response to diets low or free from EFAs were first described by Burr and Burr (2,3). A salient feature of this deficiency syndrome is decreased growth rate, particularly in pair-fed male animals. Other symptoms largely compiled from EFA-deficient rat studies include scaly dermatoses, permeability of skin to water, hair loss, tail necrosis, fatty liver, kidney damage, impaired reproduction, fetal resorption in females, testicular degeneration in males, and reduced ability to form and maintain cell membrane integrity.

BIOSYNTHESIS OF LONG-CHAIN FATTY ACIDS IN MAMMALIAN SYSTEMS: DESATURATION/ELONGATION

The shorter-chain EFAs LA and ALA serve as the initial unsaturated precursors for the in vivo biosynthesis of the longer-chain PUFAs. Metabolism of the EFAs in most tissues involves an alternating sequence of Δ^{-6}-desaturation chain elongation, and Δ^{-5} desaturation, in which two hydrogen atoms are removed from the PUFA to create a new double bond followed by the addition of two carbon atoms from glucose metabolism to lengthen the fatty acid chain (10) as shown in Fig. 2. The desaturations are catalyzed by different enzymes and the same enzymes seemingly catalyze equivalent steps in the n-3, n-6, and n-9 pathways (11). The PUFA families competitively interact in such a manner that the n-3 acids more strongly suppress the metabolism of n-6 acids than the n-6 acids suppress the metabolism of n-3 acids. Both the n-6 and n-3

acids singly or in concert strongly suppress the biosynthesis of the nonessential long-chain n-9 (20:3n-9) fatty acid.

Δ^{-6} DESATURATION OF LINOLEIC ACID (18:2n-6) The Δ^{-6} desaturase is the first step in the metabolism of LA to longer-chain polyunsaturated fatty acids. The bioconversion is carried out in the endoplasmic reticulum membranes by an aerobic mechanism. The desaturase activity is associated with the subcellular microsomal fraction of many animal species (11). To initiate the reaction, a preformed long-chain fatty acyl-CoA is required as the substrate. In the LA metabolic sequence, the Δ^{-6} desaturation to γ-linolenic acid (6,9,12-octadecatrienoic acid [GLA], 18:3n-6) is considered the rate-limiting reaction (12).

CHAIN ELONGATION OF γ-LINOLENIC ACID The microsomal chain elongation of fatty acids is a malonyl-CoA-dependent process in which a corresponding preformed fatty acyl-CoA 18:3n-6 condenses with malonyl-CoA derived from glucose metabolism to generate a β-keto derivative. The β-keto derivative is subsequently reduced to a secondary alcohol, which, upon dehydration, yields the 2-trans analog. A final reduction with NADPH (reducing equivalent) yields dihomo-γ-linolenic acid (8,11,14-eicosatrienoic acid; DGLA) with two carbons longer than the primer GLA. As there is no requirement for molecular oxygen in the elongation process, this step is classically examined under anaerobic conditions (11). Within any of the unsaturated fatty acid metabolic pathways, the rates of desaturation are generally slower than those for chain elongation (12), thus, the rate-limiting steps associated with the metabolism of LA to AA are both the Δ^{-6} desaturation and the Δ^{-5} desaturation.

Δ^{-5} DESATURATION OF DIHOMO-γ-LINOLENIC ACID (20:3n-6) The Δ^{-5} desaturation is the final step in the conversion of LA to AA and there are significant species differences in the function of this enzyme. The rodent, for instance, has an active hepatic Δ^{-5} desaturase enzyme system, whereas the enzyme activity is much lower in both the human and the guinea pig liver (10). The reason is unclear.

RELEASE OF ARACHIDONIC ACID FROM MEMBRANE PHOSPHOLIPIDS

PHOSPHOLIPASE A$_2$ (RATE-LIMITING STEP) The AA generated after the Δ^{-5} desaturation is incorporated and stored in membrane phospholipids. The release of AA from the phospholipids, which is catalyzed by the phospholipase A$_2$ (PLA$_2$) hydrolysis, sets off the series of metabolic reactions referred to as the AA metabolic cascade. The PLA$_2$ has been classified into two distinct forms: the secreted form of PLA$_2$ (sPLA$_2$) and the cytosolic form of PLA$_2$ (cPLA$_2$) based on their apparent cellular localization. The cPLA$_2$ has been purified and cloned by several groups (13–15). The enzyme is expressed in a variety of cell types such as fibroblasts, kidney mesangial cells, and platelets (16–18). The cPLA$_2$ differs from sPLA$_2$ in a number of ways. For instance, the calculated molecular mass of cPLA$_2$ is approximately 85 kDa, whereas sPLA$_2$ is 14 kDa. The cPLA$_2$ is active at low Ca^{2+} concentrations (micromolar) and is found in the cytosol, whereas the sPLA$_2$ requires high Ca^{2+} concentrations (millimolar) for activity. Because the cPLA$_2$ exhibits high selectivity for AA at the *sn*-2 position of the glycerol backbone (19), it has been implicated with initiating the inflammatory processes. In contrast, the sPLA$_2$ has no fatty acid preference; thus, its role is consistent with the normal maintenance of cell membrane homeostasis.

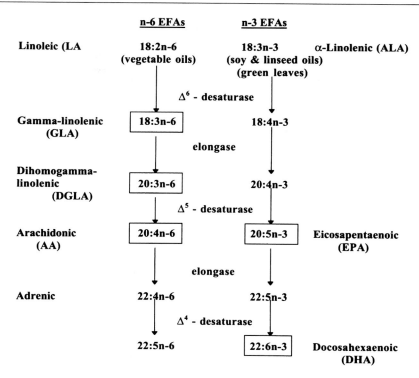

Fig. 2. Oxidative desaturation/elongation of *n*-6 and *n*-3 EFAs.

BIOSYNTHESIS OF EICOSANOIDS

THE CYCLOOXYGENASE PATHWAY One of the pathways that generate potent biological mediators from AA is the cyclooxygenase pathway. The products generated include prostaglandin E_2 (PGE$_2$), prostaglandin $F_{2\alpha}$ (PGF$_{2\alpha}$), prostaglandin D_2 (PGD$_2$), thromboxane A_2 (TXA$_2$, mainly from platelets), and prostacyclin (PGI$_2$, mainly from the vessel wall). A schematic illustration of the cyclooxygenase pathway is shown in Fig. 3. The biosynthesis of TXA$_2$ and the PGs involve three sequential steps: (1) the stimulus-induced release of AA from phospholipids by cPLA2, (2) the oxidative transformation of AA into prostaglandin endoperoxide H (PGH$_2$) and, finally, (3) the isomerization of PGH$_2$ to the respective PGs and thromboxane. Specifically, the PGH synthetases catalyze the conversion of AA and O$_2$ to PGH$_2$ *(20)*. The PGHS-1 (COX-1; cyclooxygenase-1) has been characterized and is referred to as the *constitutive* enzyme *(20)*. It is expressed in most normal cells and tissues in the absence of external stimuli. The newly characterized second isozyme, the PGHS-2 (COX-2; cyclooxygenase-2), is now referred to as the *inducible* isoform. Although COX-2 is similar to PGHS-1 in structure, it differs in its pattern of expression. For instance, it is expressed mainly in cells stimulated by a variety of factors. Both isozymes are homodimeric, heme-containing, glycosylated proteins with two catalytic sites. The isozymes have become important pharmacological targets for nonsteroidal antiinflammatory drugs (NSAIDS) *(21)*. For example, COX-2 is the relevant enzyme target of NSAIDS, which act to inhibit inflammation, fever, and pain *(21–23)*. A low concentration of aspirin, which clinically lowers the risk for mortality from cardiovascular disease *(24)*, acts via COX-1 to inhibit the biosynthesis of platelet thromboxane A$_2$. Persuasive studies have now emerged that indicate that the activity of COX-2, which is associated with inflammatory reactions, can be suppressed

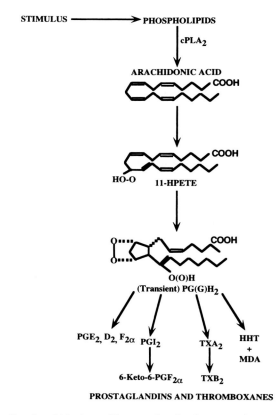

Fig. 3. Arachidonic acid cascade (cyclooxygenase pathway). TXA$_2$ = thromboxane A$_2$; PGG$_2$ = prostaglandin cyclic endoperoxide; PGH$_2$ = prostaglandin endoperoxide; PGE$_2$ = prostaglandin E$_2$; PGF$_{2\alpha}$ = prostaglandin F$_2$; PGI$_2$ = prostaglandin I$_2$ (prostacyclin).

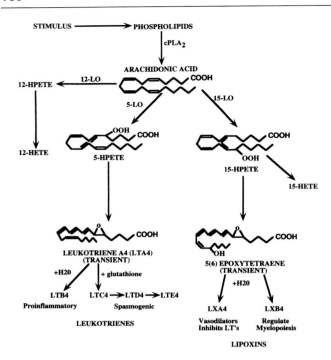

Fig. 4. Arachidonic acid cascade (lipoxygenase pathway). TXA$_2$ = thromboxane A$_4$; TXB$_4$ = thromboxane B$_4$; LTB$_4$ = leukotriene B$_4$; LTC$_4$ = leukotriene C$_4$; LTD$_4$ = leukotriene D$_4$; 12-HETE = 12-hydroxyelcosatetraenoic acid; 5-HETE = 5-hydroxyelcosatetraenoic acid; 15-HETE = 15-hydroxyelcosatetraenoic acid.

by diets supplemented with fish oil (*n*-3 PUFA) and/or vegetable oil (*n*-6 PUFA).

THE LIPOXYGENASE PATHWAY Leukotrienes (LTs) are a family of related compounds derived from the lipoxygenation of arachidonic acid in the 5-position. A schematic illustration of the lipoxygenase pathway is shown in Fig. 4.

The 5-Lipoxygenase Pathway

Generation of Leukotriene B$_4$ The 5-lipoxygenase (5-LO) enzyme catalyzes the transformation of AA to 5(*S*)-hydroperoxy-6,8,11,14-eicosatetraenoic acid (5-HPETE). The same enzyme further catalyzes the transformation of 5-HPETE to an unstable epoxide intermediate known as leukotriene A$_4$ (LTA$_4$; 5,6-oxido-7,9,11,14-eicosatetraenoic acid). These reactions are the first of two in the biosynthetic pathway for leukotriene biosynthesis. One subpathway of the 5-LO generates leukotriene B$_4$ (LTB$_4$), which is derived directly from the sequential dehydration and hydrolysis of the highly unstable precursors of 5-HPETE and LTA, respectively. Functionally, LTB$_4$ exerts very strong leukocytotropic activities. It is one of the most powerful chemotactic and chemokinetic agents, which causes neutrophil degranulation (25) and enhances binding to endothelial cells (26). It is readily biosynthesized by phagocytic cells, principally neutrophils and macrophages, upon challenge by a variety of stimuli. It has been detected in significant concentrations in inflammatory bowel disease (27) and in psoriatic skin lesions (28). Thus, LTB$_4$ appears to be a global potent inflammatory molecule.

Generation of Sulfidopeptide Leukotrienes The other subpathway of the 5-lipoxygenase includes the generation of sulfidopeptide leukotrienes C$_4$, D$_4$, and E$_4$ (LTC$_4$, LTD$_4$, and LTE$_4$). The genesis of this family of compounds was first noted when perfused

lungs were challenged with snake venom and reported to cause the release of a biologically active substance that induced a slow, long-lasting contraction of smooth muscle (29). This pathological process was named "the slow reacting substance of anaphylaxis" (SRS-A). With the identification of mediators generated from AA via the 5-lipoxygenase pathway that possessed slow-reacting properties on bronchial smooth muscle, SRS-A is now known to be induced by a mixture of LTC$_4$, LTD$_4$, and LTE$_4$ (30). The peptide leukotrienes are two to three orders of magnitude more potent than histamine as a bronchoconstrictor. Interestingly, when LTC$_4$ and LTD$_4$ are administered to human volunteers, they cause coughing, bronchoconstriction, wheezing, tightness of the chest, and a reduction in expiratory maximum airflow rate (31). Peptide leukotrienes have been detected in the sputum from asthmatics (32) and in nasal washes from allergic patients following antigen challenge (33).

The 12-Lipoxygenase Pathway The 12-lipoxygenase (12-LO) catalyzes the transformation of AA to 12-hydroperoxyeicosatetraenoic (12-HPETE) which is then reduced to 12-hydroxyeicosatetraenoic acid (12-HETE). The 12-LO activity has been identified in a variety of cells, mainly platelets (34). Functionally, 12-HETE has been reported to exert a variety of effects on cells and tissues such as its presumed involvement in the genesis of atherosceloric plaques. The 12-HETE liberated during platelet aggregation or by the vascular endothelium is known to be incorporated into the vascular endothelial phopholipids, particularly phophatidylcholine (PC), and is reported to exacerbate cell injury. 12-HETE as well as its intermediate, 12-HPETE, have been reported to inhibit vascular tissue prostacyclin biosynthesis, thus promoting platelet adhesion and aggregation.

The 15-Lipoxygenase Pathway The 15-lipoxygenase (15-LO) enzyme catalyzes the transformation of AA to 15-hydroperoxyeicosatetraenoic acid (15-HPETE) which is then reduced to the 15-hydroxyeicosatetraenoic acid (15-HETE). The presence of a mammalian 15-LO, first reported in guinea pig lung, has now been confirmed in human lung (35). The enzyme has also been demonstrated in a variety of cell types, including neutrophils, eosinophils, macrophages, and airway epithelial cells. It has also been identified in skin epidermis, human prostate, and human cornea. Two isoforms of 15-LO (15-S-LOX-1 and 15-S-LOX-2) have recently been described (36). Functionally, 15-HETE has been reported to exert varying effects in a variety of systems. For instance, both 15-HPETE and 15-HETE are considered to be immunosuppressive because they inhibit murine splenocyte proliferation induced by lipopolysaccharide. The 15-LO products have been reported to induce bronchoconstriction in airways, on the one hand, and chemotaxis of inflammatory cells on the other (37,38). 15-HETE has also been reported to modulate the activity of enzymes associated with the AA cascade (39). Overall, compelling new information continues to emerge that implicate hydroxy fatty acids once thought to be inactivation products of AA with no biological actions in a variety of biological functions.

THE BIOLOGICAL SIGNIFICANCE OF *n*-3 PUFAs

Role in Brain Function Recent studies that implicate the PUFAs, particularly the *n*-3 PUFAs, in the biology of the brain has excited great interest. Rapid brain growth is recognized as an important feature of prenatal and early postnatal periods of development. Associated with this rapid growth is the accumulation of long-chain polyunsaturated fatty acids (LCPUFA) necessary for the formation of the neural tissue. The dry weight of the human brain is predominantly lipid, of which 22% is associated with the cerebral cortex and 24% of the white mater consisting of phospholipids. Therefore, it is not surprising that the mammalian fetus and placenta are dependent on the supply of maternal EFAs that form a constituent part of brain phospholipids. The major EFA deposition in the human fetus occurs during the third trimester. Phospholipids in placental vessels and uterine vasculature are dependent on EFA supplied by the mother for eicosanoid biosynthesis. Thus, maternal preconceptional nutrition determines, in part, which specific types of fat accumulate in the conceptus and placental tissues *(40)*. Studies of several animal species and recent evidence from humans have established that brain phospholipid AA and DHA decrease when LA and ALA or only *n-3* PUFAs are deficient in the diet *(41)*. Alternatively, under the above condition, the *n-9* and *n-7* mono-MUFAs and nonessential PUFAs increase. These reports, therefore, underscore the significance of long-chain PUFAs in the brain and neural functions.

ROLE IN INFANT NUTRITION   The potential for dietary EFA deficiency has become a significant issue for the nutrition of preterm-born infants, as these infants do not receive the third-trimester intrauterine supply of DHA and AA. Even full-term infants are at risk of DHA deficiency, as most formulas are devoid of this critical EFA. Recent postmortem investigations of term infants indicate the dependency of brain cortex on diet in the FA composition. Infants who are breast fed have higher DHA and lower *n-6* PUFAs (AA) in their cortex phospholipids when compared to infants receiving cow-milk-based formulas *(42,43)*. The DHA content increases with advancing age in breast-fed infants and is proportional to the duration of human-milk feeding while the AA content remains stable. Furthermore, the dietary ratio of *n-6/n-3* PUFAs appears relevant in human infants, as the lowest DHA and highest DHA contents in brain cortex phospholipids were observed in preterm infants fed formulas with a high LA/ALA ratio. Several studies are currently being pursued at various clinical centers to evolve an appropriate *n-3/n-6* PUFA ratio to be incorporated into infant formula. There is enough evidence taken from measurements made by rod electroretinogram (ERG) and visual evoked potential (VEP) visual acuity to support the view that the dietary deficiency of *n-3* PUFAs can affect the normal eye and brain functions of preterm infants. Preterm infants require DHA in their diet because they are incapable of biosynthesizing a sufficient quantity of DHA from dietary ALA, although it is provided by soy-oil-based formula products. Compelling reports continue to emerge that indicate that *n-3* PUFA (particularly DHA) is required for optimal maturation of the nervous system and the retina in the human.

ROLE IN INFLAMMATORY/IMMUNE SYSTEMS   The products of 5-LO-catalyzed oxygenations of AA (LTB_4, LTC_4, and LTD_4) are known to participate in a variety of inflammatory diseases. This view is based on the fact that LTB_4 has been found in exudates from experimental animals and humans with chronic inflammatory disease *(44)*, as well as in lesional psoriatic skin and psoriatic scale *(45)*. Consistent with this latter view, the topical application of LTB_4 to normal human skin promotes the infiltration of polymorphonuclear leukocytes (PMN), along with other inflammatory cells into the skin epidermis. PMNs, macrophages, and mast cells are found in inflammatory diseases and the current dogma implicates these phagocytes as the sources of the leukotrienes. Studies with these cells in culture have indicated that

PMNs have the capacity to produce large amounts of LTB_4, whereas macrophages, monocytes, as well as mast cells biosynthesize larger amounts of the peptide-leukotrienes (LTC_4, LTD_4).

In Inflammatory Bowel Disease   Although the etiology of inflammatory bowel disease has not been fully delineated, local mediators consisting of AA metabolites and peptide mediators (cytokines) have been suggested as possible culprits in the pathogenesis of this disease. Because LTB_4 is associated with inflammatory processes, a number of studies have aimed at reducing local bowel LTB_4 formation by inhibiting the 5-LO. Also, because *n-3* PUFAs have been shown to inhibit LTB_4 formation in a number of systems, the hypothesis has been developed to treat patients with inflammatory bowel disease with fish oil containing *n-3* PUFAs. In a controlled and double-blind dietary study, *n-3* PUFAs was reported to exert beneficial effects in patients with ulcerative colitis but not in patients with Crohn's disease. In a more recent study, in which enteric-coated fish oil (made to minimize gastric acidity) were given to patients with Crohn's diseases, the investigators demonstrated marked reductions in the rate of relapse of the patients when compared to patients on placebo *(46)*. Although it appears that dietary supplementation of *n-3* PUFAs may be beneficial in inflammatory bowel disease, more trials are warranted in order to elucidate its mechanisms of action. The findings nonetheless suggest that suppressing the generation of bowel proinflammatory LTB_4 may attenuate the severity of the disease.

In Rheumatoid Arthritis   The recognition that *n-3* PUFAs can suppress the tissue/cellular generation of proinflammatory leukotrienes (LTB_4, LTC_4, and LTD_4) in vitro and can also ameliorate in vivo inflammatory conditions has prompted trials of fish oil (*n-3* PUFAs) in rheumatoid arthritis. In animal studies, dietary modifications containing *n-3* PUFAs has been reported to exert significant reduction in the severity of diffuse proliferative glomerulonephritis in several autoimmune strains of mice, including the NZBXNZWF, BXSB/Mpj, and MRL/lpr strains *(47)*.

In human studies, the effects of dietary fish oil supplements in patients with rheumatoid arthritis have been studied *(48)*. The effect of high-dose fish oil after stopping NSAIDs has also been studied *(49)*. An improvement in the number of tender joints on physical examination is most often observed, with some authors also reporting improvement in morning stiffness. The most striking benefits regarding tender joints and morning stiffness have been confirmed in a recent meta-analysis *(50)*. Although the overall clinical response to fish oil supplements reported in these studies are modest, these promising beneficial effects warrant more and longer-duration studies. Furthermore, it is likely that the future will reveal increasing reports of *n-3* PUFA modulation of interleukin-I (IL-1) and tumor necrosis factor (TNF)-driven disorders.

In Psoriasis   The interest in the role of *n-3* PUFAs in psoriasis, a skin disorder characterized by chronic inflammatory and hyperproliferative skin lesions, was accentuated after the report of an epidemiologic study of Eskimos in Greenland by Kromann and Green *(51)*. This report revealed a 20-fold more incidence of psoriasis among the Danish population when compared to the Greenland Eskimos. An initial study of AA metabolism in vitro by preparations from the psoriatic lesion revealed an increased formation of PGE_2, $PGF_{2\alpha}$ and 12-HETE *(52)*. A later report revealed that the psoriatic lesion contained elevated amounts of LTB_4 *(53)*. Because *n-3* PUFAs have been shown in vitro to suppress LTB_4 formation, an open-trial study to test the efficacy of dietary fish oil (Max-EPA), which is rich in *n-3* PUFAs, was investigated in a group of 18 psoriatic patients *(54)*. Each patient's diet was supplemented with sufficient fish oil to contain approximately 10.8 g of EPA, 7.2 g of DHA, and 0.6 g of AA per day. Clinical findings from these studies revealed a favorable response characterized by mild to moderate improvement of psoriatic lesional scaling, erythema, and epidermal thickness after an 8-wk dietary intake of the fish oil in approximately 60% of the 18 patients. In another open-trial study *(55)*, the investigators provided more fish oil (containing approximately 12 g of EPA/d) to 10 psoriatic patients for 6 wk and reported moderate beneficial effects in 8. Additionally, this group reported biochemical evidence of suppressed ability of PMNs from the patients to generate LTB_4 when challenged in vitro. Taken together, these two open-trial studies with dietary fish oil containing EPA and DHA exerted moderate to excellent beneficial effects to the patients.

Subsequently, in one double-blind, randomized, placebo-controlled trial study of 28 patients with stable psoriasis who received less Max-EPA (fish oil) capsules, equivalent to 1.8 g of EPA/d, for 8–12 wk, these investigators reported a lessening of itching, erythema, and scaling in the treated group when compared to the placebo group *(56)*. The findings from this double-blind, placebo-controlled trial study are consistent with the open-trial findings. However, in another double-blind, placebo-controlled study, the investigators reported that the administration of a low amount of Max-EPA (fish oil) capsules, equivalent to 1.8 g of EPA/d as in the preceding study for 8 wk, resulted in no statistical difference in the clinical manifestations of the psoriasis between the active treatment group and the placebo group *(57)*. The reason for the discrepancy in these two double-blind studies, which supplemented diets with the same amount of *n*-3 PUFA (1.8 g EPA/d), has remained unclear. The reports raise serious questions as to the source of the oils used and their preservation during the period of the study. Nonetheless, in a recent large study, 6 capsules containing a total of 1.12 g and 7.56 g of ethyl esters of EPA and DHA, respectively, were given daily to 80 members of the Finnish Psoriasis Foundation with stable plaque psoriasis. After 8 wk, approximately 72.4% of the patients who completed the study showed moderate to excellent clinical improvement in pruritus, scaling, induration, and. erythema *(58)*. Data from these dietary *n*-3 PUFA trials indicate that minimal to excellent efficacy was attained as a monotherapy for psoriasis. These promising findings have prompted the use of fish oil capsules with success as an adjunct to reduce ultraviolet-irradiation (UV-B)-induced inflammation to prolong the beneficial effects of phototherapy *(59)*. In order to evolve an effective efficacy for these *n*-3 PUFAs, it is imperative that the mechanisms of action of EPA/DHA or their 15-LO metabolites, particularly the monohydroxy fatty acids (15-hydroxyeicosapentaenoic acid [15-HEPE] and 17-hydroxydocosahexaenoic acid [17-HDoHE]), which are biosynthesized locally in the skin, be elucidated. Recent incubations using guinea pig epidermis and/or human epidermis with EPA and/or DHA in vitro revealed the generation of 15-HEPE and 17-HDoHE by epidermal 15-LO *(60,61)*. These metabolites presumably function in vivo as endogenous anti-inflammatory metabolites. The role that these metabolites play in vivo deserves further explorations.

A speculative scenario of the possible modulatory effects of EPA/DHA as constituents of the fish oil *n*-3 PUFAs on the generation of AA inflammatory metabolites generated via the 5-LO pathway of AA is shown in Fig. 5. Pathway A illustrates the dietary ingestion of vegetable oil (safflower or corn oil, containing

LA), its desaturation, and elongation into AA. The resulting AA is further metabolized in vivo by PMNs via the 5-LO into pro-inflammatory leukotrienes, particularly, LTB_4, LTC_4, and LTD_4. Pathway B illustrates the oxidative metabolism of fish oil (containing EPA/DHA) via the cyclooxygenase and lipoxygenase pathways to generate metabolites. The possible mechanisms of the reported beneficial effects of fish oil in cutaneous disorders seem consistent with the possible in vivo epidermal generation of 15-LO products of EPA (15-HEPE) and DHA (17-HDoHE). These metabolites have been shown in vitro to inhibit the generation of LTB_4 by activated PMNs from AA. The possibility that LTB_5 (a moderate competitor for LTB_4) is formed via the 5-LO after dietary intake of fish oil (containing EPA) also exists *(55)* and could possibly attenuate the pro-inflammatory effects of LTB_4. The increase in these metabolites are dose dependent after dietary intake of fish oil. It is, therefore, reasonable to speculate that increased dietary ingestion of fish oil (containing EPA/DHA) could result in increased endogenous epidermal biosynthesis of these putative anti-inflammatory monohydroxy metabolites (15-HEPE and 17 HDoHE). Local epidermal increases in these monohydroxy acids could, in turn, inhibit the local generation of the pro-inflammatory leukotrienes induced by infiltrating PMNs. Thus, the dietary intake of highly purified fish oil or its ethyl esters as a monotherapy or as adjunct with other therapeutic modalities may offer a less toxic approach to alleviating cutaneous as well as other inflammatory disorders. More trial studies are warranted.

THE BIOLOGICAL SIGNIFICANCE OF *n*-6 PUFAs

ROLE IN MEMBRANE STRUCTURE   The prevailing concept of the cell membrane is that most of the phospholipid in the membrane is present as a bimolecular sheet, with the fatty acids chains in the interior of the bilayer—"the fluid mosaic model" *(62)*. Membrane proteins are located either at the internal or external faces of the membrane or projecting from one side to the other. An important physical feature of the membrane is the degree of freedom for molecules to move around, generally described as "membrane fluidity." Thus, the membrane lipid provides a flexible structure in which a variety of membrane proteins are located, some of which are enzymes, receptors, or growth factors that modulate a variety of metabolic activities within the cell membrane.

Unsaturated fatty acids are important constituents of these membrane lipids and they are mainly esterified in the phosphoglycerides. The presence of unsaturation in the chains of the fatty acids affects their shape and their ability to pack together. For instance, saturated fatty acids pack together in crystalline arrays that give low fluidity. In contrast, the introduction of a double bond in the fatty acid chain results in less packing but increased fluidity. The stability of mammalian membranes is, therefore, highly dependent on the presence of *n*-6 essential fatty acids, a major functional role of the *n*-6 PUFAs. For instance, if the *n*-6 PUFA (AA) is replaced by the *n*-9 PUFA (20:3*n*-9), an abnormality is induced in the membrane, as in the case of essential fatty acid deficiency (EFAD). The membrane under this condition is characterized by a dysfunctional membrane that is more permeable to water and ions. Similarly, the dietary substitution of AA with EPA in the membrane phospholipid results in diminished metabolic transformation of AA into eicosanoids.

The recognition that excessive generation of 20-carbon eicosanoids with pro-inflammatory properties can result from ingestion

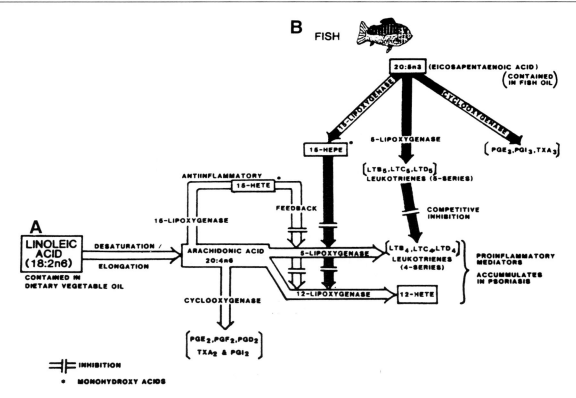

Fig. 5. Speculative regulation of inflammatory eicosanoid biosynthesis by ω-3 polyunsaturated eicosapentaenoic acid.

of shorter-chain *n*-6 PUFAs has lend itself to the unfortunate misconception that dietary *n*-6 PUFAs may be deleterious because of its metabolic transformation (via desaturation/elongation) to pro-inflammatory eicosanoids. For instance, it is believed that the dietary intake of dietary 18-carbon *n*-6 PUFAs (LA) would convert immediately to its desaturated/elongation intermediates: GLA, DGLA, and AA. It is reasoned that the resulting AA would generate excessive amounts of pro-inflammatory *n*-6 prostanoids and leukotrienes. In contrast to this exaggerated view, the likelihood of the above to occur after normal dietary ingestion of LA containing oils is small because the desaturation of LA to GLA has been reported to be minor (approx 4–20%). In other instances, the desaturation does not occur or is diminished when the Δ^{-6} desaturase is inactivated *(63,64)*, because the activity of the Δ^{-6} desaturase is influenced by nutritional, hormonal, and physiological/pathophysiological factors. Thus, under these conditions, increased dietary GLA could serve as an alternate essential PUFA, undergoing rapid elongation to DGLA. The accumulated DGLA then undergoes metabolic transformations via the cyclooxygenase and 15-LO pathways to generate PGE$_1$ and 15-hydroxyeicosatrienoic acid (15-HETrE), respectively. Both of these metabolites have been reported to exert anti-inflammatory effects in vitro and in vivo by suppressing LTB$_4$ biosynthesis.

ROLE IN INFLAMMATORY/IMMUNE SYSTEM

In Rheumatoid Arthritis There is a body of experimental evidence to support the view that eicosanoids do participate in the development and regulation of immunological and inflammatory responses. Because rheumatoid arthritis (RA) is characterized by inflammation, disordered immune regulation, and tissue injury, there is increasing interest in the role of eicosanoids in the regulation of host defense in RA patients. Furthermore, because of the

deleterious effects that can often result in the therapy of RA when NSAIDs are used excessively, there is a need for new, safe approaches to treatment of chronic RA patients. Although the modulatory role of *n*-3 PUFAs in the management of RA has been investigated, emerging evidence obtained from experiments in vitro as well as in vivo suggest that novel (*n*-6) PUFAs may also be safe and effective anti-inflammatory and immunomodulatory agents. For example, oil extracts from seeds of the evening primrose and borage plants contain relatively large amounts of GLA. In vivo, the GLA is metabolized rapidly to DGLA, resulting in increased tissue level of DHA, a precursor for the biosynthesis of the monoenoic prostanoid PGE$_1$. This prostanoid has been reported to exert anti-inflammatory and immunoregulating properties such as the suppression of diverse T-lymphocyte functions and interleukin-2 (IL-2) production *(65,66)*. PGE$_1$ has also been reported to suppress PMN leucocyte and monocyte activation. Furthermore, DGLA is also metabolized by 15-LO to 15-HETrE. This hydroxy acid has been demonstrated to suppress the biosynthesis of pro-inflammatory LTB$_4$ *(67)*. For example, the enrichment of synovial cells with DGLA in cell culture results in increased PGE$_1$ biosynthesis, on the one hand, and a marked decrease in PGE$_2$ synthesis on the other hand. These prostanoid alterations paralleled the reduction of IL-1-induced synovial cell proliferation *(68)*.

Moderate to significant reductions in the signs and symptoms of disease activity in RA patients have been observed clinically after a daily supplementation of 1.4 g of GLA (in the form of borage seed oil) for 24 wk *(69,70)*. In a double-blind placebo-controlled trial of RA patients, it was reported that after a 15-mo administration of evening primrose oil to RA patients, there was a significant improvement in subjective measures of the disease

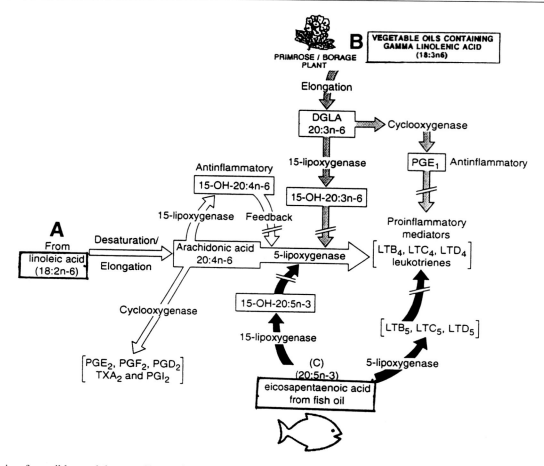

Fig. 6. Scenario of possible modulatory effects of the constituent dietary fatty acids on the generation of pro-inflammatory leukotrienes from AA.

(71). For instance, 12 mo after the dietary intake, the patients significantly reduced their NSAID intake without adversely affecting the clinical symptoms of the disease. Thus, the potential ability of PUFAs to regulate cell activation, immune responses, and inflammation is exciting at the clinical, cellular, and molecular levels. A better understanding of how fatty acids modulate the function of cells involved in host defense might lead to development of new, benign treatment for diseases characterized by acute and chronic inflammation.

In Skin

Significance of 18-Carbon Chain PUFA Two PUFAs with different carbon chain lengths play important roles in the physiology and pathophysiology of skin. For instance, the 18-carbon LA is the most abundant PUFA in human skin *(71).* One functional significance of the LA is its involvement in the maintenance of the epidermal water barrier *(72),* which is one of the major abnormalities of cutaneous EFAD. Another major functional role of LA is its involvement in the suppression of the proliferative activity of the skin epidermis. A possible mechanism for this suppressive effect was recently associated with tissue elevation of 13-hydroxyoctadecadienoic acid (13-HODE) *(73).* 13-HODE was shown to be initially incorporated into epidermal phospholipids, particularly phosphatidylinositol 4,5-bisphosphate (PtdIns 4,5P$_2$), followed by phospholipase C-catalyzed hydrolysis of

PtdIns 4,5-P$_2$ and generation of 13-HODE-containing diacylglycerol (13-HODE–DAG) *(74).* The level of 13-HODE–DAG was found to be markedly depleted in the hyperproliferative skin of the EFAD animal model. Interestingly, the depletions of 13-HODE and 13-HODE–DAG in the epidermis of EFAD animals paralleled the elevated expressions and activities of Protein Kinase C (PKC)-α and β-isozymes *(75).* Refeeding the animals with safflower oil (containing LA) replenished the epidermal level of LA, restored the tissue levels of 13-HODE and 13-HODE–DAG to normal, and selectively downregulated PKC-β expression and activity. These biochemical alterations paralleled the reversal of the hyperproliferative skin to normal. These results indicate that adequate dietary amount of LA is required to maintain adequate tissue levels of 13-HODE/13-HODE–DAG in normal epidermis.

Significance of 20-Carbon Chain PUFA The 20-carbon-AA is the second prominent PUFA in the skin epidermis. It is approximately 6–10% of the total fatty acids in the epidermal phospholipids of normal human epidermis. It functions largely as a precursor for the generation of biologically potent metabolites from AA. The AA released from epidermal membrane phospholipids by epidermal cPLA$_2$ undergoes oxidative transformations via the cyclooxygenase pathway, generating mainly prostaglandins PGE$_2$, PGF$_{2\alpha}$, and PGD$_2$ and 15-LO into 15-HETE. 15-HETE functions as a potent inhibitor of proinflammatory LTB$_4$ generation from PMNs and basophils. Consistent with this anti-inflammatory potential, 15-HETE after intralesional injections into psoriatic lesion has been reported to improve the symptoms of inflammation and hyperproliferation *(76)*.

Significance of 20-Carbon PUFA 20-Carbon PUFA (DGLA) is a metabolite of GLA rapid elongation by the epidermal elongase. When GLA is taken as a dietary supplement, beneficial effects have has been reported in patients with atopic eczema *(77)* and in the suppression of acute chronic inflammation *(78)*. A possible mode of action of dietary GLA in skin involves an initial rapid in vivo elongation to DGLA, followed, on the one hand, by the latter's oxidative metabolism via the cyclooxygenase pathway to PGE_1, and on the other hand, by the metabolism of DGLA by 15-LO enzyme into 15-HETrE *(79)*. Supplementation of human diet with borage oil (which contains GLA) has also been shown to elevate in vivo cellular levels of DGLA in human PMN phospholipids *(80)*. The elevation of DGLA in PMNs paralleled the suppression of LTB_4 generation from AA *(80)*. 15-HETrE has been shown to markedly inhibit LTB_4 generation in vitro from AA by rat basophilic leukemia (RBL-I) cells *(81)*. These in vitro effects of DGLA metabolites (PGE_1/15-HETrE) on pro-inflammatory LTB_4 generation from PMNs are consistent with the reported beneficial effects of dietary oils containing GLA on inflammatory conditions.

SUMMARY

The biological significance of polyunsaturated fatty acids (PUFAs) are associated with fatty acids termed "essential fatty acids" provided from dietary sources. The PUFAs are subdivided into two groups commonly referred to as *n*-6 PUFAs and *n*-3 PUFAs. The 18-carbon *n*-6 PUFAs undergo an alternating sequence of Δ^{-6} desaturation, chain elongation, and Δ^{-5} desaturation to yield the 20-carbon AA. The *n*-6 PUFAs serve as the important structural constituent of the cell membrane. Furthermore, the AA undergoes metabolism via cyclooxygenase and the lipoxygenase pathways to generate prostagandins, leukotrienes, and hydroxy acids. When generated in excessive amounts in vivo, these metabolites trigger deleterious inflammatory and proliferative conditions. However, when generated in moderate amounts under physiological conditions, they modulate physiological functions. Similarly, *n*-3 PUFAs must also be supplemented dietarily with fish oil (containing EPA/DHA) in adequate amounts. Sufficient dietary intake of *n*-3 PUFAs increases the tissue of EPA and DHA in phospholipids, diminishes the level of AA, and decreases excessive generation of *n*-6 PUFAs pro-inflammatory and proliferative eicosanoids.

A speculative scenario of the possible modulatory effects of the constituent dietary fatty acids from vegetable oils (mainly *n*-6 PUFAs), fish oils (mainly *n*-3 PUFAs), and their respective metabolites on the generation of pro-inflammatory leukotrienes from AA is shown in Fig. 6. It is reasonable to speculate that metabolites from both the B and C pathways could singly or in concert inhibit the in vivo generation of local tissue pro-inflammatory leukotrienes generated from AA (pathway A). These in vivo possibilities imply that the dietary intake of purified triglycerides from vegetable or fish oils, or the intake of synthetic structured triglycerides with appropriate positional esterification of *n*-6/*n*-3 PUFAs may offer an alternative therapeutic modality for alleviating inflammatory/hyper-proliferative conditions with minimal side effects.

ACKNOWLEDGMENTS

The author thanks Donnelle Yoshino for the preparation of the manuscript. Some of the studies referenced in this review were carried out in the author's laboratory and supported in part by Research Grant AM30679 from the National Institutes of Health of the United States Public Health Service.

REFERENCES

1. Aron H. Uber den Nahrwert. Biochem Z. 1918; 92:211–33.
2. Burr GO, Burr MM. A new deficiency disease produced by the rigid exclusion of fat from the diet. J Biol Chem 1929; 82:345–56.
3. Burr GO, Burr MM. On the nature of the fatty acids essential in nutrition. J Biol Chem 1930; 86:587–621.
4. Turpeinen O. Further studies on the unsaturated fatty acids essential in nutrition. J Nutr 1937; 15:351–66.
5. Burr GO, Brown JB, Kass JP, Lundberg WO. Comparative curative values of unsaturated fatty acids in fat deficiency. Proc Soc Exp Biol Med 1940; 44:242–5.
6. Quackenbush FW, Kummerow FA, Steenbock H. The effectiveness of linoleic, arachidonic, and linolenic acids in reproduction and lactation. J Nutr 1942; 24:213–24.
7. Rivers JP, Frankel TL. Essential fatty acid deficiency. Br Med Bul 1981; 37(1):59–64.
8. Holman RT, Smythe L, Johnson S. Effect of sex and age on fatty acid composition of human serum lipids. Am J Clin Nutr 1979; 32:2390–9.
9. Homan RT. The ratio of trienoic : tetraenoic acids in tissue lipids as a measure of essential fatty acid requirements. J Nutr 1960; 70:405–10.
10. Marcel YL, Christiansen K, Holman RT. The preferred metabolic pathway from linoleic acid to arachidonic acid in vitro. Biochim Biophys Acta 1968; 164:25–34.
11. Brenner RR. The oxidative desaturation of unsaturated fatty acids in animals. Mol Cell Biochem 1974; 3:41–52.
12. Crawford MA, Rivers JP, Hassam AG. Comparative studies on the metabolic equivalence of linoleic and arachidonic acids. Nutr Metab 1977; 21:189–96.
13. Leslie CC, Voelker DR, Channon JY, Wall MM, Zelarney PT. Purification and properties of an arachidonyl-hydrolyzing phospholipase A_2 from a macrophage cell line, RAW 264.7. Biochim Biophys Acta 1988; 963:476–92.
14. Kramer RM, Roberts EF, Manetta J, Putnam JE. The Ca^{2+}-sensitive cytosolic phospholipase A_2 is a 100-kDa protein in human monoblast U937 cells. J Biol Chem 1991; 266:5268–72.
15. Sharp JD, White DL, Chiou SG, Goodson T, Gamboa GC, McClure D. Molecular cloning and expression of human Ca^{2+}-sensitive cytosolic phospholipase A_2. J Biol Chem 1991; 266:14,850–3.
16. Lin LL, Lin AY, DeWitt DL. IL-1α induces the accumulation of $cPLA_2$ and the release of PGE_2 in human fibroblasts. J Biol Chem 1992b; 267:23,451–4.
17. Gronich JH, Boventre JV, Nemonoff RA. Purification of a high-molecular-mass form of phospholipase A_2 from rat kidney activated at physiological calcium concentrations. Biochem J 1990; 271:37–43.
18. Takayama K, Kudo I, Kim DK, Nagata K, Nozawa Y, Inoue K. Purification and characterization of human platelet phospholipase A_2 which preferentially hydroyzes an arachidonoyl residue. FEBS Lett 1991; 282:326–30.
19. Clark JD, Lin LL, Kriz RW, Ramesha CS, Sultzman LA, Lin AY. A novel arachidonic acid-selective cytosolic PLA_2 contains a Ca^{2+}-dependent translocation domain with homology to PKC and GAP. Cell 1991; 65:1043–51.
20. Smith WL, DeWitt DL. Prostaglandin endoperoxide H synthases-1 and -2. Adv Immunol 1996; 62:167–215.
21. Carty TJ, Marfat A. The prospect for improved medicines. (Bowman WC, Fitzgerald JD, and Taylor JB eds.) Emerging Drugs. 1996; 391–411.
22. Seibert K, Zhang Y, Leahy K, Hauser S, Masferres J, Perkins W. Pharmacological and biochemical demonstration of the role of

cyclooxygenase 2 in inflammation and pain. Proc Natl Acad Sci USA 1994; 91:12,013–7.

23. Chan CC, Boyce S, Brideau C, Ford-Hutchinson AW, Gordon R, Guay D. Pharmacology of a selective cyclooxygenase-2 inhibitor, L-745,337: a novel nonsteroidal anti-inflammatory agent with an ulcerogenic sparing effect in rat and nonhuman primate stomach. J Pharmacol Exp Ther 1995; 274:1531–7.

24. Patrono C. Aspirin as an antiplatelet drug. N Engl J Med 1994; 330:1287–94.

25. Showell HJ, Naccache PH, Borgeat P, Picard S, Valley P. Characterization of the secretory activity of LTB$_4$ toward rabbit neutrophils. J Immunol 1982; 128:811–16.

26. Bray MA, Ford-Hutchinson AW, Smith MJH. Leukotriene B$_4$: an inflammatory mediator *in vivo*. Prostaglandins 1981; 22:213–22.

27. Sharon P, Stenson WF. Production of leukotrienes by colonic mucosa from patients with inflammatory blood disease. Gastroenterology 1983; 84:1306(A).

28. Brain SD, Camp RDR, Dowd PM, Black AK, Woolard PM, Mallet, Greaves M. Psoriasis and leukotriene B$_4$. Lancet 1982; 2:762–63.

29. Feldberg W, Kellaway CH. Liberation of histamine and formation of lysolecithin-like substances by cobra venom. J Physiol 1938; 94:187–226.

30. Murphy RC, Hammarström S, Samuelsson B. Leukotriene C. A slow reacting substance from murine mastocytoma cells. Proc Natl Acad Sci USA 1979; 76:4275–9.

31. Holroyde MC, Altounyan REC, Cole M, Dixon M, Elliott EV. Bronchoconstriction produced in man by leukotrienes C and D. Lancet 1981; 2:17–8.

32. Zakrzewski JT, Barnes NC, Piper PJ, Costello JF. Quantitation of leukotrienes in asthmatic sputum. Br J Pharmacol 1985; 19:574P.

33. Creticos PS, Peters SP, Adkinson NF Jr. Neiclerio RM, Hayes EC, and Notman PS. Peptide leukotriene release after antigen challenge in patients sensitive to ragweed. N Engl J Med 1984; 310:1626–30.

34. Hamberg M, Samuelsson B. Prostaglandin endoperoxides. Novel transformations of arachidonic acid in human platelets. Proc Natl Acad Sci USA 1984; 71:3400–4.

35. Hamberg M, Hedqvist P, Radegran K. Identification of 15-hydroxy-5,8,11,13-eicosatetraenoic acid (15-HETE) as a major metabolite of arachidonic acid in human lung. Acta Physiol Scand 1980; 110(2): 219–21.

36 Takashi I, Rådmark O, Jörnvall H, Samuelsson B. Purification of two forms of arachidonate 15-lipoxygenase from human leukocytes. Eur J Biochem 1991; 202:1231–8.

37. Hunter JA, Finkbeiner WE, Nadel JA, Goetzl EJ, Holtzman MJ. Predominant generation of 15-lipoxygenase metabolites of arachidonic acid by epitheial cells from human trachea. Proc Natl Acad Sci USA 1985; 82(14):4633–7.

38. Henke D, Danilowicz RM, Curtis JF, Boucher RC, Eling TE. Metabolism of arachidonic acid by human nasal and bronchial epithelial cells. Arch Biochem Biophys 1988; 267(2):426–36.

39. Vanderhoek JY, Karmin MT, Ekborg SL. Endogenous hydroxyeicosatetraenoic acids stimulate the human polymorphonuclear leukocyte 15-lipoxygenase pathway. J Biol Chem 1985; 260(29):15482–7.

40. Galli C, Socini A. Dietary lipids in pre- and post-natal development in dietary fats and health. In: Perkins EG, Visek WJ, eds, pp. 278–301. American Oil Chemical Society, 1983.

41. Bourre JM, Durand G, Pascal G, Youyou A. Brain cell and tissue recovery in rats made deficient in *n*-3 fatty acids by alteration of dietary fat. J Nutr 1989; 119:15–22.

42. Farquharson J, Cockburn F, Ainslie PW. Infant cerebral cortex phospholipid fatty-acid composition and diet. Lancet 1992; 340:810–3.

43. Makrides M, Neuman MA, Byard RW, Gibson RA. Fatty acid composition of brain retina and erythrocytes in breast and formula fed infants. Am J Clin Nutr 1994; 60:189–94.

44. Simmons PM, Salmon JA, Moncada S. The release of leukotriene B4 during experimental inflammation. Biochem Pharmacol 1983; 32(8):1353–9.

45. Brain SD, Camp RD, Cunningham FM, Dowd PM, Greaves MW,

Black AK. Leukotriene B4-like material in scale of psoriatic skin lesions. Br J Pharmacol 1984; 83(1):313–7.

46. Belluzzi A, Brignola C, Campieri M, Peya A, Boschi S, Miglioli M. Effect of an enteric-coated fish oil preparation on relapses in Crohn's disease. N Engl J Med 1996; 334:1557–1616.

47. Robinson DR, Prickett JD, Makoul GT, Steinber AD, Colvin RB. Dietary fish oil reduces progression of established renal disease in (NZBxNZW)F1 mice and delays renal disease in BXSB and MRL/1 strains. Arthrtis Rheum 1986; 29:539–46.

48. Kremer JM, Bigauoette J, Michalek AU. Effects of manipulating dietary fatty acids on clinical manifestations of rheumatoid arthritis. Lancet 1985; 1:184–7.

49. Kremer JM, Lawrence DA, Petrillo GF, Mullaly PM, Rynes RL, et al. The effect of high dose fish oil on rheumatoid arthritis after stopping NSAIDs: clinical and immune correlates in patients with rheumatoid arthritis. Arthritis Rheum 1995; 38:1107–14.

50. Fortin PR, Lian MH, Beckett LA, Wright EAC, Ralmeys TC, Sterling RI. A meta-analysis of the efficacy of fish oil in rheumatoid arthritis. Arthritis Rheum 1992; 35:S201.

51. Kroman N, Green A. Epidemiological studies in the Upernavik district, Greenland. Acta Med Scand 1980; 208:401–6.

52. Hammarstrom A, Hamberg M, Samuelsson B, Duell EA, Strawiski M, Voorhees JJ. Increased concentration of nonesterified arachidonic acid. 12L-hydroxy-5,8,10,14-eicosatetraenoic acid, prostaglandin E$_2$ and prostagllandin F$_{2\alpha}$ in epidermis of psoriasis. Proc Natl Acad Sci USA 1975; 72:5130–4.

53. Brain S, Camp R, Dowd P, Black AK, Greaves M. The release of leukotriene B$_4$-like material in biologically active amounts from the lesional skin of patients with psoriasis. J Invest Dermatol 1984; 83:70–3.

54. Ziboh VA, Cohen KA, Ellis CN, Miller C, Hamilton TA, Kragballe K. Effects of dietary supplementation of fish oil on neutrophil and epidermal fatty acids. Arch Dermatol 1986; 122:1277–82.

55. Maurice PDL, Allen BR, Barkley ASJ, Cockbill SR, Stammers J, Bather PC. The effects of dietary supplementation with fish oil in patients with psoriasis. Br J Dermatol 1987; 117:599–606.

56. Bittner SB, Cartwright I, Tucker WFG, Bleehen SS. A double-blind randomized placebo-controlled trial of fish oil in psoriasis. Lancet 1988; 1:378–80.

57. Bjørneboe A, Smith AK, Bjørneboe GE, Thune PO, Drevon CA. Effect of dietary supplementation with *n*-3 fatty acids on clinical manifestations of psoriasis. Br J Dermatol 1988; 118:77–83.

58. Lassus A, Dahlgren AL, Halpern MJ, Santalahti J, Happonen HP. Effects of dietary supplementation with ethyl ester lipids (angiosan) in patients with psoriasis and psoriatic arthritis. J Int Med Res 1990; 18:68–73.

59. Gupta AK, Ellis CN, Tellner DC, Anderson TF, Voorhees JJ. Double-blind placebo-controlled study to evaluate the efficacy of fish oil and low-dose UVB in the treatment of psoriasis. Br J Dermatol 1989; 120:801–7.

60. Miller CC, Yamaguchi RY, Ziboh VA. Guinea pig epidermis generates putative anti-inflammatory metabolites from fish oil polyunsaturated fatty acids. Lipids 1989; 24:998–1003.

61. Miller CC, Ziboh VA. Human epidermal transforms eicosapentaenoic acid to 15-hydroxy-5,8,11,13,17-eicosapentaenoic acid: a potent inhibitor of 5-lipoxygenase. J Am Oil Chem Soc 1988; 65:474.

62. Singer SJ, Nicholson GL. The fluid mosaic model of the structure of cell membranes. Science 1972; 175:720–31.

63. Horrobin DF. The regulation of prostaglandin biosynthesis by the manipulation of essential fatty acid metabolism. Rev Pure Appl Pharmacol Sci 1983; 4:339–432.

64. Nassar BA, Huang YS, Manku MS, Das UN, Morse N, Horrobin DF. The influence of dietary manipulation with *n*-3 and *n*-6 fatty acids on liver and plasma phospholipid fatty acids in rats. Lipids 1986; 21:652–6.

65. Fantone JC, Kunkel SL, Ward PA, Zurier RB. Suppression by prostaglandin E$_1$ of vascular permeability induced by vasoactive inflammatory mediators. J Immunol 1980; 125:2591–2600.

66. Kunkel SL, Thrall RS, Kunkel RG, McCormack JR, Ward PA, Zurier RB. Supression of immune complex vasculitis by prostaglandins. J Clin Invest 1979; 64:1525–35.

67. Miller CC, McCready CA, Jones AD, Ziboh VA. Oxidative metabolism of dihomogammalinolenic acid by guinea pig epidermis. Evidence of generation of anti-inflammatory products. Prostaglandins 1988; 35:917–38.

68. Baker DG, Krakauer KA, Tate GA, Laposata M, Zurier RB. Suppression of human synovial cell proliferation by dihomo-γ-linolenic acid. Arthritis Rheum 1989; 32:1273–81.

69. Leventhal LJ, Boyce EG, Zurier RB. Treatment of rheumatoid arthritis with gammalinolenic acid. Ann Intern Med 1993; 119:867–73.

70. Belch JJF, Ansell D, Madhok AR, Dowd A, Sturrock RD. Effects of altering dietary essential fatty acids on requirements for nonsteroidal anti-inflammatory drugs in patients with rheumatoid arthritis: a double blind placebo controlled study. Ann Rheum Dis 1988; 47:96–104.

71. Chapkin RS, Ziboh VA, Marcelo CL, Voorhees JJ. Metabolism of essential fatty acids by human epidermal perparations: evidence of chain elongation. J Lipid Res 1986; 27:945–54.

72. Hansen HS, Jensen B. Essential function of linoleic acid esterified in acylglucosylceramide and acylceramide in maintaining the epidermal water permeability barrier. Evidence form feeding studies with oleate, linoleate, arachidonate, columbinate and α-linoleate. Biochim Biophys Acta 1985; 834:357–63.

73. Chapkin RS, Ziboh VA. Inability of skin enzyme preparation to biosynthesize arachidonic acid from linoleic acid. Biochem Biophys Res Commun 1984; 124:784–92.

74. Cho Y, Ziboh VA. Incorporation of 13-hydroxyoctadecadienoic acid (13-HODE) into epidermal ceramides and phospholipids: phospholipase C-catalyzed release of novel 13-HODE-containing diacylglycerol. J Lipid Res 1994; 35:255–62.

75. Cho Y, Ziboh VA. Nutritional modulation of guinea pig skin hyperproliferation by essential fatty acid deficiency is associated with selective down regulation of protein kinase C-β. J Nutr 1995; 125:2741–50.

76. Fogh K, Sogaard H, Herlin T, Kragballe K. Improvement of psoriasis vulgaris after intralesional injections of 15-hydroxyeicosatetraenoic acid (15-HETE). J Am Acad Dermatol 1988; 18:279–85.

77. Wright S, Buton JL. Oral evening primrose seed oil improves atopic eczema. Lancet 1982; ii:1120–22.

78. Tate G, Mandell BF, Laposata M, Ohliger D, Baker DG, and Schumacher HR. Suppression of acute and chronic inflammation by dietary gammalinolenic acid. J Rheumatol 1989; 16:1729–36.

79. Miller CC, Ziboh VA. Gammalinolenic acid-enriched diet alters cutaneous eicosanoids. Biochim Biophys Res Commun 1988; 154:967–74.

80. Ziboh VA, Fletcher MP. Dose-response effects of dietary γ-linolenic acid-enriched oils on human polymorphonuclear-neutrophil biosynthesis of leukotriene B_4. J Clin Nutr 1992; 55:39–45.

81. Vanderhoek JY, Bryant RV, Bailey JM. Inhibition of leukotriene biosynthesis by the leukocyte product 15-hydroxy-5,5,11,13-eicosatetraenoic acid. J Biol Chem 1980; 225:10,064–6.

CLINICAL ISSUES | IV

14 Immunological Considerations of Breast Milk

Bo Lönnerdal

INTRODUCTION

There is considerable evidence for infants in developing countries that breast-feeding prevents infection and that both incidence and prevalence of illness is considerably lower in breast-fed infants than in infants fed other diets *(1)*. There are also studies on poor socioeconomic populations in more affluent countries showing a positive effect of breast-feeding on illness prevalence *(2)*. Recently, carefully controlled studies in upper-middle-class, well-educated populations in affluent countries demonstrated a lower incidence of infections in breast-fed infants than in formula-fed infants and also that, when ill, the duration of the illness is shorter in the breast-fed infants *(3)*. Taken together, there is ample evidence that breast-feeding protects the infant against infections.

Newborn infants are highly susceptible to infection during early life, which, in large part, is the result of delayed development of the immune function. Neutrophil functions, macrophage activation by interferon-γ (IF-γ), production of secretory IgA, formation of T cells displaying the CD45RO memory phenotype, IgG antibody to T-cell-independent immunogens, and complement components have all been noted to be lower during early infancy *(4,5)*. In addition, newborn infants produce lower amounts of many cytokines, including granulocyte/macrophage colony-stimulating factor, IF-γ, interleukin (IL)-3, IL-4, IL-6, and tumor necrosis factor-α (TNF-α) than adults, reducing their capacity to respond to an infectious challenge. A supply of factors in breast milk that can augment these deficits may, therefore, be critical for the infant and may, for example, explain the markedly lower incidence of necrotizing enterocolitis (NEC) in infants fed breast milk as compared to infants fed formula or given total parenteral nutrition (TPN) *(6)*.

When attempting to dissociate the various factors associated with the process of breast-feeding and evaluate their relative importance/quantitative significance with regard to acquiring or preventing illness, it is apparent that the situation is very complex. Exposure to pathogens is an obvious factor to consider. Whereas it is well-recognized that the use of contaminated water in the preparation utensils and bottles when preparing formulas or weaning foods will expose infants not being breast-fed to bacteria, viruses, and other microorganisms, it has recently become evident that there is a risk of transmission of HIV, cytomegalovirus (CMV), and other viruses through breast milk of infected mothers. The capacity of the maternal system and breast milk components to immunologically respond to the viral challenge is not well understood.

Breast milk contains several components that directly participate in the immune function of the breast-fed infant. There are also many components that directly interact with immune factors in breast milk or more indirectly affect its responsiveness and activity. These components include cells as well as soluble substances in breast milk. This chapter will focus on a more detailed review of these factors. It should also be recognized that breast milk provides a very balanced supply of nutrients to the infant; in fact, the healthy, normal breast-fed infant is generally accepted as the "gold standard" with regard to infant nutrition. Clinical studies as well as theoretical considerations of nutrient requirements show that breast-fed infants very rarely obtain inadequate or excessive amounts of any nutrient. Because nutritional status is known to affect immune function (see other chapters), it may be implied that the parts of the immune system that are affected by nutritional status are optimized in breast-fed infants, whereas this may not be the case in infants fed other diets.

The lack of exposure of the exclusively breast-fed infants to various antigens, dietary or environmental, also warrants some consideration. The proportion of infants and children having allergy and asthma has steadily increased in the last few decades. Induction of atopic disease as well as the development of tolerance are two areas that are intimately connected with the mode of feeding, antigen exposure, and timing and duration of these events.

MATERNAL IMMUNITY: IMMUNOGLOBULINS, ANTI-IDIOTYPIC ANTIBODIES, ACTIVATED AND MEMORY T CELLS

Human milk contains considerable concentrations of antibodies, with secretory IgA (SIgA) being the predominant class *(7)*. In fact, SIgA was first isolated and characterized from breast milk and this type of IgA is considerably more resistant toward proteolytic degradation than the monomeric form *(8)*. SIgA is assembled from

From: *Nutrition and Immunology: Principles and Practice* (ME Gershwin et al. eds.), © Humana Press, Inc., Totowa, NJ

the J-chain containing IgA dimers, which are bound to a specific polyimmunoglobulin receptor, also called secretory component (SC), present in the membrane of epithelial cells of lactating women (9,10). These receptors appear abundant, as measurable concentrations of free SC are found in human milk (11), possibly suggesting facilitation of B-cell homing to mammary tissue during lactation. The SIgA antibodies in human milk are known to recognize a wide variety of microorganisms that are found in the respiratory tract and intestine. They include bacterial pathogens such as E. coli, V. cholerae, H. influenzae, S. pneumoniae, C. difficile, and Salmonella, viruses like rotavirus, CMV, HIV, influenza virus, and RSV, as well as yeasts like Candida albicans (12). The specificity of these antibodies is believed to be acquired by antigen-triggered migration of B cells from Peyer's patches in the small intestinal tract and from lymphoid tissue in the respiratory tract to the lamina propria of the mammary gland.

The mechanism behind the migration of B cells appears to be cytokine mediated; when the mucosa is challenged by microbial antigens, cytokines will be released from mononuclear cells in Peyer's patches. Their release will cause local IgM⁺ B lymphocytes to undergo isotype switching to IgA⁺ lymphocytes or transform to IgA-secreting cells (12–14). Isotype-switched cells are then transported via lymph vessels to the mammary gland, most likely the result of the influence of hormones produced during late pregnancy and early lactation. Within the mammary gland, the lymphocytes differentiate into IgA-synthesizing plasma cells that secrete dimeric IgA. Once the dimeric IgA binds to the polymeric immunoglobulin receptor on the basolateral membrane of the epithelial cell, the receptor–dimeric IgA complex will be transported to the apical side of the membrane (15). Following cleavage of the intracytoplasmic part of the receptor, secretory IgA is secreted into the milk. This so-called "enteromammary" pathway thereby provides the newborn, whose immune system is relatively immature, protection against the same mucosal pathogens to which the mother is exposed (16). Because the production of secretory IgA is low during early infancy (17), breast-fed infants provided these antibodies orally will be provided protection against enteric and respiratory pathogens, whereas formula-fed infants will not.

The quantitative significance of milk SIgA in the overall defense against infection that breast-fed infants acquire is difficult to assess. However, it has been shown that protection against cholera in breast-fed infants is correlated to milk SIgA antibody titers against V. cholerae enterotoxin and lipopolysaccharide (18). Similarly, it has been demonstrated that milk sIgA antibodies protect breast-fed infants against enterotoxigenic E. coli (ETEC) (19). These findings clearly show that antibody titers are important in the immune defense of infants. Antibody avidity, however, may also be significant in the development of immunity. Svennerholm et al. (20) have shown that whereas parenteral vaccination may boost breast milk sIgA antibodies, oral vaccines may have the opposite effect. This suggested that "oral tolerance" may not be occurring consistently, particularly as the decrease in milk sIgA antibodies after oral exposure was accompanied by an increase in serum antibody. Roberton et al. (21) explored the avidity of sIgA antibodies against the E. coli O antigen and diphtheria toxin and found a higher relative affinity index in milk samples from Swedish mothers than from Pakistani women. Although compromised nutritional status possibly could have explained this finding, no changes in titers or avidities of SIgA antibodies were found

in Guatemalan mothers before and after they were given a food supplement (440 kcal/d) for 3 mo. This suggested that there were other reasons for the differences observed between Swedish and Pakistani women. Cruz et al. (22) have shown that intestinal infections in lactating Guatemalan women, who already had antibodies in their milk against Shigella and Giardia, led to a decrease in antibody levels in most women. The magnitude and duration of the decrease varied widely among women, suggesting that factors such as the duration of the infection, infection dose, and type of microorganism may affect the milk antibody titer after an infection. Vaccination of lactating Pakistani women with whole-cell cholera vaccine increased titers but not avidities of the sIgA antibodies against cholera endotoxin (23). The authors proposed that the avidity of the milk antibodies was already high and that it was not feasible to increase it further by immunization. It is thus possible that many milk SIgA antibodies are the result of mature immune responses originating from memory cells migrating into the mammary gland. It could also explain how milk can contain antibodies against so many different bacteria and serotypes, many more than the mother can have encountered recently (24).

Anti-idiotypic IgA antibodies may also confer immunity to the newborn infant. If these antibodies survive in the gastrointestinal tract, they may elicit mucosal antibody responses targeted toward wild strains of enteric viruses, such as polioviruses. The concept of anti-idiotypic antibodies being presented to the fetus/newborn was first raised by Hanson and co-workers, who found specific secretory IgA and IgM antibodies to E. coli O antigens and poliovirus type 1 antigen in amniotic fluid, saliva, and meconium of infants at birth, indicating antigen-specific antibody production during fetal life (25). In addition, they found such antibodies in infants born to mothers with hypogammaglobulinemia or IgA deficiency, who had no IgA and/or IgM antibodies themselves (26). The authors noted that it is highly unlikely that the infants could have been exposed to poliovirus in utero, as there are no circulating wild or vaccine poliovirus strains in Sweden (where the study was done), because virtually the entire population is routinely vaccinated against polio with an inactivated virus only. They hypothesized that the antibodies may originate from transfer of maternal anti-idiotypic antibodies across the placenta and/or via breast milk. By using a poliovirus antigen–antibody system, they found anti-idiotypic antibodies against poliovirus in human serum, breast milk, and commercial Ig (27). Studies in animal models have shown that anti-idiotypic antibodies transferred from lactating dams to the pup via milk can elicit an immune response to the original antigen in the newborn (28,29). That the antibodies reached the pups through the milk was documented by injection of the anti-idiotypic antibodies to the mothers after delivery. Immunization of mice with an anti-idiotypic antibody toward poliovirus has been shown to induce an immune response consisting of antibodies reacting with both poliovirus and anti-idiotypic antibodies to poliovirus (30). This finding of induction of antibody response to infectious agents without administration of antigen has led to the suggestion of using anti-idiotypic monoclonal antibodies (Mab) as a vaccine (31). The finding of anti-id/polio in colostrum and mature breast milk is in agreement with studies showing better vaccine responses in breast-fed than in formula-fed infants (32,33), which may be the result of the additional exposure of the breast-fed infant to the anti-idiotypes present in the milk.

Leukocytes are present in breast milk, particularly in colostrum and during early lactation, when up to 3×10^6 cells/mL can be found. Neutrophils dominate with about 40–60% of the cells, whereas there are 30–50% macrophages and 5–10% lymphocytes *(34–36)*. Of the lymphocytes in human milk, T cells dominate (>80%) and they are most likely activated, as indicated by their thermostability and phenotypic expression (IL-2R, CD45RO, HLA–DR). The morphology and high motility of the macrophages suggest that they are also activated. The neutrophils in breast milk have low motility and do not respond to chemoattractants such as *N*-formyl methionyl peptides (fMLPs) *(37)*, which indicates that they may also be activated, as activated neutrophils become unresponsive to some chemoattractants, including fMLP. Keeney et al. *(38)* hypothesized that neutrophils in breast milk become activated in vivo and demonstrated that this is the case, as indicated by increased expression of CD11b, an adherence glycoprotein that is a member of the integrin family. This was further supported by reduced expression of L-selectin, an adhesion protein that is shed from the surface of activated neutrophils. Support for human milk activating the neutrophils was obtained by incubating blood neutrophils with decelled human milk; CD11b expression increased and L-selectin decreased, indicative of activation. Experiments with fractionated human milk suggested that the activation may be mediated via phagocytosis of membrane structures in milk, which reside in the particulate fraction. The function of activated neutrophils in breast milk is not yet known. It is possible, however, that they may compensate the newborn's poor capacity to recruit blood neutrophils to sites of inflammation by providing a supply of already activated neutrophils into the gastrointestinal tract and, thereby, serve an anti-inflammatory role, as suggested by Keeney et al. *(38)*.

That T cells in breast milk are activated was proposed by Wirt et al. *(36)*, who found this likely, as macrophages in human milk are activated and several immunomodulating factors such as TNF-α are present in human milk. By using flow cytometry, they found that the proportion of CD4+ T cells in breast milk is similar to that in peripheral blood, but that the proportion of CD8+ is much higher, resulting in a much lower CD4/CD8 ratio than in blood. The functional significance of this is not yet known, but the authors pointed out that most intraepithelial lymphocytes in the human small intestine are T cells expressing CD8 and it is possible that the oral and intestinal epithelial layers may have higher affinity toward CD8+ T cells than to CD4+. Thus, the environment in the infant may stimulate the transfer of maternal T cells. Wirt et al. *(36)* also found that a large proportion of the T cells in human milk showed signs of activation as indicated by phenotypic markers. Although expression of HLA-DR and CD25 (IL-2R) was found on 85% of the human milk T cells, only 10% of those in peripheral blood of adults express these markers. The presence of CD45RO indicated previous activation. Most of the CD4+ (99.8%) and the CD8+ (92%) T cells were CD45RO+, and CD45RA expression was markedly decreased, which is in agreement with switching of unprimed cells to antigen-primed or memory T cells. CD4+ cells with the CD45RA CD45RO+ phenotype are known to help antibody production (helper-cell function) and suppress antigen-specific antibody production. Wirt et al. *(36)* suggested that the low number of memory T cells in newborn may be compensated for, in part, by the transfer of maternal CD45RO+ T cells via breast milk. Studies on development of CD45RO+ T cells in exclusively breast-fed infants and formula-fed infants should provide an answer if this is the case.

ANTIMICROBIAL FACTORS

Whereas the presence of antibodies in breast milk was recognized early, it was also apparent that there are many other components in breast milk that can complement immunoglobulin-mediated defense mechanisms. Lactoferrin, an iron-binding protein, present in human milk at remarkably high concentrations (1–2 g/L or 10–20% of total protein content), was shown to have a bacteriostatic effect against *E. coli* by Bullen et al. *(39)*. It is believed that this effect of lactoferrin is the result of its strong affinity toward iron ($K_{ass}\sim10^{30}$), as this protein is present in breast milk largely in its unsaturated form and because addition of iron abolished its effect both in vitro and in vivo. Lactoferrin was subsequently also shown to be bactericidal against several pathogens that infants may be exposed to, such as *Vibrio cholerae, Salmonella, Staphylococcus,* and so forth *(40)*. Although the bacteriostatic effect of lactoferrin described by Bullen et al. *(39)* was shown to be abolished by the addition of iron, the bactericidal activity was not dependent on the iron saturation of lactoferrin *(41)*. To date, however, studies in which lactoferrin-fortified formula was used have failed to show any significant effects on the microbial flora in the infant gut *(42)*. It should be recognized, though, that *bovine* lactoferrin was used in all these studies and not human lactoferrin. It has been shown that the intestinal receptor found in human infant brush border membranes recognizes the human form and not the bovine lactoferrin, possibly explaining the lack of an effect *(43)*. Recently, lactoferrin has also been shown to have antiviral activity against both the human immunodeficiency virus (HIV) and the cytomegalovirus (CMV) in vitro *(44)*. To date, no clinical studies have been performed on this antiviral effect nor is the mechanism behind this action known.

Recently, a peptide called lactoferricin has been isolated from human (residues 20 to 37) and bovine (residues 19 to 36) lactoferrin that has strong bactericidal effects both in vitro and in animal models *(45)*. This peptide is located at the N-terminal end of lactoferrin and does not contain an iron-binding region *(46)*. It is still not known whether the bactericidal effect of human lactoferrin is the result of the formation of this peptide or if intact lactoferrin and lactoferricin act in concert. A recent study by Turchany et al. *(47)* shows that both lactoferrin and lactoferrin peptides have giardicidal activity, suggesting that this activity of lactoferrin is the result of the formation of active peptides.

Lysozyme is present in breast milk in unusually high concentrations for being an active enzyme (0.1–0.3 g/L). This enzyme can degrade the cell walls of gram-positive bacteria and has been shown to have strong antimicrobial activity in vitro. There is little evidence in vivo, however, for an involvement of lysozyme in the defense against infections in the newborn. It is possible that lysozyme and lactoferrin have synergistic effects; Ellison and Giehl *(48)* have recently demonstrated that lactoferrin can bind lipopolysaccharide (LPS) from the outer membrane of bacteria. This removal of LPS by lactoferrin opens up the outer membrane so that lysozyme gets access to the underlying proteoglycan matrix, causing lysis of the bacteria. Whether this potent synergism is in effect in vivo still remains to be explored.

Nucleotides are present in human milk in significant concentrations *(49)*, although they, up to now, have been absent in infant formulas. They are believed to boost the "salvage" pathway in the enterocytes of infants; *de novo* synthesis of nucleotides is immature in newborns and in situations of need—an additional supply of nucleotides may help nucleic acid synthesis and thereby cell growth and proliferation. An enhanced integrity of the mucosal barrier is believed to deter microorganisms from attaching and invading the host (50). Carver et al. (51) found that infants fed nucleotide-fortified formula had higher concentrations of natural-killer (NK) cells and IL-2 than infants fed formula without added nucleotides, very similar to those of exclusively breast-fed infants. That this may affect infections in infants was demonstrated by Brunser et al. (52), who found that infants in Peru who were fed nucleotide-fortified formula had a lower prevalence of infections and also a lower total number of days being sick than those fed unfortified formula.

Recently, Tanaka et al. (53) have shown that individual nucleotides, particularly AMP, can induce apoptosis in human fetal intestine in culture. These authors suggest that AMP and possibly other nucleotides via enhanced apoptosis may increase cellular proliferation and differentiation, thereby reinforcing mucosal integrity. It should be noted that the concentrations of nucleotides used in most clinical studies to date are far lower than the total concentration of nucleotides in breast milk. Human milk contains significant quantities of DNA and RNA, and Thorell et al. (54) recently showed that infant pancreatic fluid and intestine contains ample activities of the enzymes needed to degrade nucleic acids into nucleotides. Thus, the true concentration of nucleotides in the small intestine of breast-fed infants may be as high as 10 times that of preformed nucleotides. The effect of fortifying infant formula with concentrations of nucleotides similar to those expected to be available from human milk was evaluated in a recent study by Pickering et al. (55). They found that infants receiving fortified formula had higher antibody titers against *Haemophilus influenzae* type b and diphtheria after vaccinations than infants receiving control formula. Thus, it is evident that dietary factors can have a role in the response of infants to immunization.

Oligosaccharides are present in human milk in substantial concentrations and in a large number of varieties (56,57). The predominant species are lacto-*N*-tetraose, lacto-*N*-fucopentaose, sialyllactose, and disialyl-lacto-*N*-tetraose, but over 900 fucosyloligosaccharides containing up to 32 sugars and up to 15 fucose residues have been detected by time-of-flight mass spectrometry (58). This diversity is in part the result of genetic differences in enzymes involved in carbohydrate biosynthetic pathways, particularly fucosyltransferases and sialyltransferases, Lewis secretor status, and changes occurring during lactation. Most of the oligosaccharides occur in free form, but they are also linked to glycoproteins (e.g., lactoferrin, κ-casein, SIgA), glycolipids, mucins, and so forth. Many of these carbohydrate structures are identical or similar to surface-bound glycans on the small intestine mucosa, which are known receptors for adhesive bacteria (56). Thus, milk oligosaccharide structures can act as soluble "decoys" and foil attempts of pathogens to attach and invade the host's mucosa. That the carbohydrate structure itself is responsible for the activity was shown by the finding that proteolytic digestion of fractions from human milk showing inhibition of adherence of enterotoxigenic *E. coli* had no effect on activity, whereas oxidation of carbohydrates with periodate resulted in loss of activity (59).

Inhibition of adhesion of *Haemophilus influenzae* and *Streptoccus pneumoniae* to specific carbohydrate structures of human buccal epithelial cells by human milk oligosaccharides was demonstrated by Andersson et al. (60). Similarly, neutral oligosaccharides from human milk were shown to protect the infant's intestinal tract from infection by *Vibrio cholerae* (61). Cravioto et al. (62) described a milk oligosaccharide that inhibits adhesion of enteropathogenic *E. coli* to their receptors. Sialylated oligosaccharides from human milk were shown to inhibit the binding *E. coli* species, which can cause meningitis and neonatal sepsis in infants (63), and a fucosylated oligosaccharide was demonstrated to inhibit the binding of *Campylobacter jejuni* to intestinal cells (64). A study on experimental gastroenteritis has shown an inhibitory effect of human milk mucin on rotavirus replication, which is most likely mediated by the carbohydrate part of the mucin (65).

In all the above examples, it was shown, or strongly implicated, that the oligosaccharide structures inhibited binding of the bacteria to the mucosal surface. Another type of inhibitory mechanism has been demonstrated for heat-stable enterotoxin from *E. coli* (66). These authors used T84 epithelial cells and showed that the binding of heat-stable toxin is inhibited by fucosylated human milk oligosaccharides. This toxin binds to the extracellular domain of guanylyl cyclase and activates the enzyme, causing inhibition of chloride channel function and resulting net flux of fluid into the lumen, which is believed to be the major cause of secretory diarrhea (67). As washing of oligosaccharide-incubated T84 cells to remove free oligosaccharides did not diminish the inhibition of toxin-mediated guanylyl cyclase activity, it was concluded that the oligosaccharides bind to the toxin receptor, rather than to the toxin. The authors suggested that their findings represent a novel protective mechanism of milk oligosaccharides and that it may account for the inhibition of enterotoxin-induced secretory diarrhea in breast-fed infants described in vivo.

The microflora in the gut of breast-fed infants will also affect the infant's capacity to resist infection. It is well known that the bacterial population in the gastrointestinal tract of breast-fed and formula-fed infants is quite different. Several components in breast milk, among them oligosaccharides, lactoferrin, nucleotides, and lysozyme, are known to stimulate the growth of *Lactobacilli* and *Bifidobacteria,* creating a so-called "bifido-flora" (42). A predominance of these bacteria decreases the pH of the gut, because of their production of lactic acid, which, in turn, inhibits/limits the growth of many pathogens, such as *E. coli, Bacteroides, Staphylococci,* and so forth.

There are many other components of breast milk that have been shown to have antimicrobial and/or immunostimulatory activity (68). Among them are κ-casein (69), digestive fragments of casein subunits (70), lactoperoxidase (71), and polyamines (72). It should be recognized, however, that most of these activities have been demonstrated in vitro or in animal models; human studies are largely lacking.

IMMUNOMODULATING AGENTS

The finding of cytokines in human milk opened up new possibilities for components in breast milk exerting effects on various cell types. Cytokines are polypeptides that can act in autocrine/paracrine fashion by binding to specific cellular receptors, thereby affecting cell activities and/or protein synthesis. The first cytokine to be found in human milk was transforming growth factor, TGF

(73), which can cause isotype switching to IgA$^+$ B cells (discussed earlier). Tumor necrosis factor (TNF)-α was subsequently also found in breast milk, particularly in colostrum, where concentrations of approx 600 pg/mL were detected *(74).* Significantly, it was demonstrated that human milk could enhance the movement of peripheral blood neutrophils in vitro and that this mobility could be inhibited by antibodies against TNF-α *(75).* It is also possible that TNF-α may affect SC synthesis and, therefore, cellular uptake of dimeric IgA. Interleukin (IL)-1β has been quantitated in breast milk at concentrations of approx 1100 pg/mL *(76),* which is at a level that can activate T cells.

Interleukin-6, IL-8, and IL-10 have all subsequently been found in human milk, with concentrations usually being considerably higher in early milk than later during lactation *(77–79).* IL-6 is of interest, as it can affect the synthesis of IgA *(77)* as well as IgM *(80)* and activate T cells. It is also possible that IL-6 is involved in a negative-feedback control mechanism that regulates the synthesis of TNF-α in the mammary gland *(81).* IL-6 can also stimulate the terminal differentiation of IgA$^+$ B cells to plasma cells producing IgA *(82)* and enhance the production of α$_1$-antitrypsin by phagocytes *(83),* possibly explaining the presence of α$_1$-antitrypsin in breast milk and the stool of breast-fed infants *(84).* IL-8 was found in human milk as well as in cultures of human mammary gland epithelial cells when epidermal growth factor (EGF), insulin, and hydrocortisone were added *(78).* Because the supernatant culture fluid was considerably higher in IL-8 than cell lysates, it was suggested that the cells produce IL-8 and that the cytokine is released rapidly after synthesis. Similar results were obtained for IL-6, suggesting that the presence of both the cytokines is at least in part, the result of mammary gland biosynthesis. IL-8, being a chemokine, is a chemoattractant for neutrophils and it is possible that it may contribute to the recruitment of T cells and neutrophils into breast milk *(78).*

Leukocyte growth-stimulating factors (CSF) have also been found in human milk, among them macrophage CSF *(85)* and granulocyte CSF *(86).* Concentrations of these CSFs were approx 17,000 U/mL and approx 300 pg/mL, respectively. Interferon-γ (IF-γ) has also been detected in breast milk *(87),* but it has not yet been determined whether the concentrations present are at a level that would affect the immune function. Other members of the CXC and CC family have also been shown to be present in colostrum and mature milk, among them monocyte chemotactic protein 1, growth-related peptide α, and the factor called RANTES (regulated upon activation, normal T cell expressed and secreted) *(5,88).* The effects of these individual factors as well as their combined net effect on immune function, particularly in breast-fed infants, remain to be elucidated.

There are also several noncytokine immunomodulating agents in milk, such as hormones and growth factors *(89).* These hormones may act locally in the intestinal mucosa or may have systemic effects, indirectly modulating immune function of the newborn. Growth factors can also have profound effects on mucosal growth, differentiation, and physical integrity, thereby affecting the mucosal immune system. It is beyond the scope of this review to discuss these factors in detail.

ANTI-INFLAMMATORY FACTORS

It is evident that human milk contains a wide variety of cytokines and chemokines, some of them in concentrations that suggest physiological activity. Still, human milk was early found to be anti-inflammatory in that it protected against infection without providing any clinical evidence of inflammation. One possible explanation for this is that human milk also contains soluble cytokine/chemokine receptors and receptor antagonists. For example, breast milk contains soluble TNF receptor I and II, as well as IL-1 receptor antagonist, throughout the lactation period *(90).* Goldman *(12)* has noted that breast milk contains low concentrations of initiators and mediators of inflammation, and it has high concentrations of anti-inflammatory agents. One of these anti-inflammatory agents is lactoferrin, which can inhibit LPS-induced as well as TNF-α-induced release of IL-6 from fresh human monocytes or cultured monocytic cells *(91).* Both intact lactoferrin and lactoferricin (see earlier discussion) were found to be effective, with the latter being the strongest inhibitor. Expression of cell-surface receptors for TNF-α and IL-6 is rapidly downregulated by LPS, but it remains to be seen if lactoferrin receptor expression is affected. It is possible that breast-fed infants who are colonized by LPS-containing and -releasing gram-negative bacteria receive protection from lactoferrin by this inhibitory mechanism. The authors speculate that this may contribute to the well-known smaller physiologic weight loss of breast-fed infants during the first week of life as compared to formula-fed infants *(91).*

In spite of the low production of pro-inflammatory cytokines in vitro by human infant blood leukocytes (discussed earlier), sick infants do respond with increased levels of TNF-α, IL-1β, IL-6, and IL-8 *(4).* These authors therefore suggested that production of anti-inflammatory cytokines, notably IL-10, is developmentally delayed. IL-10 was a good possibility, as it inhibits the production of IL-1, IL-8, and TNF-α, limits participation of T helper-1 cells in delayed hypersensitivity, and promotes the expression of T helper-2 cell responses that enhance synthesis of IgA that protects without being proinflammatory. Strong support for an instrumental role of IL-10 in the anti-inflammatory response has been obtained from homozygous IL-10 null-gene mice, which develop lethal enterocolitis similar to NEC *(92).* Chheda et al. *(4)* showed that stimulated blood T cells and monocytes from human newborns produce less IL-10 than cells from adults. Although this might be the result of decreased production of TNF-α by infant monocytes, production of IL-10 was not affected when the cells were exposed to exogenous TNF-α. Instead, expression of TNF-α receptors was significantly reduced, suggesting that low IL-10 expression in newborns may be the result of the immaturity of the regulatory process involving TNF-α and its receptors. Because human milk has been found to contain IL-10 in concentrations that are commensurate with bioactivity, as demonstrated by inhibition of thymidine uptake by human blood lymphocytes *(79),* it is possible that IL-10 may aid in the protection of the gastrointestinal tract. Therefore, IL-10 may bridge the immunomodulating and anti-inflammatory segments of the defense system in human milk *(79).* Again, this may help explain why human milk protects against NEC.

Proteins and ligands in human milk are usually compartmentalized (i.e., they are distributed among the lipid fraction [part of milk fat globule membrane], the aqueous phase, and the casein/cell pellet) but also bound to various components within the soluble fraction *(93).* This may affect their digestive fate and biological function. The issue whether IL-10 and other cytokines can survive passage of the alimentary tract, escape digestion, and remain intact

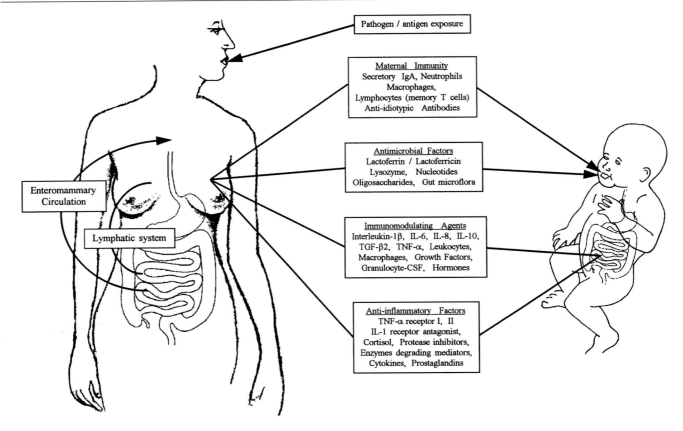

Fig. 1.   Components of breast milk that can affect the immune system of a newborn infant.

at the mucosal surface was addressed in the article of Garofalo et al. *(79)*. In their study, they found that IL-10 was distributed between the aqueous phase of breast milk and in the lipid fraction, and multiple molecular forms were detected. Infants have low acid secretion as compared to older children and adults and likewise production of pepsin and pancreatic proteases are low. These physiological conditions, coupled with the presence of protease inhibitors in human milk *(84)*, make it possible for peptide/protein components to remain in intact form in the gut. Because bile salts released some of the IL-10 from the lipids *(79)*, Garofalo et al. suggested that the total amount of IL-10 in milk that may be physiologically active in the intestine may be considerably higher than that analyzed in the aqueous phase. These observations may also explain some of the discrepancies for analyzed cytokine levels in human milk reported in the literature.

ALLERGY ASPECTS

The role of duration of breast-feeding and/or avoidance of cow-milk-based formulas during early life on the development of atopic disease has been a subject of considerable controversy. Early studies on prolonged breast-feeding demonstrated prophylaxis against atopic disease up to 3 yr of age *(94)* and a recent study by the same authors showed that the prevalence of manifest atopy, throughout follow-up to the age of 17 yr, was highest in the group that had little or no breast-feeding *(95)*. Genetic and environmental factors have strong influence on allergic disorders, with heredity having the largest effect. The reason for environmental exposure

during early infancy having an effect on sensation and subsequent development of atopy is most likely the physiological immaturity of the immune system *(95)*.

Because heredity has such a strong impact on the development of allergy, many different approaches have been used for the prophylaxis of atopy in infants with high hereditary risk. The use of an elimination diet during lactation has been shown to decrease eczema in infants at high risk *(96)*; however, it was ineffective if mothers used it during pregnancy only. It has been shown that low concentrations of cow's milk proteins can be detected in breast milk and that maternal elimination of daily products can reduce their levels significantly *(97)*.

The age for introduction of solid foods can also have an effect on atopic disease. Ferguson et al. *(98)* showed a clear association between the diversity of the infant's diet during the first months of life and the development of eczema. Delayed introduction of a single allergen has been shown to postpone, but not prevent, the respective food allergy *(95)*. In their prospective, long-term study, Saarinen and Kajosaari *(95)* found that breast-feeding for 6 mo or longer is required for prophylaxis of atopic eczema for the first 3 yr of life. However, even exclusive breast-feeding for more than 1 mo was found to be beneficial in preventing food allergy, with its peak prevalence around 3 yr of age, as well as respiratory allergy with a peak prevalence around 17 yr.

Although the study presented above and several others show a beneficial effect of breast-feeding on development of atopic disease, other studies fail to find a significant effect. In part, this is most likely due to the multitude of confounders inherent in studies of this nature. These include the lack of randomization, differences in genetic background and predisposition, environmental factors (including smoking), feeding practices, and so forth. Another confounder is the antigen load; many studies consider only the qualitative aspect ("all or none") and pay little attention to quantitative aspects (i.e., the amount of antigens in the diet of the exposed group). Antigen load may have a strong influence on whether atopy or tolerance will be the outcome. A recent large study from Finland, in which premature infants were fed breast milk or formula in a randomized fashion, there were no significant effects of diet on development of atopic disease *(99)*. It is evident that more, carefully controlled epidemiological studies are needed before conclusions can be made regarding the potential beneficial effect of breast-feeding on the development of allergy.

SUMMARY

It is evident that breast milk contains a multitude of components that can, or may, affect the immune system of the newborn infant (Fig. 1). Besides providing "optimal" nutrition (i.e., nutrients in adequate but not excessive amounts), all components of immune function that are dependent on nutrients are likely to have "optimal" physiological activity. Beyond this basic defense, breast milk components will facilitate the establishment of a microbial gut flora that will discourage many pathogens while stimulating the growth of beneficial microorganisms. Within this environment, maternal immunity will be transferred to the infant via antibodies of the SIgA type, but also anti-idiotypic antibodies, activated cells, and memory cells, thereby providing protection against the very same pathogens to which the mother has been exposed. An array of immunostimulatory components, notably cytokines, are provided in the milk and are possibly protected against proteolysis. These components will help to boost parts of the infant's immune system that have not yet been fully developed and aid in the proper response to challenges to the system. Anti-inflammatory factors in breast milk will help to modulate cytokine responses to infection, facilitating defense mechanisms without creating tissue damage and sepsis, as occurring in infants with NEC. It should be evident that it will be almost impossible to "sieve out" the components that are most important for the infant; rather, it is likely that the entire "repertoire" is needed and that many components interact synergistically. It should also be clear that it will be impossible to provide a similar system in infant formulas, even if it may be possible to add some components, thereby providing some of the benefits encountered by the breast-fed infant. Whether breast-feeding and late introduction of solids has a pronounced beneficial effect on the occurrence of atopic disease needs to be studied further, with emphasis on the induction of oral tolerance.

REFERENCES

1. Cunningham AS, Jelliffe DB, Jelliffe EFP. Breast-feeding and health in the 1980s: A global epidemiologic review. J Pediatr 1991; 118: 659–66.
2. Cunningham AS. Morbidity in breastfed and artificially fed infants II. J Pediatr 1979; 95:685–9.
3. Dewey KG, Heinig MJ, Nommsen-Rivers LA. Differences in morbidity between breast-fed and formula-fed infants. J Pediatr 1995; 126: 696––702.
4. Chheda S, Palkowetz KH, Garofalo R, Rassin DK, Goldman AS. Decreased interleukin-10 production by neonatal monocytes and T cells—relationship to decreased production and expression of tumor necrosis factor-alpha and its receptors. Pediatr Res 1996; 40:475–83.
5. Goldman AS, Chheda S, Garofalo R. Spectrum of immunomodulating agents in human milk. Int J Pediatr Hematol/Oncol 1997; 4:491–7.
6. Lucas A, Cole TJ. Breast milk and neonatal necrotising enterocolitis. Lancet 1990; 336:1519–23.
7. Goldman AS, Garza C, Johnson CA, Nichols BL, Goldblum RM. Immunologic factors in human milk during the first year of lactation. J Pediatr 1982; 100:563–7.
8. Lindh E. Increased resistance of immunogobulin dimers to proteolytic degradation after binding of secretory component. J Immunol 1985; 113:284.
9. Brandtzaeg P. Mucosal and glandular distribution of immunoglobulin components: differential localization of free and bound SC in secretory epithelial cells. J Immunol 1974; 112:1553–9.
10. Goldman AS, Chheda S, Keeney SE, Schmalstieg FC, Schanler RJ. Immunologic protection of the premature newborn by human milk. Semin Perinatol 1994; 18:495–501.
11. Sato K, Lonnerdal B. Uptake and transcytosis of free secretory component from human and bovine milk by Caco-2 cells. FASEB 1993; 7:A823.
12. Goldman AS. The immune system of human milk: antimicrobial, anti-inflammatory, and immunomodulating properties. Pediatr Infect Dis J 1993; 12:664–72.
13. Whitmore AC, Prowse DM, Haughton G, Arnold LW. Ig isotype switching in B lymphocytes. The effect of T-cell derived interleukins, cytokines, cholera toxin, and antigen on isotype switch frequency of a cloned B cell lymphoma. Int Immunol 1991; 3:95–103.
14. Schultz CL, Coffman RL. Control of isotype switching by T cells and cytokines. Curr Opin Immunol 1991; 3:350–4.
15. Mostov KE, Blobel GA. A transmembrane precursor of secretory component: the receptor for transcellular transport of polymeric immunoglobulins. J Biol Chem 1982; 257:11,816–21.
16. Telemo E, Hanson LÅ. Antibodies in milk. J Mammary Gland Biol Neopl 1996; 1:243–9.
17. Rognum TO, Thrane PS, Stoltenberg L, Vege Å, Brandtzaeg P. Development of intestinal mucosal immunity in fetal life and the first postnatal months. Pediatr Res 1992; 32:145–9.
18. Glass RI, Svennerholm AM, Stoll BJ, Khan MR, Hassain KMB, Huq MI, et al. Protection against cholera in breast-fed children by antibodies in breast milk. N Engl J Med 1983; 308:1389–92.
19. Cruz JR, Gil L, Cano F, Cáceres P, Pareja G. Breast milk anti-*Escherichia coli* heat-labile toxin IgA antibodies protect against toxin-induced diarrhea. Acta Paediatr Scand 1988; 77:658–62.
20. Svennerholm AM, Hanson LÅ, Holmgren J, Lindblad BS, Khan SR, Nilsson B, et al. Milk antibodies to live and killed polio vaccines in Pakistani and Swedish mothers. J Infect Dis 1981; 143:707–11.
21. Roberton DM, Carlsson B, Coffman K. Hahn-Zoric M, Jalil F, Jones C, et al. Avidity of IgA antibody to *Escherichia coli* polysaccharide and diphtheria toxin in breast-milk from Swedish and Pakistani mothers. Scand J Immunol 1988; 28:783–9.
22. Cruz JR, Cano F, Cáceres PP. Association of human milk SigA antibodies with maternal intestinal exposure to microbial antigens. In: Mestecky J, Blair, C, Ogra PL, eds. Immunology of Milk and the Neonate, pp. 193–9. Plenum, New York, 1991.
23. Dahlgren U, Carlsson B, Jalil F, MacDonald R, Mascart-Lemone F, Nilsson K, et al. Curr Top Microbiol Immunol 1989; 146:155.
24. Hanson LÅ, Carlsson B, Ekre HP, Jalil F, Hahn-Zoric M, Osterhaus ADME, et al. Immunoregulation mother-fetus/newborn, a role for anti-idiotypic antibodies. Acta Paediatr Scand 1989; 351:38–41.
25. Mellander L, Carlsson B, Hanson LÅ. Secretory IgA and IgM antibodies to E. coli O and poliovirus type 1 antigens occur in amniotic fluid, meconium and saliva from newborns. A neonatal immune response without antigenic exposure: a result of anti-idiotypic induction? Clin Exp Immunol 1986; 63:555–61.
26. Hahn-Zoric M, Carlsson B, Björkander J, Osterhaus ADME, Mellander L, Hanson LÅ. Presence of non-maternal antibodies in newborns of mothers with antibody deficiencies. Pediatr Res 1992; 32:150–4.

27. Hahn-Zoric M, Carlsson B, Jeansson S, Ekre HP, Osterhaus ADME, Roberton D. Anti-idiotypic antibodies to polio virus in commercial immunoglobulin preparations, human serum, and milk. Pediatr Res 1993; 33:475–80.

28. Okamoto J, Tsutsumi H, Kumar NS, Ogra PL. Effect of breast feeding on the development of anti-idiotype antibody response to F glycoprotein of respiratory syncytial virus in infant mice after post-partum maternal immunization. J Immunol 1989; 142:2507–12.

29. Stein KE, Söderström T. Neonatal administration of idiotype or anti-idiotype primes for protection against E. coli K 13 infection in mice. J Exp Med 1984; 160:1001–11.

30. Uytedehaag FGCM, Osterhaus ADME. Induction of neutralizing antibody in mice against poliovirus type II with monoconal anti-idiotypic antibody. J Immunol 1985; 134:1225–9.

31. Sacks DL. Immunization against parasitic protozoa using anti-idiotypic antibodies. Monogr Allergy 1987; 22:166–71.

32. Hahn-Zoric M, Fulconis F, Minoli J, Moro G, Carlson B, Böttiger M, et al. Antibody responses to parenteral and oral vaccines are impaired by conventional and low protein formulas as compared to breast-feeding. Acta Paediatr Scand 1990; 79:1137–42.

33. Pabst HF, Spady DW. Effect of breast-feeding on antibody response to conjugate vaccine. Lancet 1990; 336:269–70.

34. Crago SS, Prince SJ, Pretlow TG, McGhee JR, Mestecky J. Human colostral cells. I. Separation and characterization. Clin Exp Immunol 1979; 38:585–97.

35. Bertotto A, Gerli R, Fabietti G, Crupi S, Arcangeli C, Scalise F, et al. Human breast milk T cells display the phenotype and functional characteristics of memory T cells. Eur J Immunol 1990; 20:1877–80.

36. Wirt DP, Adkins LT, Palkowetz KH, Schmalstieg FC, Goldman AS. Activated and memory lymphocytes-T in human milk. Cytometry 1992; 13:282–90.

37. Thorpe LW, Rudloff HE, Powell LC, Goldman AS. Decreased response of human milk leukocytes to chemoattractant peptides. Pediatr Res 1986; 20:373–7.

38. Keeney SE, Schmalstieg FC, Palkowetz KH, Rudloff HE, Le B-M, Goldman AS. Activated neutrophils and neutrophil activators in human milk. Increased expression of CD11b and decreased expression of L-selectin. J Leukocyte Biol 1993; 54:97.

39. Bullen JJ, Rogers HJ, Leigh L. Iron-binding proteins in milk and resistance to Escherichia coli infection in infants. Br Med J 1972; 1:69–75.

40. Arnold RR, Brewer M, Gauthier JJ. Bactericidal activity of human lactoferrin: sensitivity of a variety of microorganisms. Infect Immun 1980; 28:893–8.

41. Arnold RR, Russell JE, Champion WJ, Brewer M, Gauthier JJ. Bactericidal activity of human lactoferrin: differentiation from the stasis of iron deprivation. Infect Immun 1982; 35:792–9.

42. Lönnerdal B. Effect of nutrition on microbial flora in infants—the role of lactoferrin, iron and nucleotides. In: Probiotics, other nutritional factors, and intestinal microflora, Hanson LA, Yolken RH, eds. Nestlé Nutrition Workshop series, Vol. 42. Lippincott-Raven, Philadelphia, pp. 189–201, 1999.

43. Lönnerdal B, Iyer S. Lactoferrin: molecular structure and biological function. Annu Rev Nutr 1995; 15:93–110.

44. Harmsen MC, Swart PJ, de Bethune MP, Pauwels De Clercq E, The TH, Meijer DK. Antiviral effects of plasma and milk proteins: lactoferrin shows potent activity against both human immunodeficiency virus and human cytomegalovirus in vitro. J Infect Dis 1995; 172:380–8.

45. Teraguchi S, Shin K, Ozawa K, Nakamura S, Fukuwatari Y, Tsuyuki S, et al. Bacteriostatic effect of orally administered bovine lactoferrin on proliferation of Clostridium species in the gut of mice fed bovine milk. Appl Environ Microbiol 1995; 61:501–6.

46. Yamauchi K, Tomita M, Giehl TJ, Ellison RT III. Antibacterial activity of lactoferrin and a pepsin-derived lactoferrin peptide fragment. Infect Immun 1993; 61:719–28.

47. Turchany JM, Aley SB, Gillin FD. Giardicidal activity of lactoferrin and N-terminal peptides. Infect Immunn 1995; 63:4550–2.

48. Ellison RT III, Giehl TJ. Killing of gram-negative bacteria by lactoferrin and lysozyme. J Clin Invest 1991; 88:1080–91.

49. Janas LM, Picciano MF. The nucleotide profile of human milk. Pediatr Res 1982; 16:659–62.

50. Grimble GK. Dietary nucleotides and gut mucosal defence. Gut 1994; 35:S46–S51.

51. Carver JD, Cox WI, Barness LA. Dietary nucleotide effects upon murine natural killer cell activity and macrophage activation. J Parenter Enter Nutr 1990; 14:18–22.

52. Brunser O, Espinoza J, Araya M, Cruchet S, Gil A. Effect of dietary nucleotide supplementation on diarrhoeal disease in infants. Acta Paediatr 1994; 83:188–91.

53. Tanaka M, Lee K, Martinez-Augustin O, He Y, Sanderson IR, Walker WA. Exogenous nucleotides alter the proliferation, differentiation and apoptosis of human small intestinal epithelium. J Nutr 1996; 126:424–33.

54. Thorell L. Sjöberg LB, Hernell O. Nucleotides in human milk: sources and metabolism by the newborn infant. Pediatr Res 1996; 40:845–52.

55. Pickering LK, Granoff DM, Erickson JR, Masor ML, Cordle CT, Schaller JP, et al. Modulation of the immune system by human milk and infant formula containing nucleotides. Pediatrics 1998; 101:242–9.

56. Kunz C, Rudloff S. Biological functions of oligosaccharides in human milk. Acta Paediatr 1993; 82:903–12.

57. Newburg DS. Do the binding properties of oligosaccharides in milk protect human infants from gastrointestinal bacteria? J Nutr 1997; 127:980S–4S.

58. Stahl B, Thurl S, Zeng J, Karas M, Hillenkamp F, Steup M, et al. Oligosaccharides from human milk as revealed by matrix-associated laser desorption/ionization mass spectrometry. Anal Biochem 1994; 223:218–26.

59. Ashkenazi S, Mirelman D. Nonimmunoglobulin fraction of human milk inhibits the adherence of certain enterotoxigenic Escherichia coli strains to guinea pig intestinal tract. Pediatr Res 1987; 22:130–4.

60. Andersson B, Porras O, Hanson LÅ, Lagergård T, Svanborg-Eden C. Inhibition of attachment of Streptococcus pneumoniae and Haemophilus influenzae by human milk and receptor oligosaccharides. J Infect Dis 1986; 153:232–7.

61. Holmgren J, Svennerholm AM, Lindblad M. Receptor-like glycocompounds in human milk that inhibit classical and El Tor Vibrio cholerae cell adherence (hemagglutination). Infect Immun 1983; 39:147–54.

62. Cravioto A, Tello O, Villafari H, Ruiz J, del Vedovo S, Neeser J-R. Inhibition of localized adhesion of enteropathogenic Escherichia coli to Hep-2 cells by immunoglobulin and oligosaccharide fractions of human colostrum and breast milk. J Infect Dis 1991; 163:1247–55.

63. Korhonen TK, Valtonen MV, Parkkinen J, Väisänen-Rhen V, Finne J, Orskov I. Serotypes, hemolysin production and receptor recognition of Escherichia coli strains associated with neonatal sepsis and meningitis. Infect Immun 1985; 48:486–91.

64. Cervantes LE, Newburg DS, Ruiz-Palacios GM. α-1-2 Fucosylated chains (H-2 and Lewis[b]) are the main human milk receptor analogs for Campylobacter. Pediatr Res 1995; 37:171A (abstract).

65. Yolken RH, Peterson JA, Vonderfecht SL, Fouts ET, Midthun K, Newburg DS. Human milk mucin inhibits rotavirus replication and prevents experimental gastroenteritis. J Clin Invest 1992; 90:1984–91.

66. Newburg DS, Pickering LK, McCluer RH, Cleary TG. Fucosylated oligosaccharides of human milk protect suckling mice from heat-stable enterotoxin from Escherichia coli. J Infect Dis 1990; 162:1075–80.

67. Crane JK, Azar SS, Stam A, Newburg DS. Oligosaccharides from human milk block binding and activity of the Escherichia coli heat-stable enterotoxin (Sta) in T84 intestinal cells. J Nutr 1994; 124:2358–64.

68. Lönnerdal B. Biochemistry and physiological function of human milk proteins. Am J Clin Nutr 1985; 42:1299–1317.

69. Strömquist M, Falk P, Bergström S, Hansson L, Lönnerdal B, Normark S, et al. Human milk κ-casein and inhibition of Helicobacter pylori adhesion to human gastric mucosa. J Pediatr Gastroenterol Nutr 1995; 21:288–96.

70. Parker F, Migliore-Samour D, Floch F, Zerial A, Werner GH, Jollies

J. Immunostimulating hexapeptide from human casein: amino acid sequence, synthesis and biological properties. Eur J Biochem 1984; 145:677–82.

71. Gothefors L, Marklund S. Lactoperoxidase activity in human milk and in saliva of newborn infants. Infect Immun 1975; 11:1210–5.

72. Sanguansermsri J, György P, Zilliken F. Polyamines in human and cow's milk. Am J Clin Nutr 1974; 27:859–65.

73. Noda K, Umeda M, Ono T. Transforming growth factor activity in human colostrum. Gann 1984; 75:109–12.

74. Rudloff HE, Schmalstieg FC, Mushtaha AA, Palkowetz KH, Liu SK, Goldman AS. Tumor necrosis factor-alpha in human milk. Pediatr Res 1992; 31:29–33.

75. Mushtaha AA, Schmalstieg FC, Hughes JrTK, Rajaraman S, Rudloff HE, Goldman AS. Chemokinetic agents for monocytes in human milk: possible role of tumor necrosis factor-alpha. Pediatr Res 1989; 25:629–33.

76. Munoz C, Endres S, van der Meer J, Schlesinger L, Arevalo M, Dinarello C. Interleukin-1β in human colostrum. Res Immunol 1990; 141:501–13.

77. Saito S, Maruyama M, Kato Y, Moriyama I, Ichijo M. Detection of IL-6 in human milk and its involvement in IgA production. J Reprod Immunol 1991; 20:267–76.

78. Palkowetz KH, Royer CL, Garofalo R, Rudloff HE, Schmalstieg FC, Golldman AS. Production of interleukin-6 and interleukin-8 by human mammary gland epithelial cells. J Reprod Immunol 1994; 26:57–64.

79. Garofalo R, Chheda S, Mei F, Palkowetz KH, Rudloff HE, Schmalstieg FC, et al. Interleukin-10 in human milk. Pediatr Res 1995; 37:444–9.

80. Hirano T, Akira S, Taga T, Kishimoto T. Biological and clinical aspects of interleukin 6. Immunol Today 1990; 11:443–9.

81. Rudloff HE, Schmalstieg FC, Palkowetz KH, Paskiewicz EJ, Goldman AS. Interleukin-6 in human milk. J Reprod Immunol 1993; 23:13–20.

82. Kono Y, Beagley KW, Fujihasi K, McGhee JR, Taga T, Hirano T, et al. Cytokine regulation of localized inflammation. Induction of activated B cells and IL-6 mediated polyclonal IgG and IgA synthesis in inflamed human gingiva. J Immunol 1991; 146:1812–21.

83. Perlmutter DH, May LT, Sehgal PB. Interferon β2/interleukin 6 modulates synthesis of α_1-antitrypsin in human mononuclear phagocytes and in human hepatoma cells. J Clin Invest 1989; 84:138–44.

84. Davidson LA, Lönnerdal B. Fecal α_1-antitrypsin in breast-fed infants is derived from human milk and is not indicative of enteric protein loss. Acta Paediatr Scand 1990; 79:137–41.

85. Hara T, Irie K, Saito S, Ichijo M, Yamada M, Yanai N, et al. Identification of macrophage colony-stimulating factor in human milk and mammary epithelial cells. Pediatr Res 1995; 37:437–43.

86. Gilmore WS, McKelvey-Martin VJ, Rutherford S, Strain JJ, Loane P, Kell M. Human milk contains granulocyte-colony stimulating factor (G-CSF). Eur J Clin Nutr 1994; 48:222–4.

87. Bocci V, von Bremen K, Corradeschi F, Luzzi E, Paulesu L. Presence of interferon-γ and interleukin-6 in colostrum of normal women. Lymphokine Cytokine Res 1993; 12:21–4.

88. Srivastava MD, Srivastava A, Brouhard B, Saneto R, Grohwargo S, Kubit J. Cytokines in human milk. Res Commun Mol Pathol Pharmacol 1996; 93:263–87.

89. Grosvenor CE, Picciano MF, Baumrucker CR. Hormones and growth factors in milk. Endocr Rev 1993; 14:710–28.

90. Buescher ES, Malinowska I. Soluble receptors and cytokine antagonists in human milk. Pediatr Res 1996; 40:839–44.

91. Mattsby-Baltzer I, Roseanu A, Motas C, Elverfors J, Engberg I, Hanson LÅ. Lactoferrin or a fragment thereof inhibits the endotoxin-induced interleukin-6 response in human monocytic cells. Pediatr Res 1996; 40:257–62.

92. Kühn R, Löher J, Rennick D, Rajewski K, Müller W. Interleukin-10-deficient mice develop chronic enterocolitis. Cell 1993; 75: 263–74.

93. Lönnerdal B, Woodhouse LR, Glazier C. Compartmentalization and quantitation of proteins in human milk. J Nutr 1987; 117:1385–95.

94. Saarinen UM, Kajosaari M, Blackman A, Siimes MA. Prolonged breast-feeding as prophylaxis for atopic disease. Lancet 1979; ii:163–8.

95. Saarinen UM, Kajosaari M. Breastfeeding as prophylaxis against atopic disease: prospective follow-up study until 17 years old. Lancet 1995; 346:1065–9.

96. Arshad SH, Matthews S, Gant C, Hide DW. Effect of allergen avoidance on development of allergic disorders in infancy. Lancet 1992; 339:1493–7.

97. Lilja G, Dannaeus A, Foucard T, Graff-Lönnevig V, Johansson SGO, Öhman H. Effects of maternal diet during late pregnancy and lactation on the development of atopic diseases in infants up to eighteen months of age—in vivo results. Clin Exp Allergy 1989; 19:473–9.

98. Ferguson DM, Horwood LJ, Shannon FT. Early solid feeding and recurrent childhood eczema: a 10-year longitudinal study. Pediatrics 1990; 86:541–6.

99. Lope L, et al. In: International Society for Research on Human Milk and Lactation (ISRHML 9), (in press).

15 Clinical Issues

Childhood Illnesses, Vaccinations, and Nutritional Status

NOEL W. SOLOMONS AND GERALD T. KEUSCH

THE INTERACTION OF NUTRITION AND INFECTION

The concept that malnutrition conditions the response to infectious diseases was convincingly presented by Scrimshaw et al. in 1959 (1) and updated in a World Health Organization monograph in 1968. The mechanisms by which this interaction occurred were not understood, but they were thought to be mediated by an effect of nutrition on the immune system. Most of the data reviewed at the time came from animal studies because there were only a limited number of published human investigations that examined immunological functions. In addition, these studies focused primarily on the effects of malnutrition on antibody-mediated immunity because that was the best understood immune host defense. Of particular interest to us, looking back three decades later, is the virtual lack of any reference to the potential impact of malnutrition on lymphocytes or cell-mediated immune responses, reflecting the state of understanding of basic immunological mechanisms at the time. The immune system is now known to be a complex interaction of cells with cells and soluble regulatory factors leading to immune responses mediated by both activated cells and soluble factors; this is described in greater detail elsewhere in this text. It is the specific goal of this chapter to examine the implications of nutritionally mediated alterations in immune function on the clinical response to infectious agents and vaccines.

Studies prior to the epidemic of HIV/AIDS are consistent with the concept that malnutrition adversely affects immune responses. This is one major reason why life expectancy is significantly lower in poor developing countries with a high prevalence of malnutrition, compared to wealthier and better nourished populations. Reduced life expectancy is primarily the result of the markedly increased perinatal and infantile mortality rates in the poor countries, and this is, in turn, primarily from infectious diseases. The disparity in survival between developed and developing countries continues to today. In fact, infant mortality in the Third World at the end of the 20th century, which still exceeds 150/1000 live born/year in many countries, is similar to the rates in Europe, Scandinavia, and North America in the 18th and 19th

centuries (2). Although immunization and the chemotherapeutic revolution have significantly contributed to the reduction in infectious diseases mortality in the industrialized countries, the downward trends had already become obvious before the widespread availability of vaccines or the chemotherapeutic revolution that has produced multiple classes of antibiotics, antivirals, antifungals, and antiparasitic drugs. Better living conditions, better diets, and access to health care clearly have an independent impact. Nonetheless, the more recent reductions in the under-5 mortality rate in the industrialized nations, which has been reduced a further 75% since 1960 (3), is in great part attributable to improvements in immunizations against and specific therapy of the common infectious diseases of childhood and in recovery rates from acute diarrheal dehydration.

Pelletier et al. (4) have looked carefully at the relationship between nutritional anthropometrical indices as markers of nutritional status and infant and child mortality. They conclude that weight deficits, even of a mild–moderate magnitude, are significantly associated with mortality, with as much as 50% of total-cause mortality due at least in part to undernutrition. In this chapter, we will explore this relationship and examine how nutritional status affects the clinical presentation of infectious diseases.

THE CHILDHOOD INFECTIOUS ILLNESSES

Beyond the first few months of life when maternally derived, transplacentally transported antibody and protective factors in breast milk afford some degree of protection against a variety of bacterial and viral infections, infants and children generally become more susceptible to the communicable diseases. There are two major reasons for this. First, the disappearance of maternally derived antibody-mediated immunity and, second, enhanced direct transfer of infectious agents by hand–mouth contact and close physical interactions during play and the difficulty in maintaining adequate sanitary practices in the young. Lack of immunity and ease of transmission result in ready transmission of the classical viral exanthems of childhood, including mumps, varicella, rubella, and measles. In addition, children are susceptible to enteroviruses such as poliomyelitis, classical bacterial infections such as diphtheria and pertussis, a variety of upper and lower respiratory infections, including otitis media, streptococcal pharyngitis, viral upper respiratory illnesses, and respiratory syncytial virus, pneu-

From: *Nutrition and Immunology: Principles and Practice* (ME Gershwin et al. eds.), © Humana Press, Inc., Totowa, NJ

Table 1
Reductions in Morbidity Attributed to Universal Immunization Programs in the United States

	Peak year	Cases reported		
		Cases	1992 Cases	% Reduction
Diphtheria	1921	206,939	4	99.99
Measles	1941	894,134	2,200	99.75
Mumps	1968	152,209	2,460	98.38
Pertussis	1934	265,269	3,359	98.73
Paralytic polio	1952	21,269	0	100.00
Rubella	1969	57,686	148	99.74
Congenital rubella		20,000	9	99.96
Tetanus	1923	1,560	42	97.31

mococcal and *Hemophilus influenzae* infection, and what used to be called "summer" and "winter" diarrhea, due to a variety of bacterial pathogens and rotavirus, respectively.

Before the era of universal immunization, infection with the common viral agents of childhood was essentially universal at some time during early childhood. Poliomyelitis generally presented as a summer diarrheal illness in the young and only occasionally progressed to paralytic polio; however, the frequency of infection led to a significant toll in paralytic disease. Each of these viral infections is vaccine preventable, and their occurrence and severity can be markedly reduced in both well-nourished and malnourished populations by universal application of immunization (Table 1). The serious adverse consequences of diphtheria and pertussis infection can also be prevented by prior immunization, and these two are among the earliest developed and applied vaccines throughout the world. Their incorporation into the universal childhood immunization scheme of the World Health Organization for developing countries, the Expanded Programme on Immunization (or EPI), has led to a major reduction in transmission of these infections (5,6).

However, whenever public health programs fail to achieve sufficient vaccine coverage to induce herd immunity to block transmission of these infections in the community, the incidence of infection and disease can increase sharply. This occurred in the United Kingdom two decades ago when a sharp drop in pertussis immunization occurred as a result of public antipathy to immunization related to exaggerated concerns for the adverse neurological effects of the old vaccine preparation. It also happened more recently in Russia because of the breakdown of public health services and consequent reduction in diphtheria immunization after the dissolution of the former Soviet Union. In both instances, epidemics of illness followed in a just a few years, as a new susceptible population was born. Acute respiratory and diarrheal diseases of both viral and bacterial origin are exceedingly common in all children, regardless of nutritional status (7). Many of these pathogens are actually groups of related, but antigenically distinct types, and unless immunity is group-specific, infection with one type does not protect against infection with other types. Hence, under circumstances of poverty, crowding, and limited environmental sanitation, it is predictable that children will develop a series of symptomatic respiratory and enteric infections, as they are highly likely to encounter many virulent members of these pathogenic groups of organisms. Mucosal infections with *Hemophilus influenzae*, typically type b, or various serotypes of *Strepto-*

coccus pneumoniae can disseminate and lead to bacteremia and systemic infection, including pneumonia and meningitis.

In many developing regions of the world, protozoal and helminthic diseases (usually grouped together as parasitic infections) are also common. In areas endemic for *Plasmodium falciparum*, infants and children bear the brunt of morbidity and mortality because protective immunity to this parasite is slow to develop. Malaria is, in fact, quite unusual because multiple symptomatic encounters with the parasite are required before effective resistance to clinical illness appears and, even then, recurrent infections continue to occur (8). Recurrent malaria, by means of the catabolic response and anorexia induced with each episode, accounts for a significant proportion of the growth faltering of young infants and children in malaria-endemic developing countries (9). Systemic protozoal diseases such as visceral leishmaniasis also cause a severe catabolic response that may progress to overt protein-energy malnutrition (10). The systemic helminthic infection caused by *Schistosoma mansoni* or *S. japonicum* also may result in severe malnutrition, secondary to the cirrhosis these worms induce (11). Unfortunately, none of these infections is vaccine preventable at this time.

Intestinal helminthic infections are the most common chronic infections of humans. Eggs shed in feces into the soil transmit many of these multicellular eukaryotic parasites. There, they undergo an obligatory developmental state to an infectious stages and are, subsequently, orally transmitted to a new or the same host. It is the accumulation of worms by continuing exposure and reinfection that increases the worm burden to the threshold for the appearance of symptoms. Young children are, therefore, highly vulnerable to these parasites, including *Ascaris lumbricoides*, the giant roundworm, and *Trichuris trichiura*, the whipworm. Beyond infecting at least a quarter of the world's population (some 1.5–2 billion cases), roundworms are associated with a finite mortality. It has been estimated that of the 1.3 billion people infected with *A. lumbricoides*, upward of 59 million are at risk annually for some degree of morbidity, with 12 million cases of acute illness leading to 10,000 fatal infections per year (12,13). These infections are species-specific and are limited to humans, there being no reservoir or intermediate host involved. The peak of the age–intensity curve for these two human nematodes is from 7 to 10 yr of age. Hookworm, transmitted not by oral ingestion of infectious eggs but rather by the invasion across the skin of live infectious larvae hatching from eggs deposited in soil, most commonly affects older children and young adults and results in intestinal blood loss. However, it takes time to develop a sufficient worm burden before iron-deficiency anemia develops, the most prominent manifestation of hookworm infection.

Children are also susceptible to newly "emerging" and reemerging infectious diseases *(14–16)*. These include a number of newly described hepatitis viruses, Hantavirus, Ebola, and Lassa fever viruses, malaria (already mentioned above), Group A streptococcal infection, drug-resistant tuberculosis, *Shigella dysenteriae* type 1 infection, and others. Arguably the most important emerging new infection is the human immunodeficiency virus (HIV). The major route of transmission of HIV for children is perinatal, including intrapartum and perinatal as well as postpartum via breast feeding from an HIV-infected mother *(17)*. An additional route is through injections with contaminated reused needles or blood transfusion, often employed to treat the severe anemia resulting from malaria *(18)*. Unfortunately, blood-banking practices in developing countries are often inadequate and blood remains unscreened for all transfusion-transmitted infectious agents, including HIV and hepatitis viruses. Because of its chronic nature and the frequency with which HIV infection affects the gut, malabsorption, failure to thrive, and malnutrition (referred to as "slim" disease in Africa) have become cardinal manifestations of AIDS in children as well as in adults *(15)*.

The diversity of infectious agents, the variety of routes of transmission, the serious nature of their clinical manifestations, and their interactions with nutrition account for the prominence of infectious diseases among the estimated 12–20 million young children who perish annually around the world, primarily in the poor, developing countries.

IMMUNIZATIONS

Because immunization is the most cost-effective strategy to reduce the burden of morbidity and mortality caused by infectious diseases, increasing attention has been given over the past two decades to the improvement of existing vaccines and the development of new vaccines where none have previously existed. Although considerable progress has been made, it is disappointing to note that all of the useful vaccines are not currently deployed in those countries where the disease burden is greatest because of their inability to pay the cost. Vaccine development has traditionally been carried out primarily by industry, although some of the basic research has been supported by public funds. Because of this private for-profit base of research, vaccine development has focused on the disease burden of those in the rich countries. It remains a challenge to bring the technology of vaccines to all of those who need it, and not just to those who can pay for it. Public–private initiatives are just beginning to gel around this theme, spearheaded by the World Health Organization, the World Bank, and several of the major bilateral foreign assistance agencies and nongovernmental organizations.

Among the recent victories for vaccines are the development of an acellular pertussis immunogen that is largely free of the severe adverse effects of the previously employed killed whole cell vaccine, the development of a *H. influenzae* type b (Hib) polysaccharide capsular–protein conjugate vaccine that protects against the invasive systemic complications of Hib infection, including pneumonia and meningitis *(19)*, the recent successful test of a multivalent pneumococcal polysaccharide–protein conjugate vaccine in the United States, the development of vaccines for hepatitis A and B and varicella, and a newly released reassortant rotavirus vaccine that blends the Jennerian approach of a naturally attenuated *Rhesus rotavirus* (analogous to Jenner's use of cowpox to immunize against smallpox) with the modern approach of genetically manipulated vaccine strains.

At the same time, the sad commentary is that the new pertussis vaccine is not being used in the developing world, where the cheap and more reactogenic pertussis component of standard diphtheria - tetanus-pertussis (DTP) is still employed, Hib vaccine is not available to the majority of children in developing countries, and the conjugate pneumococcal vaccine will, when licensed, be used in industrialized nations, where otitis media is the major problem, long before it reaches the developing nations, where invasive and lethal pneumonia and meningitis are common occurrences. In addition, hepatitis A vaccine is not available and only a few of the developing countries have implemented early immunization with hepatitis B vaccine, directed as much toward the reduction of adult hepatocellular carcinoma related to the virus as toward the prevention of clinical hepatitis. Varicella vaccine is slowly being implemented in the first world but will remain unavailable to the Third World for many years, and the newly licensed rotavirus vaccine, already recommended by the American Academy of Pediatrics for routine use in the United States, will present a challenge of economics to deliver to the infants of the developing nations, a million of whom die of this infection yearly.

Despite these technological successes, many challenges in vaccine development remain, especially with organisms that interact with the immune system in such a way that strong protective immune responses are not readily elicited, or because antigenic variation makes it difficult to identify useful conserved vaccine antigens. Such organisms represent particularly difficult targets for the vaccine developer, and include HIV and malaria. HIV has been difficult because it directly destroys immunological capacity and because antigenic variation so readily occurs in the surface glycoprotein targets for vaccine immunity. Malaria represents a different story, in which natural immunity is slow to develop, requires multiple encounters with the organism, which results in high morbidity and mortality while immunity is elicited, and because acquired protection dissipates readily and rapidly when the "immune" individual leaves the endemic region for relatively short periods of time. A hopeful new development has been the organization of a global collaborative network to focus on malaria vaccine development (the Multilateral Initiative on Malaria or MIM), whereas extensive work by the pharmaceutical industry and increasingly targeted research in the public sector toward an HIV vaccine offer increased promise of progress in the next few years. Few, however, would predict that a useful vaccine for either infection will result in the next decade *(20,21)*.

Molecular biology has made very significant contributions to the recent efforts in vaccine development. First, the ability to create genetically altered organisms has facilitated the task of identifying virulence factors by isolating their role in disease pathogenesis. The understanding that many virulence factors are only expressed in vivo has led to the development of appropriate models in tissue culture or in animals in order to search for in vivo expressed antigens, which then become prime targets for vaccine development. Second, selected and site-directed mutations can provide attenuated organisms or virulence molecules (e.g., biologically inactive but antigenically intact toxins involved in disease pathogenesis) for the purpose of eliciting immunity. Third, a new understanding of the function of the immune system has led to new approaches to presentation and delivery of new antigens specifically designed to activate particular limbs of the immune response. Of importance has been the development of attenuated live vaccines, carbohydrate–protein conjugates, protein subunits, and, more recently, DNA vaccines (22). Never have the prospects been better for progress. However, because the easy problems usually are solved sooner, the remaining diseases for which no useful vaccine is available generally represent the difficult cases or the orphan diseases for which little private sector resources have been made available.

An interesting case in point is the recent development of a vaccine for rotavirus (23). This is a universal infection throughout the world, targeting infants and children from 6 to 24 mo of age in developed and developing countries alike, and virtually all infants everywhere develop rotavirus infection and diarrhea. It is estimated that there are 50,000 hospitalizations annually in the United States for severe dehydration resulting from rotavirus, primarily from severe dehydration, with approximately 100 deaths. This results in an annual expenditure of around 500 million dollars for the costs of hospitalization and treatment of patients with severe rotavirus diarrhea. On top of this, a similar amount of money is lost in wages and productivity, as parents take leave from work in order to care for their sick infant. The impact on individuals in the developing world is even greater, and it is estimated that 1 million infants may die annually from rotavirus infection. Despite this toll in the developing world, the cost–benefits and affordability of this vaccine in developed countries will lead to its early implementation there, whereas developing countries will continue to experience the severe morbidity and mortality of rotavirus infection.

Four principal rotavirus serotypes affect humans, and because immunity is serotype-specific, it is necessary to have a multivalent vaccine. The first breakthrough was the discovery that a bovine rotavirus was attenuated for humans, and initial exploitation of this Jennerian opportunity produced evidence of vaccine-induced immunity. However, disease caused by the other serotypes continued unabated and this vaccine candidate was abandoned. Further work continued with a Rhesus monkey rotavirus of serotype III, which was also attenuated for humans. Rotaviruses are characterized by a segmented RNA genome, and because genetic reassortment between two different viruses occurs naturally, it was possible to create reassortants of the Rhesus rotavirus that had acquired the genes for human serotype-specific immunity. Reassortants expressing human serotype I, II, and IV were therefore combined with the serotype III native Rhesus rotavirus to create a quadrivalent vaccine that induces immunity and protects against severe infections and lethal disease resulting from all serotypes. Whereas much of the basic research underlying this vaccine was supported by public funds from the U.S. National Institutes of Health, the production and marketing of the vaccine has been transferred to industry. At present, vaccine efficacy in developing countries remains unproven; however, even if it is as effective as it has been in the United States, the current cost of the three-dose vaccine schedule will be 20–50 times greater than the per capita expenditure on health in the poor developing nations (24).

Currently recommended immunizations for children in the United States are shown in Table 2 (25,26). These recommendations are reviewed yearly, and, most recently, rotavirus vaccine has been added to the list. We may also anticipate addition of a pneumococcal polysaccharide conjugate vaccine in the near future,

if the initial safety and efficacy data are confirmed. Unfortunately, the situation in developing countries is quite different. It has taken over a decade of programmatic development by the Expanded Programme on Immunization of the World Health Organization to increase coverage of DTP, measles, polio, and bacille Calmette-Guérin (BCG) vaccines to greater than 50% in most developing countries, albeit some have done much better than this (5,6). Still, only rarely are hepatitis B and *H. influenzae* conjugate vaccines included in the national immunization plan, and nowhere is the current licensed unconjugated pneumococcal vaccine used, despite the importance of infections due to *S. pneumoniae* (19).

New vaccine-delivery techniques, such as jet injectors and national immunization days, when every age eligible infant and child is immunized regardless of prior immunization history, have helped to increase immunization coverage (27). Even in countries plagued by military insurrections, truces have been called in order to achieve maximum coverage during the national immunization campaign days. The multiple doses required for most vaccines, which require follow-up visits on a regular schedule, including the requirement for multiple injections, represent an impediment to increasing the percentage of children who receive the complete sequence of vaccine doses required for maximum induction of protective immunity. New combinations of vaccines and new adjuvants have the potential to increase compliance with full immunization in both developed and developing countries. Although these advances will help, reductions in cost are probably the most urgent need to improve vaccine coverage in the latter (28).

One of the concerns for the success of immunization programs in the Third World is the efficacy of the immunization in this setting. It is well known that nutrition impairs immune function, most particularly T-cell-mediated responses that may result in suboptimal immune response to vaccines. Indeed, vaccines have often been used as probes of the immune response in malnourished populations, with considerable evidence of an impairment in mucosal antibody-mediated immune responses and quantitatively decreased systemic antibody responses to polysaccharide versus protein antigens. However, protection derived from vaccines is a threshold phenomenon and, at any measured level of an immune response, may be conditioned by the inoculum size of the agent to which an individual is exposed. Thus, simply documenting a quantitatively diminished immune response to a vaccine does not necessarily translate into diminished protection, neither at the individual nor at the population level. This reality needs to be considered when interpreting the observations that below-standard indices of anthropometric status is associated with lower seroconversion rates or reduced titers of serum antibody and/or reduced delayed cutaneous hypersensitivity responses following vaccinations. Moreover, such reduced responses may be vaccine-specific and determined by immunogenetic factors present in that population. For example, in a recent study in Nigeria, infants and toddlers with deficits of weight-for-age had diminished postimmunization responses to BCG and poliomyelitis, but not to measles vaccination, compared to better nourished controls (29).

The relative role of nutritional deficits in conditioning poor immune responses to vaccines is not well understood. For example, tetanus toxoid is a classical protein antigen dependent on T lymphocyte help to induce an antibody immune response in mice. However, studies in severely malnourished humans suggest that tetanus toxoid still induces a level of antibody in the protective range. These studies generally examine the antibody response at

Table 2
Recommended Vaccines for Children in the United States

Vaccine	Composition	Efficacy	Adverse events
DtaP[a]	Toxoids and purified antigen	>95%	Local reactions
H. influenzae	Polysaccharide–protein conjugate	>95%	Local reactions
Hepatitis A		>95%	Local reactions
Hepatitis B	Virus subunits	>90%	Local reactions, Guillain–Barre
Measles, mumps, rubella combined	Live viruses	>95%	Encephalopathy (rare), parotitis, arthralgia
Pneumococcus	Polyvalent polysaccharide	>75%	Local reactions, fever
Rotavirus	Live viruses	>75%	Fever
Polio	Sequential inactivated and live oral virus	>95%	Rare vaccine-induced polio[b]

[a]Diphtheria and tetanus toxoids combined with acellular pertussis antigens.
[b]The new recommendation of two inactivated polio vaccine doses followed by two live oral vaccine doses is intended to reduce the frequency of vaccine-induced paralytic polio.

4 wk following primary or booster doses, and it may well be that the kinetics of the response in the malnourished host is delayed compared to that in a normally nourished host. However, for a population-based immunization program, it is not the speed with which protective immunity is achieved but rather the level of immunity achieved and its persistence over time. In the case of oral live polio vaccine, it is suspected that the presence of other enteroviruses in the intestinal tract result in competition for niche and interference with colonization of the gut by the vaccine strain. This is one explanation for the finding that the usual four-dose regimen in South India is inadequate to induce seroconversion in the majority of children; however, additional doses continue to increase the percentage that respond, independent of nutritional status.

An additional issue that remains unclear is the impact of nutritional status on the specific immune responses that develop following immunization. As an example, antibody immunity to polysaccharide antigens resides primarily in the IgG2 and IgG4 antibody subtypes, requiring a T-lymphocyte-mediated switch in isotype from IgM to the specific subtype of IgG in order to induce the most protective immune response (30). It is likely that subpopulations of T helper lymphocytes are involved in the activation of clones of B cells producing the different subtypes; therefore, differential effects of nutritional status on such subpopulations may condition the efficacy of the resulting immune response. The impact of nutrition on immune responses has not been studied to this level of sophistication and the implied questions remain unanswered.

THE "SEVENTH" IMMUNIZATION However, given the potential effect of nutrition on immune responses, including the responses to vaccines, some consideration has been given to the use of particular nutrients as potential "adjuvants" for the immune response at the time of immunization. Thus, a number of trials have given a protein supplement or vitamin A along with the vaccine in an attempt to enhance the immune response. This notion underlies the recent assertion that oral vitamin A (retinal palmitate) may represent the "seventh" immunization in the Expanded Programme of Immunization six-vaccine scheme. The basis for this is the biochemical action of vitamin A as a transcriptional gene regulator, including genes for antibody synthesis. This use of vitamin A could be a two-edged sword, however, with a presumably beneficial outcome if the response is enhanced and a detrimental one if the response is suppressed. Because this cannot be predicted a priori, field-based studies are needed to unravel the

issue, and the concurrent administration of high doses of vitamin A has been examined with respect to tetanus, measles, DPT, and poliomyelitis immunization. It should be remembered that the administration of vitamin A at the time of immunization also represents an opportunity to supplement the population with vitamin A at a point of contact that is relatively well organized by the EPI program, independent of any beneficial effect on the vaccine response *per se*.

With respect to tetanus toxoid, no effect of a supplemental dose of retinyl palmitate was demonstrated in Bangladeshi preschool children (31). When 200,000 IU of vitamin A was administered to older preschool-aged children in Indonesia 3 wk before a tetanus toxoid immunization, IgG antibody levels for tetanus were significantly enhanced in those children with pre-existing immunity for whom this was a booster injection inducing a secondary response. The experience with measles vaccination is both more extensive and more varied. In 1995, in Indonesia, Semba et al. (32) reported a 10% excess failure rate in seroconversion with measles vaccine given with 100,000 IU vitamin A in early infancy, as compared to those who had not received the supplement. In an accompanying editorial, Ross (33) commented that the "wisdom of giving vitamin A supplements with measles vaccine in programmes that vaccinate from six months (of age) is questionable." The original researchers returned to this question in a study with older (9-mo-old) Indonesian infants (34). In this study, there was a greater than 98% seroconversion rate with the concurrent administration of 100,000 IU along with measles immunization, significantly improved over the vaccine alone. Finally, in Bangladesh, Rahman et al. (35) found that 25,000 IU of retinyl palmitate, given at three monthly intervals in early life enhanced the cell-mediated skin test responses for diphtheria and tetanus toxoids and antibody responses to polio after the primary immunization series. This augmented response was seen only in those children in whom supplementation resulted in adequate circulating retinol levels. Those who received vitamin A but whose serum levels remained low generally remained anergic.

The safety of delivering high doses of vitamin A to young infants has been examined, but the results are conflicting and inconclusive. Agoestina et al. (36) in Indonesia claimed total safety and lack of adverse effects in terms of intracranial hemorrhage or increased intracranial pressure with the supplementation of 50,000 IU of retinyl palmitate compared to placebo in 2000 Indonesian children in the first semester of life. Although the rate of bulging fontanelle (5%) in those receiving vitamin A was twice that seen in the control children, this was discounted as a significant untoward or potentially harmful consequence of vitamin administration. On the other hand, Rahman et al. *(37)* observed bulging fontanelle in 5% of infants in the treatment group and 1% of those in the control group in a trial including 200 Bangladeshi infants in which 25,000 IU of vitamin A was given with the first immunizations. Another approach to improving vitamin A status in young infants has been pioneered by Stoltzfus et al. in Indonesia *(38)*, who have shown that most of a single, postpartum oral dose of 300,000 IU of retinyl palmitate given to a nursing mother is eventually delivered to the infant over the course of lactation. Administration of vitamin A to lactating women has become a standard recommendation of WHO for maternal and child health care programs in populations at risk of hypovitaminosis A. The caveat, however, is that because such a massive load of vitamin A would be teratogenic to an embryo *in utero*, it is imperative to ensure that the dose is given before there is any risk of concurrent pregnancy.

ENDEMIC MALNUTRITION

Malnutrition has often been equated with undernutrition, but its actual meaning is "bad nutrition," especially in the context of imbalanced nutrition *(39)*. This means that both polar extremes of deviation from normal intakes and status—deficient and excessive—represent a potential for malnutrition *(40)*. There are a number of dietary constituents that must be considered. First are the macronutrients; that is, substances that can be sources of energy. These include protein, carbohydrate, fat, and, in some settings, alcohol. Protein has a hierarchical use. The first priority for dietary protein is as a source of amino acids as primary building blocks for protein synthesis, including structural proteins, transporters, enzymes, hormones, regulatory and messenger proteins, antibodies, and acute-phase response proteins. Only then, do proteins normally enter into energy metabolism pathways. We recognize 13 organic compounds as essential vitamins and at least 20 elements can be classified as nutrients.

In the domain of protein and energy nutrition, there is a spectrum of manifestations related to imbalances in the diet. At the extreme end of starvation, nutritional marasmus occurs. Acute protein deficiency in excess of energy-deficiency leads to the severe edematous malnutrition syndrome, kwashiorkor. With the increased recognition of clinical markers of these deficiency states and considerable attention given to assessing nutritional status in primary health care schemes, these extreme syndromes have become less common *(41)*. The application of a more sophisticated evaluation of body composition has allowed a better characterization of a continuous scale of intermediate nutritional states. Shortness of stature, a substantial deficit of height-for-age termed stunting, is often termed "chronic" protein-energy malnutrition. This is not necessarily the case because most of the retardation of linear growth is established before 3 yr of age *(42–44)* and does not document an ongoing process *(45)*. A deficit of weight-for-height (wasting), on the other hand, can be considered to represent acute energy deficit. When there is excessive storage of energy, gradations of obesity are present. In demographic terms, wasting affects up to a quarter of the populations in some poor societies in Africa *(46)*; it is now relatively rare in Latin America and Asia, except in times of famine.

Much more common and widespread are deficiencies of micro-nutrients, including vitamins and minerals. As priorities in global public health, the nutritional anemias, hypovitaminosis A, and iodine deficiency have long represented the trinity of single-nutrient human deficiency states requiring urgent attention. Thus, these three were designated worldwide priorities at the World Summit for Children in 1990 *(47)* and designated concerns of "hidden hunger" in a technical follow-up conference in 1991 *(48)*. Recent studies have identified zinc deficiency as another critical single-nutrient deficiency affecting immune responses.

Nutritional anemia is primarily the result of iron deficiency *(49)*, although in malaria-endemic regions, the frequent bouts of clinical malaria and hemolysis contributes in a significant manner. However, iron deficiency produces a series of functional deficits beyond those ascribable to the impaired transport of oxygen to tissues *(50)*. Because of its essential role in iron metalloenzymes needed for DNA synthesis and cell replication, a critical part of the immune response as clones of responding lymphocytes must rapidly divide, iron deficiency can significantly impair immune responses. In addition, the functional role of iron in enzymes involved in oxidative metabolism and the production of antimicrobial oxygen free radicals implicates iron deficiency as a cause of reduced microbicidal capacity. In developing countries, iron deficiency is common in late infancy and the toddler years, when the burden of infection is greatest, and there is reason to believe there is a relationship between the two phenomena *(49,51)*.

Vitamin A deficiency leading to endemic hypovitaminosis A is prevalent in most developing countries, often at levels that do not lead to vitamin-A deficient eye signs or symptoms. Hypovitaminosis A is strongly associated with indices of poverty and poor sanitation, and a history of a curtailed lactation and certain dietary habits are the most powerful determinants of individual cases of vitamin A deficiency *(52,53)*. The consequences of vitamin A deficiency are most serious in preschool children, and multiple large-scale field studies have demonstrated a relationship between vitamin A nutrition and all-cause mortality, with vitamin A supplements reducing mortality by some 25–35%.

Iodine deficiency, initially identified as endemic goiter and cretinism, is a common finding in populations living away from the coast, as iodine has been leached out of most inland soils over the millennia and is present in inadequate amounts in locally produced vegetables and grains. In the past two decades, the concept of iodine deficiency as "endemic goiter" has been broadened to iodine-deficiency disorders (IDD) *(54)* to emphasize a variety of manifestations other than thyroid enlargement or cretinism. Whereas the world's population at risk of IDD is estimated to be 1 billion *(55)*, iodine deficiency has come under progressive control since the World Summit for Children, as the proportion of iodine-fortified salt consumed in developing countries had increased to 60% from <10% in 1990 *(56)*. The lack of evidence that iodine deficiency is associated with increased infectious disease risk lends further credence to substitute zinc deficiency for iodine deficiency in the action agenda, as discussed later.

It is now widely believed that marginal zinc status and overt zinc deficiency is endemic throughout the populations of developing countries *(57,58)*. Zinc is also required for DNA and protein synthesis because of its role in both DNA transcription and RNA translation *(59,60)*. Thus, zinc deficiency can restrict rapid multiplication and clonal expansion of critical cell populations in the immune response. Because of its essential role in zinc-binding finger loop domains, known as "zinc fingers," which are involved in conformational stabilization of transcription factor proteins that permit sequence-specific DNA recognition and gene expression, zinc deficiency can also limit the translation of proteins involved in host defenses *(53)*. In addition, thymus-derived peptides believed to function as thymic hormones in the differentiation of T cells are zinc metalloproteins *(61)*. At least in vitro, when these proteins are stripped of zinc they do not function as maturational signals. Zinc deficiency can specifically diminish the T-lymphocyte response by impairing the development of mature function T lymphocytes. Thus, in a number of ways, abnormal zinc nutrition can be related to heightened infection susceptibility and/or severity, and this has been shown in field studies of lower respiratory tract and diarrheal disease *(62,63)* and, more recently, malaria (Sazawal, unpublished data).

IMPROVING MICRONUTRIENT INTAKE AND STATUS OF POPULATIONS

If micronutrient status affects immune response to infection and immunization, improving intake of these nutrients can have an important impact on the burden of infectious diseases. Current public health teaching suggests four distinct (and not mutually exclusive) strategies for improving the micronutrient status of a population:

1. Supplementation *(36,64,65)*.
2. Fortification of specific foods or dietary components such as salt or sugar *(66)*.
3. Dietary change and diversification *(67,68)*.
4. Attention to remedial health conditions that interfere with micronutrient intake, absorption, or utilization.

The first three strategies are germane to the present discussion, as they represent measures aimed at enhancing the consumption of specific nutrients.

Supplementation can be undertaken with therapeutic or prophylactic intent, depending on the particular circumstances. The dosage of the supplementary nutrients can range from a fraction of the daily recommended intake to the full recommended dietary allowance (RDA), as in the over-the-counter multivitamin–mineral preparations. It must be understood, however, that the RDA is determined as the dietary levels needed to maintain healthy levels of the nutrient in the majority of a population, usually adults in industrialized nations. These levels are rarely determined for infants and children or in populations in developing countries, where local environmental or genetic factors can affect the population need. Alternatively, supplements of several multiples of the daily recommendation can be offered as in those sold in "health food" stores or sometimes prescribed by physicians, practitioners of holistic medicine, or even health authorities, whether or not evidence supports such practices.

Fortification involves the addition of micronutrients to commonly consumed foods and beverages or dietary constituents. Conventionally, at the public health level, vehicles that reach across whole populations are targets for micronutrient fortification, including salt, sugar, flour, cooking oil, and margarine *(69)*. Potable drinking water has long been exploited in the rich countries as a vehicle for fluoridation to reduce dental caries; however, water can also be fortified with iodine *(70)* and iron *(71)*. Salt has been used extensively as the vehicle for iodine and fluoride

and is also capable of bearing calcium and iron *(69)*. Sugar can be a vehicle for vitamin A and iron, and oil and margarine could be vehicles for vitamin A *(66)*. Additionally, cereal flours can be fortified with thiamin, riboflavin, niacin, folic acid, vitamin B_{12}, iron, calcium, and iodine *(69)*.

Foods and beverages other than basic staples that are consumed on a selective and voluntary basis may also provide substantial amounts of micronutrients, in part through the addition of exogenous vitamins and minerals. Many breakfast cereals provide 100% of the recommended allowances of vitamins and major minerals in a single serving with milk. In Latin America, one manufacturer fortifies its brand of corn flakes with zinc. Fruit juices and fruit drinks often contain a day's supply of vitamin C in a single serving. Foods targeted to specific populations also provide examples for the use of micronutrient fortificants. Infant formulas are fortified with iron. Milk for school programs in South America often contains iron. Similarly, the snacks served at recess breaks in elementary schools throughout developing countries are increasingly being enriched with iron, vitamin A, and other micronutrients of local public health importance.

Dietary diversification is a strategy to encourage consumers to enrich their dietary intakes of specific micronutrients by consuming foods that are rich in these nutrients. This can be accomplished either by replacing other foods or adding new foods to their diets. For instance, if one adds milk, cheese, or yogurt to a diet poor in these foods, high intakes of calcium and riboflavin are assured, and if this is not a substitution for an equivalent source, then total intakes will be increased. Similarly, ingestion of citrus fruits will raise intakes of vitamin C, whereas consumption of liver will provide increased vitamin A, iron, vitamin B_{12}, folic acid, and the majority of the B-complex vitamins. For affluent individuals in whom low micronutrient status is the result of the poor selection of food items, dietary diversification is a viable strategy for achieving an adequate intake of recommended nutrients. For the low-income inhabitants of low-income countries, the traditional fare is largely of plant origin and characterized by absent or low contents of some vitamins and minerals and poor biological availability for others. Dietary diversification to include foods of animal origin is generally an unreachable goal and it may be necessary to target the dietary change strategy to the consumption of edible plants with high micronutrient content.

Plants are sources of provitamin A carotenoids, the precursors of vitamin A. It has conventionally been considered that 6 mg of beta-carotene has the vitamin A equivalency of 1 mg of the preformed vitamin; however, when real foods with their complex matrices were the dietary form of provitamin A, the validity of this relationship was questioned *(72)*. In field studies conducted in Indonesia, de Pee et al. *(73)* showed minimal effects of cooked vegetables on vitamin A nutriture or milk content of vitamin A in lactating women. Indeed, it may take up to two to four times as many edible plants to supply the desired intake of vitamin A. Manipulating the intake of plants is also problematic for improving human iron status, and there is no solid evidence for an impact of dietary education on the prevention of iron deficiency and iron-deficiency anemia. This means that consuming more iron-containing plants or vitamin C sources is not likely to impact nutritional status of these nutrients. This is particularly relevant to improving the nutrient status of the most nutritionally vulnerable of all groups, infants and children between 6 mo and 3 yr in the weaning period, because both the acceptability of and gastric capacity for bulky vegetable dishes is lowest in this segment of the population.

ADDITIONAL CONSIDERATIONS ON UPTAKE OF MICRONUTRIENTS FROM SUPPLEMENTS There are physiological constraints on the efficacy of regimens based on high-dose supplements, as some—but not all—micronutrients can be absorbed and retained with suitable efficiency to justify this dosage format. Vitamin A and vitamin B_{12} are stored in the liver in almost limitless amounts and with long half-lives. Iron can be stored in muscle, liver, and bone marrow with high efficiency. However, most of the other water-soluble vitamins are poorly retained and are rapidly excreted or metabolized. Parenteral (injection) doses of the former three nutrients would be avidly retained; however, ample evidence shows that therapeutic parenteral administration of iron is dangerous (74). Parenteral administration of iodine is a unique story. Although the nutrient is normally stored in the thyroid gland, intramuscular injection of iodine in oil (Lipiodol, Guerbet Laboratories, France) forms a deposit of iodine in the muscle that is slowly transferred to the thyroid gland. It can be retained in this format for 2 yr or more. Unfortunately, the transmission of infectious diseases, including hepatitis B and C, HIV, and others by blood, is facilitated by the reuse of hypodermic needles in community settings.

The fractional absorption of an oral dose of the nutrients relevant to public health micronutrient programs is also variable (75). Whereas vitamin A is 70% absorbable, inorganic iron is absorbed variably, depending on the iron status of the host and total oral load. For example, from an oral dose of 60 mg of iron as ferrous sulfate, a severely iron-deficient individual or pregnant woman might take up 6 mg of the metal per dosing. This could fall to 1 mg or less in an iron-replete individual receiving a supplemental dose. Iodine in its soluble, iodide form is absorbed with high (90%) efficiency; however, an alternative form, iodine-in-oil, has a lower bioavailability (76). Folic acid has an absorption efficiency of from 30% to 60%, and vitamin B_{12}, which is absorbed from 20% to 60%, should be given with intrinsic factor in order to ensure the administered dose is maximally absorbed. Zinc derived from chemical salts in the absence of meals is absorbed with an efficiency of just 10–40%.

Consideration must be given to margins for safety, the upper limits of daily nutrient intake above which toxicity manifestations become likely (77). The margin between the recommended daily intake dosage and the highest observed safe level from nutrient to nutrient is well over 100-fold for riboflavin, 10-fold for iron, 6.5-fold for vitamin A, and 4-fold for zinc. Concomitant disease states can increase the toxicity of certain nutrients; for example, renal insufficiency and liver disease which decrease the margin of toxicity for vitamin A (78).

THE SOURCE OF UNCERTAINTIES

Despite the sound, fundamental theoretical basis for the interaction of malnutrition and infection, discussed at great length elsewhere in this book, many uncertainties remain regarding the clinical implications for human populations. One important issue is whether or not the relationship has a nutritional or a pharmacological basis (79). Current knowledge is based on cross-sectional studies in which the strength of the association between nutrition and infectious diseases are explored and longitudinal intervention studies in which nutritional status is deliberately altered and the

outcome is measured as a corresponding reduction in infection. The former approach represents a quest for associations between lesser nutritional status and greater susceptibility to an infection or its consequences; the latter seeks to establish a relationship between better nutriture and diminished infection morbidity or mortality. The stability and accuracy of the diagnostic measures for nutrient assessment are critical factors in establishing these associations, whether the individual or the group is the unit of analysis. These become substantial issues in the assessment of vitamin A, iron, or zinc status. For vitamin A, circulating retinol, which is the most commonly used index, does not represent the hepatic stores, except at the extremes of depletion and toxic excess. Moreover, infections themselves redistribute retinol from the circulating pool in the acute-phase response (80), further compounding assessment of nutritional status. Iron reserves are reflected by serum ferritin concentrations in steady-state conditions. However, ferritin is also an acute-phase reactant protein, and its measurement overestimates iron deficiency in individuals and populations with ongoing infection (81). Zinc status is most often assessed by assaying its concentration in the blood; however, there is both a poor correspondence with tissue status and variability based on technical matters and the presence of an acute-phase response that leads to reduced circulating zinc levels (82). As a consequence, the reliability of associations between nutritional status determined in the usual fashion and infections is suspect.

Interventional studies provide an opportunity to go beyond association to probable causality, by comparing the outcome variable between preintervention and postintervention periods. The interpretation of such studies is usually based on the assumption that undernourished individuals will be improved and benefit by the intervention, whereas those who are initially adequately nourished will be relatively unaffected. Unfortunately, logistic and/or cultural barriers often make nutritional assessment impossible in studies in the developing world. In some investigations, clinical manifestations of deficiency such as xerophthalmia have been used (83). In other studies, attempts to assess status have been made on just a small subsegment of the population (84,85) or, in other instances, not at all (86). Interpretation is also confounded by the general use of micronutrient supplements and variations in form and dose between studies conducted in different populations. In addition, most of the field trials have been conducted with high-dose supplements.

These problems make it difficult to resolve the questions of whether the effects of interventions detected in field trials are pharmacological or nutritional in nature and whether nutritional interventions act by reversing a pre-existing deficiency or by promoting a change across the whole population, irrespective of nutrient status.

NUTRITIONAL STATUS AND THE EXPERIENCE OF INFECTIONS

VITAMIN A Cross-sectional studies relating vitamin A status or intake to infectious diseases experience have been used to examine the effect of the nutrient on disease susceptibility. Studies from Indonesia (83), India, and Thailand (87) followed preschool children diagnosed as at-risk from hypovitaminosis A based on the presence of xerophthalmia or low retinol levels. An increased incidence of respiratory infections was documented, and in Indonesia, an increase in diarrheal incidence was noted as well. More recently, premature infants in South Africa with the lowest serum retinol levels were reported to have the highest incidence of respiratory disease (88). In older South African children, the retinol level on admission was found to be an independent risk predictor for ARI and severity (89). A study from the Sudan, in which dietary intake of vitamin A rather than any index of status was the predictive variable, found an association of increased intake and decreased rates of diarrhea and cough plus fever (90). This was observed both before and after an intervention program with high-dose vitamin A supplementation, and the intervention had no influence on the clinical findings.

Vitamin A has been employed as an adjunctive therapy with supportive hydration therapy in secretory diarrhea. In a study conducted in Bangladesh, no additional benefit on the course of noncholera watery diarrhea was observed in children randomly assigned to high-dose supplements of vitamin A compared to placebo (91). Another study carried out in 900 Indian children, aged 1–5 yr, provided high-dose vitamin A during diarrhea of 7 d duration or less (92). When stratified by their breast-feeding status at the time of admission, children who were still receiving any maternal milk derived no benefit from the vitamin A supplement. In contrast, episodes of acute diarrhea in fully weaned children were significantly less severe, shorter in duration, and less likely to become persistent in those receiving vitamin A as part of their treatment regimen.

Vitamin A has also been tested as a potential complementary treatment together with standard combined drug therapy for children with pulmonary tuberculosis. In one randomized, comparative clinical trial in children with an average circulating retinol level on admission of 18 μg/dL high-dose vitamin A had no effect on the outcome of standard therapy (93). In nontuberculous acute respiratory infection in preschool children admitted to the hospital in Guatemala with X-ray-confined pulmonary infections randomized to receive high-dose vitamin A or placebo along with appropriate antibiotics and supportive therapy, no differences in severity, duration of hospitalization, or mortality were observed between treatment groups (94). However, the national program to reduce endemic hypovitaminosis A in Guatemala by fortification of sugar may have improved baseline vitamin A status in these patients and altered their ability to respond to acute treatment with vitamin A.

Vitamin A has become a recommended adjuvant in the treatment of measles patients sick enough to be hospitalized. This is based on the results from a randomized, double-blind clinical trial carried out in Capetown, South Africa among measles patients hospitalized for severe complications. Patients in the treatment group received a total dose of 400,000 IU of water-miscible vitamin A in divided doses on the day of admission and the subsequent day. Recovery from pneumonia and diarrhea were more rapid in the supplemented group, and these children experienced a lower mortality rate (95). A subsequent retrospective comparison of outcome of patients hospitalized because of severe measles in the preperiod and postperiod of routine administration of Vitamin A was performed. The mortality rate fell from 5% to 1.6% and the duration of hospitalization and utilization of intensive care were lower after adoption of routine vitamin A for these patients (96).

To determine if vitamin A administration had any impact on less severe measles infections in the community, an outpatient study on the use of vitamin A was carried out in Zambia (97). Following a single oral dose of 200,000 IU of oil-soluble vitamin or placebo, those receiving supplementary vitamin A had less cough but they also recovered more slowly from pneumonia if it developed. Unfortunately, both the form of the supplement and the dose was altered in this study compared to the Capetown study and it is possible that this explains the difference in results. Alternatively, the lesser severity of disease in the outpatient study could preclude the detection of a difference due to the treatment.

A particularly striking effect of routine periodic administration of vitamin A has been shown to reduce all-cause mortality in infants and children in a number of studies. The initial findings were reported in 1983 from a study designed to examine the effects of vitamin administration on progression of eye disease in children with mild signs of xerophthalmia (nightblindness, Bitot's spots) at a baseline survey examination (98). At least 10 prospective, intervention studies have since been conducted and published in peer-reviewed journals, and several meta-analyses have been performed (e.g., refs. 99 and 100). Meta-analysis indicates a 25–30% reduction in all-cause mortality in subjects receiving vitamin A supplements, with the exception of two studies—one in Hyderabad, India (101) and the other from the Sudan (86). The significance of the finding is given further credence by the finding of the life-sparing effect of the vitamin A intervention, as there is excess mortality in the placebo-treatment limbs of the trials. Controversy has remained about the effects of vitamin A on infants, especially those under 6 mo of age. Of the two studies that have addressed this, one, in Indonesia, showed a reduction in mortality rates (102), whereas the second, carried out in Nepal, reported no difference in mortality between the two groups (103).

Prophylactic administration of Vitamin A has also had inconsistent effects on morbidity, with some studies finding a reduction in diarrheal or respiratory disease morbidity, whereas others using the same dose and dose interval find no effect. The effects, when found, are often based on symptom complexes not otherwise etiologically defined. For example, placebo-treated infants studied in Indonesia had an increased hospitalization rate for cough and fever (102), but there was no difference between groups in the infant cohort in Nepal (103). Some studies have been designed to detect differences in morbidity between the intervention and control groups. In one study in South India, there were no effects on childhood illness from periodic administration of high-dose vitamin A to preschool children (104). Another investigation in northeastern Brazil reported only a slight decrease in the incidence of severe episodes of diarrhea and no effect on acute respiratory illnesses as a consequence of vitamin A assignment (105). The effect is not strikingly enhanced in HIV-infected children either. For example, in a study in Durban, South Africa, 118 infants born of HIV-positive mothers were followed for up to 15 mo (mean = 8 mo) and given either an age-appropriate dose of vitamin A or a placebo at 1 and 3 mo of age and every 3 mo thereafter. Only when respiratory and diarrheal morbidity was pooled was there a significant reduction in the intervention group. Vitamin A did, however, significantly reduce diarrheal morbidity in those infants who had become HIV infected. An in-depth review of studies bearing on the hypothesis relating supplemental vitamin A to disease experience concludes the relationship to be inconsistent and the overall findings to be unremarkable (106).

IRON The relationship of iron status and iron supplements to the incidence and severity of infection is complex (107,108). In particular, there are differences of opinion regarding the adverse effect of iron deficiency on immune response and the risk of infectious morbidity and the concept that acute iron administration or iron-overload syndromes provide pathogens with needed iron and enhance infection. The accumulated experience suggests that iron deficiency generally impairs host defenses and increases infection morbidity; however, malaria replication may be increased by iron administration via increased hemoglobin synthesis, and certain organisms lacking efficient iron acquisition mechanisms are more prevalent and virulent in individuals with iron-overload syndromes.

ZINC Acute and chronic diarrheal disease are one of the leading causes of death among children under 5 yr of age. With increased understanding of the role of zinc in immune function and the evidence that zinc deficiency is common whenever protein intake is marginal, several trials of zinc supplementation to reduce morbidity have been undertaken. The design of these trials is different from the vitamin A trials because, unlike vitamin A, zinc is not stored after a bolus dose and must, instead, be continuously dosed. Although there is variation in the response from study to study, the overall impression is that zinc supplementation has advanced control of the immediate evolution of an episode of watery diarrhea and dehydration (79,108,109). In one large cohort study in India, including 937 children aged 6–35 mo, the inclusion of 20 mg/d of zinc as part of oral rehydration therapy reduced the number of watery stools and the number of days of purging (62).

Studies in three nations—India (110), Guatemala (111), and Mexico (112)–have addressed the question whether or not prophylactic zinc supplementation reduced infectious morbidity. In India, the study involved a follow-up interventional trial of the cohort enrolled in the earlier therapeutic study (62). A cohort of 570 children aged 6–35 mo were randomly assigned to a maintenance dose of 10 mg of elemental zinc daily or placebo. The subsequent incidence of dysentery and the progression of acute episodes of watery diarrhea into persistent diarrhea lasting over 14 d was reduced significantly. These effects were most pronounced in the group of children 1 yr of age and older and in those with low initial circulating zinc concentrations. In Guatemala, a cohort of rural indigenous preschoolers in a mountain village receiving either 10 mg of elemental zinc or placebo were followed (111). The intervention decreased the incidence of acute and persistent diarrhea but had no effect on acute respiratory infections over a period of 7 mo. In Mexico, a factorial design was used to study the effects of iron and zinc alone and combined (112). Preschoolers in a rural, highlands village were followed for a year while receiving four randomly assigned daily treatments: placebo; 20 mg of elemental iron alone; 20 mg of zinc alone; and a combination of iron and zinc. Both zinc-containing regimens reduced diarrheal morbidity by 40%; however, there were no differences in the experience of respiratory diseases among the four groups.

RIBOFLAVIN Although riboflavin status has been virtually ignored in public health of late, riboflavin status may be particularly important in malaria-hyperendemic regions. In a study in India, riboflavin-deficient individuals had lower parasitization of red cells, but clinical recovery from an episode of malaria was slower compared to those with better riboflavin nutrition (113). Levels of malonyldialdehyde, a circulating marker of lipid peroxidation of cell membranes, was found to be higher in malaria-infected children than in controls as well as in riboflavin-deficient than riboflavin-sufficient subjects. It is proposed that riboflavin deficiency restricts the regeneration of reduced glutathione, mak-

ing the parasitized erythrocyte more vulnerable to destructive lipid peroxidation and increasing plasma lipid hydroperoxides (114).

DIET AND CHILDHOOD DISEASES

In contrast to dietary deficiencies and supplements, the influence of the pattern of food consumption and specific nutrient and non-nutrient components in the diet on susceptibility to infectious diseases has not been systematically examined. The diet is, of course, the source of food-borne pathogens and contamination of food remains a major route for the transmission of infectious agents (115). In addition, there is increasing understanding that the pattern of consumption of foods and beverages influences susceptibility or resistance to chronic degenerative diseases, including cardiovascular, neoplastic, and inflammatory diseases (116). Although the specific dietary components involved are not known, they may include the presence or absence of chemical constituents not considered to be essential nutrients themselves. Putative protective substances include dietary fiber (cellulose, hemicellulose, lignin, pectin, oligosaccharides), phytic acid, oxalic acid, carotenoids, organic acids, phytosterols, and flavonoids (117). Among the potentially noxious substances are soluble carbohydrates, alcohols, aflatoxins, trans fatty acids, and rare earth metals. It is possible that various combinations, imbalances and interactions among these substances, perhaps interacting with the genetic constitution of individuals and/or in the presence of other environmental exposures, determine chronic disease risk. If this complex interaction of multiple factors, including diet, constitutes the risk for chronic disease, then it becomes understandable why progress has been slow in deciphering these relationships.

There may be similar relationships between diet and infectious diseases. It is known, for example, that the intestinal flora represents an ecosystem that may exclude the implantation or colonization of pathogens via niche occupancy or the production of antimicrobial substances (e.g., colicins) (118). The initial gut flora that colonizes breast-fed infants, composed primarily of *Bifidobacterium bifidis*, resists colonization by other bacteria and provides one level of protection against enteric infections. Unpasteurized fermented foods may introduce bacteria into the intestinal flora with salutary effects in older individuals and provide significant resistance to the colonization of the intestine by pathogens or assist in their clearance. This concept of using selected microbial agents as probiotics has recently been demonstrated in clinical trials in which the administration of a human colonizing strain of *Lactobacillus* successfully treated and prevented recurrence of antibiotic related diarrhea caused by *Clostridium diffiicile* (119).

Natural antioxidants in the diet may be an important part of host defenses against infections (120). As the data implicating oxidative mechanisms in infectious disease pathogenesis and pathophysiology for both bacterial (121) and viral (122) diseases increase, the significance of dietary antioxidant intake becomes more relevant. This may be the explanation for the effects of dietary vitamin A in reducing diarrheal and respiratory disease morbidity in the Sudanese (90). These dietary sources were actually provitamin A carotenoids present in local edible plants and it is at least possible that these dietary constituents were a marker for the foods with protective qualities, rather than the specific mediator of the effects.

As these effects of diet are explored, the new science of food technology and engineering presents us with many new situations in which food may plan an important role in the host–pathogen interaction. The food industry has created new chemical dietary compounds (e.g., non-nutritive sweeteners and sucrose polyesters) used as artificial fats and the synthetic capacity of the approach appears to be unlimited. Although we do not yet know how the long-term consumption of these "new foods" will alter health, it may be possible to develop components that influence microbial pathogens at least locally in the intestinal tract. It is also possible that adverse interactions among flora, pathogens, and the hereto-fore unheard of food substances being invented and introduced into the human diet will become apparent.

It is also worthwhile to point out that diet may affect the pharmacology and pharmacokinetics of therapeutic agents used in the treatment of infection. One mechanism for this is the influ-ence of food or specific constituents of diet on the absorption of drugs or their capacity to induce side effects (123,124). It is interesting that charcoal-broiled meats and cruciferous vegetables induce the metabolism of xenobiotics, whereas protein levels in the diet are strong mediators of drug clearance. Hence, diet can lead both to loss of efficacy and to unexpected toxicity of drugs.

UNDERNUTRITION AND NUTRIENT LOSSES RESULTING FROM INFECTIONS

Infections, via the inflammatory response and the production of cytokines with metabolic effects, induce both a catabolic state and an anabolic state in which metabolic priorities are reordered toward the synthesis of proteins with host defense capacity. By these (and other) mechanisms, infection is a cause of malnutrition and, indeed, it has been proposed that control of infection is one of the best ways to prevent childhood malnutrition (125). This strategy is currently reflected in international health policy (6).

Decreased intake of food, one of the most common responses to infection, is an obvious contributor to undernutrition in this setting. The effects of anorexia, mediated by the inflammatory cytokines (126,127) are compounded by the frequent cultural response of withholding of diet and food taboos, which account for both a quantitative and qualitative change in nutrient intake, respectively. Mothers have specific beliefs and practices regarding the feeding of sick children, some of which are now thought to be detrimental. For example, indigenous Peruvian mothers reduce the offering of non-breast-milk foods during diarrheal episodes (128), whereas in a Mayan-speaking mountain village in central Guatemala, mothers prefer to offer more liquid foods of presum-ably less nutrient density during episodes of both diarrhea and respiratory infections (129). Similar examples abound in the nutri-tional anthropology literature.

Maldigestion and malabsorption are additional mechanisms altering the availability of food-derived nutrients (45,130). Loss and wastage of nutrients already taken up by the body is the final mechanism by which infection promotes undernutrition. Three-quarters of total-body iron is found in the erythron; hence, bleeding is a direct mechanism of nutrient loss (131). Thus, hookworm infections produce variable, but occasionally heavy daily iron losses that result in clinically significant iron deficiency (108). For this reason, some public health workers have advocated mass drug therapy with anthelminthics as a measure to reverse iron deficiency in hookworm-endemic areas (132). Heavy infection with *Trichuris trichiura* (133) and amebic colitis and schistosomia-sis (130) are other direct causes of iron deficiency.

The activation of the acute-phase response leads to urinary losses of nutrients, including nitrogen, zinc, and iron. The impor-tance of vitamin A losses has recently been highlighted by studies in Bangladesh (134). Infants given oral vitamin A at 2, 3, and 4 mo who suffered respiratory infections during the period of supplementation failed to raise their circulating retinol levels. As a follow-up study, Peruvian children with acute diarrheal disease were studied in a metabolic ward, allowing for complete collection of excreta (135). There was no urinary vitamin A loss among healthy children, but renal loss of vitamin A proceeded at a rate of 1.44 mμmol of retinol per 24 h on d 1, 0.62 on d 2 and 0.23 on d 4, for a cumulative mean loss of 2.25 mμmol. The highest excretion of urinary vitamin A was associated with febrile episodes of diarrhea.

Acute watery diarrhea is also responsible for the loss of nutri-ents from the intestinal tract itself. Guatemalan children receiving oral rehydration fluid were shown to lose endogenous iron, zinc, and copper into the stools (136). The losses of zinc amounted to a day's requirement of the nutrient. Shigellosis is also well documented to result in protein-losing enteropathy (137).

The significance of these losses may be underestimated because of the usually short and self-limited duration of these infections. Whereas the losses in any individual episode may be inconsequen-tial for overall host nutritional status and readily repaired during convalescence, the cumulative impact of repeated infections can be severe. Although episodic, diarrhea and respiratory infections are frequent and recurrent in children in poor developing countries. In many such settings, children may experience infections during 30–40% of their first year or two of life (39). Because it takes much longer to replete the host of these losses than it does to cause them in the first place, and because the diet is often limiting in protein, energy, and micronutrients, development of clinically overt malnutrition commonly occurs. This is readily seen in the retardation in linear growth and the reduction in weight for length in infants so affected.

NUTRITIONAL INTERVENTIONS IN INFECTED INDIVIDUALS

Given these inevitable mediator-driven alterations in nutritional status during infection, the obvious question is whether or not compensatory feeding of nutrient-dense diets has any favorable impact in nutrient-wasting situations? First, solid and semisolid foods as well as oral rehydration solutions increase the fecal volume in children with watery diarrhea, although there is net gain in water and salt absorbed. Because total nutrient absorption also increases under such circumstances, it is therefore recom-mended that the caloric density of the oral rehydration fluids used to manage diarrheal episodes be increased, that breast-feeding be maintained, and that a normal diet be introduced early in the recovery regimen (138). There is a nuance to feeding associated with acute lower respiratory infections, which are known to inter-fere with alveolar diffusion of gases. Given the increase in energy consumption during infection, the increased CO_2 produced from energy metabolism can become a complicating issue. As carbohy-drate generates more CO_2 than fat, a high-fat, low-carbohydrate regimen has theoretical merit for refeeding of children with severe acute respiratory infections. Second, because the anorexia associ-ated with the production of inflammatory cytokines (which occurs coincidentally with consumption of body stores and appears to be designed to reduce voluntary work such as foraging for food in order to redirect metabolism toward the acute-phase response) appears to have been selected through evolution, there may be a danger in attempting to overcome this behavior. Some data support this concept. Monkeys infected with yellow fever viruses become anorectic and generally survive the experimental infection, but when force fed by the parenteral route, their mortality rate increases (Wannemacher, personal communication). Similarly, the use of parenteral iron to reverse the acute hypoferremia during acute infection has been shown to increase infection morbidity and mortality *(74,139)*.

There is great need to better understand the benefits and risks of feeding during infectious diseases in populations with different nutritional status at the outset, in those with protein-energy malabsorption, and in those with specific micronutrient deficiencies and in different infectious diseases so that we may assist the healing process and, in so doing, do no harm.

REFERENCES

1. Scrimshaw NS, Taylor CE, Gordon JE. Interaction of nutrition and infection. Am J Med Sci 1959; 237:367–403.
2. Caldwell P. Child survival: physical vulnerability and resilience in adversity in the European past and the contemporary Third World. Soc Sci Med 1996; 43:609–19.
3. Ebrahim GJ. Malnutrition and the child survival revolution. J Trop Pediatrics 1998; 44:126–7.
4. Pelletier DL, Frongllo EA Jr, Schroeder DG, Habicht JP. A methodology for estimating the contribution of malnutrition to child mortality in developing countries. J Nutr 1994; 124(suppl 10):2106S–22S.
5. World Health Organization/UNICEF. Joint WHO/UNICEF statement on vitamin A for measles. Wkly Epidemiol Rec 1987; 62: 133–4.
6. Campbell H, Gove S. Integrated management of childhood infections and malnutrition. A global initiative. Arch Dis Child 1996; 75:468–71.
7. Karaivanova GM. Viral respiratory infections and their role as public health problem in tropical countries. Afr J Med Sci 1995; 24:1–7.
8. Baird JK. Age-dependent characteristics of protection vs. susceptibility to *Plasmodium falciparum*. Ann Trop Med Parasitol 1998; 92:367–90.
9. Rowland MG, Cole TJ, Whitehead RG. A quantitative study into the role of infection in determining nutritional status in Gambian village children. Br J Nutr 1997; 37:441–50.
10. Pearson RD, Cox G, Jeronimo SM, Castracane J, Drew JS, Evans T, et al. Visceral leishmaniasis: a model for infection-induced cachexia. Am J Trop Med Hyg 1992; 47:8–15.
11. Warren KS. Schistosomiasis: host–pathogen biology. Rev Infect Dis 1982; 4:771–5.
12. Bundy DA. Immunoepidemiology of intestinal helminthic infections. I. The global burden of intestinal nematode disease. Trans R Soc Trop Med Hyg 1994; 88:259–61.
13. de Silva NR, Chan MS, Bundy DA. Morbidity and mortality due to ascariasis: reestimation and sensitivity analysis of global numbers at risk. Trop Med Int Health 1997; 2:519–28.
14. Le Guenno B. Emerging viruses. Sci Am 1995; 273:56–64.
15. Levander OA. Nutrition and newly emerging viral diseases: an overview. J Nutr 1997; 127(suppl 5):948S–50S.
16. Krause RM, Dimmock NJ, Morens DM. Summary of antibody workshop. The role of humoral immunity in the treatment and prevention of emerging and extant infectious diseases. J Infect Dis 1997; 176:549–59.
17. Kreiss J. Breastfeeding and vertical transmission of HIV-1. Acta Paediatr 1997; 421:113–7.
18. Binda ki Muaka P, Nzita M, Eeckels R. Malaria, anemia, and HIV-1 transmission in central Africa. Lancet 1995; 346:1294–5.
19. Mulholland K, Hilton S, Adegbola R, Usen S, Oparaugo A, Omosigho C, et al. Randomised trial of *Haemophilus influenzae* type b

tetanus protein conjugate vaccine for prevention of pneumonia and meningitis in Gambian infants. Lancet 1997; 349:1191–7.
20. Letvin NL. Progress in the development of an HIV-1 vaccine. Science 1998; 280:1875–80.
21. Kwiatkowski D, Marsh K. Development of a malaria vaccine. Lancet 1997; 350:1696–1701.
22. Nossal GJ, Lambert PH. The Jennerian heritage: new generation vaccines for all the world's children and adults. Biologicals 1997; 25:131–5.
23. Kapikian AZ, Hoshino Y, Chanock RM, Perez-Schael I. Jennerian and modified Jennerian approach to vaccination against rotavirus diarrhea using a quadrivalent rhesus rotavirus (RRV) and human–RRV reassortant vaccine. Arch Virol 1996; 12(suppl):163–75.
24. Keusch GT, Cash RA. A vaccine against rotavirus—when is too much too much? N Engl J Med 1997; 337:1228–9.
25. Adkins SB III. Immunizations: current recommendations. Am Fam Physician 1997; 56:865–74.
26. Anonymous. Recommended childhood immunization schedule—United States, 1998. Morbid Mortal Wkly Rep 1998; 47:8–12.
27. Chen RT, Orenstein WA. Epidemiologic methods in immunization programs. Epidemiol Rev 1996; 18:99–117.
28. Lambert PH, Siegrist CA. Science, medicine, and the future. Vaccines and vaccination. Br Med J 1997; 315:1595–8.
29. Adiega AA, Akinosho RO, Onyewuche J. Evaluation of immune response in infants with different nutritional status: vaccinated against tuberculosis, measles and poliomyelitis. J. Trop Pediat 1994; 40:345–50.
30. Keusch GT. Nutrition effects on response of children in developing countries to respiratory tract pathogens. Implications for vaccine development. Rev Inf Dis 1991; 13(suppl 6):S486–91.
31. Brown KH, Rajan MM, Chakroborty J, Aziz KM. Failure of a large dose of vitamin A to enhance the antibody response to tetanus toxoid in children. Am J Clin Nutr 1980; 33:212–7.
32. Sembra RD, Munasir Z, Beeler J, Akib A, Muhilal, Audet S, et al. Reduced seroconversion to measles in infants given vitamin A with measles vaccination. Lancet 1995; 345:1330–2.
33. Ross DA. Vitamin A plus measles vaccination: the downside of convenience. Lancet 1995; 345:1317–9.
34. Semba RD, Akib A, Beeler J, Munasir Z, Permaesih D, Muherdiyantiningsih, et al. Effect of vitamin A supplementation on measles vaccination in nine-month-old infants. Public Health 1997; 111: 245–7.
35. Rahman MM, Mahalanabis D, Alvarez JO, Wahed MA, Islam MA, Habte D. Effect of early vitamin A supplementation on cell-mediated immunity in infants younger than 6 months. Am J Clin Nutr 1997; 65:144–8.
36. Agoestina T, Humphrey JH, Taylor GA, Usman A, Subardja D, Hidayat S, et al. Safety of one 52-mμmol (50,000 IU) oral dose of vitamin A administered to neonates. Bull WHO 1994; 72:859–68.
37. Rahman MM, Mahalanabis D, Wahed MA, Islam MA, Habte D. Administration of 25,000 IU vitamin A doses at routine immunisation in young infants. Eur J Clin Nutr 1995; 49:439–45.
38. Stoltzfus RJ, Hakimi M, Miller KW, Rasmussen KM, Dawiesah S, Habicht JP, et al. High dose vitamin A supplementation of breast-feeding Indonesian mothers: effects on the vitamin A status of mother and infant. J Nutr 1993; 123:666–75.
39. Brown KH, Solomons NW. Nutritional problems of developing countries. Inf Dis Clin North Am 1991; 5:297–317.
40. Delpeuch F, Maire B. Obesity and developing countries of the south. Med Tropic 1997; 57:380–8.
41. Scrimshaw NS. Nutrition: prospects for the 1990s. Annu Rev Public Health 1990; 11:53–68.
42. Keller W. The epidemiology of stunting. In: Waterlow JC, ed, Linear Growth Retardation in Less Developed Countries. Nestlé Nutrition Workshop Series Volume 14, pp. 17–40. Raven, New York, 1988.
43. Martorell R, Kettel Khan L, Schroeder DG. Reversibility of stunting: epidemiological funding in children from developing countries. Eur J Clin Nutr 1994; 48:S54–7.
44. Valdez C, Mazariegos M, Romero-Abal ME, Grazioso C, Solomons

NW. Growth and growth faltering in a periurban Guatemalan community. Int Child Health 1997; 8:83–93.

45. Solomons NW, Mazariegos M, Brown KH, Klasing K. The underprivileged, developing country child. Environmental contamination and growth revisited. Nutr Rev 1993; 51:327–32.

46. Victora CG. The association between wasting and stunting: an international perspective. J Nutr 1992; 122:1105–10.

47. Anonymous. World declaration on the survival, protection and development of children. World Summit for Children. United Nations, New York. Asia-Pacific J Public Health 1990; 4:99–101.

48. Maberly GF, Trowbridge FL, Yip R, Sullivan KM, West CE. Programs against micronutrient malnutrition: ending hidden hunger. Ann Rev Public Health 1994; 15:277–301.

49. Yip R. Iron deficiency: contemporary scientific issues and international programmatic approaches. J Nutr 1994; 124:1479S–90S.

50. Beard JL. Iron metabolism: A comprehensive review. Nutr Rev 1996; 54:295–317.

51. Booth IW, Aukett MA. Iron deficiency anaemia in infancy and early childhood. Arch Dis Child 1997; 76:649–53.

52. Shankar AV, West KP Jr, Gittlesohn J, Katz J, Pradhan R. Chronic low intakes of vitamin A-rich foods in households with xerophthalmic children: a case-control study in Nepal. Am J Clin Nutr 1996; 64:242–8.

53. Shankar AH, Prasad AS. Zinc and immune function: the biological basis of altered resistance to infection. Am J Clin Nutr 1998; 63(suppl 2):447S–63S.

54. Hetzel BS. Iodine deficiency disorders (IDD) and their eradication. Lancet 1983; 2:116–29.

55. Solomons NW. There must be more than one way to skin the iodine deficiency disorders cat: novel insights from the field in Zimbabwe. Am J Clin Nutr 1998; 63:1104–5.

56. Alnwick D. Weekly iodine supplements work. Am J Clin Nutr 1998; 63:1103–4.

57. Shrimpton R. Zinc deficiency—is it widespread but underrecognized. SCN News 1993; 9:24–7.

58. Bhutta ZA. The role of zinc in health and disease: relevance to child health in developing countries. J Pak Med Assoc 1997; 47:68–73.

59. Cousins RJ. Metal elements and gene expression. Annu Rev Nutr 1994; 14:449–69.

60. Draper DE. Protein–RNA recognition. Annu Rev Biochem 1995; 64:593–620.

61. Dardenne M, Pleau JM, Savino W, Prasad AS, Bach JF. Biochemical and biological aspects of the interaction between thymulin and zinc. Prog Clin Biolog Res 1993; 380:23–32.

62. Sazawal S, Black RE, Bhan MK, Bhandari N, Sinha A, Jalla S. Zinc supplementation in young children with acute diarrhea in India. N Engl J Med 1995; 333:839–44.

63. Sazawal S, Black RE, Jalla S, Mazumdar S, Sinha A, Bhan MK. Zinc supplementation reduces the incidence of acute lower respiratory infections in infants and preschool children: a double-blind, controlled trial. Pediatrics 1998; 102:1–5.

64. Bloem MW, Hye A, Wijnroks M, Ralte A, West KP Jr, Sommer A. The role of universal distribution of vitamin A capsules in combatting vitamin A deficiency in Bangladesh. Am J Epidemiol 1995; 142: 843–55.

65. Viteri FE. Iron supplementation for the control of iron deficiency. Nutr Rev 1997; 55:195–209.

66. Nilson A, Piza J. Food fortification: a tool for fighting hidden hunger. Food Nutr Bull 1998; 19:49–60.

67. Johns T, Booth SL, Kuhnlein HV. Factors influencing vitamin A intake and programmes to improve vitamin A status. Food Nutr Bull 1992; 14:20–33.

68. Solomons NW, Bulux J. Identification and production of local carotene-rich foods to combat vitamin A malnutrition. Eur J Clin Nutr 1997; 51(suppl):S39–S45.

69. Berti PR, Leonard WR, Berti WJ. Malnutrition in rural highland Ecuador: the importance of intrahousehold food distribution, diet composition and nutrient requirements. Food Nutr Bull 1997; 18:352–62.

70. Elnagar B, Elton M, Karlsson FA, Bourdoux PP, Gebre-Medhin M. Control of iodine deficiency using iodination of water in a goitre endemic area. Int J Food Sci Nutr 1997; 48:119–28.

71. Dutra de Oliveira JE, Ferriera JF, Vasconcellos VP, Marchini JS. Drinking water as an iron carrier to control anemia in preschool children in a day-care center. J Am Coll Nutr 1994; 13:198–202.

72. Solomons NW, Bulux J. Plant sources of vitamin A and human nutriture. Nutr Rev 1993; 51:199–204.

73. de Pee S, West CE, Muhilal, Karyadi D, Hautvast JGAJ. Lack of improvement in vitamin A status with increased consumption of dark-green leafy vegetables. Lancet 1995; 346:75–81.

74. Porter KA, Blackburn GL, Bistrian BR. Safety of iron dextran in TPN: a case report. J Am Coll Nutr 1988; 7:107–10.

75. Solomons NW, Bulux J. Increased nutrient uptake in developing countries through increased bioavailability. Eur J Clin Nutr, in press.

76. Furnee CA, Pfann GA, West CE, van der Haar F, van der Heide D, Hautvast JG. New model for describing urinary iodine excretion: its use for comparing different oral preparations of iodized oil. Am J Clin Nutr 1997; 61:1257–62.

77. Hathcock JN. Vitamins and minerals: efficacy and safety. Am J Clin Nutr 1997; 66:427–37.

78. Russell RM. The impact of disease states as a modifying factor for nutrition toxicity. Nutr Rev 1997; 55:50–3.

79. Folwaczny C. Zinc and diarrhea in infants. J Trace Element Med Biol 1997; 11:116–22.

80. Thurnham DI. Impact of disease on markers of micronutrient status. Proc Nutr Soc 1997; 56:421–31.

81. Brown KH, Lanata CF, Yeun ML, Peerson JM, Butron B, Lönnerdal B. Potential magnitude of the misclassification of a populations trace element status due to infection: example from a survey of young Peruvian children. Am J Clin Nutr 1993; 58:549–54.

82. Solomons NW. On the assessment of zinc and copper nutriture in man. Am J Clin Nutr 1979; 32:856–71.

83. Sommer A, Tarwotjo I, Djunaedi E, West KP Jr, Loeden AA, Tilden R, et al. Impact of vitamin A supplementation on childhood mortality: a randomized controlled community trial. Lancet 1986; 1:1169–73.

84. Rahmathullah L, Underwood BA, Thulasiraj RD, Milton RC, Ramaswamy K, Rahmathullah R, et al. Reduced mortality among children in Southern India receiving small weekly dose of vitamin A. N Engl J Med 1990; 323:929–35.

85. Rahmathullah L, Underwood BA, Thykasuraj RD, Milton RC. Diarrhea, respiratory infections, and growth are not affected by a small weekly dose of vitamin A supplements: a masked, controlled field trial in children in southern India. Am J Clin Nutr 1991; 54:568–77.

86. Herrea MG, Nestel P, El Amin A, Fawzi WW, Mohamed KA, Weld L. Vitamin A supplementation and child survival. Lancet 1992; 340:267–71.

87. Bloem MW, Wedel M, Egger RJ, Speek AJ, Schrijver J, Saowakontha S, et al. Mild vitamin A deficiency and risk of respiratory tract diseases and diarrhea in preschool and school children in Northeastern Thailand. Am J Epidemiol 1990; 131:332–9.

88. Coutsoudis A, Adhikari M, Coovadia HM. Serum vitamin A (retinol) concentrations and association with respiratory disease in premature infants. J Trop Pediatr 1995; 41:230–3.

89. Dudley L, Hussey G, Huskissen J, Kessow G. Vitamin A status, other risk factors and acute respiratory infection morbidity in children. S Afr Med J 1997; 87:65–70.

90. Fawzi WW, Herrera MG, Willett WC, Nestel P, El Amin A, Mohamed KA. Dietary vitamin A intake and the incidence of diarrhea and respiratory infection among Sudanese children. J Nutr 1995; 125:1211–21.

91. Henning B, Stewart K, Zaman K, Alam AN, Brown KH, Black RE. Lack of therapeutic efficacy of vitamin A for non-cholera, watery diarrhoea in Bangladeshi children. Eur J Clin Nutr 1992; 46:437–43.

92. Bhandari N, Bahl R, Sazawal S, Bhan MK. Breast-feeding status alters the effect of vitamin A treatment during acute diarrhea in children. J Nutr 1997; 127:59–63.

93. Hanekom WA, Potgieter S, Hughes EJ, Malan H, Kessow G, Hussey

GD. Vitamin A status and therapy in childhood pulmonary tuberculosis. J Pediat 1997; 131:925–7.

94. Kjolhede CL, Chew FJ, Gadomski AM, Marroquin DP. Clinical trial of vitamin A as an adjuvant treatment for lower respiratory tract infections. J Pediatr 1995; 126:807–12.

95. Hussey GD, Klein H. A randomized, controlled trial of vitamin A in children with severe measles. N Engl J Med 1990; 323:160–4.

96. Hussey GD, Klein H. Routine high-dose vitamin A therapy for children hospitalized with measles. J Trop Pediatr 1993; 39:342–54.

97. Rosales FJ, Kjolhede C, Goodman S. Efficacy of a single oral dose of 200,000 IU of oil-soluble vitamin A in measles-associated morbidity. Am J Epidemiol 1996; 143:413–22.

98. Sommer A, Tarwotjo J, Hussaini G, Susanto D. Increased mortality in children with mild vitamin A deficiency. Lancet 1983; 2:585–8.

99. Beaton GH, Martorell R, Aronson KJ, Edmonston B, McCabe G, Ros AC, et al. Effectiveness of vitamin A supplementation in the control of young child morbidity and mortality in developing countries. ACC/SCN State-of-the-Art Series. Nutrition Policy Discussion Paper No. 13. Lavenham. Suffolk, UK, 1993.

100. Fawzi WW, Chalmers TC, Herrera MG, Mosteller F. Vitamin A supplementation and child mortality. A meta-analysis. JAMA 1993; 269:898–903.

101. Vijayaraghaven K, Radhaiah G, Prakasam S, Sarma KV, Reddy V. Effect of massive dose vitamin A on morbidity and mortality in Indian children. Lancet 1990; 336:1342–5.

102. Humphrey JH, Agoestina T, Wu L, Usman A, Nurachim M, Subardja D, et al. Impact of neonatal vitamin A supplementation on infant morbidity and mortality. J Pediatr 1996; 128:489–96.

103. West KP Jr, Katz J, Shrestha SR, LeClerq SC, Khatry SK, Pradhan EK, et al. Mortality of infants <6 mo of age supplemented with vitamin A: a randomized, double-masked trial in Nepal. Am J Clin Nutr 1995; 62:143–8.

104. Ramakrishan U, Latham MC, Abel R, Frongillo EA Jr. Vitamin A supplementation and morbidity among preschool children in south India. Am J Clin Nutr 1995; 61:1295–1303.

105. Barreto ML, Santos LMP, Assis AM, Araújo MP, Farenzena GG, Santos PA, et al. Effect of vitamin A supplementation on diarrhoea and acute lower respiratory infections in young children in Brazil. Lancet 1994; 344:228–31.

106. Underwood BA. Was the "anti-infective" vitamin misnamed? Nutr Rev 1994; 52:140–3.

107. Keusch GT. Micronutrients and susceptibility to infections. Ann NY Acad Sci 1990; 587:181–8.

108. Scrimshaw NS, SanGiovanni JP. Synergism of nutrition, infection, and immunity: an overview. Am J Clin Nutr 1997; 66:464S–77S.

109. Chugh K. Zinc therapy in acute diarrhea. Indian Ped 1996; 33:352.

110. Sazawal S, Black RE, Bhan MK, Jalla S, Bhandari N, Sinha A, et al. Zinc supplementation reduces the incidence of persistent diarrhea and dysentery among low socioeconomic children in India. J Nutr 1996; 126:443–50.

111. Ruel MT, Rivera JA, Santizo MC, Lönnerdal B, Brown KH. Impact of zinc supplementation on morbidity from diarrhea and respiratory infections among rural Guatemalan children. Pediatrics 1997; 99:808–13.

112. Rosado JL, Lopez P, Muñoz E, Nartinez H, Allen LH. Zinc supplementation reduced morbidity, but neither zinc nor iron supplementation affected growth or body composition of Mexican preschoolers. Am J Clin Nutr 1997; 65:13–9.

113. Das BS, Das DB, Satpathy RN, Patnaik JK, Bose TK. Riboflavin deficiency and severity of malaria. Eur J Clin Nutr 1988; 42:277–83.

114. Das BS, Thurnham DI, Patnaik JK, Das DB, Satpathy R, Bose TK. Increased plasma lipid peroxidation in riboflavin-deficient, malaria-infected children. Am J Clin Nutr 1990; 51:859–63.

115. Todd EC. Epidemiology of foodborne diseases: a worldwide review. World Health Stat Quart 1997; 50:30–50.

116. Ziegler RG. Vegetables, fruits and carotenoids and the risk of cancer. Am J Clin Nutr 1991; 53:251S–9S.

117. Messina M, Messina V. Nutritional implications of dietary phytochemicals. Adv Exp Med Biol 1996; 401:207–12.

118. Macfarlane GT, Macfarlane S. Human colonic microbiota: ecology, physiology and metabolic potential of intestinal bacteria. Scand J Gastroenterol 1997; 222(suppl):3–9.

119. Biller JA, Katz AJ, Flores AF, Buie TM, Gorbach SL. Treatment of recurrent *Clostridium difficile* colitis with *Lactobacillus* GG. J Ped Gastroenterol Nutr 1995; 21:224–6.

120. Keusch GT. Antioxidants in infection. J Nutr Sci Vit 1993; 39(suppl):S23–S33.

121. Miller RA, Britigan BE. Role of oxidants in microbial pathophysiology. Clin Microbial Rev 1997; 10:1–18.

122. Peterhans E. Oxidants and antioxidants in viral diseases: disease mechanisms and metabolic regulation. J Nutr 1997; 127(suppl 5): 962S–5S.

123. Walter-Sack I, Klotz U. Influence of diet and nutritional status on drug metabolism. Clin Pharmacokinet 1996; 31:47–64.

124. Williams L, Hill DP Jr, Davis JA, Lowenthal DT. The influence of food on the absorption and metabolism of drugs: an update. Eur J Drug Metab Pharmacokinet 1996; 21:201–11.

125. Keusch GT, Scrimshaw NS. Selective primary health care: strategies for control of disease in the developing world. XXIII. Control of infection to reduce the prevalence of infantile and childhood malnutrition. Rev Infect Dis 1986; 8:273–87.

126. Chang HR, Bistrian B. The role of cytokines in the catabolic consequences of infection and injury. J Parenteral Enteral Nutr 1998; 22:156–66.

127. Plata-Salaman CR. Cytokines and anorexia: a brief overview. Semin Oncol 1998; 25(suppl):64–72.

128. Huffman SL, Lopez de Romaña G, Madrid S, Brown KH, Bentley M, Black RE. Do child feeding practices change due to diarrhoea in the Central Peruvian Highlands? J Diarrh Dis Res 1991; 9:295–300.

129. Parker ME, Schroeder DG, Begin D, Hurtado E. Maternal preferences for consistency of complementary foods in Guatemala. Food Nutr Bull 1998; 19:6–12.

130. Keusch GT, Solomons NW. Microorganisms, malabsorption, diarrhea and dysnutrition. J Environ Pathol Toxicol Oncol 1985; 5: 165–209.

131. Worwood M. Influence of disease on iron status. Proc Nutr Soc 1997; 56:409–19.

132. Stoltzfus RJ, Dreyfuss ML, Chwaya HM, Albonico M. Hookworm control as a strategy to prevent iron deficiency. Nutr Rev 1997; 55:223–32.

133. Cooper ES, Duff EM, Howell S, Bundy DA. "Catch-up" growth velocities after treatment for Trichuris dysentery syndrome. Trans R Soc Trop Med Hyg 1995; 89:653.

134. Rahman MM, Mahalanabis D, Alvarez JO, Wahed MA, Islam MA, Habte D, et al. Acute respiratory infections prevent improvement of vitamin A status in young infants supplemented with vitamin A. J Nutr 1996; 126:628–33.

135. Alvarez JO, Salazar-Lindo E, Kohatsu J, Miranda P, Stephensen CB. Urinary excretion of retinol in children with acute diarrhea. Am J Clin Nutr 1995; 61:1273–6.

136. Ruz M, Solomons NW. Mineral excretion during acute, dehydrating diarrhea treated with oral rehydration therapy. Pediatr Res 1990; 27:179–175.

137. Bennish ML, Salam MA, Wahed MA. Enteric protein loss during shigellosis. Am J Gastroenterol 1993; 88:53–7.

138. Brown KH. Dietary management of acute diarrheal disease: contemporary scientific issues. J Nutr 1994; 124(suppl 8):1455S–60S.

139. Barry DM, Reeve AW. Increased incidence of gram-negative neonatal sepsis with intramuscular iron administration. Pediatrics 1987; 60:908–12.

16 Protein-Energy Malnutrition and Infectious Disease

Synergistic Interactions

CHRISTOPHER A. JOLLY AND GABRIEL FERNANDES

INTRODUCTION

The immune system plays a leading role in fighting off the constant bombardment of our bodies by invading pathogenic organisms, such as bacteria, fungi, viruses, toxins, and allergic compounds. Also, the immune system is intimately linked to the quality and quantity of nutrient intake (1,2). The host is defense-regulated and maintained by two branches of the immune system. One is cell-mediated immunity, carried out primarily by the CD4+ Th-1 and CD8+ T lymphocytes, which plays a pivotal role in cytotoxic responses against malignant cells and cells infected with intracellular bacteria and viruses. The other branch is humoral (antibody-mediated) immunity, of which the B lymphocyte plays a dominant role, to ward off and/or destroy extracellular pathogens. The T lymphocytes may also influence humoral immunity, as the Th-2 CD4+ T-lymphocyte subset secretes a wide variety of antibody-inducing cytokines. The Th-1 CD4+ T lymphocyte produces primarily interleukin-2 (IL-2) and interferon gamma (IFN-γ) and the Th-2 population produces primarily IL-4, -5, -6, and -10. Antibody isotype production (IgA, IgE, IgG, etc.) is dependent on the kind of cytokine produced to fight invading antigen assaults. Unfortunately, this vast array of defense mechanisms is not impregnable. Primary causes of a breakdown in these lines of defense (i.e., serious breakdown of our immune system) is either chronic or acute under nutrition and malnutrition.

The devastating consequences of malnutrition are most profound in young children and the elderly. More than 6 million (approximately 55%) children under 5 yr of age in developing countries die directly or indirectly from malnutrition (1) and 177 million children have or have had malnutrition at some point in their lives. Malnutrition can arise from either inadequate food intake or, as is the case in breast-fed children (< 18 mo old), from inadequate milk nutrient densities or deficiencies induced from a malnourished mother. The cause of this problem is multifactorial, having social, political, cultural and geographical components.

The elderly are also overwhelmingly affected by malnutrition, with approximately 33% (suffering from nutritional deficiencies) living in industrialized countries (3). Again, the etiology of this problem is multifactorial, involving social, physical, and psychological issues. Figure 1 summarizes the diverse etiologies of malnutrition, ranging from congenital defects in infants to physical and mental impairment in the elderly. Although the etiology is slightly different between malnourished young children and the elderly, both have a significant increase in the risk of infection and subsequent death resulting from these infections. In young children, the immune system is still developing its innate and acquired defense mechanisms, whereas in aging persons, immune function is, at least in part, dysregulated because of the involution of the thymus and decline in its function. Therefore (compared to healthy young adults), both young children and the elderly exhibit altered immune responses that increase their susceptibility to infection, which is exacerbated by malnutrition (5). Thus, malnutrition further suppresses the immune system, allowing the host to be vulnerable to attack and subsequent rise in chronic infections. Hence, the viscious cycle of malnutrition and the onset of chronic illness begins (Fig. 2). One rather unique aspect of malnutrition is that it alters virtually every aspect of the immune response, including lymphoid anatomy, humoral and cellular immunity, phagocytic function, and the complement system (Table 1).

Malnutrition and protein-energy malnutrition (PEM) are generally used interchangeably. However, PEM is somewhat a misnomer, as it rarely occurs without deficiencies in other essential micronutrients like select vitamins and trace minerals, making not only the etiology but the pathology quite complex. In rodent models, the majority of the defects observed in malnourished humans are induced by only limiting the amount of protein in the diet while maintaining adequate quantities of vitamins and minerals (Table 1). For example, reducing the normal 18% protein diet in weanling mice with a 5% protein diet and increasing the corn starch (to adjust for the other 13%) results in PEM symptoms while maintaining normal growth as assessed by body weight measurements. However, a 1–2% protein diet results in severe PEM and subsequent blunting (stunting) of growth (i.e., body weight) (8). It should be noted, however, that PEM caused primar-

From: *Nutrition and Immunology: Principles and Practice* (ME Gershwin et al. eds.), © Humana Press, Inc., Totowa, NJ

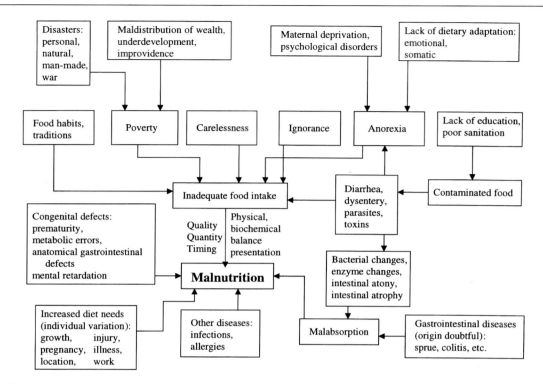

Fig. 1. Flow diagram depicting the multiple etiologies of protein energy malnutrition. (Reproduced from *ref. 4* with permission.)

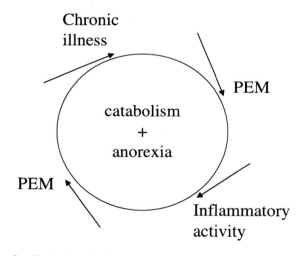

Fig. 2. Depiction of the viscious cycle of chronic infection and protein-energy malnutrition (PEM). (From *ref. 6* with permission.)

ily by extremely low protein intakes in the presence of adequate calories may not result in significant weight loss because as muscle wasting begins to occur, fat production could increase or edema develops. Therefore, biochemical measurements in the blood (e.g., serum albumin) are important values for the diagnosis of ongoing PEM.

As noted earlier, malnutrition is a global problem affecting both developing and industrialized countries. Its consequences are primarily respiratory tract infections and diarrhea, leading to a major cause of morbidity and/or mortality. Indeed, much of the recent work done in the area of PEM and immunity has also focused on the salivary and gut immune components and the

intimate role the T and B lymphocyte plays in this system. Specific emphasis has been on the production of immunoglobulin A (IgA), which plays a key role in preventing the entrance of invading microbes and allergens into the body. Here, we will review briefly the current literature on how PEM influences the immune system, allowing higher and more severe infection rates, as well as essential current treatment modalities. One important point to keep in mind is that even though the etiology of malnutrition (i.e., PEM) is quite complex, it is preventable. Additionally, if PEM is already present, it can be partially reversed, from the immune system's standpoint.

STUDIES IN THE YOUNG

PEM IN CHILDREN Two severe forms of PEM are kwashiorkor and marasmus diseases. Kwashiorkor is most prevalent in children 1–3 yr of age and is characterized by edema, hair loss, and/or discoloration and flaky skin. Marasmus exhibits similar clinical signs, but, generally, edema is not present. One dramatic feature of PEM is lymphoid atrophy. Specifically, the thymus gland becomes smaller and its cellularity is altered; furthermore, the spleen and lymph nodes show signs of altered microanatomy and ratios of immune cells within the lymphoid organs. As expected, the ultimate result is impairment of most host defense mechanisms *(3)*. Recently, Sauerwein et al. *(9)* examined the effect of kwashiorkor and marasmus in children with a mean age of 3 yr. Children in both groups showed impaired antioxidant defense mechanisms. Specifically, plasma vitamin E levels were found to be significantly reduced in the kwashiorkor groups and glutathione quantities were also lower in both kwashiorkor and marasmus, with the kwashiorkor group having the lowest, compared to healthy age-matched controls. Free radicals are important effector molecules in many physiological processes (immunity being one); however, modulat-

Table 1
Summary of the Effects of Protein-Energy
Malnutrition on Immune Functions:
Comparison Between Human and Animal Studies

	Human	Animal
Lymphoid anatomy		
Thymus	↓	↓
Spleen	↓	↓
Lymph nodes	↓	↓
Other lymphoid tissue	↓	↓
Total circulating lymphocytes	↓	↓
Humoral immunity		
Circulating B lymphocytes	↓ or N	
Serum Ig levels	↑ or N	↓
Serum Ab, response to Ag	↓	↓
Secretory IgA	↓	
Splenic plaque-forming cell responses		↓
Cellular immunity		
Circulating T lymphocytes	↓	
Delayed cutaneous hypersensitivity	↓	↓
Allograft rejection		N or ↑ or ↓
Tumor cytotoxicity		↑
Immunity to intracellular organisms	↓	
Lymphocyte proliferation		
(a) Concanavalin A	↓ or N	
(b) PHA	↓ or N	N or ↑ or ↓
(c) PWM	↑ or N	
Lymphokine production	↓	
Phagocytic function		
Monocyte chemotaxis	↓	↓
PMN chemotaxis	N	↑
PMN phagocytosis	N	
RES function		↑ or ↓
Intracellular killing	↓ or N	N
Complement	↓	↓

Note: PMN = polymorphonuclear leukocyte; RES = reticuloendothelial system; N = normal; ↓ = depressed; ↑ = increased.
Source: Adapted from *ref. 7*.

ing proxidant levels could cause further tissue damage and heighten inflammation. Furthermore, clinical indices of concomitant infection were also shown to be elevated. For example, plasma IL-6 was higher in the kwashiorkor group, and soluble tumor necrosis factor (TNF) receptors (both p55 and p75) were found to be significantly elevated in both the kwashiorkor and marasmus groups, suggesting the presence of some type of infection. Interestingly, soluble IL-6 receptor was not affected and, in general, the effects were more dramatic in the kwashiorkor group relative to the marasmus group.

In contrast, PEM children showed lower IL-6 and TNF production when peripheral blood mononuclear cells were unable to be stimulated with lipopolysaccharide *(10)*. This suggests that, at least in the peripheral blood, immune cells are impaired to the point that they do not respond to in vitro stimulation. However, the increase in inflammatory mediators, such as IL-6 in the study described earlier *(9)*, indicates that at least some aspects of the immune system are still able to respond, or that the magnitude of the immune response may not be adequate enough to ward off the invading infectious agents. The suppressed cytokine secretion

seen is in agreement with other reports showing both reduced CD4[+] and CD8[+] T-lymphocyte subsets, as well as reduced production of IgG in vitro *(3)*. Not only are the relative proportions of T-lymphocyte subsets altered but their function is also suppressed (i.e., proliferative response in vitro). Phagocytic function is also commonly found to be suppressed, in part, through the reduction in complement protein levels. Secretory IgA levels are lower as well, which enhances the risk of bacterial translocation into the body via the gut *(11)*. Decreased secretory IgA levels appear to be relatively universal, since it has been found in Indian, Thai, and Indonesian children suffering from PEM. Furthermore, suppressed IgA is not restricted to a select anatomical site, as levels were low in nasopharyngeal secretions, tears, saliva, and the duodenum *(7)*.

Studies have also found that C3 and C5 complement proteins are also reduced in PEM children *(12)*, which is now accepted to be a common feature of PEM *(13)*. Complement proteins are important to opsonize extracellular pathogens for their enhanced phagocytosis by macrophages as well as directly lyse invading organisms *(13)*. In PEM children, bacterial adherence to the trachea was enhanced, indicating that the risk of respiratory tract infection was elevated. Clearly, the mucosal defense system in PEM children is impaired, thereby increasing their risk of respiratory and gastrointestinal tract infections from both low- and high-virulent organisms. Furthermore, the anemia seen in PEM can also enhance the establishment of infectious microorganisms because the red blood cells have a complement receptor that will bind to the microorganisms, increasing their clearance primarily by the liver *(13)*.

Even moderate PEM dramatically affects the salivary and gut mucosal immune system *(14)*. Young children who were moderately malnourished (i.e., serum albumin within the normal range) showed significantly lower IgA levels in the saliva, although higher levels were in the sera. Thus, both salivary and mucosal immune components appear to become very sensitive to malnutrition and/or PEM.

PEM IN WEANLING MOUSE MODELS Many of the immunological effects of PEM in humans also develop in mice when fed an isocaloric protein-deficient diet. Woods and Woodward *(8)* found that weanling mice fed a protein-deficient diet (0.6% by weight) for 14 d induced wasting and suppressed the cell-mediated immune response to skin allograft rejection and antibody response to sheep red blood cells (SRBC). Following this same dietary protocol, the same authors showed in a subsequent study that the delayed-type hypersensitivity to SRBCs was also reduced *(15)*. Ha et al. *(16)* found that in weanling PEM mice, the gut and biliary lumen IgA levels were reduced and that serum IgA was elevated. Furthermore, Ig-producing cells were still expanding in the mucosa, albeit at a slower rate than in normal-fed control mice *(16)*. Therefore, the authors proposed that because Ig-producing cells, in terms of expansion, are relatively resistant to PEM, perhaps the ability of the mucosa to secrete IgA into the lumen was impaired. The succeeding article by Ha and Woodward showed that, indeed, the polymeric IgA receptor (pIgR) was reduced in the liver, with only minimal effects seen in the intestinal epithelium *(17)*. The pIgR is responsible for the transport of IgA into the gut lumen; these data, in conjunction with the high serum IgA, suggest that IgA transport, not synthesis, is more sensitive to PEM and that the liver is a major contributor to secretory IgA into the gut lumen. These data are in agreement with other studies in mice showing that relatively mild PEM enhances serum IgA while reducing that found in the intestinal lumen. McGee and McMurray *(18)* also found that IgA-producing spleen cells were significantly reduced in response to oral challenge with SRBCs in PEM mice. As has been found in humans, this effect reverted back to normal when the mice were fed the control diet for 3 wk *(18)*.

Interestingly, overall neutrophil function is only moderately suppressed by PEM as measured by enzyme release, bacterial phagocytosis, and subsequent killing *(19)*. In other words, the reductions were small, yet statistically significant. Similar results were seen in alveolar macrophages *(20)*. PEM did not significantly reduce macrophage killing of *Listeria monocytogenes*, production of hydrogen peroxide and superoxide anion, and production of IL-1 and TNF production. However, prostaglandin, leukotriene, and thromboxane production was further reduced, suggesting that although PEM may not significantly affect macrophage function *per se*, it may influence the macrophage's ability to modulate the immune response indirectly *(20)*.

STUDIES IN THE ELDERLY

PEM IN THE ELDERLY Both aging and PEM have cumulative effects on the immune system. Aging results in a dysregulation of the immune system, particularly the functional loss of T lymphocytes, leading to enhanced risk of infection and decreased clearance of infectious agents. In terms of the immune system, the primary effects of aging are associated with alterations in T-lymphocyte-dependent cell-mediated immunity. The onset of aging lowers $CD8^+$ T-lymphocyte numbers with only marginal effects on $CD4^+$ T-lymphocyte levels, but B lymphocytes and monocytes remain relatively unchanged. Not only does the relative proportions of T lymphocytes change, but so does their functional activity. T-Lymphocyte IL-2 secretion and subsequent proliferation is reduced, indicating a decline in T-lymphocyte function with respect to age. $CD4^+$ T-lymphocyte Th-1 cytokine production (IL-2, IFN-γ) decreases, and Th-2 cytokine production (IL-4, -5, -6, -10) increases with age. The net effect predisposes the elderly to a reduced cell-mediated immune response and increased susceptibility to certain infectious agents. On the other hand, the humoral response may be hyperactive, leading to the overproduction of certain antibodies, resulting in increased circulating autoantibody levels *(21)*. It is well established that memory T lymphocytes increase with age and naive T-lymphocytes decrease. This, in part, is the result of decreases in thymic function with age, which results in lower antibody titers in response to antigenic stimulation and/or immunization. The mechanism may, in part, involve the reduced thymulin bioactivity and the decreased size of the thymus, which could primarily cause the loss of naive T lymphocytes in the periphery with age.

Protein-energy malnutrition has similar effects as aging on the immune system, making the elderly, in some cases, as immunosuppressed as AIDS patients *(22)*. For example, aging reduces $CD8^+$, but not $CD4^+$ levels, and in the background of PEM, both $CD8^+$ and $CD4^+$ T-lymphocyte populations are reduced *(9)*. Unlike aging, PEM also suppresses B-lymphocyte and polymorphonuclear cell function *(21)*. In chronically ill PEM patients, serum IL-6 and orosomucoid was higher compared to well-nourished controls. Furthermore, peripheral blood monocyte stimulation in vitro with lipopolysaccharide (LPS) generated a higher production of IL-1β and IL-6 in PEM patients, whereas IL-10, TNF, and transforming growth factor-β (TGF-β) did not change. The end result is full-

blown immunodeficiency and increased risk of infection because of the imbalanced cytokine levels. Chronic infection gives rise to the elevated production of IL-1, TNF-α, and IL-6, thereby inducing a cachectic state in which protein breakdown increases and food intake declines. These adverse effects further exacerbate the already existing PEM. Supplementation with 400 kcal energy and 40 g protein per day for 3 mo resulted in decreased serum IL-6 levels and an increase in the anabolic hormone insulin-like growth factor-1 (IGF-1) in patients who responded to nutritional repletion (four out of seven patients) *(6)*.

In addition, PEM in the elderly can arise from either primary or secondary causes *(23)*. The primary cause of malnutrition is inadequate food intake, which manifests itself in a variety ways (refer to Fig. 1). Secondary malnutrition is the result of physiological changes occurring during aging, resulting in inadequate intake or digestion of foods (refer to Fig. 3). Specifically, the senses of taste and smell are reduced, which can make food less appealing, thereby reducing food consumption. Gastric, liver, and biliary functions are also reduced, thus decreasing the absorption of essential nutrients. The decrease in liver function may be further aggravated by various drugs and/or medications commonly taken, long term, by the elderly. Therefore, drug dosages may need to be reduced (Table 2) *(24)*. The important point is that even in the presence of adequate food availability, the decreased desire to eat or, in the case of adequate or near adequate intake, reduced nutrient absorptive processes itself may give rise to chronic PEM.

Measurement of serum albumin is commonly used as a diagnostic marker for PEM. Serum albumin less than 35 g/L is associated with a significantly decreased probability of surviving 1 yr after hospitalization *(25)*. A prospective study showed that mortality in the elderly with PEM who had been admitted as emergency cases was 41%, compared to 18% in well-nourished age-matched controls. A follow-up study also showed that infection leading to doctor visits and death were significantly reduced in the elderly who had been nutritionally repleted *(26)*. Furthermore, PEM can lead to enhanced bacterial gut translocation, resulting in intestinal and pulmonary infections *(11)*, which are commonly seen in the elderly.

The grim effects of PEM on the elderly immune system is, at least in part, reversible. Supplementation of elderly patients, showing no clinical signs of disease or infection, with a 4- to 500-kcal/d canned drink supplement containing macronutrients and micronutrients could partially restore cell-mediated immune function. Furthermore, antibody titers in response to vaccines are partially restored, indicating that supplementation prior to vaccination may prove highly effective in the elderly *(21)*. Beneficial results were also found in chronically ill, elderly PEM patients. Supplementation with 400 kcal energy and 40 g protein per day for 3 mo resulted in a higher DTH response, as was blood levels of the acute-phase protein orosomucoid, indicating improvement in immune status even after disease onset *(27)*. However, supplementation would have to continue, otherwise the immune system will revert back to its suppressed status.

Current therapeutic approaches involve the use of drugs to enhance appetite. However, these drugs are associated with ill side effects such as delirium, sedation, nausea, and so on *(28)*. Whereas pharmacologic intervention targeted at modulating serotonin and other hormone levels to control appetite does seem appealing, another adverse side effect of many drugs is decreased salivary gland function. This, in turn, may cause difficulty in

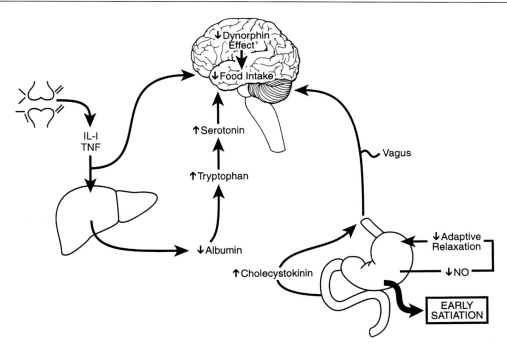

Fig. 3. Diagram of the complex relationship among the immune, digestive and neuroendocrine systems in the manifestation of the anorexia of aging. (Adapted from *ref. 27.*)

chewing and/or swallowing food, thereby exacerbating the PEM state. Therefore, it would seem that the most efficient and health-conscious method to enhance health status would be to improve dietary habits as well as provide easier access to well-balanced meals.

PEM IN AGED RODENT MODELS One current theory on the mechanisms of aging is explained based on altered antioxidant defense systems resulting in the accumulation of oxidatively damaged cell products. This mechanism is thought to play a major role in the impairment of cellular function seen in aged animals. PEM mice have been shown to have lower glutathione in their spleens, heart, and liver, which correlated with reduced splenic lymphocyte intracellular calcium mobilization and subsequent proliferation (29). Glutathione is a free-radical scavenging mole-

Table 2
Alterations in Organ Function with Respect to Aging that May Influence Nutrient Status

Organ function	Physical change	Importance to nutrition
Taste and smell	Decreased taste buds and papilla on tongue	Loss of ability to detect salt and sweet
	Decrease in taste and olfactory nerve endings	Decreased palatability causing poor food intake
	Change in taste and smell threshold	
Saliva secretion	Saliva flow may be reduced	Doubtful clinical significance
Esophageal function and swallowing	Minor changes including disordered contractions	Doubtful clinical significance
Gastric function and emptying	Decreased secretion of hydrochloric acid; intrinsic factor; and pepsin in 20% of healthy population > 60 yr of age (atrophic gastritis); rapid rate of emptying of liquids; increased proximal small bowel pH; bacterial overgrowth in bowel	Decreased bioavailability of mineral, vitamins, and proteins; decreased absorption of protein-bound vitamin B_{12} and folate; increase in bacterial folate synthesis to counteract malabsorption
Liver and biliary function	Decreased size and blood flow; minor structural and biochemical changes; activity of drug-metabolizing enzymes reduced	Rate of albumin synthesis may be decreased; drug dosages may need to be lower
Pancreatic secretion	Slightly lower bicarbonate and enzyme outputs	Doubtful clinical significance
Intestinal morphology and function	Insignificant changes in small-bowel morphology	Doubtful clinical significance
Intestinal microflora	Bacterial overgrowth in proximal small bowel in atrophic gastritis	Functional significance unknown; influences supply of water-soluble vitamins and vitamin K

Source: ref. 24.

cule that aids in protecting the cell from oxidative damage. Feeding a normal diet to the mice for only 1 wk returned glutathione levels to the normal range. Studies have found that PEM in mice suppresses the number of splenic B lymphocytes that produce anti-SRBC antibody following SRBC immunization. Interestingly, although the number of CD4$^+$ and CD8$^+$ T lymphocytes was suppressed in the peripheral blood, the relative proportions were enhanced in spleens and mesenteric lymph nodes (30), suggesting that a lymphocyte homing increase or occurrence of selective "sticking" in certain lymphoid compartments is occurring. This may offer further insight into the mechanism for unresponsiveness in cell-mediated immunity in PEM.

Protein-energy malnutrition also has site-specific influences on salivary and gastrointestinal immunity (31). Although tear volume was unaffected in adult (3 mo) and aged (16 mo) mice, the total IgA-containing cells in the lacrimal gland was suppressed in adult mice, and there was no effect of PEM in aged mice. The later lack of effect is due to the fact that aging itself reduces the number of IgA-containing cells; therefore, PEM did not show a cumulative effect with aging. Furthermore, the IgA content in tears was lower in response to PEM in adult, but not old, mice. In contrast, PEM reduced IgA in saliva in both adult and old mice. Interestingly, feeding the PEM mice a control diet reversed the PEM effects in both the salivary and intestinal immune system (31).

Studies employing the Fisher F344 rat-aging model found that whereas peritoneal macrophage production of IL-1 and TNF is reduced with aging, PEM did not affect the production of these cytokines. Furthermore, PEM did not have a cumulative effect on the suppression of monocyte function in aged rats (32). Effects on neutrophil function were quite unique. Neither aging nor PEM alone suppressed neutrophil function. However, the combination of old age and PEM suppressed neutrophil respiratory burst, exocytosis, and enzyme release (19). These studies show how diet (specifically PEM) can have different effects on the various cells of the immune system.

SINGLE-NUTRIENT DEFICIENCIES

It is almost impossible to discuss PEM without mentioning deficiencies of individual nutrients like select vitamins and/or trace minerals, which, alone or in combination, have dramatic effects on cell-mediated immunity, nonspecific immunity, and to a lesser extent, humoral immunity (33). Common immune abnormalities seen in deficiencies of pyridoxine, pantothenic acid, folic acid, vitamin B$_{12}$, biotin, thiamin, and vitamins C, A, and E include decreased lymphocyte response to in vitro stimulation and impaired antibody response (7). Pyridoxine and biotin deficiency also reduces thymic size and/or thymulin levels, whereas vitamin A deficiency results in an increased susceptibility to certain tumors (7). Iron deficiency is the most common single-nutrient deficiency. Both human and laboratory animal studies show significant reductions in complement levels and cell-mediated, humoral, and nonspecific immunity when iron deficiency is present (33). Similar effects are seen with selenium and copper deficiency (33). Among several trace mineral studies, the role of zinc on immune function and its susceptibility to infection was studied most extensively. The early studies by Fraker et al. (34,35) have established the critical role of zinc on immunity and antibody production. Our own studies in mice revealed that zinc is essential to develop cytotoxic T lymphocytes and natural-killer cells to ward off both malignancy and infectious agents (36). Also, zinc deficiency may

be quite common among the elderly (37). It is also widespread in underdeveloped countries in pregnant women as well as in young children, which often leads to diarrheal diseases (38–40). These results clearly show that insufficient quantities of only a single nutrient (vitamin or mineral) can have profound negative effects on the immune system. Furthermore, it highlights the necessity of evaluating the status of all macronutrients and micronutrients when diagnosing and, subsequently, during the treatment of immunocompromised patients.

TREATMENT

The obvious cure for PEM is renutrition or renourishment. However, several potential pitfalls should be considered. First, the introduction of well-balanced meals may not be easily tolerated by the atrophied gut mucosa and other digestive organs that are functioning suboptimally. This could result in a malabsorption syndrome, resulting in decreased transit time through the colon and leading to soft to runny stools, exacerbating the dehydration associated with diarrhea. The best example of this comes from the experiences encountered during World Wars. Prisoners of war, having been starved for up to several years, were given free access to adequate food upon return. The net result was malabsorption, which, in some cases, resulted in death. Second, introduction of minerals such as iron, selenium, zinc, and copper without the simultaneous increase in their respective binding (storage) protein could result in enhanced free-radical production and subsequent tissue damage. Third, replenishment of iron without its binding protein could exacerbate infection because many microorganisms use iron for growth. Therefore, renourishment should be carried out gradually and under the close supervision of a dietitian and physician and, in the case of the elderly, a psychologist or social worker. If renourishment does not seem to work in terms of increasing body weight and serum protein (i.e., albumin) levels, then the patient should be checked for infections and/or metabolic defects resulting in PEM (23).

Protein-energy malnutrition can initiate and/or participate in a vicious cycle of malnutrition and infection. PEM renders the body susceptible to infections of all sorts, including opportunistic ones (i.e., those that are usually successfully defended by the host). The net result is increased infection, which leads to enhanced production of the cytokines TNF and IL-6, causing cachexia, of which lack of appetite is a classic effect (41). Cachexia, in turn, results in loss of body mass (protein and fat stores) and renders the animal more susceptible to infection. Hence, the cycle continues, not only decreasing the quality of life of the patient but also increasing medical expenses, which can be financially taxing not only to family members but to our health care system in general. Amazingly, something as simple as proper diet can have dramatic effects in breaking this vicious cycle.

Although the answer is simple, the solution is extremely difficult and complex. With regard to young children in developing countries, society as a whole has to be involved to correct the deficiency. Training in effective agricultural practices is paramount to increase food productivity. Also, parents (especially breast-feeding mothers) should be educated on proper nutritional habits to provide nutritionally adequate milk for their infants and toddlers, as children are not able to take care of themselves. Similar measures should be taken for the elderly. The elderly need help not only in obtaining food but also preparing it because of debilitating chronic diseases such as rheumatoid arthritis. Furthermore, chronic illness and prolonged intake of medication leads to dental disease involving salivary gland hypofunction, resulting in difficulty in chewing and swallowing. The net effect, once again, is malnutrition (i.e., PEM), which causes impaired immunity, increasing the rate of infection, which then leads to a further reduction in food intake. Interestingly, there is common ground between the PEM seen in children and the elderly. Both groups are, in most cases, unable to help themselves adequately and rely on society for support. Perhaps, society should put forth its best efforts not only to improve the quality of life of the underprivileged and their peers but also offer help to decrease the health care expenses by optimizing the essential nutrient intake to ward off the occurrence of common infectious diseases both in children and elderly populations.

SUMMARY

Protein-energy malnutrition is a global problem primarily afflicting young children and the elderly. It does not discriminate between developing and industrialized countries. PEM results in a vast array of immunodeficiencies; however, the most notable outcome is the reduced IgA levels involved in mucosal immunity. Low IgA immunoglobulin allows the host to be highly susceptible to a wide variety of organisms, thereby increasing the risk of infection. Infection, in turn, leads to cachexia, which, in most cases, is already present as a result of PEM. Therefore, it is quite evident how the viscious cycle continues between PEM and infection. In many cases, especially in the elderly, PEM goes undetected unless proper biochemical analysis is conducted and aggressively corrected by optimal dietary intervention. Perhaps the most significant observation, normally overlooked, is that the need for adequate nutrition is involved in the life cycle. Many problems and concerns of the young (primarily infants and toddlers) are identical to that of the elderly. Furthermore, both groups require the assistance of both family and society to recognize and remedy the chronic and/or acute situation. The best treatment is a balanced diet with adequate vitamin and trace metal supplements; however, this should be approached with caution, as too aggressive a treatment regimen can be detrimental. Proper management requires the involvement of a team of health professionals, including nutritional specialists (i.e., dietitians), physicians, and/or social workers and psychologists.

REFERENCES

1. The state of the world's children 1998: A UNICEF report. Malnutrition: causes, consequences and solutions. Nutr Rev 1998; 56:115–23.
2. Fernandes G. Nutrition and immunity. Encycl Hum Biol 1991; 5:503–16.
3. Chandra RK. Nutrition and the immune system: an introduction. Am J Clin Nutr 1997; 66:460S–3S.
4. Williams SR. Nutritional deficiency diseases. In: Williams SR, ed, Nutrition and Diet Therapy, pp. 327–50. CRC, Boca Raton, FL, 1985.
5. Lesourd B. Protein undernutrition as the major cause of decreased immune function in the elderly: clinical and functional implications. Nutr Rev 1995; 53:S86–S94.
6. Cederholm T, Wretlind B, Hellstrom K, Anderson B, et al. Enhanced generation of interleukins 1β and 6 may contribute to the cachexia of chronic disease. Am J Clin Nutr 1997; 65:876–82.
7. Myrvik QN. Immunology and nutrition. In: Shils ME, Olson JA, Shike M, eds, Modern Nutrition in Health and Disease, pp. 623–62. Lea & Febiger, Philadelphia, 1994.
8. Woods JW, Woodward BD. Enhancement of primary systemic acquired immunity by exogenous triiodothyronine in wasted, protein-energy malnourished weanling mice. J Nutr 1991; 121:1425–32.
9. Sauerwein RW, Mulder JA, Mulder L, Lowe B et al. Inflammatory mediators in children with protein-energy malnutrition. Am J Clin Nutr 1997; 65:1534–9.
10. Doherty JF, Golden MHN, Remick DG, Griffin GE. Production of interleukin-6 and tumour necrosis factor-α in vitro is reduced in whole blood of severely malnourished children. Clin Sci 1994; 86:347–51.
11. Deitch EA, Winterton J, Li M, Berg R. The gut as a portal of entry for bacteremia. Ann Surg 1987; 205:681–92.
12. Chandra RK. 1990 McCollum award lecture. Nutrition and immunity: lessons from the past and new insights into the future. Am J Clin Nutr 1991; 53:1087–101.
13. Sakamoto M, Fujisawa Y, Nishioka K. Physiologic role of the complement system in host defense, disease, and malnutrition. Nutrition 1998; 14:391–8.
14. McMurray DN, Rey H, Casazza LJ, Watson RR. Effect of moderate malnutrition on concentrations of immunoglobulins and enzymes in tears and saliva of young Colombian children. Am J Clin Nutr 1977; 30:1944–8.
15. Woodward BD, Woods JW, Crouch DA. Direct evidence that primary acquired cell-mediated immunity is less resistant than is primary thymus-dependent humoral immunity to the depressive influence of wasting protein-energy malnutrition in weanling mice. Am J Clin Nutr 1992; 55:1180–5.
16. Ha CL, Paulino-Racine LE, Woodward BD. Expansion of the humoral effector cell compartment of both systemic and mucosal immune systems in a weanling murine model which duplicates critical features of human protein-energy malnutrition. Br J Nutr 1996; 75:445–60.
17. Ha CL, Woodward B. Reduction in the quantity of the polymeric immunoglobulin receptor is sufficient to account for the low concentration of intestinal secretory immunoglobulin A in a weanling mouse model of wasting protein-energy malnutrition. J Nutr 1997; 127: 427–35.
18. McGee DW, McMurray DN. The effect of protein malnutrition on the IgA immune response in mice. Immunology 1988; 63:25–9.
19. Lipschitz DA, Uduj KB. Influence of aging and protein deficiency on neutrophil function. J Gerontol 1986; 41:690–4.
20. Skerrett SJ, Henderson WR, Martin TR. Alveolar macrophage function in rats with severe protein calorie malnutrition. J Immunol 1990; 144:1052–61.
21. Lesourd BM. Nutrition and immunity in the elderly: modification of immune responses with nutritional treatments. Am J Clin Nutr 1997; 66:478S–84S.
22. Lesourd BM, Meaume S. Cell mediated immunity changes in aging, relative importance of cell subpopulation switches and of nutritional factors. Immunol Lett 1994; 40:235–42.
23. Verdery RB. The role of malnutrition in the failure to thrive syndrome. In: Watson RR, ed, Handbook of Nutrition in the Aged, pp. 304–8. CRC, Boca Raton, FL, 1985.
24. Ausman LM, Russell RM. Nutrition in the elderly. In: Shils ME, Olson JA, Shike M, eds, Modern Nutrition in Health and Disease, pp. 770–80. Lea & Febiger, Philadelphia, 1994.
25. Sullivan DH, Walls RC, Bopp MM. Protein-energy undernutrition and the risk of mortality within one year of hospital discharge: a follow-up study. J Am Geriatr Soc 1995; 43:507–12.
26. Cederholm T, Jagren C, Hellstrom K. Outcome of protein-energy malnutrition in elderly medical patients. Am J Med 1995; 98:67–74.
27. Cederholm TE, Hellstrom KH. Reversibility of protein-energy malnutrition in a group of chronically-ill elderly outpatients. Clin Nutr 1995; 14:81–7.
28. Morley JE. Anorexia of aging: physiologic and pathologic. Am J Clin Nutr 1997; 66:760–73.
29. Taylor CG, Potter AJ, Rabinovitch PS. Splenocyte glutathione and CD3-mediated cell proliferation are reduced in mice fed a protein-deficient diet. J Nutr 1997; 127:44–50.
30. Woodward BD, Miller RG. Depression of thymus-dependent immunity in wasting protein-energy malnutrition does not depend on an altered ratio of helper (CD4+) to suppressor (CD8+) T cells or on a

disproportionately large atrophy of the T-cell relative to the B-cell pool. Am J Clin Nutr 1991; 53:1329–35.

31. Sullivan DA, Vaerman JP, Soo C. Influence of severe protein malnutrition on rat lacrimal, salivary and gastrointestinal immune expression during development adulthood and aging. Immunology 1993; 78:308–17.

32. Bradley SF, Vibhagool A, Kunkel SL, Kauffman CA. Monokine secretion in aging and protein malnutrition. J Leuk Biol 1989; 45:510–4.

33. Kuvibidila S, Lolie Y, Ode D, Warrier RP. The immune response in protein-energy malnutrition and single nutrient deficiencies. In: Klurfeld DM, ed, Human Nutrition: A Comprehensive Treatise, pp. 121–55. Plenum, New York, 1993.

34. Fraker PJ, Haas SM, Leucke RW. Effect of zinc deficiency on the immune response of the young adult A/J mouse. J Nutr 1977; 107:1889–95.

35. Fraker PJ, King LE, Garvey BA, Medina CA. The immunopathology of zinc deficiency in humans and rodents. A possible role for programmed cell death. In: Klurfeld DM, ed, Human Nutrition: A Comprehensive Treatise, pp. 267–83. Plenum, New York, 1993.

36. Fernandes G, Nair M, Onoe K, Tanaka T, Floyd R, Good RA. Impairment of cell-mediated immunity functions by dietary zinc deficiency in mice. Proc Natl Acad Sci USA 1979; 76:457–61.

37. Prasad AS, Fitzgerald JT, Hess JW, Kaplan J, Peleu F, Dardenne M. Zinc deficiency in elderly patients. Nutrition 1993; 9:218–24.

38. Sazawal S, Black RE, Bhan MK, Bhandali N, Sinha A, Jolla S. Zinc supplementation in young children with acute diarrhea in India. N Engl J Med 1995; 333:839–44.

39. Prasad AS. Zinc deficiency in women, infants and children. J Am Coll Nutr 1996; 15:113–20.

40. Folwaezy C. Zinc and diarrhea in infants. J Trace Element Med Biol 1997; 11:116–22.

41. Tracey KJ. TNF and other cytokines in the metabolism of septic shock and cachexia. Clin Nutr 1992; 11:1–11.

17 Lipids, Inflammatory Cytokines, and Endothelial Cell Injury

Bernhard Hennig, Michal Toborek, and Gilbert A. Boissonneault

INTRODUCTION

LIPIDS AND ATHEROSCLEROSIS Although the mortality from coronary heart disease has declined recently, atherosclerosis and related vascular disorders are still the leading cause of death in the United States and other Western countries. The etiology of this disease is multifactorial, with hyperlipidemia, smoking, diabetes mellitus, hypertension, and obesity being well-established risk factors for the development of atherosclerosis. Dietary fat affects plasma lipids and lipoproteins and, thus, is linked to atherosclerosis *(1)*. Injury to or dysfunction of the vascular endothelium may be initiating events in the etiology of atherosclerosis.

There are numerous theories for the pathogenesis of atherosclerosis *(2)*, which include the response to injury theory *(3)*, response to modified lipoprotein theory *(4)*, response to low-density lipoprotein (LDL) retention theory *(5)*, and immunological hypothesis for atherosclerosis *(6)*. The current trend is to consider atherosclerosis as a response of the vascular wall to a variety of initiating agents and multiple pathogenic mechanisms (e.g., hyperlipidemia), contributing to the development of atheromatous plaques. It appears that the major participants in the atherosclerotic disease process include an active vascular endothelium, smooth-muscle cells, blood-borne cells such as monocytes and macrophages, and circulating lipoproteins *(7–9)*. The result is a multifactorial sequence of events involving endothelial cell injury/dysfunction and uptake of circulating blood monocytes and their differentiation into macrophages, coupled with smooth-muscle cell migration and proliferation.

There is ample evidence suggesting that serum cholesterol is a predictor of atherosclerosis and that serum cholesterol concentrations can be modified by varying the composition of dietary fat. Even though regression analysis of numerous human studies suggests that cholesterol and saturated fatty acid intake are primary determinants of serum cholesterol *(10)*, the role of dietary fat in the development of atherosclerosis remains controversial and

poorly understood *(11)*. In addition to dietary intake, biosynthesis of cholesterol represents a major input into whole-body cholesterol pools as well, and energy deprivation appears to result in the greatest decline in cholesterol synthesis, explaining, in part, the beneficial decline in circulating cholesterol concentrations observed with weight loss. Interestingly, consumption of oils, rich in polyunsaturated fatty acids, despite reducing circulating concentrations, can increase the cholesterol synthesis rate compared to other fats *(12)*.

Even though serum cholesterol appears to be a predictor of atherosclerosis and serum cholesterol concentrations can be modified by varying the composition of dietary fat, less is known about the role of specific fatty acids in atherosclerosis. The general indication is that saturated fatty acids increase, whereas polyunsaturated fatty acids decrease, serum cholesterol *(10)* and atherosclerosis, especially in some animal models *(13)*. Also, monounsaturated fatty acids appear to have no specific effect on plasma cholesterol concentrations. However, it is now known that saturated fatty acids are not equally hypercholesterolemic. For example, stearic acid and saturated fatty acids with less than 12 carbon atoms are thought not to raise serum cholesterol concentrations *(14)*. In fact, some studies suggest that stearic acid can be hypocholesterolemic *(15–17)*. This would suggest that the cholesterol-raising properties of saturated fatty acids should be attributed solely to lauric, myristic, and palmitic acids. However, these three saturated fatty acids appear to have different effects on serum total cholesterol concentrations as well. Several studies suggest that lauric acid is less, and myristic acid probably more, hypercholesterolemic than palmitic acid *(14,18)*. Furthermore, recent human studies suggest that lauric acid raises total serum cholesterol and LDL cholesterol concentrations compared with oleic acid. However, it is not as potent in increasing cholesterol concentrations as is palmitic acid *(19)*. On the other hand, in normocholesterolemic men and women, dietary palmitic and oleic acids seemed to exert similar effects on serum cholesterol and lipoprotein profiles *(20)*.

The question then arises of whether dietary saturated fats should be replaced by unsaturated fats. Unsaturated fats, especially *n*-3 or omega-3 fatty acids, may be beneficial to human health *(21,22)*,

From: *Nutrition and Immunology: Principles and Practice* (ME Gershwin et al. eds.), © Humana Press, Inc., Totowa, NJ

especially when incorporated into a low- rather than a high-fat diet (23). Diets high in n-6 and n-3 polyunsaturated fatty acids may lead to a decrease in serum cholesterol, but replacing saturated with unsaturated lipids may not be desirable because of their ability to oxidize easily. Numerous recent studies and biochemical investigations suggest that lipid-oxidation products, ingested with food or produced endogenously, represent a health risk (24). In fact, evidence supports the hypothesis that LDL undergoes oxidative modifications that increase its uptake by macrophages (4). Dietary antioxidants such as vitamin E might act as antiatherogenic agents by suppressing oxidative modification of LDL and the recruitment of monocytes into the arterial subendothelium by smooth-muscle cells (25). In fact, data from subjects with varying degrees of coronary atherosclerosis support the hypothesis that high serum polyunsaturated fatty acid levels, when insufficiently protected by antioxidants (e.g., vitamin E), may indicate a higher risk of atherosclerosis (26).

IMMUNE NATURE OF THE ATHEROSCLEROTIC PROCESS
Atherosclerosis is an inflammatory disease, and like other inflammatory diseases, it involves T cells, monocyte/macrophages, complement, and immunoglobulins. In addition, the vascular endothelium plays a central role in atherogenesis. Although many aspects of the immune nature of atherosclerotic plaque formation have been elucidated, many others remain to be discovered, including the initiating event resulting in the formation of a plaque at a specific location in the vascular tree. A number of excellent reviews addressing the immunological nature of the atherosclerotic process are available (27–33).

The initial step in plaque formation likely involves dysfunction of the vascular endothelium directly overlying the future atherosclerotic lesion. Atherosclerotic lesions occur in predictable and well-defined regions of slow blood flow, generally at vascular bifurcations or arterial branches (34). Hypertension exacerbates this response (35). Although LDL infiltration into the vascular intima is a hallmark of developing lesions, it is unclear whether this occurs prior to or following infiltration by immune T cells and monocytes. Two partially competing hypotheses addressing endothelial dysfunction and vascular inflammatory activities seek to explain these early stages of plaque formation.

The first hypothesis suggests that injury to the endothelium (e.g., caused by hypertension, blood flow irregularities, or other causes) enhances LDL passage through the endothelium. The increased rate of LDL translocation increases the intimal LDL concentration and, hence, LDL residence time. With increased residence time comes an increase in the rate of LDL oxidation (or other modification), aggregation, or association with matrix proteins (36–38). These products, particularly LDL oxidation products such as lysophospholipids (39), oxysterols (40–43), and other free-radical-containing lipid species induce changes in endothelial physiology, resulting in the initiation or perpetuation of inflammation (29,44), finally resulting in cellular infiltration, lipid, and matrix protein deposition, and ultimate mature plaque formation.

By itself, native LDL is relatively inert, as demonstrated by the effectiveness of vitamin E and other antioxidants in reducing atheroma formation in experimental hypercholesterolemia models of atherosclerosis (45,46). Macrophages (47,48) and endothelial cells (49,50) have been shown to oxidize LDL. Moreover, transition metals such as copper, present in the form of ceruloplasmin

as well as in its free, ionized form, are available to contribute to this oxidative process (51,52). Increased residence in the intima markedly augments the oxidation of LDL, and such oxidative modification greatly increases its internalization by intimal macrophages via scavenger receptors (53), resulting in foam cell formation. As internalized, oxidized lipids accumulate, they damage and possibly induce apoptosis in foam cells, resulting in the disgorgement of lipids into the intima. These oxidized lipids, as well as nonendocytosed oxidized LDL and other oxidized lipids, injure endothelial cells and further enhance permeability to serum LDL, thus perpetuating the development of this chronic inflammatory site.

An alternative, related hypothesis suggests that injurious conditions such as hypertension and slow blood flow contribute to endothelial changes; the primary change of importance is activation of stress protein hsp 60 (6). In itself, this physiologic response is not injurious; however, in the presence of anti-hsp 60 antibodies originating from immune responses directed against viral antigens, an autoimmune, antiendothelial cell response takes place in the vicinity of the developing plaque (6). This response, in turn, results in endothelial cell adhesion molecule expression with infiltration first with T cells and later with monocytes (54). The end result of the ensuing inflammatory response is the same: a marked increase in endothelial permeability to LDL, an increase in LDL residence in the intima, its oxidation and internalization by macrophages, foam cell formation, injury to foam cells and endothelial cells by exposure to oxidized lipids, death of foam cells with release of lipids into the intima (forming the beginning of the lipid core), and perpetuation of the response by continued, enhanced infiltration of LDL into the intima.

Fundamental to these hypotheses is the primary role played by the endothelium in initiation of inflammation at a defined location. A unique facet of the inflammatory response occurring in the wall of a large blood vessel, compared to other tissues, is the exposure to high concentrations of lipoproteins and lipoprotein remnants. Although all inflammatory responses involve altered endothelial permeability, only certain inflammatory responses taking place within large arteries result in atherogenesis. Without infiltration and accumulation of large amounts of cholesterol-laden LDL in the vessel wall, vessel wall inflammatory responses are transient and without lasting effect. Therefore, the immigration of copious amounts of LDL into the intima and its oxidation in situ is unique and central to the genesis of atherosclerosis.

Expression of adhesion molecules such as the E-selectins allow T cells and monocytes to migrate into the affected area of the vessel wall. The T cells bearing antigen receptors cross-reactive with endothelial hsp 60 may also directly induce inflammation of the vessel wall (6). These T cells and monocyte/macrophages, in response to hsp 60 or other antigens, or to oxidized, aggregated, or otherwise modified LDL, secrete cytokines such as tumor necrosis factor (TNF) which have direct, injurious, and proinflammatory effects on the endothelium (30,32). This chapter will focus on TNF as a modifier of endothelial function, including interactions between fatty acids and TNF (Fig. 1). Ultimately, these immune cytokines further exacerbate endothelial monolayer dysfunction, enhance endothelial permeability to LDL and other serum macromolecules, and augment recruitment of other leukocytes into the intima. Thus begins the slow, chronic inflammatory cycle resulting in atheroma formation.

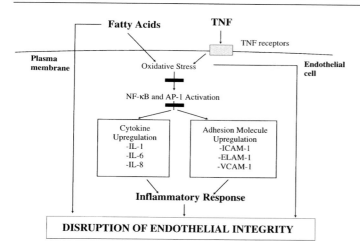

Fig. 1. Schematic diagram of the proposed mechanisms involved in lipid and inflammatory cytokine-mediated endothelial cell dysfunction. Bold bars represent pathways hypothesized to be inhibited by antioxidant and/or anti-inflammatory nutrients.

PATHOLOGICAL RESPONSES IN VASCULAR ENDOTHELIAL CELL INJURY AS AFFECTED BY SELECTED NUTRIENTS

FATTY ACIDS, LIPOPROTEINS, INFLAMMATORY RESPONSE, AND ENDOTHELIAL CELL DYSFUNCTION High levels of circulating triglyceride-rich lipoproteins (chylomicrons and very low-density lipoprotein [VLDL]) have been implicated in the injury process of the endothelium (55,56). Plasma chylomicron levels are elevated in humans after consuming a high-fat meal, and hepatic synthesis of VLDL is increased when caloric intake is in excess of body needs. Hydrolysis of triglyceride-rich lipoproteins mediated by lipoprotein lipase, a key enzyme in lipoprotein metabolism that is associated with the luminal site of endothelial cells, may be an important source of high concentrations of fatty acid anions in proximity to the endothelium (57,58). It has been hypothesized that high levels of diet-derived fatty acids can cause endothelial injury or dysfunction and thus disrupt the ability of the endothelium to function as a selective barrier (57,58). This would result in lipid deposition by allowing increased penetration of cholesterol-rich remnant lipoproteins into the arterial wall. In fact, activity of lipoprotein lipase is increased in atherosclerotic lesions (58–60). A recent report also provides evidence that lipoprotein lipase may be a chemoattractant for activated macrophages (61). Furthermore, activated lipoprotein lipase induces TNF gene expression in macrophages and TNF production by this type of cell (62). Lipoprotein lipase-derived remnants of lipoproteins isolated from hypertriglyceridemic subjects, as well as selective unsaturated fatty acids such as linoleic acid, were demonstrated to disrupt endothelial integrity (63,64).

As mentioned earlier, there is evidence that selected fatty acids, derived from the hydrolysis of triglyceride-rich lipoproteins, may be atherogenic by causing endothelial injury or dysfunction and subsequent endothelial barrier dysfunction (reviewed in *ref.* 65). In support of this hypothesis, we have shown that exposure of cultured endothelial cells to selected fatty acids (e.g., oleic acid) decreased endothelial barrier function, expressed as an increased transfer of both albumin and LDL across the endothelium (66,67).

In addition to oleic acid, we also investigated the effects of other fatty acids on endothelial barrier function (68). Albumin-bound palmitic and stearic acid had little effect on endothelial barrier function, but exposure of cell monolayers to linoleic acid produced an even greater increase in albumin transfer than did equal concentrations of oleic acid. The disruption in endothelial barrier function was exacerbated greatly in the presence of small amounts of oxidation derivatives of unsaturated fatty acids (69). Furthermore, when comparing fatty acid extracts derived from different animal fats and plant oils, the fat-induced disruption of endothelial barrier function was related to the amount of linoleic acid present in the fat source (70). These data suggest that among different fatty acids, linoleic acid may play a critical role in the pathogenesis of atherosclerosis (71). This hypothesis is supported by the fact that adipose tissue levels of linoleic acid, which reflect intake of this fatty acid over a period of time, were positively associated with the degree of coronary artery disease (72). In addition, concentrations of linoleic acid were increased in the phospholipid fractions of human coronary arteries in cases of sudden cardiac death resulting from ischemic heart disease (73). Recent research involving a population from a country with one of the highest dietary polyunsaturated/saturated fat ratios in the world has concluded that diets rich in omega-6 fatty acids may contribute to an increased incidence of atherosclerosis, hyperinsulinemia, and tumorigenesis (74).

Several mechanisms were proposed to explain injurious effects of linoleic acid on endothelial cells. Because of very low basal activity of endothelial cell elongases and delta 5 and delta 9 desaturases, arachidonic acid is not produced from linoleic acid significantly in this type of cell (75,76). Consequently, linoleic acid accumulates within endothelial cells (75,77). Moreover, linoleic acid decreases levels of intracellular ATP (78) and proteoglycans (79) and enhances elastase-like activity (80). Linoleic-acid-mediated disruption of endothelial barrier function also may be caused by its ability to inhibit gap–junctional intracellular communication (81) and to induce intracellular oxidative stress (64).

In recent years, the role of oxidative stress has gained much attention in studies of lipid-mediated and/or inflammatory cytokine-mediated endothelial cell dysfunction or injury. It is now generally accepted that oxidation of LDL plays one of the most critical roles in atherogenesis. LDL can be oxidized in the subendothelial space, which lacks many of the antioxidants present in whole blood. It is possible that LDL is oxidized by endothelial cells while passing through the endothelium (82). In fact, oxidative modifications of LDL were first characterized in vitro using endothelial cell culture model systems (83). Moreover, other major cell types present in the arterial wall, such as smooth-muscle cells and macrophages, are able to oxidize LDL in vitro (84). However, mechanisms of LDL oxidation still remain controversial. Whereas superoxide radicals appear to be involved in monocyte-mediated LDL oxidation (85), their role in endothelial-cell-stimulated LDL oxidation has been questioned. In addition, lipoxygenase may be involved in oxidative modification of LDL by endothelial cells (86). Oxidized LDL exerts several harmful effects on the endothelium. Oxidatively modified LDL is cytotoxic to endothelial cells (87), induces endothelial cell production of monocyte chemotactic protein (88) and growth factors (89), inhibits the release of endothelium-derived relaxing factor (EDRF) (90), and increases adhesiveness of leukocytes to endothelial cells (92). Interestingly, high-density lipoproteins (HDL), and mainly Apo A, can prevent cell death of endothelial cells induced by oxidized LDL *(93)*.

There is clear evidence that in humans, dietary oxidized lipids can be absorbed by the small intestine, be incorporated into chylomicrons, appear in the bloodstream, and thus contribute to the total body pool of oxidized lipids *(94)*. Including oxidized corn oil in a diet accelerated the development of fatty streaks in cholesterol-fed rabbits *(95)*, suggesting that the consumption of oxidized lipids (e.g., high-corn-oil diets) may be an important risk factor for atherosclerosis. It also has been shown that, compared with normal LDL, mildly oxidized LDL may be atherogenic because it may circulate in plasma for a period sufficiently long to enter, accumulate, and be degraded in the arterial intima *(96)*. Interestingly, when studying lipoproteins from subjects consuming different types of dietary fat (e.g., high in oleic acid or linoleic acid), only the percentage of linoleic acid in LDL correlated strongly with the extent of oxidizability and macrophage degradation of these lipoproteins *(97)*. This suggests that substitution of monounsaturated (rather than polyunsaturated) fatty acids for saturated fatty acids in the diet might be preferable for the possible prevention of atherosclerosis.

There is evidence that diets enriched with polyunsaturated fatty acids increase the susceptibility of LDL to undergo oxidative modifications *(98)*. We determined the impact of different high-fat diets on the oxidizability of LDL combined with the effect of native and/or oxidized LDL on endothelial barrier function *(99)*. Rabbits were fed diets enriched with corn oil, corn oil with added cholesterol, milk fat, chicken fat, beef tallow, or lard. Feeding rabbits a diet enriched with corn oil decreased plasma total cholesterol and LDL cholesterol. However, LDL isolated from this group of rabbits exhibited the most significant oxidizability. Moreover, oxidized LDL derived from the corn oil group significantly disrupted endothelial integrity and endothelial barrier function. On the other hand, cholesterol supplementation to the corn oil diet decreased the oxidizability of LDL and partially protected the oxidized LDL-mediated endothelial cell dysfunction, as compared with the corn oil group *(100)*. In addition, vitamin E levels in LDL isolated from the animals fed corn oil with added cholesterol were higher than those in the nonsupplemented group even though the vitamin E levels in these two diets were not different. These data suggest that there was a lower level of oxidation in the presence of added cholesterol, supporting the hypothesis that cholesterol may act as an antioxidant *(101)*. One may suggest that the antioxidant effect of cholesterol was, at least partially, mediated by the sparing of vitamin E. Our data confirm observations that diets rich in unsaturated fats contribute to decreased antioxidant status, increased oxidizability of LDL, and enhanced toxicity of oxidized LDL toward endothelial cells *(99)*. There is now in vivo evidence that oxidized LDL can injure the endothelium, compromising the function of the endothelium as a permeability barrier *(102)*. Furthermore, oleic acid may attenuate dysfunction of cultured endothelial cell monolayers mediated by oxidized LDL *(103)*.

It is widely recognized that the effects of fatty acids released from triglyceride-rich lipoproteins on endothelial cell metabolism depend largely on the degree of unsaturation. However, the role of oxidative stress is one of the controversial issues in fatty-acid-mediated injury to endothelial cells. Although oxidizability of fatty acids is linearly dependent on the degree of unsaturation *(104)*, linolenic acid appears to be less toxic to endothelial cells than the less unsaturated linoleic acid *(105)*. To test the role of oxidative stress and antioxidant protection in fatty-acid-mediated disturbances in endothelial integrity, we measured cellular oxidation in cells exposed to 18-carbon fatty acids *(106)*. Cellular oxidation was determined using a new cell-imaging technique based on reactive oxygen species-mediated conversion of 2,7-dichlorofluorescin into fluorescent 2,7-dichlorofluorescein (DCF) *(107)*. This technique allows measurement of oxidative stress in living cells. An increased DCF fluorescence emission reflects enhanced oxidative stress. Among the 18-carbon fatty acids differing in the degree of unsaturation, the most significant increase in cellular oxidation was caused by linoleic acid *(106)*. This high potency of linoleic acid to induce cellular oxidative stress may be related to the fact that it can accumulate within endothelial cells because of insufficient conversion to arachidonic acid *(75)*. Moreover, linoleic acid induced endothelial cell peroxisomal β-peroxidation, a pathway that leads to the production of hydrogen peroxide *(108)*. Other reports support our observation that linoleic acid can act as a potent oxidant within endothelial cells *(109)*.

Inflammation and any agents that provoke an inflammatory response may be the most critical risk factors in the atherosclerotic disease process *(110)*, and there is evidence that the progression of atherosclerosis includes events that are immunologically mediated *(6,48,111)*. Little is known about the interaction of nutrition (and, in particular, fatty acids) and inflammatory mediators, but there is evidence that selected nutrients can provoke an inflammatory response or, on the other hand, provide anti-inflammatory or anti-atherogenic properties *(65,112,113)*. It appears that only selected omega-3 fatty acids can reduce endothelial expression of adhesion molecules *(114–117)* and that linoleic acid can increase adhesion receptor expression *(118)*. In fact, our data strongly support the fact that selected unsaturated fatty acids (e.g., linoleic acid) and inflammatory cytokines may cross-amplify vascular endothelial cell activation, a response common to inflammation and atherosclerosis *(106)*. Others have shown that oxidatively modified LDL can augment cytokine-activated VCAM-1 gene expression in human vascular endothelial cells *(119)*, suggesting an imbalance in oxidative stress/antioxidant status as part of the mechanisms involved in these inflammatory events.

Even though numerous risk factors, including hyperlipidemia, smoking, and hypertension, seem to contribute to the development of atherosclerosis, to date it has not been possible to link these risk factors into a common pathogenic mechanism. There is evidence, however, that modulations in the level of activity of a select set of endothelial transcription factors (e.g., endothelial nuclear factor-κB [NF-κB]) may provide a mechanism for linking these seemingly diverse processes with the generation of dysfunctional endothelium and the onset of atherosclerotic lesion formation *(120,121)*. Stimuli known to activate the NF-κB complex include inflammatory cytokines, activators of protein kinase C, viruses, and oxidants *(122–124)*. Recent studies suggest a dysfunction of NF-κB by oxidized LDL *(125)*, presenting further evidence for a critical role of this transcription factor in the pathology of atherosclerosis. One may speculate that selected diet-derived fatty acids may induce endothelial oxidative stress and generate excess reactive oxygen species, which activate NF-κB and modulate endothelial gene expression. Our data support the hypothesis that linoleic acid may be atherogenic by intensifying cytokine expression and endothelial cell injury in atherosclerosis. We have recently shown that linoleic acid can activate NF-κB *(126)* and induce synthesis of adhesion molecules and inflammatory cytokines in cultured endothelial cells *(127)*. All these studies lead one to conclude that excessive consumption of oils and fats rich in linoleic acid may be proinflammatory and atherogenic and that the type of fat becomes a less significant component in the pathogenesis of atherosclerosis when one consumes a low-fat diet rich in soluble fibers and natural antioxidants.

CHOLESTEROL, LIPOPROTEINS, AND ENDOTHELIAL CELL DYSFUNCTION

Elevated serum cholesterol, particularly in the form of LDL, is a well-known risk factor for atherogenesis. It is becoming generally accepted that LDL *per se* may be relatively inert, and acquires its atherogenic qualities upon variable degrees of modification (e.g., oxidation). The oxidation of LDL is a semisequential process involving initiation of oxidation of its hydrophilic surface phospholipids; depletion of its vitamin E stores, further oxidation of surface phospholipids and apolipoprotein B and of core cholesteryl ester fatty acids; oxidation of cholesterol to various oxysterols, and formation of lipid/apo B conjugates and fragmentation of apo B. The process of LDL oxidation has been described in more detail elsewhere *(128)*. Oxidized LDL has been identified in human atherosclerotic plaque *(129,130)* and its long-term presence in vivo was demonstrated by the presence of serum antibodies directed against oxidized LDL *(131–134)*.

Cholesterol accumulation in the arterial intima is a hallmark of the atherosclerotic plaques *(27,135)*. The vast majority of this cholesterol is delivered into the intima in the form of native, nonoxidized LDL and is oxidized *in situ (128)*. Penetration of excess quantities of LDL into the intima is the result of disrupted endothelial barrier function *(136)*, potentially resulting from vascular injury *(3)*, retention *(5)* and/or modification *(4)* of LDL, or immune injury to the arterial wall caused by an autoimmune response *(6)*. Once in the intima, LDL may be oxidized by free radicals released from endothelial cells *(49,50)*, intimal monocytes *(47,48)*, and transition metals *(51,52)*. The acetic milieu within the atherosclerotic plaque is thought to contribute to the predilection to oxidation of LDL trapped in the intima *(137)*. Oxidized LDL can contribute to atherosclerotic plaque formation through a number of immune and nonimmune mechanisms *(27,30,121,135,138)*.

The fatty acid composition of LDL is known to affect its oxidizability *(99,139–143)*. Moreover, enrichment of endothelial cells with oleic acid attenuated alteration of endothelial actin microfilament architecture and barrier function caused by exposure to oxidized LDL *(144)*. As described earlier, exposure to stearic and palmitic acids had minimal effect on endothelial barrier function, whereas exposure to oleic acid caused a moderate reduction in endothelial barrier function and exposure to linoleic acid resulted in a marked reduction *(67–69)*. Enrichment with linoleic acid synergistically reduced endothelial barrier function and increased intraendothelial oxidative stress related to TNF exposure *(106)*.

Tappia and Grimble recently reported that thioglycollate-elicited peritoneal macrophages isolated from rats fed diets enriched with a variety of fats responded to TNF stimulation with different levels of interleukin-1 (IL-1) and interleukin-6 (IL-6) production *(145)*. Rats fed the corn-oil-enriched diet for 8 wk produced the greatest amounts of these cytokines. These investigators reported a direct relationship between membrane phospholipid containing linoleic or arachidonic acid in the *sn*-2 position and both IL-1 and IL-6 production. The dietary linoleic acid effects on cytokine formation were only partially related to changes in prostaglandin E_2 (PGE$_2$ or to LTB$_4$ production.

We reported that LDL from rabbits fed diets enriched with corn

oil and cholesterol was less oxidizable and had fewer detrimental effects on endothelial barrier function than LDL from rabbits fed corn-oil-enriched diets without cholesterol *(99)*. However, we also found that exposure of endothelial cells to LDL isolated from rabbits exposed to an acute intragastric dose of cholesterol resulted in a loss of barrier integrity *(146)*. In contrast, in vitro enrichment of LDL with cholesterol did not affect endothelial barrier function compared with control LDL; however, LDL enriched in vitro or in vivo with the oxysterol cholestan-3β,5α,6β-triol (Triol) reduced endothelial barrier function *(146)*.

As oxysterols are formed during LDL oxidation *(40–43)* and are found in atherosclerotic plaque *(43,147,148)*, their effects on vascular wall biology are of interest. We previously reported that a variety of oxysterols detrimentally affected in vitro measures of endothelial barrier function *(149)*, an effect that was not prevented by supplemental vitamin E *(150)*. The reduction in endothelial barrier function caused by oxysterol exposure may be related to direct toxicity. Indeed, oxysterols were shown to be cytotoxic in many cell types, including monocytes, smooth-muscle cells, and endothelial cells *(151–153)*, probably as a result of apoptosis *(154,155)*.

In addition to their cytotoxic effects, oxysterols were shown to inhibit gap–junction communication between smooth-muscle cells in culture, whereas pure cholesterol enhanced this function *(156)*. Exposure to oxysterols also had no effect on or enhanced smooth-muscle cell DNA synthesis *(157,158)*, even in the presence of cytotoxicity. Whereas smooth muscle cells were not actively attracted to oxysterols, they also were not repelled, resulting in occasional suicidal in vitro migration toward oxysterol crystals *(157)*.

Exposure to oxysterols enhanced LDL uptake by smooth-muscle cells *(159)*. Macrophages exposed to oxidized LDL accumulated oxysterols in the form of oxysterol esters *(41)*, and sterol efflux from such oxysterol-enriched macrophage foam cells was impaired *(160)*. A similar inhibition of sterol efflux was noted in oxysterol-enriched L cells *(161)*.

Therefore, oxysterols, either delivered into the intima in the core of "native" LDL *(162)* or generated *in situ* during the process of LDL oxidation in the intima, likely influence atherosclerotic plaque formation *(152)*. Following engulfment by macrophages or smooth-muscle cells, oxysterols reduce sterol efflux, thereby enhancing foam cell formation. Upon accumulation of oxysterols as intracellular oxysterol esters, foam cells succumb to their cytotoxic effects, ultimately disgorging their lipid contents into the intima *(135)*. These oxidized lipids, including oxysterols, become available to endothelial cells, resulting in disruption of endothelial barrier function and subsequent dysfunction and death of the endothelial monolayer. These endothelial effects, in turn, increase penetration of LDL into the intima, accelerating the cycle and promoting atheroma formation.

INFLAMMATORY EVENTS AND ENDOTHELIAL CELL INJURY

Injury to or dysfunction of the endothelium is believed to be one of the first events in the development of atherosclerosis, and inflammatory mechanisms are an integral part of this process *(121,163)*. Leukocyte recruitment followed by monocyte migration across the endothelium are among the earliest steps in atherogenesis *(163)*. These processes are mediated by adhesion molecules located both on endothelial cells and leukocytes. Adhesion molecules which are members of the selectin family, such as P-selectin and E-selectin (endothelial–leukocyte adhesion molecule-1 (ELAM-1), or members of the immunoglobulin super-family, such as ICAM-1 (intracellular adhesion molecule-1), ICAM-2, VCAM-1 (vascular cell adhesion molecule-1) and PECAM-1 (platelet–endothelial cell adhesion molecule-1) are present in endothelial cells in a resting state or can be expressed after TNF activation (164). In fact, there is strong evidence that increased cytokine production, namely TNF, stimulates inflammatory mechanisms within the endothelium and contributes to the development of atherosclerosis. Activated macrophages and T lymphocytes are considered to be main sources of inflammatory cytokines within the arterial wall (165). Supporting the role of TNF in atherogenesis, increased levels of TNF are detected in atherosclerotic vessels, mainly in intimal thickening (166,167). Moreover, production of TNF by circulating leukocytes is enhanced in atherosclerotic patients (168). The latter observation may be especially important because hypoxia induces high-affinity receptors for TNF in human endothelial cells in a time- and dose-dependent manner (169). Released TNF can stimulate oxidation of LDL (170) and potentiate inflammatory reactions within the endothelium of the vessel wall. Endothelial cells which exhibit both TNF receptor types (described below) (171–173) are especially prone to TNF-mediated processes. TNF can stimulate both endothelial cell upregulation of adhesion molecules and endothelial cell production of other cytokines, such as interleukins-1, -6, and -8 (IL-1, IL-6, IL-8) (174,175). TNF also exerts injurious effects on endothelial cells. For example, treatment with TNF induces endothelial cell oxidative stress (a compromised balance between production of reactive oxygen species and antioxidant protection), decreases cellular glutathione (176) and ATP (177), increases intracellular calcium, disrupts endothelial barrier function (176), activates matrix proteinases (80,178), and induces endothelial cell apoptosis (179).

Cellular effects of inflammatory cytokines, including TNF, are mediated by specific receptor(s). Two distinct TNF receptors have been isolated, cloned, and characterized. TNF-R55, also called p55, is a protein with a molecular mass of approximately 55 kDa, and TNF-R75, called p75 or p70, is a protein of approximately 75 kDa (180). Both TNF-R55 and TNF-R75 consist of extracellular, transmembrane, and intracellular domains. Although the extracellular domains of both receptors are identical in 28%, no homology exists between intracellular regions of TNF-R55 and TNF-R75. Moreover, intracellular signals generated by both receptors are different (181). The role of particular receptors in TNF-mediated effects on endothelial cell metabolism is unclear. It appears that TNF activates endothelial cells preferentially through TNF-R55. This receptor pathway controls TNF-stimulated endothelial cell expression of adhesion molecules (ELAM-1, VCAM-1, ICAM-1), class I major histocompatibility complex (I MHC) molecules (172), production of interleukins (IL-6, IL-8), synthesis of tissue factor (171), activation of sphingomyelinase with generation of ceramide (182,183), activation of NF-κB (182,183), and induction of manganese superoxide dismutase (MnSOD) (184). In addition, TNF-mediated cytotoxic effects also appear to be connected to TNF-R55 signaling (185). The role of the TNF-R75 in TNF-mediated effects is unclear. It was proposed that the TNF-R75 "presents" TNF to the TNF-R55 in nonlymphoid cells at low TNF doses (186). Thus, the TNF-R75 might promote cytotoxic effects of TNF-R55 (184). Evidence suggests that the TNF-R75 may potentiate the role of the TNF-R55 in neutrophil and endothelial cell activation (171,187,188). In contrast, it was proposed that the TNF-R75 may play a role in inactivation of TNF (189). Recent

evidence suggests that TNF-R75 may induce signals which inhibit TNF-mediated apoptosis (190). However, the only confirmed direct effect of the TNF-R75-mediated signals on cellular metabolism is stimulation of TNF-induced proliferation of activated mononuclear cells (191).

Recent evidence suggests a direct relationship between dietary fatty acids and production of inflammatory cytokines such as TNF. When plasma triglyceride-rich lipoproteins (e.g., chylomicrons and VLDL) are elevated, hydrolysis of triglycerides and, thus, release of free fatty acids by lipoprotein lipase occurs in proximity to the endothelial surface. It was shown that lipoprotein lipase, an enzyme which is associated with the luminal site of endothelial cells, can induce expression of the TNF gene and TNF production in macrophages (62,192). Although the detailed mechanism of these effects are not known, it appears that protein kinase C can be involved in lipoprotein lipase-induced TNF synthesis (192).

Although TNF is mainly generated by activated macrophages, other cell types also can produce this cytokine. Few reports indicate that endothelial cells express the TNF gene and can release this cytokine (193–195). However, only sparse information is available concerning the regulation of endothelial cell TNF gene expression and the role of locally produced TNF on endothelial cell metabolism. It was demonstrated that endothelial cell TNF production is stimulated by lipopolysaccharide (LPS) (193) or exogenous TNF (194). Evidence suggests that TNF produced by an autocrine pathway in endothelial cells may significantly influence endothelial cell metabolism. For example, autocrine secretion of TNF can mediate LPS-stimulated synthesis of nitric oxide in cultured endothelial cells (193).

OXIDATIVE STRESS AND ENDOTHELIAL CELL INJURY

Free-radical reactions, including lipid peroxidation, are considered to be important factors in the pathogenesis of a variety of pathological states, including injury to endothelial cells and the development of atherosclerosis. Free radicals, especially reactive oxygen species formed by univalent reduction of oxygen, are characterized by very high chemical activity. They can damage proteins, lipids, carbohydrates, and nucleic acids. Plasma membranes are critical targets of free-radical reactions. Reactive oxygen species can easily produce injuries to cell membranes by initiation of polyunsaturated fatty acid peroxidation, inactivation of membrane enzymes and receptors, depolymerization of polysaccharides, as well as by protein crosslinking and fragmentation. These disturbances result in changes of the membrane structure, fluidity, transport, antigenic character, and others (196). In a variety of diseases, the endothelium is very susceptible to oxidative stress and free-radical-mediated reactions. It is generally assumed that injury to the endothelium may trigger atherogenesis (197).

Reactive oxygen species can be generated as a result of inflammatory reactions which include activated neutrophils. These cells can generate large amounts of superoxide anion radicals (2 O_2 via the reaction catalyzed by NADPH oxidase:

$$2\ O_2 + NADPH \rightarrow 2\ O_2^- + NADP^+ + H^+.$$

Superoxide anion radicals can further participate in the formation of other active oxygen species. For example, dysmutation of superoxide anion radicals yields generation of hydrogen peroxide (H_2O_2) (198).

Superoxide anion radical and hydrogen peroxide are able to reduce, oxidize, damage, degrade, and inactivate a variety of enzymes and biologically important compounds. Superoxide anion radical is conjugated with its protonated form—perhydroxyl radical (HO_2), a potent oxidant, sufficiently reactive to initiate peroxidation or polyunsaturated fatty acids. Moreover, hydrogen peroxide in the presence of transition metal ions (e.g., iron and copper) may react with O_2^- to give hydroxyl radical (OH), the most reactive free radical produced in biological systems. Hydroxyl radicals can react with all organic compounds and produce site-directed damage. They can also easily induce peroxidation of unsaturated fatty acids *(198)*. Because hydrogen peroxide diffuses through cell membranes *(199)*, and superoxide anion radical is transported through membrane anion channels *(200)*, hydroxyl radicals can be formed both extracellularly and intracellularly.

Cell injury mediated by activated leukocytes is not only limited to reactions induced by reactive oxygen species. For example, activated leukocytes can release hydrolytic enzymes from lysosomes, thus causing injury to cell plasma membranes. Stimulated neutrophils also release myeloperoxidase into extracellular medium. Myeloperoxidase is an enzyme which catalyzes oxidation of a number of halides and pseudohalides. Chloride ion, a result of its high extracellular concentration, is preferentially oxidized to hypochlorous acid, a potent oxidizing agent about 100 times more reactive than hydrogen peroxide. Hypochlorous acid can exert harmful effects on sulfhydryl oxidation and hemoprotein inactivation as well as on protein and nucleic acid degradation *(201)*.

Polyunsaturated fatty acids can be oxidized not only in nonenzymatic reactions of fatty acid peroxidation but also in enzyme-mediated reactions, such as in reactions catalyzed by different lipoxygenases. Both types of fatty acid oxidation are essential in the development of atherosclerosis. However, evidence indicates that enzymatic oxidation of fatty acids and lipoproteins might be more important in the early stages of atherosclerosis *(202)*. Among different lipoxygenases, it appears that 15-lipoxygenase may be of critical significance in the development of atherosclerosis. Both 15-lipoxygenase mRNA and protein were determined in atherosclerotic lesions of humans and rabbits. Moreover, expression of 15-lipoxygenase was colocalized with epitopes of oxidized LDL *(201,203)*. Macrophages exert the high activity of 15-lipoxygenase, indicating the significance of immune reactions in enzymatic oxidation of fatty acids and lipoproteins. In reactions catalyzed by 15-lipoxygenase, linoleic acid is converted into hydroperoxyoctadecadienoic acid (13-HPODE) and arachidonic acid into hydroperoxyeicosatetraenoic acid (15-HPETE). 13-HPODE and 15-HPETE are biosynthetic precursors of more stable oxidized metabolites, such as 13-hydroxyoctadecadienoic acid (13-HODE) and 15-monohydroxyeicosatetraenoic acid (15-HETE), respectively. In support of the role of 15-lipoxygenase in atherogenesis, 13-HODE and 15-HETE were also detected in atherosclerotic lesions *(202,204)*. In addition, 13-HPODE is the major fatty acid oxidation product found in oxidized LDL *(205)*. 13-HPODE may contribute to oxidized LDL-mediated effects on endothelial cell metabolism. It was hypothesized that 13-HPODE might serve as a specific redox signal in cytokine-mediated expression of adhesion molecules in endothelial cells *(119)*.

Not only endothelial cells but also vascular smooth-muscle cells are sensitive to linoleic acid and 13-HPODE-induced metabolic disturbances. For example, both agents induce DNA synthesis, expression of *c-fos*, *c-jun*, and *c-myc*, as well as activation of mitogen-activated protein kinase (MAP kinase). A cotreatment with nordihydroguaiaretic acid, a potent inhibitor of the lipoxygen-ase system, reduced these alterations of cellular growth and pro-oncogene expression *(206)*.

Despite their several mitogenic effects, fatty acids oxidized by 15-lipoxygenase might also contribute to cell death. For example, 15-HPETE and 13-HPODE can induce apoptosis, decrease cellular viability, increase intracellular calcium, and induce DNA fragmentation in different T-cell lines *(207)*. Moreover, highly oxidized LDL, which contains significant amounts of 13-HPODE, can initiate apoptosis in arterial smooth-muscle cells, macrophages, and fibroblasts *(208)*.

GLUTATHIONE AND OXIDATIVE STRESS-MEDIATED ENDOTHELIAL CELL DYSFUNCTION   Several antioxidant systems protect cells against injury induced by free-radical and lipid peroxidation processes. Among these antioxidative mechanisms, the glutathione redox cycle appears to be one of the most effective in endothelial cells. Total glutathione content and the equilibrium between its reduced (GSH) and oxidized (GSSG) forms are believed to play one of the most important roles in the maintenance of cellular redox status. The dominant form of cellular glutathione is GSH. It is the major nonprotein sulfhydryl compound within cells which controls the regeneration of protein sulfhydryl groups from disulfide bonds *(209)*. Generally, it is accepted that modifications in the thiol contents are critical for the overall cellular redox status. This status may determine the cellular response to different stimuli. For example, cellular redox status influenced by glutathione depletion or an increase in GSSG was shown to stimulate activation of NF-κB. However, GSSG in high concentrations can inhibit NF-κB binding capacity *(210)*. Thus, for optimal activation of NF-κB, well-balanced GSSG levels are required.

Glutathione exerts its antioxidant properties not only as a nonenzymatic free-radical scavenger but also as a substrate for antioxidant enzymes, glutathione peroxidase, phospholipid hydroperoxide glutathione peroxidase, and glutathione-S-transferase. All these enzymes are involved in the detoxification of lipid hydroperoxides. However, glutathione peroxidase not only catalyzes the conversion of lipid hydroperoxides, released from membranes by phospholipase A2 *(211)*, to corresponding fatty acids, but also reduced H_2O_2 *(212)*. The glutathione redox cycle is much more effective than catalase in H_2O_2 detoxification in endothelial cell cultures *(213)*. Both enzymatic and nonenzymatic glutathione-mediated detoxification of reactive oxygen species and lipid hydroperoxides are connected with the oxidation of GSH to GSSG. The pool of GSH may be regenerated by glutathione reductase *(209)*.

Concurrent interaction between GSH and vitamin E is another important factor that determines the antioxidative functions of glutathione and endothelial cell protection against oxidative stress. Vitamin E acts as an antioxidant by donating a hydrogen atom to a lipid peroxyl radical. A lipid hydroperoxide and oxidized vitamin E are products of this reaction. Because only reduced vitamin E can serve as an antioxidant, compounds such as GSH and vitamin C are required to maintain the active form of vitamin E by reducing the oxidized form. Vitamin E-dependent inhibition of liver microsomal lipid peroxidation is approximately five times more active in the presence of GSH than in its absence *(214)*.

Because GSH is a crucial antioxidant for normal cell metabolism, an increase in cellular glutathione levels could be a potent protector of cells against oxidative damage. Although glutathione uptake is not sufficiently active within the majority of different cell types, its intracellular pool may be modulated by a variety of nutrients, including buthionine sulfoximine (BSO) and *N*-acetyl-L-cysteine (NAC). GSH is synthesized from glutamic acid, cysteine, and glycine in two ATP-dependent reactions. BSO selectively inhibits the first reaction in glutathione synthesis, catalyzed by γ-glutamylcysteine synthetase. Therefore, cellular treatment with BSO can provide a decrease in glutathione levels. On the other hand, supplementation with NAC, a cysteine prodrug, may effectively increase cellular glutathione levels. It is well established that the limiting factor in glutathione synthesis is the availability of cysteine *(215)*. There is evidence that the first step in NAC metabolism may involve extracellular deacylation to cysteine, followed by cysteine uptake *(216)*. Therefore, it is possible that NAC contribution to glutathione synthesis is mediated partially by cysteine. However, in contrast to cysteine, NAC is metabolized preferentially to glutathione but not to taurine or sulfate *(216,217)*. NAC exerts several beneficial effects on endothelial cells, including protection against chronic hyperoxia *(218)* and acute immunological reactions *(219)*, inhibition of antiproliferative effects of transforming growth factor-β1 (TGF-β1) *(220)*, and repression of interleukin-1β-mediated expression of VCAM-1 *(221)*.

Oxidized glutathione (GSSH), which is formed in antioxidant reactions involving GSH, can accumulate within cells during increased oxidative processes. Therefore, the cellular level of GSSG and especially the ratio of GSSG/GSH are considered to be valuable markers of oxidative stress *(222)*. However, excessive accumulation of GSSG can exert toxic effects to cells. Therefore, when GSSG approaches toxic levels, it may be transported out of cells or form mixed disulfides with intracellular proteins. These protective mechanisms against accumulation of GSSG can lead to depletion of total intracellular glutathione.

We observed marked disturbances in glutathione metabolism in endothelial cells exposed to selected fatty acids as well as to inflammatory cytokines such as TNF. Treatment with oleic acid, linoleic acid, or linolenic acid caused an initial decrease in endothelial cell glutathione levels, reaching the minimum after a 6-h exposure. The lowest levels of glutathione, compared both to the control and treatments specimens, were observed in cultures exposed to linoleic acid *(64)*. However, depletion of glutathione can cause a rapid increase in its synthesis in liver up to 2–3 μmol/h/g of wet liver tissue *(223)*. The short half-life (4–6 h) of utilizable glutathione in endothelial cells *(224)* also makes possible such quick regeneration of this antioxidant in this type of cells. Similar results (i.e., a decrease in intracellular glutathione also) were observed in endothelial cells exposed to TNF *(176)*.

Our results also demonstrate the significance of cysteine nutrition in fatty-acid- or TNF-mediated effects on endothelial cell glutathione metabolism and overall cellular integrity. For example, a coexposure of endothelial cells to TNF and NAC resulted in a less marked decrease in intracellular glutathione as compared to effects exerted only by TNF. In addition, such combined exposure attenuated a TNF-mediated increase in transendothelial albumin movement, indicating less enhanced disruption of endothelial barrier function *(176)*.

Although both selected dietary fatty acids such as linoleic acid and inflammatory cytokines such as TNF can induce cellular oxidative stress, evidence indicates that these agents can potentiate their injurious effects to endothelial cells. For example, combined exposure to TNF and linoleic acid cross-amplified endothelial cell oxidation measured as DCF fluorescence. Increased cellular oxidation results not only in enhanced levels of Reactive Oxygen Species (ROS) but also in depletion of antioxidants. In fact, depletion of cellular glutathione and decrease in cell and medium vitamin E contents were enhanced when endothelial cells were exposed to a combined treatment with linoleic acid and TNF *(106)*. As the consequence of these increased oxidative processes, loss of endothelial integrity also was more advanced in cells treated with linoleic acid and TNF as compared to effects of linoleic acid or TNF alone. Pretreatment with vitamin E attenuated the linoleic acid and TNF-mediated disruption of endothelial barrier integrity *(106)*. Increased intracellular calcium ($[Ca^{2+}]_i$) is another important indicator of cell injury, which may eventually lead to irreversible cell damage *(225)*. Treatment of endothelial cells with either linoleic acid or TNF caused an increase in $[Ca^{2+}]_i$ compared to controls. However, a combined cellular exposure to linoleic acid and TNF amplified this effect. A pretreatment with vitamin E attenuated elevated levels of $[Ca^{2+}]_i$ *(106)*, indicating the role of oxidative stress in the observed metabolic disturbances.

PROTECTION BY SELECTED NUTRIENTS (E.G., VITAMIN E AND ZINC) AGAINST LIPID/CYTOKINE-MEDIATED ENDOTHELIAL CELL DYSFUNCTION   The vascular endothelium is exposed directly to diet-derived oxidized lipids, hyperoxia, drugs, chemicals, and reactive oxygen metabolites released by blood-borne cells, as well as those generated within the endothelial cells. This provides an environment of increased oxidative stress that will be detrimental to the cell, especially if the overall cellular antioxidant system is inadequate. As mentioned earlier, there is increasing experimental and epidemiological evidence that oxidative modification of plasma lipoproteins (in particular, LDL) plays an important role in the development of atherosclerosis *(82,226)*. There also is evidence that certain antioxidant nutrients and adequate antioxidant enzyme activities may protect against atherosclerosis by preventing metabolic and physiologic derangements of the vascular endothelium *(71)*. This may be critical during lipid/cytokine-mediated expression of adhesion molecules and the overall inflammatory process *(227–230)*.

Several vitamins and minerals may be involved in metabolic events that protect the vascular endothelium or maintain endothelial integrity. Of particular interest are vitamin E and zinc, because both can function as antioxidants and membrane stabilizers *(71,231)*. Vitamin E is the only significant lipid-soluble, chain-breaking type of antioxidant present in human blood and all cellular membranes *(232–234)*. Primary functions of vitamin E are to terminate lipid peroxidation chain reactions generated by free radicals, particularly in membranes rich in polyunsaturated lipids *(235)*, to regulate cell proliferation *(236)* and to stabilize cell membranes *(237)*. These protective actions of vitamin E could have major implications in preventing vessel wall injury and atherosclerotic lesion formation. Data from humans suggest an inverse correlation between plasma, and especially LDL vitamin E levels, and mortality from ischemic heart disease *(238,239)*. Part of the protective mechanism of vitamin E is its ability to protect LDL from lipid peroxidation *(240–242)*. Recent studies also suggest that vitamin E has a potent inhibitory effect on LDL-induced production of adhesion molecules and adhesion of monocytes to endothelial cells via its antioxidant function and apparent direct regulatory effect on adhesion molecule expression *(243)*. Furthermore, data from subjects with varying degrees of coronary atherosclerosis support the hypothesis that high serum polyunsaturated fatty acid levels, when insufficiently protected by antioxidants (e.g., vitamin E), may indicate a higher risk of atherosclerosis (72,244,245).

The accumulated data suggest that high-fat diets may be atherogenic and that high levels of polyunsaturated lipids subject vascular endothelial cells to oxidative stress. As mentioned earlier, we have demonstrated that endothelial cells are injured by free fatty acids and, in particular, by their hydroperoxide derivatives, as evidenced by a decrease in endothelial barrier function (231). This impairment of the endothelial barrier function was greatly reduced by preenrichment of cells with vitamin E (246). In fact, endothelial cells can remain enriched with vitamin E as long as 5 d following a single vitamin E treatment, thus allowing vitamin E to be available for its biological function as a protector against cell injury (247). Vitamin E can also protect by stimulating endothelial cell proliferation in an apparent attempt to maintain endothelial integrity (150). Another possible mechanism of action of vitamin E is to prevent fatty-acid-induced peroxisome proliferation and thus the formation of excess peroxisomal hydrogen peroxide (247). In vitro studies with endothelial cells showed that hydrogen peroxide significantly damages the plasma membrane, leading to alterations in fluidity and leaks in the membrane (248). This type of injury was prevented when cultures were pretreated with vitamin E (248).

Vitamin E also may be antiatherogenic by modulating endothelial-cell-mediated prostacyclin (PGI$_2$) metabolism (249). PGI$_2$ synthesis by the vascular wall is decreased in vitamin E-deficient animals (250,251). In addition, vitamin E has been shown to restore reduced PGI$_2$ synthesis in aortic endothelial cells cultured in glucose-enriched medium (252). Thus, vitamin E may be antiatherogenic in hyperglycemic conditions such as those seen in patients with diabetes mellitus (252,253). Antiatherogenic activities of vitamin E in nonendothelial cells also may retard the overall progression of atherosclerosis. For example, vitamin E might act as an antiatherogenic agent by suppressing oxidative modification of LDL (254,255) and thus decrease the cytotoxicity of LDL to endothelial cells (256) and the recruitment of monocytes into the arterial subendothelium by smooth-muscle cells (25). Vitamin E also can modify protein kinase C activity, decrease platelet aggregation and adhesion, and inhibit the interaction of the immune system with the vasculature by preventing the expression of adhesion molecules on the surface of vascular endothelial cells (229).

Mechanisms of the protective function(s) of zinc in the pathogenesis of atherosclerosis, including vascular cell injury/dysfunction and the inflammatory response, are not clear. Epidemiological studies suggest that in some population groups, lower serum levels of zinc are inversely associated with coronary artery disease (257). Furthermore, zinc concentrations were significantly lower in atherosclerotic plaques of abdominal aortas of deceased patients with ischemic heart disease and acute myocardial infarction (258). There is evidence suggesting that zinc can act as an endogenous protective factor against atherosclerosis by inhibiting the oxidation of LDL by cells or transition metals (259). In fact, compared with zinc-adequate rats, zinc-deficient rats fed a highly unsaturated fat diet (linseed oil) had increased plasma levels of total lipids and cholesterol and an increased susceptibility of LDL to copper-induced lipid peroxidation (260). In another study, supplementary antioxidants decreased the osmotic fragility and oxidative damage of erythrocytes in zinc-deficient rats (261). More recently, we now have evidence that zinc can attenuate oxidative stress-sensitive transcription factors and IL-8 expression in activated endothelial cells (262). Because of its antioxidant and membrane-stabilizing properties, zinc appears to be crucial for protection against cell-destabilizing agents such as inflammatory cytokines and polyunsaturated lipids (263).

Zinc is an essential component of biomembranes. It is known to modify cell membranes and is required for maintenance of membrane structure and function and the activity of numerous enzymes (264,265). It has been speculated that zinc may form mercaptides with thiol groups of proteins, possibly linking to the phosphate moiety of phospholipids or interacting with carboxyl groups of sialic acids or proteins on plasma membranes, resulting in change of fluidity and stabilization of membranes (266). Zinc also participates extensively in protein, nucleic acid, carbohydrate, and lipid metabolism, as well as in the control of gene transcription and other fundamental biological processes (267). For example, isolated lysosome membranes were protected from oxidative injury in the presence of zinc (268,269), whereas zinc deficiency resulted in oxidative damage to proteins, lipids, and DNA in rat testes (270). Therefore, in addition to its function as a membrane stabilizer, zinc may have a physiological role as an antioxidant by protecting sulfhydryl groups against oxidation and inhibiting the production of reactive oxygen by transition metals (270,271). Dietary zinc deficiency was also reported to decrease plasma concentrations of vitamin E (272), suggesting that dietary zinc deficiency may increase the nutritional requirement for vitamin E necessary to maintain adequate plasma concentrations.

Little is known about the requirements and functions of zinc in maintaining the integrity of the vasculature and, particularly, the vascular endothelium. Because zinc is required for normal cellular repair processes and because atherosclerosis is believed to begin with vessel wall injury or dysfunction, a low zinc concentration may be involved in either initiation of cell injury or inadequate tissue repair, which may have important implications in the pathogenesis of atherosclerosis (71). We have shown that zinc is vital to endothelial integrity and that zinc deficiency causes a severe impairment of endothelial barrier function (273,274). Media supplemented with physiological concentrations of zinc completely restored the cell integrity. Supplementation with calcium or magnesium, however, did not restore this function, suggesting a unique role of zinc in maintaining normal endothelial integrity. There is evidence that a critical sign of zinc "deficiency" may be a compromised control of activation of transcription factors, cytokine activity, and endothelial cell inflammatory response (262). Our data support the concept that zinc can have distinct protective properties during the inflammatory response in atherosclerosis (227,263).

Pathological conditions related to increased activity of TNF, such as inflammation or infection, may significantly influence zinc metabolism. It is known that during inflammation or infection, there is an internal redistribution of zinc, with zinc being lost from some tissues such as plasma, and zinc accumulating in other tissues such as liver. The endothelium may be one tissue from which zinc is lost during the acute-phase response. It is probable that similar depletion of endothelial zinc may occur in atherosclerosis. We have shown previously that there is a depletion of cellular zinc in association with TNF-mediated endothelial cell injury, which may lead to disruption of normal membrane integrity

(275). It has been reported that intravenous injection of acetylated low-density lipoprotein or lipopolysaccharide into mice induced a decrease in serum zinc levels, probably as a result of the release of IL-1 (276). Interestingly, oral administration of probucol (a hypocholesterolemic agent with antioxidant properties) inhibited the LPS-induced fall in serum zinc levels (276). In addition to the role of zinc as an antioxidant or membrane stabilizer, cytotoxic compounds may interfere with cellular uptake or release of zinc. Cadmium has been shown to competitively inhibit zinc transport into endothelial cells, whereas equimolar concentrations of copper and magnesium were ineffective (277). Furthermore, zinc supplementation was capable of inducing a tolerance to cadmium cytotoxicity in cultured vascular endothelial cells (278). Interestingly, cadmium and TNF exhibit similar cytotoxicity (279), suggesting that TNF-mediated signaling pathways also may be shared by cadmium and prevented by zinc.

The nutritional status of the endothelium is likely to influence its response to TNF (227,280), as a marginal status of protective nutrients (e.g., zinc) may increase the susceptibility of the endothelial cell toward TNF-induced injury. Cellular enrichment with zinc has been shown to attenuate or prevent TNF-induced endothelial cell injury (275). The protective mechanism(s) of zinc against cytokine-induced injury still requires further clarification, but exciting new evidence suggests that TNF-mediated activation of transcription factors, such as NF-κB and AP-1, can be attenuated by zinc (262). It is not clear if zinc can attenuate transcription factors directly or possibly indirectly through activation of zinc-finger proteins such as A20 (Fig. 1). Interestingly, A20 has been shown to block TNF-induced signal transduction pathways and specifically to inhibit activation of NF-κB and AP-1 in carcinoma cells (281). Also, in bovine aortic endothelial cells, expression of A20 downregulated the expression of genes associated with TNF, LPS, or hydrogen peroxide-induced endothelial cell activation (282). All these studies support the hypothesis that adequate zinc nutrition may protect against inflammatory diseases such as atherosclerosis by inhibiting the activation of oxidative stress-responsive transcription factors, as well as expression of inflammatory cytokines (263).

OXIDATIVE STRESS-SENSITIVE TRANSCRIPTION FACTORS: A PROPOSED LINK AMONG LIPIDS, INFLAMMATORY CYTOKINES, ENDOTHELIAL DYSFUNCTION, AND ATHEROSCLEROSIS

Recent evidence indicates that oxidative stress may affect cellular metabolism not only by direct cell injury but also by activation of transcription factors and induction of the expression of genes regulated by these transcription factors. Evidence indicates that among transcription factors induced by oxidative stress, NF-κB may play a crucial role by its involvement in the regulation of expression of genes encoding for adhesion molecules and inflammatory cytokines. NF-κB consists of different subunits: p50 (NK-κB1), p52 (NK-κB2), p65 (RelA), and an inhibitory subunit, IκB. In the normal state, NF-κB is composed of a p50/p65 complex bound to IκB. The binding to IκB determines that this complex is inactive and remains in cytoplasm. Phosphorylation of IκB, followed by its dissociation and degradation by proteases, activates the p50/p65 complex and induces translocation of this dimer into the nucleus. Subsequently, activated NF-κB can bind to cis-acting κB sites in the promoters and enhancers of NF-κB-responsive genes (175).

Phosphorylation of IκB appears to be critical in the process of NF-κB activation. It appears that different signal transduction pathways and several different kinases are responsible for that process, depending on the type of stimuli and types of cells. For example, double-stranded RNA activates NF-κB by phosphorylation of IκB by specific double-stranded RNA-dependent protein kinase (283). Moreover, protein tyrosine kinases of the src family were identified as responsible kinases for hydrogen-peroxide-induced activation of NF-κB (210). Protein kinase C appears to be involved in lipoprotein lipase-mediated activation of NF-κB (192), and cAMP and cAMP-dependent protein kinase may play a regulatory role in activation of NF-κB by minimally modified LDL (284). Strong evidence indicates that the ceramide pathway is critical in TNF-induced NF-κB activation (182). However, the detailed signal transduction mechanisms involved in lipid-mediated activation of NF-κB have yet to be identified.

The significance of NF-κB activation on endothelial cell inflammatory response is related to the stimulation of the production of inflammatory cytokines and adhesion molecules (121). NF-κB binding sites were identified in the promotor regions of genes encoding ELAM-1, VCAM-1, and ICAM-1. Although other transcription factors, such as activating transcription factor-2 (ATF-2) or high-mobility-group protein I (Y) are required for expression of ELAM-1 and possibly for other adhesion molecules, NF-κB constitutes an important component of transcriptional regulation of these genes (175). Moreover, NF-κB regulates transcription of genes encoding for cytokines (such as IL-1, IL-6, IL-8, TNF) and growth factors. Expression of inflammatory cytokines is dependent on activated NF-κB. However, in turn, these cytokines stimulate activation of this transcription factor. Thus, inflammatory cytokines use NF-κB to amplify their own signals (123). However, to date, no evidence suggests that NF-κB activation may directly participate in fatty acid or cytokine-induced cytotoxicity (181). On the other hand, NF-κB stimulates expression of manganese superoxide dismutase (MnSOD), a potent antioxidant enzyme of mitochondrial matrix (285). It is possible that NF-κB-dependent stimulation of MnSOD protects against oxidative stress induced by fatty acids, cytokines, or other inducers of this transcription factor. This notion is supported by the observation that injury to mitochondria and production of superoxides are an integral part of TNF cytotoxicity in endothelial cells (285). Thus, activated NF-κB can lead to both harmful and protective events in endothelial cell metabolism. It appears that NF-κB is a pleiotropic regulatory activator, capable of induction of two different cellular functions, inflammatory response, and antioxidant protection. However, the regulatory mechanisms that determine the induction of the specific NF-κB related signal(s) are unknown. One may speculate that they may be dependent on the cellular microenvironment, which can be modulated by the presence of specific nutrients.

We determined effects of linoleic acid and/or TNF on activation of NF-κB in cultured endothelial cells. A short-term exposure to both linoleic acid and TNF resulted in a marked activation of NF-κB. In addition, pretreatment of endothelial cells with N-acetyl-L-cysteine or with vitamin E inhibited linoleic acid-mediated activation of NF-κB (126). Although both treatments with TNF or linoleic-acid-activated NF-κB, a combined exposure to these factors did not potentiate activation of NF-κB as compared to the cultures exposed to linoleic acid or TNF alone (106).

To establish if linoleic acid- and/or TNF-mediated activation of NF-κB may induce gene expression in endothelial cells, we transfected endothelial cells with a plasmid (pκB/TK5–CAT) encoding bacterial protein chloramphenicol acetyltransferase (CAT). This construct contained a CAT coding sequence driven by a thymidine kinase promoter containing six copies of the κB enhancer from the human TNF promoter. CAT activity was elevated and, thus, indicated active NF-κB-related transcription in cells exposed to linoleic acid and/or TNF. A pretreatment with vitamin E normalized CAT activity in linoleic acid and/or TNF treated cells *(106)*.

In addition to CAT assay, our data indicate that physiological concentrations of linoleic acid can stimulate production of inflammatory interleukins, such as IL-8, as well as expression of adhesion molecules, such as ICAM-1, at the surface of endothelial cells *(127)*. Both IL-8 and ICAM-1 are important mediators of the inflammatory process. For example, neutrophil migration across endothelial cell monolayers was shown to be partly blocked by a monoclonal antibody against IL-8 *(286)*, and both adherence and migration was inhibited by anti-ICAM-1 antibody *(287,288)*. In addition, IL-8 might exert a direct injurious effect toward endothelial cells. It was demonstrated that IL-8 increased endothelial permeability *(289)*. Thus, it is possible that selected dietary fatty acids such as linoleic acid and the induced production of IL-8 may cause massive damage to the endothelium by participating in the inflammatory process and atherogenesis. Although both IL-8 and ICAM are involved in leukocyte recruitment and their production is regulated by NF-κB, a direct relationship between these two inflammatory mediators is unclear. For example, it has been reported that IL-8 expression is not dependent on the early response cytokines (IL-1, TNF) or expression of ICAM-1 *(290)*. However, in patients with sepsis, it was reported that soluble ICAM-1, released from the membrane into circulation, significantly correlated with levels of endotoxin, TNF and IL-8 *(291)*. Thus, it appears that both IL-8 and ICAM-1 are upregulated and coexpressed under proinflammatory conditions. However, their expression might be regulated by separate mechanisms, partially related to the induction of oxidative stress and NF-κB activation.

Evidence indicates that increased cellular oxidation may also activate oxidative stress-response genes of the Immediate Early Gene (IEG) family, such as *c-jun* and *c-fos*. The Fos and Jun proteins, products of the *c-jun* and *c-fos* genes, create another potent transcription factor, AP-1. The role of *c-fos, c-jun,* and AP-1 in endothelial cell metabolism is not fully understood. However, they may be involved in induction of adhesion molecule expression *(292)*. Thus, AP-1-dependent transcription together with NF-κB-related gene regulation may contribute to the inflammatory response in atherogenesis.

SUMMARY

There is compelling evidence that the lipid environment of the vascular endothelium may profoundly influence the inflammatory response mediated by cytokines during atherosclerosis. With the discoveries of potential relationships of oxidative stress, activation of oxidative stress-sensitive transcription factors and the etiology of acute and chronic diseases, the issues of types of dietary fat (e.g., saturation/unsaturation) and the pathogenesis of atherosclerosis need to be revisited. Recent data suggest that certain diet-derived unsaturated fatty acids (e.g., linoleic acid) may be proinflammatory and, thus, atherogenic by disrupting endothelial cell integrity and that nutrients/chemicals with antioxidant properties can protect endothelial cells against lipid-mediated cell injury

(Fig. 1). This may be critical during lipid/cytokine-mediated expression of adhesion molecules and the overall inflammatory process. Recent findings that certain lipids can influence significantly the cytokine-mediated inflammatory response in atherosclerosis may open new fields in dietary intervention of atherosclerosis.

REFERENCES

1. Watkins BA, Hennig B, Toborek M. Diet and health. In: Hui YH, ed, Bailey's Industrial Oil and Fat Products, 5th ed., Volume 1 Edible Oil and Fat Products: General Applications, pp. 159–214. Wiley, New York, 1996.
2. Haudenschild CC. Pathogenesis of atherosclerosis: state of the art. Cardiovasc Drugs Ther 1990; 4:993–1004.
3. Ross R. The pathogenesis of atherosclerosis: a perspective for the 1990s. Nature 1993; 362:801–9.
4. Steinberg D, Witztum JL. Lipoproteins and atherosclerosis: current concepts. JAMA 1990; 264:3047–52.
5. Williams KJ, Tabas I. The response-to-retention hypothesis of early atherosclerosis. Arterioscler Thromb Vasc Biol 1995; 15:551–61.
6. Wick G, Romen M, Amberger A, Metzler B, Mayr M, Falkensammer G, et al. Atherosclerosis, autoimmunity, and vascular-associated lymphoid tissue. FASEB J 1997; 11:1199–207.
7. Munro JM, Cotran RS. The pathogenesis of atherosclerosis: atherogenesis and inflammation. Lab Invest 1988; 58:249–61.
8. Simionescu M, Simionescu N. Proatherosclerotic events: pathobiochemical changes occurring in the arterial wall before monocyte migration. FASEB J 1993; 7:1359–66.
9. Ross R. The pathogenesis of atherosclerosis—an update. N Engl J Med 1986; 314:488–500.
10. Hegsted DM, Ausman LM, Johnson, JA, Dallal GE. Dietary fat and serum lipids: an evaluation of the experimental data. Am J Clin Nutr 1993; 57:875–83.
11. Howell WH, McNamara DJ, Tosca MA, Smith BT, Gaines JA. Plasma lipid and lipoprotein responses to dietary fat and cholesterol: a meta-analysis. Am J Clin Nutr 1997; 65:1747–64.
12. Jones PJH. Regulation of cholesterol biosynthesis by diet in humans. Am J Clin Nutr 1997; 66:438–46.
13. Rudel LL, Parks JS, Sawyer JK. Compared with dietary monounsaturated and saturated fat, polyunsaturated fat protects African Green Monkeys from coronary artery atherosclerosis. Arterioscler Thromb Vasc Biol 1995; 15:2101–10.
14. Mensink RP. Effects of the individual saturated fatty acids on serum lipids and lipoprotein concentrations. Am J Clin Nutr 1993; 57:711S–4S.
15. Denke MA, Grundy SM. Effects of fats high in stearic acid on lipid and lipoprotein concentrations in men. Am J Clin Nutr 1991; 54:1036–40.
16. Woolett LA, Spady DK, Dietschy JM. Regulatory effects of the saturated fatty acids 6 : 0 through 18 : 0 on hepatic LDL receptor activity in the hamster. J Clin Invest 1992; 89:1133–41.
17. Hassel CA, Mensing EA, Gallaher DD. Dietary stearic acid reduces plasma and hepatic cholesterol concentrations without increasing bile acid excretion in cholesterol-fed hamsters. J Nutr 1997; 127:1148–55.
18. Hegsted DM, McGandy RB, Myers ML, Stare FJ. Quantitative effects of dietary fat on serum cholesterol in man. Am J Clin Nutr 1965; 17:281–95.
19. Denke MA, Grundy SM. Comparison of effects of lauric and palmitic acid on plasma lipids and lipoproteins. Am J Clin Nutr 1992; 56:895–8.
20. Ng TKW, Hayes KC, DeWitt GF, Jegathesan M, Satgunasingam N, Ong ASH, et al. Dietary palmitic and oleic acids exert similar effects on serum cholesterol and lipoprotein profiles in normocholesterolemic men and women. J Am Coll Nutr 1992; 11:383–90.
21. Connor WE, Connor SL. Diet, atherosclerosis and fish oil. Adv Intern Med 1990; 35:139–72.
22. Simopoulos AP. Omega-3 fatty acids in health and disease and in growth and development. Am J Clin Nutr 1991; 54:438–63.

23. Mori TA, Beilin LJ, Burke V, Morris J, Ritchie J. Interactions between dietary fat, fish, and fish oils and their effects on platelet function in men at risk of cardiovascular disease. Arterioscler Thromb Vasc Biol 1997; 17:279–86.

24. Esterbauer H. Cytotoxicity and genotoxicity of lipid-oxidation products. Am J Clin Nutr 1993; 57:779S–86S.

25. Janero DR. Therapeutic potential of vitamin E in the pathogenesis of spontaneous atherosclerosis. Free Radical Biol Med 1991; 11:129–44.

26. Kok FJ, van Poppel G, Melse J, Verheul E, Schouten EG, Kruyssen DHCM, et al. Do antioxidants and polyunsaturated fatty acids have a combined association with coronary atherosclerosis? Atherosclerosis 1991; 31:85–90.

27. Hegele RA. The pathogenesis of atherosclerosis. Clin Chim Acta 1996; 246:21–38.

28. Tschoepe D. Adhesion molecules influencing atherosclerosis. Diabetes Res Clin Pract 1996; 30(suppl):S19–S24.

29. Massy ZA, Keane WF. Pathogenesis of atherosclerosis. Semin Nephrol 1996; 16:12–20.

30. Lopes-Virella MF, Virella G. Cytokines, modified lipoproteins, and arteriosclerosis in diabetes. Diabetes 1996; 45(suppl 3):S40–4.

31. Watanabe T, Haraoka S, Shimokama T. Inflammatory and immunological nature of atherosclerosis. Int J Cardiol 1996; 54:S25–S34.

32. Mantovani A, Bussolino F, Introna M. Cytokine regulation of endothelial cell function: from molecular level to the bedside. Immunol Today 1997; 18:231–40.

33. Stemme S, Hansson GK. Immune mechanisms in atherosclerosis. Coronary Artery Dis 1994; 5:216–22.

34. DeBakey ME. Patterns of atherosclerosis and rates of progression. Atherosclerosis 1978; 3:1–56.

35. Alexander RW. Hypertension and the pathogenesis of atherosclerosis: oxidative stress and the mediation of arterial inflammatory response: a new perspective. Hypertension 1995; 25:155–61.

36. Vijayagopal P. Regulation of the metabolism of lipoprotein-proteoglycan complexes in human monocyte-derived macrophages. Biochem J 1994; 301:675–81.

37. Jimi S, Sakata N, Matunaga A, Takebayashi S. Low density lipoproteins bind more to type I and III collagens by negative charge-dependent mechanisms than to type IV and V collagens. Atherosclerosis 1994; 107:109–16.

38. Jimi S, Sakata N, Takebayashi S. Oxidized low density lipoproteins bind to collagen by negative-charge-dependent mechanisms. Ann NY Acad Sci 1995; 748:609–12.

39. Liu S-Y, Lu X, Choy S, Dembinski TC, Hatch GM, Mymin D, et al. Alteration of lysophosphatidylcholine content in low density lipoprotein after oxidative modification: relationship to endothelium dependent relaxation. Cardiovasc Res 1994; 28:1476–81.

40. Dzeletovic S, Babiker A, Lund E, Diczfalusy U. Time course of oxysterol formation during in vitro oxidation of low density lipoprotein. Chem Phys Lipids 1995; 78:119–28.

41. Brown AJ, Dean RT, Jessup W. Free and esterified oxysterol: formation during copper-oxidation of low density lipoprotein and uptake by macrophages. J Lipid Res 1996; 37:320–35.

42. Caruso D, Rasetti MF, De Angelis L, Galli G. Identification of 3β-hydroxy-5α-cholest-6-ene-5-hydroperoxide in human oxidized LDL. Chem Phys Lipids 1996; 79:181–6.

43. Breuer O, Dzeletovic S, Lund E, Diczfalusy U. The oxysterols cholest-5-ene-3β,4α-diol, cholest-5-ene-3β, 4β-diol and cholestane-3b,5α,6α-triol are formed during in vitro oxidation of low density lipoprotein, and are present in human atherosclerotic plaques. Biochim Biophys Acta Lipids Lipid Metab 1996; 1302:145–52.

44. Ross R: Cell biology of atherosclerosis. Annu Rev Physiol 1995; 57:791–804.

45. Williams RJ, Motteram JM, Sharp CH, Gallagher PJ. Dietary vitamin E and the attenuation of early lesion development in modified Watanabe rabbits. Atherosclerosis 1992; 94:153–9.

46. Wahle KWJ, Duthie GG. Lipoproteins, antioxidants and vascular disease. Eur J Clin Nutr 1991; 45:103–9.

47. Ehrenwald E, Fox PL. Role of endogenous ceruloplasmin in low density lipoprotein oxidation by human U937 monocytic cells. J Clin Invest 1996; 97:884–90.

48. Folcik VA, Aamir R, Cathcart MK. Cytokine modulation of LDL oxidation by activated human monocytes. Arterioscler Thromb Vasc Biol 1997; 17:1954–61.

49. Cominacini L, Garbin U, De Santis A, Campagnola M, Davoli A, Pasini AF, et al. Mechanisms involved in the in vitro modification of low density lipoprotein by human umbilical vein endothelial cells and copper ions. J Lipid Mediat Cell Signal 1996; 13:19–33.

50. Mabile L, Meilhac O, Escargueil-Blanc I, Troly M, Pieraggi MT, Salvayre R, et al. Mitochondrial function is involved in LDL oxidation mediated by human cultured endothelial cells. Arterioscler Thromb Vasc Biol 1997; 17:1575–82.

51. Lamb DJ, Leake DS. Acidic pH enables caeruloplasmin to catalyse the modification of low-density lipoprotein. FEBS Lett 1994; 338:122–6.

52. Ehrenwald E, Chisolm GM, Fox PL. Intact human ceruloplasmin oxidatively modifies low density lipoprotein. J Clin Invest 1994; 93:1493–501.

53. Aviram M. Modified forms of low density lipoprotein and atherosclerosis. Atherosclerosis 1993; 98:1–9.

54. Xu Q, Oberhuber G, Gruschwitz M, Wick G. Immunology of atherosclerosis: cellular composition and major histocompatibility complex class II antigen expression in aortic intima, fatty streaks, and atherosclerotic plaques in young and aged human specimens. Clin Immunol Immunopathol 1990; 56:344–59.

55. DiCorleto PE, Chisolm GM. Participation of the endothelium in the development of the atherosclerotic plaque. Prog Lipid Res 1986; 25:365–74.

56. Zilversmit DB. Role of triglyceride-rich lipoproteins in atherosclerosis. Ann NY Acad Sci 1976; 275:138–44.

57. Zilversmit DB. A proposal linking atherogenesis to the interaction of endothelial lipoprotein lipase with triglyceride-rich lipoproteins. Circ Res 1973; 33:633–8.

58. Zilversmit DB. Atherogenesis: a postprandial phenomenon. Circulation 1979; 60:473–85.

59. Ylä-Herttuala S, Lipton BA, Rosenfeld ME, Goldberg IJ, Steinberg D, Witztum JC. Macrophages and smooth muscle cells express lipoprotein lipase in human and rabbit atherosclerotic lesions. Proc Natl Acad Sci USA 1991; 88:10143–7.

60. O'Brien KD, Deeb SS, Ferguson M, McDonald TO, Allen MD, Alpers CE, et al. Apolipoprotein E localization in human coronary atherosclerotic plaques by in situ hybridization and immunohistochemistry and comparison with lipoprotein lipase. Am J Pathol 1994; 144:538–48.

61. Obunike JC, Paka L, Sivaram P, Goldberg IJ. Lipoprotein lipase can function as a monocyte adhesion protein. Atheroscler Thromb Vasc Biol 1997; 17:1414–20.

62. Renier G, Olivier M, Skamene E, Radzioch D. Induction of tumor necrosis factor a gene expression by lipoprotein lipase. J Lipid Res 1994; 35:271–8.

63. Hennig B, Chung BH, Watkins BA, Alvarado A. Disruption of endothelial barrier function by lipolytic remnants of triglyceride-rich lipoproteins. Atherosclerosis 1992; 95:235–47.

64. Toborek M, Hennig B. Fatty acid-mediated effects on the glutathione redox cycle in cultured endothelial cells. Am J Clin Nutr 1994; 59:60–5.

65. Hennig B, Toborek M, McClain CJ, Diana JN. Nutritional implications in vascular endothelial cell metabolism. J Am Coll Nutr 1996; 15:345–58.

66. Hennig B, Shasby DM, Fulton AB, Spector AA. Exposure to free fatty acid increases the transfer of albumin across cultured endothelial monolayers. Arteriosclerosis 1984; 4:489–97.

67. Hennig B, Shasby DM, Spector AA. Exposure to fatty acid increases human low density lipoprotein transfer across cultured endothelial monolayers. Circ Res 1985; 57:776–80.

68. Hennig B, Alvarado A, Ramasamy S, Boissonneault GA, Decker E,

Means WJ. Fatty acid induced disruption of endothelial barrier function in culture. Biochem Arch 1990; 6:409–17.

69. Hennig B, Enoch C, Chow DK. Linoleic acid hydroperoxide increases the transfer of albumin across cultured endothelial monolayers. Arch Biochem Biophys 1986; 248:353–7.

70. Hennig B, Ramasamy S, Alvarado A, Shantha NC, Boissonneault GA, Decker EA, et al. Selective disruption of endothelial barrier function in culture by pure fatty acids and fatty acids derived from animal and plant fats. J Nutr 1993; 123:1208–16.

71. Hennig B, Toborek M, Cader AA, Decker EA. Nutrition, endothelial cell metabolism, and atherosclerosis. Crit Rev Food Sci Nutr 1994; 34:253–82.

72. Hodgson JM, Wahlquist ML, Boxall JA, Balazs ND. Can linoleic acid contribute to coronary artery disease? Am J Clin Nutr 1993; 58:228–34.

73. Luostarinen R, Boberg M, Saldeen T. Fatty acid composition in total phospholipids of human coronary arteries in sudden cardiac death. Atherosclerosis 1993; 99:187–93.

74. Yam D, Eliraz A, Berry EM. Diet and disease, the Israeli paradox: possible dangers of a high omega-6 polyunsaturated fatty acid diet. Isr J Med Sci 1996; 32:1134–43.

75. Spector AA, Kaduce TL, Hoak JC, Fry GL. Utilization of arachidonic and linoleic acids by cultured human endothelial cells. J Clin Invest 1981; 68:1003–11.

76. Debry G, Pelletier XL. Physiological importance of ω-3/ω-6 polyunsaturated fatty acids in man. An overview of still unresolved and controversial questions. Experientia 1991; 47:172–8.

77. Hennig B, Watkins BA. Linoleic acid and linolenic acid: effect on permeability properties of cultured endothelial cell monolayers. Am J Clin Nutr 1989; 49:301–5.

78. Toborek M, Hennig B. Effect of different fatty acids on ATP levels in cultured endothelial cells. FASEB J 1992; 6:A1322.

79. Ramasamy S, Boissonneault GA, Lipke DW, Hennig B. Proteoglycans and endothelial barrier function: effect of linoleic acid exposure to porcine pulmonary artery endothelial cells. Atherosclerosis 1993; 103:279–90.

80. Toborek M, Hennig B. Vitamin E attenuates induction of elastase-like activity by tumor necrosis factor-α, cholestan-3β,5α,6β-triol, and linoleic acid in cultured endothelial cells. Clin Chim Acta 1993; 215:201–11.

81. de Haan LH, Bosselaers I, Jongen WM, Zwijsen RM, Koeman JH. Effect of lipids and aldehydes on gap–junctional intercellular communication between human smooth muscle cells. Carcinogenesis 1994; 15:253–6.

82. Steinberg D, Parthasarathy S, Carew TE, Khoo JC, Witztum JL. Beyond cholesterol: modification of low density lipoprotein that increase its atherogenicity. N Engl J Med 1989; 320:915–24.

83. Steinbrecher UP, Parthasarathy S, Leake DS, Witztum JL, Steinberg D. Modification of low density lipoprotein by endothelial cells involves lipid peroxidation and degradation of low density lipoprotein phospholipids. Proc Natl Acad Sci USA 1984; 81:3883–7.

84. Witztum JL. Role of oxidized low density lipoprotein in atherogenesis. Br Heart J 1993; 69:S12–8.

85. Hiramatsu K, Rosen H, Heinecke JW, Wolfbauer G, Chait A. Superoxide initiates oxidation of low density lipoprotein by human monocytes. Arteriosclerosis 1986; 7:55–60.

86. Parthasarathy S, Wieland E, Steinberg D. A role of endothelial cell lipoxygenase in the oxidative modification of low density lipoprotein. Proc Natl Acad Sci USA 1989; 86:1046–50.

87. Morel DW, DiCorleto PE, Chisholm GM. Endothelial and smooth muscle cells alter low density lipoprotein in vitro by free radical oxidation. Arteriosclerosis 1984; 4:357–64.

88. Navab M, Imes SS, Hama SY, Hough GP, Ross LA, Bork RW, et al. Monocyte transmigration induced by modification of low density lipoprotein in cocultures of human aortic wall cells is due to induction of monocyte chemotactic protein 1 synthesis and is abolished by high density lipoprotein. J Clin Invest 1991; 88:2039–46.

89. Rajavashisth TB, Andalibi A, Territo MC, Berliner JA, Navab M, Fogelman AM, et al. Induction of endothelial cell expression of granulocyte and macrophage colony stimulating factors by modified low density lipoprotein. Nature 1990; 244:254–7.

90. Kugiyama K, Kerns SA, Morrisett JD, Roberts R, Henry PD. Impairment of endothelium-dependent arterial relaxation by lysolecithin in modified low density lipoproteins. Nature 1990; 344:160–2.

91. Berliner JA, Territo MC, Sevanian A, Ramin S, Kim JA, Bamshad B, et al. Minimally modified LDL stimulates monocyte endothelial interaction. J Clin Invest 1990; 85:1260–6.

92. Escargueil-Blanc I, Meihac O, Pieraggi MT, Arnal JF, Salvayre R, Negre-Salvayre A. Oxidized LDLs induce massive apoptosis of cultured human endothelial cells through a calcium-dependent pathway. Arterioscler Thromb Vasc Biol 1997; 17:331–9.

93. Suc I, Escargueil-Blanc I, Troly M, Salvayre R, Negre-Salvayre A. HDL and ApoA prevent cell death of endothelial cells induced by oxidized LDL. Arterioscler Thromb Vasc Biol 1997; 17:2158–66.

94. Staprans I, Rapp JH, Pan XM, Kim KY, Feingold KR. Oxidized lipids in the diet are a source of oxidized lipid in chylomicrons of human serum. Arterioscler Thromb Vasc Biol 1994; 14:1900–5.

95. Staprans I, Rapp JH, Pan XM, Hardman DA, Feingold KR. Oxidized lipids in the diet accelerate the development of fatty streaks in cholesterol-fed rabbits. Arterioscler Thromb Vasc Biol 1996; 16:533–8.

96. Juul K, Nielsen LB, Munkholm K, Stender S, Nordestgaard BG. Oxidation of plasma low-density lipoprotein accelerates its accumulation and degradation in the arterial wall in vivo. Circulation 1996; 94:1698–704.

97. Reaven P, Parthasarathy S, Grasse BJ, Miller E, Steinberg D, Witztum JL. Effects of oleate-rich and linoleate-rich diets on the susceptibility of low density lipoprotein to oxidative modification in mildly hypercholesterolemic subjects. J Clin Invest 1993; 91:668–76.

98. Reaven P, Parthasarathy S, Grasse BJ, Miller E, Almazan F, Mattson FH, et al. Feasibility of using an oleate-rich diet to reduce the susceptibility of low-density lipoprotein to oxidative modification in humans. Am J Clin Nutr 1991; 54:701–76.

99. Hennig B, Toborek M, Boissonneault GA, Shantha NC, Decker EA, Oeltgen PR. Animal and plant fats selectively modulate oxidizability of rabbit LDL and LDL-mediated disruption of endothelial barrier function. J Nutr 1995; 125:2045–54.

100. Nicholas KN, Toborek M, Slim R, Watkins BA, Chung BH, Oeltgen PR, et al. Dietary cholesterol supplementation protects against endothelial cell dysfunction mediated by native and lipolyzed lipoproteins derived from rabbits fed high-corn diets. J Nutr Biochem 1997; 8:566–72.

101. Smith LL. Another cholesterol hypothesis: cholesterol as antioxidant. Free Radical Biol Med 1991; 11:47–61.

102. Rangaswamy S, Penn MS, Seidel GM, Chilsolm GM. Exogenous oxidized low-density lipoprotein injures and alters the barrier function of endothelium in rats in vivo. Circ Res 1997; 80:37–44.

103. Karman RJ, Garcia JG, Hart CM. Endothelial cell monolayer dysfunction caused by oxidized low density lipoprotein: attenuation by oleic acid. Prostaglandins Leukot Essential Fatty Acids 1997; 56:345–53.

104. Cosgrove JP, Church DF, Pryor WA. The kinetics of the autoxidation of polyunsaturated fatty acids. Lipids 1987; 22:299–304.

105. Hennig B, Watkins BA. Linoleic acid and linolenic acid: effect on permeability properties of cultured endothelial cell monolayers. Am J Clin Nutr 1989; 49:301–5.

106. Toborek M, Barger SW, Mattson MP, Barve S, McClain CJ, Hennig B. Linoleic acid and TNF-α cross-amplify oxidative injury and dysfunction of endothelial cells. J Lipid Res 1996; 37:123–35.

107. Mattson MP, Barger SW, Begley JG, Mark RJ. Calcium, free radicals, and excitotoxic neuronal death in primary cell culture. Methods Cell Biol 1995; 46:187–215.

108. Hennig B, Wang Y, Boissonneault GA, Alvarado A, Glauert HP. Effects of fatty acid enrichment on the induction of peroxisomal enzymes in cultured porcine endothelial cells. Biochem Arch 1990; 6:141–6.

109. Pacifici EH, McLeod LL, Peterson H, Sevanian A. Linoleic acid

hydroperoxide-induced peroxidation of endothelial cell phospholipids and cytotoxicity. Free Radical Biol Med 1994; 17:285–95.

110. Ridker PM, Cushman M, Stampfer MJ, Tracy RP, Hennekens CH. Inflammation, aspirin, and the risk of cardiovascular disease in apparently healthy men. N Engl J Med 1997; 336:973–9.

111. Mantovani A, Bussolino F, Introna M. Cytokine regulation of endothelial cell function: from molecular level to the bedside. Immunol Today 1997; 18:231–40.

112. Grimble RF. Interaction between nutrients, pro-inflammatory cytokines and inflammation. Clin Sci 1996; 91:121–30.

113. Meydani SN. Effect of (n-3) polyunsaturated fatty acids on cytokine production and their biologic function. Nutrition 1996; 12:S8–S14.

114. De Caterina R, Libby P. Control of endothelial leukocyte adhesion molecules by fatty acids. Lipids 1996; 31:S57–S63.

115. Kim DN, Eastman A, Baker JE, Mastrangelo A, Sethi S, Ross JS, et al. Fish oil, atherosclerosis, and thrombogenesis. Ann NY Acad Sci 1995; 748:474–80.

116. Weber C, Erl W, Pietsch A, Danesch U, Weber PC. Docosahexaenoic acid selectively attenuates induction of vascular cell adhesion molecule-1 and subsequent monocytic cell adhesion to human endothelial cells stimulated by tumor necrosis factor-α. Arterioscler Thromb Vasc Biol 1995; 15:622–8.

117. De Caterina R, Cybulsky MI, Clinton SK, Gimbrone MA Jr, Libby P. The omega-3 fatty acid docosahexaenoate reduces cytokine-induced expression of proatherogenic and proinflammatory proteins in human endothelial cells. Arterioscler Thromb 1994; 14:1829–36.

118. Pietsch A, Weber C, Goretzki M, Weber PC, Lorenz RL. N-3 but not N-6 fatty acids reduce the expression of the combined adhesion and scavenger receptor CD 36 in human monocyte cells. Cell Biochem Funct 1995; 13:211–6.

119. Khan BV, Parthasarathy SS, Alexander RW, Medford RM. Modified low density lipoprotein and its constituents augment cytokine-activated vascular cell adhesion molecule-1 gene expression in human vascular endothelial cells. J Clin Invest 1995; 95:1262–70.

120. Collins T. Endothelial nuclear factor-κB and the initiation of the atherosclerotic lesion. Lab Invest 1993; 68:499–508.

121. Berliner JA, Navab M, Fogelman AM, Frank JS, Demer LL, Edwards PA, et al. Atherosclerosis: basic mechanisms. Oxidation, inflammation, and genetics. Circulation 1995; 91:2488–96.

122. Baeuerle PA. The inducible transcription activator NF-κB: regulation by distinct protein subunits. Biochim Biophys Acta 1991; 1072:63–80.

123. Siebenlist U, Franzoso G, Brown K. Structure, regulation and function of NF-κB. Annu Rev Cell Biol 1994; 10:405–55.

124. Barnes PJ, Karin M. Nuclear factor-κB. A pivotal transcription factor in chronic inflammatory diseases. N Engl J Med 1997; 336:1066–71.

125. Brand K, Eisele T, Kreusel U, Page M, Page S, Haas M, et al. Dysregulation of monocytic nuclear factor-κB by oxidized low-density lipoprotein. Arterioscler Thromb Vasc Biol 1997; 17:1901–9.

126. Hennig B, Toborek M, Joshi-Barve S, Barger SW, Barve S, Mattson MP, et al. Linoleic acid activates NF-κB and induces NF-κB-dependent transcription in cultured endothelial cells. Am J Clin Nutr 1996; 63:322–8.

127. Young VM, Toborek M, Yang F, McClain CJ, Hennig B. Effect of linoleic acid on endothelial cell inflammatory mediators. Metabolism in press.

128. Berliner JA, Heinecke JW. The role of oxidized lipoproteins in atherogenesis. Free Radical Biol Med 1996; 20:707–27.

129. Aviram M, Maor I, Keidar S, Hayek T, Oiknine J, Bar-EL Y, et al. Lesioned low density lipoprotein in atherosclerotic apolipoprotein E-deficient transgenic mice and in humans is oxidized and aggregated. Biochem Biophys Res Commun 1995; 216:501–13.

130. O'Brien KD, Alpers CE, Hokanson JE, Wang S, Chait A. Oxidation-specific epitopes in human coronary atherosclerosis are not limited to oxidized low-density lipoprotein. Circulation 1996; 94:1216–25.

131. Eber B, Schumacher M, Tatzber F, Kaufmann P, Luha O, Esterbauer H, et al. Autoantibodies to oxidized low density lipoproteins in restenosis following coronary angioplasty. Cardiology 1994; 84:310–15.

132. Maggi E, Chiesa R, Melissano G, Castellano R, Astore D, Grossi A, et al. LDL oxidation in patients with severe carotid atherosclerosis: a study of in vitro and in vivo oxidation markers. Arterioscler Thromb 1994; 14:1892–9.

133. Puurunen M, Mänttäri M, Manninen V, Tenkanen L, Alfthan G, Ehnholm C, et al. Antibody against oxidized low-density lipoprotein predicting myocardial infarction. Arch Intern Med 1994; 154: 2605–9.

134. Maggi E, Marchesi E, Ravetta V, Martignoni A, Finardi G, Bellomo G. Presence of autoantibodies against oxidatively modified low-density lipoprotein in essential hypertension: a biochemical signature of an enhanced *in vivo* low-density lipoprotein oxidation. J Hypertens 1995; 13:129–38.

135. Guyton JR, Klemp KF. Development of the lipid-rich core in human atherosclerosis. Arterioscler Thromb Vasc Biol 1996; 16:4–11.

136. Nielsen LB. Transfer of low density lipoprotein into the arterial wall and risk of atherosclerosis. Atherosclerosis 1996; 123:1–15.

137. Leake DS. Does an acidic pH explain why low density lipoprotein is oxidised in atherosclerotic lesions? Atherosclerosis 1997; 129: 149–57.

138. George J, Harats D, Gilburd B, Shoenfeld Y. Emerging cross-regulatory roles of immunity and autoimmunity in atherosclerosis. Immunol Res 1996; 15:315–22.

139. Thomas MJ, Thornburg T, Manning J, Hooper K, Rudel LL. Fatty acid composition of low-density lipoprotein influences in susceptibility to autoxidation. Biochemistry 1994; 33:1828–34.

140. Bonanome A, Pagnan A, Biffanti S, Opportuno A, Sorgato F, Dorella M, et al. Effect of dietary monounsaturated and polyunsaturated fatty acids on the susceptibility of plasma low density lipoproteins to oxidative modification. Arterioscler Thromb 1992; 12:529–33.

141. Carmena R, Ascaso JF, Camejo G, Varela G, Hurt-Camejo E, Ordovas JM, et al. Effect of olive and sunflower oils on low density lipoprotein level, composition, size, oxidation and interaction with arterial proteoglycans. Atherosclerosis 1996; 125:243–55.

142. Parthasarathy S, Khoo JC, Miller E, Barnett J, Witztum JL, Steinberg D. Low density lipoprotein rich in oleic acid is protected against oxidative modification: implications for dietary prevention of atherosclerosis. Proc Natl Acad Sci USA 1990; 87:3894–8.

143. Mata P, Varela O, Alonso R, Lahoz C, De Oya M, Badimon L. Monounsaturated and polyunsaturated n-6 fatty acid-enriched diets modify LDL oxidation and decrease human coronary smooth muscle cell DNA synthesis. Arterioscler Thromb Vasc Biol 1997; 17: 2088–95.

144. Karman RJ, Garcia JGN, Hart CM. Endothelial cell monolayer dysfunction caused by oxidized low density lipoprotein: attenuation by oleic acid. Prostaglandins Leukot Essential Fatty Acids 1997; 56:345–53.

145. Tappia PS, Grimble RF. The relationship between altered membrane composition, eicosanoids and TNF-induced IL1 and IL6 production in macrophages of rats fed fats of different unsaturated fatty acid composition. Mol Cell Biochem 1996; 165:135–43.

146. Boissonneault GA, Hennig B, Wang Y, Ouyang C-M, Krahulik K, Cunnup L, et al. Effect of oxysterol-enriched low-density lipoprotein on endothelial barrier function in culture. Low-density lipoproteins. Ann Nutr Metab 1991; 35:226–32.

147. Stalenhoef AFH, Kleinveld HA, Kosmeijer-Schuil TG, Demacker PNM, Katan MB. In vivo oxidised cholesterol in atherosclerosis. Atherosclerosis 1993; 98:113–4.

148. Hultén LM, Lindmark H, Diczfalusy U, Björkhem I, Ottosson M, Liu Y, et al. Oxysterols present in atherosclerotic tissue decrease the expression of lipoprotein lipase messenger RNA in human monocyte-derived macrophages. J Clin Invest 1996; 97:461–8.

149. Boissonneault GA, Hennig B, Ouyang C-M. Oxysterols, cholesterol biosynthesis, and vascular endothelial cell monolayer barrier function. Proc Soc Exp Biol Med 1991; 196:338–43.

150. Hennig B, Boissonneault GA, Fiscus LJ, Marra ME. Effect of vitamin E on oxysterol- and fatty acid hydroperoxide-induced changes of repair and permeability properties of cultured endothelial cell monolayers. Int J Vitam Nutr Res 1988; 58:41–7.

151. Zhou Q, Smith TL, Kummerow FA. Cytotoxicity of oxysterols on cultured smooth muscle cells from human umbilical arteries. Proc Soc Exp Biol Med 1993; 202:75–80.

152. Guardiola F, Codony R, Addis PB, Rafecas M, Boatella J. Biological effects of oxysterols: current status. Food Chem Toxicol 1996; 45:193–211.

153. Ohtani K, Miyabara K, Okamoto E, Kamei M, Matsui-Yuasa I. Cytotoxicity of 7-ketocholesterol toward cultured rat hepatocytes and the effect of vitamin E. Biosci Biotechnol Biochem 1996; 60:1989–93.

154. Aupeix K, Weltin D, Mejia JE, Christ M, Marchal J, Freyssinet JM, et al. Oxysterol-induced apoptosis in human monocytic cell lines. Immunobiology 1995; 194:415–28.

155. Lizard G, Decker V, Dubrez L, Moisant M, Gambert P, Lagrost L. Induction of apoptosis in endothelial cells treated with cholesterol oxides. Am J Pathol 1996; 148:1625–38.

156. Zwijsen RML, Oudenhoven IMJ, De Haan LHJ. Effects of cholesterol and oxysterols on gap junctional communication between human smooth muscle cells. Eur J Pharmacol 1992; 228:115–20.

157. Guyton JR, Black BL, Seidel CL. Focal toxicity of oxysterols in vascular smooth muscle cell culture: a model of the atherosclerotic core region. Am J Pathol 1990; 137:425–34.

158. Jimi S, Smith TL, Kummerow FA. 26-Hydroxycholesterol-stimulated DNA synthesis in smooth muscle cells and induction of endothelial injury using a coculture technique. Biochem Med Met Biol 1990; 44:114–25.

159. Liu K, Ramjiawan B, Kutryk MJB, Pierce GN. Effects of oxidative modification of cholesterol in isolated low density lipoproteins on cultured smooth muscle cells. Mol Cell Biochem 1991; 108:49–56.

160. Gelissen IC, Brown AJ, Mander EL, Kritharides L, Dean RT, Jessup W. Sterol efflux is impaired from macrophage foam cells selectively enriched with 7-ketocholesterol. J Biol Chem 1996; 271:17,852–60.

161. Kilsdonk EPC, Morel DW, Johnson WJ, Rothblat GH. Inhibition of cellular cholesterol efflux by 25-hydroxycholesterol. J Lipid Res 1995; 36:505–16.

162. Lin CY, Morel DW. Distribution of oxysterols in human serum: characterization of 25-hydroxycholesterol association with serum albumin. J Nutr Biochem 1995; 6:618–25.

163. Ross R. The pathogenesis of atherosclerosis: a perspective for the 1990s. Nature 1993; 362:801–9.

164. Albelda SM, Smith CW, Ward PA. Adhesion molecules and inflammatory injury. FASEB J 1994; 8:504–12.

165. Tracey KJ, Cerami A. Tumor necrosis factor and regulation of metabolism in infection: role of systemic versus tissue levels. Proc Soc Exp Biol Med 1992; 200:233–9.

166. Rus HG, Niculescu F, Vlaicu R. Tumor necrosis factor-alpha in human arterial wall with atherosclerosis. Atherosclerosis 1991; 89:247–54.

167. Barath P, Fishbein MC, Cao J, Berenson J, Helfant RH, Forrester JS. Detection and localization of tumor necrosis factor in human atheroma. Am J Cardiol 1990; 65:297–302.

168. Vaddi K, Nicolini FA, Mehta P, Mehta JL. Increased secretion of tumor necrosis factor-α and interferon-γ by mononuclear leukocytes in patients with ischemic heart disease. Relevance in superoxide anion generation. Circulation 1994; 90:694–99.

169. Xing Z, Kirpalani H, Torry D, Jordana M, Gauldie J. Polymorphonuclear leukocytes as a significant source of tumor necrosis factor-1 in endotoxin-challenged lung tissue. Am J Pathol 1993; 143:1009–15.

170. Maziere C, Auclair M, Maziere JC. Tumor necrosis factor enhances low density lipoprotein oxidative modification by monocytes and endothelial cells. FEBS Lett 1994; 338:43–6.

171. Paleolog EM, Delasalle S-AJ, Burman WA, Feldman M. Functional activities of receptors for tumor necrosis factor-α on human vascular endothelial cells. Blood 1994; 84:2578–90.

172. Slowik MR, de Luca LG, Fiers W, Pober JS. Tumor necrosis factor activates human endothelial cells through the p55 tumor necrosis factor receptor but the p75 receptor contributes to activation at low tumor necrosis factor concentration. Am J Pathol 1993; 143:1724–30.

173. Bradley JR, Thiru S, Pober JS. Disparate localization of 55-kd and 75-kd tumor necrosis factor receptors in human endothelial cells. Am J Pathol 1995; 146:27–32.

174. Read MA, Neish AS, Luscinskas FW, Palombella VJ, Maniatis T, Collins T. The proteasome pathway is required for cytokine-induced endothelial-leukocyte adhesion molecule expression. Immunity 1995; 2:493–506.

175. Collins T, Read MA, Neish AS, Whitley MZ, Thanos D, Maniatis T. Transcriptional regulation of endothelial cell adhesion molecules: NF-κB and cytokine-inducible enhancers. FASEB J 1995; 9: 899–909.

176. Toborek M, Barger SW, Mattson MP, McClain CJ, Hennig B. Role of glutathione redox cycle in TNF-mediated endothelial cell dysfunction. Atherosclerosis 1995; 117:179–88.

177. Koga S, Morris S, Ogawa S, Liao H, Bilezikian JP, Chen G, et al. TNF modulates endothelial properties by decreasing cAMP. Am J Pathol 1995; 268:C1104–13.

178. Hanemaaijer R, Koolwijk P, le Clercq L, de Vree WJ, van Hinsbergh VW. Regulation of matrix metalloproteinase expression in human vein and microvascular endothelial cells. Effects of tumour necrosis factor alpha, interleukin 1 and phorbol ester. Biochem J 1993; 296:803–9.

179. Polunovsky VA, Wendt CH, Ingbar DH, Peterson MS, Bitterman PB. Induction of endothelial cell apoptosis by TNF alfa: modulation by inhibitors of protein synthesis. Exp Cell Res 1994; 214:584–94.

180. Smith CA, Farrah T, Goodwin RG. The TNF-receptor superfamily of cellular and viral proteins: activation, costimulation, and death. Cell 1994; 76:959–62.

181. Beyaert R, Fiers W. Molecular mechanisms of tumor necrosis factor-induced cytotoxicity. What we do understand and what we do not. FEBS Lett 1994; 340:9–16.

182. Kolesnick R, Golde DW. The sphingomyelin pathway in tumor necrosis factor and interleukin-1 signaling. Cell 1994; 77:325–8.

183. Wiegmann K, Shütze S, Machleidt T, Witte D, Krönke M. Functional dichotomy of neutral and acidic sphingomyelinases in tumor necrosis factor signaling. Cell 1994; 78:1005–15.

184. Wong GH. Protective roles of cytokines against radiation: induction of mitochondrial MnSOD. Biochim Biophys Acta 1995; 1271: 205–9.

185. Tartaglia LA, Rothe M, Hu Y-F, Goeddel DV. Tumor necrosis factor's cytotoxic activity is signaled by the p55 TNF receptor. Cell 1993; 73:213–16.

186. Tartaglia LA, Pennica D, Goeddel DV. Ligand passing: the 75-kDa tumor necrosis factor (TNF) receptor recruits TNF for signaling by the 55-kDa TNF receptor. J Biol Chem 1993; 268:18,542.

187. Heller RA, Song K, Fan N. Cytotoxicity by tumor necrosis factor is mediated by both p55 and p70 receptor. Cell 1993; 73:216.

188. Barbara JAJ, Smith WB, Gamble JR, Van Ostade X, Vandenabeele P, Tavernier J, et al. Dissociation of TNF-α cytotoxic and proinflammatory activities by p55 receptor- and p75 receptor-selective TNF-α mutants. EMBO J 1994; 13:843–50.

189. Van Tits LJH, Bemelmans MHA, Steinshamn S, Waage A, Leeuwenberg JFM, Buurman WA. Non-signaling function of TNF-R75: findings in man and mouse. Circ Shock 1994; 44:40–4.

190. Rothe M, Pan M-G, Henzel WJ, Ayres TM, Goeddel DV. The TNFR2-TRAF signaling complex contains two novel proteins related to baculoviral inhibitor of apoptosis proteins. Cell 1995; 83:1243–52.

191. Tartaglia LA, Goeddel DV, Reynolds C, Figari IS, Weber RF, Fendly BM, et al. Stimulation of human T-cell proliferation by specific activation of the 75-kDa tumor necrosis factor receptor. J Immunol 1993; 151:4637–41.

192. Reiner G, Oliver M, Skamene E, Radzioch D. Induction of tumor necrosis factor alpha gene expression by lipoprotein lipase requires protein kinase C activation. J Lipid Res 1994; 35:1413–21.

193. Cendan JC, Moldawer LL, Souba WW, Copeland EM, Lind S. Endotoxin-induced nitric oxide production in pulmonary artery endothelial cells is regulated by cytokines. Arch Surg 1994; 129:1296–1300.

194. Kahaleh MB, Zhou S. Induction of tumor necrosis factor (TNF) synthesis by endothelial cells upon exposure to r-TNF. Arthritis Rheum 1989; 32:S124.

195. Nagura H, Ohtani H. Expression of major histocompatibility class-II antigens by vascular endothelial cells leads to amplified immunoinflammatory processes. Acta Histochem Cytochem 1992; 25: 653–60.

196. Slater TF. Free radical mechanisms in tissue injury. Biochem J 1984; 222:1–15.

197. Hennig B, Chow CK. Lipid peroxidation and endothelial cell injury: implication in atherosclerosis. Free Radical Biol Med 1988; 4: 99–106.

198. Grisham MB, McCord JM. Chemistry and cytotoxicity of reactive oxygen metabolites. In: Physiology of Oxygen Radicals, (Taylor EA, Matuba S, Word P, eds) pp. 1–8. American Physiological Society, Washington, DC, 1986.

199. Chance B, Sies H, Bovetis E. Hydroperoxide metabolism in mammalian organs. Physiol Rev 1979; 59:527–605.

200. Lynch RE, Fridovich I. Effects of superoxide on the erythrocyte membrane. J Biol Chem 1978; 253:1838–41.

201. Ylä-Herttuala S, Rosenfed ME, Parthasarathy S, Sigal E, Särkioia T, Witztum JT, et al. Gene expression in macrophage-rich human atherosclerotic lesions. 15-lipoxygenase and acetyl low density lipoprotein receptor messenger RNA colocalize with oxidation specific lipic–protein adducts. Clin Invest 1991; 87:1146–52.

202. Kühn H, Belkner J, Zaiss S, Fahrenklemper T, Wohlfeil S. Involvement of 15-lipoxygenase in early stages of atherogenesis. J Exp Med 1994; 179:1903–11.

203. Ylä-Herttuala S, Rosenfed ME, Parthasarathy S, Glass CK, Sigal E, Witztum JT, et al. Colocalization of 15-lipoxygenase mRNA and protein with epitopes of oxidized low density lipoprotein in macrophage-rich areas of atherosclerotic lesions. Proc Natl Acad Sci USA 1990; 87:6959–63.

204. Wang T, Powell WS. Increased levels of monohydroxy metabolites of arachidonic acid and linoleic acid in LDL and aorta from atherosclerotic rabbits. Biochem Biophys Res Commun 1991; 1084: 129–38.

205. Folcik VA, Cathcart MK. Predominance of esterified hydroperoxy-linoleic acid in human monocyte-oxidized LDL. J Lipid Res 1994; 35:1570–82.

206. Rao GN, Alexander RW, Runge MS. Linoleic acid and its metabolites, hydroperoxyoctadecadienoic acids, stimulate c-Fos, c-Jun, and c-Myc mRNA expression, mitogen-activated protein kinase activation, and growth in rat aortic smooth muscle cells. J Clin Invest 1995; 96:842–7.

207. Sandstrom PA, Pardi D, Tebbey PW, Dudek RW, Terrian DM, Folks TM, et al. Lipid hydroperoxide-induced apoptosis: lack of inhibition by Bcl-2 over-expression. FEBS Lett 1995; 365:66–70.

208. Bjorkerud B, Bjorkerud S. Contrary effects of lightly and strongly oxidized LDL with potent promotion of growth versus apoptosis on arterial smooth muscle cells, macrophages, and fibroblasts. Arterioscler Thromb Vasc Biol 1996; 16:416–24.

209. Beutler E. Nutritional and metabolic aspects of glutathione. Annu Rev Nutr 1989; 9:287–302.

210. Droge W, Schulze-Osthoff K, Mihm S, Galter D, Schenk H, Eck HP, et al. Functions of glutathione and glutathione disulfide in immunology and immunopathology. FASEB J 1994; 8:1131–8.

211. Van Kuijk FJGM, Handelman GJ, Dratz EA. Consecutive action of phospholipase A2 and glutathione peroxidase is required for reduction of phospholipid hydroperoxides and provides a convenient method to determine peroxide values in membranes. J Free Radical Biol Med 1985; 1:421–7.

212. Kappus H. Lipid peroxidation: mechanisms, analysis, enzymology and biological relevance. In: Sies H, ed, Oxidative Stress, pp. 273–310. Academic, London, 1985.

213. Suttorp N, Toepfer W, Roka L. Antioxidant defense mechanisms of endothelial cells: glutathione redox cycle versus catalase. Am J Physiol 1986; 252:C671–80.

214. Leedle RA, Aust SD. The effect of glutathione on the vitamin E

215. Ruffmann R, Wendel A. GSH rescue by N-acetylcysteine. Klin Wochenschr 1991; 69:857–62.

216. Banks MF, Stipanuk MH. The utilization of N-acetylcysteine and 2-oxothiazolidine-4-carboxylate by rat hepatocytes is limited by their rate of uptake and conversion to cysteine. J Nutr 1994; 124:378–87.

217. Schroder H, Warren S, Bargetzi MJ, Torti SV, Torti FM. N-Acetyl-L-cysteine protects endothelial cells but not L929 tumor cells from tumor necrosis factor-alpha-mediated cytotoxicity. Naunyn Schmiedebergs Arch Pharmacol 1993; 347:664–6.

218. Suttorp N, Kästle S, Neuhof H. Glutathione redox cycle is an important defense system of endothelial cells against chronic hyperoxia. Lung 1991; 169:203–14.

219. Sala R, Moriggi E, Corvasce G, Morelli D. Protection by N-acetylcysteine against pulmonary endothelial cell damage induced by oxidant injury. Eur Respir J 1993; 6:440–6.

220. Das SK, White AC, Fanburg BL. Modulation of transforming growth factor-beta 1 antiproliferative effects on endothelial cells by cysteine, cystine, and N-acetylcysteine. J Clin Invest 1992; 90:1649–56.

221. Marui N, Offermann MK, Swerlick R, Kunsch C, Rosen CA, Ahmad M, et al. Vascular cell adhesion molecule-1 (VCAM-1) gene transcription and expression are regulated through an antioxidant-sensitive mechanism in human vascular endothelial cells. J Clin Invest 1993; 92:1866–74.

222. Németh I, Boda D. The ratio of oxidized/reduced glutathione as an index of oxidative stress in various experimental models of shock syndrome. Biomed Biochim Acta 1989; 48:S53–7.

223. Reed DJ, Fariss MW. Glutathione depletion and susceptibility. Pharmacol Rev 1984; 36:25S–33S.

224. Cotgreave IA, Constantin-Teodosiu D, Moldéus P. Nonxenobiotic manipulation and sulfur precursor specificity of human endothelial glutathione. J Appl Physiol 1991; 70:1220–7.

225. Mattson MP, Scheff SW. Endogenous neuroprotection factors and traumatic brain injury: mechanisms of action and implications for therapy. J Neurotrauma 1994; 11:3–33.

226. Esterbauer H, Gebicki J, Puhl H, Jürgens G. The role of lipid peroxidation and antioxidants in oxidative modification of LDL. Free Radical Biol Med 1992; 13:341–90.

227. Hennig B, Diana JN, Toborek M, McClain C J. Influence of nutrients and cytokines on endothelial cell metabolism. J Am Coll Nutr 1994; 13:224–31.

228. Faruqi R, de la Motte C, DiCorleto PE. α-Tocopherol inhibits agonist-induced monocytic cell adhesion to cultured human endothelial cells. J Clin Invest 1994; 94:592–600.

229. Offermann MK, Medford RM. Antioxidants and atherosclerosis: a molecular perspective. Heart Dis Stroke 1994; 3:52–7.

230. Grimble RF. Nutritional antioxidants and the modulation of inflammation: theory and practice. New Horiz 1994; 2:175–85.

231. Hennig B, Alvarado A. Nutrition and endothelial cell integrity: implications in atherosclerosis. Prog Food Nutr Sci 1993; 17: 119–57.

232. Machlin LJ, Bendich A. Free radical tissue damage: protective role of antioxidant nutrients. FASEB J 1987; 1:441–5.

233. Niki E. Antioxidants in relation to lipid peroxidation. Chem Phys Lipids 1987; 44:227–53.

234. DiMascio P, Murphy ME, Sies H. Antioxidant defense systems: the role of carotenoids, tocopherols, and thiols. Am J Clin Nutr 1991; 53:194S–200S.

235. Chow CK. Vitamin E and oxidative stress. Free Radical Biol Med 1991; 11:215–32.

236. Gavino VC, Miller JS, Ikharebha SO, Milo GE, Cornwell DG. Effect of polyunsaturated fatty acids and antioxidants on lipid peroxidation in tissue cultures. J Lipid Res 1981; 22:763–9.

237. Erin AN, Spirin MM, Tabidza LV, Kagan VE. Formation of alpha-tocopherol complexes with fatty acids: a hypothetical mechanism of stabilization of biomembranes by vitamin E. Biochim Biophys Acta 1984; 774:96–102.

requirement for inhibition of liver microsomal lipid peroxidation. Lipids 1990; 25:241–5.

238. Gey KF, Puska P, Jordan P, Moser UK. Inverse correlation between plasma vitamin E and mortality from ischemic heart disease in cross-cultural epidemiology. Am J Clin Nutr 1991; 53:326S–34S.

239. Regenström J, Nilsson J, Moldeus P, Ström K, Bavenholm P, Tornvall P, et al. Inverse relation between the concentration of low-density-lipoprotein vitamin E and severity of coronary artery disease. Am J Clin Nutr 1996; 63:377–85.

240. Princen HMG, van Duyvenvoorde W, Buytenhek R, van der Laarse A, van Poppel G, Gevers-Leuven JA, et al. Supplementation with low doses of vitamin E protects LDL from lipid peroxidation in men and women. Arterioscler Thromb Vasc Biol 1995; 15:325–33.

241. Jialal I, Fuller CJ, Huet BA. The effect of α-tocopherol supplementation of LDL oxidation. Arterioscler Thromb Vasc Biol 1995; 15: 190–8.

242. Devaraj S, Adams-Huet B, Fuller CJ, Jialal I. Dose-response comparison of *RRR*-α-tocopherol and all-racemic α-tocopherol on LDL oxidation. Arterioscler Thromb Vasc Biol 1997; 17:2273–9.

243. Matin A, Foxall T, Blumberg JB, Meydani M. Vitamin E inhibits low-density lipoprotein-induced adhesion of monocytes to human aortic endothelial cells in vitro. Arterioscler Thromb Vasc Biol 1997; 17:429–36.

244. Kok FJ, van Poppel G, Melse J, Verheul E, Schouten EG, Kruyssen DHCM, et al. Do antioxidants and polyunsaturated fatty acids have a combined association with coronary atherosclerosis? Atherosclerosis 1991; 31:85–90.

245. Manson JE, Gaziano JM, Jonas MA, Hennekens CH. Antioxidants and cardiovascular disease: a review. J Am Coll Nutr 1993; 12: 426–32.

246. Hennig B, Enoch C, Chow CK. Protection by vitamin E against endothelial cell injury by linoleic acid hydroperoxides. Nutr Res 1987; 7:1253–60.

247. Hennig B, Boissonneault GA, Chow CK, Wang Y, Matulionis DH, Glauert HP. Effect of vitamin E on linoleic acid-mediated induction of peroxisomal enzymes in cultured porcine endothelial cells. J Nutr 1990; 120:331–7.

248. Block ER. Hydrogen peroxide alters the physical state and function of the plasma membrane of pulmonary artery endothelial cells. J Cell Physiol 1991; 46:362–9.

249. Kunisaki M, Umeda F, Inoguchi T, Nawata H. Vitamin E binds to specific binding sites and enhances prostacyclin production by cultured aortic endothelial cells. Thromb Haemost 1992; 68:744–51.

250. Okuma M, Takayama H, Uchino H. Generation of prostacyclin-like substance and lipid peroxidation in vitamin E-deficient rats. Prostaglandins 1980; 19:527–36.

251. Chan AC, Leith MK. Decreased prostacyclin synthesis in vitamin E-deficient rabbit aorta. Am J Clin Nutr 1981; 34:2341–7.

252. Kunisaki M, Umeda F, Inoguchi T, Nawata H. Vitamin E restores reduced prostacyclin synthesis in aortic endothelial cells cultures with a high concentration of glucose. Metabolism 1992; 41:613–21.

253. Wang J, Zheu E, Guo Z, Lu Y. Effect of hyperlipidemic serum on lipid peroxidation, synthesis of prostacyclin and thromboxane by cultured endothelial cells: protective effect of antioxidants. Free Radical Biol Med 1989; 7:243–9.

254. Esterbauer H, Dieber-Rotheneder M, Striegl G, Waeg G. Role of vitamin E in preventing the oxidation of low-density lipoprotein. Am J Clin Nutr 1991; 53:314S–21S.

255. Dieber-Rotheneder M, Puhl H, Waeg G, Striegl G, Esterbauer H. Effect of oral supplementation with D-α-tocopherol on the vitamin E content of human low density lipoproteins and resistance to oxidation. J Lipid Res 1992; 32:1325–32.

256. Belcher JD, Balla J, Balla G, Jacobs Jr DR, Gross M, Jaboc HS, et al. Vitamin E, LDL, and endothelium. Brief oral vitamin supplementation prevents oxidized LDL-mediated vascular injury in vitro. Arterioscler Thromb 1993; 13:1779–89.

257. Singh RB, Gupta UC, Mittal N, Niaz MA, Ghosh S, Rastogi V. Epidemiologic study of trace elements and magnesium on risk of coronary artery disease in rural and urban Indian populations. J Am Coll Nutr 1997; 16:62–7.

258. Vlad M, Caseanu E, Uza G, Petrescu M. Concentration of copper, zinc, chromium, iron and nickel in the abdominal aorta of patients deceased with coronary heart disease. J Trace Element Electrolytes Health Dis 1994; 8:111–4.

259. Wilkins GM, Leake DS. The oxidation of low density lipoprotein by cells or ion is inhibited by zinc. FEBS Lett 1994; 341:259–62.

260. Eder K, Kirchgessner M. Concentrations of lipids in plasma and lipoproteins and oxidative susceptibility of low-density lipoproteins in zinc-deficient rats fed linseed oil or olive oil. J Nutr Biochem 1997; 8:461–8.

261. Kraus A, Roth HP, Kirchgessner M. Supplementation with vitamin C, vitamin E or β-carotene influences osmotic fragility and oxidative damage of erythrocytes of zinc-deficient rats. J Nutr 1997; 127: 1290–96.

262. Connell P, Young VM, Toborek M, Cohen DA, Barve S, McClain CJ, et al. Zinc attenuates tumor necrosis factor-mediated activation of transcription factors in endothelial cells. J Am Coll Nutr 1997; 16:411–7.

263. Hennig B, Toborek MN, McClain CJ. Antiatherogenic properties of zinc: implications in endothelial cell metabolism. Nutrition 1996; 12:711–7.

264. Bettger WJ, O'Dell BL. A critical physiological role of zinc in the structure and function of biomembranes. Life Sci 1981; 28:1425–38.

265. Bettger WJ, O'Dell BL. Physiological roles of zinc in the plasma membrane of mammalian cells. J Nutr Biochem 1993; 4:194–207.

266. Prasad AS. Clinical spectrum of human zinc deficiency. In: Prasad AS, ed, Biochemistry of Zinc, pp. 219–58. Plenum, New York, 1993.

267. Vallee B, Falchuk KH. The biochemical basis of zinc physiology. Physiol Rev 1993; 73:9–118.

268. Ludwig JC, Chvapil M. Reversible stabilization of liver lysosomes by zinc ions. J Nutr 1980; 110:945–53.

269. Pfeiffer CJ, Cho CH. Modulating effect of zinc on hepatic lysosomal fragility induced by surface-active agents. Res Commun Chem Pathol Pharmacol 1980; 27:587–98.

270. Oteiza PI, Olin KL, Fraga CG, Keen CL. Zinc deficiency causes oxidative damage to proteins, lipids and DNA in rat testes. J Nutr 1995; 125:823–9.

271. Bray TM, Bettger WJ. The physiological role of zinc as an antioxidant. Free Radical Biol Med 1990; 8:281–91.

272. Bunk MJ, Dnistrian AM, Schwartz MK, Rivlin RS. Dietary zinc deficiency decreases plasma concentrations of vitamin E. Proc Soc Exp Biol Med 1989; 190:379–84.

273. Clair J, Talwalkar R, McClain CJ, Hennig B. Selective removal of zinc from cell culture media. J Trace Element Exp Med 1995; 7:143–51.

274. Hennig B, Wang Y, Ramasamy S, McClain CJ. Zinc deficiency alters barrier function of cultured porcine endothelial cells. J Nutr 1992; 122:1242–7.

275. Hennig B, Wang Y, Ramasamy S, McClain CJ. Zinc protects against tumor necrosis factor-induced disruption of porcine endothelial cell monolayer integrity. J Nutr 1993; 123:1003–9.

276. Ku G, Doherty NS, Wolos JA, Jackson RL. Inhibition by probucol of interleukin-1 secretion and its implication in atherosclerosis. Am J Cardiol 1988; 62:77B–81B.

277. Bobilya DJ, Briske-Anderson M, Reeves PG. Zinc transport into endothelial cells is a facilitated process. J Cell Physiol 1992; 151:1–7.

278. Mishima A, Kaji T, Yamamoto C, Sakamoto M, Kozuka H. Zinc-induced tolerance to cadmium cytotoxicity without metallothionein induction in cultured bovine aortic endothelial cells. Toxicol Lett 1995; 75:85–92.

279. Kaji T, Yamamoto C, Tsubaki S, Ohkawara S, Sakamoto M, Sato M, et al. Metallothionein induction by cadmium, cytokines, thrombin and endothelin-1 in cultured vascular endothelial cells. Life Sci 1993; 53:1185–91.

280. Klasing KC. Nutritional aspects of leukocyte cytokines. J Nutr 1988; 118:1436–46.

281. Jaattela M, Mouritzen H, Elling F, Bastholm L. A20 zinc finger protein inhibits TNF and IL-1 signaling. J Immunol 1996; 156: 1166–73.

282. Cooper JT, Stroka DM, Brostjan C, Palmetshofer A, Bach FH, Ferran C. A20 blocks endothelial cell activation through a NF-κB-dependent mechanism. J Biol Chem 1996; 271:18,068–73.

283. Maran A, Maitra RK, Kumar A, Dong B, Xiao W, Li G, et al. Blockage of NF-kappa B signaling by selective ablation of an mRNA target by 2-5A antisense chimeras. Science 1994; 265:789–92.

284. Parhami F, Fang ZT, Fogelman AM, Andalibi A, Territo MC, Berliner JA. Minimally modified low density lipoprotein-induced inflammatory responses in endothelial cells are mediated by cyclic adenosine monophosphate. J Clin Invest 1993; 92:471–8.

285. Schulze-Osthoff K, Bakker AC, Vanhaesebroeck B, Beyaert R, Jacob WA, Fries W. Cytotoxic activity of tumor necrosis factor is mediated by early damage of mitochondrial functions. Evidence for the involvement of mitochondrial radical generation. J Biol Chem 1992; 267:5317–23.

286. Liu L, Mul FPJ, Kuijpers TW, Lutter R, Roos D, Knol EF. Neutrophil transmigration across monolayers of endothelial cells and airway epithelial cells is regulated by different mechanisms. Ann NY Acad Sci 1996; 31:21–9.

287. Smith CW, Rothlein R, Hughes BJ, Mariscalco MM, Rudloff HE, Schmalstieg FC, et al. Recognition of an endothelial determinant for CD18-dependent human neutrophil adherence and transendothelial migration. J Clin Invest 1988; 82:1746–56.

288. Furie MB, Tancinco CA, Smith CW. Monoclonal antibodies to leukocyte integrins CD11a/CD18 and CD11b/CD18 or intercellular adhesion molecule-1 inhibit chemoattractant-stimulated neutrophil transendothelial migration in vitro. Blood 1991; 78:2089–97.

289. Biffl WL, Moore EE, Moore FA, Carl VS, Franciose RJ, Banerjee A. Interleukin-8 increases endothelial permeability independent of neutrophils. J Trauma: Injury Infect Crit Care 1995; 39:98–103.

290. Lukacs NW, Strieter RM, Elner V, Evanoff HL, Burdick MD, Kunkel SL. Production of chemokines, interleukin-8 and monocyte chemoattractant protein-1, during monocyte : endothelial cell interactions. Blood 1995; 7:2767–73.

291. Nakae H, Endo S, Inada K, Takakuwa T, Kasai T. Changes in adhesion molecule levels in sepsis. Res Commun Mol Pathol Pharmacol 1996; 91:329–38.

292. Heller RA, Kronke M. Tumor necrosis factor receptor-mediated signaling pathways. J Cell Biol 1994; 126:5–9.

18 Nutrition and Allergy

CHRISTOPHER CHANG AND M. ERIC GERSHWIN

INTRODUCTION

Foods are often responsible for allergies. In fact, it is one of the most common complaints of patients. However, many of the incidents of intolerance to foods are not allergic in nature. Often the complaints are vague and inconsistent. Symptoms these patients describe run the gamut and include headaches, fatigue, insomnia, hives, wheezing, diarrhea, runny nose, congestion, and so on. Patients often feel that a food or food supplement is responsible for these symptoms. However, the concept that foods or food supplements may be beneficial in the treatment of allergies, asthma or other atopic disorders is widely accepted. In fact, our efforts to manipulate the immune system through dietary intervention have been in existence since the 1920s. With the increased emphasis on healthier living that has occurred in recent years, we find that this concept has certainly been more present in the public's consciousness. A large proportion of the population is taking high doses of vitamins and minerals and cutting down on salt and animal fat. The incidence of smoking has decreased. The diseases that we try to combat by diet include heart disease, cancer, diabetes, and atopic disease, among others.

In this chapter, we will evaluate foods and food supplements as they relate to the prevention or treatment of asthma, eczema, allergies, or other forms of atopy. Asthma is now known to be primarily an inflammatory condition. Failure to adequately control inflammation in the airways leads to long-term sequelae which decrease longevity and compromise quality of life (Table 1). Our increasing knowledge of the pathogenesis of allergies and asthma has allowed us to conduct studies on foods that we think may theoretically modulate the inflammatory response, such as antioxidants, fatty acids, and certain minerals. We will discuss the evolution of food through the ages and how changes in what we consume may have an effect on our illness patterns.

BREAST FEEDING AND THE DEVELOPMENT OF ATOPY

It is well known that the development of allergies begins from the time a child is born. In those individuals who are considered high risk for atopy, it is especially true that early exposure to ingested and inhalant allergens has a profound effect on the subse-

quent development of allergies. Typically, allergies present in the early months with either diarrhea, bloody stools, or other gastrointestinal complaints or with determatologic manifestations (eczema). Lately, there has been a re-emphasis on the advantage of breast-feeding in American society. However, although breast-feeding may have many other advantages, the subject of breast-feeding and the development of atopy, both in high-risk and "normal" individuals, is still controversial. The identification of individuals who are at high risk for developing atopy is important, and it may be true that dietary manipulation is only needed in this subset of patients. Risk factors for atopy include a significant family history of atopy, high cord blood IgE, and high serum IgE early in life. Amniotic fluid IgE and maternal serum IgE do not appear to be predictive for atopy (1). Other risk factors include eosinophilia in blood or nasal secretions, decreased cord blood platelets, decreased CD8 T cells, and the lambdaMS.51 marker on chromosome 11q. Increased monocyte phosphodiesterase activity has also been found to be a risk factor (2).

The idea that breast-feeding prevents allergic disease has led to the synthesis of a great number of hypoallergeneic formulas by pharmaceutical companies. How do the drug companies come up with what exactly goes into a hypoallergeneic formula if we still do not completely understand why, if, and how breast-feeding actually does prevent allergies? In fact, most formulas have simply been manufactured to mimic breast milk as closely as possible. Hypoallergeneic formulas are constructed to minimize the native protein component of artificial formulas. The theory behind the construction of a hypoallergeneic formula is to break up the proteins into smaller particles to render them less allergenic. There are two types of hypoallergeneic formulas, namely casein hydrolysates and whey hydrolysates. Only casein hydrolysates have been shown to contain peptide units that are short enough so as to lack immunogenicity. These peptide units are generally shorter than 1500 D, and these formulas have been shown to be hypoallergeneic in milk-sensitive infants. In a study by Mallet and Henocq (3), protein hydrolysate formulas were studied with respect to prevention of allergic disease. These formulas were found to have beneficial effect in preventing eczema, but not asthma. In the 177 high-atopic-risk infants studied, there was no difference in cord blood IgE or allergy family history among the various groups studied. It was found that at 1 yr of age, there was no difference in incidence of allergic episodes. At 2 yr of age, there were 18 allergic episodes in the hydrolysate group and 31 in the cow's milk group. By 4

From: *Nutrition and Immunology: Principles and Practice* (ME Gershwin et al. eds.), © Humana Press, Inc., Totowa, NJ

Table 1
Long-Term Sequelae of Uncontrolled Asthma

Thickening of the subepithelial layer and subepithelial fibrosis
Submucosal gland hypertropy
Epithelial damage and shedding
Inflammatory cell infiltration (eosinophils, lymphocytes)
Smooth-muscle hypertropy
Mucus gland and goblet cell hypertropy
Deposition of collagen
Inflammation of pulmonary vasculature

Table 2
Strategy for Decreasing Atopy in Infancy

Prolonged exclusive breast-feeding
Maternal avoidance of milk, egg, peanut, and fish during lactation
Delayed introduction of solid foods for the first 6 mo of life

yr of age, there was still a difference (11 vs 17, respectively). Marini et al. (4) studied 279 infants with high risk of atopy who underwent dietary and environmental manipulation, and they compared these with 80 high-risk infants with no intervention. Dietary manipulation consisted of maintaining exclusive and prolonged breast-feeding, followed by weaning to a hypoantigenic diet. The nonintervention group was essentially allowed to carry on with their own regimen without advice. There was a much lower incidence of atopic dermatitis, allergic conjunctivitis and rhinitis, urticaria, and gastrointestinal disorders at 1 and 2 yr of life in the intervention group.

A whey hydrolysate formula was compared to a cow's milk-based formula for weaning at 6 mo. Ninety-one high-atopy-risk infants were studied prospectively. Thirty-two subjects were given Profylac™ (ALK Laboratories, A/S Hersholm, Denmark) and 39 were weaned to cow's milk formula. Another 20 remained breast-fed. Frequency of allergic disease was the same in all three groups. However, skin allergy symptoms occurred only in the patients fed cow's milk. Unfortunately, the sample size was too small to draw conclusive evidence of the benefits of whey-based protein hydrolysates (5).

Other studies have found that breast milk has a beneficial effect on the prevention of atopic disease. In one such study, there were no significant differences in the observed development of atopic symptoms between groups of infants fed cow's milk for 3 mo, supplemented with cow's milk for the first 5 d, and groups on breast milk alone (6).

The use of a soy-based formula to decrease the manifestation of allergy symptoms in high-risk infants has also been studied. In one study, 48 high-risk infants were fed either soy or cow's milk from weaning to 9 mo of age. There did not appear in this study to be any benefit to the use of soy formulas over cow's milk formula, both in terms of immunoglobulin levels and incidence of symptoms (7).

Potential preventative effects of breast milk can be divided into the direct effects of breast milk on the intestinal tract and indirect effects related to the lifestyles of those who breast feed predominately. The direct effects include inhibition of intestinal absorption of food antigens by sIgA and maintenance of the natural protective barrier of intestinal mucosa to foreign substances (foods).

Breast milk contains high concentrations of nucleotides, which have a potential beneficial effect on the immune function of the infant. The observed effects include a heightened response to immunization-induced antibody production (8). Whether or not nucleotides have an effect on allergic symptoms or atopy has not been studied. Indirect effects are related to the lifestyles of those who practice breast-feeding. These differences include a lesser

incidence of maternal smoking in those who breast-fed. In addition, breast-feeding may lead to decreased or delayed exposure to other foods. Breast-fed infants are usually cared for at home and are, thus, less frequently exposed to problems related to day-care settings, such as viral respiratory infections.

Future directions of infant formula development may take advantage of biotechnological methods to produce formulas that can genetically exclude allergenic epitopes with tolerogenic peptides (9). As we understand more and more about the role of nutritional manipulation in the prevention or control of allergies, biotechnological tools become crucial in the formulation of new recombinant products for use in formulas or baby foods. Such methods may be used in the mimicking of breast milk in order to create a more "hypoallergeneic formula" (10).

The effect of the arachidonic pathway and ingestion of fatty acids will be discussed later. However, it is also interesting to note the relationship between linolenic acid in cord blood and the development of allergy. Intake of formula has also been found to have an effect on serum polyunsaturated fatty acid levels in infancy. In one serum study, levels of arachidonic acid and di-homo-gamma-linolenic acid at 1 and 3 mo were found to decrease from cord blood levels. The decrease was more emphasized in infants who subsequently developed atopic disease. In addition, the lower levels of arachidonic acid and di-homo-gamma-linolenic acid at 1 and 3 mo compared with cord blood were more marked in formula-fed infants than breast-fed infants (11). These results seem to contradict other studies that suggest that increasing the levels of substrates of the arachidonic acid pathway, such as linoleic acid, increase the incidence of atopic disease. Indeed, a study of phospholipid fatty acids in cord blood showed higher levels of arachidonic acid pathway substrates, including $C20:3$, arachidonic acid, $C22:4n-6$, eicosapentaenoic acid (EPA), and docosahexaenoic (DCHA) acid in infants of allergic mothers, compared with infants of nonallergic mothers. They also found a difference in the proportion of n-3 versus n-6 fatty acids in infants who developed atopy in the first 6 yr of life (12). There was no relationship noted between the atopy and the deficient conversion of omega-6 fatty acids to prostaglandin E_1 (13).

Whether or not delayed introduction of solid foods prevents asthma in high-risk individuals is, at present, a matter of controversy (14). In one study of 250 infants from atopic families, serum IgE levels or the incidence of atopy in breast-fed infants were not different from those of formula-fed infants (15). One reviewer states that there is sufficient evidence to at least suggest that there are benefits in keeping infants on breast milk alone and delaying the introduction of solid foods for this time period (16). Given the discrepancy among studies, it is clear that more studies are needed to substantiate this claim.

However, in spite of the fact that our understanding is still incomplete, we can recommend some general guidelines for finding infants with a high risk for atopy. These recommendations are shown in Tables 2 and 3.

Table 3
Foods to Avoid in High-Risk Atopic Children

Milk	Fish
Egg	Wheat
Soy	Chicken
Peanut	

MINERALS, VITAMINS, ANTIOXIDANTS, AND ASTHMA

The function of minerals in the immune system and atopy has been studied from many different angles (Table 4). Some are major minerals, such as magnesium. Some are considered trace elements, such as zinc, selenium, and manganese. Serum levels of minerals have been analyzed to see if there is an association with atopy, and in most cases no such association was found. One of the recently studied mechanisms for the development of allergies and asthma concerns the role of oxygen free radicals. Some minerals and trace elements are components of antioxidants. Naturally occurring endogenous antioxidants include glutathione, catalase, superoxide dismutase, beta-carotene, coenzyme Q10, selenium, and zinc. Antioxidants have been known to prevent cellular damage and enhance repair. The role of antioxidants in allergy has been studied extensively (17–19). It has been postulated that in inflammatory diseases such as asthma, one of the pathologic mechanisms includes the generation of free radicals by a variety of inflammatory cells, and the oxygen free radicals then cause oxidative damage to tissue. Whether or not antioxidant dietary supplements add to the protective effect of the endogenous material is not clear.

Antigen challenge, which results in chemotaxis and activation of inflammatory cells, ultimately results in the releaser of reactive oxygen species such as superoxide (O_2^-) and hydrogen peroxide (H_2O_2). These compounds are further metabolized to hypochlorous acid (HOCl) and the hydroxyl radical (OH^-) by neutrophil myeloperoxidase and ferrous ion reduction, respectively. Hydroxyl radical, in particular, is an extremely damaging entity to lung tissue. The hydroxyl radical is directly related to the increased ozone-induced airway hyperresponsiveness found in asthmatic subjects. The damage resulting from oxygen free radicals includes bronchoconstriction, increased mucus secretion, and microvascular leakage (20). Superoxide dismutase is another enzyme that helps to protect against oxygen free-radical damage. Each molecule of superoxide dismutase contains either zinc and copper (cytosolic) or manganese (mitochondria). Superoxide dismutase catalyzes the conversion of superoxide O_2^- to hydrogen peroxide, which can be converted to water, through the action of catalase. Bronchial epithelial cells of asthmatics have a decreased activity of some enzymes that protect against oxygen free-radical-mediated airway hyperresponsiveness, including superoxide dismutase, but not glutathione peroxidase and catalase. Administration of inhaled corticosteroid appeared to reverse this decrease (21). Whether or not the lower levels of antioxidant in the respiratory epithelium have a direct effect on the pathogenesis of asthma cannot be determined from this study, although the association is intriguing.

NUTRITIONAL SUPPLEMENTS AND ATOPY A recent review notes that studies that link nutrients to causes of asthma show that IgE-mediated reactions to food are a minor cause of respiratory symptoms, especially in children. Also, the authors state that the data linking supplements of specific nutrients to asthma are not valid (22). However, the popularity among the general public for vitamin and mineral supplements is growing with time, and already we see that many companies are manufacturing commercially available over-the-counter preparations.

ZINC The role of zinc in atopic dermatitis has been extensively studied. Zinc is included in creams and ointments designed for use in eczema and other irritant rashes. The role of oral zinc supplements in the treatment of viral illnesses and allergic disease is poorly defined at this time. There has been extensive research in this area and data to support a beneficial role of zinc in the treatment of allergies is not strong. Serum zinc levels were found to be low in children with atopic eczema, but the significance of this as it relates to the role of zinc supplements in eczema is not clear (23). A study of 50 children with atopic eczema found no improvement in a double-blind placebo-controlled trial involving oral zinc supplementation of 185.4 mg elemental zinc per day for 8 wk (24).

MAGNESIUM Magnesium is a key element in asthma. The effects of magnesium ions include a bronchodilator effect, an inhibition of mast cell degranulation, and neurohumoral mediator release. Magnesium may also affect capillary endothelial cell integrity (25). Magnesium has been used in the treatment of status asthmaticus. It has been utilized in intravenous perfusions or inhalation aerosols. Inhaled magnesium has been found to counteract histamine and methacholine-induced bronchoconstriction (26,27). In animal models, magnesium is a preventative medication for anaphylactic shock (28). Dietary magnesium has also been studied as a nutritional supplement in the prevention of asthma. A study of 17 asthmatic subjects who were subjected to a diet low in magnesium for two 3-wk periods, with a 1-wk period during which they took either placebo or magnesium 400-mg/d supplements was conducted. It was found that asthma symptom scores were lower in the magnesium-treated group. However, there was no difference in forced expiratory volume in one second (FEV1) between the two groups (29). A large-scale study of 2633 adults was conducted in the United Kingdom, in which magnesium intake was measured and compared to airway reactivity. An increase of magnesium intake of 100 mg/d led to a 27.7-mL increase in FEV1, after adjusting for other variables, including age, sex, and height, and a decrease in symptoms as reported by the patient (30).

Magnesium has also been studied in the treatment of seasonal allergic rhinitis. One and a half grams of magnesium in the form of magnesium picolinate was administered orally three times a day for 1 mo to subjects with hayfever. The study was a randomized, double-blind trial, with half of the 38 subjects receiving placebo. Parameters measured include number of Kleenex tissues used, intensity of rhinorrhea, number of sneezes, and incidence of watery eyes. The conclusion was that magnesium picolinate was beneficial in the maintenance or prevention of allergies. Although the differences were statistically significant, the small number studied necessitates further investigation (31). In 42 patients with manifestations of acute urticaria, magnesium levels paralleled the serum levels of histamine and IgE during the evolution of the symptoms (32).

OTHER MINERALS Studies of other minerals are scarce. In a murine study, a diet low in copper enhanced histamine-induced paw edema 15 min after challenge. Delayed hypersensitivity responses to oxozalone and sheep erythrocytes were also measured (33) and found to be enhanced by copper deprivation.

Table 4
Minerals, Trace Elements, and Antioxidants in Allergy

Mineral/vitamin	In vivo form	Suggested effects on atopy or asthma	Food sources	Adult RDA	Adverse effects
Zinc	Component of Zn–Cu–SOD–antioxidant, also of many other enzymes	May prevent eczema, used in a variety of skin creams and ointments	Meat, fish, whole grains	10–15 mg	Large doses may cause decreased lymphocyte responsiveness
Selenium	Component of glutathione peroxidase–antioxidant	Potential role in protecting against oxygen free-radical-induced lung injury	Meat, seafoods, whole grains	0.02–0.2 mg	Mucous membrane irritation, liver toxicity in acute overdoses
Magnesium	Magnesium iron	Potential role in reversing bronchospasm of acute asthma, possible effects include bronchodilation	Meat, seafoods, green vegetables, dairy products	190–240 mg	Diarrhea, renal failure
Manganese	Component of certain superoxide dismutases	Antioxidant protective effects	Whole grains, tea, nuts	1–5 mg	Central nervous system effects
Vitamin C	Antioxidant	Protects against oxidative damage caused by airborne pollutants as well as cigarette smoke	Fresh fruits, vegetables	45–60 mg	Interference with vitamin B_{12} absorption, nephrolithiasis
Vitamin E	Antioxidant	May work cooperatively with selenium as an antioxidant	Vegetable oils, cereal grains, eggs, leafy green vegetables	7–10 mg (400 IU)	Gastrointestinal disorders and creatinuria, interferes with vitamin K absorption

The element selenium is also an antioxidant. Selenium is a part of the enzyme glutathione peroxidase that is present in all cells, including erythrocytes, and, in the lung, helps protect alveolar tissue against oxygen free radicals. There were much lower amounts of selenium in whole blood and plasma in 49 patients with asthma, as compared to controls, but their glutathione peroxidase activity was normal (34). This is in contrast to a study of 12 asthmatic subjects with aspirin intolerance in which 10 of the subjects had significantly decreased glutathione peroxidase activity (35) and findings in 56 asthmatic patients compared to 59 nonasthmatic controls in which serum selenium and glutathione peroxidase levels were reduced (36). Both were unaffected by prednisone use. Platelet glutathione peroxidase activity was also found to be lower in a group of asthmatics with or without nonsteroidal anti-inflammatory drug intolerance (37). These observations have been demonstrated in several other studies (38–40).

In a study of 24 patients with asthma randomized into two groups, the group receiving a 100 mg sodium selenite supplement daily for 14 wk demonstrated a decrease in in vitro irreversible platelet aggregation induced by 5 μM ADP. In addition, clinical evaluation led to the conclusion that there was subjective improvement in the asthma condition of the group receiving selenium supplementation, when compared with the placebo group (41).

Further research has shown that dietary supplementation with selenium-enriched yeast led to an increase in whole blood levels of selenium, as well as enhancement of selenium-dependent platelet glutathione peroxidase activity. However, there was no effect on the clinical severity of atopic dermatitis in 60 patients who were randomized to receive either the selenium-enriched yeast or a placebo (42). Blood glutathione activity was also enhanced by daily selenium (0.2 mg) and vitamin E (10 mg) supplementation over a period of 8 wk. Clinical effects in 506 patients with a variety of skin disorders, including atopic dermatitis, eczema, and psoriasis, were also observed, although this study was neither placebo controlled nor blinded (43).

The role of manganese in asthma is unclear. Manganese may play a role in eosinophil recruitment, which is known to be under the control of interleukin-5 (IL-5). Manganese may facilitate the adhesion of eosinophils to vascular cell adhesion molecule via beta-1 integrin, an observation that is inhibited by IL-5 in allergic subjects but not in controls (44).

VITAMIN C AND VITAMIN E Vitamin C (ascorbic acid) and vitamin E (alpha-tocopherol) are also antioxidants and are essential components of our diet. On the premise that free radicals are potentially significant in the pathogenesis of allergy, one study looked at the effect of vitamin C on nickel- and cobalt-induced contact allergy. There was no detectable inhibition of lymphocyte proliferation and the generation of interferon-gamma in peripheral blood mononuclear cells induced by nickel and cobalt (45).

A small study of 20 patients with exercise-induced asthma revealed a potential protective effect of ascorbic acid in nine patients. The study was too small to draw any firm conclusions. Further studies would be needed to confirm these observations (46). However, in a study of 12 patients with exercise-induced asthma, ingesting 500 mg of ascorbic acid per day led to a slight improvement in forced vital capacity (FVC) and FEV1 when compared to placebo, suggesting that further studies may be helpful in delineating a potential role for vitamin C in induced asthma (47). A much larger study conducted on 77,866 women aged 34–68 took place over a 10-yr period and involved questionnaires regarding the incidence of asthma and intake of vitamin E. An association between dietary intake of vitamin E and a protective effect on asthma was observed with a relative risk of 0.53 for the group with higher vitamin E intake versus the lower-intake group (48). Another study showed that there was a higher observed FEV1 and FVC associated with increased intake of vitamin C and vitamin E (49).

By contrast, an earlier study showed no effect of vitamin C on either skin and nasal hypersensitivity to histamine and allergen (50). In a separate study, there was also no significant effect of vitamin C on mast cell degranulation and histamine release in a guinea pig model of anaphylaxis (51).

The data supporting the beneficial effects of vitamin C and E on allergy has not been promising. Unfortunately, many practitioners have been drawn into the widespread practice of recommending dietary supplements like vitamins for the treatment of a wide range of disorders, including allergy and asthma. The recommendations are, as of this time, not based on any objective placebo-controlled double-blinded studies. An even more dangerous practice is that of recommending megadoses of multiple vitamins and minerals. Other commonly recommended supplements include L-tryptophan and some of the fat-soluble vitamins, which accumulate in the body and, thus, can be harmful in large doses.

OTHER ANTIOXIDANTS Although other antioxidants besides vitamins C and E have been studied and have not been found to be of significant benefit in asthma or allergies, oxidative injury may play a role in the allergic lung disease. A study of the effect of oxygen free radicals on the levels of antioxidant in bronchoalveolar lung (BAL) fluid of guinea pigs after allergen lung challenge revealed decreased levels of antioxidants after allergic insult (52). Lipid peroxidation products were also increased in challenged animals and the levels of vitamin E were decreased. Eosinophil number in BAL fluid was increased and TNF-alpha was detected after allergen challenge as well.

FISH OIL AND ASTHMA

Dietary intake of linoleic acid leads to its enzymatic conversion to arachidonic acid. Molecular structures of the polyunsaturated fatty acids of the arachidonic pathway are shown in Fig. 1. Arachidonic acid is particularly important in allergies and asthma because of its metabolism to a collection of compounds known as the leukotrienes. The reaction is catalyzed by 5-lipoxygenase (5-Lo) and produces an intermediate known as hydroperoxyeicosatetraenoic acid (HPETE), which is then enzymatically converted to hydroxyeicosatetraenoic acid (HETE) (Fig. 2). Leukotrienes are mediators that stimulate cells to produce histologic signs of an allergic reaction, including increased vascular permeability, bronchial constriction, chemotaxis, and activation of inflammatory cells and mucus plugging. A parallel limb that produces other compounds that also have an effect on the immune system is known as the cycloxygenase pathway. Compounds generated via the cycloxygenase pathway include the prostaglandins, resulting in a cascade of cellular responses, also leading to inflammatory changes. Depending on the particular prostaglandin, these inflammatory changes include pulmonary vasodilation (PGI_2), or constriction (PGF_{2a}), bronchoconstriction (PGD_2, PGF_{2a}), or bronchodilation (PGE_2), mucus production, decreased (PGD_2/I_2) or increased (TxA_2) platelet adherence and aggregation.

The importance of the leukotrienes is the result of their pro-

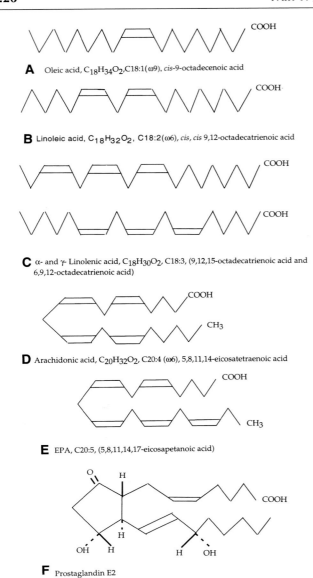

A   Oleic acid, $C_{18}H_{34}O_2$, C18:1(ω9), *cis*-9-octadecenoic acid

B   Linoleic acid, $C_{18}H_{32}O_2$, C18:2(ω6), *cis, cis* 9,12-octadecatrienoic acid

C α- and γ- Linolenic acid, $C_{18}H_{30}O_2$, C18:3, (9,12,15-octadecatrienoic acid and 6,9,12-octadecatrienoic acid)

D   Arachidonic acid, $C_{20}H_{32}O_2$, C20:4 (ω6), 5,8,11,14-eicosatetraenoic acid

E   EPA, C20:5, (5,8,11,14,17-eicosapetanoic acid)

F   Prostaglandin E2

Fig. 1. Structure of the polyunsaturated fatty acids. Essential fatty acids linoleic and linolenic acid are present in vegetable oils. Human milk generally contains higher concentrations of linoleic acid than artificial formulas.

found effects on bronchial tissues. Leukotrienes LTC4, LTD4, LTE4, previously collectively known as SRS-A (or slow reacting substance of anaphylaxis), can be released through the action of 5-LO on mast cells, mononuclear cells, phagocytes, and neutrophils. Cellular effects and target organs of these compounds are shown in Table 5. Another compound that is synthesized in vivo from arachidonic acid is platelet activating factor (PAF). PAF is an important molecule in the delayed reactions in asthma and anaphylaxis. It stimulated a variety of cells, including neutrophils, macrophages, platelets, and eosinophils, and may play a role in priming these cells for response to other stimuli.

The reason leukotrienes are so important in this discussion has to do with 20th-century American's dietary intake of fatty acids. This dietary pattern has changed significantly over the years, from past consumption of large amounts of saturated fatty acids to a health-conscious society that feeds on vegetable oils high in linoleic acid, a precursor of arachidonic acid. High intake of linoleic acid may be beneficial for heart disease, but the effects may not be so helpful in patients with asthma or allergies. A diet with a high concentration of polyunsaturated fatty acids such as linolenic acid may induce increased quantities of arachidonic acid, which may lead to increased production of the leukotrienes in certain cell types. Having shown the significance of the leukotrienes in the asthmatic condition, it would make sense to develop a therapeutic modality of asthma that would target either the production of leukotrienes or the activity of leukotrienes. In fact, the concept of using dietary modification as a way to control asthma has led to studies on fish oil and asthma. Fish oil, high in eicosapentaenoic acid, displaces arachidonic acid molecules in the oxidative metabolism of this class of polyunsaturated fatty acids. This leads to the production of by-products with a much lower potency as mediators of inflammation. Thus, the consumption of fish is thought to be helpful in the management of asthma.

The benefits of fish oil stem from its high concentration of eicosapentaenoic acid and docosahexaenoic acid (53). Eicosapentaenoic acid, once absorbed and incorporated into the cell, competes with arachidonic acid for 5-LO and, consequently, the production of leukotrienes C4, D4, and E4 as well as platelet activating factor (PAF) is reduced. The resulting metabolites theoretically are less potent than the leukotrienes in terms of their inflammatory activity, although one study demonstrated that docosahexaenoic acid and eicosapentaenoic acid inhibit cyclooxygenase pathway metabolism of arachidonic acid but do not affect the 5-LO pathway (54). Clinical studies of fish oil in asthma point to some benefit in increased consumption. A recent epidemiological study has shown that consumption of fresh, oily fish resulted in a significantly decreased risk of asthma symptoms. This study was based on food diaries and symptom questionnaires in 574 children for 6 mo. The study found no consistent trend related to the consumption of any other food (55). Broughton et al. studied the effects of n-3 polyunsaturated fat consumption on methacholine challenge testing and found that a proportionate increase in n-3 polyunsaturated fatty acid (PUFAs) consumption over 1 mo resulted in a decrease in methacholine-induced respiratory distress. The effects of changes in n-3 PUFA dietary intake could be monitored using urinary 5-series leukotriene excretion (56). A National Health and Nutrition survey of 2526 adults who completed a medical history questionnaire and diet record and performed spirometry showed a protective effect of increased dietary fish intake on FEV1, an effect that was more pronounced in nonsmokers (57).

A direct pharmacological application of the fish oil theory has been the development of medications, which more specifically target either leukotriene synthesis or receptor inhibition. An extract of fish oil lipids was found to inhibit the allergen-induced late asthmatic response in 12 of 17 subjects, but had no effect on airway conductance, total serum IgE, or histamine-induced change in airway conductance (58). Eicosapentaenoic acid supplements have failed to improve clinical status of asthma or pulmonary function in a small study of 12 patients (59). In contrast, when taken a step further, pharmacologic manipulation of the arachidonic pathway has resulted in two classes of drugs: the leukotriene pathway inhibitors and the leukotriene pathway antagonists. These drugs have clearly been shown to be beneficial in controlling asthma.

It has also been suggested that fish oil diets may have some

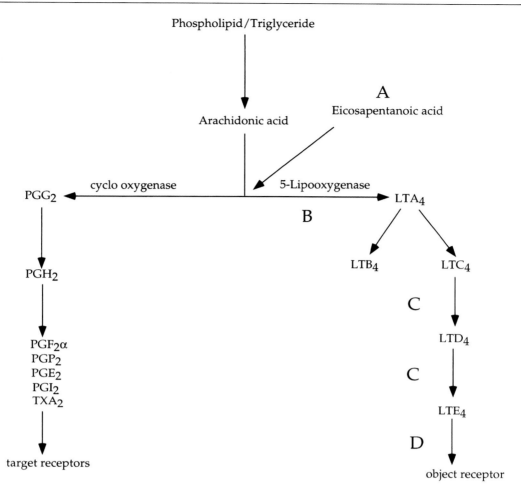

Phospholipid/Triglyceride

A

Arachidonic acid   Eicosapentanoic acid

cyclo oxygenase   5-Lipooxygenase

PGG₂ ← → LTA₄
                           B

PGH₂   LTB₄   LTC₄

                              C

PGF₂α
PGP₂   LTD₄
PGE₂
PGI₂   C
TXA₂
                              LTE₄

                              D
target receptors
                              object receptor

4 possible targets of inhibition

    1) substrate competition
    2) inhibition of synthesis
    3) inhibition of enzymatic conversion
    4) target receptor blockage

Fig. 2. Arachidonic acid metabolism and potential areas to target by "anti-inflammatory" medications and foods. Arachidonic acid is the central point in the metabolism of n-3 and n-6 polyunsaturated fatty acids. Active metabolites in asthma and atopy include the leukotrienes B4, C4, and D4 as well as the prostaglandins. Leukotrienes are produced via the 5-lipooxygenase pathway. The prostaglandins are produced by the action of cyclooxygenase on arachidonic acid. Other enzymes of the lipooxygenase pathway include 12-lipooxygenase and 15-lipooxygenase, which produced metabolites with far less activity. The effect of eicosapentaenoic acid is to compete as substrate for 5-lipooxygenase activity, leading to competitive inhibition of arachidonic acid conversion to active metabolites (**A**). Other areas of potential inhibition is to inhibit the synthesis of leukotrienes (**B**), specific enzyme inhibition (**C**), and inhibition at the receptor level (**D**).

benefit in the treatment of other forms of atopy as well. A diet high in eicosapentaenoic acid (EPA) resulted in a reduction in nasal blood flow as measured by the laser Doppler probe technique. The number of eosinophils in nasal secretion appearing after nasal challenge with ryegrass pollen was decreased in patients who ingested EPA for 8 wk at 3.5 g/d. There was no clinical correlation to these observations *(60)*. In another study, EPA supplementation led to incorporation of EPA into membrane phospholipids. Another effect seen was an inhibition of neutrophil chemotaxis and adherence to epithelial cells *(61)*. Whether or not any of these theoretical and biochemical changes result in any clinical improvements is currently still a matter of debate. Indeed, a British study of 25 pollen-sensitive subjects did not demonstrate any

clinical benefit of ingestion of 3.2 g EPA/d, in terms of wheezing, nocturnal cough, nasal symptoms, and use of medications.

FISH OIL AND ATOPIC DERMATITIS

The effect of fish oil intake on atopic dermatitis is very controversial. A study of dietary supplementation of n-3 fatty acids as compared to corn oil in 145 patients with moderate to severe atopic dermatitis showed no significant difference in clinical score of eczema as evaluated by physicians *(62)*. A separate study showed benefit in scale, erythema, and itch in a 12-wk double-blind period in which patients were randomly distributed to receive either 10 g fish oil (about 1.8 g EPA) or a placebo containing olive oil *(63)*. Late-phase cutaneous reactivity in 16 atopic individuals was studied

Table 5
Arachidonic Acid Metabolites and Their Effects on Immune Function

Fatty acid	Effects on airways	Pathway	Released by
5-HETE	Neutrophil chemotaxis and immunologic effects	Lipooxygenase pathway	Mast cells, activated alveolar macrophages
5-HPETE	Suppresses T-lymphocyte function	Lipooxygenase pathway	Mast cells, mononuclear phagocytes, neutrophils
Leukotriene B4	Polymorphonuclear cells, chemotaxis	Lipooxygenase pathway	Alveolar macrophages
Leukotriene C4, D4, E4	Bronchoconstriction, airway secretion, microvascular leakage, bronchial hyperresponsiveness	Lipooxygenase pathway	Mast cells, eosinophils
PGD_2	Bronchoconstriction, airway secretion, bronchial hyperresponsiveness, vasodilation	Cyclooxygenase pathway	Mast cells, keratinocytes
PGE_2	Airway secretion, chemotaxis, vasodilation, increased vascular permeability	Cyclooxygenase pathway	Airway epithelial cells, fibroblasts, leukocytes
PGF_{2a}	Bronchoconstriction, vascular constriction	Cyclooxygenase pathway	Alveolar macrophages, mast cells, epithelial cells, capillary endothelial cells
PGI_2	Vasodilation, increased vascular permeability	Cyclooxygenase pathway	Endothelial cells, macrophages, smooth-muscle cells
Platelet activating factor	Bronchoconstriction, airway secretion, microvascular leakage, chemotaxis, bronchial hyperresponsiveness, eosinophil chemotaxis	Acyl–CoA acyltransferase pathway	Alveolar macrophages, eosinophils, basophils, neutrophils
Thromboxane A_2	Bronchoconstriction, airway hyperresponsiveness, vasoconstrictor, platelet aggregation	Cyclooxygenase pathway	Mast cells, macrophages, platelets
Eicosapentaenoic acid	Decreases active cystinyl-leukotriene products of lipooxygenase pathway	Substrate competitor of arachidonic acid	Present in foods (fish oil)

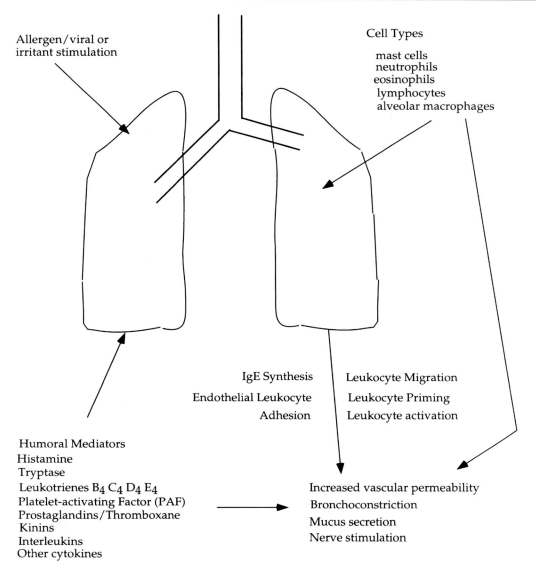

Fig. 3.   Humoral and cellular mediators of inflammation in the lung. Effects of these mediators on lung tissue are also depicted.

after ingestion of fish oil or placebo (olive oil) for 10 wk. Histologically, there was no difference in total inflammatory cell infiltration to the reaction site (64). Contrary to the situation with respect to asthma, promising data on the beneficial effects of fish oil in atopic dermatitis have not appeared (65).

TWENTIETH-CENTURY DIET AND ASTHMA

As we head into the 21st century, we have undergone a change in our diet that is based on knowledge of the biochemical and physiologic effects of certain food substances. Over the years, the health-conscious segment of our population has decreased their intake of animal fat, leading to increased consumption of margarine and vegetable oils. Although vegetable fats may be beneficial against heart disease, they contain high concentrations of omega-6 polyunsaturated fats, such as linoleic acid (66). As discussed earlier, linoleic acid is a precursor of arachidonic acid and of prostaglandin E_2. The immune effects of prostaglandin E_2 include

shifting balance of the control of IgE synthesis, by affecting T-cell generation of interferon-gamma. Thus, the shift in our diet may play a role in the increased prevalence of asthma in recent decades (67).

OBESITY AND ASTHMA: BETTER NUTRITION (OR WEIGHT CONTROL): DOES IT MEAN LESS ASTHMA (OR MORE?)

The connection between obesity and chronic disease is not a novel concept. Obesity has been linked to asthma. A correlation between triceps skinfold thickness and exercise-induced bronchospasm was observed in 13 obese and 14 control children between 6 and 10 yr of age. A cause-and-effect relationship was not characterized (68). A large study of 100,000 female nurses found a significant relationship between body mass index and asthma risk (reported at the American Lung Association/ATC 1998 International Conference.) Surveys in developed countries suggest that low income is associated with obesity. This observation parallels the occurrence of asthma in developed countries, again more common in the low-income populations.

SUMMARY AND CONCLUSIONS

As our knowledge of the immune system grows, there is the potential for the development of new modalities of therapy for allergies (Fig 3). Some of these take the form of nutritional intervention. We already have information on the effects of breast-feeding on the development of atopy. Further characterization of the components of breast milk and their effects on the immune system will help to improve the formulation of infant formulas. Identification of food substances that prevent allergies, asthma, or atopic dermatitis will help in the development of effective pharmacological agents. Such modulation has already been indirectly achieved by the development of leukotriene pathway modifiers in asthma. Clarification of the role of minerals, vitamins, and other antioxidants is essential. It is likely that the regulation of nonpharmacological products will continue to be lax or inadequate. Recommendations from the medical field regarding the use or avoidance of these materials in allergies and asthma can only come after adequate double-blind placebo-controlled studies. As with all food supplements or medications, adverse effects must always be clearly defined and the public well informed, as we must always follow the adage "first do no harm." Given the current knowledge of the effects of foods on the immune system, it is reasonable to assume that dietary modification and manipulation will have an effect on the incidence of asthma and allergies in the 21st century (69).

REFERENCES

1. Strimas JH, Chi DS. Significance of IgE level in amniotic fluid and cord blood for the prediction of allergy. Ann Allergy 1988; 61:133–6.
2. Zieger RS. Development and prevention of allergic disease in childhood. In: Middleton E, et al., eds, Allergy Principles and Practices, 4th ed., vol. 11, pp. 1137–71. 1993.
3. Mallet E, Henocq A. Long-term prevention of allergic disease by using protein hydrolysate formula in at-risk infants. J Pediatr 1992; 121:5(Pt 2):S95–S100.
4. Marini A, Agosti M, Motta G, Mosca F. Effects of a dietary and environmental prevention programme on the incidence of allergic symptoms in high atopic risk infants: three years' follow up. Acta Paediatr 1996; 414(suppl):1–21.
5. Odelram H, Vanto T, Jacobsen L, Kjellman NI. Whey hydrolysate compared with cow's milk-based formula for weaning at about 6 months of age in high allergy-risk infants: effects on atopic disease and sensitization. Allergy 1996; 51(3):192–5.
6. Piacentini GL, Boner AL, Richelli CC, Gaburro D. Artificial feeding: progresses and problems. Ann Ist Super Sanita 1995; 31(4):411–8.
7. Kjellman NI, Johansson SG. Soy versus cow's milk in infants with a biparental history of atopic disease: development of atopic disease and immunoglobulins from birth to 4 years of age. Clin Allergy 1979; 9(4):347–58.
8. Pickering LK, Granoff DM, Erickson JR, Masor ML, Cordle CT, Schaller JP, et al. Modulation of the immune system by human milk and infant formula containing nucleotides. Pediatrics 1988; 101: 242–9.
9. Lo CW, Kleinman RE. Infant formula, past and future: opportunities for improvement. Am J Clin Nutr 1996; 63(4):646S–50S.
10. Young AL, Lewis CG. Biotechnology and the potential nutritional implications for children. Pediatr Clin North Am 1995; 42(4):917–30.
11. Galli E, Picardo M, Chini L, Passi S, Moschese V, Terminali O, et al. Analysis of polyunsaturated fatty acids in newborn sera: a screening tool for atopic disease. Br J Dermatol 1994; 130(6):752–6.
12. Yu G, Kjellman NI, Buorksten B. Phospholipid fatty acids in cord blood: family history and development of allergy. Acta Paediatr 1996; 85:679–83.
13. Melnik BC, Plewig G. Is the origin of atopy linked to the deficient conversion of omega-6-fatty acids to prostaglandin E1. J Am Acad Dermatol 1989; 213(Pt 1):557–63.
14. Weiss ST. Diet as a risk factor for asthma. Ciba Found Symp 1997; 206:244–57.
15. Gordon RR, Noble DA, Ward AM, Allen R. Immunoglobulin E and the eczema–asthma syndrome in early childhood. Lancet 1982; 9:72–4.
16. Zeiger RS, Heller S, Mellon M, O'Conner R, Hamburger RN. Effectiveness of dietary manipulation in the prevention of food allergy in infants. J Allergy Clin Immunol 1986; 78:224–8.
17. Hatch GE. Asthma, inhaled oxidants, and dietary oxidants. Am J Clin Nutr 1995; 61:625S–30S.
18. Powell CV, Nash AA, Powers HJ, Primhak RA. Antioxidant status in asthma. Pediatr Pulmonol 1994; 18:34–8.
19. Sharma SC, Wilson CW. The cellular interaction of ascorbic acid with histamine, cyclic nucleotides and prostaglandins in the immediate hypersensitivity reaction. Int J Vitam Nutr Res 1980; 50:163–70.
20. Doelman CJ, Bast A. Oxygen radical in lung pathology. Free Radical Biol Med 1990; 9:381–400.
21. De Raeve HR, Thunnissen FB, Kaneko FT, Guo FH, Lewis M, Kavuru MS, et al. Decreased Cu–Zn–SOD activity in asthmatic airway epithelium: correction by inhaled corticosteroid in vivo. Am J Physiol 1997; 272:L148–54.
22. Monteleone CA, Sherman AR. Nutrition and asthma. Arch Intern Med 1997; 157(1):23–4.
23. David TJ, Gibbs AC, Sharpe TC, Wells FE. Low serum zinc in children with atopic eczema. Br J Dermatol 1984; 111:597–601.
24. Ewing CI, David TJ, Ashcroft C, Gibbs AC. Failure of oral zinc supplementation in atopic eczema. Eur J Clin Nutr 1991; 45(10):507–10.
25. Mathew R, Altura BM. Magnesium and the lungs. Magnesium 1988; 7:173–87.
26. Rolla G, Spinaci S, Arossa W, Bugiani M, Bucca C. Reduction of histamine-induced bronchoconstriction by magnesium in asthmatic subjects. Allergy 1987; 42:186–8.
27. Rolla G, Bugiani M, Arossa W, Bucca C. Magnesium attenuates methacholine-induced bronchoconstriction in asthmatics. Magnesium 1987; 6:201–4.
28. Ashkenazy Y, Zor U, Sela BA, Kusniec F, Caspi A, Feigel D, et al. Magnesium-deficient diet aggravates anaphylactic shock and promotes cardiac myolysis in guinea pigs. Magnes Trace Element 1990; 9:283–8.
29. Hill J, Britton J, Lewis S, Mickelwright A. Investigation of the effect of short-term change in dietary magnesium intake in asthma. Eur Respir J 1997; 10:2225–9.
30. Britton J, Weiss S, Tattersfield A, Lewis S, Knox A, Wisniewski A, et al. Dietary magnesium, lung function, wheezing, and airway hyperreactivity in a random adult population sample. Lancet 1994; 344:357–62.
31. Cipolla C, D'Antuono G, Lugo G, Orciara P, Occhionero T. Magnesium pidolate in the treatment of seasonal allergic rhinitis. Preliminary data. Magnes Res 1990; 3:109–12.
32. Muresan D, Flueras M, Benea V, Mosescu L, Alecu M, Nicolae I, et al. Investigations of magnesium, histamine and immunoglobulin dynamics in acute urticaria. Arch Roum Pathol Exp Microbiol 1990; 49(1):31–5.
33. Jones DG. Effects of dietary copper depletion on acute and delayed inflammatory responses in mice. Res Vet Sci 1984; 37:205–10.
34. Stone J, Hinks LJ, Beasley R, Holgate ST, Clayton BA. Reduced selenium status of patients with asthma. Clin Sci 1989; 77:495–500.
35. Malmgren R, Unge G, Zetterstrom O, Theorell H, de Wahl K. Lowered glutathione-peroxidase activity in asthmatic patients with food and aspirin intolerance. Allergy 1986; 41:43–5.
36. Flatt A, Pearce N, Thomson CD, Sears MR, Robinson MF, Beasley R. Reduced selenium in asthmatic subjects in New Zealand. Thorax 1990; 45:95–9.

37. Hasselmark L, Malmgren R, Unge G, Zetterstrom. Lowered platelet glutathione peroxidase activity in patients with intrinsic asthma. Allergy 1990; 45:523–7.

38. Pearson DJ, Suarez-Mendez VJ, Day JP, Miller PF. Selenium status in relation to reduced glutathione peroxidase activity in aspirin-sensitive asthma. Clin Exp Allergy 1991; 21:203–8.

39. Misso NJ, Powers KA, Gillon RL, Stewart GA, Thompson PJ. Reduced platelet glutathione peroxidase activity and serum selenium concentration in atopic asthmatic patients. Clin Exp Allergy 1996; 26:838–47.

40. Kadrabova J, Mad'aric A, Kovacikova Z, Podivinsky F, Ginter E, Gazdik F. Selenium status is decreased in patients with intrinsic asthma. Biol Trace Element Res 1996; 52:241–8.

41. Hasselmark L, Malmgren R, Zetterstrom O, Unge G. Selenium supplementation in intrinsic asthma. Allergy 1993; 48:30–6.

42. Fairris GM, Perkins PJ, Lloyd B, Hinks L, Clayton BE. The effect on atopic dermatitis of supplementation with selenium and vitamin E. Acta Derm Venereol 1989; 69:359–62.

43. Juhlin L, Edqvist LE, Ekman LG, Ljunghall K, Olsson M. Blood glutathione-peroxidase levels in skin disease: effect of selenium and vitamin E treatment. Acta Derm Venereol 1982; 62:211–4.

44. Werfel SJ, Yednock TA, Matsumoto K, Sterbinsky SA, Schleimer RP, Bochner BS. Functional regulation of beta 1 integrins on human eosinophils by divalent cations and cytokines. Am J Respir Cell Mol Biol 1996; 14:44–52.

45. Van Den Broeke LT, Graslund A, Larsson PH, Nilsson JL, Wahlberg JE, Scheynius A, et al. Free radicals as potential mediators of metal allergy: effect of ascorbic acid on lymphocyte proliferation and IFN-gamma production in contact allergy to Ni^{2+} and Co^{2+}. Acta Derm Venereol 1998; 78:95–8.

46. Cohen H, Neuman I, Nahum H. Blocking effect of vitamin C in exercise-induced asthma. Arch Pediatr Adoelsc Med 1997; 151: 367–70.

47. Schachter EN, Schlesinger A. The attenuation of exercise-induced bronchospasm by ascorbic acid. Ann Allergy 1982; 49:146–51.

48. Troisi RJ, Willett W, Weiss ST, Trichopoulos D, Rosner B, Speizer FE. A prospective study of diet and adult-onset asthma. Am J Respir Crit Care Med 1995; 151:1401–8.

49. Britton JR, Pavord ID, Richards KA, Knox AJ, Wisniewski AF, Lweis SA, et al. Dietary antioxidant vitamin intake and lung function in the general population. Am J Respir Crit Care Med 1995; 151: 1383–7.

50. Fortner BR Jr, Danziger RE, Rabinowitz PS, Nelson HS. The effect of ascorbic acid on cutaneous and nasal response to histamine and allergen. J Allergy Clin Immunol 1982; 69:484–8.

51. Gonzales RG, Garcia M, Perez Saad H, De la Vega AR. Comparative study of ascorbic acid and disodium cromoglycate in some models of experimental anaphylaxis. Allergol Immunopathol 1979; 7:211–6.

52. Shvedova AA, Kisin ER, Kagan VE, Karol MH. Increased lipid peroxidation and decreased antioxidants in lungs of guinea pigs following an allergic pulmonary response. Toxicol Appl Pharmacol 1995; 132:72–81.

53. Arm JP, Thien FC, Lee TH. Leukotrienes, fish-oil, and asthma. Allergy Proc 1994; 15:129–34.

54. Austen KF. The role of arachidonic acid metabolites in local and systemic inflammatory processes. Drugs 1987; 33(suppl 1):10–7.

55. Hodge L, Salome CM, Peat JK, Haby MM, Xuan W, Woolcock AJ. Consumption of oily fish and childhood asthma risk. Med J Aust 1996; 164:137–40.

56. Broughton KS, Johnson CS, Pace BK, Liebman M, Kleppinger KM. Reduced asthma symptoms with n-3 fatty acid ingestion are related to 5-series leukotriene production. Am J Clin Nutr 1997; 65:1011–7.

57. Schwartz J, Weiss ST. The relationship of dietary fish intake to level of pulmonary function in the first National Health and Nutrition Survey (NHANES I) Eur Respir J 1994; 7:1821–4.

58. Arm JP, Horton CE, Spur BW, Mencia-Huerta JM, Lee TH. The effects of dietary supplementation with fish oil lipids on the airway response to inhaled allergen in bronchial asthma. Am Rev Respir Dis 1989; 139:1395–400.

59. Kirsch CM, Payan DG, Wong MY, Dohlman JG, Blake VA, Petri MA, et al. Effect of eicosapentaenoic acid in asthma. Clin Allergy 1988; 18:177–87.

60. Rangi SP, Servonska MH, Lenathan GA, Pickett WC, Blake VA, Sample S, et al. Suppression by ingested eicosapentaenoic acid of the increases in nasal mucosal blood flow and eosinophilia of ryegrass-allergic reactions. J Allergy Clin Immunol 1990; 85:484–9.

61. Lee TH, Arm JP, Horton CE, Crea AE, Mencia-Huerta JM, Spur BW. Effects of dietary fish oil lipids on allergic and inflammatory diseases. Allergy Proc 1991; 12:299–303.

62. Soyland E, Funk J, Rajka G, Sandberg M, Thune P, Rustad L, et al. Dietary supplementation with very long-chain n-3 fatty acids in patients with atopic dermatitis. A double-blind, multicentre study. Br J Dermatol 1994; 130:757–64.

63. Bjorneboe A, Soyland E, Bjorneboe GE, Rajka G, Drevon CA. Effect of dietary supplementation with eicosapentanoic acid in the treatment of atopic dermatitis. Br J Dermatol 1987; 117:463–9.

64. Thien FC, Atkinson BA, Khan A, Mencia-Huerta JM, Lee TH. Effect of dietary fish oil supplementation on the antigen-induced late-phase response in the skin. J Allergy Clin Immunol 1992; 89:829–35.

65. Berth-Jones L, Graham-Brown RA. Placebo-controlled trial of essential fatty acid supplementation in atopic dermatitis. Lancet 1993; 341:1557–60.

66. Black PN, Sharpe S. Dietary fat and asthma: is there a connection? Eur Respir J 1997; 10:6–12.

67. Chang CC, Phinney SD, Halpern GM, Gershwin MD. Asthma mortality: another opinion—is it a matter of life and . . . bread? J Asthma 1993; 30:93–103.

68. Kaplan TA, Montana E. Exercise-induced bronchospasm in nonasthmatic obese children. Clin Pediatr 1993; 32:220–5.

69. Peat JK. Prevention of asthma. Eur Respir J 1996; 9:545–55.

19 Adverse Reactions to Foods

FRANCESCO GIUSEPPE FOSCHI, LORENZO MARSIGLI,
FRANCESCO CHIAPPELLI, MICHELLE A. KUNG, MAURO BERNARDI,
AND GIUSEPPE FRANCESCO STEFANINI

INTRODUCTION

Any symptom or sign following the intake of food is called an "adverse reaction to food" (ARF). In 1995, the European Academy of Allergy and Clinical Immunology (EAACI) published a Position Paper on ARF *(1)*, which made a thorough review of this controversial topic. More recently, a newer Position Paper has been provided by the Codex Alimentarius *(2)*.

Adverse reactions to food are thought to be common because they are reported by many patients (about 20%). Nevertheless, two studies on the general European population showed by means of elimination diets and double-blind placebo-controlled food challenges that the actual prevalence of ARF is 1.4–2.4% *(3,4)*. This means that only one out of 10 reported ARF is real!

Adverse reactions to food are broadly divided into toxic, nontoxic, and psychological (Fig. 1). Whereas toxic reactions are the result of contaminants contained in foods (e.g., poisonous, mushrooms, botulism) and, therefore, can ensue in any subject exposed to culpable food(s), nontoxic ARFs depend on a patient's sensitivity to some foods and are divided into immune-mediated and non-immune-mediated groups.

Immune-mediated ARFs (food allergy) can be further divided into IgE mediated (Type I reactions) and non-IgE mediated (involving immunoglobulins other than IgE, immune complexes and cell-mediated reaction).

Non-immune-mediated ARFs (food intolerance) can be enzymatic (e.g., lactose intolerance), pharmacological (e.g., reactions to vasoactive amines contained in some foods) and the result of additives.

Psychological reactions are usually related to former experiences; they are also referred to as food aversion and are largely psychosomatic.

In this chapter, only nontoxic ARFs will be described, as toxic reactions are best described elsewhere. Nevertheless, when dealing with ARFs, the possibility of toxic reactions should always be kept in mind.

From: *Nutrition and Immunology: Principles and Practice* (ME Gershwin et al. eds.), © Humana Press, Inc., Totowa, NJ

IMMUNE MEDIATED ARF

IMMUNOLOGIC BACKGROUND According to Gell and Coombs' classification, immunologic reactions can be divided into four types:

1. **Type I: IgE-mediated reaction.** Food specific IgE antibodies bind to high-affinity FcεRI receptors on mast cells, basophils, macrophages and dendritic cells as well as low-affinity FcεRII receptors on macrophages, monocytes, lymphocytes, eosinophis, and platelets. When food allergens penetrate the gut barrier and reach IgE bound to mast cells or basophils, preformed mediators (i.e., histamine, serotonin, tumor necrosis factor alpha) are released and induce symptoms. After IgE-mediated activation, several mediators are synthesized and amplify the immune response through the so-called late-phase reaction.

2. **Type II: Antigen–antibody-dependent cytotoxic reaction.** Antigen–antibody-dependent cytotoxic reactions are mediated by antibodies that recognize antigens on the cell surface. The complex antigen antibody can activate complement, natural-killer, or lymphocytes bearing a high-affinity immunoglobulin receptor (FcγIII, CD16). Type II reactions have been implicated in a few reports of antibody-dependent thrombocytopenia secondary to the ingestion of cow's milk.

3. **Type III: Immune complex disease (Arthus type).** In this type of reaction, inflammation is provoked by immunocomplex deposition and subsequent local cell activation. This mechanism could have a role in some food allergic patients with elevated serum levels of food antigen–antibody complexes. These immunocomplexes can also be detected in normal subjects, but further studies are needed to better define their role.

4. **Type IV: Delayed-type hypersensitivity reaction.** Lymphocytes (principally Th1 type) and macrophages are involved in hypersensitivity reactions, which occur several hours after the ingestion of food allergens. This mechanism represents a major immunological pathway in gut mucosal damage. In conditions such as celiac disease and cow's

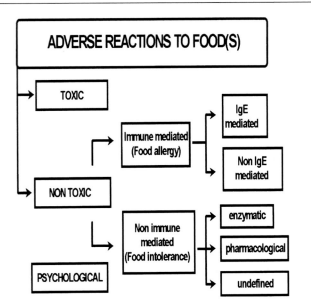

Fig. 1. Scheme of adverse reactions to food(s) according to the EAACI.

milk-induced enteropathy, delayed-type hypersensitivity reactions have been clearly demonstrated.

Gell and Coombs' classification is simple, but the immunology of ARFs is far more complex. Like all immune reactions, immune-mediated ARFs depend on the maturation of T cells. The development and maintenance of immunological memory is a fundamental aspect of immune surveillance *(5)*, which can be demonstrated across the phylogoenetic tree, in a rather primitive manner in invertebrates up to the more sophisticated manifestations we observe in higher vertebrates, including human beings *(6)*. Increased understanding of the fundamental molecular mechanisms that regulate the generation, maintenance, and functional diversity of memory immune cells is needed for the development of new and improved modes of treatment intervention for a variety of human diseases, including ARF. Immunological memory comprises a vast field of processes, which is principally, though not exclusively, concerned with that arm of the immune response, which is often referred to as antigen dependent or major histocompatibility complex (MHC) restricted. Immunological memory is also principally, though not exclusively, concerned with the fate of cells of lymphoid origin, B cells and T cells *(5,7)*. The cellular, biochemical, and molecular processes that control and regulate the maturation of B cells and T cells into memory cells are similar, although not identical, even in the case, as shown recently, of the regulation of B-cell tolerance *(8)*.

The events leading to the establishment of immune cell memory are to be deeply known. One difficulty lies in the still rather crude means at our disposal to distinguish between naïve and memory cells *(9)*. This can be achieved either by phenotypic characterization of the cell population or by monitoring certain functional responses. Inherent in both approaches are several procedural problems, such as the purity of the cell population, which is still unresolved today.

It is generally accepted that circulating T lymphocytes obtained from normal healthy donors are generally resting cells, meaning that the expression of membrane markers of activation (e.g., CD25, CD71, MHC-Dr) is <10% in the cell population. This is not the case when circulating T cells obtained from patients with some form of immune activation (e.g., food-induced immune reaction). The term "resting" signifies that the cells are positioned at the G_0/G_1 interphase of the cell cycle; the cell population is generally regarded to be fairly homogeneously resting at that stage. Upon stimulation, the cells in the population advance fairly synchronously through the initial protein synthesis phase of the cell cycle, G_1, through the DNA synthesis phase, S, through the second protein synthesis phase, G_2, and through the mitotic phase, M. Typically, the cell cycle of T cells obtained from young normal adult donors and stimulated in vitro is 20–24 h (G_1: 5–6 h, S: 9–10 h, G_2: 5–6 h, M: 1–2 h). The cells remain relatively well synchronized for about four cell divisions, and when pulsed with radioactive thymidine (^{3}H-TdR) at 72 h for a few hours (6 h to 16 h, depending upon the laboratory), a sharp peak of radioactive macromolecules is obtained, which indicates incorporation of the radiolabeled DNA precursor (note: the sharpness of the peak indicates synchronicity of the cell population). Following this burst of cell division, which may last for 7–10 days, the cell population returns to a resting state, unless further stimulation is provided. The observation that although several rounds of cell divisions occurred during that span of time, the absolute cell number of the population could remain unchanged, or actually decrease under certain experimental conditions, suggested that a significant amount of cell death may be concomitant with cell division. We now know that this is, indeed, the case because several of the molecular pathways that direct T-cell cycle traversal overlap with those that trigger the process of spontaneous cell death, apoptosis. Thus, an essential question has arisen, which seeks to determine the distinguishing mechanisms that favor T-cell maturation into a memory cell versus immune cell apoptosis *(7)*.

Naive T cells change their phenotypic and functional characteristics in a matter of hours following stimulation. Hence, the preferred terminology at this point is naive effector T cells. As naive effector T cells proceed through the several rounds of cell division, they acquire phenotypic and functional characteristics, by which we now recognize them as mature memory T cells. These cells return to a resting stage, but can be stimulated again as effector memory T cells. Indeed, there are currently two models for the generation of memory T cells: the one states that memory T cells arise from activated memory effector T cells that have reverted to the resting state, and the other states memory T cells are generated directly from naive cells, through the naive effector T cell stage *(10)*. Normal healthy young adult subjects generally have close to a 1:1 ratio of circulating naive memory T cells, as determined by phenotypic markers. Patient populations who are chronically or repeatedly exposed to a given antigen, such as a food allergen, tend to show pronounced alterations in that ratio, suggesting immune imbalance in naive and memory T cells *(11–13)*. It is possible and even probable that several but not all of the molecular mechanisms that direct naive effector T-cell proliferation should be similar to those that direct a memory effector T-cell proliferative response. It is also clear that alcohol, putatively because of its immediate and direct impact on the oral and intestinal mucosae, has polyvalent effects on these molecular events.

Phenotypically, circulating T cells of normal healthy individuals express the CD3 moiety, and either CD4 or CD8. Double positive cells, CD4 and CD8, characterize serious immunopathology in most cases. Like lymphocytes, they also express the common leukocyte antigen, CD45, but not the monocyte/macrophage marker, CD14. Thus, flow cytometric characterization of the $CD45^+CD14^-$ cell population provides a gate for lymphocyte, within which $CD3^+CD4^+$ (CD4 cells) or $CD3^+CD8^+$ (CD8 cells) cells can be found. Naive CD4 cells and naive CD8 cells only express the A restriction fragment of CD45 (CD45RA), which they lose within a few hours of stimulation. Thus, naive CD4 and naive CD8 effector cells are CD45RAdim and eventually $CD45RA^-$. As they mature, the cells acquire the 0 restriction fragment of CD45. Thus, mature memory CD4 cells and mature memory CD8 cells are defined phenotypically as $CD45RA^-$ $CD45R0^+$. Other phenotypic markers are lost by naive effector T cells (e.g., CD62L) and are gained by the cells as they attain the stage of maturity (e.g., LFAs, VLAs). Whether the conversion between the CD45RA and CD45R0 phenotype is bi-directional is unclear, meaning that CD45R0 cells may revert to a CD45RA state (14).

Functionally, as stated earlier, naive T cells are regarded as resting, although they are mobile in vivo as they migrate to peripheral lymph nodes by means in part of the homing receptor, CD62L, with which they are endowed (15). When stimulated in vitro, naive CD4 and CD8 cells become effector cells because they begin to produce cytokines, which have autocrine as well as paracrine effects. The first among these is interleukin-2 (IL-2), which can be detected as early as 24–48 h following stimulation. Interferon (IFN)-γ, IL-4, IL-5, IL-10, and other cytokines are also produced by both naive CD4 and CD8 effector cells (9,11,15–18). These cells have been referred to as TH0 cells.

Further stimulation of memory CD4 cells under well-characterized conditions generates populations capable of distinct patterns of cytokine expression (i.e., Th1: predominantly IL-2 and IFN; Th2: predominantly IL-4 and IL-5). These patterns have clearly distinct functional effects upon further maturation of CD8 cells and other cytotoxic cells (i.e., Th1), or the proliferation and maturation of B cells (i.e., Th2) and eosinophils (IL-6). Serum and other body fluids obtained from normal healthy individuals show typically low levels of Th1 or Th2 cytokines, and if any, at a rather balanced ratio. Patients with some form of immune activation have been reported to show either high Th1 cytokines or high Th2 cytokines, depending on which arm of the immune response is activated (cytotoxicity vs immunoglobulin production). Th2 cytokine (particularly IL-4) pattern has been related to IgE-mediated allergic reactions, with increased IgE synthesis and IgE-mediated responses (19).

These observations strongly suggest that Th1 and Th2-like responses in vivo play a pivotal role in determining immune effector mechanisms and clinical outcome (20–22). Moreover, additional patterns of cytokines (e.g., Th3) have been reported, which further increase the system's level of complexity.

Another pivotal role in ARF development is played by the mucosal immune system of the gastrointestinal tract, which is the main immunological organ of the human body and protects against pathogens from outside environments such as viruses, bacteria and parasites. Throughout life, an enormous quantity of potentially allergenic foods is ingested, nevertheless, only few people develop ARF. The mucosal immune system can suppress immune response to food by oral tolerance (OT), which is a specific immune-reduced responsiveness to an antigen after prior mucosal exposure. Cellular mechanism(s) producing OT are not well known, but clonal dele-

tion of T cells, clonal energy or active suppression have been proposed (23). These mechanisms can lead to a decrease in IgE synthesis and cell-mediated response, with reduction of possible secondary mucosal damage. T lymphocytes (24) and antigen-presenting cells within the gut seem to play a key role. Moreover, OT seems to be related to many factors, such as antigen type and dose, frequency of exposure, age of subjects at first antigen presentation, atopy, gut permeability, and gut flora. In particular, gut flora seems to have some influence on mucosal immune response such as IgE synthesis and Th2 regulation (25,26).

Failure of OT mechanisms are believed to lead to a variety of enteropathies including food allergy (27). In children, OT alteration is the most likely pathogenic mechanism for food sensitization. The high prevalence of food allergy in infancy could be related to immature OT with spontaneous resolution during development. In adults, responsible foods are usually vegetables, whereas in children, animal allergens are more frequently reported (milk, fish, egg). Adult vegetable hypersensitivity is due to cross-reactivity with homologous antigens shared by pollens. It is likely that sensitization starts in the airways and subsequent exposure to crossreactive food allergen induces symptoms (see the subsection Oral Allergy Syndrome for details).

FOOD ALLERGENS Although food allergens are many, only some of them have been identified using the sodium dodecylsulfate–polyacrylamide gel electrophoresis (SDS-PAGE) method. According to present allergen definitions, the following are the most important.

Cow's milk: It is the first food eaten by infants and it is the main food responsible for allergy in infancy. It contains approx. 20 proteins able to induce specific IgE synthesis, mainly caseins (80% of milk proteins) and serum proteins. Known major allergens are alpha-lactoglobulin or Bos d 4 (molecular weight, (MW) = 14.2 kDa), beta-lactoglobulin or Bos d 5 (MW = 18.3 kDa), serum albumin or Bos d 6 (MW = 67 kDa), immunoglobulin or Bos d 7 (MW = 1 60 kd) and caseins or Bos d 8 (MW ranging from 20 to 30 kd).

Egg: Major allergens of chicken's eggs are ovomucoid (Gal d 1, 28 kDa), ovalbumin (Gal d 2), and conalbumin (Gal d 3). Because of high heat stability, Gal d 1 is frequently responsible for allergic reactions resulting from cooked egg or egg derivatives added to prepared foods.

Fish: The best known fish allergen is a muscular parvalbumin from codfish, named Gad c 1 (12.3 kd). Gad c 1 is very resistant to heat and enzymatic digestion and is responsible for most allergic reactions to codfish.

Soy: Four main allergens can be extracted from soy: serum, alpha-glycine, glycinine, and aggregated glycinine.

Peanut: Two major allergens have been identified: Ara h 1 (63.5 kDa) and Ara h 2 (17 kDa). These allergens can induce a sustained IgE allergic response that usually is maintained from childhood to adult life.

Apple: In recent years, much attention has been paid to crossreactivies between vegetables and fruits. Immunoblotting studies have shown that major apple allergen Mal d 1 shows great homology with major birch allergen Bet v 1, thus explaining the so-called birch-apple syndrome (see also the subsection, Oral Allergy Syndrome).

Table 1
Enzymatic Deficiencies

Conditions	Deficiencies
Disaccharidases deficiency	Lactase, sucrase–isomaltase, glucose–galactose
Galactosemia	Galactose 1 phosphate uridyl transferase; uridine diphosphate-4-epidermase
Phenylketonuria	Phenylalanine hydroxylase
Alcohol intolerance	Aldehyde dehydrogenase
Favism	Glucose 6-phosphate dehydrogenase

Celery: Several allergenic proteins have been identified; the most important are the major allergen Api g 1, homologous to Bet v 1, and a 15 kDa protein belonging to the family of profilins.

Crustaceans: Shrimp is the most widely studied. Its major allergen, a tropomyosin called Pen a 1 (36 kDa) can also be found in other crustaceans. Pen a 1 can be responsible for crossreactions seldom observed between shrimps and dust mites.

NON-IMMUNE-MEDIATED ARF

ENZYMATIC These ARFs are the result of the lack of an enzyme with a subsequent increase in its metabolic substrate(s) that can induce symptoms in a dose-dependent fashion. The most common enzymatic ARF is lactose intolerance, resulting from lactase deficiency. Other types are uncommon. Enzymatic ARFs are listed in Table 1.

PHARMACOLOGICAL Some foods (*see* Table 2) contain substances able to provoke direct mast cell and basophil release or vasoactive amines (or their precursors) and neurotransmitters, thus mimicking allergy inflammation. Some authors indicate these reactions as "pseudo-allergies." Moreover, these mediators might enhance gut permeability and increase the passage of food through the gut barrier with possible sensitization to food allergens.

ADDITIVE Adverse reactions to food additives (listed in Table 3) are very complex and show a wide clinical spectrum (*28*). Their prevalence in the general population is actually unknown, but it can be assumed to be less than 1%, as reviewed by Wuthrich (*29*). These reactions in part overlap with pharmacological and enzymatic intolerance and many forms of pathogenesis can be hypothesized with both non-immune and immune-mediated reactions. Some additives can act as haptens, combining themselves

Table 2
Amines and Releaser Substances in Foods

Amine	Food
Histamine	Wine, fermented cheese, sardines, anchovies, spinach, canned foods, frozen fish and crustaceans, sauerkraut, tomato, sausages
Tyramine	Wine, beer, pickled herring, cheese, milk, chocolate, egg whites
Glutamate	Soy sauce, Chinese foods
Phenylethylamine	Chocolate, cheese, wine
Octopamine	Citrus fruits
Nitrite	Sausage

Table 3
Food Additives

Colorants	Azo dyes • Tartrazine (FD & C yellow #5) • Sunset yellow (FD & C yellow #6) • Ponceau (FD & C red #4) • Carmosine (FD & C red #2) Non-azo dyes • Erytrosine (FD & C red #3) • Indigotine (FD & C blue #2) • Brilliant Blue (FD & C blue #1) Chorophyll
Preservatives	Antimicrobials • Sodium benzoate/hydroxybenzoic acid • Parabens • Sorbates Antioxidant • Bisulfites/metabisulfites • Butylated hydroxyanisole and butylated hydroxytoluene (BHA/BHT) • Tocopherols • Gallates
Emulsifiers/stabilizers	Ethylene diamine tetraacetic acid (EDTA); gum arabic (acacia)
Fillers	Tragacanth; propyleneglycol alginate
Flavors/sweeteners	Vanillin; saccharin; aspartame; sorbitol, mannitol; xylitol; monosodium glutamate
Contaminants (inadvertent additives)	Toxin, biogenic amines, pharmaceutical

Modified from Weber (28).

with autologous proteins and provoking immune-mediated reactions, as in the case of tartrazine yellow. Sulfites may induce the formation of sulfur dioxide, which can, in turn, provoke bronchoconstriction. A sulfite IgE-mediated reaction has been observed. Moreover, it has been proposed that in some individuals, the deficiency of sulfite oxidase may play a role if a large quantity of sulfite is ingested. Capsules containing a single additive have been developed (Lofarma, Milan, Italy) and are available for diagnosis purposes.

CLINICAL MANIFESTATIONS OF ADVERSE REACTIONS TO FOODS

Symptoms of allergic ARF may be localized in many organs and systems (respiratory tract, skin, cardiovascular system, gut, central nervous system) or generalized. In the following subsections, the pictures arising from different systems will be discussed.

SYSTEMIC ANAPHYLAXIS Systemic anaphylaxis (SA) is the most severe from of IgE-mediated reaction and is the result of sudden IgE-mediated release of mediators (histamine, serotonin, prostaglandins, leukotriens), stored in or newly synthesized by mastcells, basophils, and eosinophils. It is very difficult to evaluate the true SA prevalence and mortality because about half of the patients admitted to the hospital with anaphylaxis do not have a previous diagnosis of food allergy and a study showed that 40% of patients were given a wrong International Classification of Disease code at the time of discharge (*30*); moreover ingestion of hidden allergens is involved (31). In the United States, up to 2500 SA and 125 deaths per year are reported (32). Death from anaphylaxis because of food allergy is more frequent than hymenoptera sting anaphylaxis (33). Death is usually related to accidental ingestion of allergic food. All foods can induce a fatal reaction, but peanuts, tree nuts, fish and shellfish (shrimp, lobster, crab, scallops, oyster), some fruit (kiwi), and seeds (cottonseed, sesame seed, psyllium) are more frequently involved. Most patients with anaphylaxis have a previous diagnosis of asthma. In highly sensitive patients, food anaphylaxis may develop not only after eating but also after contact or inhalation of responsible food. Many dramatic cases are reported in medical literature.

Latex-allergic patients may show anaphylaxis after ingestion or contact with latex crossreacting foods (chestnut, banana, and avocado (34,35). Anaphylaxis usually ensues within a few minutes from contact to culpable foods. Patients first complain of lips, tongue and mouth itching, then skin itching, laryngeal and upper and lower airways edema, bronchospasm, and vasodilation occur. Bronchospasm tends to be severe and largely refractory to beta-agonists. Secondary hypoxia and hypotension and cardiac failure lead to unrecoverable shock. Diagnosis of anaphylaxis is made on a clinical basis. Therapy relies on steroids, adrenaline, circulatory support and cardiopulmonary resuscitation. Food–exercise-induced anaphylaxis (FEIA) is an uncommon type of food anaphylaxis that arises only during physical exertion preceded by consumption of food and does not produce any symptoms at rest. Patients with FEIA show specific IgE against culpable food. Severity of anaphylaxis may vary greatly from a full-blown clinical anaphylactic picture to simple urticaria or asthma attack. Diagnosis of FEIA is best achieved following a recently published diagnostic protocol (36).

SKIN　Skin is one of the most common target organs in ARF, both immune and non-immune mediated. Gut provides a good barrier against the entry of several substances or microorganisms from the lumen; nevertheless, food antigens may cross the gut and reach the bloodstream, thus evoking reactions.

Atopic Dermatitis　Atopic dermatitis (AD) is a chronic eczematous pruritic cutaneous disease usually beginning in early infancy and very common in children (about 10%), although it can also be found in adults. It is frequently associated with seasonal rhinitis and asthma.

Atopic dermatitis itchy erythema generally begins at 3 mo of life and evolves into eczematous and crusty lesions, often with fissures. Initially, involved sites are scalp, cheeks, and ears, then lesions spread to the flexor aspect of the wrist and elbow, hands, feet, and periorbital regions. The histological appearance of AD is similar to that of classic contact dermatitis, with epidermal vesicles and dermal histiocytic and lymphoid infiltrate, thus implicating a cell-mediated hypersensitivity pathogenesis. In the skin of AD patients, CD4+ Th2 lymphocytes, IgE-bearing Langheran's cells, and eosinophil products, such as eosinophilic cationic protein (ECP) and major basic protein (MBP), can be found. Langheran's cells can act as antigen-presenting cells (37) and activate Th2 lymphocytes which can produce several cytokines (IL-4, L-5, IL-6, IL-10) with proinflammatory and chemotactic effects. The role of food(s) and IgE in AD is very controversial. About 25% of patients with AD show food-specific IgE. In a recent double-blind placebo-controlled food challenge (DBPCFC) study on children, Burks and coworkers (38) found that in about 38% of patients,

AD was provoked by food and milk, egg, peanut, soy, wheat, cod fish and catfish, and cashew.

The exact pathogenesis of AD as an ARF is not known, but it is likely that food allergens absorbed in the gut reach the skin through blood vessels and provoke mast cell activation with immediate-phase mediator release and production. Thereafter (several hours later), a late-phase reaction with infiltration develops, involving Langheran's cells, CD4+ Th2 lymphocytes, and eosinophils.

This sequence can also be seen in clinical AD: A few minutes after ingestion of culpable food(s) some patients complain of face and mouth angioedema, contact urticaria, and itching. Some hours later, eczematous skin lesion appear and/or flare up.

Intolerance mechanisms may also be important in AD, because alcoholic beverages, preservatives and dyes may worsen its course. In fact, about 20% of patients with AD have normal IgE serum levels and negative skin prick tests to common allergens. Finally, inhalants (in particular, dust mites) can play a role in inducing and/or maintaining AD lesions.

Dermatitis Herpetiformis　Dermatitis herpetiformis (DH) is a chronic and very itchy skin rash, characterized by symmetric involvement of the extensor aspects of limbs and buttocks by papulae and blisters. It could mimic AD, with a risk of misdiagnosis. DH is strongly linked to celiac disease: More than 85% of patients with DH (39) have gluten sensitive enteropathy, usually with milder intestinal lesions. Moreover patients with DH have IgG and IgA antigliadin antibodies (40). Immunohistochemical studies of skin in patients with DH have shown the presence of granular and less frequently linear deposition of dimeric IgA, neutrophils and C3 in the dermo-epidermal junction. Response to a gluten-free diet is not always complete.

Urticaria and Angioedema　Urticaria and angioedema (UA) are very common skin disorders, affecting about 15–25% of general population. Erythematous itching plaques involving the derma with subcutaneous edema characterize urticaria; angioedema occurs if deeper subcutaneous tissues are also involved. UA has a worse prognosis than urticaria alone. About one-half of patients complain of self-limiting episodes of acute UA, with fewer than 6 wk duration. In the other half, UA can have a chronic course of more than 6 mo duration. UA is related to many diseases, ranging from malignancy to infections, and therefore should not be considered a mere "allergic" disease. Differential diagnosis for UA is very complex and should never be underestimated (41). Foods can induce acute urticaria episodes, but it is not always clear whether they are responsible for chronic UA. Some authors have found food to be responsible for symptoms in 12–17% of urticaria children and adults (42,43). There are also many anecdotal reports claiming a role for preservatives in UA.

It is likely that foods and preservatives are also responsible for chronic UA, but the complexity of this disease suggests a thorough clinical evaluation of the patient before starting any allergic diagnostic procedure.

Contact Dermatitis　Contact dermatitis is a Type IV hypersensitivity reaction, mediated by sensitized T lymphocytes, characterized by inflammation and edema of those parts of the skin that have been in contact with provoking agents. Foods can also induce contact dermatitis but this is seen mainly as an occupational disease. Food patch testing can be useful in the diagnosis, together with a dietary approach. Nickel is a well-known provoking agent for contact dermatitis and is also contained in several foods (in

Table 4
Crossreactivity Between Inhalants and Vegetables

Ragweed	Melon, banana, watermelon, gourd family
Birch	Apple, hazelnut, peach, carrot, potato, cherry, fennel, celery, kiwi
Mugwort	Celery
Grass	Tomato, melon, watermelon, fennel, celery, kiwi, peanut, wheat
Hazel tree	Hazelnut

particular, fresh or canned vegetables). Avoidance of nickel-containing foods should be recommended to patients with contact dermatitis caused by nickel.

GASTROINTESTINAL TRACT

Oral Allergy Syndrome The Oral Allergy Syndrome (OAS) is one of the most common ARF in adults. Responsible foods are generally raw fruits and/or vegetables and spices, but milk and derivatives, eggs, and fish may be involved. Symptoms of OAS are mainly itching and angioedema of lips, mouth, cheeks, and pharynx, ensuing some minutes (5–30) after chewing or swallowing foods (44). Papulovesicular eruption of oral mucosa and worsening laryngeal involvement may occur. Swallowing of responsible foods may provoke gastrointestinal (abdominal pain, nausea, vomiting, diarrhea) and systemic pictures. Life-threatening reactions are not uncommon among patients with OAS: in about 13% of cases, history discloses one episode of laryngeal edema and anaphylaxis in 2.1% (45).

As is common in patients allergic to pollens: about 40% of patients with hay fever complain of oral symptoms when eating fresh fruit and vegetables (46). In particular, allergy to birch seems related to the development of OAS. Patients usually report symptoms not to one single food but to clusters of botanically related fruits and vegetables, such as nuts–apple–pear, potato–carrot, watermelon–melon–tomato and others. OAS is an IgE-mediated reaction and sensitization to vegetables relies on cross-reactivity between pollens and vegetables (Table 4). Crossreactivity is due to common allergenic epitopes shared both by vegetables and pollens (47). These epitopes have been greatly conserved during vegetal evolution because they have very important biologic functions. One of the most studied is Bet v 1, the major allergen of birch pollen, which shows a very strong homology with the apple allergen Mal d 1 (48). This finding can explain the well-known relationship between birch allergy and OAS to apple. Crossreactions involving wider clusters of fruits and vegetables may be related to the presence of profilins (49), which are present in almost all eukaryotic cells because they regulate actin polymerization. Also carbohydrates and glycoproteins seem to be involved in pollen–vegetables crossreactions.

In atopic subjects, IgE synthesized as a response to pollens and carried by the mast cells can also bind to epitopes on vegetables, thus evoking mast cell degranulation on the site of contact (i.e., oropharyngeal mucosa).

Crossreacting epitopes are very weak and can be disrupted by cooking or other food processing procedures, thus explaining the common observation that usually only raw foods elicit symptoms.

Diagnosis is based on the patient's history and finding of specific IgE, by means of serum assay and skin testing. Skin testing in OAS is best performed with fresh food, since food extracts are less reliable (50). Food challenge is rarely useful in

OAS diagnosis, as the history is usually suggestive. If needed, a challenge could be performed using milkshake-like beverages, also in a double-blind fashion. Lyophilized extracts in capsules are not useful (see the section on Diagnosis).

Lactose Intolerance Breast milk is the first eaten and usually tolerated food but lactose digestion is conserved by a minority of adults, mostly from northern countries. Lactose intolerance (LI) is therefore very common: its prevalence varies from 5% in north Europe to 90% in Africa and Asia. Moreover it can be found in diseases involving the small intestine, such as celiac spruce. Lactose is digested by lactase, a disaccharidase present in the small-gut brush border. If a lactase deficit exists, undigested lactose remaining in the gut lumen exerts an osmotic effect, provoking water retention. Moreover, intestinal bacteria can ferment lactose, producing organic acid and hydrogen. Lumen distension by gas provokes borborigmi and pain, and water retention results in diarrhea. These are the main clinical aspects of LI.

Diagnosis is best done by a H_2 breath test, which serially evaluates, in the presence of LI, the rise in hydrogen concentration in breath after lactose intake. Another way, less sensitive and specific, is to monitor blood glucose levels (also capillary) after lactose intake: A rise in blood glucose levels should rule out LI.

Because milk and lactose are widely used in food preparation, avoidance of dietary lactose, the best therapy, is very difficult to achieve. Hydrolyzed milks (containing galactose and glucose instead of lactose) and beta-galactosidase tablets are commonly available in Western countries. Patients should also be advised that the intake of up to 240 mL, of milk per day in refracted doses is usually associated with negligible symptoms (51).

Food-Sensitive Enteropathy Food-sensitive enteropathy is characterized by diarrhea, vomiting and malabsorption syndrome occurring in atopic infants. Cell-mediated hypersensitivity against cow's milk, chicken, egg, fish, and soy protein seems to be involved. The histologic appearance of the duodenum is aspecific, but there is often a good response to exclusion diet, and tolerance can be regained at the age of 1–2 yr.

Food-Sensitive Colitis Food-sensitive colitis is an acute colitis with bloody diarrhea occurring in infants of less than 1 yr of age. Histologic appearance of food-sensitive colitis is different from ulcerative colitis because of the presence of eosinophilic infiltration within the lamina propria. As in food-sensitive enteropathy, tolerance is restored before the age of 2 yr.

Eosinophilic Gastroenteritis Eosinophilic gastroenteritis is an uncommon disease characterized by peripheral eosinophilia and eosinophilic infiltration of gut layers, occurring anywhere in the gastrointestinal tract, although stomach and small intestine are more frequently involved. Symptoms are related to the extent of infiltration. If only the mucosa is involved, patients complain of abdominal pain, nausea, vomiting and diarrhea (seldom bloody); malabsorption symptoms may be present. The involvement of the gut muscle layer leads to symptoms of intestinal obstruction, whereas eosinophilic ascites is found in serosal layer infiltration. The cause is unknown, but in some patients, AFR can have some relevance, particularly those with mucosal disease, who may respond to elimination of a specific food. Muscle and serosal disease usually do not respond to dietary treatment and seldom require corticosteroids or surgery.

Celiac Disease Celiac disease is a malabsorption syndrome resulting from an abnormal immune-mediated reaction against gliadin and characterized by atrophy of small-intestine villi, hyperplasia of Lieberkuhn's cryptae, and lymphoid infiltration of the lamina propria. Gliadin is a fraction of the cereal protein gluten. Malabsorption is the result of small gut damage and depends of their extent. Thus, the clinical spectrum and malabsorption can vary widely from a severe picture with growth disturbance in children to simple lactose intolerance or iron-deficiency anemia or even an apparently unrelated clinical picture *(52)*. In CD genetic factors play an important role and patients with CD show the presence of HLA-DQ2, DQ8, and DR3 *(53)*. Moreover, association with other immunologic diseases can be found.

Intestinal lesions are likely to be provoked by T-CD4$^+$ lymphocytes that recognize gliadin expressed by enterocytes together with HLA-II antigens. Cytokine release seems to increase expression of HLA-II by enterocytes and adhesion molecules and cell proliferation within the cryptae, thus amplifying the immune response and cell damage through both cytotoxic effect and toxic mediators. Cytokines may also increase gut permeability and induce B-lymphocyte proliferation and differentiation into plasma cells with the increase in antibodies against gliadin.

Celiac disease can be strongly suspected if a patient has IgG and/or IgA antigliadin (AGA) and antiendomysium antibodies, but this must be confirmed by histological findings since positivity to AGA alone is not strictly specific *(54)*. Histologic specimens are obtained by endoscopic duodenal biopsy before and 6–12 mo after a gluten-free diet. Gluten is contained in wheat, barley, oats, and rye, but not in rice and maize. Concomitant lactose intolerance can be diagnosed by H$_2$ breath.

Strict avoidance of gluten is the best treatment for CD. This can be a difficult task to achieve, as gluten is widely present in many foods. Patients must, therefore, be carefully instructed on their diet and on availability of trade gluten-free foods. Lactose should also be avoided if lactose intolerance is present. CD symptoms usually disappear in a few weeks. If not, diet adherence must be confirmed. If symptoms do not disappear on confirmed guten-free diet, another diagnosis must be considered.

Careful follow-up of patients with CD is mandatory because malignant complications (mainly lymphomas of gastrointestinal tract) may ensue in about 10% of cases.

RESPIRATORY SYSTEM AND ARF

Rhinitis   Rhinitis due to food allergy is uncommon. It can occur several hours after the ingestion of food as a late-phase reaction or suddenly in anaphylactic reactions. Food-allergy rhinitis can also have an occupational occurrence as in rhinitis, resulting from inhalation of milk protein *(55)*. Rhinitis caused by food additives is even more uncommon.

Asthma   Although food is an uncommon cause of bronchial asthma, both immune- and non-immune-mediated reactions may ensue in the respiratory system *(56)*, more frequently in children than adults *(57)* and usually correlated to milk, egg, peanuts, and wheat hypersensitivity *(58)*.

As discussed for the oral allergy syndrome, it is well known that patients with pollen allergy also have IgE against fruits and vegetables, thus characterizing some association of pollens and clusters of vegetable foods. In countries with low concentrations of birch and mugwort, ARF are responsible only for a small percentage of perennial asthma [i.e., 4–6% in children *(59)* and 1–4% in adults *(60)*]; if concentrations are higher, about half of pollinotic patients are found to be allergic to vegetable foods *(46)*.

Respiratory symptoms as a result of ARF can be divided into acute and chronic. Acute respiratory symptoms appear in anaphy-laxis as sudden bronchial constriction: They are generally IgE mediated and lead to severe and sometimes lethal clinical pictures *(61,62)*. In other less well-defined clinical pictures, asthma can have a chronic clinical course and be associated to other symptoms such as atopic dermatitis and rhinitis.

In patients with food allergy, ingestion of culpable food may provoke release of mast cell mediators, both stored and newly synthesized, which can trigger bronchoconstriction directly and through late-phase chemotactic reactions. Leukotriens play a pivotal role. In food intolerance, some additives, such as sulfites *(63)* may directly provoke asthma or directly induce mast cell release.

The relationship between food and asthma can also rely on a mere nutritional plan. In asthmatic patients, some authors have found a protective role for tocopherols *(64)* and ascorbic acid *(65)*, others have supposed that overintake of polyunsaturated fatty acid could favor the onset of asthma *(66)*.

A particular type of food-allergy asthma is food-dependent, exercise-induced asthma, in which asthma ensues during exertion only if the patient previously ate the culpable food. In some cases, food-dependent, exercise-induced asthma may be associated with anaphylaxis (see the subsection, Systemic Anaphylaxis).

Finally, it must be taken into account that exposure to food allergens can be also the result of inhalation of food powder. This happens mainly in food processing workers. The pathogenesis is likely to be IgE mediated: workers exposed to the inhalation of food powders compared to nonexposed ones show food-specific IgE and complain more frequently of chronic respiratory symptoms *(67,68)*. Atopy seems to be a predisposing factor *(69)*. Of course, food powder can also provoke asthma by direct airway irritation *(70)*.

Diagnosis of respiratory ARF is best achieved by means of an elimination diet followed by a food challenge (as described in Diagnosis). The appearance of respiratory symptoms during food challenge can be obtained by repeated ventilatory tests after the ingestion of the food to be challenged; ventilatory tests must be performed up to 8 hours after the ingestion of the challenged food because of the presence of late respiratory reactions *(71)*. Challenge is positive if a 20% fall in FEV$_1$ occurs, with FEV$_1$ variability less than 20% after ingestion of placebo *(72)*. Also modification in aspecific airways responsiveness during challenge can be useful for diagnosis *(73)*. Although this method is less feasible, it could improve diagnosis, because challenge may only increase bronchial responsiveness without inducing constriction *(74)*.

Heiner's Syndrome   Heiner's syndrome *(75)* is a lung hemosiderosis occurring in infants and characterized by eosinophilia, frequent episodes of pneumonia, asthma, rhinitis, and gastrointestinal complaints. Patients usually show I$_J$G antibodies against cow's milk, thus suggesting a role for the ARF mechanism. The pathogenesis is unclear.

CONTROVERSIAL CLINICAL PICTURES

INTRODUCTION   As described earlier, about one-fifth of the general population report ARF; moreover, some doctors overestimate foods as a cause for many symptoms. This has led to the conviction that foods could play a role in the pathogenesis of several common and uncommon diseases of uncertain etiology and to the development of many diagnostic tools of unproven value.

In this section, we briefly report the findings on the possible relationships between foods and various diseases of uncertain etiology. Most reports deal with anecdotal observations rather than scientific confirmation by means of DBPCFC.

IRRITABLE BOWEL SYNDROME   Many relationships exist between irritable bowel syndrome (IBS) and foods. Nanda et al. found that 48.2% of patients with IBS improved their symptoms after a diet which excluded several foods (76). Many studies, reviewed in (77), mainly performed in animal, have shown that allergen challenge on gastrointestinal mucosa of a sensitized animal alters gut function through mast cell mediators release. In particular, mast cell mediators provoke an increase in gut active secretion of Cl^- and H_2O and a decrease in absorption of Na^+, Cl^- and H_2O, alter the gastrointestinal motility pattern, and increase permeability. It is noteworthy that in animal experiments in vivo, these pathophysiologic effects provoke diarrhea. According to these observations, a trial of cromolyn sodium, which inhibits mast cell release, proved useful in 60% of 101 adult patients with diet-dependent diarrheic IBS (78). The response was significantly higher in patients showing IgE toward foods responsible for their symptoms. These results have been confirmed by further studies on larger series (79). Many investigations found that colonic motility in patients with IBS differs from that in normal subjects; in particular, an enhanced preprandial motility can be observed (80). These observations imply a strong relationship between IgE-mediated ARF and diarrheic habits. IBS is a very common (15–20% of the general population) gut disorder characterized by various bowel habits (from constipation to diarrhea), bloating, abdominal pain and altered bowel feelings. Diagnosis is usually made by the exclusion of other organic causes. A role for ARF in IBS has been widely investigated. In five studies (81–83) double-blind challenge were performed to establish the role of ARF in IBS, but a causal relationship could be found only in a few patients. However, foods may be the cause in the diarrheic IBS subset through an IgE mediated mechanism and sugar malabsorption (see above).

CHRONIC FATIGUE SYNDROME AND NEUROPSYCHOLOGICAL COMPLAINTS   The Chronic Fatigue Syndrome (CFS) is a clinical entity characterized by persisting or remitting, debilitating fatigue in the absence of other defined diseases. CFS etiology is unknown, but links have been found with some conditions such as chronic viral infections, immune system alterations and oligo-elements deficiency. CFS diagnosis is mainly performed on a clinical basis (finding of fatigue associated with some minor symptoms and signs) and no specific laboratory tests are available. Extended laboratory examinations are of little, if any, value. CFS patients frequently complain of symptoms that could suggest allergies to drugs, food and inhalants and show specific IgE against inhalants or foods by serum evaluation and skin testing (84). At present, foods are not thought to have a causative role in CFS.

Medical literature reports two cases of neuropsychological complaints, confirmed by DBPCFC, provoked by food (crying and hysteria resulting from milk and EEG changes induced by beef). Neuropsychic disorder may be secondary to well-known somatic effects of ARF. There are, however, no convincing data that neuropsychological symptoms are related to ARF.

HYPERKINETIC SYNDROME   Behavior problems in children are often attributed to food by parents. In the mid seventies Feingold observed an improvement in 30–50% of hyperactive children put on an artificial colors- and flavors free diet (85). These findings gained wide popularity but were not confirmed by further studies.

Headache   The role of ARF in migraine and/or common headache is very controversial (86). Foods are able to induce vascular headache. Food amines and/or neurotransmitters (histamine, tyramine, phenylethylamine, etc.) can act directly both on blood vessels and on mast cells, leading to secondary release of their mediators (87), which can also be provoked by food allergens.

On the one hand, some authors found that hypoallergenic diets were effective in patients with headache, but elimination of skin prick test (SPT)-positive foods was not (88), whereas others showed an IgE-mediated relationship through DBPCFC (89). On the other hand, Atkins failed to demonstrate by DBPCFC any correlation between foods and migraine (90).

Although few papers studying migraine and headache by DBPCFC are available, it is likely that ARFs can provoke headache.

OTITIS SEROSA   Otitis media serosa (OMS) is a chronic inflammation on the middle ear, usually involving the Eustachian tube and mastoid cells, often leading to hearing loss. Patients (particularly children) frequently report OMS with respiratory allergy. In a few cases, OMS could be caused by food allergy, usually to dairy products, and is responsive to dietary restriction (91).

RECURRENT APHTOUS STOMATITIS   This disorder is characterized by recurrent, single or multiple mouth ulcerations that can also be severe enough to hamper chewing. They could be associated with virus infection and food-related conditions, such as oral-allergy syndrome, inflammatory bowel disease, and celiac sprue. The pathogenic mechanism is currently unknown, but ARF should be considered and eventually confirmed by accurate investigation.

HISTAMINE INTOLERANCE   Physicians in the treatment of urticaria and other not well-defined allergy-like symptoms have frequently prescribed histamine-free diets.

An example of histamine intoxication is given by scombroid poisoning. High histidine contents of spoiled fish is converted into histamine whose increase may provoke headache, vomiting, diarrhea, tachycardia, and flushes. Histamine increase is also enhanced by a secondary decarboxylase defect caused by other spoiled fish amines (such as putrescine and cadaverine). Primary decarboxylase defect is actually uncommon, and in cases other than scombroid intoxication, a histamine-free diet is not advised.

RED EYE   The prevalence of eye symptoms in food allergy has not been clearly defined: About 5% of patients with red eye show food-specific IgE. Food allergy seems to have little if any importance in the eye. Eye symptoms are mainly conjuctivitis resulting from accidental contact with food (92).

PEPTIC DISEASE   De Lazzari and co-workers (93) studied 232 patients with peptic ulcer disease and found that 21% showed total IgE serum levels above 200 kU/L. Although the clinical response to H_2 antagonists in these subjects was not related to IgE level, ulcer relapse after 6 mo was significantly lower in patients with normal circulating IgE than in patients with high circulating IgE (11.9% vs 39.5%, $p < 0.001$) (93). In patients with ulcers and hypersensitivity to inhalant allergens, some interesting studies showed an immediate reaction of the gastric mucosa after intragastric allergen provocation under endoscopic challenge; the intensity of the reaction was positively correlated to an increased number of mast cells in the gastric mucosa (94,95).

This may be indirect evidence of a possible role for foods in peptic disease, but further studies are needed.

INFLAMMATORY BOWEL DISEASE (CROHN'S DISEASE AND ULCERATIVE COLITIS)   The etiopathogenesis of Crohn's disease (CrD) and ulcerative colitis (UC) is currently unknown.

CrD and UC result from an interaction among genetic predisposing factors, immunological system alterations, and environmental influences (such as gut flora). The initial triggering factor of the inflammatory reaction remains unknown. Food allergy was suggested early as a possible trigger for the inflammatory response; however, no firm evidence has been gathered over the years to substantiate this possibility.

Relationships between nutrition and inflammatory bowel disease (IBD) have been found, thus implicating ARF in their pathogenesis. Interestingly, previous studies on mast cell number in CrD have showed contradictory results, but an increased intestinal histamine secretion in active CrD has been well demonstrated (96).

In active CrD, elemental diets have been proposed as an alternative to steroids. Although diets are less effective than steroids (97), their response rate is higher than placebo; moreover, food intolerance/sensitivities have been found in CrD patients, particularly to dairy products and some studies showed that patients eliminating culpable foods maintain remission of symptoms for a longer period than those on an unrestricted diet (98,99). These results could indicate a pathogenic role for foods in CrD, although definitive conclusions are needed. The response to elemental diet in UC is lower and ARFs do not seem to be a risk factor in this disease (100).

COLLAGENOPATHIES AND VASCULAR DISEASE Medical literature reports that foods and additives may provoke and worsen vasculitis symptoms (101), but no DBPCFC confirmations were done. Allergic patients often complain of several joint symptoms. This link seems to be the result of the presence of certain polyunsaturated fatty acids that can influence the synthesis of proinflammatory and anti-inflammatory mediators (102). A role for food has also been suspected in rheumatoid arthritis (103).

In conclusion, it must also considered that joint symptoms and vasculitis are characteristic of defined autoimmune disease (e.g., rheumatoid arthritis) as well as conditions of uncertain etiology, but with the presence of an autoimmune background, such as IBD. ARFs may be linked with these supposed or defined autoimmune diseases.

DIAGNOSIS

Careful history-taking in patients with suspect ARF can lead to a correct diagnosis and identification of culpable food. This is generally true for those who complain of obvious allergic clinical pictures (e.g., anaphylactic shock, urticaria angioedema, severe asthma, oral-allergy syndrome) ensuing after the intake of the same food(s).

In patients complaining of less well-defined clinical pictures or if their history does not disclose the food responsible for symptoms, a correct diagnosis of ARF can be achieved by dietary manipulation. Of course, physical examination should be performed in all patients suspected to have ARF, also in order to rule out other diseases (104). There are four main types of diet: simple exclusion, empirical, few foods, and hypoallergenic formula. A thorough review of dietary manipulations has been produced by Carter (105). In this authors' experience, diet diagnosis of ARF is best reached by an elimination diet (ED) (Table 5). ED is a simple diet made up of all those foodstuffs that are poorly reported as responsible for ARF and should be used for 2–6 wk. The duration depends mainly on type of symptoms, as gastrointestinal complaints may disappear within few days, whereas skin symptoms usually need 1 or 2 wk to resolve. If symptoms signifi-

Table 5
Elimination Diet

Rice	Cooked potatoes and carrots
Lamb and turkey meat	Lettuce
Peeled pears or pineapple	Olive oil
Water	Sugar
Salt	Tea

cantly decrease or even disappear, the diagnosis of ARF is very likely. However, if reported symptoms are occasional, ED is no longer useful, as no reduction and/or disappearance of symptoms can be demonstrated. After ED, diagnosis is better defined by food challenges with all eliminated foodstuffs and particularly with those believed culpable. Food challenges should not be performed if ED has not modified patient's symptoms. During challenges, patients must be told to keep a diary with challenge dates, evoked symptoms (if any), and the time between food intake and the appearance of symptoms. A list of all foods to be challenged must be given to the patient: each food must be eaten for 3 consecutive days; the suggested quantity is the normal serving dose for that food. If no symptoms arise, the food is considered safe and can, therefore, be eaten by the patient without any further restriction. If any symptoms arise, the food is considered culpable; in this case, the challenge is stopped and the patient must eat ED and safe foods (i.e., all challenged food unable to evoke symptoms) until all symptoms disappear. When the patient is again asymptomatic, challenges with other foods can be started. Also, some food and food additives can be challenged using special diagnostic jelly capsules containing lyophilized extracts. We recommend following the manufacturer's instructions carefully. Open challenges must be confirmed by DBPCFC. DBPCFC has been considered the "gold standard" in ARF diagnosis, but it can be performed only for one or few foods, it is not free from severe and even life-threatening reactions, its psychological bias is very high, and interpretation of results may be difficult (106). DBPCFC can be performed using milkshake-like beverages containing foods to be tested strongly flavored to mask the taste of the food or better the above-mentioned capsules. The choice of foods to be tested is based on the patient's history, RAST result or both.

Figure 2 shows the diagnostic flowchart of ARF. When the responsible foods have been identified, pathogenesis of ARF can be found by means of other diagnostic procedures. SPT and serum-specific IgE evaluation is useful for the diagnosis of allergic ARF. SPT have a high negative predictive value and sensitivity, but low specificity. SPT can be performed using either commercial food extracts or raw foodstuffs. This latter technique, called "prick by prick," should be avoided in patients with a previous history of severe allergic reactions due to the risk of anaphylactic shock following the prick test.

Skin-prick tests give semiquantitative results. Skin reactions evoked by foods are considered positive when the reaction size (hive diameter) is similar to that provoked by a 1 : 1000 histamine solution. Serum-specific IgE evaluation is very specific and can be achieved by different laboratory methods. Serum-specific IgE evaluation may be performed instead of SPT when the patient has skin diseases (such as eczema, urticaria, wide scars) or dermographism, is on antihistamines, or if food-induced anaphylaxis is suspected. If food additives are responsible for the patient's

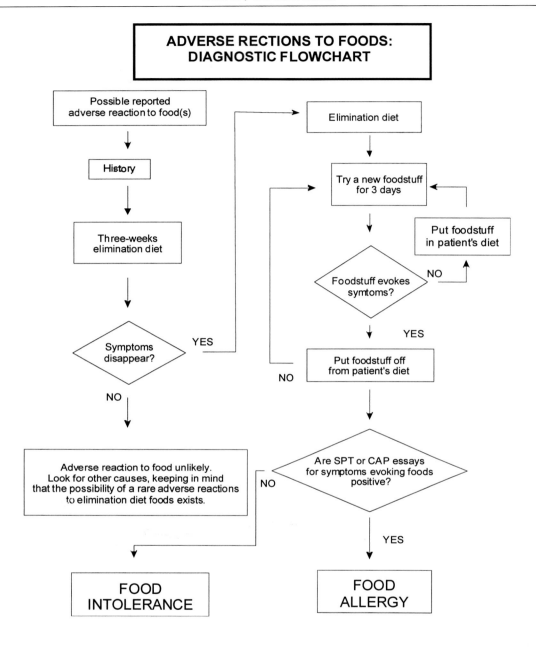

ADVERSE RECTIONS TO FOODS: DIAGNOSTIC FLOWCHART

symptoms, the evaluation for specific IgE is of no value because additives generally provoke only non-immune-mediated ARF.

Recently, Sampson and Ho *(107)* reviewed about 200 patients who underwent DBPCFC correlating challenge outcomes to several food-specific IgE concentrations. For egg, milk, peanut, and fish, the authors found the specific IgE concentration above which patients were very likely (more than 95%) to have a positive challenge. The importance of this finding is striking, because it could eliminate the need of DBPCFC in the diagnosis of IgE-mediated allergy.

Several new diagnostic tools have been proposed in ARF, such as measurement of inflammatory mediators (eosinophil cationic protein [ECP], eosinophil protein X [ECX], methylhistamine, triptase) in serum or in feces, basophil histamine release (BHR)

test, cellular allergen stimulation test (CAST), intestinal mast cell histamine release (IMCHR) test, measurement of histamine in gastric lavage fluid, intragastric provocation under endoscopic control (IPEC), and colonscopic allergen provocation (COLAP). At present, little clinical experience is available for these tests and their use is limited to research field. COLAP, in which the intestinal mucosa is challenged endoscopically with antigen extract *(107)*, seems to be very promising. Moreover, this test reduces the risk of an anaphylactic reaction that could be present in DBPCFC, but only a few foods can be tested and it is uncomfortable.

Many controversial techniques such as the cytotoxicity test, sublingual and subcutaneous provocation-and-neutralization test, change in muscular strength after sublingual food challenge (the

Table 6
Main Aspects of Dietary Treatment in ARF

Define exactly culprit foods
Always keep in mind the composition of trade foods
Evaluate the nutritional, psychological, and social impact of dietary
  exclusions
Consider crossreactivity among different foods

Table 7
Report Usual Doses of Antihistamines

Antihistamine	Preparation	Dose
Loratadine	10-mg tablets; suspension 0.1%	10–20 mg daily
Astemizole	10-mg tablets	10–20 mg daily
Cetirizine	10-mg tablets; drops 10 mg/mL	10 mg daily
Ketotiphen	2-mg slow-release tablets; syrup 2.5%	1–2 mg daily
Oxatomide	30-mg tablets; suspension 2.5%	30 mg daily

so-called DRIA test), evaluation of immune complexes, electro-acupuncture, and applied kinesiology (manual muscle strength measurement while patient holds a bottle containing the food to be tested) have been used in ARF diagnosis. The efficacy and reliability of all these techniques are unproved to date and their use must be discouraged.

TREATMENT

DIET Treatment of ARF can be dietary or pharmacological. The best treatment for any allergy and/or intolerance is exclusion or the agent responsible. This is not always possible when dealing with ARF. The main aspects of dietary treatment in ARF are listed in Table 6. Only those foods that provoke symptoms should be avoided and the best way to identify them is an elimination diet followed by challenge, as described earlier. Many nutritional and compliance problems may arise from dietary exclusion. The best example for nutritional problems is provided by infant cow's milk allergy, in which the use of milk substitutes is mandatory. These are soy milk (complete though partially antigenic) and milk hydrolysates. The latter have a composition very similar to that of human milk and are far less allergenic than cow's milk but more expensive than soy milk. Since crossreactivity between hydrolysates and cow's milk can arise, an SPT with hydrolysate is suggested before prescribing the product *(109)*.

In dietary exclusions, the problem of hidden allergens must always be kept in mind *(110)*. Several allergens (e.g., soy and milk protein, peanuts) are widely used in the preparation of trade foods so that complete exclusion can be very difficult. Patients allergic to codfish should be advised that some poultry are fed codfish-containing feed and, therefore, their meat could contain codfish allergens. If an adverse reaction to food additives is suspected, patients must be advised to read the trade food composition label carefully. Finally, the impact of dietary exclusions on the patient's psychology and social life should not be underestimated. In some cases, psychological support is warranted.

DRUG THERAPY Drug therapy in ARF is less effective than dietary exclusion. Drugs are used when the patient's compliance to diet is poor or when significant and potentially harmful dietary imbalance exists. Prescribed drugs include antihistamines, steroids, and sodium cromoglycate.

Antihistamines Newer H_1-antihistamine blockers *(111)* such as cetirizine, loratadine, ketotiphen, oxatomide, and astemizole are quite effective for skin symptoms (urticaria angioedema and itching) but are of limited efficacy for gastrointestinal complaints. In our experience, good results in a diarrheic subset of IBS can be achieved with oxatomide.

Side effects are usually dyspepsia and a very mild and often negligible sedation. The main contraindications are hepatic failure or concomitant use of drugs interfering with cytochrome P450. These conditions can reduce antihistamine clearance and provoke

accumulation, with the exception of cetirizine, which is excreted unaltered in the urine. At present, no data on the new antihistamines mizolastine and phexofenadine in the treatment of ARF are available. Table 7 reports the usual doses of antihistamines.

Steroids In ARF, steroids are mainly used, like antihistamines, in the treatment of skin symptoms. They can be applied topically in atopic dermatitis or given systemically (orally or intramuscularly) in patients complaining of urticaria angioedema poorly sensitive to antihistamines and only partially controlled by diet.

Sodium Cromoglycate Sodium cromoglycate (SC) is one of the most studied drugs in both children and adults allergic ARF. Some double-blind studies on the use of SC in children with atopic dermatitis have shown efficacy; other failed to demonstrate differences between SC and placebo.

Sodium cromoglycate has proven useful in ARF diarrhea both in children and adults. It is not possible to attribute SC efficacy to inhibition of mast cell mediators release or to reduction of intestinal permeability, which can be increased both in allergy and intolerance. Suggested doses are 750 and 2000 mg respectively for children and adults, divided in three doses per day 15–60 min before meals. In our experience, SC should be maintained for 2 mo, then repeated twice a year at the same dose and course. In ARF with main gastrointestinal symptoms, symptoms are mainly gastroenteric, SC can allow the patient to assume also culpable food(s) with great nutritional and compliance advantages.

Sodium cromoglycate has virtually no side effects; some patients complain of dyspepsia and abdominal pain. If skin symptoms coexist, antihistamines can be associated.

SUMMARY

Adverse reactions to food are those signs or symptoms occurring after ingestion of food and are classified as toxic and nontoxic (including immunomediated and nonimmunomediated reactions or food intolerance. ARF can affect several organs (skin, gut, airways, heart and blood vessels, central nervous system, and joints). Moreover, many controversy symptoms and pictures exist. Diagnosis of ARF is based on history-taking, followed by an elimination diet. If complained-about symptoms significantly decrease or disappear, the diagnosis of AFR is very likely. Diagnosis is then better defined by open food challenges with all eliminated foodstuffs and particularly with those believed culpable. Open challenges must be confirmed by double-blind, placebo-controlled food challenges because psychological bias is very high. When the responsible foods have been identified, pathogenesis of AFRs can be found by means of other diagnostic procedures, such as skin-prick tests and serum-specific IgE evaluation for allergic AFR, endoscopic biopsy for celiac disease, and H_2 breath test for lactose intolerance. Best treatment is exclusion of responsible food. If this is not possible, drug treatment with antihistamines and sodium cromoglycate can be tried.

REFERENCES

1. Bruijnzeel-Koomen C, Ortolani C, Aas K, et al. Adverse reaction to food (position paper). Allergy 1995; 50:623–35.
2. Bousquet J, Metcalfe DD, Warner JO. Food allergy position paper of the codex alimentarious. ACI Int 1997; 9(1):10–21.
3. Young E, Stoneham MD, Petruckevitch A, et al. A population study of food intolerance. Lancet 1994; 343(7):1127–30.
4. Niestijl-Janssen JJ, Kardinaal AFM, Huijbers JH, Vlieg-Boerstra BJ, Martens BPM, Ockhuizem T. Prevalence of food allergy and intolerance in the adult Dutch population. J Allergy Clin Immunol 1994; 93:446–56.
5. Huston DP. The biology of the immune system. JAMA 1997; 278(22):1804–14.
6. Chiappelli F, Franceschi C, Ottaviani E, Farné M, Faisal M. Phylogeny of the neuroendocrinimmune system: fish and shellfish as a model system for social interaction stress research in humans. Annu Rev Fish Dis 1993; 3:327–46.
7. Chiappelli F, Kung MA, Villanueva P, Ong T. Alcohol toxicity of T cell-mediated immunity in the aging population. Alcologia 1997; 9(2):81–93.
8. Fazekas de St. Groth B, Cook MC, Smith AL. The role of T cells in the regulation of B cell tolerance. Int Rev Immunol 1997; 15:73–99.
9. Horowitz MC, Friedlaender GE, Qian HY. The immune response: the efferent arm. Clin Orth Rel Res 1996; 326:25–34.
10. Farber DL. Differential TCR signaling and the generation of memory T cells. J Immunol 1998; 160:535–9.
11. Chiappelli F, Kung MA, Savage M, Villanueva P, Fiala M. Nicotine and ethanol modulation of cell-mediated immune surveillance of oral squamous cell carcinoma. Int J Oral Biol 1996; 21:19–27.
12. Cossarizza A, Kalashnikova G, Grassilli E, et al. Mitochondrial modifications during rat thymocyte apoptosis: a study at the single cell level. Exp Cell Res 1994; 214:323–30.
13. Pawelec G, Adibzadeh M, Solana R, Beckman I. The T cell in the ageing individual. Mechan Ageing Dev 1997; 1:35–45.
14. Beverley PC. Functional analysis of human T subsets defined by CD45 isoform expression. Semin Immunol 1992; 4:35–41.
15. Chiappelli F, Manfrini E, Gwirtsman HE, et al. Steroid receptor-mediated modulation of CD4+CD62L+ cell homing: Implications for drug abusers. Ann NY Acad Sci 1994; 746:421–6.
16. Chiappelli F, Manfrini E, Franceschi C, Cossarizza A, Black KL. Steroid regulation of cytokines: relevance for TH1 and TH2 shift? Ann NY Acad Sci 1994; 746:204–16.
17. Chiappelli F, Kung MA, Villanueva P, Lee P, Frost P, Prieto N. Immunotoxicity of cocaethylene. Immunopharmacol Immunotoxicol 1995; 17:399–417.
18. Delespesse G, Demeure CE, Yang LP, Ohshima Y, Byun DG, Shu U. In vitro maturation of naive human CD4+ T lymphocytes into Th1, Th2 effectors. Int Arch Allergy Immunol 1997; 113:157–9.
19. Romagnani S. The Th1/Th2 paradigm and allergic disorder. Allergy 1998; 53(46s):12–15.
20. HayGlass KT, Wang M, Gieni RS, Ellison C, Gartner J. In vivo direction of CD4 T cells to Th1 and Th2-like patterns of cytokine synthesis. Adv Exp Med Biol 1996; 409:309–16.
21. Romagnani S. Development of Th1- or Th2-dominated immune responses: what about the polarizing signal? Int J Clin Lab Res 1996; 26(2):83–98.
22. Romagnani S, Parronchi P, D'Elios MM, et al. An update on human Th1 and Th2 cells. Int Arch Allergy Immunol 1997; 113:153–6.
23. Ramsdell F, Fowlkes B. Clonal deletion versus clonal anergy: the role of the tymus in inducing self tolerance. Science 1991; 248:1342–8.
24. Husbj S, Mestechy J, Moldoveneau Z, Holland S, Elson CO. Oral tolerance in humans. T cell but not B tolerance after antigen feeding. J Immunol 1994; 152:4663–70.
25. Holt PG. Mucosal immunity in relation to the development of oral tolerance/sensitization. Allergy 1998; 53(46s):16–9.
26. Sudo N, Sawamura SA, Tanaka K, Aiba Y, Kubo C, Koga Y. The requirement of intestinal bacterial flora for development of an IgE production system fully susceptible to oral tolerance induction. J Immunol 1997; 159:1739–45.
27. Mowat AM. The regulation on immune responses to dietary proteins antigens. Immunol Today 1987; 8:93–8.
28. Weber RW. Food additives and allergy. Ann Allergy 1993; 70:183–90.
29. Wuthrich B, Adverse reaction to food additives. Ann Allergy, 1993, 71:379–84.
30. Soresen HT, Nielsen B, Nielsen JO. Anaphylactic shock occurring outside hospital. Allergy 1989; 44:288–90.
31. Sampson HA. Fatal food-induced anaphylaxis. Allergy 1998; 53(46s):125–30.
32. Yocum MW, Khan DA. Assessment of patients who have experienced anaphylaxis in north west England. Clin Exp Allergy 1996; 26:1364–70.
33. Yunginger JW. Lethal food allergy in children. N Engl J Med 1992; 327:421–2.
34. Fernandez de Corres L, Moneo J, Munoz D, et al. Sensitization from chestnuts and bananas in patients with urticaria and anaphylaxis from contact with latex. Ann Allergy 1993; 70:35–9.
35. Rodriguez M, Vega F, Garcia MT, et al. Hypersensitivity to latex, chestnut and banana. Ann Allergy 1993; 70:31–4.
36. Romano A, Di Fonso M, Giuffreda F, et al. Diagnostic work-up for food dependent, exercize induced anaphylaxis. Allergy 1995; 50:817–24.
37. Van der Heijden FL, Wierenga EA, Bos JD, et al. High frequency of IL-4 producing CD4+ allergen-specific T lymphocytes in atopic dermatitis lesional skin. J Invest Dermatol 1991; 97:389–94.
38. Burks AW, James JM, Hiegel A, et al. Atopic dermatitis and food hypersensitivity reactions. J Pediatr 1998; 132:132–6.
39. Hall RP. The pathogenesis of dermatitis herpetiformis. Recent advances. J Am Acad Dermatol 1987; 16:1129–44.
40. Chorzelski TP, Beutner EJ, Sulej J, et al. IgA antiendomisium antibody: a new immunological marker of dermatitis herpetiformis and coeliac disease. Br J Dermatol 1984; 111:395–401.
41. Charlesworth EN. Urticaria and angioedema: a clinical spectrum. Ann Allergy Asthma Immunol 1996; 76:484–96.
42. Kauppinen K, Juntunen K, Lanki H. Urticaria in children. Retrospective evaluation and follow-up. Allergy 1992; 10:281–301.
43. Sehgal VN, Rege VI. An interrogative study of 158 urticaria patients. Ann Allergy 1973; 31:279–83.
44. Ortolani C, Ispano M, Pastorello EA, et al. The oral allergy syndrome. Ann Allergy 1988; 61:47–52.
45. Ortolani C, Pastorello EA, Farioli L, et al. IgE-mediated allergy from vegetables allergens. Ann Allergy 1993; 71:470–76.
46. Bircher AJ, Van Melle G, Haller E, et al. IgE to food allergens are highly prevalent in patients allergic to pollens, with and without symptoms of food allergy. Clin Exp Allergy 1994; 24:367–74.
47. Valenta R, Kraft D. Type I allergic reactions to plant-derived food: a consequence of primary sensitization to pollen allergens. J Allergy Clin Immunol 1996; 97:893–5.
48. Ebner C, Hirschwehr R, Bauer L, et al. Identification of allergens in fruits and vegetables: IgE cross-reactivities with the important birch pollen allergens Bet v 1 and Bet v 2. J Allergy Clin Immunol, 1995; 95:962–9.
49. Valenta R, Duchene M, Pettenburger K, et al. Identification of profilin as a novel pollen allergen; IgE autoreactivity in sensitized individuals. Science 1991; 253:557–9.
50. Ortolani C, Ispano M, Pastorello EA, et al. Comparison of results of skin prick test (with fresh food and commercial extracts) and RAST in 100 patients with oral allergy syndrome. J Allergy Clin Immunol 1989; 83:683–98.
51. Suarez FL, Savaiano DA, Levitt MD. A comparison of symptoms after the consumption of milk or actose-hydrolyzed milk by people with self-reported severe lactose intolerance N Engl J Med. 1995; 333:1–4.

52. GR Corazza, G Gasbarrini. Coeliac disease in adults. Baillieres Clin Gastroenterol 1995; 9:329–50.

53. Godkin A, Jewell D. The pathogenesis of celiac disease. Gastroenterology 1998; 115:206–10.

54. Bonamico M, Ballati G, Mariani P, et al. Screening for coeliac disease: the meaning of low titers of anti-gliadin antibodies (AGA) in non-coeliac children. Eur J Epidemiol 1997; 13(1):55–9.

55. International Consensus Report on the diagnosis and management of rhinitis. Allergy 1994; 19s:5–34.

56. Bousquet J, Chanez P, Michel FB. The respiratory tract and food hypersensitivity. In: Metcalfe DD, Sampson H, eds, Food Allergy, pp. 139–49. Blackwell Scientific, Boston, 1991.

57. Monteleone CA, Sherman AR. Nutrition and asthma. Arch Int Med 1997; 157(1):23–34.

58. Hill DJ, Firer MA, Shelton MJ, et al. Manifestations of milk allergy in infancy: clinical and immunological findings. J Pediatr 1986; 109:270–6.

59. Novembre E, Veneruso G, Sabatini C, et al. Incidence of asthma caused by food allergy in childhood. Pediatr Med Chir 1987; 9:399–404.

60. Burr ML, Fehily AM, Stott NC, et al. Food-allergic asthma in general practice. Hum Nutr Appl Nutr 1985; 39:349–55.

61. Yunginger JW, Sweeney KG, Sturner WQ, et al. Fatal food-induced anaphylaxis. JAMA 1988; 260:1450–2.

62. Sampson HA, Mendelson L, Rosen JP. Fatal and near fatal anaphylactic reactions to food in children and adolescents. N Eng J Med 1992; 327:380–4.

63. Lester MR. Sulfite sensitivity: significance in human health. J Am Coll Nutr 1995; 14(3):229–32.

64. Troisi RJ, Willett WC, Weiss ST, Trichopoulos D, Rosner B, Speizer FE. A prospective study of diet and adult-onset asthma [see comments]. Am J Respir Crit Care Med 1995; 151(5):1401–8.

65. Cohen HA, Neuman J, Nahum H. Blocking effect of vitamin C in exercise-induced asthma. Arch Pediatr Adolesc Med 1997; 151(4): 367–70.

66. Chang CC, Phinney SD, Halpern GM, Gershwin ME. Asthma mortality: another opinion is it a matter of life and . . . bread? J Asthma 1993; 30: 93–103.

67. Zuskin E, Kanceljak B, Schacter EN, et al. Respiratory function and immunologic status in workers processing dried fruits and teas. Ann Allergy Asthma Immunol 1996; 77:417–22.

68. Zuskin E, Kanceljak B, Schachter EN, et al. Immunological and respiratory changes in animal food processing workers. Am J Ind Med 1992; 21:177–91.

69. De Zotti R, Larese F, Bovenzi M, et al. Allergic airway disease in Italian bakers and pastry makers. Occup Environ Med 1994; 51:548–52.

70. Zuskin E, Kanceljak B, Mustajbegovic J, et al. Immunologic findings in confectionary workers. Ann Allergy 1994; 73:521–6.

71. Onorato J, Merland N, Terral C, et al. Placebo-controlled double-blind food challenge in asthma. J Allergy Clin Immunol 1986; 78: 1139–46.

72. Bousquet JSO. Mechanisms in adverse reactions to food. The lung. Allergy 1995; 50(20s):52–5.

73. Wilson N, Silvermann M. Diagnosis of food sensitivity in childhood asthma. J R Soc Med 1985; 5s:11–6.

74. James JM, Eigenmann PA, Eggleston PA, et al. Airway reactivity changes in asthmatic patients undergoing blinded food challenges. Am J Respir Crit Care Med 1996; 153(2):597–603.

75. Heiner DC, Sears JW. Chronic respiratory disease associated with multiple circulating precipitins to cow's milk. Am J Dis Child 1969; 100:500–2.

76. Nanola R, James R, Smith H, Dudley CRD, Jewell DP. Food intolerance and the irritable bowel syndrome. Gut 1989; 30: 1099–1106.

77. Crowe SE, Perdue MH. Gastrointestinal food hypersensitivity: basic mechanism of pathophysiology. Gastroenterology 1992; 103: 1076–96.

78. Stefanini GF, Prati E, Albini MC, et al. Oral disodium cromoglycate treatment on irritable bowel syndrome: an open study on 101 subjects with diarrheic type. Am J Gastroenterol 1992; 87:55–7.

79. Stefanini GF, Saggiori A, Alvisi G, et al. Oral cromolyn sodium in comparison with elimination diet in irritable bowel syndrome, diarrheic type. Scand J Gastroenterol 1995; 30:535–41.

80. Vassallo MJ, Camilleri M, Phillips SF, et al. Colonic tone and motility in patients with irritable bowel syndrome. Mayo Clin Proc 1992; 67:725–31.

81. Jones VA, Shorthouse M, Mac Loughlan P. Food intolerance: a major factor in irritable bowel syndrome. Lancet 1982; 2:1115–7.

82. Zwetckenbaum JF, Burakof R. Food allergy and the irritable bowel syndrome. Am J Gastroenterol 1988; 83:901–4.

83. Gallo C, Vighi G, Ortolani C. Food allergy: a minor factor in irritable bowel syndrome. J Allergy Clin Immunol 1990; 85:272.

84. Straus S, Dale JK, Wright R, Metcalfe DD. Allergy and the chronic fatigue syndrome. J. Allergy Clin Immunol 1988; 81:791–5.

85. Feingold BF. Hyperkinesis and learning disabilities linked to artificial food flavors and colors. Am J Nurs 1975; 75:797–803.

86. Vaughan TR. The role of food in the pathogenesis of migraine headache. Clin Rev Allerg 1994; 12:167–80.

87. Ortolani C, ed. Atlas on mechanism in adverse reaction to foods. Allergy 1995; 50(20s):5–81.

88. Egger J, Wilson J, Carter CM, Turner M. Is migraine food allergy? A double-blind trial of oligoantigenic diet treatment. Lancet 1983; 2:865–9.

89. Mansfield LE, Vaughaln TR, Waller SF, Haverly R, Ting S. Food allergy and adult migraine: double-blind and mediator confirmation of an allergic etiology. Ann Allergy 1985; 55:129–9.

90. Atkins FM, Ball BD, Bock SA. The relationship between the ingestion of specific foods and the development of migraine headache in children. J Allergy Clin Immunol 1988; 81:125.

91. Hurst DS. Allergy management of refractory serous otitis media. Otolaryngol Head Neck Surg 1990; 102:664–9.

92. Bonini S. The eye. Allergy 1995; 50(20s):69–73.

93. De Lazzari F, Mancin O, Plebani M, et al. High IgE serum levels and "peptic" ulcers: clinical and functional approach. Ital J Gastroenterol 194; 26:7–11.

94. Romansi B, Bartuzi Z, Zbikowska-Gotz M, Staszynska M, Korenkiewicz J. Allergy to cockroach antigens in patients with peptic ulcers and chronic gastritis. Allergol Immunopathol (Madr) 1988; 16: 216–24.

95. Bagnato GF, Di Cesare E, Caruso RA, et al. Gastric mucosal mast cells in atopic subjects. Allergy 1995; 50:322–7.

96. Knutson L, Ahrenstedt O, Oblind B, Hallgren R. The jejunal secretion of histamine is increased in active Crohn's disease. Gastroenterology 1990; 98:849–54.

97. Griffiths AM, Ohlsson A, Sherman PM, Sutherland LR. Meta-analysis of enteral nutrition as a primary treatment of active Crohn's disease. Gastroenterology 1995; 108:1056–67.

98. Riordan AM, Hunter JO, Cowan RE, Crampton JR, Davidson AR, Dickinson RJ, et al. Treatment of active Crohn's disease by esclusion diet: East Anglian multicentre controlled trial. Lancet 1993; 342: 1131–4.

99. Mishkin S. Dairy sensitivity, lactose malabsorption and elimination diets in inflammatory bowel disease. Am J Clin Nutr 1997; 65:564–7.

100. Stizmann JV, Converse RL, Bayless TM, Favourable response to parenteral nutrition and medical therapy in Crohn's colitis. A report of 38 patients comparing severe Crohn's and ulcerative colitis. Gastroenterology 1990; 99:1647–52.

101. Wuthrich B. Adverse reaction to food additives. Ann Allergy 1993; 71:376–84.

102. Block WL, Kattan M, Van der Meer JW. Modulation of inflammation and cytokines production by dietary (n-3) fatty acids. J Nutr 1996; 126:1514–33.

103. Van de Laar MA, Aibers M, Bruins FG, van Dinther-Janssen AC, van der Korst JK, Meijer CJ. Food intolerance in rheumatoid arthritis. Ann Rheum Dis 1992; 51:303–6.

104. Sampson HA. Differential diagnosis in adverse reaction to food. J Allergy Clin Exp Immunol 1986; 78:212–9.

105. Carter C. Dietary manipulation of food allergy and intolerance. Clin Exp Allergy 1995; 25(1s):34–42.

106. Bock SA, Sampson HA, Atkins FM, et al. Double blind placebo-controlled food challenge (DBPCFC) as an office procedure: a manual. J Allergy Clin Immunol 1988; 82:986–7.

107. Sampson HA, Ho GD. Relationship between food-specific IgE concentrations and the risk of positive food challenges in children and adolescents. J Allergy Clin Immunol 1997; 100:216–21.

108. Bischoff SC. Colonscopic allergen provocation (COLAP) technique and results. ACI Int 1997; 9:101–9.

109. Businco L, Dreborg S, Eirnasson R, et al. Hydrolysed cow's milk formulae. Allergenicity and use in treatment and prevention. An ESPACI position paper. Pediatr Allergy Immunol 1993; 4:101–11.

110. Steinman HA. "Hidden" allergens in foods. J Allergy Clin Immunol 1996; 98:241–50.

111. Passalaqua G, Bousquet J, Bachert C, et al. The clinical safety of H1-receptor antagonists (Position Paper). Allergy 1996; 51:666–75.

20 Perioperative Feeding
Nutrition and Immunity

RONALD R. BARBOSA AND BRUCE M. WOLFE

METABOLIC RESPONSE TO INJURY

Modern surgical practice, by its name, frequently involves the care of patients who experience dramatic changes in their normal physiologic function. Such changes are most pronounced after major accidental injury, but they are also seen in a wide variety of acute and chronic surgical diseases. In addition, the diagnostic and therapeutic surgical procedures these patients must often undergo are, themselves, stressful to the human body. For convenience, a variety of physiologic perturbations such as accidental injury, major surgical procedures, or systemic manifestations of malignancy, inflammation, or infection will be referred to as "stress."

The basic element in the response to stress is a reordering of the priorities for protein synthesis to facilitate repair and recovery. Wound healing, resistance to infection, and maintenance of body structure and function all depend on responses involving new protein synthesis. Despite this, a negative nitrogen balance is universally seen in stressed patients. A starving individual experiences more whole-body protein degradation than synthesis. In the stressed state, this difference is exacerbated, creating a "protein catabolic state" in which the nitrogen balance is more negative than in the starved but unstressed state.

Virtually all patients have sufficient energy as stored fat to meet short-term energy requirements. However, an adequate supply of glucose must be continuously available to nourish tissues that are dependent on it, such as the central nervous system. The healing wound also preferentially uses glucose as an energy source. This glucose is derived largely from amino acids via gluconeogenesis, a process which contributes substantially to the nitrogen loss seen in stressed patients. Protein degradation must also occur to supply the free amino acids required by the wound and also by the liver for synthesis of the components of the acute-phase response.

The shifting of biological priorities to favor protein synthesis in the wound allows healing to progress at an unimpaired rate despite the overall protein catabolic state. Most otherwise healthy persons who are injured or who undergo major operative proce-

dures will replace the total-body protein lost in this process as they become "anabolic," an interval characterized by resumption of the ability to eat, acceleration of whole-body protein synthesis, and replacement of the net protein lost in the postinjury interval. This interval typically begins 2–3 wk after the stressful event and may last several weeks.

Prior to the development of nutrition support techniques, it was well established that if resumption of adequate nutrient intake by mouth could not be accomplished in a timely fashion after major injury, the progression of wound healing and resistance to infection would be lost. Because of a variety of factors, such as the severity of illness or injury, loss of gastrointestinal function, or other reasons for failure to achieve adequate nutrient intake, a point is reached at which the lack of appropriate nutritional substrate becomes a limiting factor in the capacity to recover from stress.

Most of the physiologic changes seen in stressed patients occur as a result of alterations in the secretion of hormones, cytokines, and other mediators. In general, the observed hormonal response is proportional to the degree of stress up to a point, at which a maximal response is seen (1). Changes in the secretion of other mediators have been less well characterized.

Plasma catecholamine levels rise soon after surgical incision (2) and are markedly elevated for 24 h, but normalize within 5 d even after major surgery, unless complications arise. Catecholamines help maintain hemodynamic stability by increasing heart rate and contractility (via $\beta 1$ receptors), and total peripheral resistance (via $\alpha 1$ receptors). Epinephrine stimulates liver gluconeogenesis and ketogenesis, lipolysis in adipose tissue, and glycogenolysis in the liver and skeletal muscle. Cortisol levels may remain normal in patients undergoing minor surgery (1), but serum levels may rise sixfold after major procedures (3). As with epinephrine, serum levels are considerably elevated for 24 h but normalize within 5 d, provided recovery is uncomplicated. Cortisol enhances gluconeogenesis in the liver and proteolysis in peripheral tissues. Glucose utilization is also decreased in peripheral tissues, inducing a state of relative insulin resistance.

In the initial 2–4 d after stress, the synergistic action of epinephrine, cortisol, and glucagon causes hyperglycemia. In hypovolemic patients, a blunted insulin response to hyperglycemia is seen. This may be secondary to inhibition of insulin secretion by norepineph-

From: *Nutrition and Immunology: Principles and Practice* (ME Gershwin et al. eds.), © Humana Press, Inc., Totowa, NJ

247

rine, which predominates by hypovolemic shock. Following volume replacement, norepinephrine secretion is diminished and insulin levels become appropriate to the level of hyperglycemia. However, a state of insulin resistance remains, possibly the result of inhibition of the pyruvate dehydrogenase complex (4). This may last for 2–3 wk or as long as stress persists. Hyperglycemia may, therefore, persist well into the course of the patient's recovery.

The mobilization of fatty acids is accelerated in response to stress, largely in response to catecholamines. These fatty acids are available for cellular uptake as fuel. However, the extent to which fatty acid oxidation increases in stress is limited, so that the majority of these mobilized fatty acids require hepatic re-esterification. Feeding additional fat to acutely stressed patients, therefore, has very limited value.

Many of the physiologic responses seen in stressed patients are secondary to cytokines elaborated following injury. Tumor necrosis factor (TNF) is secreted from a variety of cells and is thought to be a major determinant of cytokine-induced shock. TNF is proximal in the inflammatory cascade, in that it induces the release of other cytokines. It also causes vasodilation by stimulating nitric oxide synthesis. Interleukin-1 (IL-1) is also proximal in the inflammatory cascade and has effects similar to TNF. It also helps trigger the acute-phase response and has a variety of immunologic effects. IL-6 is more distal in the inflammatory cascade, but it is the main inducer of the acute-phase response and may also mediate some of the effects of TNF (5). Interferon-γ (INFγ) plays a role in the development of antigen-specific immune responses and is also important in the host response to shock and sepsis (5), although overproduction may lead to cachexia. These phenomena have been reviewed in detail (5). The interrelationships between these and other mediators are complex, so that clarification of the roles of individual cytokines and therapeutic modulation of their effects will remain exceedingly difficult.

EFFECTS OF STRESS ON IMMUNE FUNCTION

Surgeons have long known that major injuries induce an immunosuppressed state in patients. In recent years, a variety of immune deficits have been demonstrated in traumatized animals and humans. Here, they will be described briefly because a comprehensive discussion is beyond the scope of this chapter. The interested reader may refer to two thorough reviews (6,7).

Traumatic injuries usually involve the disruption of one or both of the main mechanical barriers of the body, namely the skin and the mucus membranes. This disruption invariably allows the entry of foreign microorganisms. In addition, the normal flora may gain access to areas of the body not designed to contain them, such as when anaerobic bacteria enter the peritoneal cavity through a perforated colon wall. Gut barrier function may be also compromised by other mechanisms in injured patients, such as decreased mesenteric blood flow or direct mucosal injury by endotoxin (8). The drains, catheters, and other invasive devices frequently used in critically ill patients also provide a portal of entry for pathogens.

The phagocytic system is the body's second line of defense. Various defects in this process have been shown to occur in stressed patients. These include impairments in polymorphonuclear (PMN) chemotaxis (7) as well as macrophage cytokine production (8) and superoxide generation (9). Decreased antigen presentation results (8). It is thought that these defects contribute to the increased infection rates seen after trauma, although this has not been shown definitively.

Other immune functions are also altered by major injury; Th cells are decreased in number (10,11) and express fewer IL-2 receptors on their surface (11). T-Cell function, as measured by delayed-type hypersensitivity (DTH) testing, is impaired (12). Defects in B-cell maturation and immunoglobulin synthesis also occur (13). Some of these effects may be related to increased levels of prostaglandin E_2 (PGE_2) (10), which is thought to be immunosuppressive.

PERIOPERATIVE TRANSFUSIONS, HYPOTHERMIA, AND ANESTHETICS

It has been well established that allogenic blood transfusions can produce a clinically significant immunosuppression. This was first demonstrated by Halasz et al. (14) in experiments that showed that pretransplant transfusions decrease allograft rejection in dogs. More than 70 studies in subsequent years have yielded similar results. Transfusions may also increase the risk of tumor recurrence by suppressing immune function in the recipient, although this is controversial (15).

All but one of the 24 studies reviewed by Blumberg and Heal (15) on perioperative allogeneic blood transfusion showed that it is an independent risk factor for postoperative infection. Various authors report a fourfold to fivefold increase in infection risk. This increased risk is significantly attenuated when autologous blood (15) or leukocyte-depleted allogeneic blood (16) is used. The immunologic mechanisms for the above phenomena have not been determined and are likely to be multiple and complex. Blumberg and Heal (15) have postulated that anergy secondary to the presentation of large amounts of intravenous antigen is the dominant mechanism.

Mild perioperative hypothermia increases the risk of postoperative wound infection. In a prospective randomized clinical trial in colorectal surgery patients (17), an intraoperative decrease in core body temperature from $36.6 \pm 0.5°C$ to $34.7 \pm 0.5°C$ increased the wound infection rate from 6% to 19% ($p = 0.009$) and increased the length of stay by 2.6 d ($p = 0.01$). The authors proposed that hypothermia may cause vasoconstriction in wounded tissues, thus decreasing local oxygen tension, which, in turn, impairs oxidative killing by neutrophils and weakens the wound by inhibiting collagen deposition. Intraoperative hypothermia is very common because patients are usually not actively warmed during surgery. It is recommended that patients be maintained at a core body temperature of at least 36°C to optimize the immune function of wounded tissues.

Despite the many millions of anesthetics that have been administered in the last few decades, data on the effects of anesthetic agents on immune function are equivocal at best (18). A mild inhibition of cell-mediated immunity may occur with certain agents, but the significance is unknown and results have not had good reproducibility (18). Data on the effect of anesthesia on B-cell function are sparse.

THE IMPACT OF MALNUTRITION ON SURGICAL OUTCOME

In 1936, Studley published his landmark study (19) on the outcome of 50 consecutive patients operated on for chronic peptic ulcer. In this series, patients who had lost more than 20% of their body weight preoperatively had a much higher postoperative mortality rate (33.3%) than those who did not lose as much weight (3.5%). In 1944, Cannon and others *(20)* demonstrated that hypoproteinemia can lead to impaired antibody production and increased infection rates. In 1955, Rhoads and Alexander showed that hypoproteinemic patients had increased incidences of urinary tract, respiratory, wound, and miscellaneous infections *(21)*. Seltzer et al. *(22)* found a sixfold increase in mortality in patients with serum albumin < 3.5 g/dL. Similar results have been found by others *(23,24)*. In 1974, Bistrian and colleagues *(24)* used anthropometric and biochemical measurement to draw attention to the high rate of malnutrition in general surgical patients (50%), which was underappreciated prior to that time.

The negative impact of malnutrition on clinical outcome has been confirmed by further work in recent years. A large study conducted in the Veterans Affairs (VA) population *(25)* showed that both infectious and noninfectious complications were increased in patients with severe malnutrition. Hickman and associates *(26)* found that abnormal preoperative weight was predictive of postoperative mortality. In malnourished survivors, the length of stay may be increased *(27)*. A number of other studies showing similar effects have been described in a review by Dempsey et al. *(28)*.

PREDICTING POSTOPERATIVE OUTCOME

In the last two decades, there have been a number of attempts to quantify the relationship among nutrition, immune function, and postoperative mortality and morbidity. Delayed-type hypersensitivity (DTH) testing has been useful in this regard. DTH testing involves the recognition of intracutaneously injected bacterial antigens by sensitized T cells. Individuals with intact cell-mediated immunity will have erythema and induration at the injection sites. The test is easy to perform, inexpensive, and does not require specially trained personnel.

Perioperative DTH testing has been studied extensively by Christou and colleagues *(12,29,30)*. In a study of 2202 acutely ill and elective surgical patients, 33% of patients who were anergic to five ubiquitous antigens at hospital admission developed serious infections and 31% died. In contrast, only 8% of patients normoergic to the five antigens developed serious infections and only 4% died. An analysis of the database accumulated by Christou and co-workers over 20 yr showed a similar relationship *(12)*. Anergy to the five antigens was associated with increased mortality in both elective surgical and critically ill patients when the entire cohort was examined. However, when the subgroup of elective surgical patients enrolled since 1990 was analyzed, anergy lost its predictive value entirely. Christou and colleagues attribute this to recent improvements in patient care, which decrease the total perioperative infectious challenge. However, anergy has retained its predictive value in the critically ill, who tend to have greater infectious and metabolic stressors than elective surgical patients. The absence of a DTH response in anergic patients is thought to be the result of a general immune dysfunction as well as defects in host defense in the skin and possibly the gut *(12)*. Whether or not DTH testing will have a direct clinical utility in the future is unknown. It is not currently used to guide individual patient management. Further work in critically ill patients is indicated.

The Prognostic Nutritional Index (PNI) was described in 1980 by Buzby et al. *(31)*. In this study, a variety of nutritional parameters were analyzed retrospectively in 161 gastrointestinal surgical patients. Statistical analysis was used to determine which factors were most predictive of postoperative complications. A linear prediction model was derived:

$$PNI(\%) = 158 - 16.6(ALB) - 0.78(TSF) - 0.20(TFN) - 5.8(DTH)$$

where PNI is the risk of a septic complication occurring in an individual patient, ALB is the serum albumin level (g/dL), TSF is triceps skinfold (mm), TFN is serum transferrin (mg/dL), and DTH is delayed-type hypersensitivity reactivity to three standard antigens, graded as 0 (nonreactive), 1 (<5 mm induration), and 2 (>5 mm induration). The PNI was then determined prospectively in 100 different gastrointestinal surgery patients. Those with a PNI > 50% had a significantly higher mortality and incidence of sepsis.

The original PNI study has been criticized for being retrospective and nonconsecutive and for enrolling primarily malnourished patients. Katelaris et al. *(32)* determined the PNI and other nutritional parameters in a consecutive prospective fashion in 57 patients undergoing elective abdominal or thoracic surgery, many of whom were at low risk for postoperative complications. Patients with PNI > 30% were defined as being at increased risk for postoperative complications. In this context, PNI had a sensitivity of 83% and a specificity of 73%. In a study containing only septic, malnourished patients *(33)*, PNI values were significantly lower in survivors (52.26 ± 23.72) compared to those who died (72.24 ± 15.43). A 10-d course of total parenteral nutrition (TPN) has been shown to improve PNI values *(34)*, but the study was too small to determine if postoperative outcome was also improved.

Albumin may be the single laboratory parameter that best predicts surgical outcome. Careful inspection of the equations derived by Buzby et al. *(31)* and Christou et al. *(12,29,30)* reveals that the serum albumin level plays a dominant role in the respective regression models. However, a decrease in serum albumin is not specific for malnutrition, as it may have other etiologies such as hepatic disease and increased capillary permeability.

The oldest method for evaluating nutritional status is clinical assessment by careful history-taking and physical examination. This method was first analyzed critically in a 1982 study by Baker and colleagues *(35)*. Fifty-nine patients electively admitted to a general surgical ward were classified as being of normal nutritional status, mildly malnourished, or severely malnourished by history and physical examination by two experienced clinicians. The two examiners agreed on the classification of 81% of patients. The study also demonstrated that clinical assessment was correlated with a number of objective laboratory and anthropometric measurements. The incidence of postoperative infection was increased in the malnourished groups. Baker's method of classification of patients has since been termed Subjective Global Assessment (SGA).

The largest study to date evaluating SGA in surgical patients was the VA Cooperative TPN trial *(25)*. This large randomized multicenter trial evaluated the efficacy of a preoperative course of TPN at decreasing postoperative morbidity and mortality. In this study (discussed in more detail later), TPN was found to be beneficial only in those patients classified as severely malnourished by SGA. In contrast, other workers have found clinical assessment to be a poor predictor of postoperative complications *(32)*. SGA may also not be reproducible among hospitals *(36)*. However, clinical assessment of nutritional status is likely to remain the most widely used method until a more objective model is found to be superior.

TPN IN STRESSED PATIENTS

Total parenteral nutrition was developed in 1968 by Dudrick and colleagues *(37)* as a means to feed those patients without adequately functioning gastrointestinal tracts. TPN was quickly adapted for use in premature newborns and in patients with long-term intestinal dysfunction, who would otherwise starve to death. In later years, TPN was increasingly used perioperatively in malnourished surgical patients. Supportive evidence came largely from nonrandomized studies. By the mid-1980s, it became clear that definitive evidence of the effectiveness of perioperative TPN would be needed to justify its use in light of its associated risks and cost.

In 1986, Detsky and co-workers published a meta-analysis *(36)* of the 18 controlled perioperative TPN trials conducted until that time. They noted that most of the trials were poorly designed and that only one *(38)* showed significant decreases in mortality and complication rate. Pooled estimated surgical complications and mortality rates were not significantly different between the control patients and the patients given TPN. The authors concluded that routine perioperative TPN use in unselected patients was not justified, but suggested that TPN might be useful in severely malnourished patients.

The Veterans Affairs TPN Cooperative Study *(25)* was a multicenter prospective randomized controlled clinical trial evaluating the effectiveness of perioperative TPN in surgical patients stratified by nutritional status. It was specifically designed to avoid the weaknesses of previous studies. Three hundred ninety-five malnourished patients undergoing elective abdominal or noncardiac thoracic surgery were randomized to receive TPN for 7–15 d before surgery and 3 d afterward (the TPN group) or no perioperative TPN (the control group). Patients were subdivided into three groups by nutritional state (borderline, mildly, or severely malnourished) by Subjective Global Assessment or Nutrition Risk Index. The 30-d postoperative mortality rates in the TPN and control groups were 7.3% (14/192) and 4.9% (10/203), respectively, which were not significantly different. Complication-related and overall mortality rates at 90 d were also similar between groups. Major complications occurred in 28% of patients in both groups.

A more detailed analysis showed that infectious complications were more common in the TPN group (14.1%) than the control group (6.4%; $p = 0.01$). This increase in infection rate was limited to patients classified as borderline or mildly malnourished by SGA and was compensated for by a slightly decreased incidence of noninfectious complications. In severely malnourished patients, the noninfectious complication rate was significantly lower in patients given TPN (5.3%) than in the control group (42.9%, $p = 0.03$). The overall complication rate in severely malnourished patients given TPN was also lower, but statistical significance was not reached because of the small size of this subgroup. The authors concluded that perioperative TPN was not beneficial in borderline or mildly malnourished patients and that it may actually be harmful because of the increased incidence of infections. It was suggested that these patients would be best served by prompt surgery. A clinical benefit of TPN in severely malnourished patients was implied but awaited confirmation.

The VA Cooperative Study may no longer have direct clinical application because of the advances made in TPN solutions and administration techniques since the trial was conducted. There have been concerns that the patients in the trial may have been overfed, causing an immunosuppressive effect secondary to hyperglycemia *(38a)*. Ninety-seven patients in which TPN was considered to be essential were also excluded, as it would not be ethical to randomize such patients to an unfed control group. Thus, many severely malnourished patients who would be expected to benefit most from TPN were eliminated from the trial. The amino acid mix also did not contain glutamine, which may improve outcome in patients given TPN *(39)*. These factors may have masked any benefits TPN may have had. Nevertheless, this landmark study has guided research and clinical practice more than any other TPN study conducted in surgical patients to date.

Subsequent trials have tended to substantiate the findings of the VA Cooperative Study. Brennan et al. *(40)* randomized 259 patients undergoing resection for pancreatic malignancy to receive TPN (starting on postoperative day 1) or dextrose-containing salt solutions. No benefit was seen in the TPN group and this group had a significantly higher infectious complication rate. Fan and colleagues *(41)* randomized 150 patients with hepatocellular carcinoma to receive TPN for 7 d before and 7 d after surgery in addition to their regular diet or to receive no additional therapy. Patients in the TPN groups had a lower postoperative morbidity rate, but the benefits were seen only in those with the most severe disease. Sandstrom and co-workers *(42)* estimated that perioperative TPN was a lifesaving treatment in 20% of the patients in their series, but that it tended to increase mortality in another 20%. These patients could not be identified by preoperative factors.

ENTERAL NUTRITION IN STRESSED PATIENTS

In surgical patients, total enteral nutrition (TEN) has been shown to be superior to dextrose-containing intravenous fluids at improving nutritional and laboratory parameters, such as nitrogen balance *(43)* and amino acid flux across peripheral tissues *(44)*. However, few studies have shown an improvement in clinical outcome. Moore and Jones *(45)* randomized 75 patients with severe injuries to receive TEN beginning 12 h postoperatively and continuing until oral intake was established or D5W until postoperative day 5. Patients in the enteral nutrition group had significantly fewer postoperative infections (29%) than those in the control group (9%; $p < 0.025$). However, this did not translate to a shorter length of hospital stay. In a small series of patients with severe head injuries *(46)*, enteral nutrition decreased the incidence of bacterial infections and shortened the length of stay in the Intensive Care Unit (ICU).

Other studies have shown no benefit of postoperative enteral feeding compared to standard intravenous fluids. In a small ($n = 28$) randomized controlled trial, Carr et al. *(47)* found no difference between the TEN and control groups in length of stay or number of days to oral intake. Heslin and associates *(48)* published the largest study to date ($n = 195$) comparing perioperative enteral nutrition to standard intravenous fluids. Patients undergoing surgery for upper gastrointestinal (GI) malignancy were randomized to receive intravenous fluids or enteral nutrition with an immune-enhancing formula containing arginine, RNA, and omega-3 fatty acids beginning within 24 h of operation. There were no differences in the number of minor, major, or infectious complications between groups. The length of stay and mortality rates were virtually identical. The patients in this study were relatively well nourished. The authors concluded that the routine postoperative use of TEN in patients undergoing major upper GI surgery is not indicated, a recommendation which can reasonably be extended to other types of elective surgery.

TEN VERSUS TPN

There have been many studies comparing the effects of TPN and TEN on nutritional, morphologic, and immunologic parameters in animals and humans. However, there are few randomized clinical trials showing that these two methods of nutritional support differentially affect clinical outcome. Such reports are found mostly in the trauma literature. In 1989, Moore and colleagues (49) published their series of 59 trauma patients requiring laparotomy randomized to receive either TPN or TEN beginning within 12 h of operation. Infection developed in only 17% of the TEN group compared to 37% of the TPN group. Major septic complications developed in 3% in the TEN group (one abdominal abscess) and 17% of the TPN group (two abdominal abscesses and six cases of pneumonia). This study excluded the most gravely injured patients (those with Abdominal Trauma Index [ATI] > 40). A later study by Kudsk and associates (50) included 20 such patients in a series of 98 injured patients requiring laparotomy randomized to receive TPN or TEN within 24 h of injury. Patients fed enterally developed significantly fewer pneumonias (11.8% vs TPN 31%), abdominal abscesses (1.9% vs TPN 13.3%), and overall infections. The differences in infection rates were confined to the more severely injured patients (ATI > 24).

A number of prospective randomized trials comparing postoperative TPN and TEN in high-risk surgical patients were conducted in the 1980s. Because of the considerable financial and logistical difficulties inherent to these studies, none had a large enough sample size to show a difference in clinical outcome. Moore and others combined data from eight of these into a meta-analysis (51) with numbers large enough (n = 230) to address the issue. When analyzed by intent-to-treat, patients receiving TEN developed fewer septic complications (16% vs TPN 35%; p = 0.01). This difference was significant even when patients with catheter sepsis were excluded.

EFFECTS OF TPN ON IMMUNE FUNCTION

Because the increased infection rate associated with the use of TPN (25,40,49–51) cannot be explained by catheter sepsis alone, it has been widely speculated that TPN has an immunosuppressive effect. This has been studied extensively in animals, and a number of TPN-induced alterations in immunity and intestinal morphology and function have been demonstrated.

Parenteral nutrition and/or the lack of enteral feeding has been shown to cause intestinal mucosal atrophy (52,53) and decreased microvillus height (54). Decreases in brush-border hydrolase (55) and nutrient transporter activity (56) have also been described. TPN is thought to increase intestinal permeability (54,57), although not all evidence supports this (58). Increased bacterial translocation from the lumen to mesenteric lymph nodes occurs (59,60), probably via the lymphatics (59). The bacterial overgrowth in the intestine observed after TPN administration (61,62) may contribute to this. Bacterial translocation may be important to the development of multiple-organ failure (61) and may cause regional immune defects (60), although this is controversial. Currently, there is no evidence that TPN-induced bacterial transloca-

tion is pathologic in humans. Research in this area is likely to remain active in the future.

Total parenteral nutrition may adversely affect several aspects of white blood cell function. Mitogenic responses are impaired in peripheral (63) and splenic (60) lymphocytes. Decreased $CD4^+$ and $CD8^+$ cell counts are seen in the intestine (64). Recovery of neutrophil locomotion in trauma patients is delayed by TPN (65). Pulmonary (59) and peritoneal (60) macrophage phagocytosis of *C. albicans* is impaired and superoxide production is decreased in rats given TPN. Parenteral nutrition may also affect cytokine release by inflammatory cells. In rats given intraperitoneal *E. coli*, peritoneal TNF and Il-1α levels are decreased, whereas in the systemic circulation TNF is increased and IFNγ is decreased (66).

Considerable attention has focused on the gut-associated lymphoid tissue (GALT), the primary source of mucosal immunity in humans. The GALT cell mass depends on lymphoid tissue in the Peyer patches (PP) of the small intestine (67). Precursor cells are sensitized to antigens in the PP and proliferate in the mesenteric lymph nodes. They then flow via lymphatics into the vasculature and home to the lamina propria (LP) beneath mucosal surfaces. They differentiate into plasma cells that secrete IgA into the lumen via a multistep process. IgA binds to microorganisms or toxins, preventing their attachment to epithelial cells. The GALT appears to be influenced by route of nutrition. T- and B-cell counts are decreased in the PP and LP of rats after 2 d of parenteral feeding (67). The $CD4^+$/$CD8^+$ ratio in the LP is decreased after 4 d of TPN. IgA levels in the small intestine (67) and biliary tree (64) are decreased. IgA levels in the respiratory tract are also decreased (67), which may be responsible for the impaired immune response to intranasal viral challenge seen in other studies (68,69). Many of these changes may be prevented by adding glutamine (64) or bombesin (70) to the TPN solution or reversed by enteral refeeding (68).

It must be emphasized that the vast majority of TPN-induced adverse effects on immunity have been demonstrated only in animal studies. The specific mechanisms responsible for the increased infection rates seen in human clinical trials remain unclear. Interest in this area will remain high as physicians try to clarify the role of perioperative TPN in clinical practice.

HYPERGLYCEMIA IN SURGICAL PATIENTS

The metabolic derangements that occur in the postoperative period make many surgical patients prone to hyperglycemia. As described earlier, a general catabolic state exists and levels of cortisol, glucagon, and epinephrine are increased. This promotes gluconeogenesis and glycogenolysis. A state of insulin resistance is also seen postoperatively (71,72), which may persist for up to 5 d.

Patients who are prescribed glucose-based TPN solutions are even more susceptible to hyperglycemia because of the exogenous glucose load, especially if glucose is infused at greater than 4–5 mg/kg/min (73). Hyperglycemia is the most common metabolic complication of TPN administration (74). It is a much lesser problem in enteral nutrition because of "first-pass" metabolism of glucose by the liver and because the gut is intolerant of high glucose loads because of their osmolarity.

It is well established that immune function is deranged in diabetics and that numerous mechanisms are involved. However, diabetes is, by nature, a complex and chronic disease, so that it may not be appropriate to use diabetic models to study the immune effects of hyperglycemia in nondiabetic surgical patients. Several studies demonstrate that acute hyperglycemia has immunosuppressive effects. Black et al. *(75)* reported that human IgG could be nonenzymatically glycosylated by incubation in 250 mg/dL glucose at body temperature for 8 h. The glycosylated IgG was then given to asplenic rats following *Streptococcus pneumoniae* challenge. Mean survival time was significantly less than that of control animals, indicating that glycosylation of IgG decreases its immunologic activity. Later works by the same group *(76)* showed that complement fixation by IgG is impaired when its incubation time in glucose is extended to 48 h. Glycosylation of C3 in hyperglycemic models impairs its ability to attach to the microbial surface *(77)*. Phagocytic killing is also affected by hyperglycemia. Glucose suppresses superoxide generation in normal neutrophils in concentrations as low as 270 mg/dL, possibly the result of an inhibition of phospholipase D activity *(38a)*. The respiratory burst of alveolar macrophages is depressed in rats infused with glucose to give plasma concentrations of 300 mg/dL for 3 h *(38a)*. Finally, some pathogens have unique mechanisms for flourishing in a hyperglycemic environment, such as *Candida albicans,* which expresses a glucose-inducible protein homologous to a complement receptor on phagocytes *(77)*. This protein promotes adherence of the yeast and helps it to evade phagocytosis.

GLUTAMINE

Glutamine is the most abundant amino acid in human blood, skeletal muscle, and the body as a whole *(78)*. For decades its importance was unrecognized, especially in the field of nutrition support, because the predominant biochemistry and nutrition textbooks classified it as a "nonessential" amino acid because the body can synthesize it *de novo*. Over the years, a substantial body of knowledge accumulated regarding the critical role of glutamine in a variety of tissues and the potential for glutamine depletion in the stressed state, which has led to its reclassification as "conditionally essential."

Glutamine serves as a carrier for nitrogen transfer among skeletal muscle, intestine, liver, and other tissues. As such, its serum concentration is higher than for any other amino acid (7.5 mg/ dL); in skeletal muscle, it is 30 times more concentrated. It is the most important substrate for renal ammoniagenesis. Glutamine is a key fuel source for lymphocytes *(79)*. It is a nitrogen donor for purine and pyrimidine biosynthesis and is, therefore, necessary for cell replication. It may also be needed for liver glutathione synthesis *(80)*. Glutamine also promotes liver regeneration after 70% hepatectomy in rats coinfused with glucagon and insulin *(81)*.

Marked changes in glutamine flux are seen in stressed patients. Skeletal muscle and lung *(82)* release of glutamine is increased, but serum levels are decreased because of increased uptake by a variety of tissues. Intestinal uptake of glutamine is almost doubled by a standard laparotomy, despite decreased arterial concentration and intestinal blood flow *(83)*. This is at least partially mediated by glucocorticoids, which increase glutamine uptake by the gut *(84)*, probably by increasing the activity of enterocyte mitochondrial glutaminase *(85)*. A glucocorticoid-mediated increase in renal glutaminase activity *(84)* occurs, which improves the body's ability to compensate for acidosis. Lymphocytes exhibit an increased need for glutamine as they proliferate in response to an immune challenge. In the stressed state, the increased uptake by these tissues typically overcomes the ability of the skeletal muscle and lung to supply glutamine, and total-body stores are depleted unless an exogenous source is provided.

The effects of glutamine on the gastrointestinal tract have been widely studied. It is the primary fuel for enterocytes and is one of the only nutrients that stimulates ornithine decarboxylase, the rate-limiting enzyme for enterocyte proliferation *(86)*. The gut is the primary organ of glutamine uptake, extracting 20–30% of circulating glutamine in the postabsorptive state *(87)*. Enterocytes have access to glutamine both from the gut lumen and the bloodstream. Glutamine is important in maintaining the normal architecture of the gut mucosa. In an animal model, glutaminase infusion decreases serum glutamine concentrations, causing diarrhea, villous atrophy, and intestinal mucosal ulceration and necrosis *(88)*. Glutamine increases gut mucosal integrity after abdominal irradiation in a rat model *(89)*, as measured by bacterial translocation to mesenteric lymph nodes. TPN-induced gut mucosal atrophy is attenuated by glutamine supplementation in animal models *(90–94)* and in humans *(95)*. Dipeptide forms of glutamine are as effective as free glutamine in this regard *(91–93)*. These studies described changes in a number of morphological parameters, including mucosal height, weight, thickness, protein and nucleotide content, crypt death, number of mitoses per crypt, and villous area.

Glutamine is important for the maintenance of gut immune function. Alverdy and colleagues demonstrated that glutamine is able to prevent the decreased B- and T-cell levels seen with TPN administration in a rat model *(96,97)*. TPN-induced decreases in biliary sIgA secretion were also partially attenuated. This is important because sIgA prevents bacterial adherence to mucosal cells, an initiating step for bacterial translocation. In humans, glutamine may enhance the peripheral T-cell response *(98)*. Glutamine-supplemented rats with experimentally induced *E. coli* peritonitis have increased bacterial clearance and survival *(91,94)*. In one model *(91)*, this effect was seen without a change in the number of neutrophils, macrophages, or lymphocytes in peritoneal fluid. This led to speculation that glutamine exerts its immune effect by enhancing immune cell function rather than proliferation *(91,99)*.

There is an extensive array of animal studies supporting the addition of glutamine to feeding solutions. Ziegler and Young *(100)* noted that 80% of the animal studies to date show some beneficial effect of glutamine supplementation. Data showing a positive effect on outcome in humans are much more limited. Glutamine was shown to have a clinical benefit in humans for the first time by Ziegler et al. in 1992. In this well-designed double-blind randomized controlled study *(39)*, bone marrow transplant recipients received TPN supplemented with gutamine or an isonitrogenous, isocaloric glutamine-free TPN formula. Patients in the glutamine-supplemented group had fewer clinical infections (3/ 24 vs 9/21 in the control group; $p = 0.041$) and a shorter length of stay (29 ± 1 vs 36 ± 2 d; $p = 0.017$). The incidence of microbial colonization was also significantly reduced. Another study in bone marrow transplant patients by Schloreb and Amase *(101)* found that the length of stay was decreased in the glutamine-supplemented group (26.9 ± 1.3 vs 32.7 ± 2.1 d; $p < 0.05$). In contrast to the Ziegler study, the incidence of clinical infection and bacterial colonization was unchanged. A clinical benefit of glutamine supplementation was reported in critically ill patients in a study by Griffiths and associates *(102)*. Patients who could not be given enteral nutrition were given a glutamine-supplemented or an isonitrogenous isocaloric formula. Patients in the supplemented group had a higher 6-mo survival rate (24/42 vs 14/42; $p = 0.049$).

Data from human studies demonstrating a clinical benefit are not conclusive enough to recommend the routine use of glutamine in any specific patient population except bone marrow transplant recipients. The most recent NIH/ASPEN/ASCN conference guidelines (103) do not make specific conclusions on the use of glutamine in feeding solutions. Further studies that assess the effect of glutamine on patient outcome are clearly needed. These may be more practical now that stable glutamine dipeptides are available. The theoretical and experimental basis of glutamine supplementation is quite strong, and it is expected that interest in this area will remain high.

ARGININE

Arginine was originally classified as a semiessential amino acid and is an intermediary in a number of key metabolic pathways. In the urea cycle, it is hydrolyzed to urea and ornithine by the enzyme arginase. Arginine may also be converted to nitric oxide (NO) and citrulline via the arginine deaminase pathway. This is a critical function because NO plays a key role in the regulation of vascular tone, macrophage function, and a number of other functions that are still being elucidated. Arginine is also a precursor (via ornithine) of the polyamines, which are important in cellular growth and differentiation. In the catabolic state, endogenous arginine synthesis is inadequate to meet the needs of the body, so that arginine then becomes essential.

Arginine may also affect metabolism more indirectly by influencing anabolic hormone levels. More than 30 yr ago, arginine was found to induce a rise in serum growth hormone concentration (104). This may be secondary to a suppression of hypothalamic secretion (105). Among the amino acids, it is the most potent stimulator of insulin secretion (106). Interestingly, ornithine is even more potent than arginine as a growth hormone secretagogue, but it has no effect on insulin secretion (107). Arginine is also thought to stimulate the secretion of prolactin, catecholamines, pancreatic somatostatin, and pancreatic polypeptide (108).

Specific improvements in immune function as a result of arginine supplementation were first demonstrated in rats by Barbul (109). In this study, 1% dietary arginine supplementation caused an increase in thymic weight and cellularity in both normal rats and rats subjected to femoral fracture. Thymic lymphocytes also had an increased mitogenic response to phytohemmaglutin in (PHA) and Concanavalin C (Con A). Increased peripheral blood T-lymphocyte mitogenesis has been shown in rats with a minor wound (108), healthy humans (110,111), and in patients undergoing surgery for gastrointestinal cancer (112). In mice, arginine supplementation also increases cytotoxic T-lymphocyte development and poly IC-inducible natural-killer (NK) cell activity and causes IL-2 receptor to be expressed earlier (113).

The effects of arginine supplementation on wound healing have also been studied. An increased wound hydroxyproline content was seen in rats 7 d after laparotomy (114). A higher ratio of type III/type I collagen was also seen. Hydroxyproline is found only in collagen, and type III collagen is thought to be deposited in the early stages of wound healing. Wound bursting strength is increased in rats (108). Increases in wound hydroxyproline content have been confirmed in young (110) and elderly (115) human volunteers.

Studies showing improved nitrogen balance and decreased weight loss in the arginine-fed traumatized rat have been reviewed (116). Improved nitrogen balance has also been observed in patients undergoing open cholecystectomy (117) and gastrointestinal cancer resection (112). Studies demonstrating a clinical benefit of arginine supplementation have been limited. Arginine has increased survival in burned guinea pigs (118). In a mouse study (119), survival after cecal ligation and puncture was 56% in the arginine-supplemented group compared to 20% in the standard chow group ($p < 0.02$). The investigators hypothesized that nitric oxide may play an important role, because in another experiment, the nitric oxide inhibitor NNA decreased the survival of arginine-supplemented rats from 95% to 30% ($p < 0.0001$). The utility of arginine supplementation has been questioned, because a study in a guinea pig peritonitis model (120) failed to show a benefit and higher concentrations of arginine diet actually worsened nitrogen balance and mortality. To date, there have been no human studies showing an improvement in the clinical outcome of surgical patients supplemented with arginine. Until such a benefit can be demonstrated, the addition of arginine to perioperative nutrition regimens cannot be recommended, except in the setting of a clinical trial.

OMEGA-3 FATTY ACIDS

There has been a considerable amount of interest in the use of omega-3 (N-3) fatty acids as immunomodulators. Eicosapentaenoic acid (EPA) is the principal N-3 fatty acid and is a derivative of linolenic acid. N-3 fatty acids are relatively scarce in Western diets but are found in high concentrations in fish oil. Omega-6 (N-6) fatty acids are more common in Western diets and are found in safflower oil and soybean oil. Arachidonic acid (AA) is metabolically the most important N-6 fatty acid and is a derivative of linoleic acid. AA is converted to prostaglandins of the 2-series (PGE_2, PGI_2, TXA_2) by the cyclooxygenase pathway and to leukotrienes of the 4-series (TLB_4) via the lipoxygenase pathway. In contrast, EPA is metabolized by cyclooxygenase into 3-series prostaglandins (PGE_3, PGI_3, TXB_3) and by lipoxygenase into 5-series leukotrienes.

Most immunologists believe that the E series of prostaglandins downregulate the immune system. In vitro studies show that PGE_2 suppresses a number of aspects of the immune system (121,122), including T-cell mitogenesis II-2 production, IgM synthesis, and macrophage and NK cell activity. PGE_3 does not have the same immunosuppressive properties (123). LTB_4 is a very potent chemotactic agent and is thought to be an important mediator of the inflammatory response to injury and sepsis. LTB_5 is about 10 times less potent (124). Fish-oil-supplemented diets have been shown to decrease PGE_2 production (125) and LTB_4 production (124,126) and to increase LTB_5 production (126) in humans. Decreased production of IL-1β, IL-1α, and TNF also occurs in humans (125), possibly secondary to decreased PGE_2 production.

In a burned guinea pig model, Alexander and colleagues (127) found that fish oil supplementation resulted in less weight loss, lower resting metabolic expenditure, better carbohydrate metabolism index (CMI), higher splenic weight, lower adrenal weight, and higher serum transferrin levels. However, survival was not improved. Other animal models have shown improved outcome. Rats given a regular chow diet supplemented with fish oil for 2 wk before cecal ligation and puncture had an 80% survival rate versus 50% for rats on a chow plus linoleic acid diet and 55% on a regular chow diet only (128). Fish oil supplementation also improved survival in mice given intramuscular injections of *Klebsiella pneumoniae* (129). In a prospective randomized human trial *(130)*, patients undergoing upper gastrointestinal surgery for cancer were given either a standard enteral formula or an isocaloric, isonitrogenous fish oil structured-lipid-based formula. Patients receiving the fish-oil-supplemented diet were 50% less likely to develop gastrointestinal complications (cramping, diarrhea, distention, nausea). The number of infected patients were similar between groups, but patients receiving fish oil were less likely to have multiple infections. They also had decreased serum levels of liver enzymes and had improved creatinine clearance, but these did not reach statistical significance. This was a relatively small trial ($n = 50$) and the authors recommend that a similar but larger trial be done to confirm these findings. To date, there have been no clinical trials that have demonstrated improved survival or decreased length of stay in surgical patients given a standard enteral or parenteral nutrition regimen supplemented only with N-3 fatty acids.

It has been suggested that the ratio of N-6 to N-3 fatty acids in the diet may be more important in modulating the immune system than absolute levels of either type alone *(44)*. In a rat heart allotransplant model, optimal immune function was seen in rats given a diet with an N-6/N-3 ratio of 2.1/1. Rats given fish oil (1/7.6) or safflower oil (360/1) had decreased immune function. These results suggest that a mixture of fish and safflower oils may be more beneficial than fish oil alone.

GROWTH HORMONE

Although the use of parenteral nutritional support in patients who cannot be fed enterally has beneficial and often life-saving effects, it cannot increase or even maintain body protein during the catabolic state often seen in surgical patients. This realization has led investigators to attempt to alter nitrogen metabolism by the use of anabolic hormones. The most extensively studied of these is growth hormone. Human growth hormone (GH) is an anterior pituitary peptide hormone that has a number of anabolic effects, including decreased protein catabolism with enhanced synthesis, increased fat mobilization and conversion of fatty acids to acetyl–CoA, and decreased glucose oxidation with increased glycogen deposition. GH is also thought to improve muscle strength, wound healing, and immunological function. Its anabolic effects are mediated largely by insulin-like growth factor I (IGF-1), whereas lipolytic effects are mediated by GH itself. IGF-1 production is stimulated by circulating GH and occurs in a variety of tissues, most prominently in the liver. The GH–IGF-1 axis is altered in the stressed or starved state, and increased GH levels with decreased IGF-1 levels invariably occurs *(55)*. In the unstressed fed state, the anabolic effects of GH predominate, whereas GH acts mostly as a fat-mobilizing agent in the stressed organism.

A number of studies demonstrate that providing exogenous recombinant GH improves nitrogen balance in healthy human volunteers *(131)* and surgical patients *(46,132–134)*. Positive balances of potassium *(46,131,135)* and phosphorus *(131)*, which are key intracellular components of lean body mass, are seen. There is an increase in total body weight. An elegant study by Byrne and colleagues *(136)* reported that growth hormone supplementation caused a significant gain in lean body mass with increased protein deposition but minimal body fat gain. In contrast, control patients gained a greater proportion of weight as extracellular water and fat. These findings are particularly important because they show that GH-supplemented nutritional support can preferentially increase the protein (i.e., functional) mass of the body.

The only report of improved clinical outcome and immunological function with GH administration after surgery was published in 1993 by Vara-Thorbeck and associates *(46)*. In this relatively large double-blinded randomized controlled study, patients undergoing elective cholecystectomy were given placebo ($n = 93$) or GH ($n = 87$). Delayed hypersensitivity skin testing was used to evaluate immune function. In the control group, the number of normoergic patients dropped from 56 to 40 postoperatively, whereas in the GH-supplemented group, the number of normoergic patients increased from 59 to 81. The number of anergic patients was unchanged ($n = 11$) in the control group but dropped to zero in the supplemented group. GH also prevented the postoperative decrease in IgG, IgM, and IgA seen in the control group. Wound infection occurred in 17.2% of the control patients but in only 3.4% of the patients given GH. The length of stay was also decreased (12.5 ± 7.1 d control group, 9.6 ± 3.6 d GH group; $p < 0.05$).

Growth hormone administration has been generally well tolerated in clinical studies, but metabolic side effects may occur. Blood glucose concentrations have been mildly *(46,135)* (110–160 mg/dL) or moderately *(134)* (> 200 mg/dL) increased by exogenous GH administration despite concomitant hyperinsulinemia. Uncontrolled hyperglycemia could then theoretically dampen any immunostimulatory effects that GH may have had. Up to 43% of patients given GH develop hypercalcemia (>11.0 mg/dL) and 10% may have severe hypercalcemia (>12.5 mg/dL) *(137)*. Patients with impaired renal function are particularly susceptible. Two European studies in critically ill patients showed a higher mortality in GH-supplemented patients (41.7%) than controls (18.2%) *(138)*. This led the manufacturer to recommend halting all recombinant GH use in catabolic patients. The etiology of the increased mortality rates is unknown, as the studies have not yet been published. However, interest remains high in the use of GH in patients with short-bowel syndrome and those receiving chemotherapy or radiation therapy *(139)* because of reports that GH may aid the adaptive response of the gastrointestinal tract to these conditions *(140,141)*.

BRANCHED-CHAIN AMINO ACIDS

In the 1970s and 1980s, much attention focused on the use of branched-chain amino acids (BCAA) in postoperative and critically ill patients. BCAA (leucine, isoleucine, and valine) are useful in theory because they stimulate protein synthesis and decrease protein degradation in liver and muscle, they can be oxidized peripherally for use as a fuel source, and they may serve as a substrate for gluconeogenesis *(142)*. BCAA are the only essential amino acids oxidized primarily in skeletal muscle and may prevent muscle protein wasting in the stressed state. The effects of BCAA are seen primarily in growing animals *(143)* and few data in mature animals exist.

In 1986, a symposium on the use of BCAA in injured patients was conducted and the results published *(143)*. The participants concluded that BCAA-enriched solutions lessened the caloric requirements needed to maintain nitrogen balance in animal studies. In human clinical studies, modest improvements in nitrogen metabolism parameters were seen in critically ill patients, but no major effect on outcome were seen in any group of patients. Since that time, there has been little interest in the use of BCAA-enriched nutrition regimens in the perioperative period. One animal study *(144)* showed that BCAA may reduce postoperative jejunal atrophy by increasing skeletal muscle glutamine release and intestinal glutaminase activity. A recent study in ICU patients *(142)* did show a decrease in mortality and improvements in nutritional parameters with a BCAA-enriched solution. However, most surgical nutrition researchers believe that BCAA-enriched solutions (usually 45% BCAA) offer no advantage compared to standard amino acid solutions (10–25% BCAA).

"IMMUNE-ENHANCING" FORMULAS

The increasing body of literature on the beneficial immune effects of arginine, ω-3 fatty acids, and nucleotides as dietary supplements led to the commercial development of so-called "immune-enhancing" enteral formulas containing various combinations of all three substances. Of these, the most widely studied has been Impact (Sandoz Nutrition, Basel, Switzerland), which has served as the experimental formula in at least eight human clinical trials. In these trials, Impact was shown to affect a number of immunological and physiological parameters. Senkal et al. *(145)* demonstrated that patients undergoing surgery for upper gastrointestinal cancer who were given enteral Impact did not have the increased IL-6 and TNF-α that patients given an isocaloric, isonitrogenous control diet did. This implies that Impact may attenuate the acute-phase response and decrease systemic inflammation. In the same study, patients given Impact showed mild increases in IL-2 and IL-2 receptors, which, in turn, may augment T-cell function. Schilling et al. *(146)* found that Impact patients had higher CD8+ cell count, lower CD3+ cell levels, and a lower percentage of DR+ monnocytes, macrophages, and lymphocytes when compared to patients given a relatively hypocaloric TPN solutions. The significance of these findings is unknown. Increased activated T-cell and helper T-cell levels were found in a third study *(147)*, which also showed mild increases in serum IgG and IgM. Braga and colleagues demonstrated increased small-bowel and colon microperfusion in patients given Impact perioperatively *(148)*. The same patients also had improved phagocytosis and polymorphonuclear cell respiratory burst activity and a lesser increase in C-reactive protein compared to controls.

Impact has been shown to decrease length of stay (LOS) in four studies *(146,149–151)*. However, statistical significance was not reached in one *(146)*, the control diet contained less protein and calories in another *(149)*, and in a third, it was only seen in a subgroups after a complex *post hoc* analysis *(150)*. The most promising Impact trial to date in terms of clinical outcome was conducted by Daly in upper gastrointestinal cancer patients *(151)*. In this series, patients given Impact had a significantly shorter length of stay (16 vs 22 d, $p < 0.05$) and lower rate of infection (10% vs 43%, $p < 0.05$) than control patients given a similar diet (Traumacal, Mead Johnson, Evansville, IN). A later study of burn patients *(152)* found no improvement in mortality, length of stay, or complication rate with Impact. This study is difficult to interpret because the control diet (Replete) contains ω-3 fatty acids and glutamine and, thus, may also be considered to be immunostimulatory. Finally, a large (*n* = 195) study in upper GI cancer patients found that patients given Impact beginning on postoperative day 1 did not have a better outcome than those who were given intravenous fluids only *(48)*.

Other "immune-enhancing" diets have been studied to a lesser extent. In a multicenter PCRT, Moore et al. *(153)* found that patients sustaining major torso trauma who were supplemented with Immun-Aid (which contains glutamine, arginine, nucleic acids, and N-3 fatty acids) had significantly fewer intraabdominal abscesses and multiple organ failure than patients given the control formula (Vivonex T.E.N.). In a study of burn patients fed with an experimental diet containing arginine and N-3 fatty acids, Gottschlich et al. *(154)* reported reduced wound infection rates and LOS/% burn ratio compared to patients fed with Osmolite (Ross Products, Columbus, OH) or Traumacal (which were both modified to make them isocaloric and isonitrogenous to the experimental formula). It should be noted that these two trials involved highly stressed trauma and burn patients, who may be expected to derive the greatest benefit from immune-enhancing diets. Success was lower in trials involving patients undergoing gastrointestinal cancer surgery *(145–149,151)*, in which the catabolic response is not as great.

These diets are particularly challenging to study, because they contain multiple immune-modulating agents. It is, therefore, difficult to elaborate the mechanisms for any immunological effects seen. In addition, the clinical effects have been varied. Currently, no definitive conclusions can be made regarding the use of these formulations *(103)*. However, "immune-enhancing" diets remain a promising and active area of research and it is to be hoped that a greater understanding of the specific effects of the various supplemental nutrients will clarify the role of these diets in clinical surgical practice.

RECOMMENDATIONS

In 1997, the most recent recommendations of a consensus conference of the National Institutes of Health, the American Society for Parenteral and Enteral Nutrition, and the American Society for Clinical Nutrition concerning the use of nutrition support in clinical practice were published *(103)*. The committee members concluded that there was no conclusive data to support the hypothesis that nutrition support is beneficial in critically ill patients. The rationale for nutritional support is, therefore, based more on clinical judgment than on randomized clinical trials. It is generally agreed that a critical depletion of lean body mass occurs after 14 d of starvation and that nutrition support should be initiated in patients who are not likely to resume oral feeding within 7–10 d *(103)*. The majority of such patients are readily identified by the clinician, and nutritional support should be initiated promptly to avoid protein depletion.

In severely malnourished patients who cannot tolerate an oral diet, a course of preoperative TPN may decrease postoperative complications *(25)*. The final decision for or against the use of preoperative TPN requires a clinical judgment in which the urgency of the operation, the severity of the existing malnutrition, and the expected delay until oral intake are all considered. If nutritional support is initiated before surgery, it should be continued into the postoperative period until adequate oral intake has been achieved. Most patients who receive 10 d or fewer of preoperative TPN do not replace protein stores enough to significantly improve function, and further work is needed to determine if a longer course of preoperative nutritional support is beneficial. Home enteral nutrition may be useful in this regard as a means to avoid lengthy hospitalization for the sole purpose of receiving preoperative TPN.

With the possible exception of severely traumatized patients *(46,49)*, the routine use of postoperative nutritional support in individuals expected to resume oral intake in less than 7 d has not been shown to be beneficial. Mildly or moderately malnourished patients who experience uncomplicated recovery do not seem to benefit from current postoperative nutrition support regimens. However, preliminary evidence indicates that such a benefit may be seen in severely malnourished patients *(25,41,42)*. These studies were not specifically designed to address this issue, and further trials will be necessary for confirmation.

Once the decision to provide postoperative nutrition support to a patient has been made, the clinician must then determine whether the nutrients should be given enterally or parenterally. Enteral nutrition is the preferred method of delivery because it is believed to be safer, less expensive, and more physiologic compared to TPN. It is also thought to promote gastrointestinal function and morphology and improve clinical outcome, although this has been questioned *(155)*. A nasogastric or nasojejunal feeding tube may be appropriate for patients requiring only short-term enteral access. For those requiring long-term access, feeding tubes may be introduced into the stomach or jejunum directly through the abdominal wall either at operation or postoperatively by a variety of methods *(156)*.

The specific benefits of enteral as opposed to parenteral nutrition in perioperative patients are not dependent on the provision of full nutrient support in the short term. During the first week of postoperative therapy, support of gut integrity appears to predominate over the necessity for full nutrient provision. Also, repletion of enzymes for digestion and absorption may take several days. Thus, enteral nutrition should be provided and feedings should be advanced only as tolerated. Patients should be monitored for evidence of abdominal pain, distention, and diarrhea. Aggressive enteral feeding also markedly increases blood flow to the gut, and blood volume and cardiac output must be maximized to avoid gut ischemia *(157)*.

Paralytic ileus involving the entire gastrointestinal tract is common among severely stressed patients. Enteral feeding is not tolerated or beneficial in such patients. When enteral access is unavailable or contraindicated, intravenous access must be obtained for TPN. This will typically require inserting a central venous catheter, although, in some cases, nutrients can be administered via peripheral veins, especially if the interval of postoperative nutrition therapy is expected to be fewer than 7 d. Overfeeding may be detrimental in TPN patients *(25,158)* and hyperglycemia (>200 mg/dL) in particular should be avoided due to its immunosuppressive effects *(38a,75,77,159)*. The transition to oral or enteral intake if TPN has been required is an immediate goal in all patients.

Determining the optimal amount and composition of formula to be used in the nutritional support of a given patient is a complex task. The clinician must make this decision based on a variety of factors, such as the nature and severity of illness, underlying nutritional status, cost, and availability. Because these issues have not been explored in a rigorous scientific fashion, the selection of a particular formula is usually governed by the experience and preferences of individual clinicians or institutions.

It must be emphasized that the principles which govern the current practice of perioperative nutritional support are not static but, instead, are constantly changing as new information becomes available. It is possible that the outcomes of many of the older perioperative nutrition support trials would be different if they were repeated using current standards *(103)*. Further studies are needed to determine which subgroups of patients benefit most from perioperative feeding. The potential of specific nutrients such as glutamine, arginine, N-3 fatty acids, and growth hormone to improve outcome must also be explored.

REFERENCES

1. Chernow B, Alexander R, Smallridge RC, et al. Hormonal responses to graded surgical stress. Arch Intern Med 1987; 147:1273–8.
2. Halter JB, Pflug AE, Porte D. Mechanism of plasma catecholamine increases during surgical stress in man. J Clin Endocrinol Metab 1977; 45:936–44.
3. Moore FD. Metabolic Care of the Surgical Patient. WB Saunders, Philadelphia, 1959.
4. Nygren J. Site of insulin resistance after surgery: the contribution of hypocaloric nutrition and bed rest. Clin Sci 1997; 93:137–46.
5. Chang HR, Bistrian B. The role of cytokines in the catabolic consequences of infection and injury. JPEN 1998; 22:156–66.
6. Faist E, Baue AE. Post-injury immunoregulation. In: Feliciano DV, Moore EE, Mattox KL, eds, Trauma, 3rd ed, pp. 1193–1203, Appleton & Lange, Stamford, CT, 1996.
7. Christou NV, MacLean AP, Meakins JL. Host defense in blunt trauma: interrelationships of kinetics of anergy and depressed neutrophil function, nutritional status, and sepsis. J Trauma 1980; 20:833–41.
8. Baker CC, Huynh T. Immunologic response to injury. In: Feliciano DV, Moore EE, Mattox KL, eds, Trauma, 3rd ed, pp. 1177–93. Appleton & Lange, Stamford, CT, 1996.
9. Redmond HP, Hofmann K, Shou J, Leon P, Kelly CJ, Daly JM. Effects of laparotomy on systemic macrophage function. Surgery 1992; 111:647–55.
10. Faist E, Mewes A, Baker CC, Strasser T. Prostaglandin E2 (PGE2) dependent suppression of IL-2 production in patients with major trauma. J Trauma 1987; 27:837–48.
11. Faist E, Mewes A, Strasser TH, et al. Alteration of monocyte function following major injury. Arch Surg 1988; 123:287–92.
12. Christou NV, Meakins JL, Gordon J. The delayed type hypersensitivity response and host resistance in surgical patients: 20 years later. Ann Surg 1995; 222:534–48.
13. Faist E, Ertel W, Baker CC, Heberer G. Terminal B-cell maturation and immunoglobulin synthesis in vitro in patients with major injury. J Trauma 1989; 29:2–9.
14. Halasz NA, Orloff MJ, Hirose F. Increased survival of renal homografts in dogs after injection of graft donor blood. Transplantation 1964; 2:453–8.
15. Blumberg N, Heal JM. Effect of transfusion on immune function: cancer recurrence and infection. Arch Pathol Lab Med 1994; 118:371–9.
16. Jensen LS, Andersen AJ, Christiansen PM, et al. Postoperative infection and natural killer cell function following blood transfusion in patients undergoing elective colorectal surgery. Br J Surg 1992; 79:513–6.
17. Kurz A, Sessler DI, Lenhardt R, et al. Perioperative normothermia to reduce the incidence of surgical-wound infections and shorten hospitalization. N Engl J Med 1996; 334:1209–15.
18. Roizen MF, Levy JH, Moss J. Immune responses and hypersensitivity reactions during anesthesia. In: Physiologic and Pharmacologic Bases of Anesthesia, pp. 345–60. William & Wilkins, Baltimore, MD, 1996.
19. Studley HO. Percentage weight loss: a basic indicator of surgical risk in patients with chronic peptic ulcer. JAMA 1936; 106:458–60.
20. Cannon PR, Wissler RW, Woolridge RL, Benditt EP. The relationship of protein deficiency to surgical infection. Ann Surg 1994; 120:514–25.
21. Rhoads JE, Alexander CE. Nutritional problems of surgical patients. Ann NY Acad Sci 1955; 63:269–75.
22. Seltzer MH, Bastidias JA, Cooper DM, Engler PE, Slocum B, Fletcher HS. Instant nutritional assessment. JPEN 1979; 3:157–9.
23. Reinhardt GF, Myscofski JW, Wilkens DB, Dobrin PB, Mangan

JE, Stannard RT. Incidence and mortality of hypoalbuminemic patients in hospitalized veterans. JPEN 1980; 4:357–9.

24. Bistrian BR, Blackburn GL, Hallowell E, Heddle R. Protein status of general surgical patients. JAMA 1974; 230:858–60.

25. The Veterans Affairs Total Parenteral Nutrition Cooperative Study Group. Perioperative total parenteral nutrition in surgical patients. N Engl J Med 1991; 325:525–32.

26. Hickman DM, Miller RA, Rombeau JL, et al. Serum albumin and body weight as predictors of postoperative course in colorectal cancer. JPEN 1980; 4:314–6.

27. Shaw-Stiffel TA, Zarny LA, Pleban WE, Rosman DD, Rudolph RA, Bernstein LH. Effect of nutrition status and other factors on length of hospital stay after major gastrointestinal surgery. Nutrition 1993; 9:140–5.

28. Dempsey DT, Mullen JL, Buzby GP. The link between nutritional status and clinical outcome: can nutritional intervention modify it? Am J Clin Nutr 1988; 47:352–6.

29. Christou NV. Host defense mechanisms in surgical patients: a correlative study of the delayed hypersensitivity skin test response, granulocyte function and sepsis in 2202 patients. Can J Surg 1985; 28:39–49.

30. Christou NV, Tellado-Rodriguez J, Chartrand L, et al. Estimating mortality risk in preoperative patients using immunologic, nutritional, and acute-phase response variables. Ann Surg 1989; 210:69–77.

31. Buzby GP, Mullen J, Matthews DC, Hobbs CL, Rosato EF. Prognostic nutritional index in gastrointestinal surgery. Am J Surg 1980; 139:160–6.

32. Katelaris PH, Bennett GB, Smith RC. Prediction of postoperative complications by clinical and nutritional assessment. Aust NZ J Surg 1986; 56:743–7.

33. Tellado JM, Garcia-Sabrido JL, Hanley JA, Shizgal HM, Christou NV. Predicting mortality based on body composition analysis. Ann Surg 1989; 209:81–7.

34. Smith RC, Hartemink R. Improvement of nutritional measures during preoperative parenteral nutrition in patients selected by the prognostic nutritional index: a randomized controlled trial. JPEN 1988; 12:587–91.

35. Baker JP, Detsky AS, Wesson DE, et al. Nutritional assessment: a comparison of clinical judgment and objective measurements. N Engl J Med 1982; 306:969–72.

36. Detsky AS, Baker JP, O'Rourke K, et al. Predicting nutrition associated complications for patients undergoing gastrointestinal surgery. JPEN 1987; 11:440–5.

37. Dudrick SJ, Wilmore DW, Vars HM, Rhaods JE. Long term total parenteral nutrition with growth, development, and positive nitrogen balance. Surgery 1968; 64:134–42.

38. Muller JM, Brenner U, Dienst C, Pichlmaier H. Preoperative parenteral feeding in patients with gastrointestinal carcinoma. Lancet 1982; 1:68–71.

38a. Kwoun MO, Ling PR, Lydon E, et al. Immunologic effects of acute hyperglycemia in nondiabetic rats. JPEN 1997; 21:91–5.

39. Ziegler TR, Young LS, Benfell K, et al. Clinical and metabolic efficacy of glutamine-supplemented parenteral nutrition after bone marrow transplantation. Ann Intern Med 1992; 116:821–8.

40. Brennan MF, Pisters PW, Posner M, Quesada O, Shike M. A prospective randomized trial of total parenteral nutrition after major pancreatic resection for malignancy. Ann Surg 1994; 220:436–44.

41. Fan ST, Lo CM, Lai EC, Chu KM, Liu CL, Wong J. Perioperative nutritional support in patients undergoing hepatectomy for hepatocellular carcinoma. N Engl J Med 1994; 331:1547–52.

42. Sandstrom R, Drott C, Hyltander A, et al. The effect of postoperative intravenous feeding (TPN) on outcome following major surgery evaluated in a randomized study. Ann Surg 1993; 217:185–95.

43. Hoover HC, Ryan JA, Anderson EJ, Fischer JE. Nutritional benefits of immediate postoperative jejunal feeding of an elemental diet. Am J Surg 1980; 139:153–9.

44. Grimm H, Tibell A, Norrlind B, Blecher C, Wilker S, Scwemmle K. Immunoregulation by parenteral lipids: impact of the n-3 to n-6 fatty acid ratio. JPEN 1994; 18:417–21.

45. Moore EE, Moore FA. Immediate enteral nutrition following multisystem trauma: a decade perspective. J Am Coll Nutr 1991; 10(6):633–48.

46. Vara-Thorbeck R, Guerrero JA, Rosell J, Ruiz-Requena E, Capitan LM. Exogenous growth hormone: effects on the catabolic response to surgically produced acute stress and on postoperative immune function. World J Surg 1993; 17:530–8.

47. Carr C, Ling EK, Boulos P, Singer M. Randomised trial of safety and efficacy of immediate postoperative enteral feeding in patients undergoing gastrointestinall resection. Br Med J 1996; 312:869–71.

48. Heslin MJ, Latkany L, Leung D, et al. A prospective, randomized trial of early enteral feeding after resection of upper gastrointestinal malignancy. Ann Surg 1997; 226:567–80.

49. Moore FA, Moore EE, Jones TN, McCroskey BL, Peterson VM. TEN versus TPN following major abdominal trauma-reduced septic morbidity. J Trauma 1989; 29:916–22.

50. Kudsk KA, Croce MA, Fabian TC, et al. Enteral versus parenteral feeding-effects on septic morbidity after blunt and penetrating abdominal trauma. Ann Surg 1992; 215:503–11.

51. Moore FA, Feliciano DV, Andrassy RJ, et al. Early enteral feeding, compared with parenteral, reduces postoperative septic complications—the results of a meta-analysis. Ann Surg 1992; 216:172–83.

52. Hosoda N, Nishi M, Nakagawa M, et al. Structurall and functional alterations in the gut of parenterally and enterally fed rats. J Surg Res 1989; 47:129–33.

53. Levine GM, Deren JJ, Steiger E, et al. Role of oral intake in maintenance of gut mass and disaccharide activity. Gastroenterology 1974; 67:975–82.

54. van der Hulst RR, van Kreel BK, von Meyenfeldt MF, et al. Glutamine and the preservation of gut integrity. Lancet 1993; 341:1363–5.

55. Guedon C, Schmitz J, Lerebours E, et al. Decreased brush border hydrolase activities without gross morphologic changes in human intestinal mucosa after prolonged total parenteral nutrition of adults. Gastroenterology 1986; 90:373–8.

56. Inoue Y, Espat NJ, Fronhapple DJ, Epstein H, Copeland EM, Souba WW. Effect of total parenteral nutrition on amino acid and glucose transport by the human small intestine. Ann Surg 1993; 217:604–14.

57. Li J, Langkamp-Henken B, Suzuki K, Stahlgren LH. Glutamine prevents parenteral nutrition-induces increases in intestinal permeability. JPEN 1994; 18:303–7.

58. Reynolds JV, Kanwar S, Welsh FK, et al. Does the route of feeding modify gut barrier function and clinical outcome in patients after major upper gastrointestinal surgery? JPEN 1997; 21:196–201.

59. Shou J, Lappin J, Daly JM. Impairment of pulmonary macrophage function with total parenteral nutrition. Ann Surg 1994; 219:291–7.

60. Shou J, Lappin J, Minnard EA, Daly JM. Total parenteral nutrition, bacterial translocation, and host immune function. Am J Surg 1994; 167:145–50.

61. Alverdy JC, Aoys E, Moss G. Total parenteral nutrition promotes bacterial translocation from the gut. Surgery 1988; 104:185–90.

62. Deitch EA. Bacterial translocation of the gut flora. J Trauma 1990; 30:S184–9.

63. Mainous M, Xu D, Lu Q, Berg RD, Deitch EA. Oral-TPN-induced bacterial translocation and impaired immune defenses are reversed by refeeding. Surgery 1991; 110:277–84.

64. Alverdy JA, Aoys E, Weiss-Carrington P, Burke DA. The effect of glutamine-enriched TPN on gut immune cellularity. J Surg Res 1992; 52:34–8.

65. Maderazo EG, Woronick CL, Quercia RA, et al. The inhibitory effect of parenteral nutrition on recovery of neutrophil locomotory function in blunt trauma. Ann Surg 1988; 208:221–6.

66. Lin MT, Saito H, Fukushima R, et al. Route of nutritional supply influences local, systemic, and remote organ responses to intraperitoneal bacterial challenge. Ann Surg 1996; 223:84–93.

67. King BK, Li J, Kudsk KA. A temporal study of TPN-induced changes in gut-associated lymphoid tissue and mucosal immunity. Arch Surg 1997; 132:1303–9.

68. Janu P, Li J, Renegar KB, Kudsk KA. Recovery of gut-associated lymphoid tissue and upper respiratory tract immunity after parenteral nutrition. Ann Surg 1997; 225:707–17.

69. Kudsk KA, Li J, Renegar KB. Loss of upper respiratory tract immunity with parenteral feeding. Ann Surg 1996; 223:629–38.

70. Li J, Kudsk KA, Hamidian M, Gocinski BL. Bombesin affects mucosal immunity and gut-associated lymphoid tissue in intravenously fed mice. Arch Surg 1995; 130:1164–70.

71. Nygren J, Thorell A, Efendic S, Nair KS, Ljungqvist O. Site of insulin resistance after surgery: the contribution of hypocaloric nutrition and bed rest. Clin Sci 1997; 93:137–46.

72. Thorell A, Efendic S, Gutniak M, Haggmark T, Ljungqvist O. Insulin resistance after abdominal surgery. Br J Surg 1994; 81:593–9.

73. Rosmarin DK, Wardlaw GM, Mirtallo J. Hyperglycemia associated with high, continuous infusion rates of total parenteral nutrition dextrose. Nutr Clin Pract 1996; 11:151–6.

74. Silberman H. Parenteral nutrition: nonnutritional effects and metabolic complications. In: Parenteral and Enteral Nutrition, 2nd ed, pp. 304–20. Appleton & Lange, Norwalk, CT, 1989.

75. Black CT, Hennessey PJ, Andrassy RJ. Short-term hyperglycemia depresses immunity through nonenzymatic glycosylation of circulating immunoglobulin. J Trauma 1990; 30:830–2.

76. Hennessey PJ, Black CT, Andrassy RJ. Nonenzymatic glycosylation of immunogobulin G impairs complement fixation. JPEN 1991; 15:60–4.

77. Hostetter MK. Effects of hyperglycemia on C3 and Candida albicans. Diabetes 1990; 39:271–5.

78. Krebs H. Glutamine metabolism in the animal body. In: Mora J, Palacio R, eds, Gutamine: Metabolism, Enzymology, and Regulation, pp. 1–40. Academic, New York, 1980.

79. Ardawi MS, Newshome EA. Glutamine metabolism in lymphocytes of the rat. Biochem J 1982; 208:743–8.

80. Hong RW, Rounds JD, Helton WS, Robinson MK, Wilmore DW. Glutamine preserves liver glutathione after lethal hepatic injury. Ann Surg 1992; 215:114–9.

81. Yamaguchi T, Minor T, Isselhard W. Effect of glutamine or glucagon-insulin enriched total parenteral nutrition on liver and gut in 70% hepatectomized rats with colon stenosis. J Am Coll Surg 1997; 185:156–62.

82. Souba WW, Herskowitz K, Plumley DA. Lung glutamine metabolism. JPEN 1990; 14:68S–70S.

83. Souba WW, Wilmore DW. Postoperative alteration of arteriovenous exchange of amino acids across the gastrointestinal tract. Surgery 1983; 94:342–50.

84. Souba WW, Smith RJ, Wilmore DW. Effect of glucocorticoids on glutamine metabolism in visceral organs. Metabolism 1985; 34:450–6.

85. Fox AD, Kripke SA, Berman JM, et al. Dexamethasone administration induces increased glutaminase activity in jejunum and colon. J Surg Res 1988; 44:391–6.

86. Kandil HM, Argenzio RA, Chen W, et al. L-Glutamine and L-asparagine stimulates ODC activity and proliferation in a porcine jejunal enterocyte line. Am J Physiol 1995; 269:G591–9.

87. Windmueller HG. Glutamine utilization by the small intestine. Adv Enzymol 1982; 53:202–37.

88. Baskerville A, Hambleton P, Benbough JE. Pathologic features of gutaminase toxicity. Br J Exp Pathol 1980; 61:132–8.

89. Souba WW, Klimberg VS, Hautamaki RD, et al. Oral glutamine reduces bacterial translocation following abdominal radiation. J Surg Res 1990; 48:1–5.

90. O'Dwyer ST, Smith RJ, Hwang TL, Wilmore DW. Maintenance of small bowel mucosa with glutamine-enriched parenteral nutrition. JPEN 1985; 9:579–85.

91. Furukawa S, Saito H, Inaba T, et al. Glutamine-enriched enteral diet enhances bacterial clearance in protracted bacterial peritonitis, regardless of glutamine form. JPEN 1997; 21:208–14.

92. Manzurul Haque SM, Chen K, Usui N, et al. Alanyl-glutamine dipeptide-supplemented parenteral nutrition improves intestinal metabolism and prevents increases permeability in rats. Ann Surg 1996; 223:334–41.

93. Jiang Z-M, Wang L-J, Qi Y, et al. Comparison of parenteral nutrition supplemented with L-glutamine or glutamine dipeptides. JPEN 1993; 17:134–41.

94. Inoue Y, Grant JP, Snyder PJ. Effect of glutamine-supplemented intravenous nutrition on survival after Escherichia coli-induced peritonitis. JPEN 1993; 17:41–6.

95. van der Hulst RR, van Kreel BK, von Meyenfeldt MF, et al. Glutamine and the preservation of gut integrity. Lancet 1993; 334:1363–5.

96. Alverdy JA, Aoys E, Weiss-Carrington P, Burke DA. The effect of glutamine-enriched TPN on gut immune cellularity. J Surg Res 1992; 52:34–8.

97. Burke DJ, Alverdy JC, Moss GS. Glutamine-supplemented total parenteral nutrition improves gut immune function. Arch Surg 1989; 124:1396–9.

98. O'Riordain MG, Fearon KC, Ross JA, et al. Glutamine-supplemented total parenteral nutrition enhances T-lymphocytes response in surgical patients undergoing colorectal resection. Ann Surg 1994; 220:212–21.

99. Smith RJ. Glutamine-supplemented nutrition. JPEN 1997; 21:183–4.

100. Ziegler TR, Young LS. Therapeutic effects of specific nutrients. In: Rombeau JL, Rolandelli RH, eds, Clinical Nutrition: Enteral and Tube Feeding, 3rd ed, pp. 112–38. WB Saunders, Philadelphia, 1997.

101. Schloerb PR, Amare M. Total parenteral nutrition with glutamine in bone marrow transplantation and other clinical applications (a randomized, double-blind study. JPEN 1993; 17:407–13.

102. Griffiths RD, Jones C, Palmer TEA. Six month outcome of critically ill patients given glutamine supplemented parenteral nutrition. Nutrition 1997; 13:295–302.

103. Klein S, Kinney J, Jeebjeebhoy K, et al. Nutrition support in clinical practice: review of published data and recommendations for future research directions. JPEN 1997; 21:133–56.

104. Merimee TJ, Rabinowitz D, Riggs L, Burgess JA, Rimoin DL, McKusick VA. Plasma growth hormone after arginine infusion. N Engl J Med 1967; 276:434–8.

105. Hebiguchi T, Yoshino H, Mizuno M, Koyama K. The effect of arginine supplementation on growth hormone release and intestinal mucosal growth after massive small bowel resection in growing rats. J Ped Surg 1997; 32:1149–53.

106. Floyd JC, Fajans SS, Conn JW, Knopf RF, Rull J. Stimulation of insulin secretion by amino acids. J Clin Invest 1966; 45:1487–1502.

107. Barbul A, Arginine: biochemistry, physiology, and therapeutic implications. JPEN 1986; 10:227–38.

108. Nirgiotis JG, Hennessey PJ, Andrassy RJ. The effects of an arginine-free enteral diet on wound healing and immune function in the postsurgical rat. J Ped Surg 1991; 26:936–41.

109. Barbul A, Wasserkrug HL, Seifter E, Rettura G, Levenson SM, Efron G. Immunostimulatory effects of arginine in normal and injured rats. J Surg Res 1908; 29:228–35.

110. Barbul A, Lazarou SA, Efron DT, Wasserkrug HL, Efron G. Arginine enhances wound healing and lymphocyte immune responses in humans. Surgery 1990; 108:331–7.

111. Barbul A, Sino DA, Wasserkrug HL, Efron G. Arginine stimulates lymphocyte immune response in healthy human beings. Surgery 1981; 90:244–50.

112. Daly JM, Reynolds J, Thom A, Kinsley L, Deitrick-Gallagher M, Shou J, et al. Immune and metabolic effects of arginine in the surgical patient. Ann Surg 1988; 208:512–21.

113. Reynolds JV, Daly JM, Zhang S, et al. Immunomodulatory mechanisms of arginine. Surgery 1988; 104:142–51.

114. Chyun J-H, Griminger P. Improvement of nitrogen retention by arginine and glycine supplementation and its relation to collagen synthesis in traumatized mature and aged rats. J Nutr 1984; 114:1697–1704.

115. Kirk SJ, Hurson M, Regan MC, Holt DR, Wasserkrug HL, Barbul A. Arginine stimulates wound healing and immune function in elderly human beings. Surgery 1993; 114:155–60.

116. Barbul A. Arginine: biochemistry, physiology, and therapeutic implications. JPEN 1986; 10:227–38.

117. Elsair J, Poey J, Issad H, et al. Effect of arginine chlorhydrate on nitrogen balance during the three days following routine surgery in man. Biomedicine 1978; 29:312–7.

118. Saito H, Trocki O, Liang S-L, et al. Metabolic and immune effects of supplemental arginine after burn. Arch Surg 1987; 122:784–9.

119. Gianotti L, Alexander JW, Pyles T, Fukushima R. Arginine-supplemented diets improve survival in gut-derived sepsis and peritonitis by modulating bacterial clearance: the role of nitric oxide. Ann Surg 1993; 217:644–54.

120. Gonce SJ, Peck MD, Alexander JW, Miskell PW. Arginine supplementation and its effect on established peritonitis in guinea pigs. JPEN 1990; 14:237–44.

121. Walker C, Kristensen F, Bettens F, DeWeck AL. Lymphokine regulation of activated (G1) lymphocytes. 1. Prostaglandin E2-induced inhibition of interleukin-2 production. J Immunol 1983; 130:1770–3.

122. Goodwin JS, Cueppens J. Regulation of the immune response by prostaglandins. J Clin Immunol 1983; 3:295–310.

123. Merlin J. Omega-6 and omega-3 polyunsaturates and the immune system. Br J Clin Pract 1984; 31(suppl):111–4.

124. Lee TH, Hoover RL, Williams JD, et al. Effect of dietary enrichment with eicosapentaenoic and docosahexaenoic acids on in vitro neutrophil and monocyte leukotriene generation and neutrophil function. N Engl J Med 1985; 312:1217–24.

125. Endres S, Ghorbani R, Kelley VE. The effect of dietary supplementation with n-3 polyunsaturated fatty acids on the synthesis of interleukin-1 and tumor necrosis factor by mononuclear cells. N Engl J Med 1989; 320:265–71.

126. Wachtler P, Konig W, Senkal M, Kemen M, Koller M. Influence of a total parenteral nutrition enriched with omega-3 fatty acids on leukotriene synthesis of peripheral leukocytes and systemic cytokine levels in patients with major surgery. J Trauma 1997; 42:191–8.

127. Alexander JW, Saito H, Ogle CK, Trocki O. The importance of lipid type in the diet after burn injury. Ann Surg 1986; 204:1–7.

128. Johnson JA, Griswold JA, Muakkassa FF. Essential fatty acids influence survival in sepsis. J Trauma 1993; 35:128–31.

129. Blok WL, Vogels MT, Curfs JH, Eling WM, Buurman WA, van der Meer JW. Dietary fish-oil supplementation in experimental gram-negative infection and in cerebral malaria in mice. J Infect Dis 1992; 165:898–903.

130. Kenler AS, Swails WS, Driscoll DF, et al. Early enteral feeding in postsurgical cancer patients: fish oil structured lipid-based polymeric formula versus a standard polymeric formula. Ann Surg 1996; 223:316–33.

131. Manson JMcK, Wilmore DW. Positive nitrogen balance with human growth hormone and hypocaloric intravenous feeding. Surgery 1986; 100:188–97.

132. Hammarqvist F, Stromberg C, von der Decken A, Vinnars E, Wernerman J. Biosynthetic human growth hormone preserves both muscle protein synthesis and the decrease in muscle-free glutamine, and improves whole-body nitrogen economy after operation. Ann Surg 1992; 216:184–91.

133. Jiang Z-M, He G-Z, Zhang S-Y, et al. Low-dose growth hormone and hypocaloric nutrition attenuate the protein-catabolic response after major operation. Ann Surg 1989; 210:513–25.

134. Ward HC, Halliday D, Sim AJ. Protein and energy metabolism with biosynthetic human growth hormone after gastrointestinal surgery. 1987; 206:56–61.

135. Ziegler TR, Rombeau JL, Young S, et al. Recombinant human growth hormone enhances the metabolic efficacy of parenteral nutrition: a double-blind, randomized controlled study. J Clin Endocrinol Metab 1992; 74:865–73.

136. Byrne TA, Morrissey TB, Gatzen C, et al. Anabolic therapy with growth hormone accelerates protein gain in surgical patients requiring nutritional rehabilitation. Ann Surg 1993; 218:400–18.

137. Knox JB, Demling RH, Wilmore DW. Hypercalcemia associated with the use of human growth hormone in an adult surgical intensive care unit. Arch Surg 1995; 130:442–5.

138. Pharmacia & Upjohn. *Drug Warning,* 1997.

139. Wilmore DW. Metabolic support of the gastrointestinal tract. Cancer 1997; 79:1794–1803.

140. Inoue Y, Copeland EM, Souba WW. Growth hormone enhances amino acid uptake by the human small intestine. Ann Surg 1994; 219:715–24.

141. Ziegler TR, Mantell MP, Chow JC, Rombeau JL, Smith RJ. Gut adaptation and the insulin-like growth factor system: regulation by glutamine and IGF-I administration. Am J Physiol 1996; 271:G866–75.

142. Garcia-de-Lorenzo A, Ortiz-Leyba C, Planas M, et al. Parenteral administration of different amounts of branch-chain amino acids in septic patients: clinical and metabolic aspects. Crit Care Med 1997; 25:418–24.

143. Brennan MF, Cerra F, Daly JM, et al. Report of a research workshop: branched-chain amino acids in stress and injury. JPEN 1986; 10:446–53.

144. McCauley RD, Heel KA, Hall JC. Enteral branched-chain amino acids increase the specific activity of jejuna glutaminase and reduce intestinal atrophy. J Gastroenterol Hepatol 1997; 12:429–33.

145. Senkal M, Kemen M, Homan HH, Eickhoff U, Baier J, Zumtobel V. Modulation of postoperative immune response by enteral nutrition with a diet enriched by arginine, RNA, and omega-3 fatty acids in patients with upper gastrointestinal cancer. Eur J Surg 1995; 161:115–22.

146. Schilling J, Vranjes N, Fierz W, et al. Clinical outcome and immunology of postoperative arginine, omega-3 fatty acids, and nucleotide-enriched enteral feeding: a randomized prospective comparison with standard enteral and low calorie/low fat IV solutions. Nutrition 1996; 12:423–9.

147. Kemen M, Senkal M, Homan HH, et al. Early postoperative enteral nutrition with arginine–omega-3 fatty acids and ribonucleic acid-supplemented diet versus placebo in cancer patients: an immunologic evaluation of Impact. Crit Care Med 1995; 23:652–9.

148. Braga M, Gianotti L, Cestari A, et al. Gut function and immune and inflammatory responses in patients perioperatively fed with supplemented enteral formulas. Arch Surg 1996; 131:1257–65.

149. Daly JM, Lieberman MD, Goldfine J, et al. Enteral nutrition with supplemental arginine, RNA, and omega-3 fatty acids in patients after operation: immunologic, metabolic, and clinical outcome. Surgery 1992; 112:56–67.

150. Bower GH, Cerra FB, Bershadksy B, et al. Early enteral administration of a formula (Impact) supplemented with arginine, nucleotides, and fish oil in intensive care unit patients: results of a multicenter, prospective, randomized clinical trial. Crit Care Med 1995; 23:436–49.

151. Daly JM, Weintraub FN, Shou J, Rosato EF, Lucia M. Enteral nutrition during multimodality therapy in upper gastrointestinal cancer patients. Ann Surg 1995; 221:327–38.

152. Saffle JR, Wiebke G, Jennings K, Morris SE, Barton RG. Randomized trial of immune-enhancing enteral nutrition in burned patients. J Trauma 42:793–800.

153. Moore FA, Moore EE, Kudsk KA, et al. Clinical benefits of an immune-enhancing diet for early postinjury enteral feeding. J Trauma 1994; 37:607–15.

154. Gottschlich MM, Jenkins M, Warden GD, et al. Differential effects of three enteral dietary regimens on selected outcome variables in burn patients. JPEN 1990; 14:225–36.

155. Lipman TO. Grains or veins: is enteral nutrition really better than parenteral nutrition? A look at the evidence. JPEN 1998; 22:167–82.

156. Marks JM, Ponsky JL. Access routes for enteral nutrition. Gastroenterologist 1995; 3:130–40.

157. Smith-Choban P, Max MH. Feeding jejunostomy: a small bowel stress test? Am J Surg 1988; 155:112–7.

158. Wolfe BM, Mathiesen KA. Clinical practice guidelines in nutrition support: can they be based on randomized clinical trials? JPEN 1997; 21:1–6.

159. Pomposelli JJ, Baxter JK, Babineau TJ, et al. Early postoperative glucose control predicts nosocomial Infection rate in diabetic patients. JPEN 1998; 22:77–81.

21 Alcohol and Immune Function

Francesco Chiappelli, Michelle A. Kung,
Giuseppe Francesco Stefanini, and Francesco Giuseppe Foschi

INTRODUCTION

Individuals often drink in response to stress: the more severe and chronic the stressor, the greater the alcohol consumption. Stress is commonly believed to be a factor in the development of alcoholism (alcohol dependence). Whether an individual will drink in response to stress depends on many factors, including genetic determinants, the individual's usual drinking behavior, coping strategies, expectations regarding the effect of alcohol on stress, the intensity and type of stressor, and the individual's sense of control over the stressor *(1,2)*.

What has come to be called "psychological stress" can be defined as the real or perceived lack of fit of the person within the extrinsic (outside world of the individual) or intrinsic environment (inner world of the individual), the "person–environment fit" (Scheme 1). The perception of lack of fit relates to the set of perceived and actual social roles that individuals play in everyday life: an intertwined set of rights and responsibilities that encompass the individuals' personality, social involvement, cultural background, legal status, and power position. Individuals with different resilience to psychological stress have different inner motivational strengths to overcome the lack of fit they perceive or actually experience in the reality of their everyday endeavors. Motivations in general and the motivation to use and abuse alcoholic beverages in particular rest on fundamental attributions that the individual makes (e.g., origin or locus, stability, globality). Attributions and perceived responsibility, conscious or subconscious appraisals of given situations, are critical elements of perceptions of fit and of consequential behaviors, including indulgence in alcoholic beverages.

The perception of lack of fit engenders a physiological "stress response," which has been well recognized and described since the times of Cannon and Selye: "Stress hormones" (e.g., glucocorticoids) and peptides (e.g., opioids) have a wide range of specific immunomodulatory effects, which are conserved through evolution *(3)*. This chapter discusses how alcohol directly impairs immune surveillance by means of direct effects upon cells of the immune system, and indirectly by altering psychobiological responses.

From: *Nutrition and Immunology: Principles and Practice* (ME Gershwin et al. eds.), © Humana Press, Inc., Totowa, NJ

PSYCHONEUROENDOCRINE–IMMUNE RESPONSE TO ALCOHOL

PSYCHONEUROIMMUNOLOGY Recent decades have seen the emergence of hypothesis-driven research that has convincingly demonstrated several of the interacting domains between the psychobiological and the immunobiological domains. A new scientific field, psychoneuroimmunology, has emerged that investigates the interrelationship between psychophysiology and immunophysiology. From a philosophical standpoint, psychoneuroimmunology represents the reunification of Descartes' *res extensa* (bodily functions) and *res cogitans* (the measurable functions of the "soul," the psyche). Modern trends in cognitive science refer to the same paradigm as the relationship between "action" (the physiological response) and "perception" (the information processed within the central nervous system).

Psychosocial factors clearly impact on the nervous system, on neuroendocrine responses, and on cellular and humoral immunity. Scheme 2 summarizes certain of the principal elements of psychobiological modulation of immune surveillance. The delicate balance between health and disease is threatened extrinsically by environmental factors that include external pathogens, such as alcohol and other toxic substances. Intrinsically, the ongoing processes of development and aging modulate this balance, which involves, at its core, immune surveillance processes. In brief, all aspects of the immune systems are intimately intertwined and communicate via cytokines, growth factors, complement factors and receptors, and cell populations, which, as they bring forth specific immune responses, undergo parallel processes of activation, maturation, selective migration, and, eventually, apoptosis. Structures of the lymphatic system receive direct sympathetic and parasympathetic innervation, and cells of the immune system carry specific and functional membrane receptors for most neuropeptides commonly found at sites of inflammation and pain. Most, if not all, neuropeptides identified to date are endowed with powerful immunomodulatory properties. Immune cells are endowed with hormone receptors. Thus, immune cells respond to neurobiological stimuli elicited by the brain via direct innervation and indirectly by means of the neuroendocrine system. The brain processes cognitions, memories, and emotions, and generates neurobiological signals that are recognized as significant modulatory commands of immune responses peripherally as well as centrally. Reciprocally, invasion of pathogens and inflammatory reactions peripher-

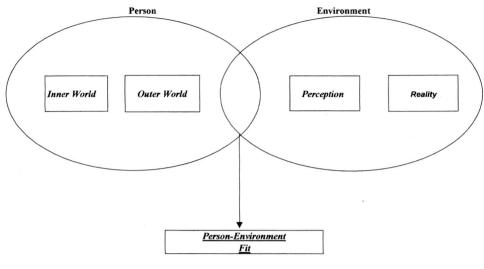

Scheme 1

ally or centrally trigger the production of cytokines, which communicate to the brain either directly or indirectly via the production of cytokines by astrocytes and other cell populations within the central nervous system. Neurobiological responses ensue that, in turn, modulate the immune response to the pathogens or the inflammation, as well as cognitions, emotions, and memories, and all other centrally mediated responses (e.g., behavior and temperature regulation) (Scheme 2) *(3–5)*.

HYPOTHALAMIC–PITUITARY–ADRENOCORTICAL–IMMUNE AXIS Several psychiatric diseases, including alcohol use and abuse, are accompanied by profound neuroendocrine disturbances that can manifest as significant alterations in cellular immune regulation. Drinking alcohol produces a physiological response akin to that consequential to stress-induced hormone release by the hypothalamus, pituitary, and adrenal glands, and activation of the sympathetic system *(6–11)*. Activation of the

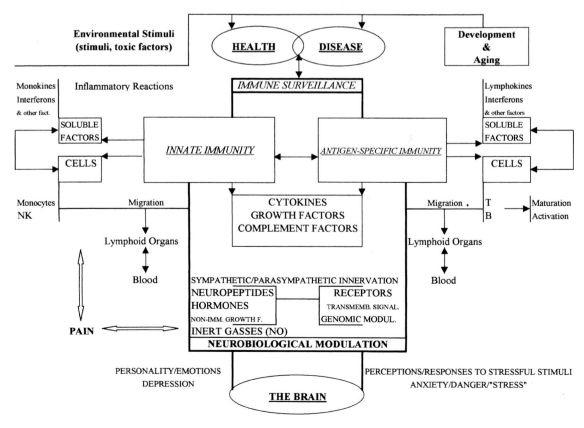

Scheme 2

hypothalamic–pituitary–adrenocortical (HPA) axis consequential to alcohol ingestion *(6,8,9)* leads to elevated circulating levels of pituitary peptides derived from the pro-opiomelanocortin gene, such as β-endorphin (βE) and adrenocorticotropin hormone (ACTH), and adrenocortical steroid, including glucocorticoids (GC). As GC increase, circulating levels of the adrenocortical androgen, dehydro-epiandrosterone (DHEA) tend to decrease *(11)* as an overall physiological energy-preservation mechanism. These changes, evident in alcohol users and abusers, are associated with changes in functional and phenotypic properties of circulating T and other immune cells, as discussed in depth in this chapter.

HYPOTHALAMIC–PITUITARY–GONADAL–IMMUNE AXIS The physiological response induced by alcohol also alters the balance of reproductive hormones. In men, alcohol impairs testosterone synthesis and interferes with normal sperm structure and movement by inhibiting the metabolism of vitamin A *(12–14)*. In women, alcohol contributes to increased production of estradiol and to decreased estradiol metabolism, resulting in elevated estradiol levels and menstrual dysfunctions *(15,16)*. Alcohol can increase the conversion of testosterone into estradiol, and post-menopausal women who drink have higher estradiol levels than abstaining women *(16,17)*, placing them at higher risk of a variety of illnesses, including breast cancer *(18)*.

Copious research has established the immunomodulatory role of gonadal hormones, which influence immunity acting at the level of primary lymphoid tissues or mature immunocompetent cells, and at the level of the hypothalamo-pituitary axis, influencing the release of hormones, which by itself also have immunoregulatory properties *(19)*. Gonadal hormones, indirectly via the HPA axis, alter the tone of the immune system and the quality and quantity of the inflammatory responses in a physiological pattern consistent with conservation and redirection of valuable energy resources toward homeostasis during times of stress *(20)*.

Cytokines, as noted earlier, are soluble mediators of immune function. These are factors that modulate the endocrine system. Interleukin-1 (IL-1), IL-6, and tumor necrosis factor-α (TNF-α), which mediate certain aspects of infammation, regulate hormone secretion from pituitary–gonadal endocrine tissues. IL-1 and IL-6 affect hormone release from anterior pituitary cells (e.g., growth hormone) and inhibit the proliferation of these cells. IL-1 and TNF-α affect granulosa cell steroidogenesis and IL-6 production *(21)*.

CELLULAR IMMUNITY AND ALCOHOL

IMMUNE SURVEILLANCE The immune system has two broad functional divisions, based on whether or not recognition of the infectious agent is directed by the major histocompatibility complex (MHC). The innate immune system is MHC unrestricted and represents the initial line of defense of the host. It consists primarily of monocytes/macrophages (Mθ) and other antigen-presenting cells, and natural-killer cells,* which act in MHC-unrestricted cytotoxicity. The antigen-dependent immune system is MHC restricted and represents the adaptive resistance of the host to a pathogen. It consists primarily of T and B lymphocytes. Humoral immunity is brought about by antibodies produced by B cells; cellular immunity is brought about by T-cell-initiated and T-cell driven events (e.g., lymphokine production, delayed hypersensitivity reaction, MHC-restricted cytotoxicity). These two intertwined branches of the immune system interact and communicate via cytokines, growth factors produced by the diverse immune cell populations. MHC-unrestricted responses form the first barrier to invading pathogens. Sustained immunity toward a given pathogen is directed and maintained by MHC-restricted processes, which, therefore, are critical to effective immune surveillance *(22)*.

Immune surveillance occurs through the concerted action of several intertwined pathways, which do not usually take place in the circulating blood lymphocytes, but in secondary lymphoid organs (e.g., spleen, lymph nodes) and body surfaces, including the oral mucosa. The oral mucosa represents the first line of defense against the cytopathic and physiopathic effects of ingested alcohol. Although more easily accessible for human studies, the immune cells found in the peripheral blood are in transit. Immune cells migrate from immune organs to other sites, and it is in that process that they are found in peripheral blood. Therefore, peripheral blood immune cells are most often used and are the optimal model system to study the immunopathic effects of alcohol, despite the fact that they represent a rather narrow window of the immune system *(22)*.

Immune cells derive from bone marrow progenitor cells *(22)*. Alcohol hampers this developmental process, and induces bone marrow damage. Alcohol-induced pathogenesis can be replicated in vitro and be shown to result, at least partly, by oxidizing ethanol-derived products, such as acetaldehyde (*vide infra*). Bone marrow Mθ appear to play an important role in the pathogenesis of alcohol-related marrow damage in vivo.

Ethanol modulates several Mθ functions, such as TNF-α production by human peripheral blood monocytes in response to stimulation in vitro by interferon-γ (IFN) in conjunction with muramyl dipeptide, by gram-negative bacterial cell-wall lipopolysaccharide (LPS) alone, or by IFN in conjunction with LPS. Down-regulation of Mθ TNF-α by ethanol was found to be independent of cell viability, but dose dependent and statistically significant in the biologically relevant, 25–150 m*M*, ethanol concentration range. That these effects were optimally obtained following a 4-h pretreatment of the Mθ with ethanol suggests that ethanol induces certain cytopathic outcomes at the membrane, cytosol or nuclear biochemistry levels, which hinder the cells' abilities to respond to future challenges. Indeed, 25 m*M* ethanol was also shown to induce Mθ constitutive production of IL-10 and of transforming growth factor-β (TGF-β) and to augment the production of these two cytokines in response to LPS or to gram-positive bacterial staphylococcal enterotoxin B (SEB). IL-10 is a potent inhibitor of Mθ TNF-α production, and TGF-β blunts several T-cell-mediated responses *(23)*. Once-only intake of a large amount of alcohol (1.12 g/kg), however, does not appear to cause measurable abnormalities in the production of IL-1, TNF-α, and IFN by peripheral blood immune cells challenged in vitro *(24)*. The validity of this study remains, however, questionable when one considers its limitation in face of the evidence already discussed.

T-CELL MATURATION Functional maturity from a resting T cell to a TH0 cell occurs, unless the cell has identified and recognized that the activation signal was improper, in which case the cell engages in apoptotic spontaneous cell death or anergy (cf. Scheme 3). T-Cell maturation leads to the production of IL-2, and soon thereafter, a variety of other cytokines (e.g., IL-4). Depending on the initial antigen and on the physiological milieu (e.g., modulatory hormones and neuropeptides), activated T cells can engage in the production of either a TH1 or a TH2 pattern

---

*NK cells actually appear to recognize target by the absence of MHC, rather than by the presence of MHC "self" plus a "nonself" molecule.

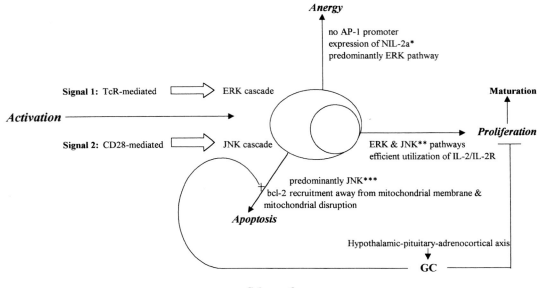

Scheme 3

of cytokines. Additional patterns of cytokines (e.g., TH3, which seems to direct the engagement of IgA production), which have now begun to be characterized, are also likely regulated during alcohol consumption, as outlined below (*vide infra*). These patterns are intimately intertwined in terms of their regulation and in terms of their relevance for the overall modulation of immune surveillance in health and disease. Cytokines of the TH1 pattern include IL-2 and IFN, participate in the regulation of cytotoxic T-cell maturation for the immune surveillance to tumor, foreign, and virally infected cells. Cytokines of the TH2 pattern include IL-4 and IL-5, whose primary role lies in fostering the maturation of B cells for the generation of immunoglobulins (*11,22,25*).

The neuroendocrine changes that accompany alcohol intake can modulate the establishment of TH1 and TH2 patterns of cytokine production. Steroids (e.g., GC, DHEA) differentially modulate the generation of Th1 and Th2 clones in mice* (*11,22,26*). The synthetic GC, dexamethasone (DEX), and DHEA modulate human normal peripheral blood T-cell maturation in vitro. DEX but DHEA blunts the ability of CD4 cells to proliferate and to produce IL-2, following stimulation with the global T-cell mitogen phytohemagglutinin (PHA) (5 µg/mL, 48 h). Both steroids fail to produce these outcomes following stimulation with the *Mycobacterium tuberculosis* purified protein derivative (TPPD), which primarily elicits a TH1 cytokine profile from human peripheral blood T cells in vitro (*27*). Thus, steroids may contribute to an alteration in the balance of TH1 and TH2 patterns of cytokines. The production of immunodetectable IL-2 by whole blood diluted in growth medium and stimulated with PHA is generally lower in older (>40 yr) compared to younger subjects (25.98 pg/mL ± 1.14 [±SD] vs 54.24 ± 1.21; $p < 0.05$). Ethyl alcohol (EtOH) (0.1%–0.2%) blunts IL-2 production[†] in both younger and older

subjects by 1.4 ± 0.05 (±SD)-fold. By contrast, production of immunodetectable IL-4 by peripheral blood cells stimulated as above is greater ($p < 0.05$) in older (3.81 pg/mL ± 0.38 [±SD]) compared to younger donors (2.72 pg/mL ± 0.70 [±SD]). Moreover, the blunting effects by 0.1% EtOH is larger ($p < 0.05$) in the samples of the older compared to the younger donors. Taken together, these data suggest that the expression of the genes for IL-4 and perhaps other TH2 cytokines are enhanced, whereas that of IL-2 and perhaps other TH1 cytokines is blunted in older individuals compared to younger donors. The data also point to differential modulation of these cytokines by EtOH in vitro among older and younger subjects (*28*).

Nicotine and EtOH, tested at concentrations approximating those found in the plasma of smokers and alcohol abusers, decrease immune surveillance of oral carcinoma by interfering with certain of the principal events involved in cell-mediated clearance of the tumor targets. Clear evidence supports a diminution of migration, a property of fully mature T cells, by fourfold to eightfold depending on the donor, as well as cytotoxicity, a property of mature CD8 T lymphocytes by nicotine when coupled with EtOH (*29*). Cocaine and the metabolic product of joint alcohol and cocaine abuse, cocaethylene* (CE) also blunt the migration of the mature

---

*It is noteworthy that patterns of cytokines are indicated as capitalized "TH1" or "TH2," but murine clones of T cells are indicated as "Th1" or "Th2."

[†]We find exceptionally high IL-2 producers are found among the aged population and exceptionally low IL-2 producers are found among the younger population. Day-to-day differences are also noted, particularly

among premenopausal women, and are putatively attributed to hormonal fluctuation during menses.

*Transesterification of cocaine in the presence of ethanol by liver microsomal carboxylesterases leads to the production of cocaethylene (ethyl-cocaine, benzoylecgonine ethyl ester). This compound, first identified in human urine samples, has important pharmacologic properties that mimic those of cocaine. Preliminary pharmacokinetic elimination studies indicate that cocaethylene's half-life ($t_{1/2}$=16 min) is about twice that of cocaine and that its steady-state volume is almost 1.5 times larger than that of cocaine in primates. In mice, cocaethylene is formed rapidly following the injection of cocaine (50 mg/kg, ip) and ethanol (3 g/kg, ip). Plasma levels peak about 15 min thereafter and decline by 90 min. Experimental administration of beverage alcohol (vodka, 1 g/kg) to human subjects followed by nasal insufflation of cocaine · HCl (100 mg) leads to the detection of urinary cocaethylene. In a group of emergency room patients whose blood contained ethanol and whose urine was positive for

T cells in vitro. Infection of autologous CD4-expressing Mφ-expressing Mθ in vitro with HIV-1$_{JR-FL}$, furthermore, significantly altered, as expected, the full maturation of stimulated T lymphocytes and the development of their migratory patterns *(30)*.

T-CELL ACTIVATION VERSUS APOPTOSIS VERSUS ANERGY Antigen presentation is initiated by the interaction of the antigen-presenting cell (principally Mθ, but astrocytes, microglia, Langerhans cells, keratinocytes, and B cells can also act in this role) and the resting T lymphocyte. Recognition occurs by the T-cell receptor (TCR) of the MHC ("self") in association with the antigen ("nonself"). The CD4 moiety on the T cells favors the interaction with Class II MHC, whereas the CD8 moiety favors the interaction with the Class I MHC molecule. These events further involve costimulatory signals, such as the interaction of CD28 with its ligand on the antigen-presenting cells, CD80 (B7.x family) *(22,31,32)*.

Phosphorylation events activate the 150-kDa isoform of phospholipase (PLC), PLC-γ1, which drives the metabolism of phosphoinositol and other membrane phospholipids for the generation of the polar lipidic product inositol triphosphate, which recruits calcium ions from intracellular stores and, thus, increases calcium fluxes. This contributes to opening specialized membrane channels (e.g., sodium, potassium, chloride), which often, but not always, leads to increasing the availability of extracellular stores of calcium and other ions to the cell. The binding of calcium to calmodulin for the activation of calmodulin-dependent kinases and phosphatases (e.g., calcineurin) further contribute to the modulation of the kinase cascade. Another product of phosphoinositol metabolism is the hydrophobic lipid diacylglycerol, which recruits cytosolic protein kinase C (PKC) to the membrane cytoskeleton, thus activating it. Activation of PKC is crucial for sustaining signal transduction. Furthermore, parallel as well as convergent tyrosine kinase cascades act as key regulatory components for the induction of phosphatidyl inositol 3-kinase for the generation of the PLC substrates, p21^{ras} proto-oncogene, a "small G-protein-like" signal transducing pathway, and the mitogen-activated kinase cascade (MAP or extracellular-signal regulated kinase [ERK]). MAP kinase phosphorylation

cocaine, plasma cocaethylene levels were found to be as high as 249 μg/L ($\approx 5 \times 10^{-7} M$). Cocaethylene *postmortem* plasma levels in joint alcohol/cocaine abusers can range from 30 μg/L to 530 μg/L.

Cocaethylene is believed to be responsible for the observed exacerbation of the acute psychoneuroendocrine toxicity of cocaine when jointly abused with alcohol. This includes a reported prolongation of the euphoria concomitant with a noticeable decrease in the unpleasant side effects that follow cocaine abuse. Cocaethylene produces significant physiopathology, including cardiovascular toxicity.

The relative short half-life of cocaethylene suggests that its effects on physiological and cellular structures occur relatively fast; the severity of the observed outcomes suggests that these effects may be relatively more prolonged compared to cocaine or alcohol alone. Animal studies indicate that cocaine and cocaethylene enhance the direct immunosuppressive effects of ethanol. Male mice (C57/B1), injected daily with cocaine or cocaethylene (20 mg/kg), were fed a liquid diet made 26% (caloric equivalent) with ethanol. The spleens from these animals were smaller and the splenocytes fewer in number compared to control animals either injected with cocaine alone or fed the ethanol diet alone. Splenocytes from the experimental mice, when stimulated with mitogens in vitro, were also less active in generating lymphokines (e.g., IFN) compared to splenocytes from control mice. More marked outcomes were obtained in the cocaethylene compared to the cocaine group. These data suggest that cocaethylene may impair the maturation of IFN-producing T cells (i.e., cells capable of TH0 and TH1 patterns of cytokines).

activates S6 ribosomal protein kinases as well as transcription factors critical to genome expression, such as *c-jun* and *c-myc (22,28)*. Several neuroendocrine products elicited as part of the physiological response to alcohol ingestion (*vide infra*) alter the phosphorylation of the T-cell receptor–CD3 complex, thus presumably altering the T cell's engagement in all subsequent phases of the response *(24)*. For example, our data show that a 15-min preincubation with human recombinant βE at the concentration range of 10^{-12}–10^{-13} *M* modulates in a bimodal pattern the phosphorylation of the γ-chain of the T-cell receptor on the TcR/CD3 complex following a 15-min stimulation with the phorbol ester, 4-β-phorbol-12,13-di-butyrate. This effect is not obtained when the N-acetylated form of βE is used, demonstrating the specific involvement of the opioid receptor on T cells. The effect of βE is specific to the CD3 complex. We also have shown that βE modulates phosphoinositol phosphate metabolism significantly *(33)*.

Alcohol may perturb signaling pathways specific to CD4+ cells, and not CD8+ cells. Both CD4 and CD8 are complexed with the protein tyrosine kinase of the *src* family; both CD4 and CD8 moieties are associated with *src* kinase p56^{lck} (lck). CD4 and CD8 are both members of the immunoglobulin gene superfamily but are significantly divergent in their structure: CD4 is a monomer, whereas CD8 consists of two distinct chains and occurs as a homodimer (α/α) or heterodimer (α/β). The relatively basic and cysteine-rich amino domain of lck interacts with the CD4's 20 cytoplasmic relatively acidic residues (408–421) and with CD8α's 10 cytoplasmic residues (194–203). This interaction is mediated by ionic forces and by cysteine residues. The CD8β chain does not contain the appropriate sequence and does not bind to lck. Upon T-cell activation, the CD4:lck complex is internalized and it dissociates. It is unclear if the homodimeric form of CD8:lck is internalized, but even if it is, it is clear that it does not dissociate. The heterodimeric form of CD8:lck is not internalized and does not dissociate. Thus, active lck kinase is released in the cytoplasmic environment only following CD4+ cell activation *(22,28,34–36)*.

The principal T-cell population affected by EtOH thus appears to be the CD4+ population *(22,28,37)*. It is possible and even probable that one of the mechanisms by which alcohol impairs CD4+ but not CD8+ cells is by perturbing the CD4:lck complex. A direct consequence of this effect could be a blunting of the process of CD4:lck internalization and dissociation. This, in turn, could result in decreased levels of cytoplasmic activated p56^{lck} in CD4 cells, following activation in the presence of alcohol and may lead to significant alteration in the kinase cascade specifically in CD4 cells.

Alternatively, alcohol could alter fundamental biochemical properties of *src* family protein tyrosine kinases. For instance, the *src* family also comprises p59^{fyn}, itself associated primarily but not exclusively with CD3, and other peptides generally implicated in the regulation of cell proliferation. The carboxyl domain of *src* family members exhibits a high degree of homology and contains the catalytic site. The N-terminal is unique to each peptide. The myristylated amino-terminal glycine of lck is immediately followed by the relatively acidic and cysteine-rich binding site for CD4 and CD8α, by a src homology 3 domain (SH3), and an SH2 domain. The catalytic domain exhibits an ATP-binding site at lysine273, a site for autophosphorylation at tyrosine394, and a site for dephosphorylation (possibly mediated by CD45 or other phosphatases) at tyrosine505. The exact sites of serine and threonine phosphorylation remain to be identified *(22,28,34–36)*.

Cocaethylene (CE) at micromolar concentrations blunts calmodulin-dependent kinase activity by up to 40%, but leaves unaltered tyrosine kinase activity and calcium flux. This finding suggests that the effects of CE are specific in the transmembrane pathway they affect and confirms, albeit indirectly, the hypothesis of specific effects of alcohol on certain kinase pathways.

T-cell activation events lead to a finely modulated activation of the cyclin-dependent kinases, which bind to appropriate cyclins and drive the cell into the proliferative response. Activated cells traverse the cell cycle and change morphology into "blast" cells, recognizable by the large cytoplasm-to-nucleus ratio and the conspicuous absence of vacuoles. Activated T cells also change phenotypically as they loose CD62L, the peripheral lymph-node homing receptor, and begin to express lymphocyte-function-associated antigens and other membrane maturation markers, such as CD45R0 instead of CD45RA. This process is initiated by the cells' expression of CD69, which controls and regulates the expression of the IL-2 gene by its action downstream to the nuclear factor of activated T cells (NAFT) and activator protein-1 (AP-1) transcription regulation complexes. Following expression of CD69, the IL-2 and CD25 genes are activated, and CD25, the α chain of the IL-2 receptor is expressed in high density on the cell membrane. The activated T cell also expresses the transferrin receptor, CD71, which is critical for the transport of iron from the extracellular environment into the cell during S-phase traversal. The expression of these and other membrane markers of activation, including the exopeptidase CD26* (dipetidyl peptidase IV) and the 4-1BB antigen of unknown function, CD137, is transient and exhibits finely controlled kinetics. Taken together, these phenotypic changes signify the beginning of the maturation process of the T cell from the naive to the memory state (22,28,38,39).

Data show a differential modulation of EtOH of the expression of the CD26 marker and of T-cell-associated CD26 enzymatic activity. Whereas increasing concentrations of EtOH enhance the expression of the marker, they progressively blunt its exopeptidase activity. We have interpreted these data as suggestive of putative EtOH-mediated alterations of the plasma membrane such that the epitope to the monoclonal anti-CD26 antibody becomes more exposed, contemporaneously with toxic effects of EtOH upon the enzymatic properties of the CD26 moiety. Aternatively, EtOH may act intracellularly by altering the synthesis and translocation of CD26 such that immunoreactive but enzymatically less active pro-forms of the moiety are expressed following treatment with EtOH (28). We have also shown that neuropeptides secreted as a result of the physiological response to alcohol ingestion have dramatic effects in exacerbating the immunotoxicity of alcohol on activated T-cells (28,37). Therefore, we have established that EtOH significantly blunts the generation of morphologically recognizable T blasts cells, the overall metabolism of the maturing T cell, the expression of the G_1/S cyclin, proliferating cell nuclear antigen (PCNA) by Western immunoblotting, ^{3}H-TDR incorporation, propidium iodide/bromo deoxyuridine (PI/BrdU) double labeling, and production of IL-2 (28,37).

Apoptotic cell death is a complex process, whose critical role in the homeostasis of cellular immunity has recently come to light. The initial signal for apoptosis is triggered in part by members of the tumor necrosis factor receptor superfamily, including the

Fas surface receptor (CD95/APO-1): when Fas interacts with the Fas ligand, transmembrane signals are initiated through the associated FADD/MORT-1 motif, which interacts with caspase-8. Caspases are proteases (hence, the suffix "ases") that have cysteine in the active site (hence, the prefix "c") as well as an exclusive requirement for aspartic acid at the cleavage site (hence, "asp"). Up to 10 caspases have been identified to date, which have been numbered based on the chronological order of publication of their respective cDNAs. Active caspases are released from cleavage from the pro-enzyme into a larger peptide (17–22 kDa) and a smaller peptide (10–12 kDa), which associate to form the active enzyme in cells undergoing apoptosis. Caspase-8 possesses two motifs near the 5'-terminal that associate with FADD, often referred to as the "death effector" domain. Activated caspase-8 may, in turn, activate other caspases or act directly upon mitochondrial permeability and metabolism. Mitochondria thus are involved in apoptosis through release of soluble molecule, such as bcl-2, which normally lies in the outer mitochondrial membrane near the inner–outer membrane contact sites where permeability pores form. The action of bcl-2 is to protect against apoptosis by preventing the opening of these pores and release of a 50-kDa protease (40). Additional events involve changes in the plasma membrane and translocation of phosphatidylserine from the inner to the outer aspect of the membrane, which can be reliably detected by its high affinity to the Ca^{2+}-dependent phospholipid-binding protein, Annexin-5 (35–36 kDa). Signals are transduced to the mitochondria as well as the nucleus and result in the activation of nucleases for the degradation of chromosomes into nucleosomal subunits. These metabolites can be detected either as fragments of increasing length on an agarose gel or as cytoplasmic content of nucleosomal proteins; whether alcohol induces apoptosis is unclear from the data obtained by our laboratory and by others (28).

T-cell stimulation by triggering through the T-cell receptor (TcR) in the absence of CD28-mediated costimulatory signals induces unresponsiveness in T cells to further stimulation, a phenomenon known as anergy (Cf., Scheme 3). Anergic T cells do not produce IL-2 when challenged. This failed response is attributable to a transcriptional defect. Anergic T cells are defective in their ability to upregulate protein binding and transactivation at two critical IL-2 DNA enhancer elements: NF-AT (a sequence that binds a heterotrimeric NFATp, Fos, and Jun protein complex) and AP-1 (that binds *Fos* and *Jun* heterodimers). The impaired DNA–protein interactions in anergic T cells is related to poor expression of the inducible AP-1 family members c-Fos, FosB, and JunB, attributable, at least in part, to a selective block in the expression of the AP-1 Fos and Jun family members in anergic T cells. Ligation of CD28 results in its phosphorylation and subsequent recruitment and activation of phosphatidylinositol 3-kinase. However, pharmacological and mutational analysis data show that disruption of phosphatidylinositol 3-kinase association with CD28 is neither necessary nor sufficient for costimulation of IL-2 production (22–28). Data obtained in alcoholics (*vide infra*) appear to support the hypothesis that alcohol use and abuse may induce anergy by blunting phospholipid metabolism.

IMMUNOPATHOLOGY OF ALCOHOL

ALCOHOL METABOLITES Metabolism is the body's process of converting ingested substances to other compounds; this results in the production of substances becoming more, and some less, toxic than those originally ingested. Metabolism involves a num-

---

*CD26 has also been proposed to be a cofactor for the penetration of HIV-1 into CD4+ cells.

ber of processes, one of which is referred to as oxidation. Through oxidation, alcohol* is detoxified and removed from the blood, preventing the alcohol from accumulating and destroying cells and organs. A minute amounts of alcohol escapes metabolism and is excreted unchanged in the breath and in urine. Until all the alcohol consumed has been metabolized, it is distributed throughout the body, affecting all tissues, including the lymphoid organs and circulating immune cells.

When alcohol is consumed, it absorbed from the stomach and intestines into the blood; it is then metabolized predominantly by specific enzymes. The tissues involved can metabolize only a certain amount of alcohol per hour, regardless of the amount that has been consumed. The rate of alcohol metabolism depends, in part, on the amount of metabolizing enzymes, which varies among individuals and appears to be genetically determined.[†] In general, after the consumption of one standard drink,[§] the amount of alcohol in the drinker's blood (blood alcohol concentration BAC) peaks within 30–45 min. Women have on average higher BAC values after consuming the same amount of alcohol as men and are more susceptible to alcoholic liver disease and a variety of alcohol-induced tissue pathologies. Indeed, women have a lower activity of these enzymes (e.g., alcohol dehydrogenase ADH, see below), thus causing a larger proportion of the ingested alcohol to remain unmetabolized. Alcohol is metabolized more slowly than it is absorbed. Because the metabolism of alcohol is relatively slow, consumption is likely to lead to accumulation in the body and intoxication (41).

The first step in the metabolism of alcohol is carried out by the enzyme alcohol dehydrogenase (ADH), which mediates the rate-limiting conversion of alcohol to acetaldehyde. This enzyme is present primarily in the liver, but a gastric mucosa form of ADH, whose putative role is to decrease the bioavailability of ingested alcohol also exists. This form ADH is significantly more active in men compared to women, and in subjects below 50 yr of age, compared to their older cohorts. Acetaldehyde is then rapidly converted to adenosine, acetate, and eventually to carbon dioxide and water. Alcohol can also be metabolized in the liver by the enzyme cytochrome P450IIE1 (CYP2E1)[¶]; this degradative

pathway becomes increasingly effective during chronic drinking (42).

NUTRITION AND PHYSIOLOGY Nutrition (i.e., diet, the type of food ingested) and the presence of food in the gastrointestinal tract influence the alcohol absorption process when alcohol is consumed (43). The rate at which alcohol is absorbed depends, in fact, on how quickly the stomach empties its contents into the intestine. The higher the dietary fat content, the more time this emptying will require and the longer the process of absorption will take. Subjects who drink alcohol while consuming a meal rich in fat, protein, and carbohydrates absorb the alcohol about three times more slowly than when they consume alcohol on an empty stomach (44). Thus, food intake contributes to reducing intoxication, but does little to affect the range or severity of alcohol-associated immune toxicity. Alcohol has a relatively high caloric value,* but alcohol consumption does not necessarily result in increased body weight. When chronic heavy drinkers substitute alcohol for carbohydrates in their diets, they actually lose weight. When chronic heavy drinkers add alcohol to an otherwise normal diet, they do not gain weight (42), probably because of an increase in resting energy expenditure and an increased lipid oxidation, probably the result of a mitochondrial alcohol-induced damage (43).

Alcohol consumption and metabolism impairs the regulation of blood sugar levels,[†] critical for the functioning of all cells, including immune cells (42). Acute alcohol consumption interferes with the three sources of glucose, the main blood sugar, and with the actions of the regulatory hormones. Alcohol consumption and metabolism also impair the regulation of available calcium stores. The main reservoirs of calcium are the bones and teeth, where its content determines their strength and their stiffness. The rest of the body's calcium is dissolved in intracellular and extracellular stores. Calcium is important for many body functions, including communication between and within immune cells. The overall calcium levels depend on how much calcium is in the diet, how much is absorbed into the body, and how much is excreted. Calcium absorption, excretion, and distribution between bones and body fluids are regulated by several hormones, namely parathyroid hormone (PTH), vitamin D-derived hormones, and calcitonin, which is made by specific cells in the thyroid. Alcohol can interfere with calcium and bone metabolism by means of a transient PTH deficiency and increased urinary calcium excretion, resulting in loss of calcium from the body, or altered vitamin D metabolism, resulting in inadequate absorption of dietary calcium. Calcium deficiency can lead to bone diseases, such as osteoporosis, characterized by a substantial loss of bone mass and, consequently, increased risk of fractures. It affects 4 to 6 million mainly older Americans, especially women after menopause. In alcoholics, the risk of osteoporosis and other calcium deficient defects is significantly increased (44,45).

Tolerance to alcohol consumption means that after continued drinking, consumption of a constant amount of alcohol produces a lesser effect or that increasing amounts of alcohol are necessary

---

*Alcohol caloric content: 7.1 cal/g (as a point of reference, 1 g of carbohydrate contains 4.5 cal and 1 g of fat contains 9 cal).

[†]Some inherited abnormalities in metabolism (e.g., flushing reaction among some persons of Asian descent) promote resistance to alcoholism. Alcohol dehydrogenase genes may be associated with differential resistance and vulnerability to alcohol.

[§]A standard drink is defined as 12 oz of beer, 5 oz of wine, or 1.5 oz of 80 proof distilled spirits, all of which contain the same amount of alcohol.

[¶]Consumption of alcohol activates the liver-specific enzyme CYP2E1, which may be responsible for transforming the common pain reliever acetaminophen ([Tylenol™] and many others) into chemicals that can cause liver damage. In alcoholics, these effects may occur with as little as 2.6 g of acetaminophen (four to five "extrastrength" pills) taken over the course of the day in persons consuming varying amounts of alcohol. Alcohol–acetaminophen hepatotoxicity is more likely to occur when acetaminophen is taken after, rather than before the alcohol has been metabolized. Alcohol consumption also affects the metabolism and the effectiveness of a wide variety of other medications. Alternate pathways of alcohol metabolism can speed up the elimination of some substances (e.g., barbiturates) and increase the toxicity of others (e.g., acetaminophen). The identification of these pathways is critical as health care providers advise patients about how alcohol–drug interactions may threaten the effectiveness of certain therapeutic medications or render them seriously harmful.

*See footnote, this page, column 1.

[†]Glucose, the principal circulating sugar, is derived from three sources: food, synthesis (manufacture) in the body, and the breakdown of glycogen, a form of glucose that the body stores in the liver. Hormones help to maintain a constant concentration of glucose in the blood. This is especially important for the brain because it cannot make or store glucose but depends on glucose supplied by the blood. Even brief periods of low glucose levels (hypoglycemia) can cause brain damage.

to produce the same effect. Metabolic tolerance, a more rapid elimination of alcohol from the body, is associated with a specific group of liver enzymes (e.g. ADH) that metabolize alcohol and that are activated after chronic drinking (44,45). Enzyme activation increases alcohol degradation and reduces the time during which alcohol is actively toxic in the body. However, certain of these enzymes also increase the metabolism of some other drugs and medications, causing a variety of harmful effects on the drinker. For example, rapid degradation of sedatives (e.g., barbiturates) can cause tolerance to them and increase the risk for their use and abuse. Increased metabolism of some prescription medications, such as those used to prevent blood clotting and to treat diabetes, reduces their effectiveness in chronic drinkers or even in recovering alcoholics. Increased degradation of the common painkiller acetaminophen precipitates liver damage in chronic drinkers (see footnote * on pg. 267, column 1) (42,46).

SPECIAL POPULATIONS

Alcoholics   Alcohol abuse leads to a complex pattern of psychopathology and physiopathology. These states include impaired cognition, coping behaviors, altered moods, and increased susceptibility to a variety of physical illnesses (e.g., chronic obstructive pulmonary disease, peptic ulcer disease, psoriasis, tobacco dependence, organic brain syndrome, malnutrition), as well as immune-mediated diseases, such as infectious diseases and cancer. Bactericidal serum activity is reduced in subjects with acute alcohol intoxication, suggesting that the complement interacts in this reaction. However, many studies on alcohol-dependent subjects have reported both raised and reduced complement levels (47). Close to 10% of alcoholics have granulocytopenia, apparently exacerbated by infections and malnutrition (48).

Alcohol also seems to impair the production of polymorphonuclear cells (neutrophils), probably by its effects upon the bone marrow (vide supra) (49), and because it inhibits several steps of neutrophil migration, from rolling to the subsequent binding to expressed adhesion molecules, to migration between endothelial cells, and to diapedesis toward the inflammatory site. The chemotaxis of neutrophils is reduced in chronic alcohol intoxication; above all, in patients with liver cirrhosis resulting from the presence of a serum leukocyte chemotaxis inhibiting factor (CIF). This factor is putatively related to C5a activation by circulating immune complexes. Alcohol does not inhibit the ability of polymorphonuclear cells (neutrophils) to destroy microorganisms, but neutrophil production of oxygen radicals and degranulation is blunted by alcohol, sharply reducing the bactericidal capacity of this cell population (50,51). This particular event could be linked to alcohol-induced changes in membrane signals and calcium homeostasis.

An activation and hyperplasia of Kupffer cells has been found in the liver in patients with alcoholic liver disease, and some studies have demonstrated an impairment in cell function at high ethanol concentrations (800 mg/dL). These effects could be the result of the direct effect of alcohol and its metabolites or mediated by the indirect effect of the endotoxins resulting from an increase in intestinal permeability. These effects could also be triggered by liver damage through the release of TGF-β, TNF-α, IL-1, IL-6, and IL-8. These cytokines may affect the endothelium of the hepatic sinusoids, stimulating endothelin production, the expression of adhesion molecules such as ICAM-1 (CD54), and the production of other pro-inflammatory cytokines with chemotactic effect. These include macrophage inflammatory protein (MIP)-1,

MIP2, and IL-8 and involve the recruitment of other leukocyte cells on the endothelium of the hepatic sinusoids and the release of free-oxygen radicals and lysosomal enzymes (52,53). This body of evidence, taken together with the elements presented earlier about the interdependence of bone and immune physiology, clearly relates to the significant effect of alcohol in bone disease.

The predisposition to infection among alcoholics with alcoholic liver disease includes impaired splenic function, as recently confirmed by an increase in the circulation of pitted cells (i.e., red cells bearing membrane abnormalities). There is no direct correlation between the number of pitted cells and the duration of alcohol abuse or the amount of alcohol ingested (54,55). Moreover, chronic alcohol exposure appears to suppress cell-mediated immunity, which may contribute to the high incidence of infections among alcohol-dependent patients. Serum neopterin, a marker of Mθ function and T-lymphocyte activation, measured in alcohol-dependent patients is significantly lower than the mean serum neopterin in matched controls. In those who abstained, the mean serum neopterin at 3 wk rose and was no longer significantly different from controls. Our findings (vide infra, 104) suggest that alcohol-dependent patients have suppressed Mθ function, which may be reversible within 3 wk of abstention.

No changes have been noted in the number of natural-killer cells (defined by flow cytometry as CD3–CD56+CD16+), whereas the effect of alcohol abuse on natural-killer (NK) function* (see footnote on pg. 163) remains controversial. The natural-killer function depends largely on the immune cells' ability to bind to the targets. The pattern of adhesion molecules expressed on the endothelium in alcohol-related liver disease may affect the type of inflammatory infiltrate and radically disrupt the pathogenesis of the liver disease. E-Selectin molecules, adhesion molecules confined to the endothelium that interact with neutrophils, natural-killer cells, and some T-lymphocyte subpopulations are noted to be increased in patients with hepatitis but not cirrhosis. Similarly, VCAM-1, an adhesion molecule that enhances the binding of T lymphocytes to the endothelium, was increased in alcoholic cirrhosis compared with alcoholic hepatitis; ICAM-1 expression was noted to be the same in both diseases. These changes result in a different inflammatory infiltrate—monocytic in cirrhosis and neutrophilic in alcoholic hepatitis.

Pro-inflammatory cytokines could play an important role in inducing the expression of adhesion molecules at the endothelial level and the increase in E-selectin could be triggered by the rise in TNF-α found in alcoholic hepatitis. The maintenance of chronic inflammation could also be caused by cytokines like IL-4, which enhance the expression of VCAM-1 on endothelial cells. As in other chronic inflammatory processes (56), there may be a switch in liver-based cytokine production that would account for the change in infiltrate in alcohol-induced hepatitis and cirrhosis. As mentioned earlier (vide supra), cytokine secretion could be the outcome of immune system activation by antigens derived from alcohol metabolism or from blood endotoxins resulting from elevated intestinal permeability. Adhesion molecules are also important in mediating cell damage because the enhanced expression of ICAM-1 on the hepatocytes of patients with alcoholic hepatitis and the raised Class 1 MHC levels combine to make these cells susceptible to lysis by CD8 positive lymphocytes.

A fall in L-selectins, adhesion molecules important for the passage through the endothelium, has been observed on both CD8+ cells and neutrophils. All these findings together with evidence of a drop in PECAM-1 (CD31), a molecule belonging to the superfamily of immunoglobulins also involved in cell migration and mostly expressed on CD45RA+ (i.e., "naïve") lymphocytes, which are typically decreased in subjects with alcoholism, help to reduce the lymphocyte recirculation required for regular immune system function. The decrease in these molecules on the CD8+ cell surface is associated with an increase in β2-integrin, a molecule also implicated in lymphocyte migration (57). Another attempt at compensation consequential to alcohol-induced immune pathology, is the observed change in the CD57 antigen usually expressed on natural-killer and T cells. This finding suggests high quantity of endotoxins present in subjects with alcoholism.

Raised blood levels of polyclonal γ-globulins, mainly IgA, IgG, and IgM, are commonly encountered in full-blown clinical forms of alcoholic liver disease, which reflects overproduction of immunoglobulins (Ig) by B lymphocytes, perhaps caused by isolated polyclonal activation of B lymphocytes and a decrease in suppressive activity by T lymphocytes (58). The enhanced intestinal permeability model and impairment in the way these antigens from the gut are sequestered by Kupffer cells in the liver could underlie this secondary hyperactivation of the humoral immune system. This entails greater plasma cell differentiation with a polyclonal increase in Ig synthesis in patients with chronic alcoholism and IgA deposits along the hepatic sinusoids. IgA levels are raised in all forms of alcoholic liver disease (ALD) and are structurally correlated with the severity of liver damage. However, a significant fall in CD5+ B lymphocytes has been observed during alcohol intake in subjects without ALD. This finding is significantly correlated to the increased secretion of Ig, suggesting that CD5+ B cells are involved in regulation.

The classification of B cells includes (CD5+CD45RA^{lo}) B1a cells, (CD5−CD45RA^{lo}) B1b cells, and (CD5−CD45RA^{hi}) B2 cells. B2 Cells usually produce antibodies against new external antigens, whereas B1a (CD5+) cells have been linked to the production of autoantibodies. Finally, B1b cells have been included in the B group because they contain CD5 mRNA (59). Recent studies have disclosed a decrease in CD5−CD45RA^{hi} (B2) cells and CD5+ CD45RA^{lo} (B1a) cells with a relative increase in CD5− CD45RA^{lo} (B1b) cells in alcoholics with ALD. The fall in B2 cells could be responsible for the inadequate response to external antigens found in subjects with alcoholism, whereas the increase in B1b cells could be a source of autoantibodies. Finally, the presence of high quantities of IgA in subjects with ALD implies that B1b cells mainly produce this type of Ig (60).

In general, in subjects with alcoholism and in ethanol-treated animals, Ig's have a shorter half-life and the activity of these antibodies seems to be impaired. Mice treated with ethanol and alcoholic subjects have a delayed response to new antigens and only develop normal antibody levels much later. However, if the antibody response is directed toward an antigen encountered prior to exposure to ethanol, the antibody response is normal. In addition, abstinent subjects with ALD present a normal or even enhanced antibody response. Circulating immune complexes containing IgA have been found in ALD subjects and correlate the severity of liver damage rather than alcohol abuse. Furthermore, IgA deposits have been detected in the renal glomeruli in over 50% of patients with alcoholism, regardless of the presence of liver damage, suggesting a significant role of IgA in inducing kidney damage (61).

In addition to an increase in immunoglobulins, patients with chronic alcoholism, especially those with liver damage, develop autoantibodies, similar to antibodies against smooth muscle (SMA), heat shock proteins, Mallory bodies (microfibrillary masses of hepatocyte), and against liver protein. The latter type of antibodies is correlated to chronic portal and periportal inflammation (62).

Acetaldehyde is one of the major intermediary metabolites of ethanol (vide supra). Injected into animals, it conjugates with proteins and stimulates the production of antibodies to these modified proteins, suggesting that acetaldehyde may act as a hapten, relatively independent from the protein carrier. The cytochrome P-4502E1 (CYP2E1), a liver microsomal enzyme, is specifically induced by ethanol and acetaldehyde (63). Recognition of these new antigens on the cell surface by specific antibodies may trigger cell lysis via complement stimulation, antibody-dependent cell-mediated cytotoxicity, and neutrophils. The finding that antibody titers against acetaldehyde adducts are also elevated in subjects with liver damage not induced by alcohol suggests that the immune response disclosed in patients with alcoholism could be the outcome rather than the cause of the damage.

Although impaired homeostasis has been implicated in the pathogenesis of liver disease, the relation between cytokine production and the metabolic activities inducing liver disease remain unknown. Nonetheless, research suggests that alcohol abuse enhances the production of TH2 cytokines at the expense of TH1 cytokines, which tends to support our in vitro observations (vide supra). We have demonstrated a correlation among serum CD30 levels, direct expression of the TH2 response, and the severity of liver disease in patients with alcoholism. These findings suggest that such an unbalanced response in these subjects could be the result of the direct effect of alcohol on cytokine production flanked by the possible interference of GCL, which tend to be raised in alcoholics. In fact, these hormones stimulate the shift toward type TH2 lymphocytes and the enhanced expression of CD30 on lymphocyte membranes.

Although alcohol-dependent subjects may produce normal amounts of IL-2, patients with alcoholic hepatitis have blood levels of TNF-α, IL-1, and IL-6 that appear to correlate with the clinical and biochemical parameters of liver damage in patients with chronic alcoholism. In vitro studies have shown that Mθ from alcoholic subjects isolated and cultured with ethanol secrete TNF-α, IL-1, and IL-6, unlike healthy controls (64,65). TNF-α receptors are expressed in high quantities in liver diseases of whatever cause and are found either only in hepatocytes or in endothelial cells of sinusoids, the epithelial cells of the bile ducts, and in Mθ infiltrate (66). The IL-6 concentration is correlated to definite factors such as serum IgA that stimulates its proliferation. Enhanced IL-6 activity has been noted in subjects with alcoholic hepatitis in relationship with the clinical and biochemical course of disease and markers of the acute-phase response such as reactive C protein (27). IgA also is able to enhance TNF-α production by Mθ in patients with alcoholism (67).

Alcohol enhances the production of chemokines, factors that attract cells of the immune system toward the tissue. Chemokines have been classified into three groups: C–X–C, C–C, and C, depending on the number and position of cysteine. The first group (C–X–C) contains IL-8, GRO-α, GRO-β, and other chemokines with chemoattractant properties mainly, but not exclusively, toward neutrophils. The second (C–C) and third (C) groups comprise substances like MCP1, MCP2, MCP3, and MIP1-α and MIP1-β which mainly work on Mθ, lymphocytes, and eosinophils.

Plasma levels of IL-8 are raised in subjects with chronic alcoholism without liver disease and even more elevated in subjects with alcoholic hepatitis (65); this cytokine also appears to be correlated with biochemical markers and the severity of liver disease. A selective increase in C–X–C chemokines has been observed in alcoholic hepatitis (68): liver tissue homogenates from patients with alcoholic hepatitis had raised IL-8 levels, whereas concentrations of GRO-α, a chemokine of the same group (which is homologous for about 40% of IL-8), were lower. However, the function of these chemokines, in this particular context, has yet to be established. Likewise, levels of the second group of chemokines (MCP1 and MIP1-α) are not elevated, even though transcription of these molecules appears increased using *in situ* hybridization techniques (68).

Alcohol abuse alters the distribution of certain T-cell subsets, including a sharp decline in circulating T lymphocytes endowed with the homing receptor to the peripheral lymph node, CD62L (*vide supra*) (69–71). Alterations in the expression of β-integrin (CD11b) were also noted on CD8+ cells from alcohol abusers (70).

At the molecular level, lymphocytes from alcoholics have significantly blunted basal and adenosine-induced levels of cAMP (72). Chronic ethanol consumption modifies polyunsaturated fatty acid (PUFA) concentrations in the plasma membranes of lymphocytes. The hypothesis that alcohol abuse induces alteration of lymphocyte activation pathways via lipid-derived second messengers (*vide supra*) was strengthened by a series of studies performed in a selected group of alcoholic patients well nourished without progressive liver damage (potentially confounding factors in the alcoholic action on immune function). In unstimulated lymphocytes samples from alcoholic patients in comparison with normal subjects, we detected a reduction in unsaturated fatty acid (mainly arachidonic) and an increase in palmitic and stearic acid molar content in phosphoinositol, phosphoinositol phosphate, and phosphoinositol diphosphate, leading to a significant decrease in the saturated/unsaturated ratio. In controls, anti-CD3 stimulation caused a marked decrease in arachidonic acid relative molar content counterbalanced by an increase in other PUFA, relative to the molar content of phosphoinositol, phosphoinositol phosphate, and phosphoinositol diphosphate fractions. After anti-CD3 stimulation, the same trend of modification in the fatty acid composition was observed in alcoholic patients, resulting in a sharp reduction of arachidonic acid relative molar content (73).

In a second series of studies, the incorporation of the [³H]-myo-inositol incorporation into the PtdIns fraction of peripheral blood lymphocytes (PBLs) from controls and alcoholics was conducted. In unstimulated lymphocytes, [2-³H]-inositol incorporation into PtdIns was similar in both groups. Following anti-CD3 stimulation, the radioactivity of the PtdIns fraction was reduced with respect to resting conditions; although in PBLs derived from controls we observed a significant decrease only a small, no significant decrease was shown in PBLs derived from alcoholic patients. In complete agreement, IPn production was similar in both controls and alcoholics in resting conditions, and following anti-CD3 stimulation, the increase in IPn production was lower in alcoholics than in controls. A further confirmation was obtained by the evaluations of the cytoplasmic free-Ca²⁺ concentration of lymphocytes from alcoholics. In alcoholics, we registered significantly lower concentrations than controls in unstimulated cells. Following anti-CD3 stimulation, in normal subjects a significant rise in cytoplasmic Ca²⁺ concentration was recorded; a similar

behavior was observed in lymphocytes from alcoholic patients, but a statistically significant lower peak levels of Ca²⁺ concentration was present in alcoholics. In the presence of EGTA, a chelator of extracellular Ca²⁺, the addiction of anti-CD3 led to a much smaller rise in Ca²⁺ concentration, but did not completely abolish the rise in Ca²⁺ concentration (74). Taken together, these observations play in favor of alcohol-dependent impairment of one of the main pathways of lymphocyte activation that usually lead to a rise in intracellular calcium concentration, via the G-protein–PLC–PtdIns pathway. In the alcoholics, the diminished Ca²⁺ release from intracellular stores and the smaller Ca²⁺ influx via IP3-dependent calcium channels is probably the result of a reduced IPn production.

Studies performed on alcoholic patients without relevant hepatic failure and/or malnutrition have not shown evidence of depressed in vitro proliferative response to mitogens such as PHA, Con-A, and to anti-CD3. These observations suggest that alternative activation patterns may compensate the impaired PLC–PtdIns pathway (75,76). There is a substantial amount of evidence that indicates that the surface CD2 glycoprotein is implicated in an alternative antigen-independent pathway. Although T-cell activation via the CD2 molecule can proceed in the absence of the TcR–CD3 complex, the latter seem to regulate the capacity of the alternative pathway to initiate clonal proliferation. CD2 membrane glycoprotein can be modulated in some lymphocytes by the contemporaneous activation of CD45RA. The function of CD45 must relate to its phosphotyrosine phosphatase activity, mainly important in the activation pathway regulated by tyrosine kinases (*vide supra*). Studies on subjects with alcoholic liver disease have shown an impairment of anti-CD2- and anti-CD3-mediated lymphocyte stimulation in the presence of an enhanced number of CD45+ T lymphocytes. Crosslinking of the CD2 and CD45 antigens modified the signal transduction directly by impairing tyrosine kinase phosphorylation and by inhibiting the mobilization of intracellular free calcium, causing the altered proliferation. A slight reduction in CD45RA+ lymphocytes in alcoholics without liver cirrhosis and a slight reduction in anti-CD3 lymphocyte proliferation. Alcohol in the absence of cirrhosis could induce an alteration in the PLC–PtdIns pathway. A common sequela, when cirrhosis is established, involves dephosphorylation of tyrosine residues of the CD3. These results suggest that malnutrition and/or relevant hepatic failure could take part in worsening the alterations that we have observed in alcoholic subjects without any hepatic pathology or malnutrition.

Fetal exposure to alcohol leads to the fetal alcohol syndrome. This condition is associated with serious anomalies in development, leading to well-recognized characteristics (craniofacial dysmorphologies, mental retardation, psychocognitive, psychosocial and behavioral problems, and altered motor performance and communication skills). Abnormal development of the neuroendocrine system is also well documented in fetal alcohol syndrome. In the context of this chapter, it is noteworthy to underscore the important immune dysfunctions found in children and adults born from alcohol-abusing parents. The T-cell system is particularly seriously impacted in these situations, and T-cell-mediated immune surveillance is reduced. Animal systems have been widely utilized to replicate and to expand the clinical observations, as well as to elucidate the underlying molecular mechanisms (77).

HIV-Seropositive and AIDS Patients   It is important to distinguish between chronic and acute exposure to alcohol: Many

HIV-infected individuals are social drinkers who drink alcoholic beverages occasionally; many others consume alcohol on a regular basis. Metabolites of alcohol, such as acetaldehyde, acetate, and adenosine, are toxic to T cells (*vide supra*). Additionally, alcohol ingestion leads to a marked pituitary–endocrine response, whose products (e.g., GC) have powerful immunosuppressive effects. Alcohol users also often coabuse cocaine: The liver metabolizes these drugs to form the ester cocaethylene (*vide supra*), whose longer half-life and immunotoxic properties make it a particularly dangerous metabolite (*see* footnote * on pg. 264, column 2). Certain of the effects of CE on immune cells in vitro were discussed above (*vide supra*). Alcohol users and HIV patients are characterized by altered pituitary–endocrine responses to a range of stimuli. This may undermine normal physiological responses, including immunoregulatory events. Last, but certainly not least, are the serious intertwined concerns rising from the epidemiological data about the rapid spread of AIDS among women and minorities, from the statistics of elevated alcohol consumption among women and among minority groups at risk for HIV infection and from the biochemical observations of sex- and ethnicity-related differences in alcohol metabolism and immunotoxicity. Recent statistics indicate that the African-American and Hispanic populations now comprise over 25% of the AIDS in California and about 45% nationwide. The fundamental trends of this pandemic have now clearly changed. The face of AIDS is now less a disease of white gay men and intravenous drug users, and more a heterosexual health threat, which strikes young women of childbearing age at an alarming rate. Consequently, pediatric AIDS has also surged to the forefront of public health concern.

Chronic ethanol ingestion predisposes to tuberculosis and bacterial pneumonia. *Mycobacterium avium* complex organisms cause bacteremia in patients with AIDS. Human Mθ and murine Kupffer cells exposed to ethanol are more permissive toward intracellular growth of *M. avium* than control mononuclear phagocytes. Ethanol also has been shown to impair the ability of human Mθ and murine Kupffer cells to respond to stimulation with TNF-α and granulocyte macrophage colony stimulating factor and to produce cytokines such as IL-1, IL-6, and TNF-α when properly stimulated. The impairment is dependent in part on a downregulation in the number of TNF receptors on the Mθ membrane. Recent evidence suggests that ethanol in nonlethal concentrations induces stress-related proteins in *M. avium,* leading to the inhibition of intracellular pathways in the Mθ and, consequently, impairing some of its functions. In summary, ethanol acts both on the host and on the mycobacterium in a complex sequence of events that influence the outcome of the infection.

We have reported *(28)* that the number of circulating CD4+ CD45RA+ and CD8+ CD38+ lymphocytes were significantly lower ($p < 0.05$) in the alcohol/cocaine coabusing group of HIV-seropositive patients (CD4+ CD45RA+: 110 cells/mm^3 blood ± 10 [±SD], CD8+ CD38+: 420 ± 60) compared to the alcohol/cocaine-free group (CD4+ CD45RA+: 180 ± 0.4, CD8+ CD38+: 650 ± 80), in the critical stage of the disease progression when patients begin to be symptomatic of opportunistic infection signifying collapse of CD4-mediated immune regulation (CD4 cell number between 500×10^3 and 200×10^3 cells/mm^3 blood). These findings, which were also shown when the data were expressed as percent lymphocytes, were not observed in any other stratification group. During the process of CD4 and CD8 cell maturation, other phenotypic markers are lost or acquired. The acquisition of CD7,

for example, has been associated with the production of certain cytokines, which signify functionally mature CD4 lymphocytes. We have noted suggestive differences in the acquisition of the CD7 marker by CD4 cells by HIV-seropositive alcohol/cocaine joint abusers, compared to alcohol/cocaine-free HIV-seropositive patients matched for CD4 cell number upon stimulation in vitro. These striking differences were evident even in the group of patients whose CD4 cell number was still relatively high. For example, a representative alcohol/cocaine using HIV-seropositive patient with 783×10^3 CD4 cells/cm^3 blood, and a CD4/CD8 ratio of 0.53 showed only 3% CD4+ CD7+ following a standard stimulation protocol in vitro (whole blood, EDTA as anticoagulant, diluted 1 : 4 with AIM-V growth medium, stimulated with PHA, 5 µg/mL, 4 d), compared to 16% of CD4+ CD7+ cells in a alcohol/cocaine-free HIV-seropositive patient, matched for CD4 cell number and CD4/CD8 ratio. For reference purposes, circulating lymphocytes from normal healthy control subjects treated in parallel show a rise in CD4+ CD7+ to 24.9%±8.3 (±SD).

In 1995/96, the Food and Drug Administration has approved the use of protease inhibitors. These compounds have good oral bioavailability and are generally well tolerated except for minor side effects (nausea, circumoral paraesthesia). The better documented to date include saquinavir (Invirase), ritonavir (Norvir), and indinavir (Crixivan). These compounds interfere with the maturation and replication of HIV by inhibiting the viral protease, the critical enzyme for processing a longer polypeptide into smaller proteins needed for incorporation the structure of the virus. The eight cleavage sites of the polypeptide constitute a template for the synthesis of a range of potential inhibitors. Only inhibitors of the Phe-Pro cleavage have shown an antiproteinase activity specific for HIV to date. Protease inhibitors lead to altered rates of selected mutant-resistant viruses. Resistance has also been noted when these inhibitors are given alone. These observations, taken together with the noted emergence of HIV-resistant strains, suggest limitations and caveats to the efficacy of these drugs, particularly when given alone. Thus, protease inhibitors are commonly administered as cocktail mixtures. Independent clinical trials with saquinavir, indinavir, and ritonavir have shown decreased viral load (plasma HIV–RNA PCR) and increased CD4 lymphocyte counts. Increased CD8 counts have also been reported but may be secondary to new CD4 cell production. A significant rise in the number of CD4 thymic emigrates, CD4+CD45RA+ (naive), as well as CD4+CD45R0+ (memory) cells has been noted in association with decreased CD38+CD4 and CD8 cells (activated) and increased proliferative and recall antigen response potential in a recent clinical trial of ritonavir in 21 HIV-seropositive patients. Until recently, the use of antiviral agents led to a transient recovery in CD4 cell number and immune competence. The recent introduction of protease-inhibitor-based therapies seems to offer the prospect of transforming HIV-seropositivity into a chronic and manageable condition. However, the clinical efficacy and the fundamental mechanisms of protease inhibitors remain to be fully elucidated. Few studies have characterized the effects of protease inhibitors upon cells of the host's immune system. This is critical because if the administration of protease inhibitors leads patients to become chronically HIV-seropositive with no symptoms or a much-delayed progression to AIDS, then it is crucial to fully characterize the patients' immunophysiological status. This knowledge should help us determine whether to continue prophylactic treatment for HIV-seropositive patients whose CD4 cell counts dropped and recovered following treatment. The effect of alcohol abuse in this context remains to be explored.

The Elderly   The young adult population today who will reach 65 yr of age ("young old") in about two decades will turn 85 yr ("oldest old") a few decades later. This is the group of "Baby Boomers" born between 1946 and 1965. The life expectancy, which was about 47 yr in the 1960s, is over 75 yr today. This change is based on several factors, which include better socioeconomic settings, better lifestyles, and better health care compared to their elders. Therefore, the percentage of elderly is expected to increase dramatically in the next half century. In the 1980s, about 11% of the U.S. population were "young old" and 1% was "oldest old"; today, 12.5% is "young old" and 1.3% is "oldest old." It is predicted that by 2050, 23% (a little less than one-fourth of the U.S. population) will be "young old" and 5% will be "oldest old." In absolute and relative numbers, the size of the elderly population will grow in the next decades from an estimated 28.6 million (12% of the total population) in 1985 to 58.8 million (20% of the total population) by 2025 (U.S. Bureau of the Census 1984). Even under the conservative assumption that current rates of alcohol consumption will continue, the sheer numbers of people who are maturing into old age means increasing numbers of elderly alcohol users. If future generations of the elderly drink more than today's older generation, the size of the problem will be even greater.

In the aged, several symptoms of alcohol use and abuse, such as musculoskeletal pain, insomnia, loss of libido, depression, anxiety, and impaired neuroendocrine regulation (1–4) as well as decreased immune competence can be confounded with conditions commonly seen among nonalcoholic older patients. Alcohol use and abuse in the elderly can also lead to increased risk of drug interactions and increased dependence on legal prescription drugs, thus further hampering immune and neuroendocrine-immune surveillance systems. Today, alcohol abuse represents the most significant drug abuse problem in the United States as well as in other industrialized and Third Word countries. In the United States alone, this situation involves over 10 million American young adults. Abusive alcohol consumption among the young adult population leads to significant social (e.g., violence, accidents, and abuse), economic (e.g., recovery programs), and health problems, as outlined earlier. Therefore, alcohol use and abuse is a critical problem of society at large, as well as a serious economic encumbrance. Consequently, it is critical to form appropriate new schemata of alcohol-induced pathology in the aging and the aged to be better positioned to address the vast array of medical situations that will present in the relatively near future (28).

CONCLUSION

The work we have outlined here demonstrates that others and we have accumulated a sizable body of data, which unquestionably indicates that alcohol impairs the maturation of T lymphocytes obtained from normal healthy young adults. Research designs performed in vivo and in vitro produce congruent results to show that alcohol can act both directly on the T cell and indirectly via certain of the hormones and neuropeptides that are secreted following alcohol ingestion. Data indicate that CD4 lymphocytes are considerably more sensitive to alcohol-mediated immunotoxicity than CD8 lymphocytes, an observation that has increasing relevance in the context of immune regulation as determined in part by the balance of TH1 and TH2 patterns of cytokines. Our

present understanding of fundamental cellular immune mechanisms allow us to formulate testable hypotheses with respect to the identification of specific molecular events and pathways, which alcohol may disturb during T-cell maturation. Research findings to date suggest that alcohol immunotoxicity may exacerbate aging-associated cellular immune depression and that interventions now being tested to recover immune resilience in the aged could be tested as well to contribute to the recovery of cellular immune responses among aging alcohol users and abusers.

Research has begun to investigate when drinking alcohol becomes a problem early or late in life. The early-onset drinker generally experiences problems with alcohol throughout life and continues to abuse it in old age. The late-onset drinker has no history of drinking difficulties but develops an abusive pattern of alcohol use as a reaction to one or more stresses of aging. Such stresses may include the death of significant others, conflict with a significant other, along with overall loss of sense of self. These distinctions aid in the correct diagnosis of alcohol dependence in the older person, which is otherwise made only about half as often as it is in the younger population. Alcohol dependence is often ignored as an Axis I differential diagnosis in the aging population. Despite the trends of longer life expectancy cited, improvements are not evident in terms of better health for the aging population. As the population's age increases, so does the proportion of age-related ailment and disease, and these health problems are exacerbated by alcohol use and abuse.

In summary, it is a timely and important societal concern as well as a scientifically relevant question to learn more about alcohol immunotoxicity in aging. Research in this domain, as well as in other domains of critical health urgency such as HIV/AIDS, will enable us to design fundamental, translational, and clinical studies aimed at elucidating and effectively acting upon health problems related to the use and abuse of alcohol by the population.

SUMMARY

Alcohol use and abuse represents the most significant drug abuse problem today among young and aging adults worldwide. Alcohol impairs normal immune responses that protect the body from disease. Chronic alcohol consumption reduces the number of infection-fighting white blood cells in laboratory animals and in alcohol users and abusers. Chronic alcohol ingestion or alcohol dependence depresses antibody production and other immune responses. Alcohol suppresses activities of certain immune system cells. The hormonal response that accompanies the use and abuse of alcoholic beverages indirectly blunts immunity. Alcohol during pregnancy can decrease immune resistance in the offspring. The relevance of these findings is discussed in the context of special populations who use and abuse alcoholic beverages, often in conjunction with other drugs.

ACKNOWLEDGMENTS

The authors acknowledge the contributions of all the colleagues, collaborators, and students who have participated in the progress of the research endeavors described here and who have been duly listed as coauthors or appropriately acknowledged in the original contribution. The authors thank the administrations of the Harbor–UCLA Medical Center, the West Los Angeles Veterans' Medical Center, the UCLA School of Dentistry, the Hospital of Faenza, Italy, the Department of Internal Medicine, Cardioangiology and Hepatology and the Department of Biochemistry "G. Moruzzi"

University of Bologna, Italy, which allowed the performance of these studies. These studies were conducted with funds obtained from the U.S. (DA07683, CA16042, AI28697, DA10442) and the Italian governments [National Research Council (C.N.R. Rome)], Ministero dell' Università e della Ricerca Scientifica e Tecnologica (Rome), Associazione Ricerca in Medicina (Bologna), and M.U.R.S.T. (40% and 60%)].

REFERENCES

1. Pohorecky LA. Stress and alcohol interaction: an update of human research. Alcoholism: Clin Exp Res 1991; 15(3):438–59.
2. Jennison KM. The impact of stressful life events and social support on drinking among older adults: a general population survey. Int J Aging Hum Dev 1992; 35(2):99–123.
3. Chiappelli F, Franceschi C, Ottaviani E, Farné M, Faisal M. Phylogeny of the neuroendocrine-immune system: fish and shellfish as a model system for social interaction stress research in humans. Ann Rev Fish Dis 1993; 3:327–46.
4. Besedovsky HO, del Rey A. Immune–neuro–endocrine interactions: facts and hypotheses. Endocr Rev 1996; 17:64–102.
5. Maier SF, Watkins LR, Fleshner M. Psychonneuroimmunology: the interface between behavior, brain and immunity. Am Psychol 1994; 49:1004–17.
6. Wand G, Froehlich JC. Alterations in hypothalamo–hypophyseal function by ethanol. In: Mueller EE, MacLeod RM, eds, Neuroendocrine Perspectives Vol 9, pp. 45–126. Verlag Publ., New York, 1991.
7. Eskay RL, Chautard T, Torda T, Hwang D. The effects of alcohol on selected regulatory aspects of the stress axis. In: Zakhari S, ed, Alcohol and Endocrine System. National Institute on Alcohol Abuse and Alcoholism, Bethesda, MD, 1993.
8. Mendelson JH, Stein S. Serum cortisol levels in alcoholic and nonalcoholic subjects during experimentally induced alcohol intoxication. Psychosom Med 1996; 28:616–26.
9. Morgan MY. Alcohol and the endocrine system. Br Med Bull 1982; 38:17–20.
10. Adinoff B, Martin PR, Bone GH, et al. Hypothalamic–pituitary–adrenal axis functioning and cerebrospinal fluid corticotropin-releasing hormone and corticotropin levels in alcoholics and recent long-term abstinence. Arch Gen Psychiat 1990; 47:325–30.
11. Chiappelli F, Manfrini E, Franceschi C, Cossarizza A, Black KL. Steroid regulation of cytokines: Relevance for TH1 → TH2 shift? Ann NY Acad Sci 1994; 746:204–16.
12. Van Thiel DH, Gavaler J, Lester R. Ethanol inhibition of vitamin A metabolism in the testes: possible mechanism for sterility in alcoholics. Science 1974; 186(4167):941–2.
13. Wright HI, Gavaler JS, Van Thiel D. Effects of alcohol on the male reproductive system. Alcohol Health Res World 1991; 15(2):110–4.
14. Leo MA, Lieber CS. Hepatic vitamin A depletion in alcoholic liver injury. N Engl J Med 1982; 307(10):597–601.
15. Mello NK, Mendelson JH, Teoh SK. An overview of the effects of alcohol on neuroendocrine function in women. In: Zakhari S, ed, Alcohol and the Endocrine System, pp. 139–69. National Institute on Alcohol Abuse and Alcoholism, Bethesda, MD, 1993.
16. Gordon GG, Lieber CS. Alcohol, hormones, and metabolism. In: Lieber CS, ed, Medical and Nutritional Complications of Alcoholism, pp. 50–90. Plenum, New York, 1992.
17. Gavaler JS, Van Thiel DH. The association between moderate alcoholic beverage consumption and serum estradiol and testosterone levels in normal postmenopausal women: relationship to the literature. Alcoholism: Clin Exp Res 1992; 16(1):87–92.
18. Willett WC, Stampfer MJ, Colditz GA, Rosner BA, Hennekens CH, Speizer FE. Moderate alcohol consumption and the risk of breast cancer. N Engl J of Med 1987; 316:1174–80.
19. Draca SR. Endocrine–immunological homeostasis: the interrelationship between the immune system and sex steroids involves the hypothalamo–pituitary–gonadal axis. Panminerva Med 1995; 37(2):71–6.
20. Torpy DJ, Chrousos GP. The three-way interactions between the hypothalamic–pituitary–adrenal and gonadal axes and the immune system. Baillieres Clin Rheum 1996; 10(2):181–98.
21. Spangelo BL, Judd AM, Call GB, Zumwalt J, Gorospe WC. Role of the cytokines in the hypothalamic–pituitary–adrenal and gonadal axes. Neuroimmunomodulation 1995; 2(5):299–312.
22. Chiappelli F, Franceschi C, Ottaviani E, Solomon GF, Taylor AN. Neuroendocrine modulation of the immune system. In: Greger R, Koepchen H-P, Mommaerts W, Winhorst U, eds., Human Physiology: From Cellular Mechanisms to Integration. Springer-Verlag, New York, 1996.
23. Szabo G, Mandrekar P, Girouard L, Catalano D. Regulation of human monocyte functions by acute ethanol treatment: decreased tumor necrosis factor-alpha, interleukin-1 beta and elevated interleukin-10, and transforming growth factor-beta production. Alcoholism: Clin Exp Res 1996; 20(5):900–7.
24. Mohadjer C, Daniel V, Althof F, Maier H. Immune status studies after one-time alcohol consumption in healthy subjects. Deutsche Med Wochenschr, 1995; 120(46):1577–81.
25. Romagnani S. Human TH1 and TH2 subjects: regulation of differentiation and role in protection and immunopathology. Int Arch All Immunol 1992; 98:279–85.
26. Snijdewint FG, Kapsenberg ML, Wauben-Penris PJ, Bos JD, Corticosteroids class-dependently inhibit in vitro Th1- and Th2-type cytokine production. Immunopharmacology 1995; 29:93–101.
27. Del Prete G, de Carli M, Mastromauro C, et al. Purified protein derivative of Mycobacterium tuberculosis and excretory–secretory antigens of Toxocara canis expand in vitro human T cells with stable and opposite (type 1 T helper and Type 2 helper) profile of cytokine production. J Clin Invest 1991; 88:346–50.
28. Chiappelli F, Kung MA, Villanueva P, Ong T. Alcohol toxicity of T cell-mediated immunity in the aging population. Alcologia 1997; 9:1–12.
29. Chiappelli F, Kung MA, Savage M, Villanueva P, Fiala M. Nicotine and ethanol modulation of cell-mediated immune surveillance of oral squamous cell carcinoma. Int J Oral Biol 1996; 21:19–27.
30. Fiala M, Newton T, Chiappelli F, et al. Divergent effects of cocaine on cytokine production by lymphocytes and monocyte/macrophages. In: Friedman H, Madden J, Sharp B, Esenstein T, eds, AIDS, Drugs of Abuse and the Neuroimmune Axis, 1996; 20:145–56.
31. Rudd CE. CD4, CD8 and the TcR-CD3 complex: A novel class of protein-tyrosine kinase receptor. Immunol Today 1990; 11:400–6.
32. Rudd CE. Upstream–downstream: CD28 cosignaling pathways and T cell function. Immunity 1996; 4:527–34.
33. Chiappelli F, Kavelaars A, Heijnen CJ. β-endorphin effects on membrane transduction in human lymphocytes. Ann NY Acad Sci 1992; 650:211–7.
34. Veillette A, Bookman MA, Horak EM, Bolen JB. The CD4 and CD8 T cell surface antigens are associated with the internal membrane tyrosine-protein kinase p56lck. Cell XX; 303–308.
35. Rudd CE, Trevillyan JM, Dasgupta JD, Wong LL, Schlossman SF. The CD4 receptor is complexed in detergent lysates to a protein-tyrosine kinase (pp58) from human T lymphocytes. PNAS 1988; 85:5190–4.
36. Rudd CE, Anderson P, Morimoto C, Streuli M, Schlossman SF. Molecular interaction, T-cell subsets and a role of the CD4/CD8:p56lck complex in human T-cell activation. Immunol Rev 1989; 111:225–65.
37. Chiappelli F, Kung MA, Lee P, Pham L, Manfrini E, Villanueva P. Alcohol modulation of T cell activation, maturation and migration. Alcoholism: Clin Exp Res 1995; 19:539–44.
38. Crabtree JR. Contingent genetic regulatory events in T lymphocyte activation. Science 1989; 243:355–61.
39. D'Ambrosio D, Cantrell DA, Frati L, Santoni A, Testi R. Involvement of p21 ras in T cell CD69 expression. Eur L. Immunol 1994; 24:616–20.
40. Martins LM, Earnshaw WC. Apoptosis: alive and kicking in 1997. Trends in Cell Biol 1997; 7:111–4.
41. Benet LZ, Kroetz DL, Sheiner LB. Pharmacokinetics: the dynamics of drug absorption, distribution, and elimination. In: Molinoff PB,

Ruddon RW, eds, Goodman and Gillman's The Pharmacological Basis of Therapeutics, 9th ed, pp. 3–27. McGraw-Hill, New York, 1996.

42. Lieber CS. Metabolic consequences of ethanol. The Endocrinologist 1994; 4(2):127–39.

43. Addolorato G, Capristo E, Greco AV, Stefanini GF, Gasbarrini G. Energy expenditure, substrate oxidation, and body composition in subject with chronic alcoholism: new findings from metabolic assessment. Alcoholism: Clin Exp Res 1997; 21(6):962–96.

44. Wallgren H. Absorption, diffusion, distribution and elimination of ethanol: effect of biological membranes. In: International Encyclopedia of Pharmacology and Therapeutics, Vol. 1, pp. 161–88. Pergamon, Oxford, 1970.

45. Jones AW, Jönsson KA. Food-induced lowering of blood-ethanol profiles and increased rate of elimination immediately after a meal. J Forensic Sci 1994; 39(4):1084–93.

46. Lieber CS. Interaction of ethanol with other drugs. In: Lieber CS, ed, Medical and Nutritional Complications of Alcoholism: Mechanisms and Management, pp. 165–83. Plenum, New York, 1992.

47. Mac Gregor RR. Alcohol and immune defense. JAMA 1986; 19:1474–9.

48. Liu YK: Effects of alcohol on granulocytes and lymphocytes. Semin Hematol 1980; 17:130.

49. Nakao S, Harada M, Knodo K, et al. Reversible bone marrow hypoplasia induced by alcohol. Am J Hematol 1991; 37:120–3.

50. Imperia PS, Chikkappa G, Phillips PG. Mechanism of inhibition of granulopoiesis by ethanol. Proc Soc Exp Biol Med 1975; 86:24.

51. Jareo PW, Preheim LC, Gentry MJ. Ethanol ingestion impairs neutrophil bacteriocidal mechanisms against *Streptococcus pneumoniae*. Alcoholism: Clin Exp Res 1996; 20:1646–52.

52. Adams DH. Leukocyte adhesion molecules and alcoholic liver disease. Alcohol Alcoholism 1994; 29:249–60.

53. Bautista AP. Chronic alcohol intoxication induces hepatic injury through enhanced macrophage inflammatory protein-2 production and intercellular adhesion molecule-1 expression in the liver. Hepatology 1997; 25:335–42.

54. Corazza GR, Adolorato G, Biagi F, et al. Splenic function and alcohol addiction. Alcoholism: Clin Exp Res 1997; 21:197–200.

55. Muller AF, Toghill J. Splenic function in alcoholic liver disease. Gut 1992; 33:1386–9.

56. Goldman M, Druet P, Gleichamann E. Th2 cells in systemic autoimmunity: insights from allogenic disease and chemically induced autoimmunity. Immunol. Today 1991; 12:223–67.

57. Mobley JL, Reynolds PJ, Shimizu Y. Regulatory mechanisms underlying T cell integrin receptor function. Semin Immunol 1993; 5:227–36.

58. Alexander GJM, Nouri-Aria KT, Eddelston ALWF. Contrasting relations between suppressor cell function and suppressor cell number in chronic liver disease. Lancet 1993; I:1291–2.

59. Kasian MT, Ikematsu H, Casali P. Identification of a novel human surface CD5– B lymphocyte subset producing natural antibodies. J Immunol 1992; 148:2690–2702.

60. Cook RT, Waldschmidt TJ, Cook BL, et al. Loss of the CD5+ and CD45RAhi B cell subset in alcoholics. Clin Exp Immunol 1996; 103:304–10.

61. Smith S, Hoy WE. Frequent association of mesangial glomerulonephritis and alcohol abuse: a study of 3 ethnic groups. Mod Pathol 1989; 2:138–43.

62. Paronetto F. Ethanol and the immune system. In: Seitz HK, Kommerell B, eds, Alcohol Related Disease in Gastroenterology. Springer-Verlag, New York, 1981.

63. Clot P, Bellomo G, Tabone M, Aricò S, Allbano E. Detection of antibodies against protein modified by hydroxyethyl free radicals in patients with alcoholic cirrhosis. Gastroenterology 1995; 108:201–7.

64. Shafer C, Ships I, Landing J, Bode JC, Bode C. Tumor necrosis factor and interleukin 6 response of peripheral blood monocytes to low concentrations of lipopolysaccharide in patients with alcoholic liver disease. J Gastroenterol 1995; 33:503–8.

65. McClain G, Hill D, Schmidt J, Diehl AM. Cytokines and alcoholic liver disease. Semin Liver Dis 1993; 13(2):170–82.

66. Volpes R, Van Den Oord JJ, De Vos R, Desmet VJ. Hepatic expression of type A and type B receptors for tumor necrosis factor. J Hepatol 1992; 14:361–9.

67. Deviere J, Content J, Denys C. Immunoglobulin A and interleukin 6 form a positive secretory feedback loop: a study of normal subjects and alcoholic cirrhotics. Gastroenterology 1992; 103:1296–301.

68. Maltby J, Wright S, Bird G, Sheron N. Chemokine levels in liver homogenates: associations between GROα and histopathological evidence of alcoholic hepatitis. Hepatology 1996; 24:1156–60.

69. Cook RT, Garvey MJ, Booth BM, Goeken JA, Stewart B, Noel M, Activated CD8 cells and HLA-Dr expressionn in alcoholics without liver disease. J Clin Immunol 1991; 11:246–53.

70. Cook RT, Waldschmidt TJ, Ballas ZK, Cook BL, Booth BM, Stewart BC, et al. Fine T cell subsets in alcoholics as determined by the expression of L-selectin, leukocyte common antigen and β-integrin. J Immunol 1994; 18:71–80.

71. Cook RT, Ballas ZK, Waldschmidt TJ, Cook BL, La Brecque DR, Byers C. Phenotypic alterations of lymphocyte fine subsets in the alcoholic: Implications for function. Adv Biosci 1993; 86:91–102.

72. Diamond I, Wrubel B, Estrin W, Gordon A. Basal and adenosine receptor-stimulated levels of cAMP are reduced in lymphocytes from alcoholic patients. Proc Natl Acad Sci USA 1987; 84:1413–6.

73. Celadon M, Biagi PL, Bordoni A, Mazzetti M, Castelli E, Stefanini GF, et al. Influence of chronic ethanol consumption on the inositol phospholipid fatty acid composition of human peripheral blood lymphocytes. Immunol Lett 1992; 34:155–60.

74. Hrelia S, Celadon M, Bordoni A, Castelli E, Foschi FG, Stefanini GF, et al. Phosphatidylinositol metabolism in lymphocytes of chronic alcoholic patients anter anti-CD3 stimulation. Immunol Lett 1995; 46:63–6.

75. Hunig T, Tiefenthaler G, Meyer zum Buscehnfelde S, Meuer S. Alternative pathway activation of T cells by binding CD2 to its cell-surface ligand. Nature 1987; 326:400–5.

76. Brown MH, Cantrell DA, Brattsand G, Crumpton MJ, Gullberg M. The CD2 antigen associates with the T cell antigen receptor CD3 antigen complex on the surface of human T lymphocytes. Nature 1989; 339:551–4.

77. Chiappelli F, Taylor AN. The fetal alcohol syndrome and fetal alcohol effects on immune competence. Alcohol Alcoholism 1995; 30: 259–63.

22 Cigarette Smoking, Substance Abuse, Nutritional Status, and Immune Function

Mari S. Golub

INTRODUCTION

Substance abuse, smoking, poor nutrition, and depressed immune function often cooccur in high-risk human populations. Studies of drug-addicted populations in the era of AIDS are beginning to bring increased attention and effort to characterizing nutritional and immune status. Similarly, more attention is being directed at nutritional and immunological status of smokers using new methodologies. However, to date, no clear hypotheses of causal biological links between tobacco smoke components, specific drugs, specific nutritional deficiencies, and specific syndromes of immune dysfunction have been proposed and tested.

CIGARETTE SMOKING

Food intake and nutrient status of smokers has been studied in detail over a number of years *(1)*. Smoking does not lead to anorexia (reduced food intake) but is associated with changes food selection, as indicated in data from NHANESII *(2)*. Smokers are characterized by a lower intake of fresh fruit and vegetables and a greater intake of fat. In terms of vitamin and mineral intake and plasma levels, vitamin C, vitamin E, and beta-carotene deficiencies have been well documented. There is also some information on folate, vitamin B_{12}, and various trace elements. It is recognized that the metabolic effects of tobacco smoke components could contribute to some of these deficiencies. Animal studies of cigarette smoke and nutrition are rare. Short-term anorexia and weight loss is a pharmacological effect of nicotine in rats *(3)*. Both increased and decreased preference for sucrose have been demonstrated in nicotine-treated rats *(4)*.

Particular attention has been given to (a) the role of nutrition in connection with low-birth-weight infants of smokers and (b) the role of reduced antioxidant nutrient intake in connection with the increased incidence of cancer and heart disease. Reduced antioxidant defense is thought to increase the impact of free radicals in causing DNA mutations that lead to cancers and oxidative damage associated with myocardial ischemia. (It is also recognized that antioxidant defense systems can be compromised by oxidant stress of tobacco smoke components.) As a result of these studies,

the National Research Council has specified a higher Recommended Daily Allowance (RDA) for vitamin C in smokers than nonsmokers.

Recently, examination of dietary antioxidant deficiency in smokers has been expanded to study immune function parameters *(5)*. Smokers and nonsmokers differed on a number of nutrient and immune status measures. However, no correlation between nutrient status and immune function were found in the smokers. Smokers had a history of 24 pack-years, and the smoking variable was quantified in terms of cigarettes/d, pack-years, and plasma nicotine and cotinine. Nutritional measures included plasma vitamin C, vitamin E, carotenes, vitamin A, and selenium, all nutrients related to antioxidant defense. Immune measures included white blood cell counts, immunoglobulin quantification, complement cascade components, and acute-phase proteins. White blood cell counts (total, neutrophils, monocytes, and lymphocytes) and acute-phase reactants (ceruloplasmin and $\alpha 1$-P1) were significantly elevated in the smokers compared to age- and sex-matched controls ($n = 160$/group). Immunoglobulins were similar in both groups, and complement C9 and Factor B were higher in the smokers. For the micronutrients, vitamin C, carotenes, and vitamin A were significantly lower in the smoker's group than controls. When linear correlations were computed between nutrient and immune measures, no significant associations were found, except for a weak (-0.189) correlation between IgG and plasma carotenes. Notably, however, vitamin A plasma concentrations were correlated with several lung function parameters. In a follow-up study, smokers and nonsmokers were not found to differ in vitamin C intake, although they did differ in plasma and leukocyte vitamin C concentrations. A marginally significant correlation was found between leukocyte vitamin C and neutrophil count. The authors suggested an effect on neutrophil function mediated by elevated myeloperoxidase activity based on previous studies, although no correlation was found between myeloperoxidase activity and plasma or leukocyte vitamin C in this study. They further suggest that these findings could indicate reduced antimicrobial action of neutrophils and increased risk of free-radical-mediated tissue damage.

In the more general literature on cigarette smoking and immune function, emphasis has been on lung macrophage function in connection with development of upper respiratory infections and

From: *Nutrition and Immunology: Principles and Practice* (ME Gershwin et al. eds.), © Humana Press, Inc., Totowa, NJ

oral and lung cancers in smokers. Mucosal immunity has also been a focus in connection with cervical cancer. In addition, general depression of immunity has been documented in a variety of human, animal, in vivo, and in vitro studies. These studies do not typically discuss possible nutritional mediation of the immune effects or interaction of smoking and nutritional variables.

Recently, studies indicate that passive smokers (i.e. those exposed to environmental tobacco smoke) demonstrate similar dietary deficiencies (6,7). However, in one study, controlling for educational level largely eliminated these differences (8). Passive smokers are also at risk of increased cancer incidence.

SUBSTANCE ABUSE

INTRODUCTION   The relationship among drug abuse, nutritional deficiency, and immune deficiency is usually conceptualized as comorbidity; that is, all three disorders occur together in some human populations. This section describes a few relevant human and animal studies, presents some additional research related to causal relationships among drug abuse, nutrition, and immunity, and suggests other potential areas for inquiry.

Although this section focuses on abuse of illegal psychoactive drugs, it is important to remember that substance abuse is a broader concept that includes, for example, anabolic steroid use by body builders and athletes, solvent abuse, purgative/emetic abuse in eating disorders, and abuse of prescription drugs like sedatives, analgesics, and tranquilizers. Each type of abuse is likely to have a different pattern of involvement with nutritional and immune deficiency. Polydrug use and associated lifestyle and socioeconomic factors are also common in these populations.

NUTRITIONAL AND IMMUNE STATUS IN POPULATIONS OF DRUG USERS   In the most complete and controlled study of this type (9), 140 men and women voluntarily entering a substance abuse program in Spain were studied. None of the subjects had concurrent organ pathology. As in other studies, this was a young population (average age 26 yr). Of the group, 31.3% were HIV positive but asymptomatic and 16.4% were heavy alcohol users. As in most other studies of drug-addict populations, all the subjects were smokers. The majority (83%) were heroin addicts, 16% were heroin and cocaine addicts, and 2% used only cocaine. In this study, nutritional status was inferred from anthropometric parameters and a diet recall interview; immune status was inferred from lymphocyte count and the delayed hypersensitivity test. Anthropometric data were compared to appropriate age and sex norms for a Spanish population.

The drug-addicted population was underweight at the time of entry into the substance abuse program, with 30% weighing less than 80% of the population mean (a criterion for malnutrition). The mean values for arm circumference and triceps skinfolds were at about the 80th percentile for the control population. Furthermore, 18% of this population was rated as severely malnourished based on a scale that included rank scores of fat and muscle mass. The mean body mass index was 20.9 ± 0.2. Calorie intake as determined by a 1-wk recall averaged 1188 ± 53 and was estimated to be 76% of the basal requirement; 66.4% of the group reported being anorexic. The women ($n = 42$) had a significantly lower body mass index than the men ($n = 98$) and generally poorer scores on all anthropomorphic and nutritional assessments. Also, patients reporting anorexia had lower values on almost all variables than those not reporting anorexia (e.g., caloric intake anorexic 1051 ± 60 vs nonanorexic 1473 ± 103, $p < 0.0001$). The severity

of drug addiction (moderate vs heavy) also related to severity of the nutritional deficits. No anthropometric or nutritional differences were found between HIV+ and HIV− groups.

Only two immune assessments, lymphocyte count and delayed-type hypersensitivity as determined by a standard tool (CMI multitest), were made. Lymphocyte counts were not depressed and, in fact, appeared elevated compared to the normal range. On the delayed type hypersensitivity DTH test, the percentages of the group classified as anergic, hypoergic, and normal differed statistically from the percentages in a group of age-matched controls ($n = 50$); 58% of the addict population was anergic as compared to 23% of the controls. Subgroups of the population were not compared for DTH results. However, no differences were found between this population and a smaller population of 18 addicts with organ pathology.

In an attempt to clarify the relationship between these variables, and, in addition, qualitative assessments of food and drink intake and social disruption, the authors conducted a stepwise logistic regression. The strongest predictor of nutritional status (score based on subjective evaluation of fat and muscle mass) was food and drink consumption. The strongest determiners of this variable were anorexia and social disruption. Anorexia, in turn, was most strongly predicted by sex (more females anorexic) and severity of addiction. These two variables were also the strongest predictors of social disruption. Immune parameters were not included in the regression. The authors concluded as follows:

> Although it has been hypothesized that drug consumption may lead to malnutrition either directly by enhancing basal energy expenditure or indirectly through infection, our results . . . point out the importance of decreased food and drink consumption.

Two other studies (10,11), also from Spain, studied male and female drug addicts during a detoxification program. Immune parameters were studied in more detail in the female addicts, whereas nutritional parameters were studied in more detail in the males.

The group of young males (20–27 yr of age) were "principally heroin addicts." Weight, body mass index and percent ideal body weight increased significantly in 24 men after 0.5–1 mo of detoxification. In 38 men completing 5–6 mo detoxification, these parameters also increased from the time of admission, but did not differ from the values after the shorter period of detoxification. As a group, about 12 kg were gained after either period of detoxification. An unexpected finding of the study was that all the men were below the 50th percentile for age-appropriate norms. The authors suggest that this was due to onset of drug use in early adolescence and subsequent stunting of linear growth.

A prospective food record questionnaire was also administered during detoxification and the intake of macronutrients, minerals, and vitamins was calculated as a percentage of recommended values. (All the men lived at home during detoxification but visited the treatment center daily.) No statistical comparisons were possible but the authors noted that "intakes of magnesium, folate and vitamin E were dramatically lower" and "intakes of energy zinc, riboflavin and vitamin B-6 were lower" than recommendations. This study indicates a rapid improvement in food intake and anthropometric measures during detoxification in these young addicts, but suggests a continuing abnormality in food selection that could require intervention.

The group of young women (21–28 yr of age) were principally

intravenous heroin addicts. Seventeen were HIV$^+$ and 19 were HIV$^-$. They were recruited for the study after 1–12 mo of participation in a detoxification program. The women gained about 10 kg body weight and body mass index increased from 17 to 21 during detoxification; HIV status did not influence recovery. An extensive assessment of immune status was conducted. Leukocyte and lymphocyte counts were within the normal range. For lymphocyte cell populations reflecting cell-mediated immunity, CD2 counts were considered normal, CD4 counts were depressed in both groups, and CD8 counts were elevated in the HIV$^+$ subgroup. For humoral immunity, CD19 counts were depressed and serum immunoglobulin concentrations increased in HIV$^+$ compared to HIV$^-$ group (no comparison to normative values was provided). Complement was considered in the normal range. (It should be noted that no statistical comparisons to normative data were provided for any immune parameter.) None of the women were considered to have a normal DTH responsiveness, and the values for the HIV$^+$ group were lower than those for the HIV$^-$ group.

Taken together, these three studies suggest that malnutrition as a result of reduced food intake is seen in young heroin addicts, along with depressed cell-mediated immunity. Upon drug withdrawal, nutritional status can normalize rapidly, but cell-mediated immunity may remain depressed.

A different approach to studying the relationship among drug abuse, nutrition, and immunity was taken in a recent study of young (16–35 yr of age) pregnant African-Americans (12). Serum samples obtained once in each trimester were analyzed for abused drugs and select vitamins and minerals. In addition, food intake data were obtained at monthly intervals and anthropometric measures were taken from medical records. White blood cell count was the only immune-related variable.

Women reporting drug use during pregnancy had a significantly higher intake of vitamin C and a significantly lower intake of iron. Protein, thiamin, niacin, and vitamin B$_{12}$ intake did not differ in these two groups. Women reporting drug use before pregnancy had significantly lower intakes of energy, protein, rag saturate fat, phosphorus, and zinc. Their prepregnancy weight, percent ideal weight, body mass index, and delivery weight were also lower; however, the mean values for both groups within a normal range (ideal body weight > 100%, body mass index > 21).

Another report (13) from this group compared a subset of drug users (determined by National Institutes of Drug Abuse standards for serum concentrations of cocaine, PCP, and marijuana in the third trimester) to nonusers. White blood cell (WBC) counts were significantly elevated in the drug-user group, whereas ferritin and folate were significantly reduced. Furthermore, vitamin B$_{12}$ and ascorbic acid were lower, although the difference was not significant ($p < 0.06$).

ANIMAL STUDIES OF THE INTERACTION BETWEEN DIET AND DRUGS IN DETERMINING IMMUNE FUNCTION

Studies in mice (14) have investigated the combined action of a low-protein diet (4% casein compared to 20% casein control) and drug administration (morphine or cocaine) on immune parameters (lymphocyte populations in spleen as determined by Fluorescence Activated Cell Sorting [FACS]). The low-protein diet was fed for 3 wk before and during an 11-wk morphine or cocaine treatment (daily ip injection). To simulate the human scenario, doses were increased during the treatment period. Two separate experiments were conducted, each with a nontreated (no injection) and an injection control group. As anticipated, cocaine alone reduced

body weight and this effect was more severe in the protein-malnourished group; morphine alone did not affect body weight, but morphine plus protein deprivation led to lower weights (not statistically significant) than untreated controls. An interesting feature of this experiment was the unanticipated effect of the intraperitoneal saline in the injection control group that led to significant reduction in spleen weight and cell number. The intraperitoneal injections also led to changes in lymphocyte subpopulations that varied with diet and experiment (cocaine or morphine). The effect of the injection control, the inconsistency of the effect across studies, and the variation in lymphocyte subpopulations of the control group (adequate protein, no injection) across experiments unfortunately leads to difficulty in interpretation of the lymphocyte subpopulation data in this well-designed study.

There were some suggested differences between the effects of cocaine under the adequate and protein-malnourished conditions. In the adequate nutrition condition, both cocaine and injection reduced the percentage of T cells and macrophages and increased the percentage of B cells. In the protein-malnourished condition, a smaller increase in B-cell percentage was also indicated as a result of both cocaine and injection. For T lymphocytes, the percentages were somewhat but not significantly decreased in the saline group and increased in the cocaine group, leading to significant group differences between saline and cocaine injected groups in total (Thy 1.2+) and CD8+ lymphocytes. The authors suggest that the effects of cocaine and saline injection may have a common origin in the activation of the adrenal cortex.

There were no suggested differences between dietary conditions on the effect of morphine on lymphocyte subpopulations. In this experiment, there was no effect of saline injection on lymphocyte subpopulations. Morphine increased the percentage of lymphocytes with B-cell markers in both the protein-adequate and protein-malnourished groups. The percentage of macrophages was also higher in the morphine group than untreated controls under the adequate-protein condition; however, this percentage was generally higher in all groups under the protein-malnourished condition.

This research group has used a mouse model to study nutrition and alcohol effects on progression of retroviral infection (15,16). Some published data concerning morphine and cocaine was located (17,18), but nutritional variables were not included in the studies.

SOME RESEARCH POTENTIALLY RELEVANT TO CAUSAL INTERRELATIONSHIPS AMONG DRUG ABUSE, NUTRITIONAL STATUS, AND IMMUNE FUNCTION

Identification of specific causal biological links among drug action, nutritional deficiency and changes in immune function is difficult. In humans, polydrug abuse, smoking, and economic and social disadvantage further complicate attempts to identify causal patterns. No examples of specific nutritional deficiencies, as is the case for alcohol and vitamin B$_6$, have emerged. Thus, few hypotheses are available to guide animal research. However, some areas of research involving two of these three variables may prove valuable in eventually generating these types of hypotheses.

Anorexic and Appetite Stimulating Effects of Abused CNS-Active Drugs A large body of research has been devoted to studying the effects of central nervous system (CNS)-active drugs on food intake. Most of this work is aimed at understanding the brain systems that regulate food intake in order to develop therapeutic appetite suppressants, rather than to develop an understanding of the nutritional consequences of drug abuse. However, these studies confirm and extend what has been observed concerning appetite in drug users and point the way to the study of reduced food intake as a major intervening nutritional variable in drug-induced immune dysfunction.

An example of such a study was performed by Vaupel and Morton (19). They conducted dose-response studies of five agents (d-amphetamine, phencylidine, Δ-9 THC, pentobarbital, and lysergic acid diethylamide (LSD)) by administering a single dosage of the drugs to 23-h food-deprived dogs and measuring food intake over the next 5 d. d-Amphetamine, LSD, and phencylidine decreased food intake, with amphetamine being by far the most potent agent. However, Δ-9 THC and pentobarbital produced increased food intake. Anorexic effects of MDMA (ecstasy) have also been demonstrated in dogs (20).

A general stimulation of food intake by opiate agents and reduction in food intake by opiate antagonists has been well documented in animal studies (21). Heroin has not been studied in this regard, and it is difficult to extrapolate from the animal studies to addict populations.

Marijuana is widely known for appetite stimulation among recreational users. It is used therapeutically to promote food intake in AIDS and cancer patients, but only antiemetic properties have been studied in clinical populations. Appetite stimulation by marijuana has proven difficult to demonstrate reliably in either laboratory animals or humans under controlled conditions (22). Poor nutritional status was not mentioned in recent reviews of the chronic effects of marijuana use (23). Poor-quality diets without accompanying nutritional inadequacies were reported in adolescent marijuana and combined alcohol–marijuana abusers (24).

Tolerance to the anorexic effects of amphetamine develops in animal models; less is known about other agents (25,26). Thus, the role of pharmacological suppression of appetite in chronic drug abusers may not be of major significance to their nutritional status. A more common situation may arise when compulsive use of drugs circumvents normal physiological and behavioral homeostatic regulation of food intake. In the case of opiate drugs, a disruption of endogenous opiate regulation of food intake could be involved.

Abused CNS Active Drug Effects on Nutrient Selection and Utilization One dimension of brain regulation of feeding is the selection of specific foods to correct nutritional imbalances. Alterations in food selection inappropriately triggered by drugs of abuse could lead to selective nutritional deficiencies. It is also possible that effects attributed to anorexia in animal studies where a single diet is available could be ameliorated in the human situation, where nutritional needs can be met by selecting from a variety of foods.

Although amphetamine generally depresses food intake, effects are greater on fat and protein than on carbohydrate in animal studies (27,28). Conversely, morphine stimulation of food intake is greater for fat compared to protein or carbohydrate in rats (29). However, in humans, sweet foods were eaten in preference to protein and fat by opiate addicts (30). Recent studies suggest that food choice alterations associated with opiate agents could be the result of changes in palatability (31). Other information concerning nutrient selection and utilization has been reviewed for opiates (heroin and morphine), cocaine, marijuana, and nicotine (32).

Comorbidity of Eating Disorders and Substance Abuse Recently, a number of studies have elucidated a relationship between substance abuse and eating disorders (33). About one-third of cocaine users have been diagnosed as having eating disorders (34); a similar percentage of persons with eating disorders are substance abusers (35). It has been suggested, but not established, that both types of disorders could result from the same underlying genetic/biochemical abnormality in some human populations (36). If this were the case, the nutritional deficiencies associated with substance abuse might be partially attributable to concurrent eating disorders.

Immune Abnormalities in Addict Populations Identification of specific syndromes of immune abnormalities in addict populations would be a valuable step in establishing animal models and determining the relative contributions of nutrition and drug action. However, chronic infection is very commonly found at a high incidence in intravenous drug abuse (37). Sharing of needles and sexual promiscuity contribute to exposure to a broad range of pathogens, and injection of various adulterants and contaminants further taxes the immune system. In addition to acute infections and chronic infectious disease, autoimmune disorders have been identified (38,39). Under these conditions, epidemiological studies are not likely to be successful in characterizing a specific pattern of immune deficiency associated with abuse of a specific drug.

Direct Effects of Drugs of Abuse on Lymphocytes The discovery of receptors for a variety of neurotransmitters and neuromodulators on circulating lymphocytes has led to study of direct pharmacological effects of CNS-active drugs of abuse on the immune system. This topic has been of particular interest in projecting the influence of drugs of abuse on the progression of AIDS. In vitro functional tests of immune effector cells, as well as in vivo assessments, have been conducted. The drugs that have received the most attention for distinct syndromes and mechanisms of action are morphine and marijuana (Δ9-THC) (see recent reviews in refs. 40 and 41). The mechanism of action of these agents may involve direct binding of the drugs to receptors on immune effector cells, and there is some indication that endogenous opiates, cannabinoids, and catecholamines play a role in normal regulation of the immune system. However, effects mediated by CNS actions are also supported by experimental data. Additional topics related to opiate, marijuana, and nicotine interactions with the immune system have been presented by Watson (42). Immunotoxic effects of amphetamine and methamphetamine (43,44), cocaine (45), PCP (46), and MDMA (47) have also been studied, usually with in vitro exposure and/or assessment, and hypotheses concerning specific lymphocyte receptors advanced.

Potentiation of Substance Abuse by Poor Nutrition A number of animal studies suggest that diet can influence the addictive properties of drugs (48). Relevant studies demonstrate changes in opiate receptor binding in food-deprived states (49) and enhanced drug self-administration in malnourished animals (50,51). Carr (52) has suggested that malnutrition produces a general "reward sensitization" (i.e., an increased sensitivity to the reinforcing properties of food as well as other rewards). An enhancement of the reinforcing characteristics of addictive drugs could promote drug use and addiction in malnourished populations. In addition to an enhanced reward value of drugs, other possible mediators of enhanced drug effects in malnourished populations could include altered hepatic drug metabolism and changes in gastrointestinal tract absorption of drugs. Thus, malnourishment could increase both exposure to illicit drugs and the effectiveness of a given exposure in promoting addiction.

The Developmental Perspective Substance abuse, malnutrition, and infection can converge *in utero* during critical developmental stages. Growth retardation and subsequent immune function defects are among the endpoints affected after prenatal administration of drugs and environmental contaminants in animal models (53), although abused drugs are little studied. The effects of prenatal malnutrition on later immune function are reviewed elsewhere in this volume. Because of generational consistencies in substance-abuse patterns, some pathways of causality for drug–nutrient–immune interactions may involve developmental exposure.

RECOMMENDATIONS

- To provide useful clinical and scientific insights, hypothesis-based studies that untangle the direction and nature of biological effects of drugs and smoking on food intake, metabolism, general debilitation, and immune function are needed.

- Information on acute and chronic effects of abused drugs and smoking need to be separated from consequences of the addiction lifestyle. In human studies, some of the variables can be taken into account by stratification if large enough populations are available. In addition, statistical models that derive probabilistic estimates of causal chains of action could be used.

- Longitudinal studies in at-risk cohorts might provide a better idea of the natural history and time-dependent development of combined substance abuse, nutritional inadequacy, and immune system dysfunction.

- Studies in populations with a high incidence of hypersensitivity and autoimmune disorders, in addition to immune deficiency syndromes, would be valuable in understanding the role of nutrition, substance abuse, and smoking.

- Animal studies of food intake and food preference in connection with chronic self-administration of addicting substances could identify specific nutrient deficiencies that are likely to influence immune function. In particular, it would be valuable to understand if nutritional deficiency syndromes varied qualitatively between drugs or between stages of addiction.

- A possible common genetic/biological mechanism for substance abuse and eating disorders should be explored, and possible links to immune function examined.

- The use of flow cytometry for enumeration of lymphocyte populations is becoming common in addict populations at risk for AIDS. Inclusion of these measures would be valuable in animal studies of drugs of abuse. Also, the legitimacy of extrapolation of flow cytometry data from animals to humans needs to be established.

REFERENCES

1. Preston A. Cigarette smoking-nutritional implications. Prog Food Nutr Sci 1991; 15:183–217.
2. Subar A, Harlan L, Mattson M. Food and nutrient intake differences between smokers and nonsmokers in the U.S. Am J Public Health 1990; 80:1323–9.
3. McNair E, Bryson R. Effects of nicotine on weight change and food consumption in rats. Pharmacol Biochem Behav 1983; 18:341–4.
4. Jias L, Ellison G. Chronic nicotine induces a specific appetite for sucrose in rats. Pharmacol Biochem Behav 1990; 35:489–91.
5. Bridges R, Chow C, Rehm S. Micronutrient status and immune function in smokers. Ann NY Acad Sci 1990; 587:218–31.
6. Sidney S, Caan B, Friedman G. Dietary intake of beta-carotene in nonsmokers with and without passive smoking at home. Am J Epidemiol 1989; 129:1305–9.
7. Emmons K, Thompson B, Feng Z, Hebert J, Heimendinger J, Linnan L. Dietary intake and exposure to environmental tobacco smoke in a worksite population. Eur J Clin Nutr 1995; 49:336–45.
8. Matanoski G, Kanchanaraksa S, Lantry D, Chang Y. Characteristics of nonsmoking women in NHANES I and NHANES I epidemiological follow-up study with exposure to spouses who smoke. Am J Epidem 1995; 142:149–57.
9. Santolaria-Fernandez F, Gomez-Sirvent J, Gonzalez-Reimers C, Batista-Lopez J, Jorge-Hernandez J, Rodriguez-Moreno R, et al. Nutritional assessment of drug addicts. Drug Alcohol Depend 1995; 38:11–8.
10. Varela P, Marcos A, Santacruz I, Ripoll S, Requejo A. Human immunodeficiency virus infection and nutritional status in female drug addicts undergoing detoxification: anthropometric and immunologic assessments. Am J Clin Nutr 1997b; 66:504S–8S.
11. Varela P, Marcos A, Santacruz I, Ripoll S, Requejo A. Effects of human immunodeficiency virus infection and detoxification time on anthropometric measurements and dietary intake of male drug addicts. Am J Clin Nutr 1997; 66:509S–14S.
12. Johnson A, Knight E, Edwards C, Oyemade U, Cole O, Westney O, et al. Selected lifestyle practices in urban African American women—relationships to pregnancy outcome, dietary intakes and anthropometric measurements. J Nutr 1994; 124:963S–72S.
13. Knight E, Hutchinson J, Edwards C, Spurlock B, Oyemade U, Johnson A, et al. Relationships of serum illicit drug concentrations during pregnancy to maternal nutritional status. J Nutr 1994; 124: 973S–80S.
14. Lopez M, Huang C, Chen G, Watson R. Splenocyte subsets in normal and protein malnourished mice after long-term exposure to cocaine and morphine. Life Sci 1991; 17:1253–62.
15. Watson R. LP-BM5, a murine model of acquired immunodeficiency syndrome: role of cocaine, morphine, alcohol and carotenoids in nutritional immunomodulation. J Nutr 1992; 122:744–8.
16. Watson R, Mohs M. Effects of morphine, cocaine, and heroin on nutrition. Prog Clin Biol Res 1989; 325:413–8.
17. Watson R, Prabhala R, Darban H, Yahya M, Smith T. Changes in lymphocyte and macrophage subsets due to morphine and ethanol treatment during a retrovirus infection causing murine AIDS. Life Sci 1988; 43:v–xi.
18. Petro R, Watson R, Feely D, Darban H. Alcohol, cocaine, murine AIDS and resistance to Giardia. In: Watson R, ed, Alcohol, Drugs of Abuse and Immunomodulation, pp. 315–30. Pergamon, New York, 1993.
19. Vaupel DB, Morton EC. Anorexia and hyperphagia produced by five pharmacologic classes of hallucinogens. Pharmacol Biochem Behav 1982; 17:539–45.
20. Nozaki M, Vaupel D, Bright L, Martin W. A pharmacological comparison of 3-methoxy-4,5-methylenedioxyamphetamine and LSD in the dog. Drug Alcohol Depend 1978; 3:153–63.
21. Cooper S, Jackson A, Kirkham T, Turkish S. Endorphins, opiates and food intake. In: Rodgers R, Cooper J, eds., Endorphins, Opiates and Behavioral Processes, pp. 143–86. Wiley, Chichester, 1988.
22. Mattes R, Engleman K, Shaw L, Essohly M. Cannabinoids and appetite stimulation. Pharmacol Biochem Behav 1994; 49:187–95.
23. Hall W, Solowij N, Lemon J. Health and psychological consequences of cannabis use. National Drug and Alcohol Research Centre, Canberra, 1997.
24. Farrow J, Rees J, Worthington-Roberts B. Health, developmental and nutritional status of adolescent alcohol and marijuana abusers. Pediatrics 1987; 79:218–23.
25. Shaw W. Long-term treatment of obese Zucker rats with LY255582 and other appetite suppressants. Pharmacol Biochem Behav 1993; 46:653–9.
26. Wolgin D. Tolerance to amphetamine anorexia: role of learning versus body weight settling point. Behav Neurosci 1983; 97:549–62.
27. Leibowitz S, Shor-Posner G, Maclow C, Grinker J. Amphetamine:

effects on meal patterns and macronutrient selection. Brain Res Bull 1986; 17:681–9.

28. Schwartz D, Hoebel B. Effect of phenylpropanolamine on diet selection in rats. Pharmacol Biochem Behav 1988; 31:721–3.

29. Marks-Kaufman R. Increased fat consumption induced by morphine administration in rats. Pharmacol Biochem Behav 1982; 16:949–55.

30. Morabia A, Fabre J, Chee E, Zeger S. Diet and opiate addiction: a quantitative assessment of the diet of non-institutionalized opiate addicts. Br J Addict 1989; 84:173–80.

31. Yeomans M, Wright P. Lower pleasantness of palatable foods in nalmefene-treated human volunteers. Appetite 1991; 16:249–59.

32. Mohs M, Watson R, Leonard-Green T. Nutritional effects of marijuana, heroin, cocaine, and nicotine. J Am Diet Assoc 1990; 90:1261–7.

33. Holderness C, Brooks-Gunn J, Warren M. Co-morbidity of eating disorders and substance abuse: review of the literature. Int J Eat Disord 1994; 16:1–34.

34. Jonas J, Gold M, Sweeney D, Pottash A. Eating disorders and cocaine abuse: a survey of 259 cocaine abusers. J Clin Psychiat 1987; 48:47–50.

35. Carlat D, Camargo C, Herzog D. Eating disorders in males: a report on 135 patients. Am J Psychiat 1997; 154:1127–32.

36. Strober M, Freeman R, Bower S, Rigali J. Binge eating in anorexia nervosa predicts later onset of substance use disorder: a ten-year prospective, longitudinal follow-up of 95 adolescents. J Youth Adolesc 1996; 25:519–32.

37. Cherubin C, Sapira J. The medical complications of drug addiction and the medical assessment of the intravenous drug user: 25 years later. Ann Intern Med 1993; 119:1017–28.

38. Fidler H, Dhillon A, Gertner D, Burroughs A. Chronic ecstasy (3,4-methylenedioxymethamphetamine) abuse: a recurrent and unpredictable cause of severe acute hepatitis. J Hepatol 1996; 25:563–6.

39. Jankovic B, Horvat J, Djordjijevic D, Ramah A, Fridman V, Spahic O. Brain-associated autoimmune features in heroin addicts: correlation to HIV infection and dementia. Int J Neurosci 1991; 58:113–26.

40. Roy S, Loh H. Effects of opioids on the immune system. Neurochem Res 1996; 21:1375–86.

41. Hollister L. Marihuana and immunity. J Psychoactive Drugs 1992; 24:159–64.

42. Watson R. Drugs of Abuse and Immune Function. CRC, Boca Raton, FL, 1990.

43. Pezzone M, Rush K, Kusnecov A, Wood P, Rabin B. Cortiscosterone-independent alteration of lymphocyte mitogenic function by amphetamine. Brain Behav Immun 1992; 6:293–9.

44. House R, Thomas P, Bhargava H. Comparison of immune functional parameters following in vitro exposure to natural and synthetic amphetamines. Immunopharmacol Immunotoxicol 1994; 16:1–21.

45. Shen M, Luo Y, Hagen K, Wu Y, Ou D. Immunomodulating activities of cocaine—evaluation of lymphocyte transformation related to other immune functions. Int J Immunopharmacol 1994; 16:311–9.

46. Khansari N, Whitten H, Fundenberg H. Phencyclidine-induced immunodepression. Science 1984; 225:76–8.

47. House R, Thomas P, Bhargava H. Selective modulation of immune function resuting from in vitro exposure to methylenedioxymethamphetamine (ecstasy). Toxicology 1995; 96:59–69.

48. Agshar K. Role of dietary and environmental factors in drug abuse. Alcohol Drug Res 1987; 1987:61–83.

49. Wolinsky T, Carr K, Hiller J, Simon E. Effects of chronic food restriction on mu and kappa opioid binding in rat forebrain: a quantitative autoradiographic study. Brain Res 1996; 706:333–6.

50. De Vry J, Donselaar I, Van Ree J. Food deprivation and acquisition of intravenous cocaine self-administration in rats: effect of naltrexone and haloperidol. J Pharmacol Exp Therap 1989; 251:735–40.

51. Carroll M, Meisch R. Increased drug-reinforced behavior due to food deprivation. Adv Behav Pharmacol 1984; 4:47–88.

52. Carr K. Feeding, drug abuse, and the sensitization of reward by metabolic need. Neurochem Res 1996; 21:1455–67.

53. Holladay S, Luster M. Developmental Immunotoxicology. In: Kimmel C, Buelke-Sam J, eds, Developmental Toxicology, 2nd ed, pp. 93–118. Raven, New York, 1994.

23 Nutrition, Immunity, and Alternative Medicine

Katherine Gundling, Andrea Borchers, and M. Eric Gershwin

INTRODUCTION

"Medicines and food have a common origin." The concept conveyed by this old Japanese proverb *(1)* is, in one form or another, central to the medical folklore of almost all cultures around the world. Modern science, however, is only now beginning to provide scientific evidence of this very concept. Until recently, nutrition science has been concerned mostly with establishing basic energy and nutrient requirements that would prevent nutritional deficiencies. Now, the focus has somewhat shifted toward the impact food can have on maintaining health and, particularly, on preventing cancer and chronic diseases. It is well accepted that certain vitamins, and particularly their antioxidant activities, can help prevent heart disease and cancer. However, a host of nonnutritive components of plant foods, especially polyphenols and phytoestrogens, have come to be recognized as "chemopreventers" [i.e., chemical compounds with the capacity to prevent certain diseases *(2,3)*].

Even substances that have not traditionally been considered as food, however, may exert beneficial or even medicinal effects when either consumed or applied. Such substances are often called "herbal remedies"; the term preferred by most scientists is "medicinal botanicals." Neither one of these names addresses the fact that although most of these compounds are of plant origin (e.g., ginseng, ginkgo, *Echinacea,* etc.), they can also be derived from animals (e.g., shark fins, bear gallbadder, etc.). "Materia medica" might be the most comprehensive alternative. We are forced to continue to use these terms somewhat interchangeably in this chapter because many publications and even government documents continue to use "herbal medicine" when really referring to materia medica. Such materia medica have been in use for millennia in different cultures, particularly in India and China, where they are integrated into elaborate medical philosophies. The next section will give a brief history of the development of the use of medicinal botanicals within the framework of these medical philosophies.

The last decades have seen a rapid rise in the use of botanical products in Western countries, including the United States, where they are most commonly consumed as dietary supplements. In view of this rising consumption, the paucity of scientific data concerning the safety and efficacy of such supplements led to concern not only in the medical community but also among US legislators. In order to set the stage for increased scientific research and better information for the public, Congress established the Office of Alternative Medicine (OAM) in 1991. The role of the OAM is to facilitate "research and evaluation of unconventional medical practices and disseminate this information to the public." One of the categories of unconventional medical practices is "Diet and Nutrition" and another category is labeled "Herbal Medicine" (*see* Table 2). Medicinal herbal products, after the passage of the DSHEA in 1994, are now included in the expanded definition of "dietary supplement" in order to give the pubic easier access to such supplements and to give manufacturers the opportunity to provide product information, for example, in accompanying literature. There is a vast array of substances marketed as dietary supplements, clearly making "herbal medicine" a misnomer. The list incudes, of course, vitamins and minerals, but also a large number of botanicals, as well as algae (e.g., Chlorella), fungi (e.g., Brewer's yeast), bacteria (e.g., *Lactobacillus acidophilus*), amino acids, and even hormones (e.g., melatonin and DHEA). It is beyond the scope of this chapter to deal with all these categories. The interactions of essential nutrients, such as vitamins and minerals, with the immune system are addressed elsewhere in this book. Among the remaining substances, several botanicals are emerging as the most likely candidates for stimulating and/or modulating the immune system. This chapter, therefore, is essentially a review of medicinal botanicals and their possible influences on the immune system. In addition, we will examine some of the data available on the usage of dietary supplements for purposes other than essential nutrient intake. We will also address some of the legal and regulatory aspects arising out of the uniqueness and complexity of medicinal botanicals.

The creation of the OAM has, despite its limited budget, given a boost to scientific research with medicinal botanicals in the United States. However, although such research is still in its

From: *Nutrition and Immunology: Principles and Practice* (ME Gershwin et al. eds.), © Humana Press, Inc., Totowa, NJ

infancy in the United States, it has been ongoing for several decades in several European countries as well as in China, Japan, and Russia. In the cases of widely known and used botanical extracts such as ginseng and *Echinacea*, the existing research spans in vitro experiments at the cellular level, in vivo studies in animal models, and controlled clinical studies with human subjects. This is also true for a compound still largely unknown in the United States but approved for clinical use in Japan, the mushroom-derived polysaccharide lentinan. Using *Echinacea*, ginseng, and lentinan as examples, the final section of this chapter will review some of the research available on the ability of medicinal botanicals to modulate various immune functions.

A BRIEF HISTORY OF HERBAL MEDICINE

Before the advent of modern pharmaceuticals, people around the world used plants, minerals, and animals as medicines (i.e., substances intended to treat or cure illness or disease). In the absence of a written language, knowledge of the medicinal properties of certain substances often resided with "specialists" and was passed orally from one generation to the next. In recent years, many ethnobotanists have attempted to preserve this traditional knowledge in writing *(4–12)*.

It is the Greeks, particularly the Hippocratic School, who are often credited with having invented rational medicine *(13,14)*. Classic Greek, as well as Persian/Arabic, medicine perceives the universe as consisting of four elements: earth, water, air, and fire *(13–15)*. Also important are the four humors: blood, yellow bile, black bile, and phlegm. Each of these humors is characterized by two out of four qualities, namely warm, moist, dry, or cold. Disease arises when the equilibrium between the humors and temperaments, of which there are also four because they arise out of the four humors (sanguine, phlegmatic, melancholic, bilious), is disturbed. The goal of therapy is to re-establish equilibrium. The rather extensive materia medica used in treatment are also characterized by the four qualities (warm, dry, moist, or cold) and are chosen accordingly.

By about 200 B.C., extensive trade existed among the Mediterranean, the Middle East, India, and China *(16,17)*. It has been suggested that the theory of the elements originated in Greece and found its way first into Ayurveda and, from there, into Chinese medicine *(17)*. In Ayurveda, besides earth, air, fire, and water, there is a fifth basic element: space. "In human beings, these five elements occur as the three *doshas,* forces that, along with the seven *dhatus* (tissues) and three *malas* (waste products), make up the human body" *(18)*. As in ancient Greek medicine, disease is attributed to an imbalance among these *doshas,* and treatment aims at re-establishing equilibrium. Such treatment relies on, among other approaches, an appropriate diet as well as a vast number of natural medicines, which also include many food items. Medicinal preparations often consist of not just one but several substances.

Trade between India and China generated cultural exchanges. It seems likely, therefore, that Ayurveda influenced Chinese medicine. In turn, many Chinese medical practices, especially acupuncture and Chinese herbal medicine, now exert a strong influence on Western medicine. Because of this special importance, a somewhat more detailed introduction to Chinese medicine seems warranted, even at the risk of oversimplifying the concepts.

Chinese medicine is one of the oldest medical traditions in the world. Its legendary origins are linked to three emperors, Fu Xi, Shen Nong, and Huang Di or the Yellow Emperor, who are said to have lived in the period between 2850 and 2600 B.C. *(17,19)*. The earliest written records of Chinese medicine, the *Shen Nong Ben Cao Jing* and the *Huang Di Nei Jing* are attributed to Shen Nong and Huang Di, respectively. However, historians now agree that these emperors are mythical figures and that the medical texts attributed to them were written at some point between 200 B.C. and A.D. 200 *(17,19)*. The *Huang Di Nei Jing* first expressed Chinese medical philosophy in its currently known form.

The most fundamental concept in the philosophy of Chinese medicine is that of yin and yang *(17,19,20)*. "Yin and yang express the idea of opposing but complementary phenomena that exist in a state of dynamic equilibrium" *(21);* that is, they always exist simultaneously, nothing is pure yin or pure yang. Another important concept is that there are five phases (earth, metal, water, wood, and fire). Some authors point to the similarity of these phases to the four basic elements of Greek medical thought and the five basic elements of Ayurveda. However, Ergil emphasizes that the Chinese concept of the five phases addresses the dynamic interactions among phenomena rather than the more static nature of material elements *(19)*.

An equally important concept in Chinese medicine is that of qi—"the idea that the body is pervaded by subtle material and mobile influences that cause most physiological functions and maintain the health and vitality of the individual" *(22)*. Just as the five phases correspond to yin (earth, water, metal) or yang (fire, wood), so different aspects of qi are linked with either yin or yang characteristics. Thus, if disease is a disturbance of qi, it also results from an imbalance between yin and yang; treatment aims to restore equilibrium. Herbal therapy is just one component of Chinese medicine; it is often used in combination with other treatment modalities.

The ancient *Shen Nong Ben Cao Jing* contains a list of about 780 herbs and also minerals and animal parts. Over the millennia, this number has risen to about 5800, compiled in the *Encyclopedia of Traditional Chinese Medicinal Substances (19)*. Like everything else, herbs have yin and yang properties. Therefore, when a disease is perceived to be the result of a yin deficiency, for example, herbs with more yin characteristics might be used for treatment. Because yin and yang are interconnected, however, and overbalance in the opposite direction is to be avoided, small amounts of herbs with yang characteristics are likely to also be added. In Chinese herbal medicine, therefore, the use of a single medicinal botanical is rare. Rather, several different plants are combined in very precise proportions, most commonly to make a tea or soup (i.e., a hot water extract) *(17)*.

Popular as some of the Chinese botanicals, such as ginkgo, ginseng, dong quai, and so forth might be today, an equally important contribution to herbal medicine has been made by Native Americans *(23,24)*. Native Americans introduced European settlers to their extensive knowledge of the medicinal properties of numerous native plants, including now widely sold botanicals such as the coneflower (*Echinacea* spp.), feverfew, goldenseal, sassafras, saw palmetto, and many more. Traditional uses of plants by American Indians brought renewed enthusiasm for herbalism back to Europe (particularly England) at the turn of the 20th century. Table 1 presents a list of the 10 top-selling botanicals in

Table 1
The 10 Top-Selling Botanicals in the United States

Common name	Latin name	Family	Origin	Sales[a]	Marketed as improving
Ginkgo	*Ginkgo biloba*	Ginkgoaceae	China, Japan	$90 million	Memory and circulation
Ginseng	*Panax ginseng, Panax quinquefolium, Eleutherococcus senticosus*	Araliaceae	East Asia, Eastern North America	$86 million	Immune function, stress
Garlic	*Allium sativum*	Liliaceae	Central Asia	$71 million	Cardiovascular health and cholesterol
Echinacea	*Echinacea purpurea, Echinacea angustifolia, Echinacea pallida*	Asteraceae = Compositae	Middle and Southwestern regions of North America	$49 million	Immune function
Goldenseal	*Hydrastis canadensis*	Ranunculaceae	Eastern North America, Northeast Europe, Northern Asia		Immune function
St. John's wort	*Hypericum perforatum*	Guttiferae	Europe, Northwest Africa, North Asia	$48 million	
Saw Palmetto	*Serenoa repens*	Palmacea	South and North America	$18 million	Prostate health
Grape seed extract	*Vitis vinifera*	Vitaceae	Transcaucasia	$10 million	Antioxidant status
Evening primrose	*Oenothera biennis*	Onagraceae	North America	$7 million	Antioxidant status, source of gamma-linolenic acid
Cranberry	*Vaccinium macrocarpon*	Ericaceae	Northeast North America	$6 million	Health of urinary tract
Valerian	*Valeriana officinalis*	Valerianaceae	Europe, Asia	$6 million	Insomnia and anxiety

Note: *The sales figures for Echinacea and Goldenseal and combined.
[a]Based only on sales from mass markets and food and drug stores.
Source: refs. *24–28.*

the United States, their Latin names, places of origin, and their advertised beneficial effects.

MEDICINAL BOTANICALS AS COMPLEMENTARY/ALTERNATIVE MEDICINE AND AS DIETARY SUPPLEMENTS

COMPLEMENTARY AND ALTERNATIVE MEDICINE

Definition of Complementary/Alternative Medicine
Medicinal botanicals constitute one of the seven categories of complementary and alternative medicine (listed in Table 2). Alternative medicine is defined as those practices explicitly used for the purpose of medical intervention, health promotion or disease prevention that are not routinely taught at US medical schools. Many of them are now paid for or supplemented! Such practices are "alternative" only in the context of conventional health care in the United States. The public is more focused on results and uses

unconventional therapies in a complementary manner to standard Western medicine *(26,27,30).* The accepted term in the United States, therefore, has become "complementary and alternative medicine" (CAM).

Worldwide Use of CAM A survey conducted with over 1500 adults in the United States in 1990 revealed that 34% of the respondents had used at least one unconventional therapy, including herbal medicine *(31).* Since then, the number of people using CAM is very likely to have increased *(32).* It is estimated that this number is now closer to at least 40%. In Great Britain, in 1992, a third of all women were thought to take some form of dietary supplement, and it was estimated that as many as 40% of the adult population had tried these products at some time *(33).* Sixty percent of British health authorities and 45% of general practitioners offer access to complementary medical practices *(34).* Nearly 50% of the participants of a survey in Australia indicated

Table 2
The Seven Categories of Alternative Medicine

Category	Definition
Alternative Systems of Medicinal Practice	Health care ranging from self-care according to folk principles, to care rendered in an organized health care system based on alternative traditions of practices
Bioelectromagnetic Applications	The study of how living organisms interact with electromagnetic (EM) fields
Diet, Nutrition, Lifestyle Changes	The knowledge of how to prevent illness, maintain health, and reverse the effects of chronic disease through dietary or nutritional intervention
Herbal Medicine	Employing plant and plant products from folk medicine traditions for pharmacological use
Manual Healing	Using touch and manipulation with the hands as a diagnostic and therapeutic tool
Mind/Body Control	Exploring the mind's capacity to affect the body, based on traditional medical systems that make up the interconnectedness of mind and body
Pharmacological & Biological Treatments	Drugs and vaccines not yet accepted by mainstream medicine

Source: ref. *29.*

that they had used at least one form of alternative medicine in the previous year.

In terms of monetary value, the botanical industry in the United States, almost nonexistent 20 yr before, had grown into a $1.5 billion industry by 1994, expecting a further growth rate of about 15% per year (35). Germany, the largest market for herbal medicine (although with less than one-fourth of the population of the United States) reportedly spent $1.9 billion on plant-based medicines (excluding homeopathic remedies) in 1994 (35). It should be noted that medicinal botanicals may be prescription medicines in Germany and, indeed, are some of the most commonly prescribed agents. In Great Britain, the market for dietary supplements such as evening primrose oil and ginseng was worth £96 million in 1992; fish oils alone added another £47 million. The total supplement market was expected to reach £750 million by the year 2000 (33).

More current estimates for the US herbal market vary from around $2 billion to $4 billion, depending to a large extent on the market segment surveyed and on the definition of "herbal product." The growth rate appears even more difficult to project; estimates range from 10% to 100% (25).

MEDICINAL BOTANICALS

Available Forms   Medicinal botanicals are offered to the consumer in a number of different forms (i.e., states of processing): in bulk (i.e., whole herbs or plants, or whole plant components such as their aerial [above-ground] part, fruits, roots, or bark), teas, tinctures, fluid extracts, and solid extracts (36). Of course, people can also grow medicinal plants in their own garden or pick them in the wild (a process called "wildcrafting"). The latter is recommended only for those with expertise; for example, hemlock, a poisonous plant, can look remarkably like parsley to the beginner's eyes. We would like to emphasize that medicinal botanicals, being whole plants, plant components, or extracts thereof, have chemical compositions that are extraordinarily complex compared to, for example, pharmaceuticals, which contain a single active ingredient.

Many Chinese herbal remedies are prepared as hot-water extracts, which can then be dried and eventually reconstituted as teas. Commercially available extracts in this country are frequently produced by alcohol extraction and are, therefore, offered in liquid forms with varying alcohol contents. The alcohol used for both extraction and storage is usually ethanol, although glycerol is becoming more popular. Of course, alcohol-extracted material can also be dried and sold in powder form, including in capsules or pills.

Composition, Potency, and Biological Activity   The method of extraction has a major impact on the composition of the final product, just as the vitamin content of food is altered by the conditions under which it is prepared. As with foods and their nutrient content, a variety of other factors can influence the final composition of medicinal botanicals:

1. The place of origin (i.e., the general growing conditions such as soil, climate, etc.);
2. The exact species used;
3. The time of harvest; and
4. The length and conditions of storage.

Given the number of factors that affect the composition of medicinal botanicals and thereby their potency and biological activity, it is not surprising that numerous studies have found wide variations in product content. In 1995, *Consumer Reports*

compared 10 ginseng products obtained over the counter. The ginsenoside content, based on the measurement of six ginsenosides, varied widely, with some preparations containing 20 times as much as others. Even those with the same labeled milligram dosage had 10-fold differences in concentration (37). This confirmed the results of several other studies on the content of ginseng products (38–40). Several samples contained none of the eight or nine ginsenosides that were tested for in these analyses (39,40). To complicate matters further, when wild and cultured *Panax ginseng* were compared, the cultured root contained a slightly higher total content of ginsenosides (known active ingredients in ginseng), yet exhibited significantly lower biologic activity than the wild variety (41). The ratio of active ingredients likely alters ginseng's biological activity, as do other unknown factors.

Standardization   It is the extraordinary variability in the content of active ingredients that has prompted the urgent demand for standardization. Most European manufacturers have been standardizing many of their herbal extracts for years, meaning that for each lot, they adjust the extraction procedure to ensure that a predetermined amount (very variable) of a known active ingredient is present in every bottle or pill.

It has to be considered, however, that standardization is only possible when several prerequisites have been met:

1. At least one active ingredient has been isolated, identified, and proven to be the—or at least one of the major—active principles;
2. This activity itself has to be well defined; and
3. It has to be shown that standardizing for a particular ingredient (which involves manipulating the extraction procedure in order to meet or exceed the required percentage of that one particular ingredient) does not alter the composition of the final product in such a way that it no longer has the desired activity.

A case in point for the first prerequisite not having been met is that of *Echinacea*. Early studies had suggested that one of the active ingredients in *E. angustifolia* and *E. pallida* was an echinacoside, which has subsequently been used for standardization of *Echinacea* extracts. However, *E. purpurea* does not contain an echinacoside and is, therefore, never standardized. Furthermore, it has since been suggested that the echinacoside does not even possess immunostimulatory activity (42). Extensive chemical analyses have identified a number of chemicals present in different *Echinacea* species and preparations, but it has as yet not been possible to identify the most active ingredient(s) for standardization purposes (43–45).

As for the second prerequisite, it is entirely possible that a particular extract contains several active principles that, individually, might be responsible for widely differing biological activities. For example, several of the ginkgolides (terpenes) of *Ginkgo biloba* are well-recognized natural antagonists of platelet-activating factor (PAF) (46). Also, some of the immunomodulatory effects of *Ginkgo biloba* have been ascribed to this PAF-antagonist activity (46–48). There is also, however, mounting evidence that *Ginkgo biloba* is beneficial in cognitive disorders, cerebral vascular insufficiency, and dementia. These effects of *Ginkgo* might be, at least in part, attributable to its antioxidant action, which appears to be mainly the result of its flavonoid constituents myricetin and quercetin (49).

Numerous medicinal botanicals have more than one active

component and exhibit several different biological activities. The question therefore becomes: Which one of them should be used for the purpose of standardization? Or should there be different standards for different biological activities?

We also mentioned the necessity to ensure that standardizing an extract for one ingredient, or group of ingredients, does not alter, lower the concentration, or altogether eliminate other components of the extracts that contribute to its effectiveness. After all, the very reasons offered by proponents of medicinal botanicals for using whole-plant extracts rather than an isolated, purified active ingredient are that:

1. Several or all of the ingredients could interact to diminish possible adverse side effects;
2. They could also act additively or even synergistically, thereby producing greater biological activity than a single ingredient; and
3. Their combination could prevent the gradual decline in effectiveness observed when single drugs are given over long periods of time.

The discipline of nutrition provides several examples for beneficial interactions of compounds, such as ascorbic acid enhancing the absorption of nonheme iron, long-chain fatty acids promoting the uptake of fat-soluble vitamins, or adequate iron status diminishing the absorption of toxic metals such as lead or cadmium. Thus, it is possible that botanical extracts contain factors that enhance or delay the absorption, digestion, or metabolism of other ingredients. Such factors might even have no known biological activity themselves (i.e., might be inert) but, nonetheless, influence the availability of active ingredients. The process of standardization could result in the reduction or loss of these factors.

Thus, although standardization is a valid concept, its practical implications do not appear to have been fully considered by the very people who seem to perceive it as the answer to all problems arising from the complexity of botanical extracts. Although it will contribute to ensuring that extracts labeled as being derived from a particular botanical contain at least a minimum amount of that botanical, standardization will not address some of the other concerns frequently brought up in the context of medicinal botanicals.

Purity and Toxicity   A major concern is the purity of botanical products. There are three possible sources of impurities in the extracts: (1) if gathered in the wild, another plant might be mistaken for the actual one; (2) another plant might intentionally be substituted for or mixed with the actual one; or (3) chemicals and/or pharmaceuticals might purposely be added to the final product. Reports of all three situations, but particularly the last one, are frequent in the literature. For example, adulteration of medicinal botanicals with aspirin, mefenamic acid, diazepam, and numerous other substances have been described (36,50–52).

Just as foods can cause allergic or other adverse reactions in some people, so can medicinal botanicals. Also, just as pharmaceuticals can cause serious side effects in some consumers, so can herbal extracts. Toxicity caused by either a component of the plant itself or of contaminants added during the processing, such as arsenic or mercury, has certainly received ample attention in the literature (53–58). It is noteworthy however, that in many cases, no attempt is made to conclusively show that a particular botanical is the actual agent that caused the toxicity or was even present in the ingested substance. Rather, the authors of many of these reports are content to indicate that because the patient was

consuming a particular botanical at the time he/she became sick, the botanical is thought to be the culprit. The botanical impurity of some extracts, their adulteration with pharmaceuticals, and, above all, the possible toxicity of some plants/their constituents are all cause for serious concern.

Finally, on the assumption that medicinal botanicals have pharmacological action, the paucity of data regarding interactions with pharmaceutical agents is of concern.

REGULATIONS GOVERNING DIETARY SUPPLEMENTS (BASED ON REFS. *59* AND *60*)   Because herbs or other botanicals are included in the definition of "dietary supplement" (*see* Table 3 for the exact definition), they fall under the same regulations and laws that are already in existence for other dietary supplements, such as vitamins and minerals.

The Food and Drug Administration (FDA) is responsible for overseeing the safety, manufacturing, and product information (labeling, package inserts, accompanying literature) of dietary supplements. The Federal Trade Commission regulates their advertising.

The DSHEA provides specific instructions as to what a product label must and must not contain. The label must include information as to the name and quantity of each ingredient. If a product does not contain what the label proclaims it does, as was shown in the case of some ginseng products, the product is fraudulent. Most important in the present context is the provision that a supplement cannot lay claim to "diagnose, cure, mitigate, treat, or prevent diseases." Those are the intended uses of FDA-approved drugs. Because dietary supplements do not require FDA approval for safety and efficacy, such claims would make the supplement an unauthorized (i.e., illegal) drug. However, the DSHEA specifically allows retailers to provide "third-party" materials to help inform consumers about any health-related benefits of dietary supplements.

As with other food products, it is the responsibility of the manufacturer to ensure that its products are safe and properly labeled prior to marketing. Once a dietary supplement is marketed, the FDA can only restrict its use or remove it from the market if it has conclusive evidence that the supplement is unsafe.

The FDA may establish Good Manufacturing Practices (GMPs) regulations concerning the preparation, packaging, and storage of dietary supplements under conditions that ensure their safety. Presently, the GMPs as established for conventional foods are in effect for dietary supplements as well. The FDA has invited public comments on whether these GMPs are adequate and is in the process of reviewing these comments.

It would appear that proper enforcement of the existing laws and regulations by the FDA would go far in addressing most of the concerns raised by the problems encountered with some botanical supplements. Nonetheless, the discussion of the necessity for stricter regulation and/or licensing of herbal medicines continues around the world (61–64).

RESEARCH ON MEDICINAL BOTANICALS

THE ROLE OF THE OFFICE OF ALTERNATIVE MEDICINE

Extensive scientific research is needed in order to determine how safe and effective medicinal botanicals are. The next step is to make the results of such scientific studies available to the public. As of now, there seems to be a major discrepancy between public interest in medicinal botanicals and the availability of good quality scientific information about them. This is, to some extent, reflected

Table 3
Defining Characteristics of a Dietary Supplement

- A product (other than tobacco) that is intended to supplement the diet that bears or contains one or more of the following dietary ingredients: a vitamin, a mineral, an herb or other botanical, an amino acid, a dietary substance for use by man (sic!) to supplement the diet by increasing the total daily intake, or a concentrate, metabolite, constituent, extract, or combination of these ingredients.
- Intended for ingestion in pill, capsule, tablet, or liquid form
- Not represented for use as a conventional food or as the sole item of a meal or diet
- Labeled as a "dietary supplement"
- Products such as an approved new drug, certified antibiotic or licensed biologic that was marketed as a dietary supplement or food before approval, certification, or license (unless the Secretary of Health and Human Services waives this provision).

Source: ref. *59.*

in the fact that there are 67 articles on *Echinacea* in Medline (as of May, 1999), but over 34,000 listings of *Echinacea* on web sites obtained through Alta Vista (an Internet information system). This is an admittedly crude methodology because it does not take into consideration that many of the journals that publish research on CAM are not, or only selectively, indexed by Medline. Nonetheless, it reflects the gap between public interest and the availability of scientific information to satisfy that interest.

The Office of Alternative Medicine (OAM) was founded in 1991 with the express goal of facilitating research and evaluation of unconventional medical practices and disseminate this information to the public. Its budget has increased from $2 million in 1992 to $20 million in fiscal year 1998. The OAM has funded 13 specialty research centers around the country to investigate complementary therapies for a variety of health conditions. Table 4 lists the funded centers and outlines their areas of study in 1998. The OAM sponsors intramural and extramural research and offers a clearinghouse of information to researchers, health professionals, and the public. The funding for research has fueled academic interest in previously understudied areas as diverse as immunologic properties of medicinal herbs, complementary methods of pain control, aging, and chiropractic therapies. Results of such research are made available to the media, which, in turn, inform the public, increasing awareness of the issues.

IMMUNOMODULATION BY SELECTED MEDICINAL BOTANICALS Despite such beginnings of research in the United States on CAM, in general, and medicinal botanicals, in particular, a vast majority of the existing literature reports the results of studies that were conducted by Chinese, Japanese, Russian, and German as well as other European scientists. Here, we want to briefly review some of the available literature concerning medicinal botanicals and their immunomodulatory activities. We have chosen *Echinacea purpurea* and *Panax ginseng* because they are among the 10 top-selling herbs in the United States, they are marketed as being able to strengthen the immune system, and they are among the most extensively studied medicinal botanicals. The third example, lentinan, has some properties that make it quite distinct from both *Echinacea* and ginseng. Unlike those two, lentinan is a purified compound, isolated from an actual food item, namely shiitake mushrooms (*Lentinus edodes*). It has been extensively researched since 1969, when the first indications became available that it had potent antitumor activities. It is now approved for clinical use in Japan, but it is still largely unknown in the United States. Furthermore, lentinan research, or at least research on similar mushroom compounds, encompasses some aspects that have, to date, been almost completely ignored in the

study of other medicinal botanicals, namely their absorption, tissue distribution, and metabolism.

Purple Coneflower (Echinacea spp.) The narrow-leaved purple coneflower (*Echinacea angustifolia*) has long been used by Native Americans as a general immunostimulant and as a disease-specific treatment *(24,66).* It was introduced by Native Americans to European settlers who subsequently took what they thought was *E. angustifolia* back to Europe. It turned out, however, that the actual species they introduced in Europe was *E. purpurea,* which has since become one of the most popular medicinal botanicals there as well as in the United States *(36,66).* For medicinal purposes, besides *E. purpurea* and *E. angustifolia,* a third species, *E. pallida,* is commonly used.

What the American consumer calls *Echinacea* can be any one of the three above-mentioned species or a combination of two or even of all three of them, which should, of course, be indicated on the label. Furthermore, many *Echinacea* preparations, including Echinacin®, one of the best-known European brands that has also been used in numerous studies, are extracts of both root and above-ground parts, whereas, in other instances, either the root only or the above-ground parts only are used. There are substantial differences between the chemical composition of *Echinacea* roots and that of *Echinacea* aerial parts *(44).*

Several laboratories have found that various ethanol extracts of the roots of *E. purpurea,* as well as *E. angustifolia* and *E. pallida,* stimulated in vitro the phagocytic activities of mouse macrophages *(42,67,68).* Polysaccharides isolated from either *E. purpurea* cell cultures or the whole plant had similar effects *(69–71).* In addition, isolated polysaccharides increased the cytotoxic activity of macrophages against tumor targets compared to media controls *(69,71).* Furthermore, incubation of mouse macrophages with *E. purpurea*-derived polysaccharides resulted in increased production of oxygen radicals as well as of the cytokines interleukin-1 (IL-1), interferon-β_2 (IFN-β_2), and tumor necrosis factor-α (TNF-α), further attesting to the ability of *E. purpurea* and/or one of its constituents to activate macrophages *(69,70).*

Whereas one study found that *E. purpurea* had a slight stimulatory effect on the proliferation of purified mouse T cells but did not activate B cells *(70),* another study reported no effect on T cells but a modest increase in B cell proliferation *(69).*

Human macrophages incubated in vitro with either a lyophilized and reconstituted fresh-pressed juice or a reconstituted dried juice (both commercially available) produced the cytokines TNF-α, IL-1, and IL-10 at levels comparable to, or higher than, those seen with lipopolysaccharide (LPS) stimulation, whereas their IL-6 production was higher than in controls but lower than

Table 4
The 13 Clinical Research Centers Supported by the OAM

Research center	Specialty	Project(s)
The Center for Addiction and Alternative Medicine Research, the Hennepin County Medical Center and University of Minnesota Medical School, Minneapolis, MN	Addictions	Study the use, applicability, and effectiveness of alternative treatments for substance abuse
Complementary and Alternative Medicine Program (CAMPS) at the Stanford Center for Research in Disease Prevention, Stanford University, Palo Alto, CA	Aging	Evaluate the effectiveness of alternative therapies for improving functional capacity and quality of life for the elderly
Center for Alternative Medicine Research in Asthma and Immunology, University of California, Davis, CA	Asthma, allergy and immunology	Identify and evaluate alternative medical treatments for asthma
University of Texas Center for Alternative Medicine (UT-CAM) Research in Cancer, University of Texas, Houston, TX	Cancer	Study the effectiveness of biopharmacological–herbal therapies in preventing and treating cancer
Consortial Center for Chiropractic Research, Palmer Center for Chiropractic Research, Davenport, IA	Chiropractic	Examine the effectiveness and validity of chiropractic therapies for musculoskeletal conditions
The Center for Alternative Medicine Research at Beth Israel Hospital, Harvard Medical School, Boston, MA	General medical conditions	Investigate alternative medical practices in the treatment of common chronic medical conditions
Bastyr University AIDS Research Center Bothel, WA	HIV and AIDS	Describe current patterns of use of CAM in patients with HIV and AIDS and examine their effectiveness
University of Virginia Center for the Study of Complementary & Alternative Therapies (CSCAT), University of Virginia School of Nursing, Charlottesvile, VA	Pain	Examine the effectiveness, safety, and cost of alternative medical therapies in the management of acute and chronic pain
Center for Alternative Medicine Pain Research and Evaluation (CAMPRE) at the University of Maryland School of Medicine, Baltimore, MD	Pain	Review the scientific literature on CAM therapies in pain management and create a research database of the existing scientific articles
Center for Research in Complimentary and Alternative Medicine for Stroke and Neurological Disorders, Kessler Institute for Rehabilitation, West Orange, NJ	Stroke and neurological conditions	Evaluate effectiveness and validity of CAM therapies for the rehabilitation of stroke, spinal cord, and traumatic brain injury patients
Center for Complementary & Alternative Medicine Research in Women's Health at the Columbia University College of Physicians and Surgeons, New York, NY	Women's health	Review the existing literature on the use of CAM therapies in promoting women's health in order to formulate a research agenda
University of Michigan, Ann Arbor, MI[a]	Cardiovascular disease	
University of Arizona, Tucson, AZ[a]	Pediatrics	

[a]More precise information was unavailable at the time of writing.
Source: ref. *65.*

that seen with LPS *(72).* Incubation of human macrophages with a purified polysaccharide from *E. purpurea* cell culture also induced the production of TNF-α, IL-1, and IL-6. In addition, this polysaccharide increased the motility of human polymorphonuclear cells (PMN) as well as their cytotoxic activity against staphylococci and stimulated the proliferation of human lymphocytes *(73).* Both natural-killer (NK) activity and antibody-dependent cell cytotoxicity were higher after treatment with an *E. purpurea*/RPMI homogenate compared to untreated controls in peripheral blood mononuclear cells (PBMC) isolated from either healthy subjects or patients with chronic fatigue syndrome (CFS) or acquired immunodeficiency syndrome (AIDS) *(74).*

In vivo, ethanolic root extracts of *E. purpurea* significantly increased the phagocytic activity of both liver and spleen macrophages in mice treated three times daily for 2 d by gavage *(42).* Intravenous (iv) treatment of mice with a polysaccharide isolated from *E. purpurea* cell culture significantly increased the survival

rate of normal as well as immunosuppressed mice infected with lethal dosages of *Candida albicans* or *Listeria monocytogenes* *(71,75).*

In human subjects, an alcohol extract of *Echinacea purpurea* roots administered either iv or orally resulted in a significant increase in the phagocytic activity of granulocytes *(76,77).* In contrast to the results obtained in vitro, iv injection of a polysaccharide from *E. purpurea* did not significantly increase the levels of TNF-α, IL-1β, or IFN activity in human serum or plasma, although monocytes and PMN were induced to migrate into the peripheral blood *(73).*

In vitro and in vivo, in mice as well as in humans, *E. purpurea* extracts or isolated polysaccharides are neither toxic nor mutagenic *(78,79).* In humans, only paleness, slight and transient tachychardia, and equally transient influenza-like symptoms are the worst side effects reported after iv injection of an *E. purpurea* extract *(77),* whereas oral ingestion of an *E. purpurea* extract produced only slightly more side effects than the placebo. In both cases, the most common side effects were headaches, nausea, and fatigue *(80)*.

In a placebo-controlled, double-blind study with 180 patients with upper respiratory infections, those given a liquid extract from the root of *E. purpurea* experienced significantly fewer and lighter symptoms of shorter duration than placebo-treated patients *(81)*. Another placebo-controlled, double-blind clinical study with a liquid extract containing *Echinacea angustifolia* taken orally by 646 volunteers demonstrated the effectiveness of the medicinal botanical in diminishing the frequency of upper respiratory infections when administered prophylactically *(80)*. A similar extract also significantly reduced the severity and duration of symptoms in patients with upper respiratory infections compared to patients receiving placebo *(82)*.

Taken together, the results of in vitro and in vivo studies with *Echinacea* suggest that it has the capacity to stimulate the nonspecific component of the immune system. The occasional results suggesting an effect of *E. purpurea* on specific cellular immunity are too variable to allow any conclusions at this point.

Panax Ginseng   Ginseng, more specifically the root of *Panax ginseng* C. A. Meyer, has a long tradition of use in China as well as various other Asian countries. It is usually harvested after 2–6 yr of cultivation. Depending on its age and the type of processing it undergoes, it is classified into fresh ginseng, white ginseng, and red ginseng. Fresh ginseng is less than 4 yr old and can be consumed in the fresh state. White ginseng is 4–6 yr old and is peeled, then dried. Red ginseng is at least 6 yr old and acquires its red color when steamed, after which it is also dried *(83)*. Every year, over 1 million pounds of ginseng are imported into the United States. Sales of ginseng alone account for at least 15% of what Americans spend on medicinal botanicals, making it one of the top-selling botanicals in the United States *(84)*. One commonly finds that "ginseng" refers to the species *Panax ginseng* C. A. Meyer. However, another member of the genus *Panax,* American ginseng (Latin: *P. quinquefolium*) and even a member of an entirely different genus, Siberian ginseng (*Eleutherococcus senticosus*), are also sometimes called simply "ginseng."

Many of the chemical constituents of both genera have been identified, including 28 ginsenosides and 7 eleutherosides *(85–88)*. These are thought to be the active ingredients of *P. ginseng* and *P. quinquefolium* and of *Eleutherococcus senticosus,* respectively. Total ginsenoside or eleutheroside content is, therefore, used for the purpose of standardization. Nonetheless, the total ginsenoside content, as well as that of individual ginsenosides, varies widely among different commercially available ginseng preparations.

The similarity of shape between the root and the human figure inspired ginseng's traditional use as a general tonic and antiaging supplement. It should be pointed out that a vast majority of clinical studies on *P. ginseng* focus on its performance-enhancing ("ergogenic") effects, either physical or mental (i.e., on its effects on the cardiovascular system or the central nervous system). However, its effects on the immune system have also garnered increasing attention. Here, we will review only studies concerning its immunomodulatory activities. We will limit ourselves to studies performed either with whole-root extract or with isolated ginsenosides of *P. ginseng,* excluding those involving other purified components or other ginseng species.

In vitro, the effect of an extract from whole *P. ginseng* on mouse macrophages has, to our knowledge, only been investigated in terms of their ability to inhibit *C. albicans* growth *(89)*. The

addition of a spray-dried aqueous extract of *P. ginseng* to the culture medium markedly reduced the ^{3}H–glucose incorporation of *C. albicans* cocultured with murine macrophages. In vitro, an isolated ginsenoside, Rg1, increased the IL-1 production by mouse peritoneal macrophages but had no effect on their phagocytic activity or that of PMNs compared to media controls *(90)*. The ethanol-insoluble fraction of a hot-water extract of *P. ginseng* generated killer cells that killed both KN-sensitive and nonsensitive targets and also increased the proliferation of murine spleenocytes compared to media controls *(91)*.

In vitro proliferation of murine spleen cells was also significantly enhanced by a hot-water extract from wild, but not from cultured *P. ginseng* roots compared to media-treated controls *(41)*. Some concentrations of a hot-water extract of red ginseng induced a slight but significant enhancement of murine spleen-cell proliferation compared to media alone, although higher concentrations were inhibitory *(92)*.

In humans, a *P. ginseng* homogenate in RPMI increased the in vitro NK activity as well as the antibody-dependent cell cytotoxicity in PBMC isolated from either healthy volunteers or from CFS or AIDS patients compared to media controls *(74)*. The in vitro proliferation of PBMC from elderly subjects was enhanced by the combination of an isolated ginsenoside, Rg1, with phytohemagglutinin (PHA) compared to PHA alone. In young subjects, however, the combination of PHA and Rg1 decreased the proliferation seen with PHA alone *(93)*.

In vivo, a spray-dried aqueous extract of *P. ginseng* root administered orally prolonged the survival of C3H/He J, but not C3H/He N, mice infected with *C. albicans (89)*. Because C3H/He J mice are characterized by a functional deficiency of their macrophages and C3H/He N mice are normal, these results suggested that macrophage activation plays an important role in the protective effect of *P. ginseng* against *C. Albicans* infection. Oral administration of a hot-water extract of red ginseng resulted in significantly increased NK activity compared to that of untreated mice *(92)*. Intraperitoneal injections of an ethanol extract of *P. ginseng* resulted in significantly higher NK activity in ginseng-treated compared to vehicle-treated mice and was also able to slightly increase the NK activity of mice that were immunosuppressed with cyclophosphamide *(94)*. In the same study, *P. ginseng* significantly improved the recovery of mice after challenge with *L. monocytogenes* compared to vehicle-treated mice. Taken together, these results suggested that the stimulation of NK activity might be one mechanism by which *P. ginseng* increases host resistance against *L. monocytogenes* infection. Mice treated intraperitoneally with an isolated ginsenoside, Rg1, also showed higher NK activity than mice treated with phosphate-buffered saline (PBS) *(90)*, whereas an extract of total *P. ginseng* saponins had no effect on NK activity *(95)*.

An increase of the percentage of T cells in murine spleen cells has been reported both after oral administration of a hot-water extract of wild (but not cultured) *P. ginseng (41)* and after ip injection of Rg1 *(90)*. The number of antigen-reactive T lymphocytes and the cell-mediated immune response were also enhanced by ip administration of Rg1 to mice *(90)*. Oral administration of a hot-water extract of red ginseng to Balb/c mice increased not only the cytotoxic activity of T cells but also the antibody formation against sheep red blood cells (SRBC) *(92)*. On the other hand, an extract of total saponins had no effect on antibody production in virus-infected CBA mice *(95)*. Yet, ip administration of Rg1 resulted in an increase in the number of plaque-forming cells against SRBC in healthy ICR mice compared to saline-injected animals (90).

In a randomized placebo-controlled clinical trial involving 60 volunteers taking either an aqueous or a standardized extract of *Panax ginseng* or placebo, both extracts significantly increased the chemotaxis of PMNs as well as their phagocytosis and intracellular killing compared to placebo treatment. The NK activity and CD4 cell count also were higher after ginseng treatment than after placebo treatment (96). A second randomized placebo-controlled clinical trial conducted by the same research group investigated the effects of a standardized *P. ginseng* extract given in conjunction with vaccination against influenza (97). The difference in antibody titers against the vaccine and NK activity between the ginseng-treated and the placebo groups were highly significant. The ginseng-treated group also had significantly fewer common colds than did the placebo group.

Taken together, the research on *Panax ginseng* strongly suggests that it not only can strengthen the nonspecific arm of the immune system, such as the activities of macrophages, PMNs, and NK cells, but is also capable of enhancing the specific immune response (e.g., antibody production by B cells and helper T-cell activation).

Lentinan   A new class of biological response modifiers is attracting increasing attention among Western scientists, namely mushroom-derived polysaccharides and proteoglycans. In the late 1960s, Japanese researchers, spurred by folklore indicating that mushrooms had medicinal properties, began studying mushrooms, then fractionating and eventually isolating substances with antitumor activities (98). Lentinan is a polysaccharide isolated from the fruit body of the shiitake mushroom (*Lentinus edodes*). It is a single, fully purified substance, more specifically a $\beta(1–3)$ glucan with $\beta(1–6)$ branches. Its molecular weight is variously reported as between 600,000 and 1,000,000 Da. In mouse studies, it is almost always injected intraperitonally or, occasionally, intravenously. In humans, it is almost invariably injected intravenously. The properties and activities of lentinan have been studied for almost 30 years. The available research up until 1982 was reviewed by two of the leading investigators in the field (99) and will be only briefly summarized here.

In 1969, lentinan was discovered to be effective against mouse sarcoma 180 inoculated into Swiss albino mice (100). In the following years, it was shown to have antitumor effects in allogeneic, syngeneic, and autochthonous tumors in various species of mice (99, and references therein). Lentinan increased the phagocytic activity of mouse macrophages in vitro (101) and increased their cytotoxic response in vitro (102) and in vivo, although considerable differences were observed among the various mouse strains tested (103–105).

The suppression of the antitumor effect of lentinan by antilymphocyte serum indicated early on that T cells played an important role in the antitumor mechanism of lentinan in mice (106). This was confirmed by the lack of effect by lentinan on tumor growth in thymectomized mice, as opposed to the almost complete regression of tumors in lentinan-treated mice that had not undergone thymectomies (107). In tumor-bearing mice with impaired T-cell-dependent antibody responses by B cells, yet unimpaired T-cell-independent antibody responses, lentinan restored the T-cell-dependent B-cell activity. This pointed to the involvement of helper T cells in the anticancer activity of lentinan (108). On the other hand, enhanced generation of cytotoxic T lymphocytes

(CTL) induced by lentinan treatment both in vitro and in vivo suggested that the lentinan antitumor mechanism also depends on cytotoxic T cells (109,110). Since then, experiments involving the depletion of T-cell subsets have confirmed that both helper and cytotoxic T cells participate in the antitumor mechanism of lentinan in mice (111,112). However, in nude mice who are almost completely devoid of T cells and in whom, therefore, lentinan alone does not exert its usual antitumor effect, a tumor-specific helper-T-cell clone alone was able to restore the antitumor effect of lentinan (112).

In addition to its effects on macrophages and T cells, lentinan also augmented the humoral response in oxazolone-sensitized mice compared to mice that had not received lentinan. Both the total antibody response and the IgG levels were higher in lentinan-treated mice than in controls, both 7 and 14 d after sensitization (113).

Further effects of lentinan on the murine immune system include the ability to activate the alternative pathway of the complement system (114,115) and to induce several acute-phase proteins (116). These two activities do not, however, correlate with the antitumor activity of lentinan.

Numerous clinical studies with lentinan are mentioned in the literature; most of them, however, are in Japanese. In most accessible studies, lentinan is given in combination with some form of chemotherapy and is injected intravenously at doses of either 1 or 2 mg/patient once a week. In a randomized controlled clinical trial involving a total of 285 patients with advanced or recurrent gastric cancer, the combination of lentinan with either 5-fluorouracil or tegafur significantly prolonged the survival time compared to treatment with one of the chemotherapeutic agents alone (117). In another randomized controlled study with a total of 145 patients with inoperable or recurrent gastric cancer, lentinan combined with tegafur significantly increased the survival time and rate compared to tegafur alone (118).

In two studies involving 13 and 39 patients, respectively, with various advanced (stage III or IV) cancers, lentinan in combination with one of several chemotherapeutic agents significantly prolonged the survival time in some patients. Those patients who responded to lentinan treatment had a significantly greater increase (about 2.5-fold) in their killer-T-cell/suppressor-T-cell ratio in peripheral blood than those patients in whom lentinan was ineffective (119,120).

There are some indications, however, that lymphocyte subset changes in peripheral blood do not necessarily correlate with the lymphocyte subset changes actually occurring in the tumor (121). Twelve out of a total of 24 gastric cancer patients received iv administration of lentinan twice before surgery. Inexplicably, the first injection was given anywhere from 9 to 3 d before surgery. The second injection, however, was received the day before the surgery by all treated patients. In the lentinan-treated group, there was increased infiltration of NK cells and monocytes into the tumor tissue compared to the control group. In the peripheral blood and the lymph nodes, however, there were no differences in the distribution of these two cell types between the lentinan-treated and the control groups.

Thirty-three gastric cancer patients in various stages of the disease participated in another study at least 6 mo after they had undergone gastrectomy (122). In contrast to the most commonly used dosage regime, these patients received 2 mg of lentinan iv either at 2- or 4-wk intervals. An increase of more than 50%

above baseline in IL-1β production by their macrophages was observed in about 70% of the patients. It took longer for this increase to achieve significance in those receiving lentinan only every 4 wk than in patients treated with lentinan every 2 wk.

Taken together, these results suggest that lentinan affects every aspect of the immune system either directly or indirectly (i.e., by stimulating cells, which, in turn, contribute to the activation of other cells, resulting in the ultimate destruction of the target tumor cells). Whereas the cells involved in the antitumor mechanism of lentinan have been studied quite extensively, research on the cytokines involved is still somewhat sparse.

Another line of investigation is almost completely absent from research not only on lentinan but also on *Echinacea* and ginseng, namely their absorption, tissue distribution, and metabolism. In the case of lentinan, at least one English publication exists on the lentinan concentrations in the blood of 10 healthy human volunteers and 3 patients with advanced gastric *(123)*. Twenty-four hours after the iv administration of a dose of 4 mg of lentinan to five volunteers, 71±21 ng/mL were detected in their blood by the Limulus Colorimetric Test. In five further volunteers, a dose of 2 mg of lentinan resulted in blood levels of 53±11 ng/mL 24 h later. In the three cancer patients who received 1 mg of lentinan, peak concentrations of 51, 73, and 71 ng/mL, respectively, were reached at the end of a 2-h drip infusion. Their 24-h level was approximately 20 ng/mL. In all three groups, lentinan was still detected in the blood even 3 d after the infusion.

Two other β(1–3) glucans isolated from mushrooms, GRN from *Grifola frondosa* and SSG from *Sclerotinia sclerotiorum,* with structures and antitumor activities similar to those of lentinan have been used in studies on blood clearance and tissue distribution of β(1–3) glucans in mice *(124–126)*. Two iv injections of metabolically labeled ^{3}H–SSG given on successive days were cleared quite rapidly from the blood and deposited mostly in the liver, kidney, and spleen, where the label remained high for at least 5 wk, even though Kuppfer cells in the liver metabolized the ^{3}H–SSG into fragments of much lower molecular weight than the native ^{3}H–SSG *(126)*. ^{3}H–SSG injected intraperitoneally also was distributed mostly to the liver, kidney, and spleen within 48 h after its administration and remained constant in those tissues for at least 4 wk *(125)*. Interestingly, ^{3}H–SSG was not effectively incorporated into PEC even after ip injection, and the majority of the ^{3}H–SSG recovered from the spleen and liver also was in the extracellular fraction. After multiple dosages over periods of up to 35 wk, both SSG and GRN remained high in the blood, although significant amounts of glucans were also found in the liver and spleen *(124)*. Such results agree with the finding that weekly administration of lentinan is sufficient to see an effect and that even intermittent injections (every 2 or 4 wk) still produce some measurable results.

Some of the research available on lentinan addresses yet another issue that appears to be ignored in the studies done with *Echinacea* and *P. ginseng,* namely the fact that different mouse strains as well as different people might not respond equally to medicinal botanicals. Numerous reports on the differences in the way various mouse strains and also people respond to lentinan are found in the literature *(102,103,119,120)*. Two biological activities of lentinan, the induction of acute-phase proteins (APP) and particularly the induction of a vascular dilatation hemorrhage (VDH) response, appear to correlate with the host responses to lentinan *(127)*. Tests on the F$_1$ hybrids obtained by crosses of strains either sensitive or resistant to lentinan as well as on backcross progeny indicated that both the APP and the VDH response were controlled by a single gene. Resistance to induction of APP but sensitivity to induction of VDH by lentinan were the dominant traits *(116,128)*.

SHORTCOMINGS OF RESEARCH ON MEDICINAL BOTANICALS The preceding examples illustrate some of the problems in the existing research on medicinal botanicals. These problems arise, on the one hand, from the different chemical composition of botanical preparations due to the use of (1) different plant species, (2) different plant parts (e.g., whole plant, root, aerial part), and (3) different extraction methods (e.g., alcohol, hot water, pressed juice). On the other hand, further complications are created by the fact that botanicals are administered by various routes (e.g., oral, intraperitoneal, intravenous, intramuscular, subcutaneous) and to numerous different animal strains that might be more or less responsive to the botanical studied.

One of the leading scientists in *Echinacea* research, Hildebert Wagner, and his colleagues accurately wrote: "Without knowing a preparation's chemical composition, extrapolation of the results obtained with that preparation to others is impossible" *(129)*. Reproducibility, of course, also becomes severely limited. The research team headed by Wagner, therefore, has long urged the use of high-performance liquid chromatography fingerprints in order to document the exact chemical composition of an extract so as to be able to correlate specific chemical constituents with observed immunomodulatory activities and to obtain reproducible results *(42,43,67)*. Questions such as how the route of administration and characteristics of the animal model impact the effectiveness of a particular botanical will have to be addressed by research as extensive and detailed as that performed with lentinan.

More extensive research is also needed in several other areas. Although occasionally animal studies, at least, are conducted over fairly long periods of time (e.g., ref. *124*), data, especially clinical data, on the effects of long-term use of medicinal botanicals are still mostly unavailable. It would seem particularly urgent to address the question of whether the long-term use of immunostimulatory compounds is advisable for healthy people or even for people with compromised immune function as a result of old age or actual disease. The use of such immunostimulatory preparations in people with autoimmune diseases is unwise.

Research on the absorption, blood clearance, tissue distribution, metabolism, and excretion of botanical extracts are also urgently needed. Difficult as it might be, it is by no means impossible to obtain metabolically labeled plant components, as was shown with SSG. Even an entire *Ginkgo biloba* tree has been grown in an environment enriched with radioactive ^{14}C-acetate in order to obtain a metabolically labeled extract from its leaves *(130)*. The identification of metabolites of substances from botanical extracts is equally important. It is entirely possible that metabolites of certain chemical constituents in botanical extracts, and not those constituents themselves, are the proximate mediators of one or several of the botanical's biological activities. The identification of such metabolites would be helpful in furthering our understanding of the modes of action of the particular botanical.

SUMMARY

Medicinal botanicals have been used for thousands of years by cultures around the world and continue to be one of the main therapeutic approaches in, for example, Chinese medicine. They are also rapidly gaining popularity in the United States, where their status as dietary supplements and the concomitant lack of regulation and/or lack of enforcement of existing regulation have raised numerous concerns. These concerns center around the issues of the efficacy and safety of medicinal botanicals and are the result of such findings as (a) the complete absence of active ingredients in some samples, (b) the adulteration of some products with either other botanical or pharmaceutical substances, (c) the actual toxicity of either the botanical itself or contaminants introduced during its manufacture, and (d) potential for interaction with pharmaceutical agents.

Standardization of extracts is often proposed as a solution to the problem of lack of active ingredients. We hope to have shown, however, that standardization itself is not devoid of problems. Ultimately, all these concerns need to be addressed either by the increased enforcement of existing regulations by the FDA or the creation of new, more stringent laws—which then also have to be enforced in order to be effective.

Equally as important as an appropriate legal framework within which to ensure the safety of medicinal botanicals in terms of their purity and potency is the creation of a solid basis of scientific knowledge that determines safety and efficacy in terms of their biological activities. The OAM has been created in order to not only facilitate such research, but also to disseminate the knowledge gained thereby to the interested public.

Examples of studies conducted with *Echinacea purpurea, Panax ginseng,* and lentinan show that at least three medicinal botanicals used for millennia by Native Americans and several Asian cultures, respectively, for their "tonic" qualities indeed have immunomodulatory activities. The examples further show that scientific research with medicinal botanicals is not only possible but has already led to clinical applications of at least one compound. Nonetheless, the obvious lack of kinetic data on absorption, blood clearance, tissue distribution, metabolism, and excretion, as well as of data concerning the long-term effects of medicinal botanicals, underscores the need for further intensive research.

REFERENCES

1. Mizuno T. Preface. Food Rev Int 1995; 11:3–4.
2. Potter JD, Steinmetz K. Vegetables, fruit and phytoestrogens as preventive agents. In: Stewart BW, McGregor D, Kleihues P, eds, Principles of Chemoprevention, pp. 61–90. IARC, Lyon, 1996.
3. Stavric B. Role of chemopreventers in human diet. Clin Biochem 1994; 27:319–32.
4. Sezik E, Tabata M, Yesilada E, Honda G, Goto K, Ikeshiro Y. Traditional medicine in Turkey I. Folk medicine in north-east Anatolia. J Ethnopharmacol 1991; 35:191–6.
5. Sezik E, Zor M, Yesilada E. Traditional medicine in Turkey II. Folk medicine in Kastamonu. J Pharmacognosy 1992; 30:233–9.
6. Tabata M, Sezik E, Honda G, Yesilada E, Goto K, Ikeshiro Y. Traditional medicine in Turkey III. Folk medicine in east Anatolia; Van and Bitis Provinces. J Pharmacognosy 1994; 32:3–12.
7. Yesilada E, Honda G, Sezik E, Tabata M, Goto K, Ikeshiro Y. Traditional medicine in Turkey IV. Folk medicine in the Mediterranean subdivision. J Ethnopharmacol 1993; 39:31–8.
8. Yesilada E, Honda G, Sezik E, et al. Traditional medicine in Turkey V. Folk medicine in the inner Taurus Mountains. J Ethnopharmacol 1995; 46:133–52.
9. Joly LG, Guerra S, Séptimo R, et al. Ethnobotanical inventory of medicinal plants used by the Guaymi Indians in Western Panama. Part II. J Ethnopharmacol 1990; 28:191–206.
10. Cox PA. Saving the ethnopharmacological heritage of Samoa. J Ethnopharmacol 1993; 38:181–8.
11. Rivera D, Obón C. The ethnopharmacology of Madeira and Porto Santo Islands, a review. J Ethnopharmacol 1995; 46:73–93.
12. González-Tejero MR, Molera-Mesa J, Casares-Porcel M, Martínez Lirola MJ. New contributions to the ethnopharmacology of Spain. J Ethnopharmacol 1995; 45:157–65.
13. Phillips ED. Aspects of Greek Medicine. St. Martin's, New York, 1973.
14. Longrigg J. Greek Rational Medicine: Philosophy and Medicine from Alcmaeon to the Alexandrians. Routledge, New York, 1993.
15. Fleurentin J. Ethnopharmacologie et rhumatologie. Rev Rhum 1991; 58:22–8S.
16. Madihassan S. A comparative study of Greek and Chinese alchemy. Am J Chin Med 1979; 7:171–81.
17. Hyatt R. Chinese Herbal Medicine: Ancient Art and Modern Science. Schocken Books, New York, 1978.
18. Zysk KG. Traditional Ayurveda. In: Micozzi MS, ed, Fundamentals of Complementary and Alternative Medicine, p. 234. Churchill Livingstone, New York, 1996.
19. Ergil KV. China's Traditional Medicine. In: Micozzi MS, ed, Fundamentals of Complementary and Alternative Medicine, pp. 185–223. Livingstone, New York, 1996.
20. Bresler DE. Chinese Medicine and Holistic Health. In: Hastings AC, Fadiman J, Gordon JS, eds, Health for the Whole Person. The Complete Guide to Holistic Medicine, pp. 407–26. Westview, Boulder, CO, 1980.
21. Ergil KV. China's Traditional Medicine. In: Micozzi MS, ed, Fundamentals of Complementary and Alternative Medicine, p. 194. Churchill Livingstone, New York, 1996.
22. Ergil KV. China's Traditional Medicine. In: MS M, ed, Fundamentals of Complementary and Alternative Medicine, p. 195. Churchill Livingstone, New York, 1996.
23. Vogel VJ. American Indian Medicine. University of Oklahoma Press, Oklahoma City, 1970.
24. Foster S, Duke JA. A Field Guide to Medicinal Plants: Eastern and Central North America. Houghton Mifflin, Boston, 1990.
25. Scimone A, Scimone A. US sees the green in herbal supplements. Chem Market Reporter 1998; July 13:FR3–4.
26. Thomson WAR. Medicines from the Earth: a Guide to Healing Plants. Harper & Row, New York, 1983.
27. Tierra M. The Way of Herbs. Pocket Books, New York, 1990.
28. Duke JA. The Green Pharmacy: New Discoveries in Herbal Remedies for Common Diseases and Conditions from the Nation's Foremost Authority on Heaing Herbs. Rodale, Emmaus, PA, 1997.
29. www.altmed.od.nih.gov/oam. Office of Alternative Medicine: Fields of Practice: National Institutes of Health/OAM, 1992.
30. Delbanco TL. Bitter herbs: mainstream, magic, and menace. Ann Intern Med 1994; 121:803–4.
31. Eisenberg DM, Kessler RC, Foster C, Norlook FE, Calkins DR, Delbanco TL. Unconventional Medicine in the United States. N Engl J Med 1993; 328:246–52.
32. Gordon JS. Alternative medicine and the family physician. Am Fam Physician 1996; 54:2205–12.
33. Levi J. Vitamins, fish oils and a tonic for profit. Accountancy 1992; 110:40.
34. Smith I. More than pin money. Health Serv J 1996; 106:24–5.
35. Marwick C. Growing use of medicinal botanicals forces assessment by drug regulators. JAMA 1995; 273:607–9.
36. Wuest JR, Gossel TA. The Pharmacist's Guide to Nutritional Products and Natural Medicinals. Health Media of America, San Diego, CA, 1995.
37. Anon. Herbal roulette. Consumer Reports 1995:698–705.
38. Cui J, Garle M, Eneroth P, Björkhem I. What do commercial ginseng preparations contain? Lancet 1994; 344:134.
39. Liberti LE, Der Marderosian A. Evaluation of commercial ginseng products. J Pharm Sci 1978; 67:1487–9.
40. Soldati F, Sticher O. HPLC separation and quantitative determination of ginsenosides from *Panax ginseng, Panax quinquefolium* and from ginseng drug preparations. Planta Med 1980; 38:348–57.
41. Mizuno M, Yamada J, Terai H, Kozukue N, Lee YS, Tsuchida H.

Differences in immunomodulating effects between wild and cultured *Panax ginseng*. Biochem Biophys Res Commun 1994; 200:1672–8.

42. Bauer R, Jurcic K, Puhlmann J, Wagner H. Immunologische Invivo und In-vitro-Untersuchungen mit Echinacea-Extrakten. Arzneimittelforschung 1988; 38:276–81.

43. Bauer R, Khan IA, Wagner H. Neue Möglichkeiten zur Standardisierung von Echinacea-Extrakten. Sci Pharm 1986; 54:145.

44. Bauer R, Remiger P. TLC and HPLC Analysis of alkamides in *Echinacea* drugs. Planta Med 1989; 55:367–71.

45. Jentsch J. Auftrennung und partielle Charakterisierung niedermolekularer Aminoverbindungen aus Echinacea-Extrakt. Sci Pharm 1986; 54:195.

46. Braquet P, Hosford D. Ethnopharmacology and the development of natural PAF antagonists as therapeutic agents. J Ethnopharmacol 1991; 32:135–9.

47. Braquet P. Proofs of involvement of PAF-acether in various immune disorders using BN 52021 (Ginkgolide B): a powerful PAF acether antagonist isolated from *Ginkgo biloba* L. Adv Prostagl Thrombox Leukot Res 1986; 16:179–98.

48. Vilain B, Lagente V, Touvay C, et al. Pharmacological control of the in vivo passive anaphylactic shock by the PAF-acether antagonist compound BN 52021. Pharmacol Res Commun 1986; 18(suppl): 119–26.

49. Oyama Y, Fuchs PA, Katayama N, Noda K. Myricetin and quercetin, the flavonoid constituents of *Ginkgo biloba* extract, greatly reduce oxidative metabolism in both resting and Ca(2+)-loaded brain neurons. Brain Res 1994; 635:125–9.

50. Abt AB, Oh JY, Huntington RA, Burkhart KK. Chinese herbal medicine induced acute renal failure. Arch Intern Med 1995; 155:211–2.

51. Gertner E, Marshall PS, Filandrinos D, Potek AS, Smith TM. Complications resulting from the use of Chinese herbal medications containing undeclared prescription drugs. Arthrit Rheum 1995; 38:614–7.

52. Huang WF, Wen KC, Hsiao ML. Adulteration by synthetic therapeutic substances of traditional Chinese medicines in Taiwan. J Clin Pharmacol 1997; 37:344–50.

53. Ferguson JE, Chalmers RJ, Rowlands DJ. Reversible dilated cardiomyopathy following treatment of atopic eczema with Chinese herbal medicine. Br J Dermatol 1997; 136:592–3.

54. Heki U, Fujimura M, Ogawa H, Matsuda T, Kitagawa M. Pneumonitis caused by saikokeisikankyou-tou, an herbal drug. Intern Med 1997; 36:214–7.

55. Kao WF, Hung DZ, Tsai WJ, Lin KP, Deng JF. Podophyllotoxin intoxication: toxic effect of Bajiaolian in herbal therapeutics. Hum Exp Toxicol 1992; 11:480–7.

56. Kang-Yum E, Oransky SH. Chinese patent medicine as a potential source of mercury poisoning. Vet Hum Toxicol 1992; 34:235–8.

57. Senanayake N, Sanmuganathan PS. Acute intravascular hemolysis in glucose-6-phosphate dehydrogenase deficient patients following ingestion of herbal broth containing Acalypha indica. Trop Doct 1996; 26:32.

58. Tai YT, But PP, Yound K, Lau CP. Cardiotoxicity after accidental herb-induced aconite poisoning. Lancet 1992; 340:1254–6.

59. www.vm.cfsan.fda.gov/~dms/dietsupp.html. Dietary Supplement Health and Education Act of 1994: FDA, 1995.

60. www.cfsan.fda.gov/~dms/supplmnt.html. An FDA Guide to Dietary Supplements: Kurtzweil P, 1998.

61. DeSmet PA. Should herbal medicine-like products be licensed as medicines. Br Med J 1995; 310:1023–4.

62. Vautier G, Spiller RC. Safety of complementary medicines should be monitored. Br Med J 1995; 311:633.

63. Saw HM. Safety of complementary medicines should be monitored. Br Med J 1996; 312:122.

64. Abbot NC, White AR, Ernst E. Complementary medicine. Nature 1996; 381:361.

65. www.altmed.od.nih.gov/oam. Office of Alternative Medicine: CAM Research Centers: National Institutes of Health/OAM, 1998.

66. Hobbs C. Echinacea: a literature review. Botany, history, chemistry, pharmacology, toxicology, and clinical uses. Herbalgram 1994; 35–48.

67. Bauer R, Remiger P, Jurcic K, Wagner H. Beeinflussung der Phagozytose-Aktivität durch Echinacea-Extrakte. Z Phytother 1989; 10:43–8.

68. Tympner K-D. Der immunologische Wirkungsnachweis von Pflanzenextrakten. Z Angew Phytother 1981; 5:181–4.

69. Stimpel M, Proksch A, Wagner H, Lohmann-Matthes M-L. Macrophage activation and induction of macrophage cytotoxicity by purified polysaccharide fractions from the plant *Echinacea purpurea*. Infect Immun 1984; 46:845–9.

70. Luettig B, Steinmüller C, Gifford G, Wagner H, Lohmann-Matthes M-L. Macrophage activation by the polysaccharide arabinogalactan isolated from plant cell cultures of *Echinacea purpurea*. J Natl Cancer Inst 1989; 81:669–75.

71. Steinmüller C, Roesler J, Gröttrup E, Franke G, Wagner H, Lohmann-Matthes M-L. Polysaccharides isolated from plant cell cultures of *Echinacea purpurea* enhance the resistance of immunosuppressed mice against systemic infections with *Candida albicans* and *Listeria monocytogenes*. Int J Immunopharmacol 1993; 15:605–14.

72. Burger RA, Torres A, Warren RP, Caldwell VD, Hughes BG. Echinacea-induced cytokine production by human macrophages. Int J Immunopharmacol 1997; 19:371–9.

73. Roesler J, Emmendörfer A, Steinmüller C, Luettig B, Wagner H, Lohmann-Matthes M-L. Application of purified polysaccharides from cell cultures of the plant Echinacea purpurea to test subjects mediates activation of the phagocytic system. Int J Immunopharmacol 1991; 13:931–41.

74. See DM, Broumand N, Sahl L, Tilles JG. In vitro effects of echinacea and ginseng on natural killer and antibody-dependent cell cytotoxicity in healthy subjects and chronic fatigue syndrome or acquired immunodeficiency syndrome patients. Immunopharmacology 1997; 35:229–35.

75. Roesler J, Steinmüller C, Kinderlein A, Emmendörfer A, Wagner H, Lohmann-Matthes M-L. Application of purified polysaccharides from cell cultures of the plant Echinacea purpurea to mice mediates protection against systemic infections with *Listeria monocytogenes* and *Candida albicans*. Int J Immunopharmacol 1991; 13:27–37.

76. Möse JR. Zur Wirkung von Echinacin auf Phagozytoseaktivität und Natural Killer Cells. Medwelt 1983; 51/52:1463–7.

77. Jurcic K, Melchart D, Holzmann M, et al. Zwei Probandenstudien zur Stimulierung der Granulozyten-Phagozytose durch *Echinacea*-Extrakt-haltige Präparate. Z Phytother 1989; 10:67–70.

78. Mengs U, Clare CB, Poiley JA. Toxicity of *Echinacea purpurea*. Arzneimittelforschung 1991; 41:1076–81.

79. Schimmer O, Abel G, Behninger C. Untersuchungen zur gentoxischen Potenz eines neutralen Polysacchards aus Echinacea-Gewebekulturen in menschlichen Lymphozytenkulturen. Z Phytother 1989; 10:39–42.

80. Schmidt U, Albrecht M, Schenk N. Pflanzliches Immunstimulans senkt Häufigkeit grippaler Infekte. Natur- und GanzheitsMedizin 1990; 3:277–81.

81. Bräunig B, Dorn M, Limburg E, Knick E. Echinaceae purpureae radix: zur Stärkung der körpereigenen Abwehr bei grippalen Infekten. Z Phytother 1992; 13:7–13.

82. Dorn M. Milderung grippaler Infekte durch ein pflanzliches Immunstimulans. Natur- und Ganzheitsmedizin 1989; 2:314–9.

83. Yun T-K. Experimental and epidemiological evidence of the cancer-preventive effects of *Panax ginseng* C. A. Meyer. Nutr Rev 1996; 54:S71–81.

84. Gillis NC. Panax ginseng pharmacology: a nitric oxide link? Biochem Pharmacol 1997; 54:1–8.

85. Hou JP. The chemical constituents of ginseng plants. Comp Med East West 1977; 5:123–45.

86. Liu GX, Xiao PG. Recent advances on ginseng research in China. J Ethnopharmacol 1992; 36:27–38.

87. Shibata S. Some recent studies on ginseng saponins. International Gerontological Symposium. Singapore, 1997, pp. 183–97.

88. Hikino H, Takahashi M, Otake K, Konno C. Isolation and hypoglyce-

mic activity of eleutherans A, B, C, D, E, F, and G: glycans of *Eleutherococcus senticosus* roots. J Nat Prod 1986; 49:293–7.

89. Akagawa G, Abe S, Tansho S, Uchida K, Yamaguchi H. Protection of C3H/He J mice from developement (sic!) of *Candida albicans* infection by oral administration of Juzen-taiho-to and its component, ginseng radix: possible roles of macrophages in the host defense mechanisms. Immunopharmacol Immunotoxicol 1996; 18:73–89.

90. Kenarova B, Neychev H, Hadjiivanova C, Petkov VD. Immunomodulating activity of ginsenoside Rg1 from *Panax ginseng*. Jpn J Pharmacol 1990; 54:447–54.

91. Yun YS, Lee YS, Jo SK, Jung IS. Inhibition of autochthonous tumor by ethanol insoluble fraction from *Panax ginseng* as an immunomodulator. Planta Med 1993; 59:521–4.

92. Jie YH, Cammisuli S, Baggiolini M. Immunomoduatory effects of *Panax ginseng* C. A. Meyer in the mouse. Agents Actions 1984; 15:386–91.

93. Liu J, Wang S, Liu H, Yang L, Nan G. Stimulatory effect of saponin from *Panax ginseng* on immune function of lymphocytes in the elderly. Mech Ageing Dev 1995; 83:43–53.

94. Kim JY, Germolec DR, Luster MI. *Panax ginseng* as a potential immunomodulator: studies in mice. Immunopharmacol Immunotoxicol 1990; 12:257–76.

95. Yeung HW, Cheung K, Leung KN. Immunopharmacology of Chinese medicine 1, ginseng induced immunosuppression in virus-infected mice. Am J Chin Med 1982; 10:1–4.

96. Scaglione F, Ferrara F, Dugnansi S, Falchi M, Santoro G, Fraschini F. Immunomodulatory effects of two extracts of *Panax ginseng* C. A. Meyer. Drugs Exp Clin Res 1990; 16:537–42.

97. Scaglione F, Cattano G, Alessandria M, Cogo R. Efficacy and safety of the standardised extract G115 for potentiating vaccination against the influenza syndrome and protection against the common cold. Drugs Exp Clin Res 1996; 22:65–72.

98. Chihara G. The antitumor polysaccharide Lentinan: an overview. In: Aoki T, Urushizaki I, Tsubura E, eds, Manipulation of Host Defense Mechanisms, pp. 1–16. Excerpta Medica, Princeton, NJ, 1981.

99. Hamuro J, Chihara G. Lentinan, a T-cell-oriented immunopotentiator: its experimental and clinical applications and possible mechanism of immune modulation. In: Fenichel RL, Chirigos MA, eds, Immune Modulating Agents and Their Mechanisms, pp. 409–36. Marcel Dekker, New York, 1985.

100. Chihara G, Maeda YY, Hamuro J, Sasaki T, Fukuoka F. Inhibition of mouse sarcoma 180 by polysaccharides from Lentinus edodes (Berk.) Sing. Nature 1969; 222:687–8.

101. Abel G, Szöllösi J, Chihara G, Fachet J. Effect of lentinan and mannan on phagocytosis of fluorescent latex microbeads by mouse peritoneal macrophages: a flow cytometric study. Int J Immunopharmacol 1989; 11:615–21.

102. Kerékgyártó C, Virág L, Tankó L, Chihara G, Fachet J. Strain differences in the cytotoxic activity and TNF production of murine macrophages stimulated by lentinan. Int J Immunopharmacol 1996; 18:347–53.

103. Hamuro J, Röllinghoff M, Wagner H. Induction of cytotoxic peritoneal exudate cells by T-cell immune adjuvants of the β(1–3) glucan-type lentinan and its analogues. Immunology 1980; 39:551–9.

104. Herlyn D, Kaneko Y, Powe J, Aoki T, Koprowski H. Monoclonal antibody-dependent murine macrophage-mediated cytotoxicity against human tumors is stimulated by lentinan. Jpn J Cancer Res 1985; 76:37–42.

105. Ladányi A, Tímár J, Lapis K. Effect of lentinan on macrophage cytotoxicity against metastatic tumor cells. Cancer Immunol Immunother 1993; 36:123–6.

106. Maeda YY, Hamuro J, Chihara G. The mechanisms of action of anti-tumour polysaccharides. I. The effects of antilymphocyte serum on the anti-tumour activity of lentinan. Int J Cancer 1971; 8:41–6.

107. Maeda YY, Chihara G. The effects of neonatal thymectomy on the antitumour activity of lentinan, carboxymethylpachymaran and zymosan, and their effects on various immune responses. Int J Cancer 1973; 11:153–61.

108. Haba S, Hamaoka T, Takatsu K, Kitagawa M. Selective suppression of T-cell activity in tumorbearing mice and its improvement by lentinan, a potent anti-tumor polysaccharide. Int J Cancer 1976; 18:93–104.

109. Hamuro J, Röllinghoff M, Wagner H. β(1–3) glucan-mediated augmentation of alloreactive murine cytotoxic T-lymphocytes in vivo. Cancer Res 1978; 38:3080–5.

110. Hamuro J, Wagner H, Röllinghoff M. β(1–3) glucans as a probe for T cell specific immunne adjuvants II. Enhanced in vitro generation of cytotoxic T lymphocytes. Cell Immunol 1978; 38:328–35.

111. Suzuki M, Kikuchi T, Takatsuki F, Hamuro J. Curative effects of combination therapy with lentinan and interleukin-2 against established murine tumors, and the role of CD8-positive T cells. Cancer Immunol Immunother 1994; 38:1–8.

112. Suzuki M, Iwashiro M, Takatsuki F, Kuribayashi K, Hamuro J. Reconstitution of anti-tumor effects of lentinan in nude mice: roles of delayed-type hypersensitivity reaction triggered by CD4-positive T cell clone in the infiltration of effector cells into tumor. Jpn J Cancer Res 1994; 85:409–17.

113. Fachet J, Abel G, Erdei J, Josupova S, Chihara G. Effect of lentinan on different types of immune responses including anaphylactic shock. In: Urushizaki I, Aoki T, Tsubura E, eds, Host Defense Mechanisms Against Cancer, pp. 183–94. Excerpta Medica, Princeton, NJ, 1981.

114. Hamuro J, Hadding U, Bitter-Suermann D. Solid Phase activation of alternative pathway of complement by β-1,3-glucans and its possible role for tumour regressing activity. Immunology 1978; 34:695–705.

115. Suzuki T, Ohno N, Saito K, Yadomae T. Activation of the complement system by (1-3)-β-D-glucans having different degrees of branching and different ultrastructures. J Pharmacobio-Dyn 1992; 15:277–85.

116. Maeda YY, Sakaizumi M, Moriwaki K, Yonekawa H. Genetic control of the expression of two biological activities of an antitumor polysaccharide, lentinan. Int J Immunopharmacol 1991; 13:977–86.

117. Taguchi T, Furue H, Hattori T, et al. Cooperative phase studies of lentinan. In: Periti P, Grassi GG, eds, Current Chemotherapy and Immunotherapy: Proceedings of the 12th International Congress of Chemotherapy, Florence, Italy, pp. 1210–1. American Society for Microbiology, Washington, DC, 1982.

118. Taguchi T, Kaneko Y. Lentinan: an overview of experimental and clinical studies of its action against cancer. In: Urushizaki I, Aoki T, Tsubura E, eds, Host Defense Mechanisms Against Cancer, pp. 221–9. Excerpta Medica, Amsterdam, 1981.

119. Matsuoka H, Yano K, Seo Y, Saito T, Tomoda H, Tsurumoto S. Usefulness of lymphocyte subset change as an indicator for predicting survival time and effectiveness of treatment with the immunopotentiator lentinan. Anticancer Res 1995; 15:2291–6.

120. Matsuoka H, Seo Y, Wakasugi H, Saito T, Tomoda H. Lentinan potentiates immunity and prolongs the survival of patients. Anticancer Res 1997; 17–19.

121. Takeshita K, Watanuki S, Iida M, et al. Effect of lentinan on lymphocyte subsets of peripheral blood, lymph nodes, and tumor tissues in patients with gastric cancer. Surg Today (Jpn J Surg) 1993; 23: 125–9.

122. Takeshita K, Hayashi S, Tani M, Kando F, Saito N, Endo M. Monocyte function associated with intermittent lentinan therapy after resection of gastric cancer. Surg Oncol 1996; 5:23–8.

123. Yajima Y, Satoh J, Fukuda I, Kikuchi T, Toyota T. Quantitative assay of lentinan in human blood with the Limulus Colorimetric Test. Tohoku J Exp Med 1989; 157:145–51.

124. Miura NN, Ohno N, Aketagawa J, Tamura H, Tanaka S, Yadomae T. Blood clearance of (1-3)-β-D-glucan in MRL *lpr/lpr* mice. FEMS Immunol Med Microbiol 1996; 13:51–7.

125. Suda M, Ohno N, Adachi Y, Yadomae T. Tissue distribution of intraperitoneally administered (1-3)-β-D-glucan (SSG), a highly branched antitumor glucan, in mice. J Pharmacobio-Dyn 1992; 15:417–26.

126. Suda M, Ohno N, Hashimoto T, Koizumi K, Adachi Y, Yadomae

T. Kupffer cells play important roles in the metabolic degradation of a soluble antitumor (1-3)-β-D-glucan, SSG, in mice. FEMS Immunol Med Microbiol 1996; 15:93–100.

127. Takatsuki F, Namiki R, Kikuchi T, Suzuki M, Hamuro J. Lentinan augments skin reaction induced by bradykinin: its correlation with vascular dilatation and hemorrhage responses and antitumor activities. Int J Immunopharmacol 1995; 17:465–74.

128. Maeda YY, Sakaizumi M, Moriwaki K, Chihara G, Yonekawa H. Genetical control on lentinan-induced acute phase responses and vascular responses. Folia Histochem Cytobiol 1992; 30:207–10.

129. Melchart D, Linde K, Worku F, et al. Results of five randomized studies on the immunomodulatory activity of preparations of Echinacea. J Alt Compar Med 1995; 1:145–60.

130. Moreau JP, Eck CR, McCabe J, Skinner S. Absorption, distribution et élimination de l'extrait marqué de feuilles de Ginkgo biloba chez le rat. Presse Méd 1986; 15:1458–61.

24 Obesity and Immunity

PAUL A. DAVIS AND JUDITH S. STERN

INTRODUCTION

Obesity is defined as an excessive accumulation of body fat stores caused by a mismatch between energy intake and energy expenditure. A clinical definition of obesity is a body mass index (weight/height^2) exceeding 30. A major consequence of obesity and, therefore, a major reason for the intense efforts to understand it are the increased health risks associated with obesity (*see* Fig. 1 for risk stratification by weight and height). Obese subjects have been reported to be significantly more susceptible to coronary heart disease, hypertension, and diabetes mellitus relative to normal, nonobese subjects. Unfortunately, data from national surveys indicate that the prevalence of obesity in the United States has markedly increased (Fig. 2).

As obesity and resultant attempts at weight reduction are an increasingly significant public health concern not only in the United States but other developed countries, a great deal of research has focused on obesity. The majority of this research has centered on the finding and then detailing of the mechanisms responsible for body weight control, weight gain, and, finally, the mechanisms responsible for the negative associations between obesity and health. The nature and identity of both the short-term and long-term mechanisms that match energy in to energy out over a lifetime and their failure or absence in obesity have been, as noted above, the subject of intense scrutiny. The results of these studies have thus far indicated that multiple mechanisms exist that monitor, regulate, or influence body weight. Moreover, it is recognized that not only is our inventory of weight regulatory systems incomplete, but the nature of their interactions that ultimately lead to the development of obesity is far from completely understood. For example, an as-yet incompletely resolved question regarding all forms of obesity is the extent to which obesity is a result of overeating versus reduced energy expenditure *(1)*. The relative importance of these two factors is as yet undefined and only very incompletely addressed in many forms of human obesity *(2,3)*. One reason for the difficulties encountered in obesity research is our incomplete inventory of systems involved, combined with only a rudimentary understanding of how the mechanisms by which the pathways that have been identified participate

From: *Nutrition and Immunology: Principles and Practice* (ME Gershwin et al. eds.), © Humana Press, Inc., Totowa, NJ

in the regulation of body weight work. In addition, there is increasing evidence that these signaling pathways as well as effectors serve multiple functions, not just body weight regulation alone. Disentangling these has been and will continue to be a formidable challenge.

One area of potentially great importance, which reflects the potential complexity that results from the crosstalk between systems, is the interrelationship between obesity and the immune system. The recent explosion in the identification of the signaling systems involved in body weight has opened a new era in obesity research. As will be detailed later, this explosion has also presented us with exciting new opportunities in the field of obesity and its interaction with the immune system. The literature on obesity and its effect on/interaction with the immune system is relatively small. In general, studies of immunologic function in obese humans and experimental animals have indicated that excess adiposity is associated with impairments in host defense mechanisms. We will review several studies that have sought to characterize these differences. This chapter will be divided into several sections. One section will very briefly introduce the immune system. Another section will then deal with experimental studies using human beings as subjects. A following section will discuss experimental studies that have employed animals. We will end with a section that summarizes several exciting observations and findings in disparate fields that represent potentially major opportunities or directions for moving not only studies of obesity and its effects on the immune system but also the overall field of nutrition and health forward.

BRIEF OVERVIEW OF THE IMMUNE SYSTEM

The immune system represents a exceedingly diverse and dynamic collection of cells that provide a defense system to protect the host body from biologically based attacks. The fundamental role of this system is to identify and then to either neutralize and or kill those entities that the systems identify/perceive as foreign or nonself. These include bacteria, viruses, and fungi as well as host cells that have damaged or suffered a mutation. As the field of immunology represents a burgeoning literature, we will make no attempt to describe in any detail the current state of understanding regarding the multiplicity of pathways and cells involved in providing immunoprotection. A simplified approach to the immune system suggests that it can be viewed as consisting of two parts. One part consists of those mechanisms that provide passive and

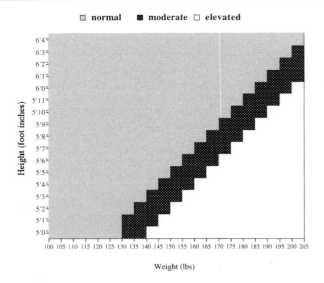

□ normal   ▩ moderate   □ elevated

Fig. 1. The relationship between BMI (weight/height²) and health risk. As BMI increases, risk increases with BMI's between 26 and 27 (■) carrying moderate health risks and those above (□) increasing with further increases in BMI.

or generic defense against the nonself. These include phagocytic cells such as polymorphonuclear leukocytes as well as those structures and components that provide a barrier to entry of foreign material such as the skin and the various different mucous membranes. Another part encompasses those cells that provide an active, recognition-based defense system. This active system relies on a prior exposure to an invader to elicit an initial response and then, upon re-exposure, the "memory" of this invader provokes a rapid and massive mobilization of cells that either directly and specifically recognize or secrete molecules that do so and these processes then rapidly neutralize/kill the nonself entity. The cells composing this active immune defense system are predominantly

lymphocytes. The lymphocytes can be further subdivided into two types of lymphocytes. One family is the B cell that, upon suitable stimulation and/or exposure, secrete antibodies directed at epitopes, recognition sites, on the nonself entity that are recognized as foreign. The other lymphocyte type are the T cells, which provide cell-based defense mechanisms as well as being intimately involved in the process of generating the B-lymphocyte-derived antibody responses. This multiplicity of systems provides multiple potential targets for examining/quantifying changes in or the response to various alterations. However, the linkage of these markers to the overall status of the immune system or immunocompetence remains an area of ongoing and active research and debate. Thus, the interpretation of any study that makes use of a marker or markers to demonstrate alterations as a function of obesity must be done with caution.

HUMAN STUDIES ON IMMUNITY AND OBESITY

Several reports have indicated that obesity results in immune dysfunction. Obese subjects have been reported to have a greater incidence of infections as well as infection-related mortality. These reports have led to efforts to characterize the nature of these defects and/or to overify and examine them in various animal models of obesity. For example, MacMurray et al. *(4)* studied aspects of humoral, secretory, and cell-mediated immunologic status in a group of 22 adults with severe, uncomplicated obesity. Normal concentrations of serum immunoglobulins (IgG, IgA, IgM, IgD) and complement components (C3, C4) were found. Levels of secretory IgA and lysozyme in the tears of obese patients did not differ from normal-weight controls. The obese individuals had circulating subpopulations of T and B lymphocytes that were the same as controls. No effect of obesity was detected on the response of lymphocytes to stimulation in vitro with polyclonal T- and B-cell mitogens. All but two of the obese patients responded to one or more of the recall skill test antigens employed. These authors concluded that severe overweight alone, uncomplicated by diabetes or hyperlipidemia, is not associated with significant immuno-

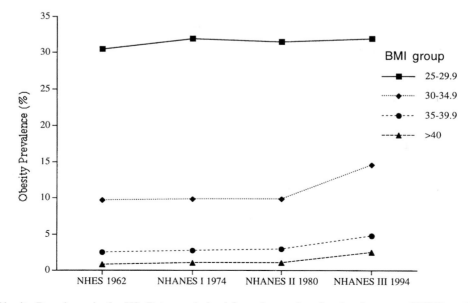

Fig. 2. Changes in Obesity Prevalence in the US. Data are derived from the results of national surveys (NHES, and NHANES I, II & III). The data are presented divided into 4 different BMI ranges ranging from preobese (25–29.9,′) to morbidly obese (> 40; π)

logic dysfunction. In another study, Nieman et al. *(5)* studied the effect of moderate energy restriction (4.19–5.44 MJ or 1200–1300 kcal/d). They measured body composition and immune function before and after a 12-wk diet intervention period for 13 obese (42.3 ± 0.8% body fat) and 10 nonobese (21.2 ± 1.0%) healthy, normoglycemic, premenopausal females. Measures of both innate and adaptive immune function measures (mitogen-stimulated lymphocyte proliferative response, monocyte and granulocyte phagocytosis, and oxidative burst) indicated that despite large differences in body fat mass between the obese and nonobese groups, immune function, as measured in this study, was similar between groups. Noteworthy was finding that relatively moderate weight loss (9.9 ± 1.4 kg) appeared to cause significant immune system functional decreases relative to the nonobese in several measures of T, B, monocyte, and granulocyte function. The authors reported that these data did not support any association of mild-to-moderate obesity with alterations in immune function. In contrast, in a study not designed to look directly at the issues of obesity and immunity, the immune response to immunization against the hepatitis B virus was decreased by increasing age, obesity, smoking cigarettes, and, not surprisingly, having a medical condition that compromises the immune system.

Another study, with the purpose of exploring the nature of the effect of anorexia nervosa on the immune system, examined T lymphocytes, including CD4+ and CD8+ phenotypes, in patients with anorexia nervosa, and, for comparison, in dieting obese subjects *(6)*. Fink and co-workers reported that CD8+ counts were low in anorectics, both before and after weight gain, and in obese subjects after (but not before) dieting.

In a different type of study examining another aspect of the cellular immune process, the in vitro release of macrophage migration inhibitory factor (MIF) by lymphocytes was examined in nonhyperglycemic obese patients *(7)*. The authors reported that MIF release by cells from nonhyperglycemic obese subjects was 36 ± 17% of control values.

Tanaka and co-workers directly investigated whether obesity affects immunity by studying obese subjects body mass index ([BMI] > 30 kg/m²) whose health was uncomplicated by any other disorder, including hyperglycemia *(8)*. They compared mitogen-induced blastogenic response of peripheral blood lymphocytes in 34 obese subjects (mean ± S.E.; BMI: 38.4 ± 2.0 kg/m²) and 35 nonobese controls (BMI: 21.3 ± 0.4 kg/m²) who were matched for age and sex. Mean (± S.E.) intracellular incorporation of [3H]–thymidine, upon stimulation of T lymphocytes with either phytohemagglutinin (PHA) or concanavalin-A (Con A) and B lymphocytes with pokeweed mitogen, was significantly diminished in obese subjects compared to nonobese controls, suggesting that obese subjects have underlying immune impairment in responsiveness of lymphocytes.

Zalevskaia and Blagosklonnaia also examined the influence of obesity and a decrease of the body weight in the patients when treated with a low-calorie diet on several indices of cellular immunity *(9)*. Absolute and relative T- and B-lymphocyte content, monocyte lysosome content, and granulocyte phagocytic activity were examined in the peripheral blood of 27 obese patients and 30 normal subjects. They also reported that an impairment of cellular immunity was present in the obese patients that was reversed upon body weight reduction.

Finally, Chandra and Kutty *(10)* in a study involving obese children reported that 38% of obese children and adolescents

showed a variable impairment of cell-mediated immune responses in vivo and in vitro and reduction of intracellular bacterial killing by polymorphonuclear leukocytes. However, the authors found that the obese group had a higher incidence of iron deficiency and moderately lower serum zinc concentrations and that the immunologic changes correlated with the presence of subclinical deficiencies of trace minerals.

In summary, the bulk of the studies in humans seem to suggest that a variable and apparently modest immune system impairment exists in obese humans. However, the evidence is diffuse and rendered less convincing because, as has been noted by Chandra and Kutty *(10)*, obese subject groups are much more likely to have subclinical deficiencies which may, in fact, be driving the immunologic changes noted. It is likely that the variations in immunocompetence are also significantly influenced by the differing definitions of obesity employed to stratify and/or recruit the subjects examined.

ANIMAL STUDIES ON IMMUNITY AND OBESITY

A large part of the data that link obesity to immune system alterations has been derived from animal studies. The obvious differences between animal models and humans combined with the difficulties in extrapolating results obtained in an animal model versus the case in humans makes a suggestive but nonconclusive case for alterations in the immune system in obesity.

In a direct test of the obesity–immune system interrelationship, Conge et al. studied the ability to resist infections by *Salmonella typhimurium* and *Klebsiella pneumoniae* upon inoculation in mice that were obese via potentially different mechanisms *(11)*. They employed three different models of obesity: gene-based obesity (i.e., ob/ob and db/db mutants), obesity induced by a high-fat diet, and obesity caused by gold thioglucose (aurothioglucose) injection. Kebsiella infection was aggravated in all types of obesity, whereas Salmonella infection was aggravated only in genetically diabetic and dietary-obese mice. Thus, the two kinds of genetically obese mice showed an important functional decrease in splenic lymphocytes, but the third model of obesity (i.e., aurothioglucose-obese mice who were more resistant than controls) indicated that the etiology of the obesity plays a determining role in the nature of its effect on the immune system.

In another study using a mouse genetic model of obesity (db/db), Bennett and co-workers reported that the steady-state levels of peripheral blood B cells and CD4-expressing T cells were dramatically reduced *(12)*. Colony assays performed using marrow from db/db indicated that db/db marrow had a deficit in lymphopoietic progenitors. Moreover, db/db mice were also unable to fully recover the lymphopoietic population following irradiation insult.

In an animal study that did not directly address the issue of obesity and immunity, Moriguchi et al. studied the ability of food restriction to alter several indices of immune competence in young (11 wk old) and adult (33 wk old) female lean (+/?) and obese (ob/ob) C57BL/6J mice *(13)*. Food restriction in the obese mice had a greater effect on body weight accumulation, tail length accretion, and organ weight than in lean mice. Splenocyte mitogen responses as an indicator of the status of the immune system were generally not altered with age in lean or obese mice fed *ad libitum*. However, food restriction augmented these responses in lean mice, but had no effect or reducing them in obese mice. The authors concluded that genetic obesity largely eliminates the immunopotentiating effects of food restriction, indicating that the immune system differs in some manner between lean and obese subjects.

Thus, the animal-model-based studies provide evidence that there exists an alteration in the immune system in obese animals. Again, the limitations of the studies reported preclude a firm conclusion that obesity alters immunocompetence.

IMMUNITY AND OBESITY: POTENTIAL INTERRELATIONSHIPS VIA OVERLAPPING SIGNALS AND SYSTEMS

LEPTIN   The mechanisms that could potentially link obesity and immunity appear to be mediated by a variety of molecules and receptors. A major recent finding in obesity is the discovery of the leptin/leptin receptor system and its involvement in weight control (14). As the obesity-associated increased incidence of infection, diabetes, and cardiovascular disease account for most obesity-related morbidity and mortality, the potential exists that altered expression of leptin or of functional leptin receptors may initiate and/or promote these conditions. Loffreda et al. have indicated that exogenous leptin upregulated not only phagocytosis but the production of pro-inflammatory cytokines as well (15). Moreover, levels of leptin thought to reflect adipose tissue mass have recently been demonstrated to have effects on cells that do not appear to be directly connected to body weight. In particular, leptin appears to be involved in the production of multiple blood cell lineages by acting on the regulated expansion and differentiation of hematopoietic precursors that originate from self-renewing hematopoietic stem cells. Expression analysis by Bennet et al. has revealed that the leptin receptor is expressed in both human and murine hematopoietic stem cell populations and that leptin is expressed by hematopoietic stroma (12). Furthermore, they have demonstrated that leptin provides a proliferative signal in hematopoietic cells. The proliferative effects of leptin seem to be at the level of a multilineage progenitor, as shown by leptin's ability to increase myelopoiesis, erythropoiesis, and lymphopoiesis. Further support for leptin and the leptin receptor's involvement comes from an analysis of db/db mice, in which the leptin receptor is truncated. These mice have steady-state levels of peripheral blood B cells and CD4-expressing T cells that are dramatically reduced and their marrow has a deficit in lymphopoietic progenitors. The deficit in lymphopoiesis in db/db mice was further illustrated by this mouse's inability to fully recover the lymphopoietic population following irradiation insult. In other studies, Mikhail and co-workers (16) have also shown that leptin significantly stimulates the proliferation and differentiation of yolk sac cells and fetal liver cells, and leptin alone increased the number of macrophage and granulocyte colonies. Losato et al. have demonstrated a direct linkage between leptin and the immune system by using anti-leptin monoclonal antibodies to show that leptin receptors are present in the plasma membrane of immune cells located in the lamina propria of the small intestine (17). Finally, in a different animal model of obesity, Yamashita and others (18) have shown that the leptin receptor in the obese Zucker fatty (fa/fa) rats not only exhibits a slightly reduced leptin-binding affinity but also exhibits a reduced ability for signal transduction. This alteration may account for the immune system defects found, as noted in the Zucker rat.

Weigle has suggested that adipocyte via leptin release is a major unrecognized participant in not only energy balance and insulin action but host defense and reproduction, and he has suggested that this new insight may provide new approaches for understanding several important human diseases (19). However, as cautioned by Sinha and Caro in their review of the clinical aspects of leptin, in spite of the strong correlation between body fat and leptin levels, there is great heterogeneity in leptin levels at any given index of body fat (20). This heterogeneity presumably reflects the complexity and multiple-organ systems linked by the leptin-signaling system and makes any demonstration of a leptin-level function linkage difficult.

GROWTH HORMONE   Another bridge connecting obesity and immunity is provided by the growth hormone (GH) system. In vivo studies in experimental animals and in vitro studies using human lymphocytes have indicated that GH is important for the development and function of the immune system. Evidence for a relationship between GH and immunity can be seen in an animal model, the dwarf Snell mice, which has been shown to exhibit an underdevelopment of the thymus along with severe immunodeficiencies that are preventable by GH treatment (21). In humans, the evidence is not so clear. In growth-hormone-deficient children, contradictory data on the immune status have been reported. Span et al. have investigated indices of cellular immunity in 22 adult patients with proven growth hormone deficiency in comparison to those in 100 healthy volunteers (22). Cellular immunity as assessed using total leukocyte count, percentage lymphocytes, and percentage and absolute numbers of CD3, CD4, CD8, CD19, and CD3– CD56+ (NK) cells revealed a statistically significantly lower percentage and absolute number of NK cells ($p < 0.001$). Except for a trend toward an increased CD4/CD8 ratio, no other statistically significant differences for B and T lymphocytes could be observed.

Leidy et al. examined the development and sex-related changes in the hypothalamic–pituitary GH axis in lean and obese Zucker male and female rats (23). They reported that GH content at 10 and 12 wk was decreased in obese male rats relative to lean rats. Spontaneous GH secretion was dramatically reduced in obese animals when compared to sex-matched lean rats. The GH peak amplitude and mean GH concentration were decreased in obese male rats, whereas in obese female rats, the number of GH peaks, peak amplitude, baseline GH, and mean GH concentration were all decreased compared to lean female rats.

Aging in humans is associated not only with diminished immune responsiveness but also decreased lean body mass and increased percent body fat. Spontaneous and stimulated GH secretion, as well as circulating IGF-I and IGFBP-3 levels, are significantly decreased with advancing age. The extent to which these age-related changes in GH and IGF-I contribute to alterations in body composition and function remains an area of active investigation. For example, GH treatment of GH-deficient adults or elderly men with reduced IGF-I levels with exogenous GH increases plasma IGF-I, nitrogen retention, and lean body mass while decreasing percent body fat. GH secretion is markedly blunted in obesity. In humans, metabolic changes such as obesity and fasting can modulate pulsatile GH release. Riedel et al. have reported that 24-h mean GHs are basically higher in normal subjects (1.1 ± 0.6 mU/L) relative to overweight subjects (0.4 ± 0.2, $p < 0.01$ vs. normal) and that the GH pulse amplitudes were increased by fasting in normal subjects but not in obese subjects (24).

Finally, Wu et al. have demonstrated that GH is synthesized and secreted by mononuclear leukocytes by identifying the presence of

GH messenger RNA (mRNA) in both normal and abnormal human lymphoid tissues by reverse transcription–polymerase chain reaction (RT-PCR) and nonisotopic *in situ* mRNA hybridization (25).

ALPHA-MELANOCYTE STIMULATING HORMONE Another example of findings that support a close relationship between obesity and immunity are the data regarding the mouse gene in which the agouti (A) coat color gene produces not only hairs that are entirely yellow but also a syndrome of juvenile-onset obesity, insulin resistance, and premature infertility (26). A clue to the mechanism of agouti-induced obesity came from another mouse coat color mutation, extension, which results from an inactivation of the receptor for alpha-melanocyte stimulating hormone (α-MSH) (27). Further studies subsequently demonstrated that agouti-induced obesity is caused by interference with signaling pathways activated by α-MSH or related ligands (28). Melanocortins, melanocyte-stimulating hormones (MSH), and adrenocorticotropic hormones (ACTH) are homologous natural peptides derived from pro-opiomelanocortin that modulate fever, inflammation, and immunity (29,30). For example, during fever, endogenous melanocortins exert antipyretic effects by acting on melanocortin receptors located within the brain, suggesting a protective counterregulatory role of the central melanocortin system. Melanocortin receptors (MCR), a group of five G-protein-associated subtypes, are also found in myelogenous and lymphoid tissues, various endocrine and exocrine glands, adipocytes, and autonomic ganglia. Of most relevance here is the fact that the agouti protein represents an endogenous inhibitor of MCI-R as well as potentially other MCR subtypes.

UNCOUPLING PROTEINS The recent discoveries regarding the identification of a family of uncoupling proteins that appear to be involved in body weight regulation has energized the field of obesity research. The family of mitochondrial uncoupling proteins play important roles in generating heat and burning calories by creating a pathway that allows dissipation of the proton electrochemical gradient without coupling to any other energy-consuming process. This pathway has been implicated in the regulation of body temperature, body composition, and glucose metabolism. Compared to the limited distribution of UCP1, which makes it unlikely to be involved in body weight management in large mammals, the UCP2 gene is widely expressed in adult human tissues, including lymphoid tissues (in particular, macrophages). These findings suggest that UCP2 has a unique role not only in body weight regulation but also in the immune response (31). Again demonstrating the complexity of the system, leptin appears to modulate UCP2 expression. Zhou et al. have reported that in animals infused with a recombinant adenovirus containing the leptin cDNA, the levels of mRNAs encoding enzymes of mitochondrial and peroxisomal oxidation rose twofold to threefold, whereas leptin overexpression increased UCP-2 mRNA by more than 10-fold in epididymal, retroperitoneal, and subcutaneous fat tissue of normal, but not of leptin-receptor-defective obese rats (32).

SLEEP As a final integrative section, the combination of two data sets suggests an interrelationship between the immune system and obesity. The two differing sets of observation that provide this evidence are (1) the set of observations that indicate that there exists an increased level of sleep disturbances in the obese (33,34) and (2) other studies that have linked sleep disturbances with immune system and cytokine changes (35,36).

The primary observation lending credence to this association is the report by Vgontzas and co-workers examining sleep disturbance subjects. Sleep-disturbed subjects when examined showed a significantly elevated TNF-α in sleep apneics and narcoleptics compared to that in normal subjects (37). Plasma IL-1β concentrations were not different between sleep-disorder patients and controls, whereas IL-6 was markedly and significantly elevated in sleep apneics compared to normal controls. The primary factor influencing TNF-α values was the extent of nocturnal sleep disturbance, whereas the determinant for IL-6 levels was body mass index (37).

Other studies have shown that sleep disturbances are very prevalent in obese subjects. For example, Kronholm et al. (38) have reported that obese twins had higher nocturnal motor activity levels, less quiet sleep, and more habitual snoring than did their nonobese cotwins and that the differences in sleep were associated with obesity-related factors. They concluded that relatively moderate obesity is associated with the disruption of the physiological structure of sleep that cannot be attributed to either snoring or breathing disturbances. Veldhuis and Iranmanesh (39) have studied interrelationship of sleep and obesity with an emphasis on GH secretion by the pituitary gland. They were particularly interested in its regulation by the dominant hypothalamic regulatory peptides, GH-releasing hormone (GHRH), and somatostatin. They reported strongly negative correlation with obesity (+1.5 kg/m² BMI increase, −50% in the amount of GH secreted per day) and that deep sleep (stages 3 and 4) is accompanied by a markedly increased pulsatile GH secretion. They felt that the combined defects in GHRH release and somatostatin excess were the most plausible pathophysiology of sleep disturbances accompanying obesity. As noted earlier, GH levels are intimately involved in immune system function.

SUMMARY AND CONCLUSIONS

In summary, this review has sought to provide an examination of the state of the existing literature in terms of both animal models and human subjects dealing with the interaction of obesity and the immune system. The evidence *in toto* provides only modest support for a downward effect of obesity on the immune system, immunocompetence. Given the multiple, redundant systems that appear to be involved, the defects that result from the interaction of body weight and immunity are unfortunately likely to be subtle. However, the recent and ongoing explosion of discoveries that have provided insights at a molecular level into the identity of the pathways that comprise the body's regulatory system(s) provide suggestive evidence of a tight interdigitation of body weight control and the immune system. The current lack of solid evidence in this area, obesity's status as a major public health concern, is combined with what appears to be an area on the verge of revolution in the understanding of its regulation and interaction (i.e., signaling systems for immune and body weight systems). These factors should lead to an increasing scrutiny and understanding of the interrelationships between immune system and body weight.

REFERENCES

1. Vilberg TR, Keesey RE. Reduced energy expenditure after ventromedial hypothalamic lesions in female rats. Am J Physiol 1984; 247:R183–8.

2. Leibel RL, Rosenbaum M, Hirsch J. Changes in energy expenditure resulting from altered body weight. N Engl J Med 1995; 332:621–8.

3. Lichtman SW, Pisarska K, Berman ER, et al. Discrepancy between self-reported and actual caloric intake and exercise in obese subjects. N Engl J Med 1992; 327:1893–8.

4. McMurray DN, Beskitt PA, Newmark SR. Immunologic status in severe obesity. Int J Obesity 1982; 6:61–8.

5. Nieman DC, Nehlsen-Cannarella SI, Henson DA, et al. Immune response to obesity and moderate weight loss. Int J Obesity Relat Metab Disorders 1996; 20:353–60.

6. Fink S, Eckert E, Mitchell J, Crosby R, Pomeroy C. T-lymphocyte subsets in patients with abnormal body weight: longitudinal studies in anorexia nervosa and obesity. Int J Eat Disorders 1996; 20:295–305.

7. Hirokawa J, Sakaue S, Tagami S, et al. Identification of macrophage migration inhibitory factor in adipose tissue and its induction by tumor necrosis factor-alpha. Biochem Biophys Res Commun 1997; 235:94–8.

8. Tanaka S, Inoue S, Isoda F, et al. Impaired immunity in obesity: suppressed but reversible lymphocyte responsiveness. Int J Obesity Relat Metab Disorders 1993; 17:631–6.

9. Zalevskaia AG, Blagosklonnaia IV. Various indicators of cellular immunity in obesity. Effect of low-calorie diet. Probl Endokrinol (Mosk) 1981; 27:35–8.

10. Chandra RK, Kutty KM. Immunocompetence in obesity. Acta Paediatr Scand 1980; 69:25–30.

11. Conge GA, Gouache P, Joyeux Y, Goichot J, Fournier JM. Influence of different types of experimental obesity on resistance of the mouse to infection by *Salmonella typhimurium* and *Klebsiella pneumoniae*. Ann Nutr Metab 1988; 32:113–20.

12. Bennett BD, Solar GP, Yuan JQ, Mathias J, Thomas GR, Matthews W. A role for leptin and its cognate receptor in hematopoiesis. Curr Biol 1996; 6:1170–80.

13. Moriguchi S, Kato M, Sakai K, Yamamoto S, Shimizu E. Exercise training restores decreased cellular immune functions in obese Zucker rats. J Appl Physiol 1998; 84:311–7.

14. Auwerx J, Staels B. Leptin. Lancet 1998; 351:737–42.

15. Loffreda S, Yang SQ, Lin HZ, et a. Leptin regulates proinflammatory immune responses. FASEB J 1998; 12:57–65.

16. Mikhail AA, Beck EX, Shafer A, et al. Leptin stimulates fetal and adult erythroid and myeloid development. Blood 1997; 89:1507–12.

17. Lostao MP, Urdaneta E, Martinez-Annso E, Barber A, Martinez JA. Presence of leptin receptors in rat small intestine and leptin effect on sugar absorption. FEBS Lett 1998; 423:302–6.

18. Yamashita T, Murakami T, Iida M, Kuwajima M, Shima K. Leptin receptor of Zucker fatty rat performs reduced signal transduction. Diabetes 1997; 46:1077–80.

19. Weigle DS. Leptin and other secretory products of adipocytes modulate multiple physiological functions. Ann Endocrinol (Paris) 1997; 58:132–6.

20. Sinha MK, Caro JF. Clinical aspects of leptin. Vitam Horm 1998; 54:1–30.

21. Wit JM, Kooijman R, Rijkers GT, Zegers BJ. Immunological findings in growth hormone-treated patients. Horm Res 1993; 39:107–10.

22. Span JP, Pieters GF, Smals AG, Koopmans PP, Kloppenborg PW. Number and percentage of NK-cells are decreased in growth hormone-deficient adults. Clin Immunol Immunopathol 1996; 78:90–2.

23. Leidy JW Jr, Romano TM, Millard WJ. Developmental and sex-related changes of the growth hormone axis in lean and obese Zucker rats. Neuroendocrinology 1993; 57:213–23.

24. Riedel M, Hoeft B, Blum WF, von zur Muhlen A, Brabant G. Pulsatile growth hormone secretion in normal-weight and obese men: differential metabolic regulation during energy restriction. Metabolism 1995; 44:605–10.

25. Wu H, Devi R, Malarkey WB. Localization of growth hormone messenger ribonucleic acid in the human immune system—a Clinical Research Center study. J Clin Endocrinol Metab 1996; 81:1278–82.

26. Carpenter KJ, Mayer J. Physiologic observations on yellow obesity in the mouse. Amer J Physiol 1958; 193:499–504.

27. Robbins LS, Nadeau JH, Johnson KR, et al. Pigmentation phenotypes of variant extension locus alleles result from point mutations that alter MSH receptor function. Cell 1993; 72:827–34.

28. Lu D, Willard D, Patel IR, et al. Agouti protein is an antagonist of the melanocyte-stimulating-hormone receptor. Nature 1994; 371: 799–802.

29. Tatro JB. Receptor biology of the melanocortins, a family of neuro-immunomodulatory peptides. Neuroimmunomodulation 1996; 3:259–84.

30. Rothwell NJ. CNS regulation of thermogenesis. Crit Rev Neurobiol 1994; 8:1–10.

31. Fleury C, Neverova M, Collins S, et al. Uncoupling protein-2: a novel gene linked to obesity and hyperinsulinemia. Nature Genet 1997; 15:269–72.

32. Zhou YT, Shimabukuro M, Koyama K, et al. Induction by leptin of uncoupling protein-2 and enzymes of fatty acid oxidation. Proc Natl Acad Sci USA 1997; 94:6386–90.

33. Kripke DF, Ancoli-Israel S, Klauber MR, Wingard DL, Mason WJ, Mullaney DJ. Prevalence of sleep-disordered breathing in ages 40–64 years: a population-based survey. Sleep 1997; 20:65–76.

34. Grunstein RR. Metabolic aspects of sleep apnea. Sleep 1996; 19:S218–20.

35. Everson CA. Sustained sleep deprivation impairs host defense. Am J Physiol 1993; 265:R1148–54.

36. Born J, Lange T, Hansen K, Molle M, Fehm HL. Effects of sleep and circadian rhythm on human circulating immune cells. J Immunol 1997; 158:4454–64.

37. Vgontzas AN, Papanicolaou DA, Bixler EO, Kales A, Tyson K, Chrousos GP. Elevation of plasma cytokines in disorders of excessive daytime sleepiness: role of sleep disturbance and obesity. J Clin Endocrinol Metab 1997; 82:1313–6.

38. Kronholm E, Aunola S, Hyyppä MT, et al. Sleep in monozygotic twin pairs discordant for obesity. J Appl Physiol 1996; 80:14–9.

39. Veldhuis JD, Iranmanesh A. Physiological regulation of the human growth hormone (GH)-insulin-like growth factor type I (IGF-I) axis: predominant impact of age, obesity, gonadal function, and sleep. Sleep 1996; 19:S221–4.

25 Diabetes and Immunity

Manuel E. Baldeón and H. Rex Gaskins

INTRODUCTION

Diabetes mellitus is a metabolic disease characterized by alterations in insulin production, insulin action, or a combination of both, leading to abnormal hyperglycemia (1–3). Diabetes is a chronic disease that has no cure and is an increasing major public health problem (4). The chronic nature of diabetes frequently leads to debilitating complications resulting primarily from nonenzymatic glycation of nerves and blood vessels supplying organ systems (1–3). For example, diabetes is the main cause of blindness in the United States and accounts for approximately 25% of chronic renal failure (3). Diabetes has also been associated with premature death from cardiovascular diseases (4,5). Total social and medical costs in the United States for people with diabetes exceeds $92 billion per year (3). Over 90% of the cases of diabetes are thought to be genetically encoded and are classified as either type 1 (insulin-dependent diabetes mellitus) or type 2 (non-insulin-dependent diabetes mellitus) diabetes. Type 2 diabetes comprises the majority of cases and is typically late in onset, associated with obesity, and characterized by insulin resistance (1–3). Approximately 15.3 million North Americans have type 2 diabetes (3).

Type 1 diabetes, accounting for approximately 10% of all cases of diabetes, is characterized by the destruction of insulin-producing pancreatic β cells and has two major forms. Immune-mediated type 1 diabetes results from selective autoimmune destruction of β cells with disease onset typically between 5 and 15 yr of age, although disease can also arise in adults of any age (3). Idiopathic type 1 diabetes refers to rare forms of the disease that have no known cause (3). The incidence of autoimmune diabetes varies by geographic location and is most common among people of northern European descent (2,4). For example, disease incidence ranges from 1 to 2 cases per 100,000 persons per year in Japan to more than 40 cases per 100,000 persons per year in Finland. In the United States, approximately 1 million individuals have type 1 diabetes (3).

The etiology of type 1 diabetes remains elusive, with both genetic and environmental risk factors (viral infections, diet) being associated with the development of the disease. The genetic component appears to consist primarily of genes controlling immune responsiveness. For example, disease is associated with certain allelic variations of genes in the major histocompatibility complex (MHC) of humans and rodents (6–8). Intensive research is underway to define the mechanisms by which MHC susceptibility genes influence diabetes pathogenesis. Viral infections, toxins, and dietary components have each been implicated as putative environmental risk factors (1,2). Precisely how these ubiquitous risk factors contribute to either onset or progression of disease is not known. However, both genetic predisposition and exposure to environmental risk factors appear to be necessary for disease onset (2,3).

The recognition that diet might modulate onset or progression of type 1 diabetes opens exciting possibilities of preventing and potentially treating this disease. However, a much better understanding of the relationship between diet and the autoimmune process is required. Herein, available evidence demonstrating the modulatory effects of diet in the natural history of autoimmune diabetes is summarized. That body of research forces consideration of intestinal responses to lumenal antigens, especially during development, and possible mechanisms by which protective or deleterious dietary components might modulate the autoimmune process. Accordingly, the latter half of the chapter considers unanswered mechanistic issues, with the goal of providing a conceptual framework to experimentally clarify the relationship between diet and type 1 diabetes.

THE AUTOIMMUNE NATURE OF TYPE 1 DIABETES

Autoimmune β-cell destruction is thought to begin long before clinical presentation of hyperglycemia and to progress through distinct stages (9). The temporal pattern of β-cell loss is not precisely defined and likely varies among individuals.

Although the insults that initiate β-cell destruction are unknown, there is abundant evidence that inflammatory T lymphocytes and macrophages mediate the autoimmune attack (Fig. 1; refs. 10–13). Similar to other autoimmune diseases, it has been proposed that an imbalance between T-helper (Th)-cell cytokine profiles leads to the development of β-cell reactive inflammatory Th1 cells (Fig. 1; refs. 14 and 15). Th1 cytokines (e.g., interferon-gamma [IFN-γ], interleukin-2 (IL-2), and IL-12) are thought to promote inflammation and Th2 cytokines (e.g., IL-4, IL-5, and IL-10) are thought to antagonize inflammation (15). Soluble proteins synthesized and secreted by islet-infiltrating inflammatory cells, including cytokines (interferons, interleukins), perforin, and proteases, have been implicated as mediators of β-cell destruction (2).

From: *Nutrition and Immunology: Principles and Practice* (ME Gershwin et al. eds.), © Humana Press, Inc., Totowa, NJ

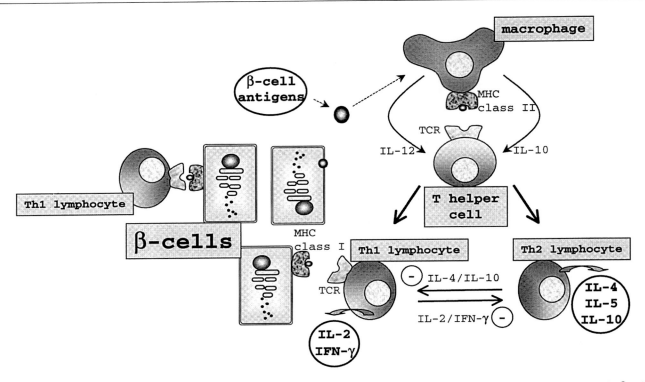

Fig. 1. Schematic representation of the autoimmune process underlying the selective destruction of insulin-producing pancreatic β cells in type 1 diabetes. Beta-cell antigens are processed and presented by macrophages in the context of MHC class II molecules to T helper cells bearing T-cell receptors specific for β-cell antigens. In susceptible individuals, T helper cells would promote a diabetogenic Th1 cell response characterized by the secretion of inflammatory interleukin-2 (IL-2) and interferon-gamma (IFN-γ). Th1 cytokines inhibit Th2 cell production of IL-4, IL-5, and IL-10. Activated Th1 cells target β-cell autoantigens complexed with MHC class I molecules, leading to β-cell destruction.

Further research is needed to conceive molecular-based therapeutic strategies to prevent immune-mediated alterations and preserve β-cell integrity during prediabetes.

DIET AND TYPE 1 DIABETES: AVAILABLE EVIDENCE

The importance of diet as a possible environmental modulator of type 1 diabetes has been supported by human studies and by research with rodent models of autoimmune diabetes (16–19). Consideration of the role of diet in human type 1 diabetes has been primarily a debate on the possibility that early exposure to cow's milk may contribute to disease onset (20,21). Establishing a definitive link between infant and early childhood diets and disease is complicated by confounding issues such as the duration of breast-feeding, the effects of bioactive factors in breast milk, feeding patterns, and the nutrient composition of the diet.

THE ROLE OF BREAST-FEEDING Short duration of breast feeding and early infant exposure to alternative milks or foods have been identified as significant risk factors for type 1 diabetes in epidemiological as well as time-series studies (21,22). Patients with type 1 diabetes were more likely to have been breast-fed for less than 3 mo and to have been exposed to cow's milk before 4 mo of age (19). Early cessation of breast-feeding was correlated with early introduction of cow's milk; however, the weaning diet was not always specified (19). In a single study that controlled for ethnicity, birth order, and family income, people with type 1 diabetes were exposed earlier (before 3 mo of age) to cow's milk

or solid foods than were control subjects (23). This association was observed only in high-risk individuals harboring a human leukocyte antigen (HLA, human MHC) DQB1 genetic marker (23). However, the percentage of breast-fed individuals and the duration of breast-feeding were similar between control subjects and persons with type 1 diabetes (23).

Despite evidence that breast-feeding may protect against diabetes, limited research has examined the effects of breast milk or its absence on the development of either systemic or intestinal immune responsiveness in infants. Breast milk provides cellular and immune factors that protect the newborn against infection, and nursing delays exposure to potential diabetogenic diet components (24). Immune-related factors are typically abundant in "early milk," when the neonatal immune system is functionally immature (25). For example, breast milk contains macrophages, immunoglobulin-secreting B lymphocytes and immunoglobulins, T lymphocytes and cytokines (Table 1; refs. 26–37). Maternal cells have been detected in neonatal intestinal mucosa, mesenteric lymph nodes, blood, lungs, liver, and spleen (27). Not understood are mechanisms whereby maternal cells gain access into the intestinal mucosa or how these cells might influence the neonatal immune system (27).

In addition, growth factors in breast milk, including epidermal growth factor, insulin, insulin-like growth factors, polyamines, and glucocorticosteroids, promote intestinal development and the formation of effective mucosal barrier function (25,38). Thus, infants who are weaned early are deprived of key developmental signals as well as immune-related bioactive factors, and they have

Table 1
Immune-Related Components in Human Breast Milk

Components	Approximate numbers or concentrations	Refer.
Cells	1×10^6/mL	
Macrophages	75% of mononuclear cells	28
Lymphocytes	25% of mononuclear cells	
B cells: IgG, IgA, IgM	20% of lymphocytes	29
T cells	80% of lymphocytes	
αβ T cells		30
γδ T cells		31
Cytokines		
Interleukins		
IL-1β	1130 pg/mL	32
IL-6	150 pg/mL	33
Interferons		
IFN-γ	400 ng/mL	34,35
Others		
TGF-β	1300 ng/mL	36
TNF-α	600 pg/mL	37

Note: Total cell yield, proportion of individual cell types, and cytokine production vary among donors *(35)*.

the added burden of precocious exposure to antigenic or perhaps diabetogenic dietary components. Endocytosis and protein uptake are characteristically enhanced in immature enterocytes *(39)*. Exposure to protein antigens at a time when gastrointestinal mucosal barrier functions are immature could predispose to disturbances in intestinal immune responsiveness or alter the development of oral tolerance *(25,40)*. These considerations expose numerous potentially critical questions that have not been addressed adequately or at all in the context of diet and type 1 diabetes.

COW'S MILK AND TYPE 1 DIABETES IN HUMANS The "milk hypothesis" postulates that early exposure to cow's milk proteins may trigger diabetes *(41–45)*. Abnormal immunity to cow's milk protein has been reported for humans and for the common rodent models of autoimmune diabetes, the diabetes-prone BioBreeding (BBdp) rat, and the nonobese diabetic (NOD) mouse *(44,46,47)*. For persons with type 1 diabetes, both humoral and cellular immune responses to cow's milk antigens have been reported (reviewed in Ref. *21*). Based on these studies, The American Academy of Pediatrics has recommended avoidance of intact dietary cow's milk in infants genetically at risk to develop type 1 diabetes and has asked for prospective trials to study the role of diet in disease prevention in at-risk children *(48)*.

The "milk hypothesis" has been controversial *(20,21)*. Several epidemiological studies from various research groups support a possible link between early cow's milk consumption and diabetes, whereas others fail to find such a relationship *(19–21,49–51)*. Recall bias and differences in laboratory methods (e.g., measurement of diabetes-associated serum bovine albumin antibodies) have been cited as major reasons for the conflicting results *(21,50)*. In a meta-analysis of 17 case-control studies, a moderate effect was observed for exposure to breast milk substitutes or cow's milk before 3 mo of age and the development of type 1 diabetes *(50)*. Fourteen of those studies were retrospective and relied on long-term maternal recall and only three studies used existing infant diet records. When evaluated separately, none of the three studies that used existing infant diet records supported an associa-

tion between milk and diabetes *(52–54)*. The authors of that meta-analysis conclude that the moderate relationship between infant diet and risk of type 1 diabetes could be explained by bias in the long-term recall of the infant diet *(50)*.

Unequivocal documentation that diet influences the development of type 1 diabetes in genetically susceptible individuals would require the identification and recruitment of suitably matched groups of prediabetic individuals (at-risk population and controls) who could be asked to consume defined diets over a period of years *(55)*. The Trial to Reduce IDDM in the Genetically at Risk (TRIGR) was designed to determine if avoidance of intact cow's milk protein during the first 6 mo of life reduces the development of type 1 diabetes in children with MHC alleles associated with diabetes or first-degree relatives of people with diabetes *(56)*. This study, now underway in Finland and other European countries, is a blinded, randomized, and prospective trial that uses the casein hydrolysate-based infant formula Nutramigen® (Mead-Johnson Inc., Evansville, IN, USA) for weaning of exclusively breast-fed infants at risk for diabetes. Nutramigen prevents diabetes in NOD mice, possibly by promoting the development of regulatory T cells that hinder the destructive autoimmune process *(57)*.

RODENT MODELS OF AUTOIMMUNE DIABETES The availability of rodent models for autoimmune diabetes has facilitated greatly studies to define the role of diet in the onset or progression of disease. However, BBdp rats *(58,59)* and NOD mice *(60–63)* have certain immunologic alterations that have not been identified in patients with type 1 diabetes. For example, BBdp rats are severely lymphopenic and lack normal cytotoxic T-lymphocyte activity *(58,59)*. NOD mice have elevated numbers of T lymphocytes and exhibit antigen-presenting cell and suppressor T-cell abnormalities *(60,61)*. In addition, inbred rodents are typically maintained in pathogen-free environments. Intestinal antigens, including dietary components, may provoke immune responsiveness more readily under pathogen-free versus conventional environmental conditions. Despite these and perhaps other yet-to-be-defined features that distinguish disease in rodent models and humans, inbred animals that spontaneously develop autoimmune diabetes are extremely valuable and offer outstanding advantages to evaluate the catalytic role of diet in autoimmune diabetes.

COW'S MILK AND AUTOIMMUNE DIABETES IN RODENT MODELS Overall, dietary inclusion of intact or hydrolyzed casein, a major protein fraction of cow's milk, appears to prevent or delay the onset of diabetes development in BBdp rats and NOD mice (Table 2; ref. *64–68*). For example, a semipurified diet containing 10% skim milk powder and 20% casein inhibited the development of diabetes in NOD female mice *(64)*. Similarly, skim milk powder and several other milk components, including lactalbumin and hydrolyzed lactalbumin, have variable and generally low diabetogenic effects in the BBdp rat *(17,20)*. Because of their protective nature, casein or hydrolyzed casein-based diets are often used as negative control diets when evaluating diabetogenic plant-based diets in rodent models of diabetes *(16–18,64)*.

PLANT-BASED DIETS AND AUTOIMMUNE DIABETES IN THE DIABETES-PRONE BIOBREEDING RAT The most conclusive evidence for a direct modulatory role of diet in the development of autoimmune diabetes comes from studies of animals fed plant-based diets. Cereal-based standard diets such as the NIH-07 diet (Ziegler Brothers, Gardner, PA, USA) promote diabetes

Table 2
Comparative Effects of Diabetogenic and Nondiabetogenic Diets on the Natural Course
of Autoimmune Diabetes in Diabetes-Prone Biobreeding (BBdp) Rats and Nonobese Diabetic (NOD) mice

	BBdp rat		NOD mouse	
	Cereal-based diet	*Casein-based diet*	*Cereal-based diet*	*Casein-based diet*
Diabetes incidence	62–80%	0–12%	30–95%	0–44%
Time of onset	Early	Late	Early	Late
Degree of insulitis	Severe	Mild to absent	Severe	Mild to absent

Note: Data summarized from refs. *17, 18, 64, 69,* and *71.*

development in both BBdp rats and NOD mice (Table 2). BBdp rats fed cereal-based diets exhibited earlier onset of diabetes and a greater degree of islet inflammation than did BBdp rats fed diabetes-protective casein- or hydrolyzed casein-based diets *(69).* A clear cause-and-effect relationship between diet and diabetes is further demonstrated by dose-response studies with BBdp rats fed diabetogenic cereal-based diets. Beginning at 30% inclusion to a hydrolyzed casein-based diet, increasing doses of the cereal-based NIH-07 diet increased diabetes incidence and the degree of insulitis in BBdp rats *(69).* Dietary control of diabetogenesis is not restricted to a period early in life in BBdp rats, as long-term daily exposure to either NIH-07 or hydrolyzed casein-based diets from early puberty to late adolescence (50–100 d) is important for either the development or prevention of diabetes, respectively *(17,18,69).* Delaying the time of exposure of hydrolyzed casein-fed rats to a diabetogenic cereal-based diet decreased both diabetes incidence and the severity of insulitis *(69).* Similarly, rats fed a diabetogenic cereal-based diet early in life and then switched to a protective hydrolyzed casein-based diet exhibited a lower incidence of diabetes, with insulitis severity being similar to that of BBdp rats fed the hydrolyzed casein-based diet throughout the study *(69).*

Diabetogenic cereal-based diets such as NIH-07 contain as much as 82% plant materials *(71).* Feeding hydrolyzed casein-based diet supplemented with individual components of the NIH-07 diet to BBdp rats demonstrated that wheat bran, corn, brewer's yeast, and fish meal are low diabetogens, whereas whole ground wheat, wheat gluten, soybean meal, soy flakes, and soy flour are moderate-to-high diabetogens *(17).*

PLANT-BASED DIETS AND AUTOIMMUNE DIABETES IN THE NONOBESE DIABETIC MOUSE Studies with the NOD mouse also clearly demonstrate a modulatory role of diet in the development of autoimmune diabetes (Table 2). Similar to the BBdp rat, NOD female mice maintained on a complex natural-ingredient, cereal-based diet (diet 86, New Zealand Stockfoods) exhibited a higher diabetes incidence than did animals fed Pregestimil® (Mead-Johnson Inc.), a hypoallergenic infant formula containing casein hydrolysate and lacking vegetable meal *(70).* Supplementation of diet 86 with vitamin E, polysaturated sardine oil, or saturated coconut oil did not affect its diabetogenic effects *(70).*

Coleman and co-workers *(64)* demonstrated that NOD/Lt female mice fed a natural-ingredient, cereal-based diet (Old Guilford 96W, OG96W; Emory Morse, Guilford, CT, USA) exhibited a significantly higher incidence of diabetes compared to NOD females receiving either of two semisynthetic, casein-based diets, AIN-76 *(71)* or Pregestimil. Pregestimil also completely abrogated

insulitis in OG96W-fed and AIN-76-fed mice. Chloroform–methanol extractions of the 96W diet indicated that the diabetes-promoting factor(s) in this diet may be lipid or peptide *(64).* As observed with BBdp rats, delaying exposure to diabetogenic dietary components delayed the onset of diabetes in NOD mice *(64).*

In summary, it is clear from studies with the BBdp rat and NOD mouse that diet composition is a critical determinant of diabetes development, with cereal-based diets generally promoting disease and semipurified diets based on cow's milk proteins preventing or delaying the onset of diabetes (Table 2). Wheat- or soy-derived proteins are candidate diabetogens in the plant-based animal diets. The animal-model studies also demonstrate the important finding that the age interval critical for exposure to diabetogenic dietary components may extend through puberty *(64,69).* Given our current knowledge base, it remains necessary to fully consider the unique genetic and environmental characteristics that typify rodent models when comparing results from those studies to the human situation (Table 3).

DIET AND TYPE 1 DIABETES: MECHANISTIC CONSIDERATIONS

Most of the research relating diet as an important environmental modulator of type 1 diabetes has focused on identification of diabetogenic foods. Much less research has evaluated possible mechanisms by which dietary factors could modulate the immune system to either target or protect pancreatic β cells. Experimental evidence to date, primarily from rodent models, favors at least three putative mechanisms of dietary modulation of autoimmune diabetes—molecular mimicry, dietary modulation of cytokine profiles, or direct effects of diet on pancreatic β-cell growth or metabolism (Table 4). Several other mechanistic issues, including antigen sampling by the intestine, trafficking of lymphocytes in gut and pancreas, and oral tolerance, deserve further experimental consideration relative to the relationship between diet and type 1 diabetes.

MOLECULAR MIMICRY A frequently considered mechanism by which dietary factors could trigger autoimmune diabetes is antigenic or "molecular" mimicry between environmental and host-cell proteins. For example, an antigenic determinant from a dietary protein resembling a component of the pancreatic β-cell could elicit an immune response against self, leading eventually to β-cell destruction *(76).* The molecular mimicry hypothesis implies that autoreactive lymphocytes remain present even in the absence of the originating antigen and that the mimicking epitope is sufficiently similar to allow cross-recognition but different enough to break tolerance *(20,21).*

Table 3
Current Information Regarding Dietary
Modulation of Autoimmune Diabetes Development

Human data
  Possible association between short duration of breast-feeding or early cow's milk consumption with type 1 diabetes development is controversial.
  Most human studies focus only on early exposure to cow's milk proteins.
  Mechanisms underlying dietary modulation of diabetes development are poorly understood.

Animal studies
  Diet greatly regulates diabetes development in genetically susceptible inbred animals.
    Cereal-based diets promote high diabetes incidence.
    Semipurified diets based on casein or hydrolyzed casein prevent or delay the onset of diabetes.
  Exposure to diabetogenic foods as late as puberty still induces diabetes.
  Mechanisms underlying dietary modulation of diabetes development are poorly understood.

Note: Data summarized from refs. *19, 20, 64,* and *69.*

Table 4
Putative Mechanisms of Dietary Modulation of Autoimmune Diabetes

Molecular mimicry *Milk-based diet*	*Immune response modulation*		*Direct effects on pancreatic β-cells*	
	Cereal-based diet	*Casein-based diet*	*Cereal-based diet*	*Casein-based diet*
Evidence for crossreactivity between milk protein epitopes and β-cell antigens	Inflammatory Th1 cytokine profile (*see* Fig. 1)	Anti-inflammatory Th2 cytokine profile	Lower total islet mass Greater MHC class I expression in islets	Greater total islet mass Lower MHC class I expression in islets

Note: Data summarized from refs. *24, 69,* and *72–75.*

There are several examples of the role of molecular mimicry in animal models of autoimmune diseases, including experimental allergic encephalitis in rabbits, adjuvant arthritis in rats, and Theiler's murine encephalitis (76). Similarly, in humans, molecular mimicry has been implicated in rheumatic fever, Chagas' disease, celiac disease, myasthenia gravis, and type 1 diabetes (76).

Five pancreatic β-cell proteins have been identified as important target antigens primarily in rodent autoimmune diabetes: insulin, glutamic acid decarboxylase, heat-shock protein 65, and islet-cell cytoplasmic autoantigens ICA512/IA-2 and ICAp69 (77). Of these, ICAp69 has been associated with dietary antigenic mimicry in autoimmune diabetes. Islet-cell antigen p69 is a neuroendocrine protein of unknown function (23). High ICAp69 mRNA and protein expression has been detected in pancreatic β cells, the brain, and testis in humans and rodents (78).

Autoreactivity to ICAp69 has been demonstrated in North American and European persons with type 1 diabetes as well as in rodent models (73,77,79,80). Both humoral and cellular immune responses against ICAp69 have been detected in newly diagnosed diabetic children, and anti-ICAp69 autoantibodies have been detected in diabetic and prediabetic subjects (73,80,81).

Islet cell antigen p69 shares sequence homology with bovine serum albumin (BSA), a dietary milk protein of possible importance to the development of type 1 diabetes (42,45,46). Homologies span regions at amino acid positions 151–157, 198–203, and 397–404 of BSA (80). The structural similarities between BSA and β-cell ICAp69 underlie the hypothesis that the autoimmune process triggered by dietary milk results from crossreactivity to these proteins (74). In susceptible individuals, exposure to cow's milk proteins could generate BSA-reactive T lymphocytes with the potential to target β cells expressing ICAp69. In support of this idea, T lymphocytes from children with recent onset diabetes exhibit specific sensitization to BSA and to the BSA-encoded epitope ABBOS peptide (amino acids 152–169 of BSA; ref. 75). However, abnormal humoral and cellular immune responses to BSA and specifically to the ABBOS epitope in patients newly diagnosed for type 1 diabetes has not been confirmed in all studies (82–84).

DIETARY MODULATION OF CYTOKINE PROFILES Dietary antigens may influence the cytokines synthesized by T cells with specificities for β-cell antigens and, thus, generate either diabetogenic or protective T-cell clones. Studies with BBdp rats demonstrate that cytokine profiles in islets can be modulated by diet (69). BBdp rats fed a diabetogenic cereal-based diet exhibited high IFN-γ and low IL-10 and T-cell growth factor (TGF)-β mRNA expression within islets, characteristic of a Th1-cell cytokine profile, whereas BBdp rats fed a protective hydrolyzed casein-based diet exhibited low IFN-γ and high TGF-β expression, characteristic of a Th2-cell-mediated response (69). Oral administration of insulin to 6-wk-old female NOD mice has been associated with the generation of IL-4-secreting regulatory Th2 cells and diabetes prevention (85).

DIETARY MODULATION OF β-CELL GROWTH AND FUNCTION In regard to possible direct effects of diet on β-cell functions, there is evidence indicating that the degree of metabolic stimulation exerted on β cells by diet may alter β-cell antigenicity. For example, treatment of BBdp rats early in life with agents that directly affect β-cell activity, such as insulin or glucose, decrease diabetes incidence (86,87). The protective effect observed with prophylactic insulin in BBdp rats and NOD mice has lead to the "β-cell rest" hypothesis, which states that insulin therapy induces a "quiescent" functional state in the β-cell characterized by a reduced expression of cellular autoantigens *(88–90)*. This phenomenon may also be evoked relative to the metabolic demands exerted by specific diets.

A more direct effect of diet on pancreatic pathology is demonstrated by decreases in total islet mass provoked by diabetogenic diets. Total islet area was lower in NIH-07-fed BBdp rats than in hydrolyzed casein-fed rats prior to insulitis onset *(19,69)*. That this diet–islet interaction occurs before classic insulitis likely indicates a direct effect of diet on islet growth that is independent of the presence of autoreactive immune cells.

Another indication of possible direct effects of diet on islet pathology is the modulation of MHC class I expression observed in BBdp rat islets. At 5 d of age, islet MHC class I expression was similar in cereal-fed BBdp rats and hydrolyzed casein-fed rats *(91)*. However, beginning at 25 d of age, islet MHC class I expression was significantly elevated in cereal-fed BBdp rats but not in hydrolyzed casein-fed BBdp rats *(91)*. Upregulation of local MHC class I expression reached a plateau by 50 d of age when the number of normal islets began to decline *(91)*. Enhanced MHC class I expression in cereal-fed BBdp rats apparently occurred independent of lymphocytic infiltration, as administration of silica, an agent known to deplete macrophages and halt insulitis, did not abrogate enhanced MHC class I expression *(91,92)*. Dietary modulation of islet MHC expression would likely lead to local infiltration of reactive leukocytes. Because MHC class I cell-surface expression is generally dependent on the inclusion of peptide antigens *(93)*, β-cell "self" proteins would presumably be the only source of class I peptides in noninfected animals responding to diabetogens in cereal-based diets.

ANTIGEN SAMPLING BY THE INTESTINE The first step in the induction of a mucosal immune response is the regulated transport of antigens across the epithelial barrier (Fig. 2). Controlled uptake of macromolecules enables the mucosal immune system to sample antigens present in the gut lumen. The primary physiologic route of antigen sampling is through specialized epithelial cells that line the Peyer's patches, the membranous epithelial cells (M cells; Fig. 2; ref. *94)*. This process mediates the production of secretory IgA, the predominant component of adaptive immunity at mucosal surfaces *(95)*.

Intestinal enterocytes are also able to take up and transport antigens by endocytosis and vesicular trafficking *(96)*; however, neither the functional role of this process nor the molecules involved are well defined. Although considerable evidence indicates that intestinal epithelial cells are capable of presenting antigens in the context of MHC class I or class II molecules, it is not clear if or how endocytosis contributes to the process *(97,98)*. Likewise, the functional consequences of epithelial antigen presentation are poorly understood *(97,98)*.

Under normal conditions, nonimmune and immune factors limit nonspecific transport of antigens across the epithelium (Fig. 2). Intestinal enterocytes, for example, are sealed by tight junctions that normally exclude antigenic molecules (Fig. 2). The pore size at tight junctions has been estimated to be approximately 5 nm, allowing passage of small peptides while preventing the passage of large macromolecules *(99)*. Under pathologic conditions such as infection and acute inflammation, tight junctions could open sufficiently to allow the passage of luminal antigens *(100,101)*.

The state of functional maturity also appears to affect the degree of both intracellular and intercellular antigen transport through the epithelium *(96,102)*. For example, nonspecific transport of horseradish peroxidase through vesicular compartments of enterocytes, and ovalbumin through tight junctions have been observed *(96)*. The efficacy of nonimmune factors limiting epithelial antigen transfer, including gastric acidity, proteolytic digestion, mucus secretion, and peristalsis, is also subject to the state of intestinal development *(96,102)*. Nonspecific transport of luminal antigens either through epithelial cells or between tight junctions would expose these antigens to antigen-presenting cells in the lamina propria and thereby potentially elicit humoral or cellular immune responses (Fig. 2). Further characterization of antigenic transport in the developing intestine may warrant particular attention relative to the generation or breakdown of intestinal tolerance, prior to diabetes development.

A finite window of susceptibility early in life is characteristic of autoimmune diabetes in humans and in animal models of disease *(18,19,103,104)*. Similarly, food-related intestinal diseases appear more common during early developmental periods. For example, food protein enteropathy is a disease of infancy and childhood in which a hypersensitivity reaction to food proteins produces varying degrees of damage to the intestinal mucosa, resulting in mucosal dysfunction *(105,106)*. Cow's milk enteropathy early in infancy is one of the best examples of food protein enteropathy *(105)*. Milk protein enteropathy usually resolves with increasing age, indicating that immaturity of the intestine could have an important role in this disease. It has been suggested that macromolecules present in cow's milk may be more adherent to the surface of immature epithelial cells than to mature cells, thus facilitating their uptake in infants *(107)*. Other immune-related enteropathies such as celiac disease, allergic enteropathy, and autoimmune enteropathy are also characterized by the presence of immature epithelia *(108)*.

TRAFFICKING OF LYMPHOCYTES IN GUT AND PANCREAS Lymph, containing activated intestinal immune cells, flows through lymphatic vessels toward the mesenteric lymph nodes for further division and differentiation *(95)*. Lymphatics from the upper gastrointestinal tract are intimately connected with pancreatic lymphatics (Fig. 3; ref. *109)*. Some of the duodenal lymphatic channels pass through the pancreas and are indistinguishable from the lymph vessels of the pancreas itself *(109)*. This contiguous arrangement could facilitate the mixture of intestinal and pancreatic lymph, thereby providing immune cells common exposure to inductive microenvironments, perhaps leading to common phenotypes. Related to this possibility, a human "diabetogenic" T-cell line from the pancreas bound specifically to both pancreatic and intestinal mucosal endothelium *(110)*. Further studies demonstrated induction of mucosal vascular addressin (MadCAM-1) and peripheral vascular addressin (PNAd) on vessels in inflamed islets of NOD mice, and accumulation within islets of lymphocytes expressing the α4β7 mucosal and L-selectin homing receptors *(111)*. Those observations point to the possibility that vascular addressins and lymphocyte homing receptors, which are normally involved in lymphocyte trafficking to mucosal surfaces, may also mediate the infiltration of leukocytes into pancreatic islets *(110,111)*.

The anatomical proximity and shared lymphatic systems of the intestine and pancreas could facilitate intestinal modulation of

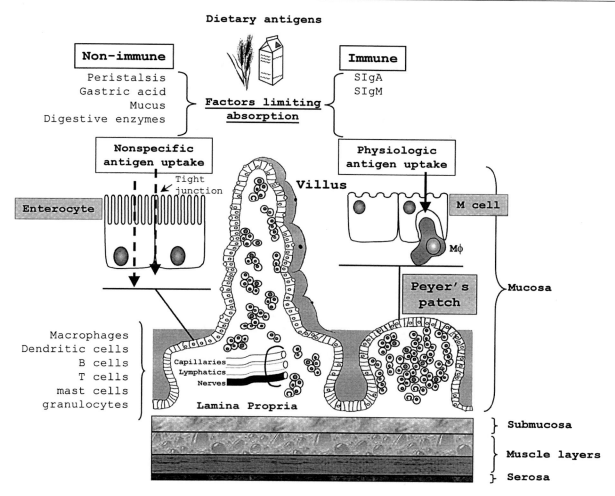

Fig. 2. Routes of antigen translocation through the small intestinal epithelium. Antigen uptake is normally limited by immune and nonimmune factors present in the gut lumen and by the distinct anatomical structure of the intestinal epithelium. Selective antigen sampling is carried out by membranous epithelial cells (M cells) covering the Peyer's patches. M cells are in close contact with immune cells like macrophages (Mφ) present in the Peyer's patches. Abnormal nonspecific antigen uptake during inflammation or intestinal immaturity can also occur through enterocytes and tight junctions.

insulitic cytokine profiles. For example, the characteristic insulitic Th1 cytokine profile observed in the BBdp rat can be shifted toward a Th2 cytokine profile by the oral administration of lipo-polysaccharide (LPS) or an endotoxin-free glycoprotein preparation from *Escherichia coli (112)*. A similar, but less pronounced shift in cytokine secretion was observed with parenteral bacterial vaccines such as diphtheria toxoid or tuberculosis, indicating that mucosal-induced modulation of autoreactive immune cells was greater than the modulation induced by the parenteral route *(112)*. Systematic studies addressing the physiology and the molecular and cellular biology of lymphocyte trafficking in the gut and pancreas are needed, specifically as affected by diet and intestinal antigens.

ORAL TOLERANCE Distinguishing harmful and innocuous external agents is a critical function of the intestinal immune system. This function is particularly important early in life when antigenically complex foods begin to challenge the intestinal immune system. Animal studies indicate that humoral- or cell-mediated immune unresponsiveness can be induced by enteral administration of antigens *(113)*. For example, feeding of myelin basic protein (MBP) to an inbred rat model of experimental autoimmune encephalomyelitis generated regulatory T cells that were able to suppress autoimmune responses in the brain *(114)*. Similarly, oral administration of insulin to NOD mice suppressed diabetes *(85,115)*. Oral administration of insulin has been associated with the generation of regulatory T cells that migrate to the pancreas and pancreatic lymph nodes where they secrete IL-4, leading to the suppression of autoreactive Th1 cells *(85)*. Further, it has been suggested that the enhanced cell-mediated immune response to β-lactoglobulin present in newly diagnosed type 1 diabetes patients is the result of a generalized failure to develop tolerance to dietary antigens *(116)*. Whether tolerance or immune responsiveness develops in response to particular intestinal antigens depends on several variables, including animal type, age at feeding, amount of antigen fed, frequency of feeding, and the presence or absence of adjuvants *(113,117)*. Several recent review articles provide thorough discussions of the important topic of oral tolerance *(118–120)*, another area of research that needs to be expanded

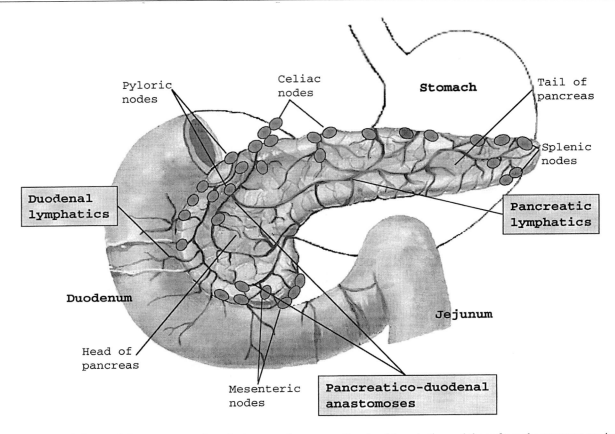

Fig. 3. Lymphatic drainage of the upper gastrointestinal tract and pancreas. Duodenal lymphatics and those from the pancreas are intimately related forming frequent anastomoses *(94)*. This proximity facilitates the flow of lymphocytes from the lamina propria in the intestine to the pancreas and vice versa.

to better understand the relationship between diet and type 1 diabetes.

SUMMARY

The realization that diet might modulate type 1 diabetes onset or disease progression generates promise for novel approaches to the prevention or treatment of this disease. However, the identification of diabetogenic foods has proven difficult and the topic is controversial. Although certain diabetogenic plant-derived components have been identified in rodent models of autoimmune diabetes, the role of specific dietary antigens as modulators of type 1 diabetes in humans is less clear. Several issues associated with feeding patterns and precocious exposure to oral antigens must be considered when assessing the role of diet in the development of tolerance in infants at risk for type 1 diabetes. For example, early cessation of breast-feeding simultaneously removes breast milk bioactive factors critical for normal intestinal maturation—both morphologic growth and immunologic development—and introduces novel antigens present in breast milk substitutes such as cow's milk. Immature epithelial barrier function may allow abnormal translocation of luminal antigens, including dietary proteins or peptides, and result in the generation of autoreactive lymphocytes that target pancreatic β cells expressing self proteins with cross-reactive epitopes. Further studies are clearly needed to identify and characterize potential food diabetogens. In addition, with gut-

associated lymphoid tissue harboring the cells that primarily respond to and mediate the effects of diabetogenic foods, it is necessary to experimentally determine how the mucosal immune system may contribute to onset or progression of autoimmune diabetes.

REFERENCES

1. Sherwin RS. Diabetes mellitus. In: Bennett JC, Plum F, eds, pp. 1258–77. Cecil Text Book of Medicine. Saunders, Philadelphia, 1996.
2. Rossini AA, Greiner DL, Friedman HP, Mordes JP. Immunopathogenesis of diabetes mellitus. Diabetes Rev 1993; 1:43–75.
3. Gavin JR III, Alberti KGMM, Davidson MB, DeFrozo RA, Drash A, Gabbe SG, et al. The expert committee on the diagnosis and classification of diabetes mellitus. Report of the expert committee on the diagnosis and classification of diabetes mellitus. Diabetes Care 1997; 20:1183–97.
4. Bingley PJ, Gale EAM: Rising incidence of IDDM in Europe. Diabetes Care 1989; 12:289–95.
5. Funk JL, Feingold KR. Disorders of the endocrine pancreas. In: McPhee SJ, Lingappa VR, Ganong WF, Lange JD, eds, Pathophysiology of Disease, Appleton & Lange, pp. 367–92. Stamford, CT, 1995.
6. Trucco M, Dorman JS. Immunogenetics of insulin-dependent diabetes mellitus in humans. CRC Crit Rev Immunol 1989; 9:201–45.
7. Baisch JM, Weeks T, Giles R, Hoover M, Stastny P, Capra JD. Analysis of HLA-DQ genotypes and susceptibility in insulin-dependent diabetes mellitus. N Engl J Med 1990; 322:1836–41.

8. Weatheral D: Genetic control of diabetes mellitus. Diabetologia 1992; 35:S1–S7.

9. Thai A-C, Eisenbarth GS. Natural history of IDDM. Diabetes Rev 1993; 1:1–14.

10. Bach JF. Insulin-dependent diabetes mellitus as an autoimmune disease. Endocr Rev 1994; 15:516–42.

11. Castano L, Eisenbarth GS. Type 1 diabetes: a chronic autoimmune disease of human, mouse, and rat. Annu Rev Immunol 1990; 8:647–79.

12. Shehadeh NN, Lafferty KJ. The role of T-cells in the development of autoimmune diabetes. Diabetes Rev 1993; 1:141–51.

13. Wilson SB, Kent SC, Patton FT, Orbans T, Jackson RA, Exley M, et al. Extreme Th1 bias of invariant Va24JaQ T cells in type 1 diabetes. Nature 1998; 391:177–81.

14. Trembleau S, Germann T, Gately MK, Adorini L. The role of IL-12 in the induction of organ-specific autoimmune disease. Immunol Today 1995; 16:383–6.

15. Rabinovitch A. Immunoregulatory and cytokine imbalances in the pathogenesis of IDDM: therapeutic intervention by immunostimulation? Diabetes 1994; 43:613–21.

16. Leiter EH. The role of environmental factors in modulating insulin dependent diabetes. In: DeVries RRP, Cohen IR, Van Rood JJ, eds, The Role of Micro-organisms in Non-infectious Diseases, pp. 39–55. Springer-Verlag, London, 1990.

17. Scott FW. Food, diabetes, and immunology. In: Forse RA, Bell SJ, Blackburn GL, Kabbash LG, eds. Diet, Nutrition and Immunity, pp. 73–95. CRC, Boca Raton, FL: 1994.

18. Scott FW. Food-induced type 1 diabetes in the BB rat. Diabetes Metab Rev 1996; 12:341–59.

19. Gerstein HC: Cow's milk exposure and type 1 diabetes mellitus. Diabetes Care 1994; 17:13–9.

20. Scott FW, Norris JM, Kolb H. Milk and type 1 diabetes examining the evidence and broadening the focus. Diabetes Care 1996; 19:379–83.

21. Hammond-McKibben D, Dosch H-M. Cow's milk, bovine serum albumin, and IDDM: can we settle the controversies? Diabetes Care 1997; 20:897–901.

22. Karges W, Dosch H-M: Environmental factors: cow milk and others. In: Palmer JP, ed, Diabetes Prediction, Prevention and Genetic Counseling in IDDM, pp. 167–80. Wiley, Chichester, 1996.

23. Kostraba JN, Cruickshanks KJ, Lawler-Heavener J, Jobin LF, Rewers MA, Gay EC, et al. Early exposure to cow's milk and solid foods in infancy, genetic predisposition, and risk of IDDM. Diabetes 1993; 42:288–95.

24. Newburg DS, Street JM. Bioactive materials in human milk: milk sugars sweeten the argument for breast-feeding. Nutr Today 1997; 32:191–210.

25. Hanson LA, Hahn-Zoric M, Wiedermann U, Lundin S, Dahlman-Hoglund A, Saalman R, et al. Early dietary influence on later immunocompetence. Nutr Rev 1996; 54:S23–S30.

26. Ellis LA, Mastro AM, Picciano MF. Do milk-borne cytokines and hormones influence neonatal immune cell function? J Nutr 1997; 127:985S–88S.

27. Jan CL. Cellular components of mammary secretions and neonatal immunity: a review. Vet Res 1996; 27:403–17.

28. Ozkaragoz F, Rudloff HB, Rajaraman S, Mushtaha AA, Schmalstieg FC, Goldman AS. The motility of human milk macrophages in collagen gels. Pediatr Res 1988; 23:449–52.

29. Slade HB, Schwartz SA. Antigen-driven immunoglobulin production by human colostral lymphocytes. Pediatr Res 1989; 25:295–9.

30. Eglinton BA, Robertson DM, Cummins AG. Phenotype of T cells, their soluble receptor levels, and cytokine profile of human milk. Immunol Cell Biol 1994; 72:306–13.

31. Bertotto A, Gerli R, Castellucci G, Scalise F, Vaccaro R. Human milk lymphocytes bearing the γδ T-cell receptor are mostly δ TCS1-positive cells. Immunology 1991; 74:360–3.

32. Munoz C, Endres S, van der Meer J, Schlesinger L, Arevalo M, Dinarello C. Interleukin 1β in human colostrum. Res Immunol 1990; 141:505–13.

33. Rudloff HE, Schmalstieg FC Jr, Palkowetz EJ, Goldman AS. Interleukin-6 in human milk. J Reprod Immunol 1993; 23:13–20.

34. Bocci V, von Bremen K, Corradeschi F, Luzzi E, Paulesu L. Presence of interferon-γ and interleukin-6 in colostrum of normal women. Lymphokine Cytokine Res 1993; 12:21–4.

35. Skansen-Saphir U, Lindfors A, Andersson U. Cytokine production in mononuclear cells in human milk studied at the single-cell level. Pediatr Res 1993; 34:213–16.

36. Saito S, Ichijo S, Ishizaka S, Tsujii T. Transforming growth factor-β (TGF-β) in human milk. Clin Exp Immunol 1993; 94:220–4.

37. Rudloff HE, Schmalstieg Jr, FC, Mushtaha AA, Palkowetz KH, Liu SK, Goldman AS. Tumor necrosis factor-α in human mik. Pediatr Res 1992; 31:29–33.

38. Donovan SM, Odle J. Growth factors in milk as mediators of infant development. Annu Rev Nutr 1994; 14:147–67.

39. Heyman M, Crain-Denoyelle AM, Desjeux JF. Endocytosis and processing of protein by isolated villus and crypt cells of the mouse small intestine. J Pediatr Gastroenterol Nutr 1989; 9:238–45.

40. Arvola T, Rantala I, Martinen A, Isolauri E. Early dietary antigens delay the development of gut mucosal barrier in pre-weaning rats. Pediatr Res 1992; 32:301–5.

41. Glerum M, Robinson BH, Martin JM. Could bovine serum albumin be the initiating antigen ultimately responsible for the development of insulin dependent diabetes mellitus? Diabetes Res 1989; 10: 103–7.

42. Martin JM, Trink B, Daneman D, Dosch H-M, Robinson B. Milk proteins in the etiology of insulin-dependent diabetes mellitus (IDDM). Ann Med 1992; 23:447–52.

43. Dosch H-M, Karjalainen J, Morkowski J, Martin JM, Robinson BH. Nutritional triggers of IDDM. Ped Adoles Endocrinol 1991; 21: 202–17.

44. Dosch H-M, Karjalainen J, Morkowski J, Martin JM, Robinson BH. Nutritional triggers of IDDM. In: Levy-Marchal C, Czrnichow P, eds, Epidemiology and Etiology of Insulin-Dependent Diabetes in the Young, pp. 202–17. Karger, Basel, 1992.

45. Dosch H-M. The possible link between insulin dependent (juvenile) diabetes mellitus and dietary cow milk. Clin Biochem 1993; 26:307–8.

46. Tainio V-M, Savilahti E, Arjomaa P, Salmenpera L, Perheentupa J, Siimes MA. Plasma antibodies to cow's milk are increased by early weaning and consumption of unmodified milk, but production of IgA and IgM cow's milk antibodies is stimulated even during exclusive breast-feeding. Acta Paediatr Scand 1988; 77:807–11.

47. Beppu H, Winter WE, Atkinson MA, Maclaren NK, Fujita K, Takahashi H. Bovine albumin antibodies in NOD mice. Diabetes Res 1987; 6:67–9.

48. Drash AL, Kramer MS, Swanson J, Udall JN. Work group on cow's milk protein and diabetes mellitus. Infant feeding practices and their possible relationship to the etiology of diabetes mellitus. Pediatrics 1994; 94:752–4.

49. Norris JM, Beaty B, Klingensmith G, Yu L, Hoffman M, Chase P, et al. Lack of association between early exposure to cow's milk protein and β-cell autoimmunity. Diabetes autoimmunity study in the young (DAISY). JAMA 1996; 276:609–14.

50. Norris JM, Scott FW. A meta-analysis of infant diet and insulin-dependent diabetes mellitus: do biases play a role? Epidemiology 1996; 7:87–92.

51. Dosch H-M. Association of exposure to cow's milk protein and β-cell autoimmunity. JAMA 1996; 276:1799.

52. Kyvik KO, Green A, Svendsen A, Mortensen K. Breast-feeding and the development of type 1 diabetes mellitus. Diabet Med 1992; 9:233–5.

53. Samuelson U, Johansson C, Ludvigsson J. Breast-feeding seems to play a marginal role in the prevention of insulin-dependent diabetes mellitus. Diabetes Res Clin Pract 1993; 19:203–10.

54. Patterson CC, Carson DJ, Hadden DR, Waugh NR, Cole SK. A case-control investigation of perinatal risk factors for childhood IDDM in Northern Ireland and Scotland. Diabetes 1994; 17:376–81.

55. Gerstein HC, Simpson JR, Atkinson S, Taylor DW, Vandermeulen

J. Feasibility and acceptability of a proposed infant feeding intervention trial for the prevention of type 1 diabetes. Diabetes Care 1995; 18:940–2.

56. Akerblom HK, Savilahti E, Saukkonen TT, Paganus A, Virtanen SM, Teramo K, et al. The case for elimination of cow's milk in early infancy in the prevention of type 1 diabetes: the Finnish experience. Diabetes Metab 1994; 9:269–78.

57. Karges W, Hammon-McKibben D, Cheung RK, Visconti M, Shibuya N, Kemp D, et al. Immunological aspects of nutritional diabetes prevention in NOD mice: a pilot study for the cow's milk-based IDDM prevention trial. Diabetes 1997; 46:557–64.

58. Mordes JP, Bortell R, Doukas J, Rigby M, Whalen B, Zipris D, et al. The BB/WOR rat and the balance hypothesis of autoimmunity. Diabetes Metab Rev 1996; 12:103–9.

59. Bellgrau D, Lagarde AC. Cytotoxic T-cell precursors with low-level CD8 in the diabetes-prone Biobreeding rat: implications for generation of an autoimmune T-cell repertoire. Proc Natl Acad Sci USA 1990; 87:313–7.

60. Zipris D, Crow AR, Delovitch TL. Altered thymic and peripheral T-lymphocyte repertoire preceding onset of diabetes in NOD mice. Diabetes 1991; 40:429–35.

61. Serreze DV, Leiter EH. Genetic and pathogenic basis of autoimmune diabetes in NOD mice. Curr Opin Immunol 1994; 6:900–6.

62. Serreze DV, Gaskins HR, Leiter EH. Defects in the differentiation and function of antigen presenting cells in NOD/Lt mice. J Immunol 1993; 150:2534–43.

63. Serreze DV, Leiter EH. Defective activation of T suppressor cell function in nonobese diabetic mice. Potential relation to cytokine deficiencies. J Immunol 1988; 140:3801–7.

64. Coleman DL, Kuzava JE, Leiter EH. Effect of diet on incidence of diabetes in nonobese diabetic mice. Diabetes 1990; 39:432–6.

65. Issa-Chergui D, Guttmann RD, Seemayer TA, Kelley VE, Colle EC. The effect of diet on the spontaneous insulin-dependent diabetic syndrome in the rat. Diabetes Res 1988; 9:81–6.

66. Scott FW, Elliot RB, Kolb H. Diet and autoimmunity: prospects of prevention of type 1 diabetes. Diabetes Nutr Metab 1989; 2:61–73.

67. Klandorf H, Chirra AR, DeGruccio A, Girman DJ. Dimethyl sulfoxide modulation of diabetes onset in NOD mice. Diabetes 1989; 38:194–7.

68. Hoorfar J, Buschard K, Dagnaes-Hansen F. Prophylactic nutritional modification of the incidence of diabetes in autoimmune non-obese diabetic (NOD) mice. Br J Nutr 1993; 69:597–607.

69. Scott FW, Cloutier HE, Kleemann R, Woerz-Pagenstert U, Rowsell P, Modler HW, et al. Potential mechanisms by which certain foods promote or inhibit the development of spontaneous diabetes in BB rats. Dose, timing, early effect on islet area, and switch in infiltrate from Th1 to Th2 cells. Diabetes 1997; 46:589–98.

70. Elliot RB, Reddy SN, Bibby NJ, Kida K. Dietary prevention of diabetes in the non-obese diabetic mouse. Diabetologia 1988; 31:62–4.

71. American Institute of Nutrition Ad Hoc Committee on Standards for Nutritional Studies. Report of the AIN Ad Hoc Committee on standards for nutritional studies. J Nutr 1977; 107:1340–8.

72. Miyazaki I, Cheung RK, Gaedigk R, Hui MF, VanderMeulen J, Rajotte RV, et al. T Cell activation and anergy to islet cell antigen in type 1 diabetes. J Immunol 1995; 154:1461–9.

73. Martin S, Kardorf J, Schulte B, Lampeter EF, Gries FA, Melchers I, et al. Autoantibodies to the islet antigen ICA69 occur in IDDM and in rheumatoid arthritis. Diabetologia 1995; 38:351–5.

74. Karjalainen J, Martin JM, Knip M, Ilonen J, Robinson BH, Savilahti E, et al. A bovine albumin peptide as a possible trigger of insulin-dependent diabetes mellitus. N Engl J Med 1992; 327:302–7.

75. Cheung RK, Karjalainen J, VanderMeulen J, Singal D, Dosch H-M. T cells from children with insulin-dependent diabetes are sensitized to bovine serum albumin. Scand J Immunol 1994; 40:623–8.

76. Dyrberg T. Molecular mimicry in autoimmune disease. In: DeVries RRP, Cohen IR, Van Rood JJ, eds, The Role of Micro-organisms in Non-infectious Diseases, pp. 156–65. Springer-Verlag, London, 1990.

77. Bosi E, Bonifacio E, Bottazzo GF. Autoantigens in IDDM. Diabetes Rev 1993; 1:204–14.

78. Karges W, Pietropaolo M, Ackerley CA, Dosch H-M. Gene expression of islet cell antigen p69 in human, mouse, and rat. Diabetes 1996; 45:513–21.

79. Roep BO, Duinkerken G, Schreuder GMT, Kolb H, de Vries RRP, Martin S. HLA-associated inverse correlation between T cell and antibody responsiveness to islet autoantigen in recent-onset insulin-dependent diabetes mellitus. Eur J Immunol 1996; 26:1285–89.

80. Miyazaki I, Gaedigk R, Hui MF, Cheung RK, Morkowski J, Rajotte RV, et al. Cloning of human and rat p69, a candidate autoimmune target in type 1 diabetes. Biochim Biophys Acta 1994; 1227:101–4.

81. Pietropaolo M, Castano L, Babu S, Buelow R, Kuo Y-L, Martin S, et al. Islet cell autoantigens 69 kD (ICA69): molecular cloning and characterization of a novel diabetes associated autoantigen. J Clin Invest 1993; 92:359–71.

82. Levymarchal C, Karjalainen J, Dubois F, Karges W, Czernichow P, Dosch H-M. Antibodies against bovine albumin and other diabetes markers in French Children. Diabetes Care 1995; 18:1089–94.

83. Atkinson MA, Bowman MA, Kao K-J, Campbell L, Dush PJ, Shah SC, et al. Lack of immune responsiveness to bovine serum albumin in insulin-dependent diabetes. N Engl J Med 1993; 329:1853–8.

84. Krokowski M, Caillat-Zucman S, Timsit J, Larger E, Pehuet-Figoni M, Bach JF, et al. Anti-bovine serum albumin antibodies: genetic heterogeneity and clinical relevance in adult-onset IDDM. Diabetes Care 1995; 18:170–3.

85. Ploix C, Bergerot I, Fabien N, Perche S, Moulin V, Thivolet C. Protection against autoimmune diabetes with oral insulin is associated with the presence of IL-4 type 2 T-cells in the pancreas and pancreatic lymph nodes. Diabetes 1998; 47:39–44.

86. Gotfredsen CF, Buschard K, Frandsen EK. Reduction of diabetes incidence of BB rats by early prophylactic insulin treatment of diabetes-prone animals. Diabetologia 1989; 28:933–5.

87. Buschard K, Jorgensen M, Aaen K, Block T, Josefsen K. Prevention of diabetes mellitus in BB rats by neonatal stimulation of beta cells. Lancet 1990; 335:134–5.

88. Aaen K, Rygaard J, Josefsen K, Petersen H, Brogren CH, Horn T, et al. Dependence of antigen expression on functional state of beta-cells. Diabetes 1990; 39:697–701.

89. Muir A, Peck A, Clare-Salzler M, Song Y-H, Cornelius J, Luchetta R, et al. Insulin immunization of nonobese diabetic mice induces a protective insulitis characterized by diminished intraislet interferon-γ transcription. J Clin Invest 1995; 95:628–34.

90. Bjork E, Kampe O, Grawe J, Hallberg A, Norheim I, Karisson FA. Modulation of beta-cell activity and its influence on islet cell antibody (ICA) and islet cell surface antibody (ICSA) reactivity. Autoimmunity 1993; 16:181–8.

91. Li XB, Scott FW, Park YH, Yoon J-M. Low incidence of type 1 diabetes in BB rats fed a hydrolyzed casein-based diet associated with early inhibition of non-macrophage dependent hyperexpression of MHC class I molecules on β-cells. Diabetologia 1995; 38:1138–47.

92. Oschilewski U, Kiesel U, Kolb H. Administration of silica prevents diabetes in BBdp rats. Diabetes 1985; 34:197–9.

93. Ortiz-Navarrete V, Hammerling GJ: Surface appearance and instability of empty H-2 class I molecules under physiological conditions. Proc Natl Acad Sci USA 1991; 88:3594–7.

94. Savidge TC. The life and times of an intestinal M cell. Trends Microbiol 1996; 4:301–6.

95. Elson CO, Mestecky JF. The mucosal immune system. In: Blaser MJ, Smith PD, Ravdin JI, Greenberg HB, Guerrant RL, eds, Infections of the Gastrointestinal Tract, pp. 153–62. Raven, New York, 1995.

96. Walker AW, Sanderson IR. The enterocyte and antigen transport. In: Auricchio S, Ferguson A, Troncone R, eds., Mucosal Immunity and the Gut Epithelium: Interactions in Health and Disease, pp. 18–31. Karger, Basel, 1995.

97. Matsumoto S, Setoyama H, Umesaki Y. Differential induction of major histocompatibility complex molecules in mouse intestine by bacterial colonization. Gastroenterology 1992; 103:1777–82.

98. Brandeis JM, Sayegh MH, Gallon L, Blumber RS, Carpenter CB. Rat intestinal epithelial cells present major histocompatibility complex allopeptides to primed T cells. Gastroenterology 1994; 107:1537–42.

99. Atisook K, Madara JL. An oligopeptide permeates intestinal tight junctions at glucose-elicited dilatations: implications for oligopeptide absorption. Gastroenterology 1991; 100:719–24.

100. Bloch KJ, Bloch DB, Sterns M, Walker WA. Intestinal uptake of macromolecules. VI. Uptake of protein antigen in vivo in normal rats and rats infected with *Nippostrongylus brasiliensis* or subject to mild systemic anaphylaxis. Gastroenterology 1979; 77:1038–44.

101. Ramage JK, Stainsz A, Scicchitano R, Hunt RH, Perdue MH. Effect of immunologic reactions on rat intestinal epithelium: correlation of increased permeability to chromium 51-labeled ethylene-diamine-tetraacetic acid and ovalbumin during acute inflammation and anaphylaxis. Gastroenterology 1988; 94:1368–75.

102. Insoft RM, Sanderson IR, Walker WA. Development of immune function in the intestine and its role in neonatal diseases. Pediatric Clin North Am 1996; 43:551–71.

103. Virtanen SM, Saukkonen T, Savilahti E, Ylonen K, Rasanen L, Aro A. and the Childhood Diabetes Finland Study Group. Diet, cow's milk protein antibodies and the risk of IDDM in Finnish children. Diabetologia 1994; 37:381–7.

104. Elliot RB, Martin JM. Dietary protein: a trigger of insulin dependent diabetes in the BB rat? Diabetologia 1984; 26:297–9.

105. Kuitunen P, Visakorpi J, Savilahti E, Pelkonen P. Malabsorption syndrome with cow's milk intolerance: clinical findings and course in 54 cases. Arch Dis Child 1975; 50:251–6.

106. Ament M, Rubin C. Soy protein: another cause of flat intestinal lesion. Gastroenterology 1972; 62:227.

107. Stern M, Pang KY, Walker WA. Food proteins and gut mucosal barrier. II. Differential interaction of cow's milk proteins with the mucous coat and the surface membrane of adult and immature rat jejunum. Pediatr Res 1984; 18:1252–57.

108. Sanderson IR, Walker WA. Uptake and transport of macromolecules by the intestine: possible role in clinical disorders: an update. Gastroenterology 1993; 104:622–9.

109. Netter FH, Cliffton EE, Popper H. Normal anatomy of liver, biliary tract and pancreas. In: Oppenheimer E, ed., The Ciba Collection of Medical Illustrations of Digestive System. Part II, pp. 2–31. CIBA, New York, 1967.

110. Hanninen A, Salmi M, Simell O, Jalkanen S. Endothelial cell-binding properties of lymphocytes infiltrated into human diabetic pancreas: Implications for pathogenesis of IDDM. Diabetes 1993; 42:1656–62.

111. Hanninen A, Taylor C, Streeter PR, Stark LS, Sarte JM, Shizuru JA, et al. Vascular addressins are induced on islet vessels during insulitis in nonobese diabetic mice and are involved in lymphoid cell binding to islet endothelium. J Clin Invest 1993; 92:2509–15.

112. Kolb H, Worz-Pagenstert U, Kleemann R, Rothe H, Rowsell P, Scott FW. Cytokine gene expression in the BB rat pancreas: natural course and impact of bacterial vaccines. Diabetologia 1996; 39:1448–54.

113. Mowat AM. The regulation of immune responses to dietary protein antigens. Immunol Today 1987; 8:93–8.

114. Khoury SJ, Hancock WW, Weiner HL. Oral tolerance to myelin basic protein and natural recovery from experimental autoimmune encephalomyelitis are associated with down regulation of inflammatory cytokines and differetial upregulation of transforming growth factor-β, interleukin 4, and prostaglandin E expression in the brain. J Exp Med 1992; 176:1355–64.

115. Zhang ZJ, Davidson LE, Eisenbarth G, Weiner HL. Suppression of diabetes in NOD mice by oral administration of porcine insulin. Proc Natl Acad Sci USA 1991; 88:10,252–6.

116. Vaalara O, Klemetti P, Savilahti E, Reijonen H, Ilonen J, Akerblom HK. Cellular immune response to cow's milk β-lactoglobulin in patients with newly diagnosed IDDM. Diabetes 1996; 45:178–82.

117. Strobel S. Dietary manipulation and induction of tolerance. J Pediatr 1992; 121:S74–9.

118. Weiner HL, Friedman A, Miller A, Khoury SJ, Al-Sabbagh A, Santos L, et al. Oral tolerance: immunologic mechanisms and treatment of animal and human organ-specific autoimmune diseases by oral administration of autoantigens. Annu Rev Immunol 1994; 12:809–37.

119. Brandtzaeg P. Mechanisms of gastrointestinal reactions to food. Environ Toxicol Pharmacol 1997; 4:9–24.

120. Strober W, Kelsall B, Marth T. Oral tolerance. J Clin Immunol 1998; 18:1–30 (review).

26 Nutritional Modulation of Autoimmune Diseases

Claudio Galperin, Gabriel Fernandes, Ricardo M. Oliveira, and M. Eric Gershwin

INTRODUCTION

Diet therapy for autoimmune diseases generally has been considered quackery; yet an overwhelming number of patients, namely those suffering from autoimmune rheumatic diseases, spend nearly one billion dollars annually on this and related unconventional therapies *(1)*. Food and drink have had enormous psychological and even ritualistic importance in virtually all cultures. For no other reason, the potential role of specific foods and dietary therapies has swung in and out of medical fashion for centuries. Although in the past few years, an increasing number of well-conducted studies emerged reporting favorable results using dietary manipulation in animal models of autoimmune disorders, the grounds for its clinical application are still being paved. Notably, as its potential benefits are currently being investigated, the unrestrained use of dietary manipulation in a clinical setting is not invariably harmless. Following folk-belief, many patients will turn to fad diets when faced with chronic and long-term diseases. Besides substantial economic hardship, many of them may develop or aggravate nutritional deficiencies by limiting food intake to what is regarded as a "miracle food." It is therefore time for the combined efforts of the scientific community—such as the establishment of the National Institutes of Health Office of Alternative Medicine—to objectively investigate these issues, pursuing ways to expand available health care resources while protecting our patients from unnecessary hazards. Herein, available evidence demonstrating the modulatory effects of diet in the natural history of selected autoimmune disorders is discussed.

SPECIFIC NUTRIENTS AND THEIR RELATIONSHIP TO AUTOIMMUNE DISEASES

TRACE MINERALS

Iron It is generally accepted that iron deficiency is the most common nutritional insufficiency in the world, for which iron deficiency anemia is one of the most prevalent presentations. Anemia is a frequent finding in patients with chronic inflammatory autoimmune diseases and may arise from different mechanisms.

From: *Nutrition and Immunology: Principles and Practice* (ME Gershwin et al. eds.), © Humana Press, Inc., Totowa, NJ

Although autoimmune mediated hemolysis might be the cardinal factor in some patients with systemic lupus erythematosus (SLE), shortened erythrocyte survival accounts for most cases of the usually mild anemia seen in patients with rheumatoid arthritis (RA). The latter, usually defined as anemia of chronic disease (ACD), has abnormalities of iron handling, but the anemia is usually not one characteristic of iron deficiency. Although also marked by decreased serum iron and total iron-binding capacity, unlike true iron deficiency states, iron stores are normal or even increased. Studies have also disclosed that a cytokine-mediated failure of the bone marrow to increase red blood cell production in response to erythropoietin, associated with an impaired release of iron from the reticuloendothelial system, are the most likely underlining mechanisms *(2)*. Less commonly, true iron deficiency anemia resulting from poor dietary intake or gastrointestinal blood loss secondary to medication might occur in such patients. Distinguishing a true iron deficiency anemia from ACD has important therapeutic implications because the latter only seldom improves by iron administration alone. Likewise, erythropoietin can correct anemia in ACD but cannot overcome the anemia of iron deficiency. The more reliable ways of demonstrating iron deficiency in patients with chronic inflammatory diseases, such as RA, include showing the absence of stainable iron in bone marrow aspirates and correction of the anemia following iron therapy. Serum levels of transferrin receptor, which are commonly increased in patients with iron deficiency but only rarely in patients with ACD, might also help to distinguish between ACD and iron-deficiency anemia and to identify iron deficiency in subjects with chronic inflammation.

Numerous investigators have observed the deposition of large amounts of iron in the synovial tissue of patients with RA and have associated them with the occurrence of persistent joint inflammation *(3,4)*. It has been hypothesized that excessive iron deposits may catalyze the formation of reactive oxygen species and, therefore, contribute to inflammation and tissue injury in RA *(5)*. The body of evidence to support this contention includes the following:

1. Intravenous infusion of iron has been shown to produce synovitis in murine models *(6)* and to precipitate flares of joint inflammation, with evidence of oxygen free-radical

reaction products in serum and synovial fluid, in patients with RA *(7,8)*.

2. Degradation of hyaluronate in RA synovial tissue can be completely inhibited by iron chelators *(9)*.

3. Proliferation of fibroblasts, a major finding in rheumatoid synovial tissue, appears to be mediated by cytokines produced by infiltrating immune cells *(10)*. It has been shown that ferric nitrilotriacetate increased the production of collagenase and prostaglandin (PG) E_2, as well as the number of rabbit synovial fibroblasts in vitro *(11)*.

4. Iron stimulates in vitro DNA synthesis by synovial cells and exerts an additive effect on the activity of human cytokines (interleukin-1β [IL-1β], IL-7, tumor necrosis factor-α [TNF-α], interferon-γ [IFN-γ]) for RA synovial cell proliferation *(12)*.

5. Suppression of fibroblasts growth parallels increased synthesis of PGE_2 and is reversed by the addition of inhibitors of PGE_2 synthesis *(13)*. PG endoperoxide synthetase is an iron-dependent enzyme critical for the generation of PG species *(14)*. As PGE_2 is an endogenous mediator of IL-1 production, it is conceivable that impaired PG production secondary to iron deficiency could also affect the production of this cytokine.

Altogether, these studies provide compelling evidence that excessive quantities of iron in the synovium may play a role in the pathogenesis of RA.

Zinc   Zinc is an essential cofactor in approximately 200 enzymes that are known to participate in many metabolic processes, including synthesis and degradation of carbohydrates, protein, lipids, and nucleic acids. This element has also been shown to play an important role in antioxidant protection and immunity.

Plasma zinc levels were found to be reduced in patients with many chronic inflammatory autoimmune diseases, including RA *(15)*. The modifications in zinc status produced by inflammatory processes, however, appear to be different from the one observed in zinc-deficient subjects, like those with alcoholic cirrhosis, diabetes, or renal insufficiency. Recent data point toward to the occurrence of a redistribution of this element within the body compartments, characterized by a decrease in plasma zinc concentrations, and an increase in zinc concentrations in mononuclear leukocytes, urine, and synovial fluid *(15)*. These modifications significantly correlate to the degree of inflammation, and the zinc status in patients with chronic inflammatory diseases is rather insensitive to zinc nutritional intake. Because of its pharmacological proprieties, zinc administration has also been proposed for the treatment of immune and inflammatory disorders. The use of supplementation in these instances is based on the assumption that there is at least a functional deficiency of zinc in these diseases.

The clinical effects of zinc supplementation in RA were first examined by Simkin in 1976 *(16)*. This author reported clinical improvement in patients suffering from chronic refractory RA by using 660 mg/d of zinc sulfate. These results, however, could not be confirmed by several subsequent trials *(15,17–19)*. Noteworthy, the fad of zinc supplementation has proved not to be exempt from side effects. Significant impairment of lymphocyte and neutrophil functions *(20)* and a potentially harmful increase of the low- to high-density lipoprotein (LDL/HDL) ratio *(21)* have been described in healthy adults under excessive intake of zinc (≥150 mg/d, a 10-fold excess of the recommended dietary allowance).

Copper   Copper is an essential nutrient for a large number of critical metabolic and immunologic functions. Most free copper is rapidly complexed in the plasma to ceruloplasmin, an acute-phase reactant that increases nonspecifically in response to inflammation. Copper, along with zinc, is also a constituent in cytoplasmic superoxide dismutase (SOD). Both ceruloplasmin and SOD possess antioxidant proprieties and have been shown to play an essential protective role against the free-radical-mediated tissue damage observed in inflammatory states *(22)*. In this context, it is interesting to note that copper bracelets were used by the ancient Greeks to relieve aches and pains and, for the present, as a folk remedy for RA. Although uncontrolled observations account for mild improvement in some of these patients, many side effects have been reported and it is unlikely that copper compounds would play any relevant role in RA therapy *(23)*. Elevated copper levels have been observed in both serum and synovial fluid in patients with RA, with most studies showing a positive correlation with disease activity *(24,25)*. Normalization of levels along with acute-phase reactants have also been reported following pharmacological control of disease *(25)*. Hence, data thus far indicate that increased serum copper values in patients with RA are most likely to be determined by the activity and extent of the inflammatory process, rather than by dietary factors.

Selenium   Selenium is involved in several important biological pathways relevant to autoimmune diseases. In RA, for instance, part of the destructive process that takes place in the inflamed joint space is related to neutrophil activation and, consequently, pathological generation of oxygen-derived free radicals. A protective role of selenium against pathology characterized by free-radical injury has been reported. This property is attributed to its involvement in the enzyme glutathione peroxidase (GSH-Px), which is active in the detoxification of damaging oxygen derivatives, and reduction of lipid hydroperoxides in cellular membranes *(26)*. Selenium also participates in several steps of both the cycloxygenase and lipoxygenase pathways of the arachidonic acid cascade; GSH-Px contributes in the reduction of PGG_2, enhancing the production of comparatively less potent inflammatory mediators such as prostacyclin and tromboxane A_2 *(27)*. In platelets and, perhaps in polymorphonuclear (PMN) leukocytes, GSH-Px mediates the conversion of 12-hydroperoxyeicosatetraenoic acid (12-HPETE) to the inactive metabolite 12-hydroeicosatetraenoic acid (12-HETE) *(28)*.

Immunomodulatory proprieties of selenium have been reported on both humoral and cell-mediated responses. In animal models, selenium deficiency has been shown to reduce the ability of T and B cells to proliferate in response to stimulation with various mitogens and antigens, whereas selenium supplementation increases these responses *(29)*. Accordingly, in vivo studies in humans demonstrated enhancement of cell-mediated immune response by selenium supplementation in elderly subjects and in patients requiring total parenteral nutrition *(30,31)*.

The antiinflammatory and immunomodulatory proprieties of selenium prompted studies in RA, juvenile RA, psoriatic arthritis, and SLE. Most selenium-supplementation trials, however (usually using organic selenium compounds), failed to demonstrate any significant improvement in any of these diseases, even when their deficient selenium status was corrected *(32,33)*. Interestingly, although selenium supplementation (250 μg/d) significantly increases selenium concentration in serum and red blood cells of both RA and control subjects *(32,33)*, it does not increase selenium levels in PMN leukocytes from patients with RA, as it does in PMN from control subjects *(34)*. Moreover, although selenium supplementation has been shown to substantially increase GSH-Px activity in serum, red blood cells, and platelets from RA patients, in PMN leukocytes the increase was not sufficient to reach the levels of controls *(26)*. Given the important role of PMN leukocytes in the inflammatory process observed in RA, these findings are in consonance with the lack of beneficial effect of selenium supplementation in controlled studies among patients with RA.

VITAMINS

Vitamin C (Ascorbic Acid) Ascorbic acid is essential for the synthesis of collagen, the main extracellular protein of connective tissue. Its deficiency, such as seen in patients with scurvy, accounts for inadequate synthesis of collagen and consequent impairment of wound healing and capillary fragility. Scurvy lesions in the skin can, at times, mimic those seen in autoimmune-mediated cutaneous vasculitis, highlighting the importance of a proper differential diagnostic *(35)*. Decreased synthesis of collagen, however, is not a key feature in any of the autoimmune diseases.

Low levels of ascorbic acid, in plasma, blood cells, and synovial fluid have been described in patients with RA, irrespective to drug therapy. In the 1940s, vitamin C was used to treat RA; nevertheless, no effects were seen on the clinical course of RA or on laboratory parameters of inflammation when large vitamin C supplements were given to normalize its serum levels *(36)*. Therefore, there is no evidence to support this form of therapy in patients with RA.

Vitamin B$_6$ (Pyridoxine) Low vitamin B$_6$ levels in the circulation is a well-described metabolic abnormality in patients with RA *(37)*. Low plasma levels of pyridoxal-5'-phosphate (PLP), the metabolically active form of B$_6$, has also been described in these patients *(38)* and appear to be related to the degree of inflammation and the levels of inflammatory cytokines, such as TNF-α *(37)*. Given its role as a cofactor in numerous enzymatic reactions, an altered availability of B$_6$ has been hypothesized to have an important effect on the balance of protein synthesis and degradation. Low levels of vitamin B$_6$ have also been postulated to impair the immune response *(39)*.

Reduction in muscle mass, the main storage compartment for PLP, is well known to occur in RA *(40)* and animal data suggest that the PLP level in plasma is a good reflection of the PLP in the muscle. Nevertheless, there are not conclusive data on whether lower plasma levels of B$_6$ and PLP truly reflect cellular deficiency. Vitamin B$_6$ administration in patients with RA, including those with low serum levels of PLP, failed to show any clinical improvement in disease *(38)*. Today, there is little reason to suspect that vitamin B$_6$ might be of any help in the treatment of RA or other autoimmune disease, especially in the light of potential toxicity *(41)*.

Vitamin E In addition to the damage mediated on cartilage and other joint components, oxygen-derived species can also cause peroxidation of cell membrane lipids. Vitamin E (α-tocopherol) is the major lipid-soluble antioxidant found in the sera and within the cells. By donating its phenolic hydrogen atom to peroxyl radicals and converting it to a hydroxiperoxide, α-tocopherol may terminate the chain reaction of free-radical damage to the cell membrane. By virtue of this property, vitamin E is critical for the proper function of the immune system. Although peroxidative damage has been associated with the loss of certain T-cell-receptor activities *(42)*, human lymphocytes have been shown to be protected from lipid peroxidation when cultured with vitamin E *(43)*.

Data from studies assessing the plasma levels of vitamin E in patients with RA are not uniform. Some studies found a normal baseline *(44,45)*, whereas others reported significantly lower levels *(46,47)* when compared to normal individuals. Significantly, lower concentrations of α-tocopherol in the synovial fluid, relative to those of paired serum samples, have been observed in patients with RA *(45,48)*. In one study, multiple-regression analysis indicated that the depletion of α-tocopherol was largely independent of the concomitant lower concentrations of cholesterol, triacylglycerol, and low-density lipoprotein in the inflamed joint *(48)*. At least in vitro, the antioxidant activity of vitamin E is regenerated by electron donation from vitamin C *(49)*. Because vitamin C levels are low in RA joint fluid, it has been hypothesized that this is caused by local consumption of α-tocopherol. Nonetheless, the question on whether low levels of α-tocopherol in the synovium contributes to oxidative damage of the joint or are an indirect marker of the local oxidative stress remains to be properly addressed.

Fish oil preparations utilized in clinical trials of RA (discussed later in this chapter) are enriched in α-tocopherol, which prevents the peroxidation of its polyunsaturated fatty acids (PUFA). Because the degree of unsaturation of the cell membrane increases the risk for lipid peroxidation and generation of toxic-free radicals, the α-tocopherol requirement depends on the amount of PUFA consumed. Data from several studies, however, demonstrate that despite the substantial increase in the consumption of fish oil PUFA, the amount of α-tocopherol added to fish oil capsules is usually sufficient to prevent deficiencies in cellular and plasma levels of vitamin E *(44, 49, 50)*. The clinical beneficial effects of dietary fish oil supplementation in RA does not depend on the antioxidizing properties of the low dose of α-tocopherol (10.3– 12.9 mg daily) in fish oil capsules *(44,50)*. In fact, aside from subjective parameters, no significant clinical improvement could be observed even when patients with RA were supplemented with 1200 mg of α-tocopherol a day *(51)*.

It has been recently postulated that excessive production of free radicals may also play a role in the pathogenesis of autoimmune-mediated systemic sclerosis (SSc) *(52)*. Oxidized low-density lipoproteins (LDL) is highly immunogenic and can (1) activate T lymphocytes, (2) increase the release of IL-1β, (3) enhance the proliferation of smooth-muscle cells by enlarging the expression of platelet-derived growth factor by these cells, and (4) induce the expression of genes for cellular adhesion molecules in endothelial cells [216]. Alpha-tocopherol is the main antioxidant of normal LDL. In one study, LDL from patients with SSc were shown to be more susceptible to oxidation than those from healthy control subjects *(53)*. This difference, however, could not be attributed to the α-tocopherol content of LDL. In accordance to previous studies, the endogenous concentration of α-tocopherol was not reduced in the plasma of SSc patients *(54)*.

HISTIDINE Several studies have demonstrated a selective low level of serum histidine in the serum of patients with RA when compared with normal subjects *(55)*. The extent of reduction of histidine levels has been shown to correlate with the degree of disease activity as assessed by clinical and laboratory parameters. Available in health food stores, L-histidine has empirically been used to treat patients with RA. Placebo-controlled trials, however, failed to demonstrate any convincing benefits of a dietary supplement of L-histidine in RA *(56)*.

FOOD CONSTITUENTS: DO THEY TRIGGER OR IMPROVE AUTOIMMUNE DISEASES?

Diet has been hypothesized to affect selected autoimmune diseases by two possible mechanisms that are not mutually exclusive (57). First, food-related antigens might induce hypersensitivity responses leading to autoimmune-related symptoms. Second, nutritional factors might alter inflammatory and immune responses and, consequently, modulate the course of selected autoimmune diseases.

FOOD HYPERSENSITIVITY The belief that food-related antigens might provoke hypersensitivity responses leading to autoimmune-disease-related symptoms is not a recent one (58). This thesis has gained some support from sporadic but convincing case reports of the reproducible onset of a selected rheumatic syndrome shortly after ingestion of certain aliments.

For a response to food to be linked plausibly to a hypersensitivity reaction, food antigens would have to cross the gastrointestinal barrier and circulate in antigenic form until recognized by effector or intermediary cells in the immune system. Although large molecules with antigenic proprieties are known to have very limited access to the circulation, some food antigens do cross the gastrointestinal barrier and circulate not only as food antigens but also as immune complexes. The M cell, a specialized epithelial cell that covers the intestinal lymphoid tissue, being free from glycocalyx, is in direct contact with the intestinal contents. These cells, by active pinocytosis, randomly pick up foreign antigenic material from the intestinal lumen and present it to macrophages and lymphocytes beneath them (59). Antigenic molecules may also succeed in passing through the intestinal mucosa in a less controlled manner through gaps in the epithelium caused by allergic, infectious, or toxic processes. Noteworthy, nonsteroidal anti-inflammatory drugs (NSAIDs), largely used for symptomatic management of pain, might lead to a loss of intestinal integrity, thus facilitating food-antigen absorption. Because no reliable laboratory test is available, the diagnosis of food hypersensitivity still rests mostly on clinical grounds. A particular food antigen is believed to be the cause of arthritis or other autoimmune-related symptom if a double-blinded oral provocation results in a flare up of the clinical symptom within 48 h of the challenge. In this chapter, food hypersensitivity is used as an umbrella term for adverse reactions to food.

Food Hypersensitivity Associated with Inflammatory Arthritis Several clinic observations suggest an association between food intake and inflammatory (rheumatoid or rheumatoid-like) arthritis. Most of these studies, however, lack a rigorous control and, for that reason, definitive conclusions cannot be drawn from them. In the few adequately controlled studies available, only a minority of patients with alleged food-induced rheumatic symptoms could be confirmed. In a series of 16 patients who claimed to have food-related arthritis, only 3 convincingly demonstrated objective symptoms following a double-blinded, encapsulated food challenge (60). In one patient, the particular symptoms triggered by ingestion of milk or dairy products were accompanied by increased levels of IgG4 anti-α-lactalbumin, and delayed skin and cellular reactivity to milk. The other two patients had their symptoms triggered by ingestion of shrimp and exposure to nitrates, respectively. All three patients had nonerosive, rheumatoid factor negative disease. The exact prevalence of this syndrome is largely unknown. It is possible that many of these cases are underreported, in that patients may not necessarily be aware of possible sensitivities to commonly ingested foods in the diet. The small number of documented cases in the literature, however, suggests that the syndrome is probably rare.

Food Hypersensitivity Associated with Systemic Lupus Erythematosus In the late 1970s, alfalfa meal was shown to significantly reduce plasma cholesterol levels and induce regression of atherosclerotic lesions in cholesterol-fed monkeys and rabbits. Subsequent studies indicated that ingestion of alfalfa seeds was also associated with reduction in plasma cholesterol in humans. In one study, however, after a prolonged ingestion of alfalfa seeds, one human volunteer developed clinical and serologic features of SLE (61). Following the cessation of the dietary supplement of alfalfa seeds, these abnormalities reverted to normal. Because alfalfa sprouts had become an increasingly popular diet constituent in humans, further studies were undertaken to investigate potential side effects of their ingestion, in particular the induction of autoimmunity. These studies confirmed the effect of alfalfa in triggering an SLE-like syndrome in normal monkeys fed with alfalfa seeds and in reactivating disease in susceptible animals (62). Isolated reports also suggest a similar role of alfalfa in inducing or reactivating human SLE. A nonprotein amino acid, L-canavanine, has been proposed as the alfalfa component for the triggering SLE-like syndrome. Canavanine is the principal free amino acid of a number of legumes such as clover and alfalfa, and it has also been reported to be a constituent of several food crops, including onions and soybeans. Interestingly, most of the toxic proprieties of L-canavanine appear to be destroyed by heating or cooking, which might explain why humans have not been affected more adversely by its toxicity (63). Altered synthesis of messenger RNA and resultant altered protein transcription have been hypothesized as the mechanisms by which L-canavanine induces the generation of autoantibodies (63). Nevertheless, the exact pathogenic mechanism by which L-canavanine induces or exacerbates SLE is yet to be elucidated; it is also conceivable that the available data may be nothing more than an epiphenomenon.

Food Hypersensitivity Associated with Other Autoimmune Diseases Walnut extracts have been shown to conspicuously exacerbate Behçet's syndrome within 48 h of its ingestion (64). In ex vivo studies, lymphocytes from these patients exhibited significantly decreased reactivity to both walnut extract and Candida antigens, which were associated with an increase in frequency and severity of their symptoms. Although it has been suggested that this transient suppression of lymphocyte reactivity may be responsible for the deleterious effects on the course of the disease, the mechanism by which English walnuts induce exacerbation of Behçet's syndrome remains unknown. Hypersensitivity to different foods has been hypothesized to be the cause of at least some cases of palindromic rheumatism and, in one instance, has been documented to occur secondary to sodium nitrate present in food preservatives (65). Very seldom, mostly through anecdotal reports, food hypersensitivity has been also implicated as a cause of vasculitis. In 1929, Alexander and Eyermann reported six cases of Henoch–Shoenlein purpura, which improved when certain foods were excluded and recurred when those foods were reintroduced (66). Clearly, much more data are needed to prove these assertions.

Eosinophilia–Myalgia Syndrome L-Tryptophan (LT) is an essential amino acid found in meats, dairy products, and some vegetable protein sources. Marketed as an over-the-counter food supplement in the United States since 1974, this preparation achieved increasing popularity among health professionals and nutrition enthusiasts as a natural remedy for depression, insomnia, and premenstrual symptoms. However, the clinical data that support its use are scant and, at times, conflicting. In fall 1989, an outbreak of eosinophilia and severe myalgia was recognized and associated with the ingestion of tryptophan (67); this syndrome became known as eosinophilia–myalgia syndrome (EMS). Within 6 mo after the initial description, 1511 cases (including 38 fatal cases) were reported to the Centers for Disease Control and Prevention (CDC). Intensive epidemiological investigation established that all traceable EMS cases were linked to the ingestion of adulterated LT produced by a single manufacturer. From chemical analysis of the implicated LT, it is likely that identified contaminants such as 1,1'-ethylidenebis (tryptophan) play a role in the pathogenesis of EMS, although the mechanism of action remains unclear (68).

In the acute phase, most patients present with features common to autoimmune disorders, particularly SSc; they include debilitating myalgia, severe fatigue, arthralgia, sclerodermalike skin changes, pulmonary infiltrates with cough, or dyspnea. Several therapeutic interventions, including the use of corticosteroids, amitriptyline, acetaminophen, methotrexate, cyclosporine, colchicine, and plasmapheresis, have been used with variable results. Overall, although improvement of most of the symptoms has been reported in more than 60% of the patients 2 yr after the onset of the syndrome, a significant number of patients continue to have symptoms of moderate to extreme severity (69).

DIETARY THERAPY Although a few autoimmune diseases are believed to be primarily caused by a B-cell dysfunction, most destructive organ-specific autoimmune diseases are probably initiated by Th-1 cells. The cytokines produced by them activate macrophages and stimulate the production of complement-fixing antibodies, actions that can mediate inflammation and tissue injury. Because Th-2 cells produce anti-inflammatory cytokines that inhibit macrophage functions and delayed-type hypersensitivity reactions, it has been hypothesized that such cells may function as natural regulators of autoimmune diseases (70). Although glucocorticoids and cytotoxic drugs have been important agents in improving the outcome and survival of patients with autoimmune diseases, they carry their own risk of drug-induced morbidity and mortality. It has also become apparent that these medications are not the final answer in disease management because some forms of autoimmune diseases have the potential to relapse or be treatment resistant. For these reasons, the pursuit of effective, less toxic therapeutic alternatives is critical. Part of such efforts relies on the potential use of dietary intervention as an adjuvant strategy to allow for lower drug doses and shorter periods of treatments. Diet therapy for autoimmune diseases can be divided in two modalities: (1) elimination therapy, which includes both removal of selected foods from the diet and fasting, and (2) supplementation therapy, in which foods are added to the diet.

Elimination Therapy

Animal Studies Calorie restriction (CR) is known to increase the life-span and diminish histological evidence of tissue damage in different models of autoimmune diseases. For instance, it significantly ameliorates the immune-complex-mediated glomerulonephritis and prolongs the life-span in the lupus prone (NZB × NZW)F$_1$ (B/W) mice (71). Recently, an increasing number of studies begun to shed light on the potential mechanisms for CR modulating autoimmunity. Calorie restriction increases glucocorticoid levels in calorie-restricted mice in a circadian manner (72),

which presumably drives an increase of IL-2R and T-cell growth factor (TGF-β) expression. Also, glucocorticoid receptor responses to stress has been shown to fall steadily with age, and this decline is attenuated by CR, which also maintains higher free-plasma corticosterone (CORT) during aging (73). Together with the observation of elevated dexamethasone (DEX)-stimulated programmed cell death (PDC or apoptosis) in lymphocytes from calorie-restricted (or ω-3-fed) animals, these studies provide a new working hypothesis in which ω-3 and/or CR increases CORT levels and synthesis of CORT in thymic tissue, enhancing negative selection of CD4⁻CD8⁻ (potentially autoreactive cells) (74).

The survival of lymphocytes is carefully regulated in order to maintain a dynamic balance between host defense and aggression toward self. The termination of a physiological immune response, like the deletion of autoreactive T cells during their maturation, is achieved by virtue of a tightly regulated PDC process. Triggered by a variety of external stimuli (such as crosslinking of the T-cell receptor or the fas/APO receptor), this process leads to the activation of catabolic intracellular enzymes, consequent degradation and disintegration of the cell, and, eventually, its ingestion and elimination by adjacent normal cells (75). Several lines of evidence indicate that a defect in the ability to eliminate self-reactive T or B cells, caused by dysregulated PDC, is an important common denominator in autoimmune disorders. Nevertheless, the way toward which this disarrangement progresses is still difficult to be determined. From one direction, it has been shown that transgenic mice that constitutively express Bcl-2 (which prevents or delays PDC in response to a number of apoptotic stimuli) show clinical signs of human autoimmune disease; likewise, SLE patients present increased expression of Bcl-2, which parallels the severity of clinical symptoms (76). Converse to such indication of deficient apoptosis, increased expression of the soluble form of the fas cell-surface receptor and accelerated rate of apoptosis in vitro have also been associated to disease activity in human SE (77). In this respect, a relevant aspect placing PDC in the core of pathogenic interest is its possible role in the generation of autoantibodies. Antigenic forms of DNA have been demonstrated to participate in the pathogenesis of SLE by reacting with circulating antibodies and, eventually, causing immune-complex-mediated tissue injury, such as glomerulonephritis. However, the mechanism by which macromolecular DNA and other autoantigens become available in the extracellular space, and therefore accessible to circulating antibodies, is not thoroughly understood. Consistent evidence indicates that nuclear proteins targeted in autoimmune diseases are cleaved and released during apoptosis (78–80), which may thus provide the source of extracellular antigens to drive the immune response and, ultimately, the formation of potentially pathogenic immune complexes. Although this puzzling scenario remains to be clarified, it has been shown that a number of dietary manipulations can improve the course of experimental autoimmune disease while modulating PCD. To some extent, CR normalizes PDC in MRL/lrp mice (which have markedly reduced PDC) and increases the expression of fas in calorie-restricted B/W mice (81). The elucidation of the operating role of PDC in maintaining a balanced ratio between Th-1 and Th-2-like T cells is of capital importance. Ultimately, it will solidify the conceptual framework to implement nutrition strategies designed to produce both anti- and pro-inflammatory cytokines, avoiding increased susceptibility to infection while preventing the rise of autoimmune disorders.

Human Data The utilization of different diets as a strategy to treat autoimmune diseases has been the subject of numerous studies and endless speculation in both the lay and the scientific literature. The role of dietary manipulations, such as the use of foods free of additives, preservatives, fruit, red meat, herbs, dairy products, and alcohol, remains controversial partially because existing trials are not able to provide clear-cut results (82–85). The impediment of such trials is that not only is compliance difficult to achieve, but "blinding" of the trial and placebo diets poses a major problem. Moreover, the trial design might be inappropriate if the population in the study is heterogeneous and only a small number of patients are capable of being improved. In this context, studies with individual patients who have exacerbations of their symptoms on a sufficient number of occasions when exposed to the alleged offending food provides more compelling evidence that, in fact, selective patients might experience the benefits of certain dietary manipulations in which the offending food is excluded. In general, however, especially until methodological impediments can be overcome, patients should be encouraged to follow balanced and healthy diets and to avoid elimination diets and fad nutritional practices that can lead to, or increase, pre-existent nutritional deficiencies (1).

Since ancient times, fasting has been used as part of religious rites and as an attempt to treat a variety of diseases. Although anecdotal reports that fasting can improve arthritic conditions have been made for several decades, it has been only in the last 15 yr that controlled studies have yielded results that support this claim. In 1979, Sköldstam et al. reported objective improvement in RA in 5 of 15 patients fasting for 7–10 d, whereas only 1 of 10 control subjects improved (86). Equivalent results were subsequently presented by several other investigators (87,88). There has been evidence suggesting that such improvement might have been generated by reduced gastrointestinal permeability to food and/or bacterial antigens, decreased neutrophil function, depressed lymphocyte response to antigenic stimuli, or increased cortisol concentrations during fasting (89–92). However, the exact mechanism by which fasting improves RA symptoms is yet to be fully understood. In a controlled trial conducted by Kjeldsen–Kragh et al., 7–10 d of fasting, followed by an individually adjusted vegetarian diet for a year, resulted in a sustained advantage for the diet group (88). Nonetheless, in the vast majority of the studies, the antirheumatic effects obtained from fasting disappears shortly after eating is reinstated, irrespective of the diet that the patients return to, whether ordinary Western diet, lactovegetarian diet, or strict vegetarian diet (vegan) (86,90,93,94). Complete fasting for periods beyond 1 wk is considered unsafe (even for patients with no complicating disorders), with potential risk for protein-energy malnutrition and renal and cardiac complications. The absence of convincing evidence that sustained benefit can be achieved after resuming normal diets, together with the lack of any data supporting that long-lasting antirheumatic effects can be achieved by repeated periods of fasting, precludes this modality of therapy from being recommended.

Supplementation Therapy Among dietary supplements, the most extensively investigated in autoimmune diseases are the omega-3 (ω-3) and omega-6 (ω-6) polyunsaturated fatty acids. Recently, there has been also increasing experimental and clinical data supporting the use of oral feeding antigens as an attempt to treat autoimmune disorders. These strategies will be the focus of discussion in the following subsections. The use of vitamins and trace elements as an attempt to treat autoimmune disorders were discussed earlier in this chapter.

Polyunsaturated Fatty Acids The fatty acids found in the cellular membranes are substrates for the production of prostaglandin (PG) and leukotriene (LT) species fundamental for many biological activities, including modulation of the inflammatory and immune responses. Omega-3 (ω-3) and omega-6 (ω-6) fatty acids can only be originated from diet and are considered essential because their deficiency can result in growth retardation and death. It is now well established that the comparison of phospholipids in cellular membranes is determined by nutritional intake and that alterations in dietary lipids can cause major changes in the synthesis of lipid-derived mediators of inflammation. By far, the most common fatty acid constituents in the Western diet are the ω-6 fatty acids, predominantly from terrestrial sources. This represents a great departure from the nutritional habits throughout most of human evolution, which were characterized by consumption of a higher percentage of polyunsaturated fat, more ω-3 fatty acids (derived from plants or fish oil), more fiber, and less total fat than the present Western diet (95). This relatively recent change in dietary patterns has been speculated to be an important factor on the development of some major chronic diseases of the industrialized society. Epidemiological studies, for example, have shown a reduced incidence of myocardial infarction, asthma, diabetes mellitus, and psoriasis in Greenland Eskimos compared with European controls (96). In a recent study from the Faroe Islands, it was reported that RA takes a milder course in this population than the one seen in other Nordic countries (97). A continuously evolving amount of evidence suggest that these findings are, at least in part, attributed to a high dietary intake of marine oils containing ω-3 polyunsaturated fatty acids (PUFA).

In Western societies, arachidonic acid (AA) [20 : 4, ω-6] is predominantly present in cellular membranes, and leads to the formation of the most potent PGs ("2" series: via the action of cyclooxygenase), and LTs ("4" series: via the action of 5-lipoxygenase). Marine polyunsaturated ω-3 fatty acids, such as eicosapentaenoic acid (EPA) [20 : 5, ω-3] and docosahexaenoic acid (DHA) [22 : 6, ω-3], competitively inhibits the utilization of AA and becomes a substrate for the production of alternative biologically active products through the cyclooxygenase and 5-lipoxigenase cellular metabolic pathway. As a result, an increase generation of PGs of the "3" series and LTs of the "5" series occur, both of which with considerable less pro-inflammatory effects than the corresponding AA metabolites. LTB_5, for instance, which is usually undetectable in humans consuming a Western diet, has only approximately 10% of potency of LTB_4. Platelet-activating-factor-acether (PAF-acether) generation of stimulated monocytes is also significantly diminished after fish oil (FO) ingestion (98). This is of considerable interest in the context of inflammation because PAF can stimulate endothelial cell generation of TNF and is 1000 times more potent than histamine in inducing vascular permeability (99). Alteration of the cell-membrane composition by PUFA may also result in changes in the signaling pathways critical for regulation of immune responses, and cell adhesion. Of particular interest, eicosanoids modulate the immune system by either directly by stimulating target cells or indirectly by modulating the production of other soluble regulatory factors such as cytokines (100). Normal individuals given a diet enriched with fish oil have been shown to exhibit significantly reduced monocyte production of IL-1 and, to some extent, TNF (101).

Omega-3 Fatty Acids

ANIMAL STUDIES The beneficial effects of dietary supplementation with marine ω-3 fatty acids has been demonstrated in some (102), but not all, (103) models of chronic inflammatory autoimmune diseases. The most striking results have been observed in New Zealand Black × New Zealand White F1 hybrid mice (NZB/W), which spontaneously develop SLE-like features, such as hemolytic anemia, antinuclear autoantibodies, and glomerulonephritis. NZB/W mice fed a diet rich in EPA experience notably lower levels of proteinuria, significantly lower levels of antibodies binding native DNA, and a greatly improved rate of survival (103). The beneficial effect on glomerulonephritis has been observed even if dietary supplements are withheld until after the kidney disease is established (102). Importantly, FO reduction of autoimmune disease severity in NZB/W mice does not result in the reduction of immune competence, at least not in terms of susceptibility to bacterial, yeast, or viral attack (104).

The immune system is exquisitely sensitive to chronic changes in dietary micronutrient and macronutrient levels, and a correlation between increased life-span and maintenance of naive T cells has been demonstrated. Unlike naive T cells, memory T cells have previously been exposed to antigenic stimulation and generally display an immune response of greater magnitude. Relative to calorie-restricted animals, *ad libitum* feeding increases inflammatory cells such as macrophages, as well as memory T cells, which are an important source of inflammatory cytokines (e.g., IL-1, IL-6, TNF-α, and IL-10) in RA and SLE. The T cell plays an important role in both the type and magnitude of immune response. Specifically, the CD4+ T cell can be functionally divided in two subsets: Th-1 and Th-2. The Th-1 cells produce IL-2 and interferon-γ (INF-γ), which enhances cell-mediated immunity, and Th-2 cells produce IL-4, IL-5, IL-6, and IL-10, which favor humoral (antibody-mediated) immunity. It is not yet established whether ω-3 lipids are able to modify the development of either Th-1 or Th-2-like cells. Nonetheless, fish-oil-fed B/W mice (another animal model of SLE) showed decreased IL-1β, IL-6, and TNF-α mRNA in kidney tissue when compared to polyunsaturated vegetable-fat (corn oil)-fed mice (81). In addition, TGF-β1, TGF-β2, and TGF-β3 isoform mRNA, as well as fibronectin and ICAM-1 mRNA, were also found to be significantly decreased in the kidney of FO-fed mice relative to corn-oil-fed mice with renal disease (81).

Clearly, in both healthy humans and rodents, dietary FO suppresses immune function (105). At least some of these immunosuppressive/anti-inflammatory properties have been directly linked to the ω-3 and fatty acids EPA and DHA. Both EPA and DHA, fed for 10 d to younger healthy C57Bl/6 mice, suppressed mitogen-induced T-cell IL-2 secretion and subsequent lymphoproliferation, which was preceded by blunted diacylglycerol and ceramide formation (106). This is important because both diacylglycerol and ceramide are positive regulators of T-cell proliferation. Also, the prolonged survival and amelioration of disease in ω-3 fed B/W mice is accompanied by increased antioxidant enzyme levels and decreased free-radical formation in both liver and kidney tissues (107).

HUMAN DATA Because the murine strains discussed herein provide a good model for SLE in several respects, the use of

marine lipids has been postulated to be of therapeutic value for human SLE. This assumption, unfortunately, has been only seldom, and inadequately, tested to date. A placebo-controlled study of 39 patients with lupus failed to demonstrate significant improvement in disease activity after 12 mo of fish oil administration (108). Nonetheless, the heterogeneous population enrolled in this study make the results difficult to interpret. In another study, using a double-blind, crossover design, the effect of EPA was evaluated in 17 patients with moderately active SLE for a period of 6 mo (109). Significant improvement of clinical and serological parameters were observed in the treated group after 3 mo, but at 6 mo no differences could be observed between this and the group control, suggesting a short-lived effect of EPA on SLE. The small number of patients in this study along with a relatively short-term follow-up precludes definitive conclusions from being drawn.

The extraordinary spectrum of anti-inflammatory and immunomodulatory effects exerted by ω-3 fatty acid supplementation in animals and humans justifies, in great part, the excitement shared by researchers in this field with regard to its potential use in the management of human autoimmune diseases. Nevertheless, the establishment of the practical usefulness of essential fatty acids in the treatment of human SLE will wait until prospective, long-term, adequately controlled studies are conducted.

In 1985, Kremer et al. pioneered the systematic study of PUFA supplementation (EPA and DHA) in patients with RA, showing a significant improvement in the number of tender joints and morning stiffness in the treated group (110). Since then, several other studies have been carried out, most of them reporting similar findings to Kremer's original study (111–119). The details of these studies are summarized in Table 1. Altogether, they indicate that ω-3 fatty acid supplementation exerts significant, albeit modest, anti-inflammatory effects in patients with RA. These beneficial effects appear to be dose dependent, more consistently observed after 18–24 wk of fish oil administration and, in some instances, accompanied by a decrease of LTB$_4$ and/or IL-1 and an elevation of LTB$_5$. In the studies in which the stated outcome measured was the ability of patients to reduce or discontinue their NSAID therapy, a modest sparing effect was observed.

Dietary supplementation with ω-3 fatty acids in the doses utilized in most clinical trials is a fairly expensive modality of treatment. Although not associated with significant toxicity, large amounts of fish oil consumption carries potential risk for obesity, vitamin A and D toxicity, and vitamin E deficiency. These considerations acquire particular relevance in the light of the fact that the benefits of this therapy have not been clearly established. If the NSAID-sparing effect observed in some studies is confirmed by further well-designed clinical trials, the use of ω-3 fatty acids might represent a safer alternative than NSAIDs in RA, specially for patients with gastric irritation or renal impairment. Raynaud's phenomenon, a condition marked by increased vascular reactivity to cold exposure, can exist as a primary disorder or as part of the constellation of symptoms observed in the autoimmune-mediated systemic sclerosis (scleroderma). Episodes of blanching or cyanosis of the fingers are the most characteristic clinical features. Infarction of tissue at the fingertip, however, may also lead to digital pitting scars or frank gangrene. DiGiacomo et al. observed that some of the biological effects of ω-3 fatty acids in cardiovascular disease could potentially benefit such patients (120). These effects include decrease plasma viscosity, a more favorable

Table 1
Studies of Dietary Fish Oil Supplementation in Rheumatoid Arthritis

Study	No. of patients	Study design	Type of fish oil ingested and daily dose	Duration of fish oil ingestion	Placebo (control group)	Clinical results	Impact on IL and/or LT production
Kremer et al. (1985) (110)	37	Prospective, double-blinded, placebo-controlled	1.8 g EPA and 0.9 g DHA	12 wk	Paraffin wax	Significant improvement in tender joints and morning stiffness	NA
Kremer et al. (1987) (113)	33	Prospective, double-blinded, crossover	2.8 g EPA and 1.8 g DHA	14 wk	Olive oil	Significant improvement in tender joints and interval to fatigue onset	↓ LTB$_4$ ↑ LTB$_5$
Sperling et al. (1987) (114)	12	Prospective, blinded	3.6 g EPA and 2.4 g DHA	6 wk	—	Significant decrease in joint pain index	↓ LTB$_4$
Cleland et al. (1988) (115)	44	Prospective, double-blinded, placebo-controlled	3.2 g EPA and 2.0 g DHA	12 wk	Olive oil	Significant improvement in tender joints and grip strength	↓ LTB$_4$
Kremer et al. (1990) (111)	49	Prospective, double-blinded, placebo-controlled	27 mg/kg EPA and 18 mg/kg DHA or 54 mg/kg DHA and 36 mg/kg DHA	24 wk	Olive oil	Significant improvement in tender joints, grip strength (both groups), and morning stiffness (only in the higher-dose fish oil group).	↓ LTB$_4$ ↓ IL-1
Van der Tempel et al. (1990) (116)	16	Prospective, double-blinded, crossover	?	12 wk	Coconut oil	Significant improvement in tender joints and morning stiffness	↓ LTB$_4$ ↑ LTB$_5$
Nielsen et al. (1992) (117)	51	Prospective, double-blinded, placebo-controlled	2.0 g EPA and 1.2 g DHA	12 wk	Fat composition as the average Danish diet	Significant improvement in tender joints and morning stiffness	NA
Lau et al. (1993) (118)	64	Prospective, double-blinded, placebo-controlled	1.7 g EPA and 1.1 g DHA	1 yr	Air-filled capsules	Significant reduction of the requirement for NSAID usage	NA
Geusens et al. (1994) (119)	90	Prospective, double-blinded, placebo-controlled	152 mg/kg EPA and 32 mg/kg DHA or 305 mg/kg EPA and 65 mg/kg DHA	1 yr	Olive oil	Significant improvement in the patient's and physician's assessment of pain, grip strength, and reduction in the need of NSAIDs (only in the higher-dose fish oil group)	NA
Kremer et al. (1995) (112)	66	Prospective, double blinded, placebo-controlled	130 mg/kg EPA	30 wk	Corn oil	Significant improvement in tender joints, morning stiffness, patient's and physician's assessment of global arthritic activity, and reduction in the need of NSAIDs	↓ IL-1β

vascular response to ischemia, a reduced vasospastic response to catecholamines and angiotensin, increase levels of tissue plasminogen activator, and increased endothelial-dependent relaxation of arteries in response to bradykinin, serotonin, adenosine diphosphate, and thrombin. A single prospective, double-blind controlled study of the effect of dietary supplements of 3.96 g of EPA and 2.64 g of DHA was conducted in 32 patients with primary or secondary Raynaud's phenomenon for 3 wk (120). Significant improvement in the patients with primary, but not secondary, Raynaud's phenomenon was observed in the group ingesting fish oil supplementation, with regard to the time interval to the onset of Raynaud's phenomenon triggered by hand immersion in cold-water baths. The mechanism of these benefit was not clarified in this study and, clearly, much more controlled trials are needed before ω-3 could be recommended for this condition.

Omega-6 Fatty Acids Besides ω-3, other fatty acids have been found to exhibit anti-inflammatory and immunomodulatory effects in experimental models and in preliminary clinical trials. Gamma-linoleic acid (GLA) [18 : 3, ω-6], a fatty acid found in seeds from the evening primrose (EPO) and borage plants, has been the focus of substantial investigation. GLA is a precursor of other ω-6 fatty acids, including AA, and may be converted by an elongase enzyme to dihomogamma-linoleic acid (DGLA) [18 : 3, ω-6]. In humans, the delta 5 desaturase that converts DGLA to AA is inefficient. In view of the fact that GLA is rapidly converted to DGLA, concentrations of AA do not increase appreciably. Hence, DGLA competes with AA for cyclooxygenase, reducing the generation of prostanoids derived from arachidonate. Whereas AA leads to the formation of PGs of the "2" series, DGLA, as a substrate for cyclooxygenase, generates prostaglandins of the "1" series, for which it has been shown to hold beneficial anti-inflammatory and antithrombotic properties. Although the biologic activities of corresponding members of the monoenoic ("1" series) and dienoic ("2" series) are qualitatively similar in many instances, in some respects they differ considerably. For example, PGE$_1$ inhibits aggregation of human platelets in vitro, whereas PGE$_2$ does not influence this activity. Also, PGE$_1$ is much more effective than PGE$_2$ in increasing levels of cAMP in human synovial cells in culture and in suppressing synovial cell proliferation (121). Along with the influence on PGs generation, it is of considerable importance that DGLA cannot be converted to inflammatory leukotrienes by 5-lipoxygenase. Instead, DGLA is converted to hydroperoxyl DGLA, which has the additional aptitude to inhibit 5-lipoxygenase activity. Independent of its role as a prostaglandin precursor, DGLA may have an important role in regulating immune responses by suppressing IL-2 production by human peripheral blood mononuclear cells (PBMC) (122), and proliferation of IL-2-dependent T lymphocytes (123).

ANIMAL STUDIES AND HUMAN DATA Gamma-linoleic acid dietary supplementation has been shown to suppress acute and chronic inflammation, as well as joint tissue injury, in a number of experimental animal models (124,125). In ex vivo studies, addition of DGLA to human synovial cells grown in tissue culture inhibits interleukin-1β-stimulated growth fivefold, compared with cell growth in medium supplemented with AA (126). When measured up against cells in control medium, those incubated with DGLA displayed a 14-fold increase in PGE$_1$ and a 70% decrease in PGE$_2$ levels.

Studies of dietary supplementation with GLA in humans have yielded somewhat mixed results (Table 2). The use of EPO in short-term studies (12 wk), with a small number of patients with RA, have been conducted without any apparent clinical benefit (127,128). GLA, in the form of EPO, was also utilized in a 12-mo placebo-controlled, double-blinded study (129). Forty-nine patients with active RA were randomly allocated in three groups receiving 540 mg of GLA, 240 mg of EPA, and 450 mg of GLA per day, or an inert oil as placebo. In both treated groups, reduction of pain, together with a reduction or even termination of NSAIDs therapy, was reported. Nevertheless, no significant objective changes in clinical or laboratory parameters were demonstrated. Pullman-Moore et al. (130) used a higher dose of GLA (1.1 g/d), in the form of borage seed oil, to treat seven patients with active RA for 12 wk. The authors reported significant clinical improvement in morning stiffness and in the number of swollen and tender joints. Although it is possible that the larger dose of GLA utilized could explain the apparent favorable results, the lack of a placebo control in this study makes this assumption impossible to assess. More recently, two prospective double-blinded, placebo-controlled studies observed significant clinical improvement in RA patients taking GLA (131,132). Although well conceived with regard to the study design, the limited number of patients and follow-up duration (131,132), possible interference by concomitant use of other medications (132), and a high number of dropouts (132) underlined the necessity, as the authors of these articles state, of further controlled studies.

Because phosphatidylinositol (PI), a critical source of AA, is remarkably insensitive to dietary modification of ω-3 PUFA, it has been hypothesized that alternative strategies to replace PI could displace a more significant amount of cell membrane AA and, therefore, exert a more potent anti-inflammatory and immunomodulatory effect (133). It has been recently demonstrated that dietary *Platycladus orientalis* seed oil, which is rich in 5,11,14-eicosatrienoic acid and 5,11,14,17-eicosatetraenoic acid, alters the fatty acid composition of PI in the cell membrane (134), displacing a significant amount of AA (133). Moreover, *P. orientalis* seed oil was shown to suppress antierythrocyte autoantibodies and to significantly prolong the survival of NZB mice, suggesting that the use of unique exotic oils might have a place in the nutritional therapy of autoimmune-mediated diseases. No clinical studies with such derivatives have been reported to date.

In summary, convincing clinical evidence supporting the use of ω-6 fatty acids in autoimmune diseases is yet to be demonstrated. The choice of an appropriate placebo for clinical studies on both EPO and fish oil has been the focus of evolving dispute. Because some fatty acids, such as olive oil, are thought to have potentially significant immunologic effects (135), it has been hypothesized that some of the so-called "placebo fatty acids" utilized in different studies could produce beneficial effects. The controversial issue of the ideal placebo dietary intervention to compare with EPO or fish oil has not yet been settled.

Mucosal Tolerance The observation that orally fed antigens can suppress immune responses was first recognized long before the era of modern immunology. As early as 1911, Wells described that systemic anaphylaxis in guinea pigs could be prevented by previous feeding of hen's egg proteins (136). Eighty-seven years later, mucosal tolerance by oral or nasal antigen administration has been successfully employed to prevent a number of experimental autoimmune disease models, including experimental allergic encephalomyelitis (137), experimental autoimmune uveoretinitis (138), experimental insulin-dependent diabetes mellitus (139),

Table 2
Studies of Dietary Evening Primrose/Borage Seed Oil Supplementation in Rheumatoid Arthritis

Study	No. of patients	Study design	Daily dose of GLA from evening primrose or borage seed oil	Duration of evening primrose or borage seed oil ingestion	Placebo (control group)	Clinical results
Hansen et al. (1983) (127)	20	Open, uncontrolled	360 mg GLA[a]	12 wk	—	No objective improvement on disease activity
Belch et al. (1988) (129)	49	Prospective, double-blinded, placebo-controlled	540 mg GLA[a] or 450 mg GLA[a] and 240 mg EPA	12 mo	Paraffin	Significant reduction of the requirement for NSAID usage; no objective improvement on disease activity
Jäntti et al. (1989) (128)	20	Prospective, Placebo-controlled	750 mg GLA[a]	12 wk	Olive oil	No objective improvement on disease activity
Pullman-Moore et al. (1990) (130)	7	Open, uncontrolled	1.1 g GLA[b]	12 wk	—	Significant improvement in tender joints and morning stiffness
Brzeski et al. (1991) (132)	40	Prospective, double-blinded, placebo-controlled	540 mg GLA[a]	24 wk	Olive oil	Significant improvement in morning stiffness
Leventhal et al. (1993) (131)	37	Prospective, double-blinded, placebo-controlled	1.4 g GLA[b]	24 wk	Cotton seed oil	Significant improvement in tender and swollen joints

[a]From evening primrose oil.
[b]From borage seed oil.

experimental autoimmune myasthenia gravis *(140)*, experimental autoimmune thyroiditis *(141)*, and collagen-induced arthritis *(142)*. Lately, it has also been used in clinical trials as an attempt to treat human multiple sclerosis *(143)*, Hashimoto's thyroiditis *(144)*, and rheumatoid arthritis *(145)*.

Oral tolerization takes advantage of an expedient the body uses to prevent immune reactions to the food we eat: foreign proteins that enter the body through the digestive system suppress immune responses to those proteins instead of provoking them. Two mechanisms have been proposed to explain the immunologic basis for tolerance induction depending on the dose of antigen administered: Selective expansion of cells producing immunosuppressive cytokines (lower doses) and anergy/deletion of specific T cells (higher doses). *Low doses* of orally administered antigen are taken up by mucosal-associated antigen-presenting cell that preferentially stimulate regulatory T cells; these cells, in turn, mediate suppression of the specific immune response in the target organ via the secretion of suppressive cytokines such as TGF-β, IL-4, and IL-10 *(146)*. This process, termed antigen-driven bystander suppression, implies that an orally administered protein can downregulate organ-specific autoimmune disease as long as it is a constituent of the target tissue and is capable of inducing regulatory T cells *(146)*. In other words, the regulatory T cells generated following oral tolerization are triggered in an antigen-specific fashion but are suppressed in an antigen-nonspecific fashion when they encounter the fed autoantigen at the target organ. Such a scenario poses an appealing conceptual answer to overcome a major problem that hampers the designing of T-cell-specific therapy for autoimmune diseases; according to it, it is no longer necessary to know the specific nature of the disease-relevant autoantigen. Unlike low doses, *high doses* of orally administered antigen appear to pass through the gut and enter the systemic circulation, either as an intact or as a processed protein, thus inducing unresponsiveness of T-cell function primarily through clonal anergy/deletion *(70)*.

Rheumatoid Arthritis   Among autoimmune diseases, RA has been one of the most scrutinized with regard to oral tolerance investigation. Type II collagen is the most abundant structural protein of cartilage and immunization of animals with the native protein causes an arthritis morphologically resembling rheumatoid arthritis *(142)*. Patients with RA manifest immune responses to native type II collagen *(147)*, but whether this reactivity participates in the primary pathogenesis of the disease or reflects tissue degradation is currently unknown. Oral administration of native type II collagen has been shown to significantly ameliorate two animal models of rheumatoid arthritis induced by type II collagen or complete Freund's adjuvant *(148)*. In these models, suppressor T cells triggered in rats by oral administration of collagen appear to travel to the joints, and there they prevent other types of T cells from being activated and causing inflammation. More recently, Trentham et al. reported dramatic improvement in a double-blind, placebo-controlled study of RA patients taking daily liquid doses of chicken collagen for 3 mo *(145)*. Although providing encouraging results, the clinical design of this study demands cautious enthusiasm. This study lacked an initial drug-free period that would prevent misinterpretation with regard to the interfering effect of previous medications. Moreover, because the natural history of RA is notoriously remitting and exacerbating, studies with a longer follow-up and a larger number of patients should be performed in order to access whether these results are truly reliable.

Experimental Autoimmune Encephalomyelitis   Chronic relapsing experimental autoimmune encephalomyelitis (EAE), induced in mice by the injection of myelin basic protein (MBP) or myelin proteolipid protein (PLP), is a T-cell-mediated autoimmune demyelinating disease of the central nervous system (CNS) that serves as an animal model for multiple sclerosis (MS). A variety of tolerance regimens, using CNS myelin proteins, have been used to prevent development of acute EAE *(149,150)* and, occasionally, to improve its course once relapsing EAE is established *(151)*. Interestingly, by means of bystander suppression, PLP peptide-induced EAE can be inhibited by feeding MBP, and MBP-specific T-cell clones from orally tolerized animals also suppress PLP-induced disease *(70)*. This prevention has been shown to be accompanied by reduced antigen-specific T-cell proliferation and IL-2 and IFN-γ production, with concomitant increased IL-4 production *(152)*, indicating suppressed Th-1 responses in tolerized rats. Accordingly, in tolerized rats, cells, upon restimulation with MBP in vitro, reveal increase levels of TGF-β and IL-4 mRNA, reflecting an IL-4-mediated Th-1 to Th-2 switch *(70)*. More recently, a novel mechanism for monocyte chemotactic protein (MCP)-1 as a regulatory factor of oral tolerance has been described *(153)*. Oral administration of PLP increased MCP-1 expression in the intestinal mucosa, Peyer's patch, and mesenteric lymph nodes; this resulted in downregulation of mucosal IL-12 expression with a concomitant increase in IL-4 mucosal expression. Functionally, MCP-1 upregulation was shown to regulate oral tolerance induction by the ability of antibodies to MCP-1 to inhibit tolerance induction. The anti-MCP abrogation of tolerance induction also resulted in restoration of mucosal IL-12 expression as well as peripheral antigen-specific T-helper-cell 1 responses.

Based on the evidence that EAE pathogenesis is related to a tolerance failure to myelin components, bovine myelin has been used as an attempt to treat MS. In one study, T-cell lines were generated from patients with relapsing–remitting MS; the frequency of TGF-β-secreting T-cell lines after MBP and PLP stimulation was greater in myelin-treated patients than in nonfed patients *(154)*. In spite of showing that oral myelin antigen administration was able to modulate the cytokine secretion profile in patients with MS, these promising observations will have to be tested in large, double-blind studies in order to determine whether such findings are translated into clinical improvement of this disease.

Experimental Autoimmune Uveoretinitis   Experimental autoimmune uveoretinitis (EAU) is a T-lymphocyte-mediated inflammation of the uveal tract and retina that serves as an animal model of human autoimmune posterior uveitis. S-Antigen (S-Ag) and interphotoreceptor retinol-binding protein (IRBP) are the two major autoantigens within retinal extracts (RE) that are potent inducers of EAU. Tolerance to S-Ag-induced EAU has been achieved in susceptible animals by oral administration of milligram quantities of S-Ag *(138)* or via the upper respiratory tract with microgram doses of antigen *(155)*. Intranasal administration of S-Ag and/or IRBP to Lewis rats prior to immunization with RE successfully suppresses both severity and incidence of clinical EAU and histopathological changes *(155)*. This suppression is accompanied by reduced antigen-specific delay hypersensitivity response activity but maintained T-cell-dependent (IgG2a) antibody responses. As expected, suppression of RE-induced EAU is not achieved with administration of a non-retinal-specific autoantigen such as MBP. Recently, it has been showed that mucosal tolerance induction is also possible after immunization with RE in EAU *(156)*. At the present time, no clinical trials investigating the oral or nasal administration of retinal antigens in human auto-immune posterior uveitis have been reported.

Experimental Autoimmune Myasthenia Gravis Experimental autoimmune myasthenia gravis (EAMG) is a well-established animal model, which can be induced in various animal species and strains with the acethylcholine receptor (AChR) and represents an experimental counterpart of human myasthenia gravis (MG) *(157)*. The abnormality in MG is a deficiency of AChRs at neuromuscular junctions due to an antibody-mediated autoimmune attack. Oral and nasal administration of AChR to Lewis rats prior to immunization with AChR results in prevention or a marked decrease of the severity of EAMG and suppression of AChR-specific B-cell responses and AChR-reactive T-cell function *(158,159)*. *In situ* hybridization with radiolabeled cDNA probes has been used to identify mononuclear cells expressing mRNA for the proinflamatory cytokine IFN-γ, the B-cell stimulating IL-4, and the immunosuppressive TGF-β *(158,160)*. Oral and nasal tolerance was accompanied by decreased numbers of AChR-reactive IFN-γ and IL-4 mRNA-expressing cells and strong upregulation of TGF-β mRNA-positive cells in lymphoid organs when compared to nontolerized EAMG control rats. These results suggest that although IFN-γ and IL-4 are central effector molecules in the development of EAMG, induction of tolerance to EAMG is, at least partly, determined by TGF-β-producing cells. Presently, there are no available data on clinical trials using oral tolerance strategy to treat human MG.

Experimental Insulin-Dependent Diabetes Mellitus Experimental insulin-dependent diabetes mellitus (IDDM) is an autoimmune disease that is characterized by destruction of insulin-producing β cells in the pancreatic islets. Insulin is an autoantigen in human and selected animal model IDDM. It has recently been reported that islet-infiltrating cells isolated from nonobese diabetic (NOD) mice model of IDDM are enriched for insuline-specific T cells, with the epitopes on residues 9–23 of the B chain being immune dominant in this spontaneous response *(161)*. Oral and nasal administration of insulin, insulin B chain or insuline peptide B (9–23) to some *(162,163)*, but not all, animal models of IDDM *(164)* results in a marked delay or suppression of insulinitis and a decrease incidence of diabetes. When T-cell lines derived from a NOD mice model of IDDM are analyzed after insuline exposure, this protective effect is accompanied by reduced T-cell proliferative response to insuline or insuline B chain, a decrease in IFN-γ expression, and an increase in IL-4, TGF-β, and IL-10 expression *(162,163)*. Recently, it has been demonstrated that the ability of splenocytes from insuline-treated NOD mice to suppress the adoptive transfer of diabetes to nondiabetic mice by T cells of diabetic mice *(162)*; this was shown to be caused by small numbers of CD8 γ/δ T cells. Although the benefit of mucosal tolerance induction has not yet moved from experimental disease into clinical grounds, these findings unfold a conceptual strategy in which induction of regulatory cells by nasal or oral insulin administration could be effective for the prevention or treatment of human IDDM.

SUMMARY

Autoimmune diseases are believed to be caused by the failure of the immune system to distinguish between self, for which there exists a state of natural immune tolerance, and nonself. The failure

of immune tolerance often results in adverse consequences, including tissue and organ destruction dependent on abnormalities of both humoral and cell-mediated responses. The current therapy of autoimmune diseases is nonspecific and limited by drug toxicity and unpredictable relapses. In the lure of circumventing at least some of these constraints, nutritional strategies to modulate the course of autoimmune diseases has been under continuous and intense assessment. Although scant evidence suggests that certain food components may trigger or aggravate autoimmune-related symptoms, a continuously evolving body of data support the existence of an important place for nutrition and diet as an auxiliary approach to treat autoimmune diseases. At the present time, calorie restriction, supplementation of ω-3 and ω-6 fatty acids, and orally fed antigens are known to exert an extraordinary range of anti-inflammatory and immunomodulatory effects in animal models for a number of autoimmune diseases, including a significant increase in the life-span and diminished histological evidence of tissue damage. The mechanism by which these is achieved is also continuously being unfolded as it becomes clear the nutritional influence on (1) PG and LT production, (2) cytokine gene expression, (3) T- and B-cell apoptosis, and (4) free-radical damage to the cell membrane. Clinical trials applying nutritional strategies are, by far and large, less encouraging than experimental studies. These studies, however, have to be critically evaluated. For instance, the trial design might be inappropriate if the population in the study is heterogeneous and only a small number of patients are capable of being improved. Clearly, a larger number of well-conducted studies are needed before we can safely move from experimental disease into clinical grounds. Therefore, until more conclusive studies are available, patients with autoimmune diseases should be discouraged from "miracle diets" and self-administration of over-the-counter collagen, vitamins, and trace element pills—a practice that is more likely to cause frustration than provide relief.

REFERENCES

1. Panush RS. American College of Rheumatology position statement: diet and arthritis. Rheum Dis Clin North Am 1991; 17:443–4.
2. Means RT, Krantz SB. Progress in understanding the pathogenesis of the anemia of chronic disease. Blood 1992; 80:1639–47.
3. Blake DR, Gallagher PJ, Potter AR, Bell MJ, Bacon PA. The effect of synovial iron on the progression of rheumatoid disease. A histological assessment of patients with early rheumatoid synovitis. Arthritis Rheum 1984; 495–501.
4. Morris CJ, Blake DR, Wainwright AC, Steven MM. Relationship between iron deposits and tissue damage in the synovium: a ultrastructural study. Ann Rheum Dis 1986; 45:21–6.
5. Blake DR, Hall ND, Bacon PA, Dieppe PA, Halliwell B, Gutteridge JM. The importance of iron in rheumatoid disease. Lancet 1981; 2:1142–4.
6. De Sousa M, Dynesius-Trentham R, Mota-Garcia F, da Silva MT, Trentham DE. Activation of rat synovium by iron. Arthritis Rheum 1988; 31:653–61.
7. Blake DR, Lunec J, Ahern M, Ring EF, Bradfield J, Gutteridge JM. Effect of intravenous iron dextran on rheumatoid synovitis. Ann Rheum Dis 1985; 44:183–8.
8. Winyard PG, Blake DR, Chirico S, Gutteridge JM, Lunec J. Mechanism of exacerbation of rheumatoid synovitis by total-dose iron-dextran infusion: in vivo demonstration of iron promoted oxidant stress. Lancet 1987; 1:69–72.
9. Schenk P, Schneider S, Miehlke R, Prehm P. Synthesis and degradation of hyaluronate by synovia from patients with rheumatoid arthritis. J Rheumatol 1995; 22:400–5.

10. Gitter BD, Labus JM, Lees SL, Scheetz ME. Characteristics of human synovial fibroblast activation by IL-1β and TNFα. Immunology 1989; 66:196–200.

11. Okazaki I, Brinckerhoff CE, Sinclair JF, Sinclair PR, Bonkowsky HL, Harris ED Jr. Iron increases collagenase production by rabbit synovial fibroblasts. J Lab Clin Med 1981; 97:396–402.

12. Nishiya K. Stimulation of human synovial cell DNA synthesis by iron. J Rheum 1994; 21:1802–7.

13. Korn JH, Halushka PV, LeRoy EC. Mononuclear cell modulation of connective tissue function: suppression of fibroblast growth by stimulation of endogenous prostaglandin production. J Clin Invest 1980; 65:543–54.

14. Sherman AR. Influence of iron on immunity and disease resistance. Ann NY Acad Sci 1990; 587:140–6.

15. Peretz A, Neve J, Jeghers O, Pelen F. Zinc distribution in blood components, inflammatory status, and clinical indexes of disease activity during zinc supplementation in inflammatory rheumatic diseases. Am J Nutr 1993; 690–4.

16. Simkin PA. Oral zinc sulphate in rheumatoid arthritis. Lancet 1976; 2:539–42.

17. Job C, Menkes CJ, Delbarre F. Zinc sulfate in the treatment of rheumatoid arthritis. Arthritis Rheum 1980; 23:1408–9.

18. Rasker JJ, Kardaun SH. Lack of beneficial effect of zinc sulfate in rheumatoid arthritis. Scand J Rheum 1982; 11:168–70.

19. Sorenson JR. An evaluation of altered copper, iron, magnesium and zinc concentrations in rheumatoid arthritis. Inorg Prospec Biol Med 1978; 2:1–16.

20. Chandra R. Excessive intake of zinc impairs immune response. JAMA 1984; 252:1443–6.

21. Hooper PL, Visconti L, Gary PJ, et al. Zinc lowers high-density lipoprotein cholesterol levels. JAMA 1980; 244:1960–1.

22. Gutteridge JMC. Ceruloplasmin: a plasma protein, enzyme and antioxidant. Ann Clin Biochem 1978; 15:293–6.

23. Sorenson JR, Hangarter W. Treatment of rheumatoid and degenerative diseases with copper complexes. A review with emphasis on copper-salicylate. Inflammation 1977; 2:217–38.

24. Honkanen VEA, Lambert-Allardt CH, Vesterinen MK, et al. Plasma zinc and copper concentrations in rheumatoid arthritis: influence of dietary factors and disease activity. Am J Clin Nutr 1991; 54:1082–6.

25. Brown DH, Buchanan WE, El-Ghobarey A, Smith WE, Teape J. Serum copper and its relationship to clinical symptoms in rheumatoid arthritis. Ann Rheum Dis 1979; 38:174–6.

26. Tarp U. Selenium and the selenium-dependent glutathione peroxidase in rheumatoid arthritis. Danish Med Bull 1994; 41:264–74.

27. Spallholz JE, Boyland LM, HS L. Advances in understanding selenium's role in the immune system. Ann NY Acad Sci 1990; 587:123–39.

28. Redanna P, Whelan J, Burgess JR, et al. The role of vitamin E and selenium on arachidonic acid oxidation by way of the 5-lipoxygenase pathway. Ann NY Acad Sci 1989; 570:136–45.

29. Turner RJ, Wheatley LB, Beck NEG. Stimulatory effect of selenium on mitogen response in lambs. Vet Immunol Imunopathol 1985; 8:119–24.

30. Peretz A, Nève J, Desmedt J, Duchateau J, Dramaix M, Famaey JP. Lymphocyte response is enhanced by supplementation of elderly subjects with selenium-enriched yeast. Am J Clin Nutr 1991; 53:1323–8.

31. Peretz A, Nève J, Duchateau J, et al. Effects of selenium supplementation on immune parameters in gut failure patients on home parenteral nutrition. Nutrition 1991; 7:215–21.

32. Tarp U, Overvad K, Thorling E, Graudal H, Hansen JC. Selenium treatment in rheumatoid arthritis. Scand J Rheumatol 1985; 4:364–8.

33. Tarp U, Hansen JC, Overvad K, Thorling EB, Tarp BD, Graudal H. Glutathione peroxidase activity in patients with rheumatoid arthritis and in normal subjects: effects of long-term selenium supplementation. Arthritis Rheum 1987; 30:1162–6.

34. Tarp U, Stengaard-Pedersen K, Hansen JC, Thorling EB. Glutathione redox cycle enzymes and selenium in severe rheumatoid arthritis: lack of anti-oxidative response to selenium supplementation in polymorphonuclear leucocytes. Ann Rheum Dis 1992; 51:1044–9.

35. Warshauer DM, Hayes ME, Shumer SM. Scurvy, a clinical mimic of vasculitis. Cutis 1984; 34:539–41.

36. Hall MG, Darling RC, Taylor FHC. The vitamin C requirement in rheumatoid arthritis. Ann Intern Med 1939; 13:415–23.

37. Roubenoff R, Roubenoff RA, Selhub J, et al. Abnormal vitamin B6 status in rheumatoid arthritis cachexia. Association with spontaneous tumor necrosis factor a production and markers of inflammation. Arthritis Rheum 1995; 1:105–9.

38. Schumacher HR, Bernhard FW, Gyorgy P. Vitamin B6 levels in rheumatoid arthritis: effect of treatment. Am J Clin Nutr 1975; 28:1200–3.

39. Rall LCR, Meydani SN. Vitamin B6 and immune competence. Nutr Rev 1993; 51:217–25.

40. Roubenoff R, Roubenoff RA, Cannon JG, et al. Rheumatoid cachexia: cytokine driven hypermetabolism accompanying reduced body cell mass in chronic inflammation. J Clin Invest 1994; 93:2379–86.

41. Schaumburg H, Kaplan J, Windebank A. Sensory neuropathy from pyridoxine abuse. N Engl J Med 1983; 309:445–8.

42. Grever MR, Thompson VN, Balcerzac SP, Sagone AL Jr. The effect of oxidant stress on human lymphocyte cytotoxicity. Blood 1980; 56:284–8.

43. Topinka J, Binkova B, Sram RJ, Erin AN. The influence of alpha-tocopherol and pirytinol on oxidative DNA damage and lipid peroxidation in human lymphocytes. Mutat Res 1989; 225:131–6.

44. Tulleken JE, Limburg PC, Muskiet FA, Rijswijk MK. Vitamin E status during fish oil supplementation in rheumatoid arthritis. Arthritis Rheum 1990; 33:1416–9.

45. Wasil M, Hutchinson DCS, Cheesman P, Baum H. Alpha-tocopherol status in patients with rheumatoid arthritis: Relationship to antioxidant activity. Biochem Soc Trans 1992; 20:277S.

46. Honkanen V, Kontinnen YT, Mussalo-Rauhamaa H. Vitamins A and E, retinol binding protein and zinc in rheumatoid arthritis. Clin Exp Rheum 1990; 7:465–9.

47. Situnayake RD, Thurnham DI, Kootathep S, et al. Chain breaking antioxidant status in rheumatoid arthritis: clinical and laboratory correlates. Ann Rheum Dis 1991; 50:81–6.

48. Fairburn K, Grootveld M, Ward RJ, et al. Alpha-tocopherol, lipids and lipoproteins in knee-joint synovial fluid and serum from patients with inflammatory joint disease. Clin Sci 1992; 83:657–64.

49. Doba T, Burton GW, Ingold KU. Anti-oxidant and co-oxidant effect of vitamin C. Biochem Biophys Acta 1985; 835:298–303.

50. Scherak O, Kolarz G. Vitamin E and rheumatoid arthritis. Arthritis Rheum 1991; 34:1205–6.

51. Kolarz G, Scherak O, Shohoumi M, et al. Hochdosiertes Vitamin E bei chronicher Polyarthritis: Eine multizentriche Doppelblindstudie gegeuber Diclofenac-Natrium. Aktuel Rheumatol 1990; 15:223–37.

52. Murrel DF. A radical proposal for the pathogenesis of scleroderma. J Am Acad Dermatol 1993; 28:78–85.

53. Bruckdorfer KR, Hillary JB, Bunce T, Vancheeswaran R, Black CM. Increased susceptibility to oxidation of low-density lipoproteins isolated from patients with systemic sclerosis. Arthritis Rheum 1995; 38:1060–7.

54. Herrick AL, Rieley F, Schofield D, Hollis S, Braganza JM, Jayson MI. Micronutrient antioxidant status in patients with primary Raynaud's phenomenon and systemic sclerosis. J Rheumatol 1994; 21:1477–83.

55. Gerber DA. Low free serum histidine concentration in rheumatoid arthritis: a measure of disease activity. J Clin Invest 1975; 55:1164–73.

56. Pinals RS, Harris ED, Burnett JB, Gerber DA. Treatment of rheumatoid arthritis with L-histidine: a randomized, placebo-controlled double blind trial. J Rheumatol 1977; 4:414–9.

57. Panush RS. Does food cause or cure arthritis? Rheum Dis Clin North Am 1991; 17:259–72.

58. Turnbull JA. Food allergens in connection with arthritis. Boston Med Surg J 1924:438–40.

59. Darlington LG, Ramsey NW. Review of dietary therapy for rheumatoid arthritis. Br J Rheumatol 1993; 32:507–14.

60. Panush RS. Food induced ("allergic") arthritis: clinical and serologic studies. J Rheumatol 1990; 17:291–4.

61. Malinow MR, Bardana EJ, Goodnight SH. Pancytopenia during ingestion of alfalfa seeds. Lancet 1981; 1:615.

62. Malinow MR, Bardana EJ, Pirofsky B, Craig S, McLaughlin P. Systemic lupus erythematosus-like syndrome in monkeys fed with alfalfa sprouts: Role of a non-protein amino acid. Science 1982; 216:415–7.

63. Montanaro A, Bardana EJ Jr. Dietary aminoacid-induced systemic lupus erythematosus. Rheum Dis Clin North Am 1991; 17:323–32.

64. Marquardt JC, Snyderman R, Oppenheim JJ. Depression of lymphocyte transformation and exacerbation of Behçet's syndrome by ingestion of English walnuts. Cell Immunol 1973; 9:263–72.

65. Epstein S. Hypersensitivity to sodium nitrate: a major causative factor in case of palindromic rheumatism. Ann Allergy 1969; 27:343–9.

66. Alexander HL, Eyermann CH. Allergic purpura. JAMA 1929; 92:2092–4.

67. Hertzman PA, Blevins WL, Mayer J, Greenfield B, Ting M, Gleich GJ. Association of the eosinophilia–myalgia syndrome with the ingestion of tryptophan. N Engl J Med 1990; 322:869–73.

68. Mayeno AN, Lin F, Foote CS, et al. Characterization of "peak E," a novel amino acid associated with eosinophilia–myalgia syndrome. Science 1990; 250:1707–8.

69. Hertzman PA, Clauw DJ, Kaufman LD, et al. The eosinophilia–myalgia syndrome: status of 205 patients and results of treatment 2 years after onset. Ann Intern Med 1995; 122:851–5.

70. Xiao B-G, Link H. Mucosal tolerance: a two-edged sword to prevent and treat autoimmune diseases. Clin Immunol Immunopathol 1997; 85:119–28.

71. Fernandes G, Friend P, Yunis EJ, Good RA. Influence of dietary restriction on immunologic function and renal disease in (NZB × NZW)F1 mice. Proc Natl Acad Sci USA 1978; 75:1500–4.

72. Sabatini F, Masoro EJ, McMahan CA, Kuhn RW. Assessment of the role of the glucocorticoid system in aging processes in the action of food restriction. J Gerontol Biol Sci 1991; 46:171–9.

73. Sapolsky RM, Krey LC, Mc Ewen BS. The neuroendocrinology of stress and aging: the glucocorticoid cascade hypothesis. Endocr Rev 1986; 7:284–301.

74. Wilder RL. Neuroendocrine–immune system interactions and autoimmunity. Ann Rev Immunol 1995; 13:307–8.

75. Graninger WB, Smolen JS. Should the clinician have interest in the deregulation of apoptosis in autoimmunity? Br J Rheumatol 1998; 36:1244–6.

76. Gatenby PA, Irvine M. The bcl-2 proto-oncogene is overexpressed in systemic lupus erythematosus lymphocytes. J Autoimmun 1994; 7:623–31.

77. Emlen W, Niebur J, Kadera R. Accelerated in vitro apoptosis of lymphocytes from patients with systemic lupus erythematosus. J Immunol 1994; 152:3685–92.

78. Utz PJ, Hottelet M, Schur PH, Anderson P. Proteins phosphorylated during stress-induced apoptosis are common targets for autoantibody production in patients with systemic lupus erythematosus. J Exp Med 1997; 185:843–54.

79. Rosen A, Casciola-Rosen L, Ahearn J. Novel packages of viral and self-antigens are generated during apoptosis. J Exp Med 1995; 181:1557–61.

80. Casiano CA, Martin SJ, Green DR, Tan EM. Selective cleavage of nuclear autoantigens during CD95 (Fas/APO-1)-mediated T cell apoptosis. J Exp Med 1996; 184:765–70.

81. Fernandes G, Jolly CA. Nutrition and autoimmune disease. Nutr Rev 1998; 56(1):S161–9.

82. Beri D, Malaviya AN, Shandilya R, Singh RR. Effect of dietary restrictions on disease activity in rheumatoid arthritis. Ann Rheum Dis 1988; 47:69–72.

83. Panush RS, Carter RL, Katz P, Kowsari B, Longley S, Finnie S. Diet therapy for rheumatoid arthritis. Br J Rheumatol 1995; 34:270–3.

84. Kavanaghi R, Workman E, Nash P, Smith M, Hazleman BL, Hunter JO. The effects of elemental diet and subsequent food reintroduction on rheumatoid arthritis. Br J Rheumatol 1995; 34:270–3.

85. Darllington LG, Ramsey NW, Mansfield JR. Placebo-controlled, blind study of dietary manipulation therapy in rheumatoid arthritis. Lancet 1986; i:238–76.

86. Skoldstam L, Larsson L, Lindström FD. Effects of fasting and lactovegetarian diet on rheumatoid arthritis. Scand J Rheumatol 1979; 8:249–55.

87. Trang LE, Lovgren O, Bendz R, Mjos O. The effect of fasting on plasma cyclic adenosine-3',5'-monophosphate in rheumatoid arthritis. Scand J Rheumatol 1980; 9:229–33.

88. Kjeldsen-Kragh J, Haugen M, Borchgrevink CF, et al. Controlled trial of fasting and one-year vegetarian diet in rheumatoid arthritis. Lancet 1991; 338(8772):899–902.

89. Holm G, Palmblad J. Acute energy depravation in man: effect on cell-mediated immunological reactions. Clin Exp Immunol 1976; 25:207–11.

90. Hafstrom I, Ringertz B, Gyllenhammar H, Palmblad J, Harms-Ringdahl M. Effects of fasting on disease activity, neutrophil function, fatty acid composition, and leukotriene biosynthesis in patients with rheumatoid arthritis. Arthritis Rheum 1988; 31:585–92.

91. Sundqvist T, Lindstrom F, Magnusson KE, Skoldstam L, Stjernstrom I, Tagesson C. Influence of fasting on intestinal permeability and disease activity in patients with rheumatoid arthritis. Scand J Rheumatol 1982; 11:33–8.

92. Uden AM, Trang L, Venizelos N, Palmblad J. Neutrophil functions and clinical performance after total fasting in patients with rheumatoid arthritis. Ann Rheum Dis 1983; 42:45–51.

93. Lithell H, Bruce A, Gustafsson IB, et al. A fasting and vegetarian diet treatment trial on chronic inflammatory disorders. Acta Derm Venereol 1983; 63:397–403.

94. Skoldstam L. Fasting and vegan diet in rheumatoid arthritis. Scand J Rheumatol 1986; 15:219–21.

95. Eaton SB, Konner M. Paleolithic nutrition: A consideration of its nature and current implications. N Engl J Med 1985; 312:283–9.

96. Kromann N, Green A. Epidemiological studies in the Upernavik District, Greenland. Acta Med Scand 1980; 208:401–6.

97. Recht L, Helin P, Rasmussen JO, Jacobsen J, Lithman T, Schersten B. Hand handicap and rheumatoid arthritis in a fish-eating society (the Faroe Islands). J Intern Med 1990; 227:49–55.

98. Lee TH, Hoover RL, Williams JD, et al. Effect of dietary enrichment with eicosapentaenoic and docosaexaenoic acids on in vitro neutrophil functions. N Engl J Med 1985; 312:1217–24.

99. Humphrey DM, McManase L, Satouchi K, Hanahan DJ, Pinckard RN. Vasoactive properties of acetyl glyceryl ether phosphorylcholine and analogs. Lab Invest 1982; 46:422–7.

100. Endres S, Cannon JG, Ghorbani R, et al. In vitro production of IL 1 beta, IL 1 alpha TNA and IL 2 in healthy subjects: distribution, effects of cycloxygenase inhibitors and evidence of independent gene regulation. Eur J Immunol 1989; 19:2327–33.

101. Endres S, Ghorbani R, Kelley VE, et al. The effects of dietary supplementation with ω-3 polyunsaturated fatty acids on the synthesis of interleukin-1 and tumor necrosis factor by mononuclear cells. N Engl J Med 1989; 320:265–71.

102. Robinson DR, Prickett JD, Makaoul GT, Steinberg AD, Colvin RB. Dietary fish oil reduces progression of established renal disease in (NZB × NZW) F1 mice and delays renal disease in BXSB and MRL/1 strains. Arthritis Rheum 1986; 29:539–46.

103. Prickett JD, Trentham DE, Robinson DR. Dietary fish oil augments the induction of arthritis in rats immunized with type II collagen. J Immunol 1984; 132:725–9.

104. Rubin RH, Wilkinson RA, Xu I, Robinson DR. Dietary marine lipids does not alter susceptibility of (NZB × NZW) F1 mice to pathogenic microorganisms. Prostaglandins 1989; 38:251–62.

105. Meydani SN. Effect of (n-3) polyunsaturated fatty acids on cytokine production and their biologic function. Nutrition 1996; 12:S8–14.

106. Jolly CA, Jiang Y-H, Chapkin RS, McMurray DN. Dietary (n-3)

polyunsaturated fatty acids suppress murine lymphoproliferation, interleukin-2 secretion, and the formation of diacylglycerol and ceramide. J Nutr 1997; 127:37–43.

107. Chandrasekar B, Fernandes G. Decreased proinflammatory cytokines and increased antioxidant enzyme gene expression by ω-3 lipids in murine lupus nephritis. Biochem Biophys Res Commun 1994; 200:893–8.

108. Moore GF, Yarboro C, Sebring NG, et al. Eicosapentaenoic acid (EPA) in the treatment of systemic lupus erythematosus (SLE). Arthritis Rheum 1987; 30:S33.

109. Westberg C, Tarkowski A. Effect of MaxEPA in patients with SLE. A double-blind, crossover study. Scand J Rheumatol 1990; 19: 137–43.

110. Kremer JM, Bigauotte J, Michalek A, et al. Effect of manipulating dietary fatty acids on clinical manifestations of rheumatoid arthritis. Lancet 1985; 1:184–7.

111. Kremer JM, Lawrence DA, Jubiz W, et al. Dietary fish oil and olive oil supplementation in patients with rheumatoid arthritis. Clinical and immunologic effects. Arthritis Rheum 1990; 33:810–20.

112. Kremer JM, Lawrence DA, Petrillo GF, et al. Effects of high-dose fish oil on rheumatoid arthritis after stopping nonsteroidal antiinflammatory drugs. Clinical and immune correlates. Arthritis Rheum 1995; 38:1107–14.

113. Kremer JM, Jubiz W, Michalek A, et al. Fish oil fatty acid supplementation in active rheumatoid arthritis, a double blinded, controlled cross over study. Ann Intern Med 1987; 106:497–503.

114. Sperling RI, Weinblatt M, Robin JL, et al. Effects of dietary supplementation with marine fish oil on leukocyte lipid mediator generation and function in rheumatoid arthritis. Arthritis Rheum 1987; 30: 988–97.

115. Cleland LG, French JK, Betts WH, Murphy GA, Elliott MJ. Clinical and biochemical effects of dietary fish oil supplements in rheumatoid arthritis. J Rheumatol 1988; 15:1471–5.

116. van der Tempel H, Tulleken JE, Limburg PC, Muskiet FA, van Rijswijk MH. Effects of fish oil supplementation in rheumatoid arthritis. Ann Rheum Dis 1990; 49:76–80.

117. Nielsen GL, Faarvang KL, Thomsen BS, et al. The effects of dietary supplementation with n-3 polyunsaturated fatty acids in patients with rheumatoid arthritis: a randomized, double blind trial. Eur J Clin Invest 1992; 22:687–91.

118. Lau CS, Morley KD, Belch JJ. Effects of fish oil supplementation on non-steroidal anti-inflammatory drug requirement in patients with mild rheumatoid arthritis—a double blind placebo controlled study. Br J Rheumatol 1993; 32:982–9.

119. Geusens P, Wouters C, Nijs J, Jiang Y, Dequeker J. Long-term effect of omega-3 fatty acid supplementation in active rheumatoid arthritis. A 12-month, double-blind, controlled study. Arthritis Rheum 1994; 37:824–9.

120. DiGiacomo RA, Kremer JM, Shah DM. Fish oil supplementation in patients with Raynaud's phenomenon: a double-blind controlled prospective study. Am J Med 1989; 86:158–64.

121. Callegari PE, Zurier RB. Botanical lipids: potential role in modulation of immunologic responses and inflammatory reactions. Rheum Dis Clin North Am 1991; 17:415–25.

122. Santoli D, Zurier RB. Prostaglandinn E (PGE) precursor fatty acids inhibit human IL-2 production by a PGE-independent mechanism. J Immunol 1989; 143:1303–9.

123. Santoli D, Phillips PD, Colt TL, Zurier RB. Suppression of interleukin 2-dependent human T cell growth by E-series prostaglandins (PGE) and their precursors fatty acids: evidence for a PGE-independent mechanism of inhibition by the fatty acids. J Clin Invest 1990; 85:424–32.

124. Tate G, Mandell FB, Laposata M, et al. Suppression of acute and chronic inflammation by dietary gamma-linoleic acid. J Rheumatol 1989; 16:1729–34.

125. Kunkel SL, Ogawa H, Ward PA, Zurier RB. Suppression of chronic inflammation by evening primrose oil. Prog Lipid Res 1982; 20: 885–8.

126. Baker DG, Krakauer KA, Tate G, Laposata M, Zurier RB. Suppres-

sion of human synovial cell proliferation by dihomogamma-linoleic acid. Arthritis Rheum 1989; 1273–81.

127. Hansen MT, Lerche A, Kassis V, Lorenzen I, Sondergaard J. Treatment of rheumatoid arthritis with prostaglandin E1-precursors cis-linoleic acid and gammalinoleic acid. Scand J Rheumatol 1983; 12:85–8.

128. Jäntti J, Seppälä E, Vapaatalo H, Isomaki H. Evening primrose oil and olive oil in treatment of rheumatoid arthritis. Clin Rheumatol 1989; 8:238–44.

129. Belch JJ, Ansell D, Madho R, O'Dowd A, Sturrock RD. Effects of altering dietary essential fatty acids on requirements for non-steroidal anti-inflammatory drugs in patients with rheumatoid arthritis: a double blind placebo control study. Ann Rheum Dis 1988; 47:96–104.

130. Pullman-Moore S, Laposata M, Lem D, et al. Alteration of the fatty acid profile and the production of eicosanoids in human monocytes by gamma-linoleic acid. Arthritis Rheum 1990; 33:1526–33.

131. Leventhal LJ, Boyce EG, Zurier RB. Treatment of rheumatoid arthritis with gamma-linoleic acid. Ann Intern Med 1993; 119:867–73.

132. Brzeski M, Madhok R, Capell HA. Evening primrose oil in patients with rheumatoid arthritis and side-effects on non-steroidal anti-inflammatory drugs. Br J Rheumatol 1991; 30:370–2.

133. Lai LTY, Naiki M, Yoshida SH, German JB, Gershwin ME. Dietary *Platycladus orientalis* seed oil suppresses anti-erythrocyte autoantibodies and prolongs survival of NZB mice. Clin Immunol Immunopathol 1994; 71:293–302.

134. Berger A, Fenz R, German JB. Incorporation of dietary 5,11,14,17-eicosatetraenoate into various mouse phospholipid classes and tissues. J Nutr Biochem 1993; 4:409–20.

135. Calder PC. Fatty acids, dietary lipids and lymphocyte functions. Biochem Soc Trans 1995; 23:302–9.

136. Wells H. Studies on the chemistry of anaphylaxis. III. Experiments with isolated proteins, especially those of hen's egg. J Infect Dis 1911; 9:147–51.

137. Higgins P, Weiner HL. Suppression of experimental autoimmune encephalomyelitis by oral administration of myelin basic protein and its fragments. J Immunol 1988; 140:440–5.

138. Nussenblatt RB, Caspi RR, Mahdi R, et al. Inhibition of S-antigen induced experimental autoimmune uveoretinitis by oral induction of tolerance with S-antigen. J Immunol 1990; 144:1689–95.

139. Zhang ZJ, Davidson L, Eisenbarth G, Weiner HL. Suppression of diabetes in nonobese diabetic mice by oral administration of porcine insulin. Proc Natl Acad Sci USA 1991; 88:10,252–6.

140. Wang Z-Y, Qiao J, Link H. Suppression of experimental autoimmune myasthenia gravis by oral administration of acetylcholine receptor. J Neuroimmunol 1993; 44:209–14.

141. Peterson KE, Braley-Mullen H. Suppression of murine experimental autoimmune thyroiditis by oral administration of porcine thyroglobulin. Cell Immunol 1995; 166:123–30.

142. Courtenay JS, Dallman MJ, Dayan AD, Martin A, Mosedale B. Immunization against heterologous type II collagen induces arthritis in mice. Nature 1980; 283:666–8.

143. Weiner HL, Mackin GA, Matsui M, et al. Double-blind pilot trial of oral tolerization with myelin antigens in multiple sclerosis. Science 1993; 259:1321–4.

144. Lee S, Scherberg N, DeGroot LJ. Induction of oral tolerance in human autoimmune thyroid disease. Thyroid 1998; 8:229–34.

145. Trentham DE, Dynesius-Trentham RA, Orav EJ, et al. Effects of oral administration of type II collagen on rheumatoid arthritis. Science 1993; 261:1727–30.

146. Weiner HL, Friedman A, Miller A, et al. Oral tolerance: immunologic mechanisms and treatment of animal and human organ-specific autoimmune diseases by oral administration of autoantigens. Annu Rev Immunol 1994; 12:809–37.

147. Tarkowski A, Klareskog L, Carlsten H, Herberts P, Koopman WJ. Secretion of antibodies to types I and II collagen by synovial tissue cells in patients with rheumatoid arthritis. Arthritis Rheum 1989; 32:1087–92.

148. Nagler-Anderson C, Bober LA, Robinson ME, Siskind GW, Thorbecke GJ. Suppression of type II collagen-induced arthritis by intra-

gastric administration of soluble type II collagen. Proc Natl Acad Sci USA 1986; 83:7443–6.

149. Bitar DM, Whitacre CC. Suppression of experimental autoimmune encephalomyelitis by oral administration of myelin basic protein. Cell Immunol 1988; 112:364–70.

150. Higgins PJ, Weiner HL. Suppression of experimental autoimmune encephalomyelitis by oral administration of myelin basic protein and its fragments. J Immunol 1988; 140:440–5.

151. Meyer AL, Benson JM, Gienapp IE, Cox KL, Whitacre CC. Suppressive of murine chronic relapsing experimental autoimmune encephalomyelitis by the oral administration of myelin basic protein. J Immunol 1996; 157:4230–8.

152. Kennedy KJ, Smith WS, Miller SD, Karpus WJ. Induction of antigen-specific tolerance for the treatment of ongoing, relapsing autoimmune encephalomyelitis: a comparison between oral and peripheral tolerance. J Immunol 1997; 159:1036–44.

153. Karpus WJ, Kennedy KJ, Kunkel SL, Lukacs NW. Monocyte chemotactic protein 1 regulates oral tolerance induction by inhibition of T helper cell 1 related cytokines. J Exp Med 1998; 187:733–41.

154. Fukaura H, Kent SC, Pietrusewicz MJ, Khoury SJ, Weiner HL, Hafler DA. Antigen-specific TGF-β1 secretion with bovine myelin oral tolerization in multiple sclerosis. Ann NY Acad Sci 1996; 778:251–7.

155. Laliotou B, Liversidge J, Forrester JV, Dick AD. Interphotoreceptor retinoid binding protein is a potent tolerogen in Lewis rats: suppression of experimental autoimmune uveoretinitis is retinal antigen specific. Br J Ophthalmol 1997; 81:61–7.

156. Kreutzer B, Laliotou B, Cheng YF, Liversidge J, Forrester JV, Dick AD. Nasal administration of retinal antigens maintains immunosuppression of uveoretinitis in cyclosporin-A-treated Lewis rats: future treatment of endogenous posterior uveoretinitis? Eye 1997; 11: 445–52.

157. Ma CG, Zhang GX, Xiao BG, Link J, Olsson T, Link H. Suppression of experimental autoimmune myasthenia gravis by nasal administration of acetylcholine receptor. J Neuroimmunol 1995; 58(1):51–60.

158. Ma CG, Zhang GX, Xiao BG, et al. Mucosal tolerance to experimental autoimmune myasthenia gravis is associated with down-regulation of AChR-specific IFN-gamma-expressing Th1-like cells and up-regulation of TGF-beta mRNA in mononuclear cells. Ann NY Acad Sci 1996; 778:273–87.

159. Drachman DB, Okumura S, Adams RN, McIntosh KR. Oral tolerance in myasthenia gravis. Ann NY Acad Sci 1996; 778:258–72.

160. Wang ZY, Link H, Ljungdahl A, et al. Induction of interferon-gamma, interleukin-4, and transforming growth factor-beta in rats orally tolerized against experimental autoimmune myasthenia gravis. Cell Immunol 1994; 157:353–68.

161. Daniel D, Wegmann DR. Protection of nonobese diabetic mice from diabetes by intranasal or subcutaneous administration of insulin peptide B-(9-23). Proc Natl Acad Sci USA 1996; 93(2):956–60.

162. Harrison LC, Dempsey-Collier M, Kramer DR, Takahashi K. Aerosol insulin induces regulatory CD8 gamma delta T cells that prevent murine insulin-dependent diabetes. J Exp Med 1996; 184:2167–74.

163. Polanski M, Melican NS, Zhang J, Weiner HL. Oral administration of the immunodominant B-chain of insulin reduces diabetes in a co-transfer model of diabetes in the NOD mouse and is associated with a switch from Th1 to Th2 cytokines. J Autoimmun 1997; 10:339–46.

164. Mordes JP, Schirf B, Roipko D, et al. Oral insulin does not prevent insulin-dependent diabetes mellitus in BB rats. Ann NY Acad Sci 1996; 778:418–21.

27 Autoimmune Diseases of the Digestive Tract

Thomas P. Prindiville and Mary C. Cantrell

INTRODUCTION

Inflammatory bowel disease (IBD) comprises a group of clinical idiopathic entities that involve primarily the small bowel and/or colon and, less frequently, may involve any part of the gastrointestinal tract. Broadly speaking, the designation of IBD refers to any inflammatory process involving the luminal gastrointestinal tract. These disorders can be divided into specific diseases with known causes and an idiopathic group of diseases that embraces two conditions that may or may not be related: ulcerative colitis (UC) and Crohn's disease (CD). Although the major idiopathic diseases are grouped in these two categories, they may represent multiple diseases. Other inflammatory bowel diseases exist, such as indeterminate colitis, collagenous colitis, microscopic colitis, celiac disease, nongranulomatous chronic idiopathic enterocolitis, tropical sprue, and celiaclike illnesses. Additionally, these conditions are overshadowed or masked by enteric infectious diseases that have similar presentations and manifestations. Interestingly, the frequency of the disease location correlates with the highest concentration of luminal biota.

Soluble mediators of inflammation are the effectors of the disease process. The resulting mucosal edema, hyperemia, increased permeability, ulceration, altered motility, stricture, abscess, and fistula formation eventuate in the loss of absorptive capacity and other sequelae. Therefore, these diseases have significant nutritional importance that is much broader in scope than just the malnutrition and the mineral and vitamin deficiencies that result from the chronic inflammatory process. Ingested food substances have often been suspect in the etiology of IBD. Although not proven, they may contribute to causation. Consequently, modification of diet as a therapy has been proposed and is the subject of continuing studies. The chronic inflammatory process results in numerous disease complications and the potential for repeat surgical resections that produce an altered physiology. As a result of these surgical necessities, short-bowel syndrome, rapid transit syndromes, bacterial overgrowth, and gastroparesis frequently occur. Each of these conditions has important nutritional considerations. Short-bowel syndrome has stimulated the science of intestinal adaptation and the specific roles of growth hormones, diet types, and glutamine. Finally, the sequelae of the disease process and resultant surgery leave many patients supported by total parenteral nutrition (TPN). Inflammatory bowel disease is the primary indication for parenteral nutrition in the United Kingdom and contributes to 15% of TPN recipients in the United States *(1)*.

EPIDEMIOLOGIC AND DEMOGRAPHIC FEATURES

Ulcerative colitis and Crohn's disease share similar epidemiological and demographic features. They are worldwide in distribution with geographic tendencies and may be less common or underreported in less developed countries *(2)*. The incidence of ulcerative colitis appears stable, perhaps even decreasing, whereas that of Crohn's disease is increasing. Patients commonly fall into the younger age groups and there is no sex predominance *(2)*. Decreased intake of dietary fiber and excessive ingestion of refined sugars, food additives, and chemically processed fats (margarine) have been implicated, but the evidence is far from conclusive. Those affected by the disease tend to reside in urban and more industrialized areas and may be of any ethnic group *(3)*. Whether the two diseases represent related responses to a common etiological agent or are totally unrelated remains to be determined. The annual incidence of ulcerative colitis varies from 1.5 to 13 per 100,000 with an average prevalence of 80 per 100,000. An average annual incidence of 8 and a prevalence of 96 per 100,000 are consistently quoted as the midrange. The incidence of Crohn's disease varies from 4 to 8 per 100,000 population at risk. Midrange numbers are 5 for incidence and 60 for prevalence per 100,000 population at risk. A combined incidence and prevalence of 13 and 130 per 100,000, respectively, are obtained assuming that prevalence is 12 to 15 times the annual incidence. The national prevalence is 396,000 to 495,000 for the year 1990 *(4)*.

INDIRECT COST OF ILLNESS Although there are no systematic studies of the cost of these illnesses, if one uses third-party payer's cost and the midrange numbers for prevalence in the total 1990 US population, the estimated costs for both diseases is 1–1.2 billion dollars. When adjusted for productivity losses, it is estimated that the 1990 annual economic cost of IBD is 1.8–2.6 billion dollars *(5,6)*. Several studies comparing UC patients with

From: *Nutrition and Immunology: Principles and Practice* (ME Gershwin et al. eds.), © Humana Press, Inc., Totowa, NJ

control subjects have noted significant differences in work capacity. In other studies of ulcerative colitis, 20% of the patients had some level of work disability. At 5 yr or more after diagnosis, 15–24% of the patients with Crohn's disease were disabled compared to 4.4% of the controls. Evidence from various sources indicates that 5–10% of inflammatory bowel disease patients experience work disability annually (5,6).

GENETIC INFLUENCES   Ulcerative colitis and Crohn's disease are not classic genetic disorders. However, multiple familial occurrences are noted in both idiopathic groups (7). The single strongest risk factor for Crohn's disease is having a relative with Crohn's disease. A relative, especially a sibling, increases the risk of developing the disease by 30-fold. First-degree relatives of patients with CD have approximately a 12–15 times greater risk. Patients with Crohn's disease are confronted with an offspring risk of 10.4% (8–11). Additionally, there is a strong statistical concordance for disease location and disease behavior (12). Initially, a high degree of concordance in monozygotic twins was reported; however, recent studies cast doubt on this association (13). Ulcerative colitis is more common in families of probands with ulcerative colitis and Crohn's disease is more common in families or probands with Crohn's disease, but the two disorders are intermingled in approximately 25% of inflammatory bowel disease families (14). A Crohn's disease locus on chromosome 16 has been identified and may show an association with families with two or more affected siblings (15). The human leukocyte antigen (HLA) locus has been the subject of multiple studies with controversial results. Recent studies suggest the susceptibility locus is outside this gene region (16). Ankylosing spondylitis is an established autosomal genetic disorder in inflammatory bowel disease patients with the HLAB27 haplotype (17). The association of IBD with such genetic disorders as psoriasis and Turner syndrome as well as the familial occurrence of both ulcerative colitis and Crohn's disease with primary sclerosing cholangitis (PSC) further suggest genetically mediated mechanisms.

DIAGNOSIS AND MANIFESTATIONS   Because the etiologies for these diseases are unknown and there are no serological or "gold standard" markers for the diseases, the diagnosis is made by clinical parameters after patterns of gastrointestinal involvement are established. These are commonly demonstrated by endoscopy or, in some cases, by contrast studies. Infectious etiologies are ruled out by conventional culture techniques. The endoscopic biopsy or surgically derived tissues demonstrate specific histologic findings. The endoscopic dogma for visualized mucosal involvement has limitations, with numerous exceptions, especially in colitis patients (18).

Both diseases are recurrent throughout the life of the patient. There is no currently available cure and the diseases have both intestinal and extraintestinal manifestations. The clinical intestinal manifestations are abdominal pain, diarrhea, bleeding, weight loss, bowel obstruction, episodic fevers, fistula formation, toxic megacolon, perforation, and the late development of carcinoma. Extraintestinal manifestations include arthritis, erythema nodosum, anemia, vitamin B_{12} deficiency, iritis, episcleritis, growth retardation, addiction, depression, incomplete sexual maturation, sclerosing cholangitis, cirrhosis, metabolic bone disease, kidney stones, pyoderma gangrenosa, vitamin deficiencies, and malnutrition.

Ulcerative colitis is a superficial mucosal inflammatory process involving the colon and/or rectum. Microscopic findings are crypt abscesses, crypt distortion, depletion of mucus-secreting cells, ulceration, and acute and chronic inflammatory infiltration of the mucosa. The anatomic distribution of inflammation usually begins in the rectum and extends proximally for variable distances without skip areas. The clinical course is quite variable and may be acute, fulminant, recurrent, or chronic and indolent. It is usually characterized by periods of active disease and remissions. The terminology is based on its distribution (e.g., ulcerative proctitis or ulcerative proctocolitis).

In Crohn's disease, the inflammation is transmural and may involve any or all of the luminal gastrointestinal tract or just the small bowel, colon, rectum, or perineum. Inflammation extends into the submucosa, producing edema, lymphoid hyperplasia, a tendency for granuloma formation, lymphangiectasia, fibrosis, and fistula and stricture formation. The earliest visible mucosal involvement is the aphthous-type ulcer, penetrating fissure ulcers, and linear "rake" ulcers. Dominant clinical manifestations are abdominal pain, diarrhea, fever, intestinal obstruction, fistula formation, and malnutrition. The terminology is based on disease distribution and the nature of the inflammatory reaction (e.g., regional enteritis, terminal ileitis, ileocolitis, granulomatous colitis, granulomatous proctitis, superficial inflammatory, fibrosing, and fistulizing. Commonly, Crohn's disease is segmental in distribution, involving, classically, the terminal ileum, isolated segments of small bowel or colon, and rectum. The eponym, Crohn's disease, is most convenient; however, the first disease case series was reported by Dalziel in 1913. The clinical course is almost always chronic, at times punctuated by acute exacerbations. Spontaneous remissions have been reported to be as high as 42% (19).

Extraintestinal manifestations are frequently associated with both diseases. Many of these afflictions may precede the clinical onset of IBD by months or years. In the case of Crohn's disease, so-called "miliary or metastatic" lesions involving other abdominal viscera, skin, and lung may also occur on rare occasions.

AUTOIMMUNITY AND INFLAMMATORY BOWEL DISEASE

Because enteric pathogens and toxin-producing bacteria cannot be demonstrated and the disease process has a chronic relapsing course, the inflammatory response is assumed to be inappropriate, a failure to downregulate or an autoreactive disease process. Consequently, the B- and T-lymphocyte functions in these diseases have attracted considerable attention. In spite of numerous studies to date, the assumed autoreactive or autoimmune disease process has not been conclusively demonstrated.

ANTIBODIES   Serum from patients with IBD contain antibodies to surface antigens from mucus-secreting colonic epithelial cells, allogeneic fetal colon tissue, colonic epithelium from germ-free rats, gastric parietal cells, small-bowel mucosal cells, milk proteins, the lipopolysaccharides from *E. coli* 014, and many human serum proteins. These antibodies are also found in normal individuals and in various other disorders. There is no correlation between the presence and titer of these antibodies and the presence or extent of IBD or the level of its activity. The antibodies are of low affinity and are difficult to demonstrate by blotting methods (20,21). Immunoglobulin levels follow no consistent pattern in IBD and serum concentrations of IgA, IgG, IgM, and IgE are generally normal. Furthermore, there is no consistent pattern of immunoglobulin production by immunocytes in the involved tissue in either Crohn's disease or ulcerative colitis, although mucosal-derived antibodies have been shown to be directed to cytoplasmic proteins of luminal microorganisms (22).

It is of interest that ulcerative colitis and Crohn's disease occur in patients with IgA deficiency, common variable immune deficiency, primary acquired hypogammaglobulinemia, and thymic alymphosplasia, as isolated instances. Furthermore, patients with IBD are not exceptionally vulnerable to "exotic infections." It is, therefore, likely that humoral immune disturbances are secondary to the pathogenic process.

Perinuclear antineutrophil cytoplasmic antibodies (pANCA) are increased in many patients with IBD, especially patients with the extraintestinal manifestations of sclerosing cholangitis (18). The putative target for these antibodies is the subject of numerous studies (24–28) and include cathepsin, histone, lactoferrin, and multiple other novel antigens. The potential utility of the pANCA antibody, despite its disease overlap, lies in the ability to define a subset of patients with IBD (28).

In one family, a unique disease syndrome of autoimmunity manifest by autoantibodies to enterocytes, smooth muscle, thyroid and islet-cells was associated with an enteropathy, progressive diarrhea, and autoimmune hepatitis. Antibody reactivity to hemidesmosomal protein was demonstrated by immunofluorescence and Western blotting. Treatment required TPN and continual immune suppression (29).

T-CELL REPERTOIRE AND FUNCTION Large numbers of T cells infiltrate the mucosa in the areas of disease activity and are, therefore, likely to be important. In animal models of multiple sclerosis and in humans with multiple sclerosis, cloned infiltrating T cells demonstrating clonal expansion and a restricted T-cell-receptor (TCR) repertoire suggest a specific TCR-type association with the autoreactive disease. These cloned T lymphocytes have proven useful in defining the autoantigens and their epitopes (30). The peripheral blood lymphocytes and mucosal T cells from patients with IBD also demonstrate clonal expansion. However, individual patients differ in TCR expression, as do the different diseases (31–34). These diverse T-cell responses are predictable when one considers the nonobese diabetic (NOD) mouse model for diabetes in which T-cell responses are restricted early in life, but as the disease progresses, the expression is more diverse (35). Additionally, with the mucosal inflammatory disease, a generalized leak exposes the immune system to multiple luminal microbes and by-products. The end result is a very complex mixture of reactive T cells.

Cloned mucosal T-cell lines derived from IBD patients reveal low-grade autoreactivity and reactivity to a variety of bacterial antigens (31). T Cells reactive to bacteria were more frequent in IBD patients when compared to controls (36). Studies evaluating the responses of intestinal T cells from patients with IBD to putative food antigens have not been reported.

Sequencing of the TCR variable region of similar T-cell families in cloned mucosal T cells from patients with Crohn's disease indicates sequence variation. These findings suggest a luminal superantigen response rather than clonal expansion to a specific antigen.

An important role for lamina propria T cells is also supported by the predominance of activated CD4+, CD45RO+ cells in the tissue and reports of diminished inflammatory activity in IBD patients with AIDS as their CD4 count decreases (37).

CYTOKINES Reviews of the various cytokines, their function, inhibition, and genetics are significantly complex, voluminous, and important. These pro-inflammatory agents play a significant role as effectors of injury to the mucosa. Briefly, the cytokine profiles of activated mucosal lymphocytes suggest that ulcerative colitis and Crohn's disease are different diseases. Crohn's disease is characterized by high expression of interferon gamma and ulcerative colitis by increased interleukin-5. Interleukin-1, interleukin-6, and tumor necrosis factor-α are increased in the sera of patients with both diseases. Cytokine secretion from normal-appearing Crohn's tissue is likewise increased, suggesting a genetically determined abnormal cytokine response (38,39).

EXPERIMENTAL MODELS

DISEASE MECHANISMS Insights into possible mechanisms of disease in humans have come from several recent animal studies. Knockouts of the T-cell receptors, HLA class II, interleukin-2 (IL-2), and IL-10 are associated with spontaneous development of colitis (40). Knockouts of T-cell growth factor (TGF)-α demonstrate an increased severity in experimentally induced colitis when compared to control (41). In animal models of disrupted cahedrin function, inflammatory bowel disease results, presumably from a resultant weakened barrier (42). HLA B27 transgenic mice develop intestinal inflammation and arthritis in a manner similar to patients with that phenotype (43). This model of disease is dependent on luminal microbial populations (44). Likewise, in other animal models of induced disease, a more severe and prolonged disease is associated with luminal bacteria as compared to germ-free animals (45). These studies emphasize the importance of the integrity of the epithelial barrier to luminal products and a protection from bacterial translocation.

DIETARY STUDIES Animal models of inflammatory bowel disease have also demonstrated their utility in dietary studies. Tanaka et al. evaluated the beneficial effect of elemental diet in a rat model of granulomatous enteritis. Rats fed an elemental diet demonstrated less macroscopic and microscopic damage when compared to control rats. The elemental diet inhibited the numbers of macrophages and IL-2R positive T cells in Peyer's patches. NO levels and calcium-independent NOS activity was decreased, suggesting that the elemental diet decreases T-cell activation and reduces the production of nitric oxide and the generation of oxygen free radicals (46).

The role of a glutamine-enriched elemental diet on gut epithelial proliferation and portal endotoxemia in an experimental model of IBD in guinea pigs was studied by Fujita and Sakuri (47). Portal vein endotoxin levels in the glutamine-enriched group were reduced by 60%. Tissue ornithine decarboxylase activities were the same, indicating that the reduced endotoxemia was not secondary to a glutamine effect on epithelial proliferation. This beneficial effect was attributed to some other putative aspect of mucosal integrity.

Prophylactic glutamine modulation of the inflammatory activities of IL-8 and TNF-α was studied in TNBS-induced colitis. Glutamine-fed animals demonstrated less inflammation by microscopic examination. IL-8 and TNF-α concentrations in the glutamine groups were lower than the control. These beneficial effects were concentration dependent, with a 4% glutamine group demonstrating less disease severity and bacterial translocation than the 2% glutamine group (48).

NUTRITIONAL ASPECTS IN INFLAMMATORY BOWEL DISEASE

DIET AND THE RISK OF IBD Diet in IBD patients continues to generate significant interest. Epidemiologic studies of the effect of pre-illness diet demonstrate several potential risk factors. High sucrose consumption and high fat intake, especially animal fat and cholesterol, were associated with an increased risk of developing IBD. Lactose had no effect; however, fructose, increased fluid intake, magnesium, vitamin C, and fruits had a negative association and an increased vegetable consumption was negative for Crohn's disease only (49). Other similar studies have demonstrated an association of increased intake of carbohydrates, starch, refined sugars, and fast-food ingestion with an increased incidence of IBD. Coffee and increased fiber ingestion were associated with a protective effect (50,51). Epidemiologic studies in Japan have revealed important findings because the incidence of the disease correlates with the changes in dietary preferences. The Western diet (bread for breakfast, butter, margarine, cheese, meats, ham, and sausage) has been linked to an increased incidence of IBD (52,53).

Patients who have had repeated flares of their disease often lose function of significant areas of absorptive surfaces. Malnutrition and specific nutrient deficiencies occur in IBD patients secondary to malabsorption, protein-losing enteropathy, decreased caloric intake, bacterial overgrowth, and rapid transit syndromes. General nutritional support and replacement of vitamin and mineral losses are a significant component in management of patients with IBD. However, the use of diet as therapy for IBD is controversial.

DIET AS THERAPY The universal problem with all studies of therapies for Crohn's disease is sample size, heterogeneous patient populations, and significant numbers of patient withdrawals. Because of the heterogeneous nature of the Crohn's population and high rate of spontaneous remission, it has been estimated that at least 480 patients would be necessary for a valid trial of any therapy in Crohn's disease. Because the precise cause is not known, it is unlikely that a shotgun approach consisting of various diets would demonstrate benefit. These problems are more pronounced in the use of elemental or polymeric diets as a therapy for the induction of remission in Crohn's disease patients. An additional problem is the variability in the diet composition. Historically, patients were treated with various diets and TPN to prepare them for surgery; some patients responded with disease remission. Following these observations, initial diet studies were encouraging. These findings and the assumption that dietary factors may play a role in pathogenesis have resulted in numerous studies for induction of disease remission. This approach has demonstrated the greatest utility in the pediatric population, where growth failure represents a common serious problem unique to this group. The etiology for growth failure is most likely inadequate intake and enteral loss. Nutritional supplementation by either route restores body composition and reverses linear and ponderal growth failure (54–56). Growth failure and delayed sexual maturation are significant effects of IBD in the pediatric age group and may precede the diagnosis of IBD. The role of elemental diet in the management of Crohn's disease has its most beneficial effect in this setting. Several studies demonstrate the utility of elemental diets on growth and sexual maturation. Various strategies have been employed; TPN, supplemental liquid formula enteral feeding

Table 1
Meta-Analysis: Steroids Versus Diet in Crohn's Disease

Author	Date	No. of trials	No. of patients	Significant benefit
Grifiths	1995	8	413	Steroids > diet
Fernandez	1995	16	419	Steroids > diet
Messori	1996	7	353	Steroids > diet

or intermittent nasogastric tube feeding at night, and elemental diet 1 mo out of every 4 mo, all demonstrated marked benefit. Although the mechanisms are unknown, both supplemental methods have been shown to induce remission by CDIA scores.

DRUG THERAPY IN IBD Drug therapy for induction and maintenance of remission in Crohn's disease is problematic. One could expect a similar scenario for the use of specialized diets as therapy of IBD. From the numerous drug trials that exist, several types of specific treatment protocols have been subjected to meta-analysis. In an evaluation of single-drug therapy that included 7 trials for induction (767 patients) and 5 trials for maintenance (796 patients) of remission in Crohn's disease, single-drug therapy demonstrated a 11–29% advantage (RD = 0.13–0.33) (57). However, no therapeutic advantage was found for a single drug over placebo for maintenance of remission. Similar linear relapse rates were seen with time, 10% at 3 mo and 75% at 36 mo.

Steinhart et al. evaluated trials that utilized sulfasalazine and mesalamine for maintenance of remission by meta-analysis. Ten randomized prospective trials of 1022 patients demonstrated a decreased risk after 12 mo of therapy and a less apparent effect at 6 mo. When individual drugs were evaluated, a benefit was found only for mesalamine (58). The beneficial effects of azothioprine and 6-mercaptopurine were evaluated in a meta-analysis of nine randomized trials, four with active disease and two for maintenance of remission. A significant benefit was demonstrated compared to placebo odds ratio (OR) 3.09 (95% CI 2.45–3.91) and a steroid-sparing effect was demonstrated; active disease (OR 3.69 CI 1–21.5) and quiescent disease (OR 4.64 CI 1.5–13.2) (59).

DEFINED FORMULA DIET AS THERAPY FOR CROHN'S DISEASE Although many prospective randomized trials have evaluated the utility of elemental diets in Crohn's disease patients, the efficacy of enteral nutrition as primary therapy of active Crohn's disease is controversial. Three meta-analysis studies reviewed all clinical trials and graded the quality of each total enteral nutrition trial that was compared to corticosteroids for induction of remission. The grading of remission by definition was quite variable, consisting of the reduction of a score or CDIA index; no studies verified mucosal healing. Rates of clinical remission of active Crohn's disease, based on the intention-to-treat principle, were extracted from the studies by independent reviewers. The numbers of patients and studies evaluated are compared (Table 1).

In all three meta-analysis studies corticosteroid therapy was more beneficial in inducing remission than any type of dietary therapy. The pooled odds ratio for remission for all types of enteral diets compared to steroids in one study was 0.35 (95% CI 0.23–0.53), with the other two studies demonstrating similar odds ratios. The relative risk of treatment failure was significantly lower in the steroid group than in the diet group: (a) method of Mantel–Haenszel: resistance transfer factor (RTF) = 0.35, 95% confidence interval, 0.23–0.53; $P = 0.001$; and (b) method of Der Simonian and Laird: RTF = 0.43; 95% confidence interval, 0–0.94; $p = 0.03$. A separate analysis was carried out in which only the subgroup of patients who were not intolerant to diet were evaluated; this analysis also showed a superiority of steroids over diet (60).

Remission rates were 57.7% and 79.4% for nutrition therapy and corticosteroids, respectively. Although this exhaustive statistical evaluation demonstrates the increased benefit of corticosteroids, there was a high rate of remission in the nutritionally managed group. This remission rate was much higher than what has been noted in the placebo response rates of trials evaluating drug treatments (18–42%). Total enteral nutrition, therefore, does demonstrate a benefit. However, total enteral nutrition may be complementary to steroids for induction of remission and may be more beneficial in preventing disease recurrence. These meta-analysis studies did not evaluate specific regions, such as colon compared to small-bowel disease, or specific disease behavior. It has been suggested that small-bowel disease is more responsive to enteral nutrition. From nonrandomized open-label studies, the remission induction rate of elemental diet therapy in Japan is approximately 80%, demonstrating radiographic and mucosal healing. The differences between these studies and the meta-analysis studies are considered to be the result of duration, composition, and criteria for remission. To prevent relapse and rehospitalization, home enteral nutrition is now widely used in Japan. The therapeutic effect is observed in patients with ileal involvement, and over 1200 kcal/d is more effective than a lower amount (61).

NONELEMENTAL DIET FOR THERAPY IN CROHN'S DISEASE Elemental diets are unpalatable compared to nonelemental diets. Theoretically, the benefit of elemental diets is less antigenicity overall and lower fat content. The effects of purified and complex diets were studied in an animal model of methotrexate-induced enteritis. The complex diet resulted in less diarrhea and reversed the morphologic effects of methotrexate on the small bowel. These data support the beneficial effects of complex diets in small-bowel inflammation (62). The meta-analysis study by Griffiths, in which 134 patients were compared, showed no difference in the efficacy of elemental versus nonelemental formulas (pooled odds ratio, 0.87; 95% confidence interval, 0.41–1.83). This study was limited by sample size; however, no advantage of elemental feedings compared with a polymeric formulation could be demonstrated (63).

In the Fernandez meta-analysis study, subgroup analyses were conducted on the basis of the type of diet administered. Peptide-based diets were significantly inferior to steroids (pooled OR, 0.32; CI, 0.20–0.52). There was a trend toward lower remission rate after elemental diets than after steroids (pooled OR, 0.44; CI 0.17–1.12). Pooled OR for whole-protein-based diets compared with elemental diets was 1.28 (CI 0.40–4.02). The benefit of steroid therapy is more demonstrable when peptide-based diets are administered, and less so with either elemental or whole-protein-based diets (63).

Prospective randomized controlled trials of diet therapy compared to placebo or mesalamine have not been conducted.

FISH OIL, OMEGA-3 FATTY ACIDS The beneficial role of fish oils in maintaining intestinal epithelial integrity in experimental models for IBD has been studied by several investigators. Marotta et al. evaluated the mucosal lipid composition in a hamster model of colitis treated with a supplemental fish oil diet. The diet, rich in eicosapentaenoic acid, attenuated the colitis. The mucosal

lipid profiles were similar to normal control animals (64). The protective effect was attributed to maintaining this profile and the integrity of the mucosal cell membranes, and, possibly, a reduction of the pro-inflammatory arachidonic acid metabolites or an undetermined anti-inflammatory effect.

The effect of enteral diets supplemented with either fish oil or indigestible oligosaccharides with sulfasalazine was studied by Grisham et al. (65). All forms of elemental diets reduced mucosal injury and inflammation as compared to control. The reductions were comparable to animals treated with sulfasalazine. The use of indigestible oligosaccharides induced the production of short-chain fatty acids by bacteria. The magnitude of improvement was not statistically significant (65).

A complementary human study evaluated the effects of omega-3 fatty acids on the production of TNF and IL-1β. A diet of α-linolenic acid was associated with significant reductions of peripheral blood lymphocyte (PBL) TNF and IL-1β production. The exact mechanism of action of this beneficial effect of omega-3 fatty acid in this animal model of IBD has not been elucidated (66). The benefit of a fish-oil (eicosapentaenoic acid)-enriched diet was demonstrated in a study by Empey et al. (67). An eicosapentaenoic-acid-enriched diet was compared with saturated and polyunsaturated fatty-acid-enriched diets in an animal model of colitis. The protective effect of the fish-oil-enriched diets occurred in the presence of enhanced prostaglandin E (PGE) synthesis and was manifest by returning ileal fluid absorption to control levels. The other diets did not demonstrate this effect. Eicosapentaenoic acid competition with arachidonic acid and altered biosynthesis was the proposed mechanism (67).

Eicosanoids have been proposed as modulators of inflammation by several lines of evidence. Increased levels of prostaglandins and leukotrines in IBD correlate with disease activity (68,69). The effect of omega-3 fatty acid is to partially displace arachidonic acid from cell-membrane phospholipids and impair arachidonic acid formation (70). Additionally, they reduce the synthesis of pro-inflammatory cytokines and interfere with membrane signal transduction (71,72). Furthermore, omega-3 fatty acid decreases mucosal arachidonic acid in patients with Crohn's disease (73). In animal models of IBD, this putative beneficial effect involves enhanced membrane integrity, cytokine downregulation, competition with arachidonic acid, and altered eicosanoid biosynthesis.

Fish oil has a high concentration of eicosanoids (omega-3 fatty acids). Several prospective studies have compared fish oil to standard therapy in patients with Crohn's disease. The results are controversial, with one study reporting effective therapy and the other no benefit (74,75). Although both studies randomized patients to placebo and fish oil, there were many differences that may account for the findings. Significant differences in the patient's disease status at the initiation of the therapy existed. One study evaluated patients that were immediate postcorticosteroid suppression, whereas in the other, patients were required to have at least 3 mo remission prior to therapy. The types of fish oils were different: (1) Verum (2 capsules three times a day) 1 gram of an ethylester fish oil concentrate (50% eicosapentaenoic acid, 30% docosahexaenoic acid); (2) A time-release capsule three times a day containing 500 mg of a marine lipid concentrate in free-fatty-acid form (40% eicosapentaenoic acid, 20% docosahexaenoic acid, the remaining 40% was a mixture of omega-7 fatty acids [17%], omega-0 fatty acids [16%], and omega-6 fatty acids [7%]). The high dose (6 g) was compared to the low dose (3 g). Relapse rates

Table 2
Omega-3 Fatty Acids in Ulcerative Colitis

Author	Year	Type[a]	No. of patients	Duration	Washout	Duration	Effect
McCall	1989	PS	10	3 mo			Improved symptoms, improved histology score, steroid sparing
Solomon	1990	OT	10	2 mo			Improved symptoms, improved histology score, steroid sparing
Hawthorne	1991	RBC	87	1 yr			Modest steroid sparing; no benefit as maintenance therapy
Aslan	1991	RBPCC	11	3 mo	2 mo	3 mo	↓Disease activity 56% fish oil versus 4% placebo, p < 0.05
Stenson	1992	RBPCC	18	4 mo	1 mo	4 mo	Improvement histology score, steroid sparing
Loeschke	1996	RBPC	64	2 yr			Did not prevent relapse

[a]PS = pilot study; OT = open trial; RBC = randomized blind control; RBPCC = randomized blind placebo control crossover; RBPC = randomized blind placebo control.

were 70%, 70%, and 28%, 59% in the fish oil and placebo groups, respectively. Both trials were conducted for 1 yr and studied responses in 204 and 78 patients, respectively. The distribution of disease location in the two populations were not comparable. The groups of patients responding to the fish oil diet consisted of a higher percentage of small-bowel disease (51%, 58% compared to 11%, 19%) and a higher percentage of combined small-bowel/colon disease (89%, 85%, compared to 68%, 61%).

ULCERATIVE COLITIS AND OMEGA-3 FATTY ACIDS THERAPY Randomized prospective drug-therapy trials in groups of patients with ulcerative colitis were evaluated by a recent meta-analysis study. This evaluation included 11 trials for induction and 5 trials for maintenance of remission. Patient populations were 468 and 343 for induction and maintenance, respectively. Induction of therapy with drugs was accomplished in 37–48% of patients. Maintenance of remission was 21% at 6 mo and 46% at 1 yr (76). Prospective clinical trials designed to demonstrate the potential beneficial effects of omega-3 fatty acids in patients with ulcerative colitis are displayed in Table 2 (77–82).

With the exception of one trial, the beneficial effects were not convincingly favorable and benefit was generally expressed as steroid sparing. These studies involved small numbers of patients with the longest study interval of 2 yr duration, demonstrating no benefit in preventing disease relapse (82).

In the small study by Aslan et al. in which the remission rate of 56% was seen in the fish oil group compared to 4% for placebo, the beneficial effects were determined by symptom score and visualized healing (80).

In ulcerative colitis, the use of fish oil has demonstrated a steroid-sparing effect and a moderate decrease in disease activity.

SHORT-CHAIN FATTY ACIDS Bacteria in the lumen produce short-chain fatty acids from undigested carbohydrates. The colon epithelial cells actively take up and convert the short-chain fatty acids through beta lipolysis and the Krebs cycle for energy utilization. Short-chain fatty acids are the preferential fuel of colonocytes. A defective utilization has been suggested as a cause of epithelial cell dysfunction and a metabolic basis for ulcerative colitis (83). This theory was evaluated by prospective trials designed to demonstrate the benefit of administered short-chain fatty acids in patients with ulcerative colitis. Uniformly, these trials reveal no benefit in ulcerative colitis (84–88). These data suggest that the theory for a metabolic defect as a cause for ulcerative colitis may be incorrect. Alternately, the supply of short-chain fatty acids may be adequate and the problem may be the cellular uptake or metabolism. Subsequently, the uptake and metabolism of short-chain fatty acids by isolated colonocytes derived from patients with ulcerative colitis was evaluated and found not to be impaired (89). Additionally, short-chain fatty acids have been evaluated as a therapy of pouchitis and found to have no demonstrable beneficial effect (90).

NUTRITIONAL THERAPY OF CROHN'S FISTULA Prospective randomized studies of the effects of TPN and bowel rest on the closure of fistulas have not been conducted. Data derived from retrospective studies demonstrate lower mortality rates. Fistulas that arise from active Crohn's lesions have lower spontaneous closure rates and much lower sustained closure at 3 mo (17%) (91). However, postoperative fistulas at anastamotic sites respond with higher spontaneous closure and permanent closure rates (92).

ACUTE FULMINANT COLITIS The effect on cytokine and insulinlike growth factor (IGF) in the fasting state was evaluated by comparing fed and fasted states in a mouse-induced experimental model of inflammatory bowel disease. In the fasted group, the colitis activity score was reduced. IL-1β mRNA and IGF-1 mRNA were elevated in the fed animals. Tumor necrosis factor-α mRNA was not significantly different in the groups. The demonstrated beneficial effect of fasting is attributed to a decreased expression of IL-1β and IGF-1 mRNA in the colon (93).

Patients hospitalized for severe acute flares of ulcerative colitis and Crohn's disease are managed by restricted oral intake. Two prospective randomized trials have evaluated this clinical practice by comparing use of TPN and bowel rest with regular diet. No differences in duration of hospital stay and surgery rates were demonstrated (94).

Another study compared enteral nutrition and TPN with similar findings. Adverse events were less common in the enteral-treated group (95). These trials demonstrate that bowel rest as a treatment modality for the management of acute fulminant inflammatory bowel disease is not necessary.

BONE DISEASE The effect of circulating inflammatory mediators on linear growth was studied in a nutritionally controlled rat colitis model. Experimental colitis resulted in decreased linear bone growth independent of nutritional intake. Circulating interleukin-6 derived from intestinal inflammation was elevated and may have contributed to the suppression of bone growth (96).

Decreased linear bone growth complicates chronic inflammatory bowel disease in children, and in adults, significant osteopenia and an increased fracture rate are noted. Deficiencies in vitamin D are usually common in patients with IBD and these deficiencies are not related to inadequate absorption of vitamin D (97). However, supplementation with oral vitamin D (1000IU/d) reduces loss of bone density when compared to patients not receiving supplementation (98). Intake of oral calcium has been studied in IBD patients compared to a control population revealing a moderate decrease in calcium uptake that was not associated with a decreased bone density (99). Calcium hemostasis has been found to be normal and there was no correlation with current or past steroid use. Bone markers of osteoclastic activity, specifically, urinary levels of pyridinoline, deoxypyridinoline, and type 1 collagen carboxy terminal peptide were elevated, supporting selectively increased bone reabsorption (100). Other investigators have also concluded that the decreased bone density did not correlate with steroid use or length of resected bowel (101). Differences in the magnitude of bone disease have been noted in metabolic studies comparing ulcerative colitis and Crohn's disease that seem to be related to steroid use and sex but not the length of bowel resection (102). Evaluation of circulating factors by culturing fetal rat parietal bone with sera from patients with IBD demonstrated significant differences with Crohn's disease sera when compared to control and ulcerative colitis sera. Decreased bone dry weight and calcium content did not correlate with IL-6 levels, disease activity, or measures of bone metabolism. Other, yet to be identified, circulating pro-inflammatory cytokines appear to affect osteoblasts and bone formation (103).

EFFECTS OF DIARRHEA ON LUMINAL NUTRITION

Protracted diarrhea has significant morphologic effects on the mucosal surface in IBD patients, which is associated with low serum albumin, increased bacterial translocation, and increased mortality. Many of the mucosal morphological effects of protracted diarrhea are abrogated with parenteral nutrition (104). Severe protracted diarrhea in young children can be attributed to agents, epithelial defects, and autoimmune mechanisms, which appear to be distinct when compared to adult inflammatory bowel disease (105). Chronic diarrhea results in low serum zinc levels. Zinc supplementation has demonstrated significant beneficial effects in a randomized controlled trial in children with chronic diarrhea (106). Additionally, levels of vitamin A are decreased in children with chronic diarrhea (107). In experimental animals with induced zinc deficiency, the levels of inducible nitrous oxide synthetase was increased and diarrhea occurred when challenged with IL-1α injections (108).

In experimental guinea pig models of malnutrition, the role of zinc was evaluated by studying the response of the host to milk allergens. Malnutrition was associated with increased milk immune responses that were abrogated by zinc administration (109).

ZINC DEFICIENCY IN IBD

Zinc deficiency results from diarrhea and contributes to continual diarrhea. Zinc supplementation results in restoration of intestinal morphologic characteristics, restores brush border hydrolases, and results in increased secretory antibody responses and enhanced T-cell responses (110).

In a large retrospective study, vitamins and trace elements were found to be deficient in 85% of patients with Crohn's disease and 68% of patients with ulcerative colitis. The predominant deficiencies, in order, were iron, calcium, protein, zinc, cyanocobalamine, and folic acid (111). Zinc is necessary for all human growth and for transcription of all genetic material. Zinc deficiency has been incriminated in multiple-disease entities that result in increased bacterial mucosal translocation, malnutrition, growth failure, decreased secretory immunoglobulin production, and altered cellular immunity. Zinc deficiency is found in patients with inflammatory bowel diseases, malabsorption, protein-losing enteropathy, and steatorrhea (112). Zinc deficiency in IBD patients results in alopecia, eczematoid, and psoriaform skin lesions (113). Oral manifestations of zinc deficiency in patients with Crohn's disease are oral ulcers, chelitis, fissures, cobblestone plaques, polypoid defects, perioral erythema, and pyostomatitis vegetans. Zinc supplementation resolves these problems (114). Compared to control patients, zinc absorption has been found to be significantly decreased in patients who were malnourished with moderate disease activity. These effects were attributed to the malnourished state (115). Zinc metabolism was studied in pediatric IBD patients and significant occurrences of low zinc levels, abnormal zinc loading tests, and decreased urinary excretion were detected. These abnormalities were more commonly seen in children with growth retardation; however they were also found in children with normal growth (116).

GROWTH FACTORS

Intestinal growth factors are involved in mediating the healing and recovery process in the inflamed bowel. Increased keratinocyte growth factor mRNA is present in IBD patients (117). Likewise, administration of keratinocyte growth factor in animal models decrease the severity of inflammation (118). Transforming growth factors α and β mRNAs are both increased in active IBD (119,120). The role of these transforming growth factors on epithelial cell proliferation and maintenance of the epithelial barrier have important implications for future therapies.

SURGICAL RESECTION AND THE SHORT-BOWEL SYNDROME

The malabsorptive state that exists after extensive bowel resection is referred to as the short-bowel syndrome (121,122). Important variables are the extent of resection, the region resected, and the age of the patient. Resection of the ileocecal valve in altered intestinal motility with increased small-bowel transit, gastroparesis, and a tendency for bacterial overgrowth (123). Resection of 40–50% of the small bowel is usually tolerated. However, when the terminal ileum and ileoceocal valve are removed, short-bowel syndrome may result from resection of less than 40% of the small bowel. Frequently, TPN is necessary to provide interim nutrition until adaptation occurs and the patient's absorptive status can be determined. Beneficial factors that have been identified with discontinuation of TPN are small-bowel length of more than 35 cm and a jejunoileal anastomosis, presence of a colon, and an ileocolonic anastomosis (124). With large resections and the successful discontinuation of TPN, some degree of malnutrition and vitamin and mineral deficiencies frequently occur. The absorption of vitamin B_{12} in relation to the magnitude of bowel resection was evaluated in 75 patients undergoing ileorectal anastomosis for complications of the disease. Universal vitamin B_{12} deficiency occurred with resections of 60 cm or more. However, with resections of 10 cm including the ileoceocal valve, 38% of the patients had impaired vitamin B_{12} absorption (125). Steatorrhea frequently occurs and is commonly associated with deficiencies of fat-soluble vitamins A, D, E, and K. The most common mineral deficiencies are zinc, magnesium, and calcium.

Adaptation starts within hours after resection, with increased expression of gene products. Continual changes occurring throughout the first year are manifest by structural and functional changes in the residual bowel. The magnitude of this response is related to the extent of the resection. Cellular changes result in increased absorptive function of both nutrient and fluids. Structural changes are characterized by epithelial hyperplasia, increased villus length, bowel dilatation, and elongation. The process is stimulated by enteral feeding, and atrophy may result with enteral nutrient exclusion. The important trophic factors effecting these changes are glutamine, soluble fibers, short-chain fatty acids, epidermal growth factor, gastrin, proglucagon-derived peptides, enteroglucagon, ileal proglucagon, glucagonlike peptide 2, epidermal growth factor, insulinlike growth factor I, pancreaticobiliary secretions, and other yet to be identified factors (126). Stimulated adaptation was studied by Byrne et al. (127,128) in 47 TPN-dependent patients with short-bowel syndrome treated with a high-carbohydrate, low-fat diet supplemented with glutamine and growth hormone. Forty percent of these patients were weaned off TPN and the nutritional requirements of an additional 40% were significantly reduced (127,128). These studies suggested that intervention with diet and growth hormones can accentuate adaptation at a time when the adaptive process is usually not active. Subsequently, a randomized study designed to compare the individual components of growth hormone, glutamine, and a low-fat, high-carbohydrate diet did not support these findings (129).

PROTEIN MALNUTRITION   Significant protein malnutrition is common in IBD patients. Data support multifactorial causes related to decreased nutritional intake, increased metabolism, drug therapy, malabsorption, increased nutritional requirements, and increased enteral loss. Fecal alpha-1 antitrypsin (AAT) excretion has proven to be an accurate and reliable indicator of enteral protein loss. An altered mucosal barrier manifested by increased enteric loss has been documented in patients with IBD and AIDS compared with controls (130,131). Resting-energy expenditure in hospitalized patients was found to be 11% higher than the normal population and associated with less than ideal body weight. As the inflammatory disease activity decreased, the resting energy expenditure also decreased (132). Animal studies of induced malnutrition and inflammation secondary to enteric pathogens demonstrate significant morphological and functional changes. In malnourished animals, body weight, bowel weight, and jejunal and ileal mucosal weight are decreased. Morphologic changes reveal decreased mucosal villus height, crypt depth, disaccharidase activity, mucosal protein, and DNA content (133). Protein malnutrition may impair immune responsiveness by modifying the general immune response, decreasing cellular immune responses, and decreasing the synthesis of secretory IgA (134,135). Substrate utilization, nitrogen balance, and body composition in malnourished patients with IBD having difficulty gaining weight is altered when compared to healthy subjects. With parenteral nutrition in IBD patients, a normal accumulation of carbohydrates, protein, and a depletion of fat occurs. Concurrently, increases are noted in extracellular body weight, body cell mass, plasma T3, and insulin secretion (136).

BACTERIAL OVERGROWTH   Bacterial overgrowth is a common finding in many bowel disease entities, especially those associated with motility disturbances, stricture formation, and loss of the ileocecal valve. Bacterial overgrowth increases intestinal permeability, decreases brush border enzyme function, competes for cyanocobalamine, and is associated with increased bacterial translocation (137). Patient manifestations are usually increased abdominal pain, diarrhea, polyarthritis, malaise, and, occasionally,

a neutrophilic vasculitis (138,139). In a retrospective study of bacterial overgrowth in children with short-bowel syndrome supported by TPN, a high incidence of bacterial overgrowth was noted. All patients that remained TPN dependent had significant bacterial overgrowth. In the group of patients in which TPN weaning was successful, 23 of 42 children had bacterial overgrowth associated with intestinal inflammation. The presence of bacterial overgrowth may complicate weaning, prolong the need for TPN, and perpetuate intestinal inflammation (140).

SUMMARY

Idiopathic inflammatory disease involving the gastrointestinal system are assumed to be autoreactive or inappropriate immune responses because agents and documented cellular or mucosal defects have not been defined. The immune response at the mucosal level in the various diseases is extremely complex and may represent many different diseases; to date, the inciting event for the increased mucosal inflammatory response has not been defined. Theoretically, a two-component or double-hit scenario is most likely. A defect in mucosal permeability exists, exposing the host to an antigen challenge that bypasses M-cell-mediated tolerance mechanisms. The host response to luminal contents is accentuated or there is a failure to downregulate this immune response.

All current conventional therapies are directed nonspecifically at suppression of the cell-mediated response and the pro-inflammatory mediators of inflammation.

Epidemiological studies suggest dietary factors are important although no putative food substances have been identified. Molecular and immune mechanistic studies involving specific food substances need to be conducted. Patients with IBD progressively develop problems that are associated with disease duration and extent. Micronutrient and macronutrient deficiencies commonly contribute to the morbidity of the disease process. The use of elemental diets has been shown to downregulate the inflammatory response in experimental animals; however, as a therapy, a beneficial effect is difficult to assess in humans. Although diet as a therapy has been the subject of enormous effort, conventional drug therapy has proven to be more effective with induction and maintenance of disease remission. In the pediatric population, where growth disturbances and bone disease are significant problems, nutrition as therapy plays a significant role. As IBD progresses and complications of the disease become more manifest, nutritional factors, management, and support become critical.

REFERENCES

1. Howard L, Ament M, Fleming CR, Shike M, Steiger E. Current use and clinical outcome of home parenteral and enteral nutrition therapies in the United States. Gastroenterology 1995; 109:355–65.
2. Shivananda S, Lennard-Jones J, Logan R, et al. Incidence of inflammatory bowel disease across Europe: is there a difference between north and south? Results of the European Collaborative Study on Inflammatory Bowel Disease (EC-IBD). Gut 1996; 39:690–7.
3. Russel MG, Stockbrugger RW. Epidemiology of inflammatory bowel disease: an update. Scand J Gastroenterol 1996; 31:417–27.
4. Caulkins BM. Digestive Diseases in the United States: Epidemiology and Impact, Inflammatory Bowel Disease, pp. 510–50. National Institutes of Health, Bethesda, MD, 1994.
5. Hay JW, Hay HA. Inflammatory bowel disease: cost-of-illness. J Clin Gastroenterol 1992; 14:309–17.
6. Hay AR, Hay JW. Inflammatory bowel disease: medical cost. J Clin Gastroenterol 1992; 14:318–27.

7. Kirshner JS. Familial occurrences of ulcerative colitis. Ann Intern Med 1963; 59:133–44.

8. Sachar DB. Crohn's disease: a family affair. Gastroenterology 1996; 111:813–5.

9. JCW Lee JL-J. Inflammatory bowel disease in 67 families each with three or more affected first-degree relatives. Gastroenterology 1996; 111:587–96.

10. Peeters M, Nevens H, Baert F, et al. Familial aggregation in Crohn's disease: increased age-adjusted risk and concordance in clinical characteristics. Gastroenterology 1996; 111:597–603.

11. Colombel JF, Grandbastien B, Gower-Rousseau C, et al. Clinical characteristics of Crohn's disease in 72 families. Gastroenterology 1996; 111:604–7.

12. Bayless TM, Tokayer AZ, Polito JM II, Quaskey SA, Mellits ED, Harris ML. Crohn's disease: concordance for site and clinical type in affected family members—potential hereditary influences. Gastroenterology 1996; 111:573–9.

13. Thompson NP, Driscoll R, Pounder RE, Wakefield AJ. Genetics versus environment in inflammatory bowel disease: results of a British twin study. Br Med J 1996; 312:95–6.

14. Akolkar PN, Gulwani-Akolkar B, Heresbach D, et al. Differences in risk of Crohn's disease in offspring of mothers and fathers with inflammatory bowel disease. Am J Gastroenterol 1997; 92:2241–4.

15. Hugot JP, Laurent-Puig P, Gower-Rousseau C, et al. Mapping of a susceptibility locus for Crohn's disease on chromosome 16. Nature 1996; 379:821–3.

16. Satsangi J, Welsh KI, Bunce M, et al. Contribution of genes of the major histocompatibility complex to susceptibility and disease phenotype in inflammatory bowel disease. Lancet 1996; 347:1212–7.

17. Kidd BL, Wilson PJ, Evans PR, Cawley MI. Familial aggregation of undifferentiated spondyloarthropathy associated with HLA-B7. Ann Rheum Dis 1995; 54:125–7.

18. Bernstein CN. On making the diagnosis of ulcerative colitis. Am J Gastroenterol 1997; 92:1247–52.

19. Meyers S, Janowitz HD. "Natural history" of Crohn's disease. An analytic review of the placebo lesson. Gastroenterology 1984; 87:1189–92.

20. Cantrell M, Prindiville T, Gershwin ME. Autoantibodies to colonic cells and subcellular fractions in inflammatory bowel disease: do they exist? J Autoimmun 1990; 3:307–20.

21. Khoo UY, Bjarnason I, Donaghy A, Williams R, Macpherson A. Antibodies to colonic epithelial cells from the serum and colonic mucosal washings in ulcerative colitis. Gut 1995; 37:63–70.

22. Macpherson A, Khoo UY, Forgacs I, Philpott-Howard J, Bjarnason I. Mucosal antibodies in inflammatory bowel disease are directed against intestinal bacteria. Gut 1996; 38:365–75.

23. Eggena M, Targan SR, Iwanczyk L, Vidrich A, Gordon LK, Braun J. Phage display cloning and characterization of an immunogenetic marker (perinuclear anti-neutrophil cytoplasmic antibody) in ulcerative colitis. J Immunol 1996; 156:4005–11.

24. Uesugi H, Ozaki S, Sobajima J, et al. Prevalence and characterization of novel pANCA, antibodies to the high mobility group non-histone chromosomal proteins HMG1 and HMG2, in systemic rheumatic diseases. J Rheumatol 1998; 25:703–9.

25. Sobajima J, Ozaki S, Uesugi H, et al. Prevalence and characterization of perinuclear anti-neutrophil cytoplasmic antibodies (P-ANCA) directed against HMG1 and HMG2 in ulcerative colitis (UC). Clin Exp Immunol 1998; 111:402–7.

26. Sobajima J, Ozaki S, Osakada F, et al. Novel autoantigens of perinuclear anti-neutrophil cytoplasmic antibodies (P-ANCA) in ulcerative colitis: non-histone chromosomal proteins, HMG1 and HMG2. Clin Exp Immunol 1997; 107:135–40.

27. Sobajima J, Ozaki S, Okazaki T, et al. Anti-neutrophil cytoplasmic antibodies (ANCA) in ulcerative colitis: anti-cathepsin G and a novel antibody correlate with a refractory type. Clin Exp Immunol 1996; 105:120–4.

28. Keren DF, Goeken JA. Autoimmune reactivity in inflammatory bowel disease. Clin Lab Med 1997; 17:465–81.

29. Lachaux A, Bouvier R, Cozzani E, et al. Familial autoimmune enteropathy with circulating anti-bullous pemphigoid antibodies and chronic autoimmune hepatitis. J Pediatr 1994; 125:858–62.

30. Utz U, Biddison WE, McFarland HF, McFarlin DE, Flerlage M, Martin R. Skewed T-cell receptor repertoire in genetically identical twins correlates with multiple sclerosis. Nature 1993; 364:243–7.

31. Prindiville TP, Contrell MC, Matsumoto T, Brown WR, Ansari AA, Kotzin BL, Gershwin ME. Analysis of function, specificity and T cell receptor expression of cloned mucosal T cell lines in Crohn's disease. J Autoimmun 1996; 9:193–204.

32. Probert CS, Chott A, Turner JR, et al. Persistent clonal expansions of peripheral blood CD4+ lymphocytes in chronic inflammatory bowel disease. J Immunol 1996; 157:3183–91.

33. Gulwani-Akolkar B, Akolkar PN, Minassian A, et al. Selective expansion of specific T cell receptors in the inflamed colon of Crohn's disease. J Clin Invest 1996; 98:1334–54.

34. Nakajima A, Kodama T, Yazaki Y, et al. Specific clonal T cell accumulation in intestinal lesions of Crohn's disease. J Immunol 1996; 157:5683–8.

35. Kaufman DL, Clare-Salzler M, Tian J, et al. Spontaneous loss of T-cell tolerance to glutamic acid decarboxylase in murine insulin-dependent diabetes. Nature 1993; 366:69–72.

36. Duchmann R, Marker-Hermann E, Meyer zum Buschenfelde KH. Bacteria-specific T-cell clones are selective in their reactivity towards different enterobacteria or H. pylori and increased in inflammatory bowel disease. Scand J Immunol 1996; 44:71–9.

37. Yoshida EM, Chan NH, Herrick RA, et al. Human immunodeficiency virus infection, the acquired immunodeficiency syndrome, and inflammatory bowel disease. J Clin Gastroenterol 1996; 23:24–8.

38. Reimund JM, Wittersheim C, Dumont S, et al. Mucosal inflammatory cytokine production by intestinal biopsies in patients with ulcerative colitis and Crohn's disease. J Clin Immunol 1996; 16:144–50.

39. Reimund JM, Wittersheim C, Dumont S, et al. Increased production of tumour necrosis factor-alpha interleukin-1 beta, and interleukin-6 by morphologically normal intestinal biopsies from patients with Crohn's disease. Gut 1996; 39:684–9.

40. Mombaerts P, Mizoguchi E, Grusby MJ, Glimcher LH, Bhan AK, Tonegawa S. Spontaneous development of inflammatory bowel disease in T cell receptor mutant mice. Cell 1993; 75:274–82.

41. Egger B, Procaccino F, Lakshmanan J, et al. Mice lacking transforming growth factor alpha have an increased susceptibility to dextran sulfate-induced colitis. Gastroenterology 1997; 113:825–32.

42. Hermiston ML, Gordon JI. Inflammatory bowel disease and adenomas in mice expressing a dominant negative N-cadherin. Science 1995; 270:1203–7.

43. Taurog JD, Maika SD, Simmons WA, Breban M, Hammer RE. Susceptibility to inflammatory disease in HLA-B27 transgenic rat lines correlates with the level of B27 expression. J Immunol 1993; 150:4168–78.

44. Rath HC, Herfarth HH, Ikeda JS, et al. Normal luminal bacteria, especially Bacteroides species, mediate chronic colitis, gastritis, and arthritis in HLA-B27/human beta2 microglobulin transgenic rats. J Clin Invest 1996; 98:945–53.

45. Onderdonk AB, Hermos JA, Bartlett JG. The role of the intestinal microflora in experimental colitis. Am J Clin Nutr 1977; 30:1819–25.

46. Tanaka S, Miura S, Kimura H, et al. Amelioration of chronic inflammation by ingestion of elemental diet in a rat model of granulomatous enteritis. Dig Dis Sci 1997; 42:408–19.

47. Fujita T, Sakurai K. Efficacy of glutamine-enriched enteral nutrition in an experimental model of mucosal ulcerative colitis. Br J Surg 1995; 82:749–51.

48. Ameho CK, Adjei AA, Harrison EK, et al. Prophylactic effect of dietary glutamine supplementation on interleukin 8 and tumour necrosis factor alpha production in trinitrobenzene sulphonic acid induced colitis. Gut 1997; 41:487–93.

49. Reif S, Klein I, Lubin F, Farbstein M, Hallak A, Gilat T. Pre-illness dietary factors in inflammatory bowel disease. Gut 1997; 40:754–60.

50. Persson PG, Ahlbom A, Hellers G. Diet and inflammatory bowel disease: a case-control study. Epidemiology 1992; 3:47–52.

51. Tragnone A, Valpiani D, Miglio F, et al. Dietary habits as risk factors for inflammatory bowel disease. Eur J Gastroenterol Hepatol 1995; 7:47–51.

52. Dietary and other risk factors of ulcerative colitis. A case-control study in Japan. Epidemiology Group of the Research Committee of Inflammatory Bowel Disease in Japan. J Clin Gastroenterol 1994; 19:166–71.

53. Kitahora T, Utsunomiya T, Yokota A. Epidemiological study of ulcerative colitis in Japan: incidence of familial occurrence. The Epidemiology Group of the Research Committee of Inflammatory Bowel Disease in Japan. J Gastroenterol 1995; 30(suppl 8):5–8.

54. Seidman E, LeLeiko N, Ament M, et al. Nutritional issues in pediatric inflammatory bowel disease. J Pediatr Gastroenterol Nutr 1991; 12:424–38.

55. Seidman EG, Roy CC, Weber AM, Morin CL. Nutritional therapy of Crohn's disease in childhood. Dig Dis Sci 1987; 32:82S–8S.

56. Directors ABI. Guidelines for the use of parenteral and enteral nutrition in adult and pediatric patients. J Parenteral Enteral Nutr 1993; 17:1S–51S.

57. Salomon P, Kornbluth A, Aisenberg J, Janowitz HD. How effective are current drugs for Crohn's disease? A meta-analysis. J Clin Gastroenterol 1992; 14:211–5.

58. Steinhart AH, Hemphill D, Greenberg GR. Sulfasalazine and mesalazine for the maintenance therapy of Crohn's disease: a meta-analysis. Am J Gastroenterol 1994; 89:2116–24.

59. Pearson DC, May GR, Fick GH, Sutherland LR. Azathioprine and 6-mercaptopurine in Crohn disease. A meta-analysis. Ann Intern Med 1995; 123:132–42.

60. Messori A, Trallori G, D'Albasio G, Milla M, Vannozzi G, Pacini F. Defined-formula diets versus steroids in the treatment of active Crohn's disease: a meta-analysis. Scand J Gastroenterol 1996; 31:267–72.

61. Hiwatashi N. Enteral nutrition for Crohn's disease in Japan. Dis Colon Rectum 1997; 40:S48–53.

62. Marks SL, Cook AK, Griffey S, Kass PH, Rogers QR. Dietary modulation of methotrexate-induced enteritis in cats. Am J Vet Res 1997; 58:989–96.

63. Griffiths AM, Ohlsson A, Sherman PM, Sutherland LR. Meta-analysis of enteral nutrition as a primary treatment of active Crohn's disease. Gastroenterology 1995; 108:1056–67.

64. Marotta F, Chui DH, Safran P, Rezakovic I, Zhong GG, Ideo G. Shark fin enriched diet prevents mucosal lipid abnormalities in experimental acute colitis. Digestion 1995; 56:46–51.

65. Grisham MB DS, Garleb KAZ, Specian RD. Sulfasalaziine of enteral diets containing fish oil or oligosaccharides attenuate chronic colitis in rats. Inflam Bowel Dis 1996; 2:178–88.

66. Caughey GE, Mantzioris E, Gibson RA, Cleland LG, James MJ. The effect on human tumor necrosis factor alpha and interleukin 1 beta production of diets enriched in n-3 fatty acids from vegetable oil or fish oil. Am J Clin Nutr 1996; 63:116–22.

67. Empey LR, Jewell LD, Garg ML, Thomson AB, Clandinin MT, Fedorak RN. Fish oil-enriched diet is mucosal protective against acetic acid-induced colitis in rats. Can J Physiol Pharmacol 1991; 69:480–7.

68. Gould SR. Assay of prostaglandin-like substances in faeces and their measurement in ulcerative colitis. Prostaglandins 1976; 11:489–97.

69. Sharon P, Stenson WF. Enhanced synthesis of leukotriene B4 by colonic mucosa in inflammatory bowel disease. Gastroenterology 1984; 86:453–60.

70. Lee TH, Hoover RL, Williams JD, et al. Effect of dietary enrichment with eicosapentaenoic and docosahexaenoic acids on in vitro neutrophil and monocyte leukotriene generation and neutrophil function. N Engl J Med 1985; 312:1217–24.

71. Endres S, Ghorbani R, Kelley VE, et al. The effect of dietary supplementation with n-3 polyunsaturated fatty acids on the synthesis of interleukin-1 and tumor necrosis factor by mononuclear cells. N Engl J Med 1989; 320:265–71.

72. Endres S. n-3 polyunsaturated fatty acids and human cytokine synthesis. Lipids 1996; 31 (suppl):S239–42.

73. Hillier K, Jewell R, Dorrell L, Smith CL. Incorporation of fatty acids from fish oil and olive oil into colonic mucosal lipids and effects upon eicosanoid synthesis in inflammatory bowel disease. Gut 1991; 32:1151–5.

74. Lorenz-Meyer H, Bauer P, Nicolay C, et al. Omega-3 fatty acids and low carbohydrate diet for maintenance of remission in Crohn's disease. A randomized controlled multicenter trial. Study Group Members (German Crohn's Disease Study Group). Scand J Gastroenterol 1996; 31:778–85.

75. Belluzzi A, Brignola C, Campieri M, Pera A, Boschi S, Miglioli M. Effect of an enteric-coated fish-oil preparation on relapses in Crohn's disease. N Engl J Med 1996; 334:1557–60.

76. Kornbluth AA, Salomon P, Sacks HS, Mitty R, Janowitz HD. Meta-analysis of the effectiveness of current drug therapy of ulcerative colitis. J Clin Gastroenterol 1993; 16:215–8.

77. McCall TB, O'Leary D, Bloomfield J, O'Morain CA. Therapeutic potential of fish oil in the treatment of ulcerative colitis. Aliment Pharmacol Ther 1989; 3:415–24.

78. Salomon P, Kornbluth AA, Janowitz HD. Treatment of ulcerative colitis with fish oil n–3-omega–fatty acid: an open trial. J Clin Gastroenterol 1990; 12:157–61.

79. Hawthorne AB, Daneshmend TK, Hawkey CJ, et al. Treatment of ulcerative colitis with fish oil supplementation: a prospective 12 month randomised controlled trial. Gut 1992; 33:922–8.

80. Aslan A, Triadafilopoulos G. Fish oil fatty acid supplementation in active ulcerative colitis: a double-blind, placebo-controlled, crossover study. Am J Gastroenterol 1992; 87:432–7.

81. Stenson WF, Cort D, Rodgers J, et al. Dietary supplementation with fish oil in ulcerative colitis [see comments]. Ann Intern Med 1992; 116:609–14.

82. Loeschke K, Ueberschaer B, Pietsch A, et al. n-3 fatty acids only delay early relapse of ulcerative colitis in remission. Dig Dis Sci 1996; 41:2087–94.

83. Roediger WE. The colonic epithelium in ulcerative colitis: an energy-deficiency disease? Lancet 1980; 2:712–5.

84. Vernia P, Cittadini M, Caprilli R, Torsoli A. Topical treatment of refractory distal ulcerative colitis with 5-ASA and sodium butyrate. Dig Dis Sci 1995; 40:305–7.

85. Patz J, Jacobsohn WZ, Gottschalk-Sabag S, Zeides S, Braverman DZ. Treatment of refractory distal ulcerative colitis with short chain fatty acid enemas. Am J Gastroenterol 1996; 91:731–4.

86. Steinhart AH, Hiruki T, Brzezinski A, Baker JP. Treatment of left-sided ulcerative colitis with butyrate enemas: a controlled trial. Aliment Pharmacol Ther 1996; 10:729–36.

87. Scheppach W. Treatment of distal ulcerative colitis with short-chain fatty acid enemas. A placebo-controlled trial. German-Austrian SCFA Study Group. Dig Dis Sci 1996; 41:2254–9.

88. Breuer RI, Soergel KH, Lashner BA, et al. Short chain fatty acid rectal irrigation for left-sided ulcerative colitis: a randomised, placebo controlled trial. Gut 1997; 40:485–91.

89. Clausen MR, Mortensen PB. Kinetic studies on colonocyte metabolism of short chain fatty acids and glucose in ulcerative colitis. Gut 1995; 37:684–9.

90. Wischmeyer P, Pemberton JH, Phillips SF. Chronic pouchitis after ileal pouch–anal anastomosis: responses to butyrate and glutamine suppositories in a pilot study. Mayo Clin Proc 1993; 68:978–81.

91. Yamazaki Y, Fukushima T, Sugita A, Takemura H, Tsuchiya S. The medical, nutritional and surgical treatment of fistulae in Crohn's disease. Jpn J Surg 1990; 20:376–83.

92. Blackett RL, Hill GL. Postoperative external small bowel fistulas: a study of a consecutive series of patients treated with intravenous hyperalimentation. Br J Surg 1978; 65:775–8.

93. Savendahl L, Underwood LE, Haldemann KM, Ulshen MH, Lund PK. Fasting prevents experimental murine colitis produced by dextran sulfate sodium and decreases interleukin-1 beta and insulin-like growth factor I messenger ribonucleic acid. Endocrinology 1997; 138:734–40.

94. McIntyre PB, Powell-Tuck J, Wood SR, et al. Controlled trial of

bowel rest in the treatment of severe acute colitis. Gut 1986; 27:481–5.

95. Gonzalez-Huix F, Fernandez-Banares F, Esteve-Comas M, et al. Enteral versus parenteral nutrition as adjunct therapy in acute ulcerative colitis. Am J Gastroenterol 1993; 88:227–32.

96. Koniaris SG, Fisher SE, Rubin CT, Chawla A. Experimental colitis impairs linear bone growth independent of nutritional factors. J Pediatr Gastroenterol Nutr 1997; 25:137–41.

97. Vogelsang H, Schofl R, Tillinger W, Ferenci P, Gangl A. 25-hydroxyvitamin D absorption in patients with Crohn's disease and with pancreatic insufficiency. Wien Klin Wochenschr 1997; 109:678–82.

98. Vogelsang H, Ferenci P, Resch H, Kiss A, Gangl A. Prevention of bone mineral loss in patients with Crohn's disease by long-term vitamin D supplementation. Eur J Gastroenterol Hepatol 1995; 7:609–14.

99. Silvennoinen J, Lamberg-Allardt C, Karkkainen M, Niemela S, Lehtola J. Dietary calcium intake and its relation to bone mineral density in patients with inflammatory bowel disease. J Intern Med 1996; 240:285–92.

100. Bjarnason I, Macpherson A, Mackintosh C, Buxton-Thomas M, Forgacs I, Moniz C. Reduced bone density in patients with inflammatory bowel disease. Gut 1997; 40:228–33.

101. Staun M, Tjellesen L, Thale M, Schaadt O, Jarnum S. Bone mineral content in patients with Crohn's disease. A longitudinal study in patients with bowel resections. Scand J Gastroenterol 1997; 32:226–32.

102. Jahnsen J, Falch JA, Aadland E, Mowinckel P. Bone mineral density is reduced in patients with Crohn's disease but not in patients with ulcerative colitis: a population based study. Gut 1997; 40:313–9.

103. Hyams JS, Wyzga N, Kreutzer DL, Justinich CJ, Gronowicz GA. Alterations in bone metabolism in children with inflammatory bowel disease: an in vitro study. J Pediatr Gastroenterol Nutr 1997; 24:289–95.

104. Peret Filho LA, Brasileiro Filho G, Penna FJ. Morphological changes of the jejunal mucosa in protracted diarrhea and their correlation with disease duration, weight loss and serum albumin levels. Braz J Med Biol Res 1997; 30:1067–73.

105. Mursh SH. The molecular basis of intractable diarrhoea of infancy. Baillieres Clin Gastroenterol 1997; 11:413–40.

106. Roy SK, Tomkins AM, Akramuzzaman SM, et al. Randomised controlled trial of zinc supplementation in malnourished Bangladeshi children with acute diarrhoea. Arch Dis Child 1997; 77:196–200.

107. Velasquez-Melendez G, Roncada MJ, Toporovski J, Okani ET, Wilson D. Relationship between acute diarrhoea and low plasma levels of vitamin A and retinol binding protein. Rev Int Med Trop Sao Paulo 1996; 38:365–9.

108. Cui L, Takagi Y, Wasa M, et al. Induction of nitric oxide synthase in rat intestine by interleukin-1 alpha may explain diarrhea associated with zinc deficiency. J Nutr 1997; 127:1729–36.

109. Darmon N, Pelissier MA, Candalh C, et al. Zinc and intestinal anaphylaxis to cow's milk proteins in malnourished guinea pigs. Pediatr Res 1997; 42:208–13.

110. Folwaczny C. Zinc and diarrhea in infants. J Trace Element Med Biol 1997; 11:116–22.

111. Rath HC, Caesar I, Roth M, Scholmerich J. Nutritional deficiencies and complications in chronic inflammatory bowel diseases. Med Klin 1998; 93:6–10.

112. Jameson S. Zinc status in pregnancy: the effect of zinc therapy on perinatal mortality, prematurity, and placental ablation. Ann NY Acad Sci 1993; 678:178–92.

113. Krasovec M, Frenk E. Acrodermatitis enteropathica secondary to Crohn's disease. Dermatology 1996; 193:361–3.

114. Ficarra G, Cicchi P, Amorosi A, Piluso S. Oral Crohn's disease and pyostomatitis vegetans. An unusual association. Oral Surg Oral Med Oral Pathol 1993; 75:220–4.

115. Valberg LS, Flanagan PR, Kertesz A, Bondy DC. Zinc absorption in inflammatory bowel disease. Dig Dis Sci 1986; 31:724–31.

116. Nishi Y, Lifshitz F, Bayne MA, Daum F, Silverberg M, Aiges H. Zinc status and its relation to growth retardation in children with

chronic inflammatory bowel disease. Am J Clin Nutr 1980; 33:2613–21.

117. Finch PW, Pricolo V, Wu A, Finkelstein SD. Increased expression of keratinocyte growth factor messenger RNA associated with inflammatory bowel disease. Gastroenterology 1996; 110:441–51.

118. Zeeh JM, Procaccino F, Hoffmann P, et al. Keratinocyte growth factor ameliorates mucosal injury in an experimental model of colitis in rats. Gastroenterology 1996; 110:1077–83.

119. Babyatsky MW, Rossiter G, Podolsky DK. Expression of transforming growth factors alpha and beta in colonic mucosa in inflammatory bowel disease. Gastroenterology 1996; 110:975–84.

120. Babyatsky MW, deBeaumont M, Thim L, Podolsky DK. Oral trefoil peptides protect against ethanol- and indomethacin-induced gastric injury in rats. Gastroenterology 1996; 110:489–97.

121. Christl SU, Scheppach W. Metabolic consequences of total colectomy. Scand J Gastroenterol 1997; 222 (Suppl):20–4.

122. Hove H, Mortensen PB. Influence of intestinal inflammation (IBD) and small and large bowel length on fecal short-chain fatty acids and lactate. Dig Dis Sci 1995; 40:1372–80.

123. Scolapio JS, Camilleri M, Fleming CR. Gastrointestinal motility considerations in patients with short-bowel syndrome. Dig Dis 1997; 15:253–62.

124. Carbonnel F, Cosnes J, Chevret S, et al. The role of anatomic factors in nutritional autonomy after extensive small bowel resection. J Parenter Enteral Nutr 1996; 20:275–80.

125. Behrend C, Jeppesen PB, Mortensen PB. Vitamin B12 absorption after ileorectal anastomosis for Crohn's disease: effect of ileal resection and time span after surgery. Eur J Gastroenterol Hepatol 1995; 7:397–400.

126. Vanderhoof JA, Langnas AN. Short-bowel syndrome in children and adults. Gastroenterology 1997; 113:1767–78.

127. Byrne TA, Morrissey TB, Nattakom TV, Ziegler TR, Wilmore DW. Growth hormone, glutamine, and a modified diet enhance nutrient absorption in patients with severe short bowel syndrome. J Parenter Enteral Nutr 1995; 19:296–302.

128. Wilmore DW, Lacey JM, Soultanakis RP, Bosch RL, Byrne TA. Factors predicting a successful outcome after pharmacologic bowel compensation. Ann Surg 1997; 226:288–92; 292–3 (discussion).

129. Scolapio JS, Camilleri M, Fleming CR, et al. Effect of growth hormone, glutamine, and diet on adaptation in short-bowel syndrome: a randomized, controlled study. Gastroenterology 1997; 113:1074–81.

130. Becker K, Lindner C, Frieling T, Niederau C, Reinauer H, Haussinger D. Intestinal protein leakage in the acquired immunodeficiency syndrome. J Clin Gastroenterol 1997; 25:426–8.

131. Miura S, Yoshioka M, Tanaka S, et al. Faecal clearance of alpha 1-antitrypsin reflects disease activity and correlates with rapid turnover proteins in chronic inflammatory bowel disease. J Gastroenterol Hepatol 1991; 6:49–52.

132. Dolz C, Raurich JM. Energy expenditure of patients with Crohn's disease. Course study during hospitalization. Rev Esp Enferm Dig 1995; 87:702–6.

133. Butzner JD, Gall DG. Effects of chronic protein-calorie malnutrition on small intestinal repair after an acute bacterial enteritis: a study in infant rabbits. Pediatr Res 1988; 23:408–13.

134. McMurray DN, Rey H, Casazza LJ, Watson RR. Effect of moderate malnutrition on concentrations of immunoglobulins and enzymes in tears and saliva of young Colombian children. Am J Clin Nutr 1977; 30:1944–8.

135. Higgens CS, Matthews JB, Allan RN. Delayed hypersensitivity skin reactivity of patients with Crohn's disease: relationship with percentage ideal body weight and change after surgery. Hum Nutr Clin Nutr 1983; 37:143–6.

136. Muller MJ, Schmidt LU, Korber J, von zur Muhlen A, Canzler H, Schmidt FW. Reduced metabolic efficiency in patients with Crohn's disease. Dig Dis Sci 1993; 38:2001–9.

137. Riordan SM, McIver CJ, Thomas DH, Duncombe VM, Bolin TD, Thomas MC. Luminal bacteria and small-intestinal permeability. Scand J Gastroenterol 1997; 32:556–63.

138. Jorizzo JL, Apisarnthanarax P, Subrt P, et al. Bowel-bypass syndrome without bowel bypass. Bowel-associated dermatosis–arthritis syndrome. Arch Intern Med 1983; 143:457–61.

139. Leung FW, Drenick EJ, Stanley TM. Intestinal bypass complications involving the excluded small bowel segment. Am J Gastroenterol 1982; 77:67–72.

140. Kaufman SS, Loseke CA, Lupo JV, et al. Influence of bacterial overgrowth and intestinal inflammation on duration of parenteral nutrition in children with short bowel syndrome. J Pediatr 1997; 131:356–61.

28 Diet and Allograft Rejection

RICHARD V. PEREZ AND STEVEN KATZNELSON

INTRODUCTION

Transplantation has become an accepted mode of therapy for irreversible failure of different organs. In recent years, advances in surgical techniques, critical care medicine, and the development of better immunosuppressive protocols have led to improved results in transplantation. Kidney, liver, pancreas, heart, and lung transplants can be performed with an expected 75–93% 1-yr graft survival rate *(1)*. As the indications for transplantation continue to broaden and as more successful immunosuppressive modalities develop, the transplant population will continue to increase. An understanding of the unique metabolic and nutritional needs of this patient population will enable us to counsel these patients better and intervene therapeutically, if necessary.

Considering the diversity of patients receiving the various thoracic or intra-abdominal transplanted organs, the large number of disease processes leading to organ failure, and the different degrees of surgical stress involved with each individual operation, it is difficult to generalize when discussing the nutritional management of these patients. Immunosuppressive protocols also differ from organ to organ, as well as among transplant centers. Nevertheless, because all transplant recipients must receive immunosuppression for life, there are observations that can be made that are applicable to all.

Several reviews on the general principles of the nutritional management of patients before and after solid organ transplantation have been recently published *(2–6)*. This review will focus on the specific role of nutritional intervention aimed at modulating the immune response to an allograft. The ultimate goal is the optimization of nutritional support as one component in the overall immunosuppressive therapy used in the prevention of acute and chronic allograft rejection.

IMMUNOLOGY OF ACUTE AND CHRONIC ALLOGRAFT REJECTION

ACUTE REJECTION   Our understanding of acute allograft rejection is incomplete, although advances during the last decade have more clearly elucidated the cellular and molecular events involved in the initiation and mediation of this process. Both alloantigen-

From: *Nutrition and Immunology: Principles and Practice* (ME Gershwin et al. eds.), © Humana Press, Inc., Totowa, NJ

specific and nonspecific components contribute to the immune response, which can be divided into four phases: alloantigen recognition, lymphocyte activation, clonal expansion, and allograft inflammation (Table 1). For a more extensive discussion of acute rejection, see the recent reviews by Valente, Coffman, Suthanthiran, and Krensky *(7–10)*.

Initiation of the immune response involves T-lymphocyte recognition of alloantigen presented by antigen-presenting cells (APC). This process involves internalization of alloantigen by the APC, proteolysis, and processing of the antigen into allopeptides that are then expressed on the cell surface in the antigen-binding groove of class II major histocompatibility complex (MHC) molecules. This MHC-bound allopeptide is recognized by the lymphocyte at the T-cell receptor (TCR), a heterodimer complex with associated membrane proteins necessary for activation of the T cell.

Recent evidence has shown that the activation of T lymphocytes involves two signals. The first signal, as described above, involves engagement of the allopeptide presented by an APC with the TCR complex. Binding of the allopeptide will initiate a cascade of cytosolic signal transduction pathways involving protein tyrosine kinases. T-Cell activation and proliferation and production of cytokines will not occur without a second, costimulatory signal that involves binding of membrane-associated proteins on the APC with their complementary ligands on the T cell. A number of costimulatory molecules on the APC have been identified, the two most prominent being B7 and CD40, that bind to T-cell membrane proteins CD28 and CD40-ligand, respectively.

T-Cell expansion and the subsequent localized inflammatory response within the allograft is analogous to a classical delayed-type hypersensitivity reaction. Initial recruitment of inflammatory cells to the allograft involves enhanced expression of adhesion molecules L-selectin by host leukocytes and P- and E-selectin by activated allograft endothelium. Firm adhesion of leukocytes to the endothelium is facilitated by integrins (LFA-1 and VLA-4 released by inflammatory cells) that interact with their respective ligands (ICAM-1, -2, -3, VCAM-1) expressed by the activated endothelial cells. Antigen-specific and nonspecific T cells, B cells, and macrophages infiltrate the rejecting allograft and cause subsequent release of inflammatory cytokines such as interleukin-1, tumor necrosis factor-α, and interferon-γ, important mediators of this response. Finally, nonspecific inflammatory molecules,

Table 1
Molecular and Cellular Events in Acute Allograft Rejection

Alloantigen recognition	Lymphocyte activation	Clonal expansion	Graft infiltration
APC allopeptide processing and presentation in context of MHC molecule	First signal: binding of allopeptide at TCR complex Second signal: costimulatory molecule engagement	Expression of adhesion molecules at graft site	Graft infiltrating cells secrete cytokines (IL-1, TNF-α, interferon-γ)
T-Cell recognition of MHC-bound allopeptide at TCR site	Induction of cytosolic signal transduction pathways	Recruitment of inflammatory cells to allograft	Release of nonspecific inflammatory mediators (lipid metabolites, chemokines, etc.)

including the chemokines, lipid mediators derived from arachidonic acid and the complement, have been shown to be active in the acute rejection process.

It is possible that dietary intervention may influence cellular interactions involving many of these mediators and, thus, ameliorate the rejection response.

CHRONIC REJECTION   Chronic allograft rejection is the major barrier to long-term survival of all allografts. Its incidence varies among organs, from an estimated 5% in liver to 40–50% in heart and lung allografts (10). The pathogenesis is not completely understood, but it is thought to be secondary to both alloantigen-dependent and alloantigen independent factors (Table 2). Antigen-dependent factors such as acute rejection, poor HLA matching, and prior alloantigen sensitization have been shown to be associated with chronic rejection in renal allograft patients (11,12). Non-antigen-dependent factors contributing to chronic rejection include ischemia/reperfusion injury, hypercholesterolemia, cytomegalovirus infection, and drug toxicity. Pathologic findings common to all organs include increased extracellular matrix accumulation with interstitial fibrosis as well as evidence of endothelial injury with subsequent smooth-muscle proliferation and obliterative vasculopathy. This appears to be mediated by both macrophages and lymphocytes (13–15.).

The hallmark of chronic allograft rejection is occlusive vascular changes leading to chronic ischemia, fibrosis, and atrophy of parenchymal cells. Renal allografts exhibit tubular atrophy and thickening of the glomerular basement membrane. Chronic hepatic rejection is characterized by obliterative vasculopathy of medium-sized and large hepatic arterioles with bile duct loss (16). Chronic cardiac rejection presents with diffuse coronary artery atherosclerosis, and lung allografts present with obliteration of graft bronchioles. Chronic allograft rejection is uniformly progressive, with no effective treatment except retransplantation.

Table 2
Contributing Factors
to Chronic Rejection/Allograft Vasculopathy

Alloantigen dependent	Alloantigen independent
Acute rejection	Ischemia–reperfusion injury
Poor HLA match	Hypercholesterolemia
Prior sensitization	Drug toxicity
	Suboptimal immunosuppression
	Late cytomegalovirus infection

Many similarities exist between chronic allograft vasculopathy and atherosclerosis of native vessels. As such, dietary or pharmacologic interventions such as reduction of serum cholesterol may have a beneficial effect. We will discuss such dietary interventions in both experimental and clinical transplantation studies later in this chapter.

METABOLIC SIDE EFFECTS OF IMMUNOSUPPRESSIVE AGENTS

All of the immunosuppressive agents currently in use have an effect on nutrient metabolism or intake (Table 3). The following medications are used to varying degrees in all thoracic and abdominal transplants.

Corticosteroids are a mainstay in the immunosuppressive therapy after transplantation. The large initial doses given perioperatively are usually rapidly tapered over a period of weeks to months. Because of the side effects and complications of long-term corticosteroid use, many centers attempt to discontinue corticosteroids sometime in the first year posttransplantation; however, this discontinuance has been associated with an increased risk of rejection is some patients. Therefore, a significant number of transplant recipients remain on low-dose oral prednisone indefinitely. There are several mechanisms of glucocorticoid action, but the dominant effect appears to be the inhibition of macrophage acute-phase reactant and cytokine production, which is an important component of lymphocyte activation during allograft rejection. Important steroid-induced metabolic alterations include increased protein catabolism, especially with high doses, increased appetite, sodium retention, insulin resistance with hyperglycemia, hyperlipidemia, and calciuria.

The introduction of *cyclosporine* into clinical transplantation in 1980 was a significant breakthrough resulting in improved graft survival after kidney, heart, liver, and pancreas transplantation. It has a relatively selective inhibitory action on T-lymphocyte interleukin-2 production without significant bone marrow suppression. This inhibitory action of cyclosporine occurs by binding of cyclosporine to the cytoplasmic protein, calcineurin, which is necessary for the activation of several T-cell activation genes, including interleukin-2. Cyclosporine, however, is not without side effects, the most common being nephrotoxicity and hypertension. It has also been shown to contribute to posttransplant hyperlipidemia, hyperkalemia, hypomagnesemia, and glucose intolerance.

Tacrolimus, otherwise known as FK506 or Prograf, is a macrolide antibiotic with immunosuppressive properties similar to, but

Table 3
Nutritional and Metabolic Side Effects of Commonly Used Immunosuppressive Agents

Medication	Immunosuppressive mechanism	Metabolic side effect
Prednisone	Inhibition of macrophage cytokine and acute-phase reactant production	Hyperglycemia, sodium and fluid retention, calcium wasting, hyperlipidemia
Cyclosporine	Inhibition of T-lymphocyte IL-2 production	Nausea, gastritis, hyperkalemia, hypertension, hyperlipidemia, hyperglycemia, hyperuricemia, hypomagnesemia
Azathioprine	Inhibition of DNA synthesis (purine analog)	Nausea, decreased taste, anemia
Antilymphocyte antibodies	Lymphocyte cytotoxicity	Fever, anorexia, diarrhea
Mycophenolate mofetil	Inhibition of DNA synthesis Inhibition of adhesion molecule expression	Nausea, anorexia, gastritis, diarrhea, anemia
Tacrolimus	Inhibition of T-lymphocyte IL-2 production	Nausea, diarrhea, hyperkalemia, hypomagnesemia, hypertension, hyperglycemia

much more potent than cyclosporine. Although biochemically distinct from cyclosporine, its mechanism of action is similar (i.e., via inhibition of calcineurin). The side-effect profile is also similar to that of cyclosporine and includes nephrotoxicity and neurotoxicity. Tacrolimus may cause more gastrointestinal symptoms than cyclosporine, including mild nausea and diarrhea, and is probably more diabetogenic. Unlike cyclosporine, however, tacrolimus is not associated with significant hypercholesterolemia.

Azathioprine (Imuran), a derivative of 6-mercaptopurine, is a purine analog antimetabolite that has been used in clinical transplantation since the early 1960s. It is generally well tolerated by most patients but can result in nausea, vomiting, altered taste acuity, and liver dysfunction. It also can be a very potent bone marrow suppressant, requiring frequent monitoring for leukopenia. The development of newer more potent immunosuppressants in recent years has led to a significant decrease in the use of azathioprine.

Mycophenolate mofetil (CellCept) is an inhibitor of inosine monophosphate dehydrogenase, the rate-limiting enzyme involved in *de novo* purine synthesis. Lymphocytes are more dependent on *de novo* purine synthesis than other cells that are able to utilize "salvage" pathways. Thus, mycophenolate mofetil has a selective effect of inhibiting the proliferation of lymphocytes. It also has an inhibitory effect on the expression of adhesion molecules necessary for lymphocyte–endothelial cell interactions. The effectiveness of this agent was initially shown in large clinical renal transplant trials (17,18) and is now being evaluated for other organs. The side effects of mycophenolate mainly involve the gastrointestinal tract, including esophagitis, gastritis, and diarrhea.

The development of *antilymphocyte antibody* preparations has contributed to improved clinical outcomes in transplantation. These preparations are used by some centers prophylactically for the prevention of rejection in the early posttransplant induction phase of immunosuppression. They are also used in the treatment of acute rejection episodes not responsive to high-dose corticosteroid therapy. The most widely used polyclonal antilymphocyte preparations have similar side effects, including a virus-like syndrome of fever, myalgias, and anorexia. The more potent monoclonal antibody, OKT-3, directed against the CD3 lymphocyte cell-surface marker commonly causes a severe cytokine-release syndrome characterized by high fever, pulmonary edema, and diarrhea. These side effects usually occur after the first two or three doses, during which time nutritional intake may be markedly reduced. Subsequent doses are usually well tolerated.

EXPERIMENTAL DIETARY IMMUNOMODULATION IN TRANSPLANTATION

FATTY ACIDS Multiple studies of dietary intervention in transplantation have involved dietary lipids, specifically polyunsaturated fatty acids. The metabolism and immunosuppressive properties of these fatty acids have been well documented and discussed elsewhere (see Chapter 13). Although multiple mechanisms have been proposed, the immunosuppressive effect of these dietary lipids appears to be mediated via alterations in arachidonic acid metabolism. The metabolites of arachidonic acid, particularly certain prostaglandins and leukotrienes, have both immunosuppressive and immunostimulatory properties (19,20). Several investigators (19,21–23) have demonstrated prolongation of experimental skin, kidney, and cardiac allograft survival with polyunsaturated fatty acid-enriched diets.

Omega-3 fatty acids, the major component of fish oil, have been shown by some investigators to be particularly immunosuppressive in various models of experimental transplantation (24–27), although one study failed to show a benefit (28). The possible mechanisms of the beneficial effect of fish oil are multiple, affecting both lymphocytes and macrophages, and have been recently reviewed (29). The immunomodulating effects of fish oil include inhibition of lymphocyte proliferation, cytokine production, and cytotoxicity. Fish oil also has been shown to have multiple effects on macrophage function, including alteration of phagocytosis, chemotaxis, antigen presentation, and modulation of secretory products, including cytokines, nitric oxide, and oxygen free radicals. A particular beneficial effect relevant to transplantation is the inhibition of lymphocyte–endothelial cell adhesion (30).

Another strategy that has incorporated dietary intervention is the use of fatty acids to potentiate the immunosuppressive effects of other agents. Dietary immunomodulation of cyclosporine-induced immunosuppression has been most extensively studied. This agent may be particularly suited for dietary immunomodulation because of evidence suggesting that one mechanism of cyclosporine-induced immunosuppression involves alteration of arachidonic acid metabolism (31). Improved immunosuppression

Table 4
Potential Beneficial Nutritional Interventions in Organ Transplantation

Clinical setting	Nutritional intervention	Possible protective mechanism
Ischemia–reperfusion injury	Vitamins A, C, and E	Antioxidants
Acute rejection	Polyunsaturated fatty acids	Production of immunosuppressive prostaglandins and leukotrienes; inhibition of cytokine production
	ω-3 Fatty acids	Lymphocyte, macrophage inhibition; modulation of cytokine, nitric oxide, and free-radical production; inhibition of adhesion molecule expression
	HMG-CoA reductase inhibitors	Inhibit NK cells; inhibit lymphocyte cytotoxicity
	Vitamins A, C and E	Antioxidants
Chronic rejection	ω-3 Fatty acids	(See above)
	L-arginine	Enhanced nitric oxide production
	HMG-CoA Reductase inhibitors	Inhibits smooth-muscle proliferation
	Vitamins A, C, and E	Antioxidant
	Vitamin B/folic acid	Decreases serum homocysteine levels

has been demonstrated with the use of a prostaglandin E_1 (PGE$_1$) analog in combination with cyclosporine *(32)*. Accordingly, dietary supplementation with the arachidonic acid precursor, linoleic acid, was shown to augment the immunosuppressive effect of cyclosporine, prolonging graft survival in a rodent heart transplant model *(33)*. Omega-3 fatty acid supplementation, most commonly in the form of fish oil, has also been used to augment the immunosuppressive effect of cyclosporine *(34)*. Dietary supplementation with fish oil has the added benefit of ameliorating cyclosporine-induced nephrotoxicity, possibly by altering the production of intrarenal prostaglandins *(35)*.

Dietary fatty acids have also been used as a means of potentiating the immunosuppressive effects of blood transfusions. The immunosuppressive effects of blood transfusions have been well documented *(36)*. Transfusions have been shown to mediate their effect by increasing the production of immunosuppressive arachidonic acid metabolites, such as prostaglandin E_2 *(37,38)*. Augmentation of transfusion-induced immunosuppression with the use of dietary omega-6 arachidonic acid precursors has been demonstrated and long-term tolerance attained in a rat model of heart transplantation *(33,39)*. The omega-3 and -9 fatty acids have also been shown to be immunosuppressive, although the mechanism is not completely understood and may be completely independent of prostaglandin production *(40,41)*. Recently, short-chain fatty acids have been shown to have an immunomodulating effect on transfusions in models of transplantation *(42)*. The rationale behind the use of short-chain fatty acids, particularly butyric acid, is their ability to enhance gene transcription of immunosuppressive mediators such as PGE$_2$, as has been previously shown *(43)*.

A unique approach to modulation of the immune response to an allograft is via modification of donor tissue immunogenicity by dietary manipulation. Schreiner showed that kidneys transplanted from rat donors fed a diet deficient in essential fatty acids sustained less acute rejection than kidneys from control-diet-fed donors *(44)*. The mechanism was thought to be a lack of tissue macrophages (dendritic cells) in the renal allograft resulting from decreased production of leukotriene B$_4$, a potent chemotactic substance. Comparable studies, however, in the same *(45)* and in a different rat strain combination did not demonstrate a benefit of essential fatty acid-deficient diets administered to kidney donors *(46)*. A similar strategy of dietary immunomodulation of the donor was recently reported by Ishikawa et al. in a porcine model of liver

transplantation *(47)*. In this study, livers transplanted from fasted donors showed prolonged survival when compared to those from fed controls. The protective effect of donor fasting in this study was postulated to be secondary to inactivation of the macrophage population of the hepatic allograft. These results differ somewhat from those reported by Sadamori et al. in a previous study using the same model *(48)*. Here, livers from fasted donors did poorly after transplantation. However, if intravenous glucose was provided during the fasted state, posttransplant allograft survival was markedly improved. The donor liver level of glycogen storage and ATP generation after reperfusion were thought to be important nutritionally dependent factors that influenced outcome.

CHOLESTEROL-LOWERING PROTOCOLS Several animal studies have suggested a relationship between hypercholesterolemia and chronic transplant vasculopathy *(49–53)*, although this relationship has been questioned by at least one study *(54)*. It has been hypothesized that high cholesterol levels may initiate growth-factor-mediated proliferation of the transplant vascular walls, upregulate class II antigen expression, and act as a chemoattractant, drawing circulating lymphoid cells to the graft. These factors may be important in the initiation and propagation of both acute and chronic allograft rejection. To our knowledge, treatment of hypercholesterolemia by dietary means alone has not been studied in animal models of acute or chronic rejection. One study, however, used a surgical partial ileal bypass to lower serum cholesterol in a rabbit cardiac transplant model of graft vasculopathy *(55)*. In this model, lowering of serum cholesterol partially mitigated the fatty intimal proliferation of graft vasculopathy, suggesting a possible cholesterol-dependent and -independent mechanism.

A number of studies have demonstrated a reduction in acute or chronic rejection with the use of the cholesterol-lowering agents 3-hydroxy-3-methylglutaryl coenzyme A (HMG-CoA) reductase inhibitors in experimental transplantation. These agents have been used extensively in clinical practice with effective reduction in serum cholesterol level, incidence of myocardial infarction, and cardiovascular mortality in nontransplant patients *(56)*. The immunomodulatory effects of these agents was first noted in clinical heart transplant recipients who had a reduction in acute rejection episodes with the use of the HMG-CoA reductase inhibitor pravastatin *(57)*. Subsequent animal studies have shown a decrease in chronic allograft vasculopathy in models of rat heart *(58,59)* and liver *(60)* transplantation; however, the effect may be via a choles-

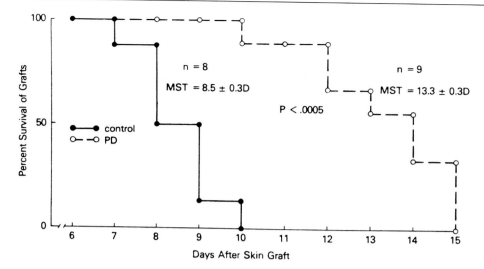

Fig. 1. Improved skin graft survival with protein-deficient diets. (Adapted from ref. *72*.)

terol-independent mechanism. Another study also recently demonstrated that pravastatin protects murine pancreatic islet isografts from immune-mediated primary nonfunction *(61)*. The immunosuppressive effects of the HMG-CoA reductase inhibitors are multiple and include inhibition of natural-killer cells *(62)*, monocyte chemotaxis *(63)*, T-lymphocyte cytotoxicity/proliferation *(64,65)*, and B-lymphocyte activation *(66)*. These cholesterol-lowering medications may also have a synergistic effect with cyclosporine in the treatment of chronic vasculopathy, as has recently been shown in a rat femoral artery transplant model *(67)*. Subsequent reports of the clinical use of cholesterol-lowering agents in heart *(57)*, kidney *(68)*, and liver *(69)* patients will be discussed later in the chapter.

PROTEIN The immunodeficient state resulting from chronic protein malnutrition has been well documented *(70,71)*. The effect of protein malnourishment on allograft survival is not completely known. Utilizing a rat skin allograft model, Austin demonstrated that protein-caloric restriction resulted in a significant increase in graft survival as well as a decrease in cytotoxic alloantibody production *(72;* Fig. 1). Conversely, other studies in similar rodent models of skin allografts have failed to show a beneficial effect of protein-caloric malnourishment on allograft survival *(73,74)*. The evidence, therefore, is not compelling that restriction of protein would confer a beneficial effect on allograft survival in the clinical setting and, in fact, could render a patient more susceptible to problems with wound healing or infection.

Nutritional modulation of the immune response with dietary supplementation of specific amino acids has been examined in models of infection, trauma, wound healing, and cancer *(75)*. Dietary amino acids in models of transplantation have been limited mostly to studies using arginine. This well-studied amino acid has potent endocrine effects stimulating the production of growth hormone, prolactin, insulin, and insulin-like growth factor, all of which have potent immunostimulatory effects *(76)*. Interestingly, arginine supplementation as part of an "immuno-enhancing" diet was shown to significantly prolong cardiac allograft survival in a model of transfusion-induced immunosuppression *(41)*. The overall immunosuppressive effect of this arginine-enriched diet may have been the result of other components in the study diet,

such as omega-3 fatty acids, or to the enhanced production of immunosuppressive mediators, as was suggested by Levy et al.

Recent attention has been focused on the role of arginine in models of chronic rejection resulting from vasculopathy of the allograft. The pathogenesis of this vascular lesion is thought to be similar to that of the atherosclerotic intimal hyperplasia of native vessels. The protective effect of L-arginine, a precursor to nitric oxide, in models of native intimal hyperplasia has been demonstrated *(77,78)*. Nitric oxide maintains active vasodilator tone in normal blood vessels, in contrast to atherosclerotic vessels, where the activity of nitric oxide is impaired, leading to decreased endothelium-dependent vasodilation and intimal thickening. Dietary L-arginine restores vascular relaxation, reduces the release of superoxide radicals, and inhibits the production of intimal lipid plaques *(79,80)*. The importance of nitric oxide as a protective molecule in a model of chronic allograft rejection was recently demonstrated *(81)*. Using gene knockout mice deficient in inducible nitric oxide synthase, this study showed that nitric oxide suppressed neointimal smooth-muscle accumulation in a heterotopic cardiac transplant model of chronic vasculopathy. In another study using a rat aortic allograft model, Shears et al. demonstrated the suppressive effect of nitric oxide on graft vasculopathy *(82)*. In this study, inhibitors of nitric oxide synthase significantly worsened the vascular lesion, whereas enhanced nitric oxide production via gene transfer completely suppressed allograft vasculopathy. Further evidence to support a possible protective effect of nitric oxide on chronic rejection is a recent study of dietary L-arginine supplementation in a rabbit cardiac allograft model *(83)*. In this study, L-arginine (2.5% added to drinking water for 5 wk) increased plasma nitric oxide levels and attenuated transplant vasculopathy possibly by modulation of vascular smooth-muscle cell response to mitogens such as insulin-like growth factor-1 and interleukin-6. The potential benefit of L-arginine supplementation in the development or treatment of chronic rejection in clinical transplantation warrants further investigation.

A limited number of studies have examined the potential beneficial effect of the amino acid glutamine on allograft function in models of intestinal transplantation. Glutamine is a preferred fuel of the normal enterocyte that improves intestinal structure and function (84). The efficacy of glutamine, given either enterally or intravenously, has been shown to improve mucosal structure, glucose absorption, and bacterial translocation in nonimmunosuppressed (85,86) and cyclosporine-treated rats after small-bowel transplantation (87). The effect of glutamine supplementation on allograft immunogenicity and/or frequency of intestinal allograft rejection has not been examined.

NUCLEOTIDES   Dietary nucleotides have been shown to be necessary for normal humoral and cell-mediated immunity (88–90). As such, one strategy for induction of immunosuppression in experimental models of transplantation has been the administration of nucleotide-free diets (90). Van Buren et al. have shown that nucleotide-free diets alone will prolong murine cardiac allograft survival (91) and, when administered with cyclosporine, will result in synergistic prolongation of rat cardiac allograft survival (92). Nucleotide restriction was shown to primarily inhibit T-helper-lymphocyte function in this model (93). To date, this strategy has not been used in clinical transplantation, possibly because of the increased susceptibility to infection observed with dietary nucleotide restriction.

VITAMINS

Antioxidants   Organs to be transplanted are subjected to a period of cold ischemia during preservation and warm ischemia during subsequent surgical implantation. As such, transplantation is a clinically pertinent model of ischemia–reperfusion injury. This immune-mediated injury is characterized by leukocyte interaction with the endothelial surface of the allograft, with the release of acute-phase reactant cytokines, adhesion molecules, arachidonic acid metabolites, MHC antigens, and oxygen free radicals (94). Resident macrophages within the allograft may also be important in this process. In an attempt to minimize the injury mediated by reactive oxygen species, several investigators have used antioxidant vitamins, mainly C (ascorbic acid) and E (α-tocopherol), in experimental models of transplantation related ischemia–reperfusion injury. Antioxidant administration within the organ preservation solution (95) or intravenously to the donor (96) has been shown to be effective in models of kidney and pancreas transplantation, respectively. Dietary vitamin supplementation of either ascorbic acid or α-tocopherol to the recipient, in combination with low-dose cyclosporine, was shown to delay allograft rejection in a rat cardiac allograft model (97). Oxygen-derived free-radical injury was determined to contribute to the rejection process in this model. Vitamin E as a dietary supplement has also recently been shown to ameliorate rejection in the immunologically incompatible setting of xenotransplantation (98). Both low (150 mg/kg/chow)- and high (8000 mg/kg/chow)-dose vitamin E-fed animals sustained a reduction in leukocyte-mediated microvascular rejection in a rat to hamster model of pancreatic islet cell xenotransplantation.

These studies stress the importance of strategies to lessen the injury of ischemia–reperfusion at the time of transplantation and in the possible prevention of acute rejection. Another important aspect of ischemia–reperfusion injury is its possible role in the subsequent development of chronic allograft rejection (94). The enhanced expression of leukocyte chemotactants and adhesion molecules seen with reperfusion injury are the same molecules seen at the endothelial surface expressed in chronic rejection (99). Additionally, oxygen free-radical species have been shown to directly induce the proliferation of vascular endothelial smooth-muscle cells (100). Ischemic injury has been correlated with the

development of chronic rejection in experimental (101,102) and clinical transplantation (103). The effect of long-term antioxidant therapy on allograft function or the vasculopathy of chronic rejection is unknown. ONe recent preliminary report suggests a possible effect of vitamin C (but not vitamin E) in ameliorating the severity of transplant coronary artery disease in a rodent model of cardiac transplantation (104). It is clear that the potential benefit of antioxidative therapy in the setting of chronic vasculopathy needs further investigation. This is underscored by the known safety and efficacy of these agents used clinically (105) and by the increasing evidence of their protective effect against native coronary artery disease (106,107).

Vitamin A   The retinoids encompass a range of compounds related to vitamin A and are known antioxidants, but they have been studied mainly for their immunopotentiating properties, including enhanced delayed-type hypersensitivity, antibody production, and cytotoxicity (108,109). These immunostimulatory properties as well as an inhibitory effect on keratinization in epithelial cells have made these compounds particularly effective in the treatment of dermatologic cancers and other skin disorders (110). Transplant recipients on chronic immunosuppression therapy have been noted to have an increased incidence of malignancies, the most common being malignant skin lesions (111–113). Consequently, there has been interest in the use of retinoids in transplant recipients. The possible interference with ongoing immunosuppression regimens and potential precipitation of rejection by vitamin A has resulted in a number of studies addressing this concern. Studies in experimental models of skin (114,115), kidney (116), and cardiac transplantation (117) have shown that vitamin A compounds do not compromise the immunosuppressive effect of standard steroid-, cyclosporine-, or azathioprine-based protocols. The effect of vitamin A on the newer agents such as tacrolimus and mycophenolic acid are not known; however, it is probably that these compounds can be cautiously used in immunosuppressed recipients with premalignant or malignant skin lesions.

Vitamin B_6/B_12 and Folic Acid   Recent attention has been focused on hyperhomocysteinemia as a risk factor for the development of atherosclerosis (118). Preliminary clinical studies have also suggested that hyperhomocysteinemia may also be a risk factor for transplant vasculopathy/chronic rejection (119). There have been no controlled studies regarding dietary interventions in experimental models of transplantation; however, clinical studies in nontransplant patients have shown that vitamin B_6/B_{12} and folic acid supplementation will decrease serum homocysteine levels. The early clinical experience with vitamin supplementation and homocysteine levels will be discussed separately in the clinical kidney and heart transplant sections to follow.

NUTRITIONALLY RELATED CLINICAL STUDIES IN TRANSPLANTATION

KIDNEY

Fatty Acids   As early as 1974, Uldall et al. reported a beneficial effect of polyunsaturated linoleic acid supplementation (as sunflower seed oil) in an uncontrolled study in renal transplantation (120). This led the same center to perform a controlled trial of polyunsaturated fatty acid supplementation (primrose oil, 74% linoleic acid) in recipients of cadaveric renal allografts (121). In this prospective, double-blinded study of 90 patients, graft survival in the fatty-acid-fed group was superior during the first 3–4 mo

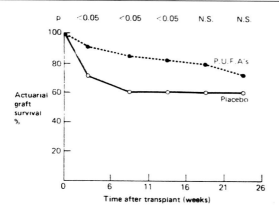

Fig. 2. Improved short-term kidney allograft survival with dietary polyunsaturated fatty acid supplementation. (Adapted from ref. *121.*)

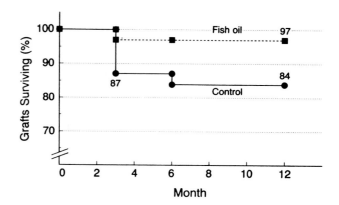

Fig. 4. Effect of dietary fish oil supplementation on renal allograft survival. (Adapted from ref. *122.*)

posttransplant, but by 6 mo, the difference in survival no longer reached statistical significance (Fig. 2).

Several clinical studies have assessed the potential benefit of omega-3 fatty acid supplementation in recipients of renal allografts. Early studies demonstrated that dietary fish oil improved renal function in stable patients *(122)* and in those with renal dysfunction resulting from chronic vascular rejection *(123)*. Subsequent studies examined the use of fish oil prophylactically at the time of transplant or shortly thereafter. Berthoux et al. randomized patients to receive 9 g of fish oil/d starting on d 3 after transplantation and continuing for 1 yr *(124)*. Fish oil supplementation improved renal blood flow and function, but no difference was seen regarding rejection episodes between groups. Van der Heide et al. subsequently showed improved hemodynamics, blood pressure control, renal function, and fewer rejection episodes in patients receiving fish oil (6 g/d for 1 yr) after transplantation *(122;* Fig. 3). The improved rejection rate observed in fish-oil-treated patients did not result in a significant difference in allograft survival (Fig. 4). Others confirmed a beneficial effect of fish oil when started at the time of transplant *(125)*, but fish oil was of little value when started 16 wk after transplant *(126)*.

Cholesterol-Lowering Protocols As was discussed earlier with models of experimental transplantation, recent evidence has suggested a causative role of hypercholesterolemia in the pathogenesis of acute and chronic allograft rejection. Clinical reports in

renal transplantation have also established an association between cholesterol levels and allograft rejection, although this relationship remains controversial. Separate studies by Dimeny et al. and Isoniemi et al. have demonstrated that elevations in serum cholesterol levels may be associated with the development of chronic rejection in kidney transplant recipients *(127,128)*. Dimeny et al. also reported that patients with high pretransplant total cholesterol levels had a higher rate of acute rejections in the first 6 mo posttransplant *(129)*.

Dietary treatment of hypercholesterolemia has proven to be safe and is the standard first line of therapy. In general, most patients are instructed to comply with the American Heart Association Step II Diet as recommended by the National Cholesterol Education Program *(130)*. However, it has been shown that dietary therapy alone may be inadequate in a significant percentage of transplant patients *(131)*. As such, many patients will require pharmacologic intervention in the posttransplant setting.

All of the clinically available antihyperlipidemic agents have been used successfully to treat posttransplant hyperlipidemia *(132)*. Each of the commonly used agents such as nicotinic acid, fibric acid derivatives, and bile acid resins have adverse side effects in the transplant setting, thus limiting their usefulness. The HMG-CoA reductase inhibitors have been shown to be effective in reducing lipid levels after kidney transplantation *(133–135)* and their immunosuppressive properties make them particularly attractive in the transplant setting. The clinical usefulness of these agents has recently been reported in a prospective randomized pilot study in cadaveric kidney transplantation *(68)*. Forty-eight patients were randomized to a group taking pravastatin at 20 mg/d or to a control group. All patients in this study were maintained on a double immunosuppressive regiment with prednisone and cyclosporine. The pravastatin-treated patients had decreases in acute rejection episodes and in the use of both OKT3 and solumedrol antirejection therapy. In addition, the patients treated with pravastatin had a significant inhibition of natural-killer-cell cytotoxicity. The decreased rejection associated with pravastatin could not be ascribed solely to differences in total cholesterol levels between groups, suggesting a possible cholesterol-independent immunomodulatory effect of pravastatin. The effect of these agents on long-term patient or graft outcome has not yet been established.

Antioxidant Vitamins Despite significant evidence showing a benefit of antioxidant vitamins in the prevention of ischemia–

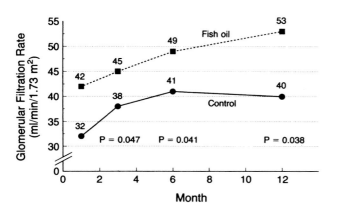

Fig. 3. Improved renal allograft filtration rate with dietary fish oil supplementation. (Adapted from ref. *122.*)

reperfusion injury and related allograft rejection in experimental transplantation, few clinical studies have addressed this issue. Rabl et al. were the first to report a prospective, double-blinded study of intravenous pretreatment with antioxidants (vitamins C, E, and A) in 30 recipients of cadaveric renal allografts *(136)*. The patients receiving vitamin pretreatment had lower levels of lipid peroxidation after transplantation and improved early allograft function when compared to controls. A similar clinical study showed a benefit of a single intraoperative intravenous dose of vitamin C (500 mg) prior to reperfusion of the allograft in renal transplantation *(137)*. To date, we are aware of no studies using dietary antioxidant supplementation in clinical renal transplantation. The advantage of a more sustained vitamin supplementation in this setting has become more apparent recently with the demonstration of reperfusion-induced free-radical activity in the renal allograft still present days after transplantation *(138)*. As previously discussed, sustained dietary antioxidant supplementation may be effective short-term treatment of the ischemia–reperfusion injury at the time of transplantation; however, a possible more important benefit may be in the prevention or treatment of allograft vasculopathy secondary to chronic rejection. In view of recent evidence demonstrating a benefit of dietary antioxidants in atherosclerotic disease in nonimmunosuppressed patients *(106)*, the possible potential protective effect of these agents against the development of chronic allograft vasculopathy warrants further investigation.

Vitamin B/Folate   The significance of hyperhomocysteinemia as a risk factor for the development of coronary artery, cerebrovascular, and peripheral vascular disease in the general population has recently been established *(118)*. It has been suggested that renal transplant recipients have an increased risk of arteriosclerotic outcomes *(139)* and have been reported to have an increased prevalence of hyperhomocysteinemia *(140–142)*. Reduction in plasma homocysteine levels can be achieved with dietary folic acid and vitamin B_6/B_{12} supplementation *(119)*. Whether interventions aimed at lowering plasma homocysteine levels will have an effect on arteriosclerotic vascular disease in these patients is not known. The role of hyperhomocysteinemia as a risk factor for chronic transplant vasculopathy is also not known, but is a question currently being investigated.

HEART   Current immunosuppression protocols have resulted in significant improvements in cardiac transplantation, with reported 5-yr patient survival approaching 80% *(143)*. The main indications for transplantation include cardiomyopathy and ischemic heart disease. The main limitation to further improvement in survival is allograft coronary vasculopathy, a probable manifestation of chronic rejection. Nutritional studies are lacking in this patient population, with the exception of those focused on the pretransplant malnourished state of these patients *(144,145)* or on strategies to lower cholesterol levels *(132)*.

Cholesterol-Lowering Protocols   Hypercholesterolemia is observed in 60–80% of patients after cardiac transplantation *(146,147)*. Several clinical studies have shown a relationship between hypercholesterolemia and the development of allograft vasculopathy *(148–150)*. In contrast, other studies have found no relationship between cholesterol levels and graft vasculopathy *(54,151)*; therefore, this relationship remains controversial.

Dietary management of hypercholesterolemia has been shown to be largely ineffective as the sole therapeutic intervention after cardiac transplantation *(152)*. As was discussed earlier in the renal transplantation section, HMG-CoA reductase inhibitors have been

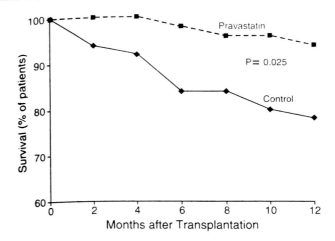

Fig. 5.   Beneficial effect of HMG-CoA reductase inhibitor in clinical cardiac transplantation. (Adapted from ref. *57*.)

used because of their dual actions of reducing lipid levels *(153,154)* and suppressing the immune response.

The first clinical report suggesting an immunomodulatory effect of HMG-CoA reductase inhibitors in transplant recipients originated in the heart transplant literature *(57)*. In a prospective randomized trial of the sue of pravastatin early after heart transplantation, patients receiving daily pravastatin therapy had an increased 1-yr survival that coincided with a decrease in clinically severe acute rejection episodes (Fig. 5). This group of patients was also followed to assess the effect of pravastatin on the incidence and progression of allograft vasculopathy. The total number of patients found to have allograft vasculopathy by angiography or autopsy was less in the pravastatin-treated group than in the control group. In a subgroup of patients, intracoronary ultrasound showed that pravastatin-treated patients had less progression of allograft vasculopathy than control patients. In another, more recent prospective randomized study with a 4-yr follow-up, the HMG-CoA reductase inhibitor simvastatin was compared to dietary measures alone in 72 cardiac transplant recipients *(155)*. Simvastatin treatment resulted in a decrease in cholesterol levels, less allograft vasculopathy progression, and higher long-term survival.

Consistent with the previous similar study in kidney patients, the decreased incidence of rejection associated with pravastatin use could not be ascribed solely to differences in total cholesterol levels between groups. This suggests that the immunomodulatory effect of pravastatin is cholesterol-level independent.

Antioxidant Vitamins   The beneficial effect of antioxidant vitamin supplementation after renal transplantation has been previously discussed. Logeril reported the use of dietary vitamin E supplementation in 20 clinically stable heart transplant recipients *(156)*. Improved immunosuppression, decreased cyclosporine nephrotoxicity, and reduction in thrombotic complications were noted with vitamin E supplementation. The antithrombotic effect was thought to be secondary to decreased platelet aggregation in the vitamin E-treated patients.

Vitamin B/Folate   As previously discussed, hyperhomocysteinemia has been shown to be a risk factor for the development of atherosclerotic complications in the general population and in patients who have undergone renal transplantation. Similar studies in patients after cardiac transplantation are few; however, recent

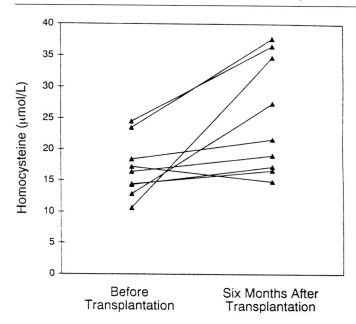

Fig. 6. Increased serum homocysteine levels in patients after cardiac transplantation. (Adapted from ref. *157*.)

reports have suggested that elevated plasma homocysteine levels are common after cardiac transplantation (*157*, Fig. 6). The development of transplant coronary vasculopathy has also been noted to correlate with plasma homocysteine levels in one study (*158*). Interventions aimed at decreasing homocysteine levels and possibly reducing the incidence of coronary vasculopathy have not been reported after cardiac transplantation.

LIVER Although the first reported successful clinical liver transplant was in 1963, it was not until the 1980s that transplantation became an accepted therapeutic option for patients with end-stage liver disease. The past decade has been significant for progressive improvement in outcomes, with current 1-yr patient survival rates of 85% being reported by some centers (*159,160*). Patients with advanced liver disease are often malnourished because of a loss of functional hepatocyte mass resulting in a decrease in protein synthesis and impairment in the delivery of nutrients to the liver secondary to extrahepatic shunting of portal blood flow (*161–163*). A hormonal imbalance characterized by increased levels of insulin, glucagon, epinephrine, and cortisol all contribute to a state of catabolism associated with liver failure. Furthermore, salt, water, and protein intolerance in these patients makes nutritional support prior to transplantation somewhat difficult. Nutritional intervention in the setting of chronic liver dysfunction has been well studied and the goals of such therapy include limitation of catabolism, correction of vitamin/mineral deficiencies, and maintenance of metabolic balance (*164,165*).

Restoration of normal hepatic function after transplantation provides a setting in which postoperative aggressive nutritional intervention is possible. Optimization of nutritional support during the posttransplantation period has been studied. Reilly reported the first randomized prospective clinical trial comparing total parenteral nutritional (TPN) support with nontreated control patients (*166*). In this study, TPN was tolerated immediately postoperatively, improved nitrogen balance, and shortened the number of days spent in the intensive care unit. Solutions high in branch-

chain amino acids, which have been suggested to be of particular benefit in nontransplant patients with liver dysfunction and encephalopathy (*167*), had no added benefit in this study when compared to standard TPN. A subsequent study showed that enteral feeding administered via jejunal tube within 18 h postoperatively was well tolerated, of comparable efficacy to TPN, and had the potential benefit of decreasing postoperative complications and costs (*168*). Another randomized prospective study suggested that early enteral tube feedings improved some posttransplant outcomes, including infectious complications, when compared to standard oral diet (*169*).

Cholesterol-Lowering Protocols Specific dietary intervention aimed at decreasing acute or chronic rejection has not been reported in liver transplantation. One recent study (*69*), however, has focused on the potential immunosuppressive effects of the cholesterol-lowering agents HMG-CoA reductase inhibitors, as was discussed previously in heart and kidney transplantation. This study showed that posttransplant hyperlipidemia is less frequent in liver allograft recipients than in kidney or cardiac recipients. However, the HMG-CoA reductase inhibitor pravastatin did reduce serum cholesterol levels and inhibited natural-killer-cell function in these patients. Pravastatin did not have an effect on acute rejection episodes after liver transplantation, as was previously shown for both renal and cardiac transplantation.

Antioxidant Vitamins Much of the literature regarding ischemia–reperfusion injury in experimental models has focused on the liver (*94,170*). The large population of resident macrophages in the liver with the capacity to release oxygen free radicals and acute-phase cytokines makes this organ particularly susceptible to reperfusion injury at the time of transplantation. Clinical studies have confirmed the presence of increased oxygen free-radical species as potential mediators of reperfusion injury in liver recipients (*171,172*). One study measured circulating levels of antioxidants in patients about to undergo liver transplantation (*173*). Pretransplant levels of antioxidants vitamin A, vitamin E, and beta-carotene were depressed in these patients. On reperfusion of the liver allograft, vitamin A and E levels fell further and were associated with the adverse hemodynamic effects observed with ischemia–reperfusion injury. These studies support the experimental data suggesting that liver transplant patients are susceptible to free-radical-induced reperfusion injury and have lowered antioxidant defenses at the time of transplantation. Surprisingly, there is a lack of clinical studies using antioxidant therapy as a means of ameliorating this injury. Clinical trials with antioxidant vitamins are warranted.

LUNG Lung transplantation has only recently become a therapeutic option for patients with end-stage pulmonary disease. The first successful lung transplantation was performed in 1983 (*174*) and the most common indications for transplantation include chronic obstructive pulmonary disease, pulmonary fibrosis, and cystic fibrosis. Patients with end-stage pulmonary disease have been shown to be significantly malnourished, possibly the result of increased basal metabolic rate, higher work of breathing, and a cachexia that is poorly understood (*175,176*). Aggressive nutritional support aimed at achieving caloric intake above the calculated maintenance requirements will improve nutritional parameters and respiratory function (*177,178*). Significant malnutrition in patients who undergo lung transplantation has been shown in a retrospective study of 35 patients (*179*). In this study, patients with cystic fibrosis, emphysema, and other types of bronchiectasis were found to be particularly nutritionally depleted preoperatively. Nutritional status improved postoperatively, with most patients achieving normal nutrition within 1 yr after transplantation.

Despite the evidence indicating that patients who undergo lung transplantation are nutritionally depleted, there are no controlled trials examining preoperative and postoperative dietary intervention in this setting. It is probable that active nutritional support will improve the preoperative status of patients undergoing lung transplantation and contribute to improvements in outcomes. The effect of diet on lung allograft rejection is another factor that needs to be investigated. Finally, an important problem in lung transplantation is a significant incidence of ischemia–reperfusion injury secondary to the release of acute-phase reactants from infiltrating neutrophils, natural-killer cells, lymphocytes, and the large population of alveolar macrophages within the allograft (180). Early graft failure, with a 3-mo mortality as high as 25%, can be attributed in part to reperfusion injury (181). The role of nutritional support by interventions such as antioxidant vitamin supplementation, as has been discussed for other allografts, warrants further investigation in the setting of lung transplantation.

PANCREAS Advances in surgical technique and immunosuppressive protocols have led to significant improvements in the results of pancreas transplantation for patients with insulindependent diabetes. Patient and allograft survival is now comparable to the other major solid organ transplants. Most patients have return of normal bowel function within 3–4 d after surgery and, therefore, are not usually placed on any form of nutritional support after transplantation. Thus, to our knowledge, there have been no reports of nutritionally related clinical studies after pancreas transplantation. The pancreas allograft is very susceptible to both ischemia–reperfusion injury and acute rejection. It is possible that nutritional modification to ameliorate rejection or reperfusion injury, as has been discussed with the other organ allografts, may also be useful after pancreas transplantation.

SMALL INTESTINE Intestinal transplantation has achieved limited success and is performed in only a relatively small number of institutions. The main limitations to the success of the procedure are technical complications, frequent bacterial and viral infections, and difficulty in the diagnosis and treatment of allograft rejection (182–184). Nutritional management of patients after intestinal transplantation is particularly challenging and has been recently reviewed (185,186). The first week after transplantation is characterized by a significant limitation of nutrient absorption by the allograft as it recovers from ischemia and preservation injury. During this period, parenteral nutrition is important and bowel rest essential for intestinal anastomotic healing. The next 2–3 wk is characterized by normal carbohydrate and amino acid absorption, but impaired fat absorption as a result of the lack of adequate intestinal lymphatic drainage (187,188). During this time, an enteral diet, low in fat and free of long-chain triglycerides, is initiated. Lymphatic regeneration and recannulization occurs by 4–6 wk, at which time the enteral diet is normalized and parenteral nutrition weaned. The effect of nutritional supplementation on acute or chronic allograft rejection has not been addressed in intestinal transplantation.

SUMMARY

The clinical field of solid organ transplantation has undergone tremendous expansion in recent years. Advances in surgical techniques and the development of improved immunosuppression

strategies have led to both improved clinical outcomes and the application of transplantation to a broader group of patients with end-stage organ failure. Despite these significant advances, the adverse side effects of present immunosuppressive protocols compromise the quality of life for organ transplant recipients. Although clinical experience is not extensive, this chapter has supported the premise that nutritional immunomodulation may be a means of improving current immunosuppressive protocols. The data presented here suggest that dietary intervention may have a protective effect on the allograft in the setting of ischemia–reperfusion injury, acute rejection, and graft vasculopathy resulting from chronic rejection. Further studies will define optimal strategies of nutritional support as one component in the overall immunosuppressive therapy aimed at maximal prolongation of allograft survival.

REFERENCES

1. The US Scientific Registry of Transplant Recipients and The Organ Procurement and Transplantation Network. 1997 Annual Report: Transplant Data 1988–1996. Compiled by The United Network for Organ Sharing, Richmond, VA and The Department of Health and Human Services, Rockville, MD, 1997.
2. Hasse J. Diet therapy for organ transplantation: a problem-based approach. Nursing Clin North Am 1997; 32:863–80.
3. Driscoll D, Palombo J, Bistrian B. Nutritional and metabolic considerations of the adult liver transplant candidate and organ donor. Nutrition 1995; 11:255–63.
4. Kirby D. Enteral nutrition in immunocompromised patients. Nutr Clin Pract 1997; 12:S25–7.
5. Lowell J. Nutritional assessment and therapy in patients requiring liver transplantation. Liver Transplant Surg 1996; 2:79–88.
6. Perez R. Managing nutrition problems in transplant patients. Nutr Clin Pract 1993; 8:28–32.
7. Valente J, Alexander J. Immunobiology of renal transplantation. Surg Clin North Am 1998; 78:1–26.
8. Coffman T. Inflammatory response to allografts. In: Norman D, Suki W, eds, Primer on Transplantation, pp. 33–42. American Society of Transplant Physicians, Thorofare, NJ, 1998.
9. Suthanthiran M, Strom T. Mechanisms and management of acute renal allograft rejection. Surg Clin North Amer 1998; 78:77–94.
10. Krensky A. Immune response to allografts. In: Norman D, Suki W, eds, Primer on Transplantation, pp. 21–32. American Society of Transplant Physicians, Thorofare, NJ, 1998.
11. Massy Z, Guijarro C, Wiederkehr M, Ma J, Kasiske B. Chronic renal allograft rejection: immunologic and nonimmunologic risk factors. Kidney Int 1996; 49:518–24.
12. Matas A. Chronic rejection in renal transplant recipients—Risk factors and correlates. Clin Transplant 1994; 8:332–5.
13. Hancock W. Basic science aspects of chronic rejection: induction of protective genes to prevent development of transplant arteriosclerosis. Transplant Proc 1998; 30:1585–9.
14. Sayegh M, Carpenter C. Tolerance and chronic rejection. Kidney Int 1997; 58:S11–4.
15. Tilney N, Kusaka M, Pratschke J, Wilhelm M. Chroinc rejection. Transplant Proc 1998; 30:1590–4.
16. Lowes J, Hubscher S, Neuberger J. Chronic rejection of the liver allograft. Gastroenter Clin North Am 1993; 22:401–20.
17. European Mycophenolate Mofetil Cooperative Study Group, Placebo-controlled study of mycophenolate mofetil combined with cyclosporin and corticosteroids for prevention of acute rejection. Lancet 1995; 345:1321–5.
18. Sollinger H, for the U.S. Renal Transplant Mycophenolate Mofetil Study Group. Mycophenolate mofetil for the prevention of acute rejection in primary cadaveric renal allograft recipients.Transplantation 1995; 60:225–32.
19. Foegh M, Alijani M, Helfrich G, et al. Fatty acids and eicosanoids in organ transplantation. Prog Lipid Res 1986; 25:567–72.

20. Kinsella J, Lokesh B. Dietary lipids, eicosanoids and the immune response. Crit Care Med 1990; 18:594–620.

21. Kort W, Weijman I, Westbrock D. Effect of stress and dietary fatty acids on allograft survival in the rat. Eur Surg Res 1979; 11:434–44.

22. Mertin J. Effect of polyunsaturated fatty acids on skin allograft survival and primary and secondary cytotoxic response in mice. Transplantation 1976; 21:1–4.

23. Ring J, Seifert J, Mertin J, Brendel W. Prolongation of skin allografts in rats by treatment with linoleic acid. Lancet 1974; 2:1331–2.

24. Grimm H, Tibell A, Norrlind B, Schott J, Bohle R. Nutrition and allorejection impact of lipids. Transplant Immunol 1995; 3:62–7.

25. Grimminger F, Grimm H, Fuhrer D, et al. ω-3 Lipid infusion in a heart allotransplant model: shift in fatty acid and lipid mediator profiles and prolongation of transplant survival. Circulation 1996; 93:365–71.

26. Otto D, Kahn D, Hamm M, Forrest D, Wooten J. Improved survival of heterotopic cardiac allografts in rats with dietary n-3 polyunsaturated fatty acids. Transplantation 1990; 50:193–8.

27. Sarris G, Mitchell S, Billingham M, Glasson J, Cahill P, Miller C. Inhibition of accelerated cardiac allograft arteriosclerosis by fish oil. J Thorac Cardiovasc Surg 1989; 97:841–55.

28. Yun K, Fann J, Sokoloff M, et al. Dose response of fish oil versus safflower oil on graft arteriosclerosis in rabbit heterotopic cardiac allografts. Ann Surg 1991; 214:155–67.

29. Calder PC. Immunomodulatory and anti-inflammatory effects of n-3 polyunsaturated fatty acids. Proc Nutr Soc 1996; 55:737–74.

30. Khalfoun B, Thibault G, Bardos P, Lebranchu Y. Docosahexaenoic and eicosapentaenoic acids inhibit in vitro human lymphocyte–endothelial cell adhesion. Transplantation 1996; 62:1649–57.

31. Whisler R, Lindsey J, Proctor K, Morisaki N, Cornwell D. Characteristics of cyclosporine induction of increased prostaglandin levels from human peripheral blood monocytes. Transplantation 1984; 38:377–81.

32. Zhao H, Aziz S, Kasahara K, et al. Improved immunosuppression using cyclosporine with 15 methyl prostaglandin E₁. Surg Forum 1984; 35:382–4.

33. Perez R, Munda R, Alexander JW. Augmentation of donor-specific transfusion and cyclosporine effects with dietary linoleic acid. Transplantation 1989; 47:937–40.

34. Kelley V, Kirkman R, Bastos M, Barrett L, Strom T. Enhancement of immunosuppression by substitution of fish oil for olive oil as a vehicle for cyclosporine. Transplantation 1989; 48:98–102.

35. Elzinga L, Kelley V, Houghton D, Bennett, W. Modification of experimental nephrotoxicity with fish oil as the vehicle for cyclosporine. Transplantation 1987; 43:271–4.

36. Opelz G, Terasaki P. Improvement of kidney-graft survival with increased numbers of blood transfusions. N Engl J Med 1978; 299:799–803.

37. Lenhard V, Gemsa D, Opelz G. Transfusion-induced release of prostaglandin-E2 and its role in activation of T-suppressor cells. Transplant Proc 1985; 17:2380–2.

38. Waymack J, Gallon L, Barcelli U, Trocki O, Alexander JW. Effect of transfusions on immune function. III. Alterations in macrophage arachidonic acid metabolism. Arch Surg 1987; 122:56–60.

39. Perez R, Munda R, Alexander JW. Dietary immunoregulation of transfusion-induced immunosuppression. Transplantation 1989; 45:614–7.

40. Alexander JW, Valente J, Greenberg N, et al. Dietary ω-3 and ω-9 fatty acids uniquely enhance allograft survival in cyclosporine-treated and donor-specific transfusion-treated rats. Transplantation 1998; 65:1304–9.

41. Levy A, Alexander JW. Nutritional immunomodulation enhances cardiac allograft survival in rats treated with donor-specific transfusion and cyclosporine. Transplantation 1995; 60:812–5.

42. Perez R, Johnson J, Hubbard NE, et al. Selective targeting of Kupffer cells with liposomal butyrate augments portal venous transfusion-induced immunosuppression. Transplantation 1998; 65:1294–8.

43. Perez R, Stevenson F, Johnson J, et al. Sodium butyrate upregulates Kupffer cell PGE2 production and modulates immune function. J Surg Res, 1998; 78:1–6.

44. Schreiner G, Flye W, Brunt E, Korber K, Lefkowith J. Essential fatty acid depletion of renal allografts and prevention of rejection. Science 1988; 240:1032–3.

45. Lawen J, Yu W, Cook H, Wright J. The failure of donor essential fatty acid deficiency to prevent allograft rejection in rats. Transplantation 1993; 56:1269–70.

46. Wiederkehr J, Pollak R. Essential fatty acid deficiency and cardiac allograft survival in histoincompatible rats. Transplantation 1989; 48:718–20.

47. Ishikawa T, Yagi T, Ishido N, et al. Effect of nutritional procurement for the donor liver on Kupffer cell activation in porcine liver transplantation. Transplant Proc 1997; 29:3357.

48. Sadamori H, Tanaka N, Yagi T, Inagaki M, Orita K. The effects of nutritional repletion on donors for liver transplantation in pigs. Transplantation 1995; 60:317–21.

49. Alonso D, Starek P, Minick C. Studies on the pathogenesis of artheroarteriosclerosis induced in rabbit cardiac allografts by the synergy of graft rejection and hypercholesterolemia. Am J Pathol 1977; 87:415–42.

50. Mennander A, Tikkanen M, Raisanen-Sokolowski A, Paavonen T, Ustinov J, Hayry P. Chronic rejection in rat aortic allografts, IV: effect of hypercholesterolemia in allograft arteriosclerosis. J Heart Lung Transplant 1993; 12:123–32.

51. Russell P, Chase C, Colvin R. Accelerated atheromatous lesions in mouse hearts transplanted to apolipoprotein-E-deficient recipients. Am J Pathol 1996; 149:91–9.

52. Shi C, Lee W, Russell M, et al. Hypercholesterolemia exacerbates transplant arteriosclerosis via increased neointimal smooth muscle cell accumulation: studies in apolipoprotein E knockout mice. Circulation 1997; 96:2722–8.

53. Tanaka H, Sukhova G, Libby P. Interaction of the allogeneic state and hypercholesterolemia in arterial lesion formation in experimental cardiac allografts. Arerioscler Thromb 1994; 14:734–45.

54. Adams D, Karnovsky M. Hypercholesterolemia does not exacerbate arterial intimal thickening in chronically rejecting rat cardiac allografts. Transplant Proc 1989; 21:437–9.

55. Esper E, Glagov S, Karp RB, et al. Role of hypercholesterolemia in accelerated transplant coronary vasculopathy: results of surgical therapy with partial ileal bypass in rabbits undergoing heterotopic heart transplantation. J Heart Lung Transplant 1997; 16:420–35.

56. Shepherd J, Cobbe S, Ford I, for the West of Scotland Coronary Prevention Study Group. Prevention of coronary heart disease with pravastatin in men with hypercholesterolemia. N Engl J Med 1995; 33:1301–7.

57. Kobashigawa J, Katznelson S, Laks H, et al. Effect of pravastatin on outcomes after cardiac transplantation. N Engl J Med 1995; 333:621–7.

58. Maggard M, Ke B, Wang T, Kaldas F, Seu P, Busuttil R, et al. Effects of pravastatin on chronic rejection of rat cardiac allografts. Transplantation 1998; 65:149–55.

59. Meiser B, Wenke K, Thiery J, et al. Simvastatin decreases accelerated graft vessel disease after heart transplantation in an animal model. Transplant Proc 1993; 25:2077–9.

60. Kakkis J, Ke B, Dawson S, et al. Pravastatin increases survival and inhibits natural killer cell enhancement factor (NKEF) in liver transplanted rats. J Surg Res 1997; 69:393–8.

61. Arita S, Une S, Ohtsuka S, et al. Prevention of primary islet isograft nonfunction in mice with pravastatin. Transplantation 1998; 65:1429–33.

62. McPherson R, Tsoukas C, Baines MG, et al. Effects of lovastatin on natural killer cell function and other immunological parameters in man. J Clin Immunol 1993; 13:439–44.

63. Kreuzer J, Bader J, Jahn L, Hautmann M, Kubler W, Von Hodenberg E. Chemotaxis of the monocyte line U937: dependence on cholesterol and early mevalonate pathway products. Atherosclerosis 1991; 90:203–9.

64. Katznelson S, Wang X, Chia D, et al. The inhibitory effects of pravastatin on natural killer cell activity in vivo and on cytotoxic T lymphocyte activity in vitro. J Heart Lung Transplant 1998; 17:335–40.

65. Chakrabarti R, Engleman EG. Interrelationships between mevalonate metabolism and the mitogenic signaling pathway in T lymphocyte proliferation. J Biol Chem 1991; 266:12,216–21.

66. Rudich SM, Mongini P, Perez R, Katznelson S. HMG-CoA reductase inhibitors Pravastatin and Simvastatin inhibit human B lymphocyte activation. Transplant Proc 1998; 30:992–5.

67. Katznelson S, Berryman E, Griffey S, Perez R, Gregory C. Combined therapy with pravastatin and cyclosporin decreases arterial intimal thickening in a model of severe vascular immune injury. Transplantation 1998; 65:S38.

68. Katznelson S, Wilkinson A, Kobashigawa J, et al. The effect of pravastatin on acute rejection after kidney transplantation—a pilot study. Transplantation 1996; 61:1469–74.

69. Imagawa D, Dawson S, Holt C, et al. Hyperlipidemia after liver transplantation: natural history and treatment with the hydroxythylglutaryl–coenzyme A reductase inhibitor Pravastatin. Transplantation 1996; 62:934–42.

70. Cooper W, Good R, Mariani T. The effects of protein insufficiency on immune responsiveness. Am J Clin Nutr 1974; 27:647–64.

71. Law D, Dudrick S, Abdou N. The effect of dietary protein depletion on immunocompetence: the importance of nutritional repletion prior to immunologic induction. Ann Surg 1974; 179:168–73.

72. Austin E, Brennan M, Rosenberg S. Effects of protein-calorie restriction on the immune response to skin allografts in the rat. Transplantation 1980; 30:219–25.

73. Jose D, Good R. Quantitative effects of nutritional protein and calorie deficiency upon immune response to tumors in mice. Cancer Res 1973; 33:807–12.

74. Purkayastha S, Kapoor B, Deo M. Influence of protein deficiency on homograft rejection and histocompatibility antigens in rats. Indian J Med Res 1975; 63:1150–4.

75. Alexander JW. Specific nutrients and the immune response. Nutrition 1995; 11:229–32.

76. Barbul A. Arginine: biochemistry, physiology, and therapeutic implication. J Parenter Enter Nutr 1986; 10:227–38.

77. McNamara D, Bedi B, Aurora H, et al. L-Arginine inhibits balloon catheter-induced intimal hyperplasia. Biochem Biophys Res Commun 1993; 193:291–6.

78. Boger R, Bode-Boger S, Brandes R, et al. Dietary L-arginine reduces the progression of atherosclerosis in cholesterol-fed rabbits: comparison with Lovastatin. Circulation 1997; 96:1282–90.

79. Boger R, Bode-Boger S, Mugge A, et al. Supplementation of hypercholesterolemic rabbits with L-arginine reduces the vascular release of superoxide anions and restores NO production. Atherosclerosis 1995; 117:273–84.

80. Cooke J, Singer, A, Tsao P, Zera P, Rowan R, Billingham M. Antiatherosclerotic effects of L-arginine in the hypercholesterolemic rabbit. J Clin Invest 1992; 90:1168–72.

81. Koglin J, Glysing-Jensen T, Mudgett J, Russell M. Exacerbated transplant arteriosclerosis in inducible nitric oxide-deficient mice. Circulation 1998; 97:2059–65.

82. Shears II L, Kawaharada N, Tzeng E. Inducible nitric oxide synthase suppresses the development of allograft arteriosclerosis. J Clin Invest 1997; 100:2035–42.

83. Lou H, Kodama T, Wang Y, Katz N, Ramwell P, Foegh M. L-Arginine prevents heart transplant arteriosclerosis by modulating the vascular cell proliferative response to insulin-like growth factor-1 and interleukin-6. J Heart Lung Transplant 1996; 15:1248–57.

84. Souba W, Smith R, Wilmore D. Glutamine metabolism by the intestinal tract. J Parenter Enter Nutr 1985; 9:608–17.

85. Frankel W, Zhang W, Alfonso J, et al. Glutamine enhancement of structure and function in transplanted small intestine in the rat. J Parenter Enter Nutr 1993; 17:47–55.

86. Zhang W, Frankel W, Singh A, Laitin E, Klurfeld D, Rombeau J. Improvement of structure and function in orthotopic small bowel transplantation in the rat by glutamine. Transplantation 1993; 56:512–7.

87. Zhang W, Frankel W, Bain A, Choi D, Klurfeld D, Rombeau J. Glutamine reduces bacterial translocation after small bowel transplantation in cyclosporine-treated rats. J Surg Res 1995; 58:159–64.

88. Jyonouchi H. Nucleotide actions on humoral immune responses. J Nutr 1994; 124:138S–43S.

89. Rudolph F, Kulkarni A, Fanslow W, Pizzini R, Kumar S, Van Buren C. Role of RNA as a dietary source of pyrimidines and purines in immune function. Nutrition 1990; 6:45–52.

90. Van Buren C, Kulkarni A, Rudolph F. The role of nucleotides in adult nutrition. J Nutr 1994; 124:160S–4S.

91. Van Buren C, Kulkarni A, Schandle V, Rudolph F. The influence of dietary nucleotides on cell-mediated immunity. Transplantation 1983; 36:350–2.

92. Van Buren C, Kim E, Kulkarni A, Fanslow W, Rudolph F. Nucleotide-free diet and suppression of immune response. Transplant Proc 1987; 19:57–9.

93. Van Buren C, Kulkarni A, Fanslow W, Rudolph F. Dietary nucleotides, a requirement for helper/inducer T lymphocytes. Transplantation 1985; 40:694–7.

94. Land W, Messmer K. The impact of ischemia/reperfusion injury on specific and non-specific, early and late chronic events after organ transplantation. Transplant Rev 1996; 10:108–27.

95. Demirbas A, Bozoklu S, Ozdemir A, Bilgin N, Haberal M. Effect of alpha tocopherol on the prevention of reperfusion injury caused by free oxygen radicals in the canine kidney autotransplantation model. Transplant Proc 1993; 25:2274.

96. Ikeda M, Sumimoto K, Urushihara T, Fukuda Y, Dohi K, Kawasaki T. Prevention of ischemic damage in rat pancreatic transplantation by pretreatment with alpha tocopherol. Transplant Proc 1994; 26:561–2.

97. Slakey D, Roza A, Pieper G, Johnson C, Adams M. Delayed cardiac allograft rejection due to combined cyclosporine and antioxidant therapy. Transplantation 1993; 56:1305–9.

98. Vajkoczy P, Lehr H, Hubner C, Arfors K, Menger M. Prevention of pancreatic islet xenograft rejection by dietary vitamin E. Am J Pathol 1997; 150:1487–95.

99. Duijvestijn A, Kok M, Miyasaka M, Vriesman P. ICAM-1 and LFA-1/CD18 expression in chronic renal allograft rejection. Transplant Proc 1993; 25:2867.

100. Rao G, Berk B. Active oxygen species stimulate vascular smooth muscle cell growth and proto-oncogene expression. Circ Res 1992; 70:593–9.

101. Wanders A, Akyurek M, Waltenberger J, et al. Ischemia-induced transplant arteriosclerosis in the rat. Arterioscler Thromb Vasc Biol 1995; 15:145–55.

102. Yilmaz S, Paavonen T, Hayry P. Chronic rejection of rat kidney allografts: II. The impact of prolonged ischemia on transplant histology. Transplantation 1992; 53:823.

103. Gaudin P, Rayburn B, Hutchins G, et al. Peritransplant injury to the myocardium associated with the development of accelerated arteriosclerosis in heart transplant recipients. Am J Surg Pathol 1994; 18:338–46.

104. Valentine-von Kaeppler H, Dai X, Hoang K, et al. Effect of antioxidant vitamins on transplant atherosclerosis in the Zucker rat model: evidence for oxidative stress in the pathophysiology? Transplantation 1998; 65:S40.

105. Halliwell B. Free radicals, antioxidants, and human disease: curiosity, cause, or consequence? Lancet 1994; 344:721–4.

106. Enstrom J, Kanim L, Klein M. Vitamin C intake and mortality among a sample of the United States population. Epidemiology 1992; 3:194–202.

107. Stephens N, Parsons A, Schofield P, et al. Randomized controlled trial of vitamin E in patients with coronary disease: Cambridge heart antioxidant study (CHAOS). Lancet 1996; 347:781–6.

108. Jurin M, Tannock I. Influence of vitamin A on immunological response. Immunology 1972; 23:283–7.

109. Medawar P, Hunt R. Anti-cancer action of retinoids. Immunology 1981; 42:349–53.

110. Elias P, Williams M. Retinoids, cancer, and the skin. Arch Dermatol 1981; 117:160–8.

111. Koranda F, Dehmel E, Kahn G, Penn I. Cutaneous complications in immunosuppressed renal homograft recipients. JAMA 1974; 229:419–24.

112. Penn I, Halgrimson C, Starzl T. De novo malignant tumors in organ transplant recipients. Transplant Proc 1971; 3:773–8.

113. Walder B, Robertson M, Jeremy D. Skin cancer and immunosuppression. Lancet 1971; 2:1282–3.

114. Haick A, Johnson D, Raju S. Vitamin A does not alter immunosuppressive properties of simultaneously administered steroids. Am J Surg 1981; 47:533.

115. Neifeld J, Lee H, Hutcher N. Lack of effect of vitamin A on corticosteroid induced immunosuppression. J Surg Res 1975; 19:225–8.

116. Schweizer R, Bartus S. Vitamin A and immunosuppression of allografts in dogs and rabbits. J Surg Res 1975; 19:229–32.

117. Kelly GE. Effect of retinoid therapy on rat cardiac allograft survival. Transplantation 1987; 44:451–3.

118. Boushey C, Beresford S, Omen G, Motulsky A. A quantitative assessment of plasma homocysteine as a risk factor for vascular disease. Probable benefits of increasing folic acid intakes. JAMA 1995; 274:1049–57.

119. Bostom A, Gohh R, Beauliew A, et al. Treatment of hyperhomocysteinemia in renal transplant recipients: a randomized, placebo-controlled trial. Ann Intern Med 1997; 127:1089–92.

120. Uldall P, Wilkinson R, McHugh M, et al. Unsaturated fatty acids and renal transplantation. Lancet 1974; 2:514 (letter).

121. McHugh M, Wilkinson R, Elliott R, et al. Immunosuppression with polyunsaturated fatty acids in renal transplantation. Transplantation 1977; 24:263–7.

122. van der Heide JJ, Bilo H, Donker J, Wilmink J, Tegzess A. Effect of dietary fish oil on renal function and rejection in cyclosporine-treated recipients of renal transplants. N Engl J Med 1993; 329:769–73.

123. Sweny P, Wheeler D, Sui S, et al. Dietary fish oil supplements preserve renal function in renal transplant recipients with chronic vascular rejection. Nephrol Dialysis Transplant 1989; 4:1070–5.

124. Berthoux F, Guerin C, Burgard G, Berthoux P, Alamartine E. One-year randomized controlled trial with omega-3 fatty acid-fish oil in clinical renal transplantation. Transplant Proc 1992; 24:2578–82.

125. Maachi K, Berthoux P, Burgard G, Burgard G, Alamartine E, Berthoux F. Results of a 1-year randomized controlled trial with omega-3 fatty acid fish oil in renal transplantation under triple immunosuppressive therapy. Transplant Proc 1995; 27:846–9.

126. Bennett W, Carpenter C, Shapiro M. Delayed omega-3 fatty acid supplements in renal transplantation: a double-blind, placebo-controlled study. Transplantation 1995; 59:352–6.

127. Dimeny E, Fellstrom B, Larsson E, Tufveson G, Lithell H. Hyperlipoproteinemia in renal transplant recipients: is there a linkage with chronic vascular rejection? Transplant Proc 1993; 25:2065–6.

128. Isoniemi H, Nurminen M, Tikkanen MJ, et al. Risk factors predicting chronic rejection of renal allografts. Transplantation 1994; 57:68–72.

129. Dimeny E, Tufveson G, Larsson E, Lithell H, Siegbahn A, Fellstrom B. The influence of posttransplant lipoprotein abnormalities on the early results of renal transplantation. Eur J Clin Invest 1993; 23:572–9.

130. Grundy SM. National Cholesterol Education Program. Second report of the expert panel on detection, evaluation, and treatment of high blood cholesterol in adults (Adult Treatment Panel II). Circulation 1994; 89:1329–36.

131. Knight R, Vathsala A, Schoenberg L, et al. Treatment of hyperlipidemia in renal transplant patients with gemfibrozil and dietary modification. Transplantation 1992; 53:244–5.

132. Kobashigawa J, Kasiske B. Hyperlipidemia in solid organ transplantation. Transplantation 1997; 63:331–8.

133. Yoshimura N, Oka T, Okamoto M, Ohmori Y. The effects of pravastatin on hyperlipidemia in renal transplant recipients. Transplantation 1992; 53:94–9.

134. Cheung A, DeVault G Jr, Gregory M. A prospective study on treatment of hypercholesterolemia with lovastatin in renal transplant patients receiving cyclosporine. J Am Soc Nephrol 1993; 3:1884–91.

135. Kasiske B, Tortorice K, Heim-Duthoy K, Goryance J, Rao K. Lovastatin treatment of hypercholesterolemia in renal transplant recipients. Transplantation 1990; 49:95–100.

136. Rabl H, Khoschsorur G, Colombo T, et al. A multivitamin infusion prevents lipid peroxidation and improves transplantation performance. Kidney Int 1993; 43:912–7.

137. Hower R, Minor T, Schneeberger H, et al. Assessment of oxygen radicals during kidney transplantation: effect of radical scavenger. Transplant Int 1996; 9:S479–82.

138. Hughes D, McLean A, Roake J, Gray D, Morris P. Free oxygen species (FOS), FOS-scavenging enzyme P-selectin and monocyte activity in cell populations aspirated from early human renal allografts. Transplant Proc 1995; 28:2879.

139. Kasiske B, Guijarro C, Massy Z, Wiederkehr M, Ma J. Cardiovascular disease after renal transplantation. J Am Soc Nephrol 1996; 7:158–65.

140. Bostrom A, Gohh R, Tsai M, et al. Excess prevalence of fasting and PML hyperhomocysteinemia in stable renal transplant recipients. Arterioscl Thromb Vasc Biol 1997; 17:1894–900.

141. Massy Z, Chadefaux-Vekemans B, Chevalier A, et al. Hyperhomocysteinemia: a significant risk factor for cardiovascular disease in renal transplant recipients. Nehrol Dialysis Transplant 1994; 9:1103–8.

142. Arnadottir M, Hultberg B, Vladov V, Nilsson-Ehle P, Thysell H. Hyperhomocysteinemia in cyclosporine-treated renal transplant recipients. Transplantation 1996; 61:509–12.

143. Kaye M. The Registry of the International Society for Heart Transplantation: Fourth Official Report—1987. J Heart Transplant 1987; 6:63–7.

144. Grady K, Herold L. Comparison of nutritional status in patients before and after heart transplantation. J Heart Transplant 1988; 7:123–7.

145. Frazier O, Van Buren C, Poindexter S, Waldenberger F. Nutritional management of the heart transplant recipient. J Heart Transplant 1985; 4:450–2.

146. Keogh A, Simons L, Spratt P, et al. Hyperlipidemia after heart transplantation. J Heart Transplant 1988; 7:171–5.

147. Miller L, Schlant R, Kobashigawa J, Kubo S, Renlund D. 24th Bethesda Conference: cardiac transplantation: Task Force 5: complications. J Am Coll Cardiol 1993; 22:41–54.

148. Eich D, Thompson J, Ko D, Hastillo A, Lower R, Katz S, et al. Hypercholesterolemia in long-term survivors of heart transplantation: an early marker of accelerated coronary artery disease. J Heart Lung Transplant 1991; 10:45–9.

149. Johnson M. Transplant coronary disease: nonimmunologic factors. J Heart Lung Transplant 1992; 11:S124–32.

150. Sharpless L, Caine N, Mullins P, et al. Risk factor analysis for the major hazards following heart transplantation: rejection, infection and coronary occlusive disease. Transplantation 1991; 52:244–52.

151. Uretsky B, Murali S, Reddy P, et al. Development of coronary artery disease in cardiac transplant patients receiving immunosuppressive therapy with cyclosporine and prednisolone. Circulation 1987; 76:827–34.

152. Ballantyne C, Radovancevic B, Farmer J, et al. Hyperlipidemia after heart transplantation: Report of a 6-year experience with treatment recommendations. J Am Coll Cardiol 1992; 19:1315–21.

153. Kobashigawa J, Murphy F, Stevenson L, et al. Low-dose lovastatin safely lowers cholesterol after cardiac transplantation. Circulation 1990; 82:IV-281–3.

154. Vanhaecke J, Van Cleemput J, Van Lierde J, Daenen W, De Geest H. Safety and efficacy of low dose simvastatin in cardiac transplant recipients treated with cyclosporine. Transplantation 1994; 58:42–5.

155. Wenke K, Meiser B, Thiery J, et al. Simvastatin reduces graft vessel disease and mortality after heart transplantation: a four-year randomized trial. Circulation 1997; 96:1398–402.

156. Lorgeril M, Boissonnat P, Salen P, et al. The beneficial effect of dietary antioxidant supplementation on platelet aggregation and cyclosporine treatment in heart transplant recipients. Transplantation 1994; 58:193–5.

157. Gupta A, Moustapha A, Jacobsen D, et al. High homocysteine, low folate, and low vitamin B6 concentrations: prevalent risk factors for vascular disease in heart transplant recipients. Transplantation 1998; 65:544–50.

158. Miner S, Ross H, Langman I, et al. Total plasma homocysteine concentrations are strongly correlated with whole blood cyclosporine levels and angiographic coronary artery disease in heart transplant patients. Transplantation 1998; 65:S27.

159. Busuttil R, Shaked A, Millis JM, et al. One thousand liver transplants: lessons learned. Ann Surg 1994; 219:490–9.

160. The U.S. Multicenter FK506 Liver Study Group. A comparison of tacrolimus (FK 506) and cyclosporine for immunosuppression in liver transplantation. N Engl J Med 1994; 331:1110–5.

161. Plevak D, DiCecco S, Wiesner R, et al. Nutritional support for liver transplantation: identifying caloric and protein requirements. Mayo Clin Proc 1994; 69:225–30.

162. DiCecco S, Wieners E, Wiesner R, et al. Assessment of nutritional status of patients with end-stage liver disease undergoing liver transplantation. Mayo Clin Proc 1989; 64:95–102.

163. Hehir D, Jenkins R, Bistrian B, et al. Nutrition in patients undergoing orthotopic liver transplantation. J Parenter Enter Nutr 1985; 9:695–700.

164. Hiyama D, Fischer J. Nutritional support in hepatic failure: current thought in practice. Nutr Clin Pract 1988; 3:96–105.

165. Latifi R, Killam R, Dudrick S. Nutritional support in liver failure. Surg Clin North Am 1991; 71:567–76.

166. Reilly J, Mehta R, Teperman L, et al. Nutritional support after liver transplantation: a randomized prospective study. J Parenter Enteral Nutr 1990; 14:386–91.

167. Morgan M. Branched chain amino acids in the management of chronic liver disease: facts and fantasies. J Hepatol 1990; 11:133–41.

168. Wicks C, Somasundaram S, Bjarnason I, et al. Comparison of enteral feeding and total parenteral nutrition after liver transplantation. Lancet 1994; 344:837–40.

169. Hasse J, Blue L, Liepa G, et al. Early enteral nutrition support in patients undergoing liver transplantation. J Parenter Enter Nutr 1995; 19:437–43.

170. Lehr H, Messmer K. Rationale for the use of antioxidant vitamins in clinical organ transplantation. Transplantation 1996; 62:1197–9.

171. Biasi F, Bosco M, Chiappino I, et al. Oxidative damage in human liver transplantation. Free Radical Biol Med 1995; 19:311–7.

172. Galley H, Richardson N, Howdle P, Walder B, Webster N. Total antioxidant capacity and lipid peroxidation during liver transplantation. Clin Sci 1995; 89:329–32.

173. Goode H, Webster N, Howdle P, et al. Reperfusion injury, antioxidants and hemodynamics during orthotopic liver transplantation. Hepatology 1994; 19:354–9.

174. Toronto Lung Transplant Group. Unilateral lung transplantation for pulmonary fibrosis. N Engl J Med 1986; 314:1140–5.

175. Wilson D, Rogers R, Sanders M, Pennock B, Reilly J. Nutritional intervention in malnourished patients with emphysema. Am Rev Respir Dis 1986; 134:672–7.

176. Hunter A, Carey M, Larsh H. The nutritional status of patients with chronic obstructive pulmonary disease. Am Rev Respir Dis 1981; 124:376–81.

177. Wilson D, Rogers R. Basal O_2 consumption and metabolic rate is elevated in severe COPD. Chest 1986; 89:517S.

178. Whitaker J, Ryan C, Buckley P, et al. The effects of refeeding on peripheral and respiratory muscle function in malnourished chronic obstructive pulmonary disease patients. Am Rev Respir Dis 1990; 142:283–8.

179. Madill J, Maurer J, De Hoyos A. A comparison of preoperative and postoperative nutritional states of lung transplant recipients. Transplantation 1993; 56:347–50.

180. Adoumie R, Serrick C, Giaid A, Shennib H. Early cellular events in the lung allograft. Ann Thor Surg 1992; 54:1071–9.

181. Hosenbud J, Novick R, Breen T, Keck B, Daily P. The Registry of the International Society for Heart and Lung Transplantation: Twelfth Official Report—1995. J Heart Lung Transplant 1995; 14:805–15.

182. Reyes J, Bueno J, Kocoshis S, et al. Current status of intestinal transplantation in children. J Pediatr Surg 1998; 33:243–54.

183. Langnas A, Shaw B, Antonson D, et al. Preliminary experience with intestinal transplantation in infants and children. Pediatrics 1996; 97:443–8.

184. Grant D. Current results of intestinal transplantation. International Transplant Registry. Lancet 1996; 347:1801–3.

185. Reyes J, Tzakis A, Todo S, et al. Nutritional management of intestinal transplant recipients. Transplant Proc 1993; 25:1200–1.

186. Staschak-Chicko S, Altieri K, Funovits M, et al. Eating difficulties in the pediatric small bowel recipient: the role of the nutritional management team. Transplant Proc 1994; 26:1434–5.

187. Hale D, Waldorf K, Kleinschmidt J, et al. Small intestinal transplantation in nonhuman primates. J Pediatr Surg 1991; 26:914–20.

188. Watson A, Lear, P. Montgomery, A., et al. Water, electrolyte, glucose and glycine absorption in rat small intestinal transplants. Gastroenterology 1988; 94:863–9.

29 Food Toxicology and Immunity

LINDA RASOOLY AND NOEL R. ROSE

INTRODUCTION

Food is an extremely complex matrix consisting of thousands of natural components, many of which have not been characterized. In addition, it may contain food additives (such as colorings, texturizers, flavoring agents, etc.), pesticide residues, drugs used in food-producing animals, chemical pollutants (such as lead and arsenic), microbial contaminants, and substances produced by cooking. As stated by Katsonis et al. *(1)*, "Food in general is more complex and variable in composition than are all the other substances to which humans are exposed. However, there is nothing to which humans have greater exposure despite the uncertainty about its chemical identity, consistency, and purity."

Interaction between the body and the environment occurs on many levels and produces many effects on the host. Of the components of the body, the immune system is the first line of defense against invading organisms and potentially damaging pathogenic products. As a result, the immune system is prominently affected whenever a toxic substance enters the body. One of the major pathways of encounter between the body and toxic materials is through food. Paradoxically, food, which is essential to maintain a healthy organism, is also the possible carrier of pathogenic micro-organisms as well as the toxic materials they produce. In addition, constituents and contaminants of food can cause toxic effects directly, or indirectly through breakdown products.

There are many sources of the toxins found in foods. Among them are bacteria, fungi, viruses, environmental pollutants, and side products of food processing and preparation. Of these toxins, the ones that have been demonstrated to have a direct effect on the immune system are those produced by bacteria and fungi as well as excess nutrients such as iodine. These will be discussed in further detail in this chapter.

Large amounts of any toxin may have lethal effects on the host, with dramatic impact on the cells of the immune system. Smaller amounts, however, often result in subtle immunomodulatory effects. Chronic, long-term exposure even to a low level of toxic materials can cause changes in the immune system that lead to dysregulation with possible pathogenic outcomes.

The genetic basis of many immune-mediated diseases, among them the autoimmune diseases (i.e., diseases where the immune system attacks the organism itself), has been well documented. The effect of the environment on the development of these diseases, however, has been less well characterized. Yet, it has been estimated that only about half of the risk of the disease is attributable to the genetic contributions of the host. The other 50%, which may tip the balance between health and disease, may be due to the effect of the environment. The principal route by which we are exposed to the environment is through the food we eat, and so the potential damage contributed by the contents of food is great. We have an opportunity to reduce our chances of developing immune-mediated disease by limiting the risk that is contributed by the environment by controlling the types of food we ingest.

In this chapter, we will discuss some of the best studied examples of toxins found in our food supply that affect the immune system, including their source, their mode of action, and their participation in pathogenic processes.

TOXINS IN FOOD

BACTERIAL TOXINS Food-borne microbial diseases afflict over 69 million Americans each year *(2)*. Despite concerns about the safety of food additives, pesticide residues, and other contaminants, bacterial contamination of the food remains the greatest food-borne risk *(1)*. Whereas some of the bacteria that may contaminate our food supply are directly pathogenic, others produce toxins that remain in the food even after the organism that produced them is no longer present. A list of the most common food-borne bacteria that produce toxins is summarized in Table 1.

Of the food-borne pathogens, the microorganisms with the capacity to produce superantigens are the ones most commonly associated with effects on the immune system. Superantigens are a group of 20–30-kDa proteins that stimulate T-cell proliferation by simultaneously binding to two molecules on two separate cells: the Vβ portion of the T-cell receptor, which is distinct from the peptide-binding groove *(3,4)*, and the major histocompatibility complex (MCH) class II molecule on B cells, monocytes, and other antigen-presenting cells. Thus, superantigens form a bridge between T cells and antigen-presenting cells, causing activation and proliferation of T cells (reviewed in ref. 5). A large portion of the T cells (up to 20% of peripheral T cells) may be activated because the response is not restricted to the antigen-specific T cells. The subsequent massive release of cytokines can lead to disease.

The sources of superantigens are both bacterial and viral. Major sources of superantigens are *Staphylococcus aureus, Streptococ-*

From: *Nutrition and Immunology: Principles and Practice* (ME Gershwin et al. eds.), © Humana Press, Inc., Totowa, NJ

Table 1
Some of the Common Food-Borne Toxin-Producing Bacteria

Organism	Toxins produced	Source of contamination
Escherichia coli	Enterotoxins	Fecal contamination
Clostridium botulinum	Botulinum toxins A–G	Canned and cured food
Staphylococcus aureus	Enterotoxins	Human carriers (nasal passages)
Clostridium perfringens	Enterotoxins	Fecal contamination
Bacillus cereus	Exotoxins and enterotoxins	Soil and dust

Source: Modified from ref. 1.

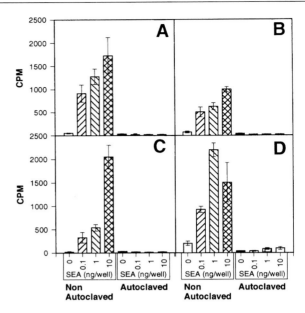

Fig. 1. Detection of SEA in four different foods using a T-cell proliferation assay. Lewis rat lymphocytes were isolated from heparinized blood and purified on Ficoll–Paque. Lymphocytes were incubated at 1×10^6 cells/mL with food samples for 2 d. ^{3}H-thymidine was added and plates were harvested 24 h later and radioactivity was measured. Food was homogenized, diluted 10-fold in phosphate-buffered saline and tested in the presence or absence of different concentrations of SEA, either directly or following autoclaving for 40 min at 121°C. A = Hot dog; B = potato salad; C = mushrooms; D = milk. Data are mean ± SEM.

cus pyogenes, and Mycoplasma arthriditis, but additional bacterial species have also been reported to produce superantigens (6). Viruses have also been reported to produce superantigens, among them are viruses affecting humans such as Epstein–Barr virus and rabies virus (6).

Because of their potent activation of a large proportion of T cells, superantigens have been incriminated in several diseases. In addition to causing food poisoning (such as S. aureus enterotoxin A), superantigens are responsible for toxic shock syndrome characterized by fever and hypotension, which can be fatal. They have also been implicated in autoimmune disease (7–9).

The uptake of superantigens from the intestinal tract into the bloodstream results in the direct activation of a large portion of the T cells (irrespective of their antigen specificity) followed by a major release of cytokines. Because the presence of natural autoreactive lymphocytes has frequently been reported even in normal individuals, the indiscriminate activation of T cells encompasses autoreactive lymphocytes that have the potential of producing autoimmune disease. Indeed, superantigens have been proposed as possible instigators of several autoimmune diseases, among them rheumatic heart diseases, Kawasaki disease, autoimmune thyroiditis, rheumatoid arthritis, and multiple sclerosis (6).

S. aureus Enterotoxin A in T-cell Proliferation and Autoimmunity Staphylococcal enterotoxins (SE) are a family of five major serological types (SEA through SEE) of heat-stable, emetic proteins encoded by five genes that share 50–85% homology at the predicted amino acid level. Of the staphylococcal enterotoxins, SEA is one of the most common causes of gastroenteritis (vomiting and diarrhea) resulting from food contamination. SEA is an extremely potent gastrointestinal toxin; amounts as low as 100 ng are sufficient to cause symptoms of intoxication (10). It is a highly stable, single-chain polypeptide of 29 kDa.

S. aureus enterotoxin A has two separate biological functions. It acts as an enterotoxin on gastrointestinal cells, causing gastroenteritis. It also acts as a superantigen with effects on the immune system (11). SEA, like other superantigens, has the ability to cause a non-antigen-specific activation of T lymphocytes and, subsequently, B cells. Upon exposure of normal rat lymphocytes to food contaminated with SEA, high levels of proliferation were observed (Fig. 1). The ability of SEA to cause proliferation was totally abolished following heat treatment (such as autoclaving) of the food samples (Fig. 1) as a result of toxin denaturation and the loss of the native structure necessary for the binding to MHC class II and the T-cell receptor.

S. aureus enterotoxin A does not activate all Vβ T-cell receptor domains. Specifically, T cells with receptors containing the Vβ 5.3, 6.3, 6.4, and 6.9 families were reported to become stimulated by SEA; others were not (12). There is a close correlation between the enterotoxin and superantigen functions of SEA. In most cases, when superantigen activity is abolished by SEA mutations, enterotoxic activity is also lost (13). Heat treatment of SEA, which leads to loss of superantigen activity, is correlated with loss of SEA recognition by anti-SEA antibodies (14).

Like many other superantigens, SEA has been associated with autoimmunity. A T-cell line isolated from a diabetic patient showed reactivity to a peptide similar to SEA (15) and has been implicated as a pathogenic agent in an experimental autoimmune disease, allergic encephalomyelitis (16,17), a murine model of multiple sclerosis. SEA has the capacity of activating autoreactive T cells that induce autoimmune disease directly (18) and autoreactive T cells able to transfer diabetes in rats (19).

The effect of SEA on the development of autoimmune disease could be by direct stimulation of autoreactive lymphocytes through the crosslinking of the MHC class II product to the T-cell receptor or through production of cytokines (such as interleukin [IL]-1 and IL-2) and antibodies (20–22). In one report, the action of SEA on autoimmunity was to suppress autoimmune diabetes, possibly by activating CD4+ regulatory T cells (23). Thus, SEA and other superantigens are environmental factors that, upon exposure in a genetically susceptible individual, can result in autoimmune disease.

FUNGAL TOXINS Fungal toxins (mycotoxins) represent a large group of materials produced, in most part, by species of

Aspergillus and *Fusarium*. They include aflatoxins, ochratoxin, patulin, and fumonisins, which are potent carcinogens, trichothecenes, which are hematopoietic toxins, and zearalenones, which have estrogenic effects *(1)*.

Of the mycotoxins, trichothecenes have been the ones most commonly associated with immunotoxicity. Trichothecenes are a family of secondary metabolites produced by species of *Fusarium* and related fungi *(24)* that have long been known to cause severe toxicoses in both humans and farm animals following ingestion of moldy cereal grains. They are sesquiterpenoid compounds (i.e., they contain 15 carbon atoms) with molecular weights of 200–400 Da. They are characterized by a tricyclic skeleton, a cyclic apoxide, and different substitutions at carbons 3, 4, 7, 8, and 15, which give them different toxic properties *(25)*.

The production of trichothecenes is highly dependent on such ecological factors as humidity, temperature, soil composition, and pH *(25)*. Trichothecene toxicoses typically occur following wet and cold periods, which are the most favorable conditions for mold growth and toxin production.

Trichothecenes are resistant to food processing and high temperatures, which enables them to permeate human foods as well as animals feeds. They were first described by Brian and McGowan *(26)*, who isolated them while investigating a fungistatic agent, which they named glutinosin. This agent caused severe skin irritation on contact and was the first metabolite of the trichothecene type to be identified.

Trichothecenes were implicated in many outbreaks of human and animal diseases. Stachybotriotoxicosis, which caused the death of thousands of horses in the Soviet Union, was described in the 1930s *(27)*, red mold toxicosis in the early twentieth century in Japan *(27,28)*, and the "turkey X disease" in Britain. In the 1940s *(29)*, trichothecenes were identified as the causative agent in alimentary toxic aleukia in the Soviet Union, where it caused the death of 10% of the population in the Orenburg district. Interest in trichothecenes was renewed in the early 1980s when the U.S. government accused the Soviet Union, Vietnam, and Laos governments of using trichothecenes for chemical warfare in regions where "yellow rain" was reported *(27,30)*. This accusation resulted from the finding of extremely high levels of trichothecenes in blood, urine, and internal tissues of putative attack victims.

Exposure to high levels of trichothecenes produces nausea, vomiting, and diarrhea, and may result in death. However, consumption of lesser amounts was reported to diminish immunity and decrease resistance to pathogens *(31)*. Indeed, trichothecenes have been reported to have suppressive effects on all aspects of the immune system, including total antibody levels, antigen-specific antibody and T-cell responses, the number of circulating T and B cells, macrophage–effector cell function, mitogenic responses in vitro, graft rejection, resistance to infection, and direct damage to lymphoid organs *(27,31–33)*.

Vomitoxin in IgA Glomerulonephritis Vomitoxin was first isolated from Ohio corn infected by *Fusarium (34)*. In the isolation procedure, each fraction was tested for the presence of an emetic material by administration to pigs. The active compound was characterized as a trichothecene with a molecular weight of 296 Da and was named vomitoxin because of its emetic effect on swine. The compound was also detected by Yoshizawa and Morooka in a culture of *Fusarium graminearum* at the same time *(35)*.

Concern about the presence of vomitoxin in crops used for food production arises for two reasons. First, even though vomitoxin is

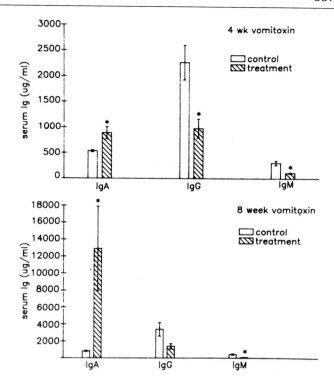

Fig. 2. Effect of feeding 25 ppm vomitoxin for 4 and 8 wk on total serum immunoglobulins in B6C3F1 mice. Data are mean ± SEM and are representative of three experiments. The asterisk (*) indicates significantly different (*p* < 0.05) from matching controls.

not as toxic as other trichothecenes, it is the major contaminant of cereals worldwide *(36)*. Second, vomitoxin is resistant to processing of grains during food preparation. Heating to 350°C, milling, and baking were not able to remove vomitoxin from food products. Thus, the widespread contamination of cereal grains with vomitoxin, combined with its resistance to processing, enables vomitoxin to persist in the human and animal food supply.

In terms of immunotoxicity, ingestion of vomitoxin causes dysregulation of serum immunoglobulin production by decreasing IgG and IgM and increasing IgA and IgE serum levels (Fig. 2) *(37,38)*. The increased serum IgA levels may result from the stimulatory effect of vomitoxin on IgA-producing B cells in the Peyer's patches (PP). This stimulatory effect was observed as an increase in the size and frequency of the germinal centers in the PP subsequent to vomitoxin feeding, as well as in the increase in the percentage of membrane IgA-bearing B cells *(39)*. The activation of IgA-producing B cells could result from the inhibition of apoptosis of helper T cells *(40)* and the activation of cytokine production in the PP *(41)*.

Following hyperelevation of serum IgA, glomerular IgA deposition occurs (Fig. 3) *(42)*. The symptoms of the glomerular deposition are very similar to human IgA nephropathy. This immune-mediated disease, the most common glomerulonephritis worldwide, is of unknown etiology. The similarity of the vomitoxin-induced disease to human IgA glomerulonephritis is further supported by increased levels of serum IgA immune complexes as well as hematuria found in vomitoxin-fed mice *(43)*. Another similarity between the vomitoxin-induced IgA glomerulonephritis and human IgA nephropathy is the male predilection; in both

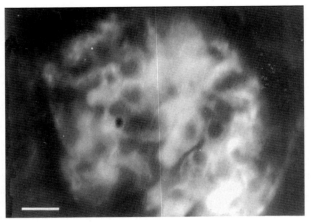

Fig. 3. Accumulation of glomerular IgA in kidneys of control mouse (top panel) and vomitoxin fed mouse (bottom panel). Kidney sections of control and vomitoxin-fed mice were stained with anti-IgA fluorescein isothiocyanate (FITC) conjugate. Bar size is 10 μM.

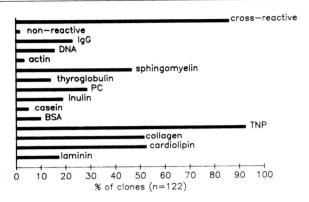

Fig. 4. Reactivity of IgA-producing clones that were isolated from B6C3F1 mice fed vomitoxin. Data are presented as percentage of total clones screened. Crossreactive = reacted to more than one antigen.

diseases, males were more susceptible than females to IgA glomerulonephropathy (44). These findings suggest the possibility that vomitoxin could be an etiologic factor in human IgA nephropathy.

The IgA that is produced at high levels in vomitoxin-fed mice is polyspecific and autoreactive (38,45,46). When IgA-producing cells were isolated from the PP of vomitoxin-fed mice, more than 80% of the IgA-producing clones secreted highly crossreactive IgA antibodies that reacted with several self and nonself antigens (Fig. 4). A similar polyspecificity was observed in IgA that was isolated from the glomerular IgA deposits (46).

In conclusion, ingestion of vomitoxin, which is present in many human and animal food products, may serve as an etiologic agent, leading to the development of IgA glomerulonephritis. This pathogenic mechanism is initiated with the vomitoxin-induced dysregulation of IgA, leading to increased autoreactive polyspecific serum IgA antibodies. These IgA antibodies form immune complexes with self and foreign antigens in the serum and are deposited in the kidneys. The immune complexes cause IgA glomerulonephritis resulting in kidney damage and, often, death.

EXCESS NUTRIENTS Although many nutrients are required for normal function, excessive amounts of some nutrients can lead to toxic effects. Examples are excess iron and some of the vitamins and minerals. Despite many reports, very little information is available on the mechanisms of immunotoxicity resulting from excess nutrients.

Iodine is a trace element required for maintenance of health. It is primarily obtained through seafood and grain products as well as from salt in countries where salt is iodinated, such as the United States. The main concentration of iodine is in the hormones produced by the thyroid gland. The thyroid gland actively traps the iodide from the circulation and, therefore, contains approximately 80% of the total-body iodide. The iodide is used to generate the thyroid hormones, whose role is to stimulate the basal rate of metabolism, oxygen consumption, and heat production. Whereas a lack of dietary iodine clearly results in the formation of a goiter, the effect of excess dietary iodine has been less well studied. The involvement of iodine in autoimmune thyroiditis is now a topic of active research.

Iodine in Autoimmune Thyroiditis In many countries, the levels of iodine ingested in the food exceeds the recommended level. Although the recommended daily allowance (RDA) for a person per day is 150 μg, in countries where the salt is iodinated, the actual consumption may be as much as fourfold higher (47).

A connection between higher levels of iodine ingestion and autoimmune thyroiditis has been demonstrated in several animal models. Excess dietary iodine accelerated development of thyroid-associated lymphoid tissue in BB rats (48) and increased the incidence of spontaneous thyroiditis in BB rats, chickens, and hamsters (49–51).

In humans, epidemiological evidence suggests an increased incidence of thyroiditis associated with iodine supplementation (52–54). Another, stronger connection between iodine and human thyroiditis is the striking finding that patients who receive amiodarone, an antianginal and antiarrhythmic agent that contains 37% of its weight in iodine, show significantly increased titers of antibody to thyroglobulin (55).

Our investigation of the effect of excess dietary iodine on autoimmunity concentrated on findings in human patients as well as studies of a mouse model. In the human disease, we have been able to demonstrate the importance of iodination to the ability of human lymphocytes to proliferate in response to human thyroglobulin (56) (Fig. 5). Lymphocytes from both normal controls and thyroiditis patients proliferated in response to normal thyroglobulin but not to a thyroglobulin preparation lacking iodine (nontoxic goiter thyroglobulin). Upon iodination of this thyroglobulin, however, the proliferative response was restored. The finding that artificially iodinated nontoxic goiter thyroglobulin causes prolifer-

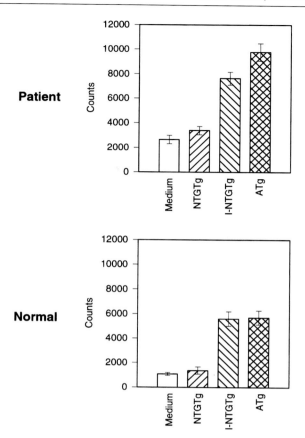

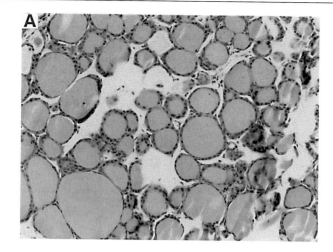

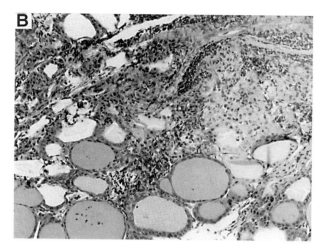

Fig. 5. Proliferation of lymphocytes from a thyroiditis patient (top panel) and a normal individual (bottom panel) in response to in vitro iodinated thyroglobulin. Results are presented in counts of ³H-uptake by proliferating lymphocytes. NTGTg = nontoxic goiter thyroglobulin (no iodination); Atg = amiodarone thyroglobulin (high iodination); I-NTGTg = nontoxic goiter thyroglobulin iodinated in vitro. Data are mean ± SEM.

Fig. 6. Iodine-induced lesions in NOD-H-2[h4] mice. Histological staining of thyroids from control mouse (top panel) and iodine-treated mouse (bottom panel).

ation (Fig. 5) provides direct evidence of the critical role that iodine plays in the antigenicity of thyroglobulin in humans.

The NOD-H-2[h4] mouse is a new model for autoimmune thyroiditis in which the animals spontaneously develop thyroiditis in a low incidence, but supplementation of iodine in the drinking water markedly increases the percentage of positive mice *(57)*. Following 8 wk of supplemental iodine ingestion, treated mouse thyroids showed extensive thyroid lesions with lymphocytic infiltration (Fig. 6). Treated mice had elevated levels of thyroglobulin-specific IgG2b autoantibody, which correlated with the appearance of lesions *(57,58)*. The appearance of thyroglobulin-specific IgG2b was gradual and differences between iodine-treated and control groups became apparent as early as 2 wk after initiation of iodine treatment (Fig. 7) *(58)*. The appearance of thyroglobulin-specific IgG2b suggests that iodine induces a so-called Th3 response involving the production of T-cell growth factor (TGF) β by T cells, as IgG2b is largely dependent on the production of that cytokine.

In addition to the IgG2b thyroglobulin-specific antibody, the development of thyroiditis correlated with a vigorous response to thyroglobulin by spleen cells *(58)*. The ability of splenic lymphocytes from untreated NOD-H-2[h4] mice to proliferate to thyroglobulin was significantly higher than three other mouse strains. The proliferation of spleen cells from mice fed iodine for 8 wk was

even further increased to more than double the values of control mice *(58)*.

In summary, we demonstrated the importance of iodine in both the human and the murine thyroiditis models. In the human disease, the ability of T cells to recognize self thyroglobulin was dependent on iodination of this autoantigen, suggesting a role for iodine in autoantigenicity of thyroglobulin. The murine model provides confirmatory findings exemplifying the importance of the interaction between the genetic background and environmental stimulus to result in autoimmune disease. In the NOD-H-2[h4] mouse, the genetic background favors autoantigen (thyroglobulin) recognition, resulting in increased proliferation of T cells compared to other mouse strains. When the environmental stimulus (excess dietary iodine) is added to the genetic predisposition, autoimmune disease is enhanced, as manifested by thyroid lesions, autoantibody levels, and a greatly increased T-cell proliferation to autoantigen. Thus, whereas a minimal amount of iodine is needed to maintain normal metabolism and function, excess iodine leads to autoimmune thyroid disease in individuals with a susceptible genetic background.

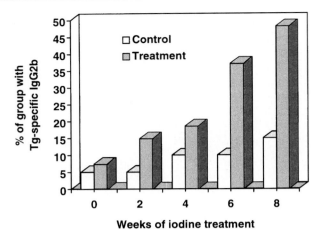

Fig. 7. The appearance of Tg-specific IgG2b serum antibodies in NOD-H-2^h4 mice. Mice were given either plain water (control group) or water with 0.05% iodine (treatment group) for 8 wk and bled at biweekly intervals. Serum was analysed by enzyme-linked immuno-sorbent assay.

SUMMARY

Despite the overall safety of our food supply, several food components have an etiologic role in immune-mediated diseases. Contamination of food with bacteria and the resultant production of bacterial toxins in the food are of special concern when superantigens are produced. Bacterial superantigens, which may cause gastroenteritis because of their direct toxic effects, are also strong activators of the immune response. Nonspecific lymphocytic proliferation may lead to toxic shock as a result of massive production of cytokines and to autoimmune disease resulting from the stimulation of autoreactive cells.

Fungal toxins, the mycotoxins, which are produced in great amounts during periods of rain when mold can grow, have been implicated in many human and animal diseases. Of the mycotoxins, the trichothecenes were most commonly involved with diseases primarily affecting the immune system. At high concentrations, trichothecenes can be lethal or cause severe toxic effects. However, at lower doses and prolonged exposure, dietary trichothecenes produce more subtle effects on the immune system. Vomitoxin, a trichothecene toxin produced by *Fusarium graminearum*, causes IgA dysregulation, resulting in the appearance of autoreactive polyspecific IgA antibodies, glomerular IgA deposition, and the development of a glomerulonephritis strikingly similar to the human IgA glomerulonephritis. Because vomitoxin is a common food contaminant whose levels in the food are not regulated and is resistant to heating, it may be an important etiologic agent in human IgA glomerulonephritis.

In terms of micronutrients, iodine is a trace element that is required for normal metabolism. However, consumption of excess dietary iodine has been linked to human and animal thyroid abnormalities and the appearance of autoimmune reactions directed against the thyroid. In our studies of human thyroiditis, we have been able to demonstrate the involvement of iodine in increasing the autoantigenic properties of thyroglobulin. In the NOD-H-2^h4 mouse, we found that iodine acts in concert with a genetic predisposition to enhance the development of autoimmune thyroiditis. Murine iodine-induced autoimmune thyroiditis involves the gener-

ation of thyroglobulin-specific IgG2b antibodies (which correlate with thyroid lesions) and increased T-cell proliferation to murine thyroglobulin. Thus, iodine-induced murine autoimmune thyroiditis in the NOD-H-2^h4 mouse is an example of an autoimmune disease for which the combination of genetic susceptibility and an environmental stimulus (excess dietary iodine) results in autoimmune disease.

ACKNOWLEDGMENTS

The authors' research on the NOD-H2^h4 mouse was supported in part by NIH research grant #DK42174. The collaboration of Dr. C. Lynne Burek is gratefully acknowledged.

REFERENCES

1. Kotsonis FN, Burdock GA, Flamm WG. Food toxicology. In: Klaassen CD ed, Casarett & Doull's Toxicology. The Basic Science of Poisons, 5th ed., pp, 909–49. McGraw-Hill, 1975 New York.
2. Archer DL, Young FE. Contemporary issues: disease with a food vector. Clin Microbiol Rev 1988; 1:377–98.
3. Marrack P, Kappler J. The staphylococcal enterotoxins and their relatives. Science 1990; 248:705–11.
4. Karp DR, Teletski CL, Scholl P, Geha RS, Long EO. The a1 domain of the HLA-DR molecule is essential for high-affinity binding of the toxic shock syndrome toxin-1. Nature 1990; 346:474.
5. Scherer MT, Ignatowics L, Winslow GM, Kappler JW, Marrack P. Superantigens: bacterial and viral proteins that manipulate the immune system. Annu Rev Cell Biol 1993; 9:101–128.
6. Kotb M. Superantigens in human diseases. Clin Microbiol Newslett 1997; 19:145–50.
7. Kotb M. Role of superantigens in the pathogenesis of infectious diseases and their sequelae. Curr Opin Infect Dis 1992; 5:364–74.
8. Acha-Orbea H. Bacterial and viral superantigens: roles in autoimmunity? Ann Rheum Dis 1993; 52:16.
9. Schlievert PM. Role of superantigens in human diseases. J Infect Dis 1993; 167:997–1002.
10. Everson ML, Hinds MW, Bernstein RS, Bergdoll MS. Estimation of human dose of Staphylococcal enterotoxin A from a large outbreak of staphylococcal food poisoning involving chocolate milk. J Food Microbiol 1988; 7:311–6.
11. Frieman SM, Tumang JR, Crow MK. Microbial superantigens as etiopathogenic agents in autoimmunity. Rheum Dis Clin North Am 1993; 19:207–22.
12. Schad EM, Zaitseva I, Zaitsev VN, Dohlsten M, Kalland T, Schlievert PM, et al. Crystal structure of the superantigen staphylococcal enterotoxin type A. EMBO J 1995; 14:3292–301.
13. Harris TO, Grossman D, Kappler JW, Marrack P, Rich RR, Betley MJ. Lack of complete correlation between emetic and T-cell-stimulatory activities of staphylococcal enterotoxins. Infect Immun 1993; 61:3175–83.
14. Stelma GN, Bradshaw JG, Kauffman PE, Archer DL. Thermal inactivation of mitogenic and serological activities of staphylococcal enterotoxin A at 1210C. IRCS Med Sci 1980; 8:629.
15. Neophytou PI, Roep BO, Arden SD, Muir EM, Duinkerken G, Kallan A, et al. T-cell epitope analysis using subtracted expression libraries (TEASEL): application of a 38-kDA autoantigen recognized by T cells from an insulin-dependent diabetic patient. Proc Natl Acad Sci USA 1996; 93:2014–8.
16. Soos JM, Hobeika AC, Butfiloski EJ, Schiffenbauer J, Johnson HM. Accelerated induction of experimental allergic encephalomyelitis in PL/J mice by a non-V beta 8-specific superantigen. Proc Natl Acad Sci USA 1995; 92:6082–6.
17. Rott O, Mignon-Godfroy K, Fleischer B, Charreire J, Cash E. Superantigens induce primary T cell responses to soluble autoantigens by a non-V beta specific mechanism of bystander activation. Cell Immunol 1995; 161:158–65.
18. Schiffenbauer J, Johnson HM, Butfiloski EJ, Wegrzyn L, Soos JM.

Staphylococcal enterotoxins can reactivate experimental allergic encephalomyelitis. Proc Natl Acad Sci USA 1993; 90:8543–6.

19. Ellerman KE, Like AA. Staphylococcal enterotoxin-activated spleen cells passively transfer diabetes in BB/Wor rat. Diabetes 1992; 41:527–32.

20. Al-Daccak R, Mehindate K, Poubelle PE, Mourad W. Signalling via MHC class II molecules selectively induces IL-1 beta over IL-1 receptor antagonist gene expression. Biochem Biophys Res Commun 1994; 201:855–60.

21. Nielsen M, Svejgaard A, Ropke C, Nordahl M, Odum N. Staphylococcal enterotoxins modulate interleukin 2 receptor expression and ligand-induced tyrosine phosphorylation of the Janus protein-tyrosine kinase 3 (Jak3) and signal transducers and activators of transcription (Stat proteins). PNAS 1995; 92:10,995–9.

22. Crow MK, Zagon G, Chu Z, Ravina B, Tumang JR, Cole BC, et al. Human B cell differentiation induced by microbial superantigens: unselected peripheral blood lymphocytes secrete polyclonal immunoglobulin in response to Mycoplasma arthritidis mitogen. Autoimmunity 14:23–32.

23. Kawamura T, Nagata M, Utsugi T, Yoon JW. Prevention of autoimmune type I diabetes by CD4+ suppressor T cells in superantigen-treated non-obese diabetic mice. J Immunol 151:4362–70.

24. Bamburg JR, Strong FM. 12,13-Epoxitrichothecenes. In: Kadis S, Ciegler A, Ajl SJ, eds, Microbial Toxins Vol. VII, pp. 207–92. Academic, London, 1971.

25. Vidal DR. Properties immunosuppressives des mycotoxines du groupe des trichothecenes. Bull Inst Pasteur 1990; 88:159–92.

26. Brian PW, McGowan JC. Biologically active metabolic products of the mold *Metarrhizium glutinosum* S. Pope. Nature 1946; 157:334.

27. Bamburg JR. Biological and biochemical actions of trichothecene mycotoxins. In: Hahn FE, eds, Progress in Molecular and Subcellular Biology, Vol. 8, pp. 41–110. Springer-Verlag, Berlin, 1983.

28. Matsuoka Y, Kubota K. Studies on mechanisms of diarrhea induced by fusarenone-X, a trichothecene mycotoxin from *Fusarium* species. Toxicol Appl Pharmacol 1981; 57:293–301.

29. Joffe AZ. Alimentary toxic aleukia. In: Kadis S, Ciegler A, Ajl SJ, eds, Microbial Toxins, Vol. VII, pp. 139–89. Academic, London, 1971.

30. Watson SA, Mirocha CJ, Hayes AW. Analysis for trichothecenes in samples from southeast asia associated with "yellow rain." Fund Appl Toxicol 1984; 4:700–17.

31. Corrier DE. Mycotoxins: mechanisms of immunosuppression. Vet Immunopathol 1991; 30:73–87.

32. Pestka JJ, Bondy GS. Alteration of immune function following dietary mycotoxin exposure. Can J Physiol Pharmacol 1990; 68:1009–16.

33. Pestka JJ, Forsell JH. Inhibition of human lymphocyte transformation by the macrocyclic trichothecenes roridin A and verrucarin A. Toxicol Lett 1988; 41:215–22.

34. Vesonder RF, Ciegler A, Jensen AH. Isolation of the emetic principle from Fusarium-infected corn. Appl Microbiol 1973; 26:1008–10.

35. Ueno Y. Trichothecenes: chemical, biological and toxicological aspects. In: Ueno Y, ed, Developments in Food Science Vol 4, Elsevier, Amsterdam, 1983.

36. Hietaniemi V, Kumpulainen J. Concents of Fusarium toxins in finnish and imported grains and feeds. Food Addit Contamin 1991; 8:171–82.

37. Pestka JJ, Dong W. Serum IgE hyperelevation in B6C3F1 mice following pulsed dietary exposure to the trichothecene vomitoxin. FASEB, 1992, Anaheim, CA.

38. Rasooly L, Pestka JJ. Vomitoxin-induced modulation of serum IgA, IgM, and IgG reactive with natural gut and self antigens. Food Chem Toxicol 1991; 30:499–504.

39. Pestka JJ, Dong W, Warner RL, Rasooly L, Bondy GS, Brooks KH. Elevated membrane IgA+ and CD4+ (T helper) populations in murine peyer's patch and splenic lymphocytes during dietary administration of the trichothecene vomitoxin (deoxynivalenol). Food Chem Toxicol 1990; 28:409–20.

40. Pestka JJ, Yan D, King LE. Flow cytometric analysis of the effects of in vitro exposure to vomitoxin (deoxynivalenol) on apoptosis in murine T, B and IgA+ cells. Food Chem Toxicol 1994; 32:1125–36.

41. Yan D, Zhou HR, Brooks KH, Pestka JJ. Potential role for IL-5 and IL-6 in enhanced IgA secretion by Peyer's patch cells isolated from mice acutely exposed to vomitoxin. Toxicology 1997; 122:145–58.

42. Pestka JJ, Tai JH, Witt MF, Dixon DE, Forsell JH. Suppression of immune response in the B6C3F1 mouse after dietary exposure to the fusarium mycotoxins deoxynivalenol (vomitoxin) and zealenone. Food Chem Toxicol 1987; 25:297–304.

43. Dong W, Sell JE, Pestka JJ. Quantitative assessment of mesangial immunoglobulin A (IgA) accumulation, elevated circulating IgA immune complexes, and hematuria during vomitoxin-induced IgA nephropathy. Fund Appl Toxicol 1991; 17:197–207.

44. Greene DM, Azcona-Olivera JI, Pestka JJ. Vomitoxin (deoxynivalenol)-induced IgA nephropathy in the B6C3F1 mouse: dose response and male predilection. Toxicology 1994; 92:245–60.

45. Rasooly L, Pestka JJ. Polyclonal autoreactive IgA increase and mesangial deposition during vomitoxin-induced IgA nephropathy in the BALB/c mouse. Food Chem Toxicol 1994; 32:329–36.

46. Rasooly L, Abouzied MM, Brooks KH, Pestka JJ. Polyspecific autoreactive IgA secreted by hybridomas derived from Peyer's patches of vomitoxin-fed mice: characterization and possible pathogenic role in IgA nephropathy. Food Chem Toxicol 1994; 32:337–48.

47. Fradkin JE, Wolff J. Iodine-induced thyrotoxicosis. Medicine 1983; 62:1–20.

48. Mooij P, de Wit HJ, Dreshage HA. An excess of dietary iodine accelerates the development of a thyroid-associated lymphoid tissue in autoimmune prone BB rats. Clin Immunol Immunopathol 1993; 69:189–98.

49. Allen EM, Appel MC, Braverman LE. The effect of iodide ingestion on the development of spontaneous lymphocytic thyroiditis in the diabetes-prone BB/W rat. Endocrinology 1986; 118:1977–81.

50. Bagchi N, Brown TR, Urdanivia E, Sundick RS. Induction of autoimmune thyroiditis in chickens by dietary iodine. Science 1985; 230:325–7.

51. Follis RH. Further observations on thyroiditis and colloid accumulation in hyperplastic thyroid glands of hamsters receiving excess iodine. Lab Invest 1964; 13:1590.

52. Beierwaltes WH. Iodide and lymphocytic thyroiditis. Bull All India Inst Med Sci 1969; 3:145.

53. Harach HR, Escalante DA, Onativia A, Outes JL, Day ES, Williams ED. Thyroid carcinoma and thyroiditis in an endemic goitre region before and after iodine prophylaxis. Acta Endocrinol (Copenhagen) 1985; 108:55.

54. Boukis MA, Koutras DA, Souvatzoglou A, Evangelopoulou A, Vrontakis M, Moulapoulous SD. Thyroid hormone and immunologic studies in endemic goiter. J Clin Endocrinol Metab 1983; 57:859.

55. Gomez-Balaguer M, Caballero E, Costa P, Gilsanz A, Bernat E, Uriel C, et al. Amiodarone thyroid autoimmunity relationship? In: Drexhage HA, Wiersinga WM, eds, The Thyroid and Autoimmunity. Elsevier Science, New York, 1986.

56. Rasooly L, Rose NR, Saboori AM, Ladenson PW, Burek CL. Iodine is essential for human T cell recognition of human thyroglobulin. Autoimmunity 1998; 27:213–219.

57. Rasooly L, Burek CL, Rose NR. Iodine-induced autoimmune thyroiditis in NOD-H-2^{h4} mice. Clin Immunol Immunopathol 1996; 81: 287–92.

58. Rasooly L, Vladut-Talor M, Hill SL, Burek CL, Rose NR. Iodine-induced thyroiditis in the NOD-H-2^{h4} mouse: the role of dose, autoantibody isotype and T cell proliferation, submitted.

30 Interactions Between Nutrition and Immunity

Lessons from Animal Agriculture

KIRK C. KLASING AND TATIANA V. LESHCHINSKY

INTRODUCTION

Basic and applied research on the interactions between nutrition and the immune system has been a focal point for animal nutritionists for more than 50 yr. Economics and concerns about food safety and animal welfare shape the types of questions considered by researchers concerned with animal husbandry. As in human nutrition, a primary goal is to determine the impact of diet on the immune system and, consequently, the incidence of diseases controlled by, or caused by, the immune system. In modern agriculture, animals are almost always fed scientifically formulated diets that provide the required levels of nutrients at a minimal cost. Nutrient requirements set by the National Research Council and other organizations are based typically on levels that maximize growth rates and reproductive performance and prevent signs of deficiency. As in human nutrition, these standards are minimum requirements and rarely consider immunity or optimal health. Because optimizing animal health increases the wholesomeness of the human food supply and improves profits of animal producers, considerable research effort has been devoted to identifying nutrients that benefit the immune system when supplemented at levels above requirements. This research extends from basic laboratory-based experimentation at the mechanistic level to controlled field-based studies at the population level. Human nutritionists should be particularly interested in the results of these field studies because they offer a chance to look directly at the impact of highly controlled nutritional interventions on the resistance to infectious challenges in animals. Studies with poultry are particularly illuminating because diets differing in the level of only a single nutrient are fed to hundreds of thousands of birds living in very identical environments during the majority of their growth and development. These studies clearly demonstrate the dynamics of nutritional immunomodulation on the incidence of diseases at the population level. The first section of this chapter reviews the impact of specific nutrients on the immune system and the impact

of these changes on the susceptibility of animals to infectious diseases.

Recently, animal nutrition research has also focused on the impact of an immune response on nutrient requirements of animals. Clearly, the immune system is central to maintaining homeostasis and serves as both a sensory system that detects insults to homeostasis and a control system that orchestrates local and systemic responses directed toward re-establishing homeostasis. The cellular and metabolic sequelae that accompanies an immune response redirects nutrients away from physiological processes important for growth and reproduction toward processes important in host defense. These events can markedly impact the nutritional needs of an animal. Animal nutritionists are determining dietary changes that permit more cost-effective nutrition during periods of clinically identifiable infectious diseases and also when husbandry and sanitation practices are substandard. The second section of this chapter considers the quantitative effects of an immune response on nutritional requirements of animals.

Studies with agriculturally important animals almost always pertain to growing or reproducing physiological states. Limited research has considered nonreproducing mature animals. Consequently, the animal literature is not very relevant to adult humans living at close to maintenance conditions (i.e., most adults). Furthermore, the fractional rate of growth and the reproductive output of economically important animals are often an order of magnitude greater than those of humans. These vast differences in physiological states must be kept in mind when interpreting the results of animal nutrition studies for human applications. A second caveat of applying the animal literature on nutrition and immunity to humans is the premier importance of minimizing infectious diseases relative to those with a metabolic, autoimmune, or hypersensitivity etiology. This emphasis is due to the importance of limiting the transfer of infectious diseases through animal food products.

IMPACT OF NUTRITION ON IMMUNITY

Our knowledge of nutrition of poultry and livestock is relatively mature, including a very complete listing of the required nutrients, a quantitative accounting of the minimal level of each nutrient that is needed to maximize production characteristics, and the

From: *Nutrition and Immunology: Principles and Practice* (ME Gershwin et al. eds.), © Humana Press, Inc., Totowa, NJ

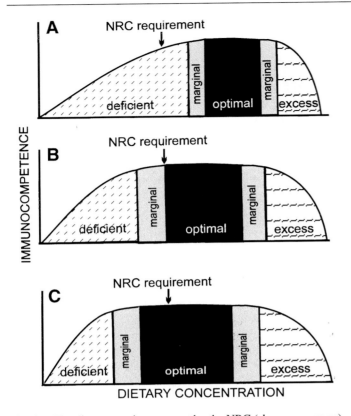

Fig. 1. The dietary requirements set by the NRC (shown as arrows) are usually based on levels that maximize growth and reproduction and prevent known deficiency pathologies. Optimal immunocompetence may occur at nutrient levels that are higher then the NRC requirement (panel A), equal to the NRC requirement (panel B), or less than the NRC requirement (panel C).

1. *Direct regulation by nutrients.* Some essential and nonessential nutrients influence regulatory decisions during an immune response by modifying intercellular or intracellular communication pathways. Examples of these nutrients include polyunsaturated fatty acids and vitamins E, A, and D.

2. *Indirect modulation mediated by the endocrine system.* Most hormones have regulatory influences on the immune system and the levels of many hormones are responsive to dietary factors. For example, the amount of calories consumed and the protein-to-calorie ratio influence the somatotropic axis and the levels of insulin, glucagon, and glucocorticoids. These hormones, in turn, modulate the immune system.

3. *Regulation by availability of substrates.* A steady supply of nutrients is needed for the clonal proliferation of lymphocytes, leukopoiesis, and the synthesis of their secretory products. Nutrients are also needed by the liver for the secretion of acute-phase proteins. Severe deficiencies of many trace nutrients cause impairments in the development of the immune system and negatively influence immunocompetence. However, moderate deficiencies during the postnatal period are usually not detrimental to the immune system because of its high priority for substrates when they become limiting in body fluids.

4. *Modulation of the pathology caused by an immune response.* Some nutrients, especially those that serve as antioxidants (e.g., vitamin E), limit the pathology that results from effector functions of leukocytes.

5. *Nutritional immunity.* The immune system orchestrates a decrease in the concentration of some nutrients in the blood and other body fluids. Low levels of some nutrients, especially iron, impair the replication of pathogens in host tissues.

Several other potential mechanisms described in the literature using laboratory rodents include nutrient interactions (e.g., amino acid antagonisms and imbalances) and nutrient toxicities. Animal nutritionists have not explored the implications of these mechanisms to a great extent because they are not typically encountered with scientifically formulated diets utilizing typical feed ingredients.

In the following subsections, these five mechanisms are discussed in further detail, with particular reference to their impact on immunocompetence and disease incidence in poultry and livestock. Practical experience and epidemiological data demonstrate the difficulty of setting specific nutrient levels that optimize immunity because immunomodulatory impacts of nutrients typically shift the types of disease prevalent in a population. Thus, animal nutritionists utilize the immunomodulatory impact of nutrients as a management tool to aid in ameliorating specific disease problems of high prevalence.

DIRECT REGULATION BY NUTRIENTS Dietary manipulation of a few nutrients results in immunoregulatory consequences resulting from direct regulatory effects of that nutrient on leukocytes. The literature is replete with examples where a nutrient modulates the rates of proliferation, cytokine production, or differentiation of specific leukocyte populations in vitro (*1*). In most instances, these in vitro observations have little relevance to nutrition because augmentation of a complete diet with additional

levels and bioavailabilities of the essential nutrients supplied by feedstuffs. However, in many cases, it is not known if the requirement values that maximize productivity in healthy, unchallenged animals are optimal for immunocompetence and disease resistance (Fig. 1). With almost 40 nutrients required by vertebrates and more than 20 interrelated immune cell types and effector mechanisms, the number of possible interactions is imposing. The complexity of these interactions has prompted animal nutritionists to base dietary management for the purpose of influencing immunocompetence on a solid mechanistic foundation instead of only on empirical observations. Basic research in laboratory animals has identified many general mechanisms through which the immune system is influenced by nutrition. Animal nutritionists concerned with optimizing disease resistance have focused on these diverse mechanisms to determine nutrient levels that optimize immune responsiveness and minimize specific infectious and noninfectious diseases.

Nutritionists commonly think of required nutrients as substrates for the synthesis of macromolecules or for provision of energy. However, in practical diets fed to animals, these substrate functions of nutrients are not the only, or even the most important, mechanisms through which nutrition affects immunity. The following mechanistic categories are somewhat arbitrary but provide a conceptual framework for this complex area:

amounts of a nutrient has relatively minor effects on its plasma and tissue concentrations. However, there are a few important exceptions in which a nutrient has important immunoregulatory effects that occur above their established requirement. Furthermore, some nutrients that are not categorized as "essential" can have important modulatory actions on the immune system. In fact, nutrients for which there is no acknowledge requirement have some of the most significant modulatory impacts on the immune system.

Polyunsaturated Fatty Acids One of the best examples of this situation is the role of long-chain polyunsaturated fatty acids (PUFAs) in regulating the immune response. The mechanisms by which PUFAs modulate the immune system through modifying cellular communication, membrane fluidity, and second messenger elaboration has been covered in Chapter 13. Experiments in chickens demonstrates that both the absolute amount of n-3 PUFAs and the ratio of dietary n-3 to n-6 fatty acids are important considerations (2–5). Supplementation of grain-based diets with low levels (1.5–3%) of fish oil enhance antibody responses following some types of antigens but decrease inflammatory and cell-mediated responses. In general, these changes can be interpreted in a shift from a Th_1 to Th_2 response to antigens. This shift in immune response has proven to be advantageous for enhancing antibody titers following some types of vaccination.

Very large field trials have been conducted in poultry, which provide an opportunity to examine how the immunomodulatory actions of PUFAs actually translate into changes in the incidence of natural infections. For example, a trial with 960,000 chicks was conducted at a single commercial production facility to compare a corn–soybean-meal-based diet supplemented with 0.26 g/kg of eicosapentanoic and docosahexaenoic acids from menhaden fish to a diet containing the same amount of supplemental animal fat. In this trial, disease incidence was determined from the records of the United States Department of Agriculture (USDA) inspector that observed the slaughtering and processing of the birds in the processing plant. Dietary n-3 fatty acids significantly decreased the incidence of septicemia of all causes by 25% and the incidence of cellulitis, which is usually the result of *E. coli*-induced inflammation of scratches in the skin, by 18%. Conversely, the incidence of tumors, both spontaneous and from Marek's disease virus, increased by 24%. This study clearly shows that the modulatory actions of dietary PUFAs on the immune system result in a change in the spectrum of disease problems that occur in the field. Thus, dietary PUFAs may be thought of as nonpharmacological immunomodulators that change the incidence diseases in animal populations. The decision to include n-3 PUFAs in the diet is dependent on the specific infectious disease processes that are a problem in a flock at any given time.

Vitamin E Most metabolic effects of vitamin E are mediated by its antioxidant properties, particularly in regard to reactive oxygen intermediates (ROI). These molecules are produced as a result of normal metabolism by all cells as well as during the immune response, primarily by neutrophils and monocytes. Traditionally, ROI have been considered highly destructive molecules. However, recent studies showed that ROI are also involved in activation of gene expression. At least two transcriptional factors, NF-κB and AP-1, which are activated by a redox-dependent process, are involved in the regulation of viral gene expression, cytokine synthesis, and the acute inflammation reaction (6–10). Many antioxidants, including vitamin E and vitamin E-related com-

pounds, inhibit NF-κB activation by ROI and activate AP-1 (6,9). Vitamin E inhibits NF-κB activation by decreasing the activity of protein kinase C, which phosphorylates I-κB, an inhibitory component associated with NF-κB (11). Lander (7) suggested that endogenous scavengers of free radicals must not not only quench but must also modify the chemical nature and transport of ROI.

Vitamin E can affect both the lipoxygenase and cyclooxygenase pathways of arachidonic acid metabolism (12). Supplementation with 300 mg/kg (approximately 30 × the National Research Council (NRC) requirement) of vitamin E depresses prostaglandins (PGE_2 and PGF_2), and thromboxane B_2 levels in chicken tissues (13). In vitro PGE_2 inhibits interleukin (IL)-2 production, T-cell mitogenesis, and IgM synthesis; therefore, its suppression by vitamin E could be a mechanism by which vitamin E regulates immune response. ROI also regulate PGE_2 synthesis by activating the inducible form of cyclooxygenase (14). Thus, it is not clear which of the mechanisms is primarily responsible for vitamin E immunoregulation.

In animal models (pigs, dogs, calves, chickens, mice), almost every aspect of the immune system has been shown to be altered by the dietary level of vitamin E, including resistance to infection, specific antibody responses, number of splenic plaque-forming cells, in vitro mitogenic responses of lymphocytes, and phagocytic index (15,16). In our studies (17), dietary vitamin E supplementation of chickens increased antibody production against killed infectious bronchitis virus (IBV), but not live IBV vaccine in young chicks. Moderate dietary vitamin E (50 IU/kg) increased antibody production to sheep red blood cells, whereas higher levels (100 and 200 IU/kg) did not. Recruitment of heterophils after lipopolysaccharide (LPS) injection was also enhanced by moderate but not high levels of dietary vitamin E. Mitogen-induced lymphocyte proliferation and acute-phase protein production (hemopexin and α1-acid glycoprotein) were not increased with vitamin E supplementation.

Several studies have demonstrated increased food conversion, decreased mortality, and an increase in immunocompetence in chickens, pigs, and cattle supplemented with high levels of vitamin E (16,18). For example, Tengerdy and Nockels (19) showed that dietary supplementation with 300 mg/kg (30 times the NRC requirement) increased the protection of chicks against *E. coli*, decreasing mortality from 40% to 5%. Part of this protection may be the result of an increase in passive immunity caused by high levels of vitamin E supplementation (20). In a field test conducted by a commercial chicken producer, 1,524,000 birds were fed a diet with either 33 IU/kg or 249 IU/kg dietary treatment (16). This high level of supplementation did not improve weight gain or mortality, but the incidence of clinically identifiable infections was markedly decreased at the time the birds underwent USDA inspection at slaughter. The vitamin E-supplemented group had 25% less septicemia and 61% less cellulitis and other inflammatory lesions. However, other studies do not show improvements either in performance or in immunocompetence. Sell et al. (21) showed that supplementation with 300 IU/kg of diet did not alleviate the effects of *E. coli* infection on performance, livability, and incidence and severity of lesions in young turkeys.

It has been postulated that inconsistencies in vitamin E studies result from differences in the degree of disease challenge, status of other antioxidants in the diet, breed, environmental conditions (stress, husbandry), and in vitro assay conditions. Kennedy et al. (22) tried to eliminate the possible effects of dietary differences, breed, and degree of disease challenge in their trial performed with approximately 3 million commercial broiler chickens fed either high (163 mg/kg) or moderate (44 mg/kg) levels of vitamin E. Their study showed no significant effect of vitamin E supplementation in the healthiest and fastest-growing flocks. However, slower-growing birds benefited from the high level of vitamin E, probably the result of improved immunocompetence and resistance to subclinical infections (22). In a follow-up study with over 1.5 million chickens, McIlroy et al. (23) demonstrated that birds exposed to subclinical Infectious Bursal disease benefited from vitamin E (178 IU/kg) with decreased morbidity, whereas birds without this viral infection did not significantly benefit from vitamin E supplementation.

As shown by McIlroy and others, the beneficial effect of vitamin E supplementation is present only when there is a challenge to the host defense system. It is possible that a balance between ROI and antioxidants determines the immunomodulating properties of vitamin E. ROI production usually increases during stress or infection, which could cause excessive tissue damage. In this case, the antioxidative properties of vitamin E may be protective and immunomodulating. High doses of vitamin E, however, may prevent the formation of, or may modify ROI necessary for, the regulation of gene expression and, thus, suppress or alter immune responses.

Other Nutrients   Vitamin A, β-carotene, and vitamin D also have regulatory actions on leukocytes that have practical applications in animal nutrition. The direct regulatory action of these fat-soluble vitamins on leukocytes has been described in vitro and in vivo. A variety of studies in chickens, pigs, and cattle have indicated that the immunomodulatory roles of Vitamin A, β-carotene, and vitamin D occur at levels that are considerably greater than current requirement recommendations (NRC) based on the prevention of deficiency-related pathology (18). Retinoic acid, acting through its specific receptor, is important in regulating the recruitment of cells into lymphocyte and macrophage lineages (24,25). The dietary level of vitamin A that maximizes growth and feed efficiency of broiler chickens (500 μg/kg) is insufficient for optimal development of the immune system. In growing chicks and poults, levels 5-fold to 20-fold higher are necessary to maximize indices of both cell-mediated and antibody-mediated immunity and minimize the incidence of infectious diseases (26–28).

A wide variety of other nutrients have been suggested to have immunoregulatory actions (e.g., chromium, arginine, glutamine) based on laboratory experiments. However, the results of these experiments have not usually been confirmed in large field trials and manipulations of the dietary levels of these nutrients for the purpose of modulating the immune system have not been adopted by animal agriculture.

INDIRECT REGULATION MEDIATED BY THE ENDO-CRINE SYSTEM   The immune system is not an autonomous system; it is influenced by other physiological systems (29–31). Leukocytes have receptors for and are regulated by most of the hormones involved in homeostasis, including the nutritionally responsive hormones insulin, glucagon, corticosterone, growth hormone, insulin-like growth factor-1, thyroxin, and the catecholamines. In vitro, the concentration of these hormones can impact leukocytes during the critical early phase of antigen recognition and commitment to cell cycling. The balance of these hormones also influences the specific cytokine secretion patterns of T_h lymphocytes and accessory cells, which presumably determine the type of immune response initiated. Furthermore, they affect the amount of pro-inflammatory cytokines produced during an infectious challenge. For example, growth hormone dampens the amount of tumor necrosis factor-α released in response to LPS in pigs and cattle (33–35). A change in the balance of hormones originating from the endocrine system is readily induced by a wide variety of dietary factors, including the amount of food consumed, meal pattern, and ratio of protein to energy in the diet.

The antibody response to vaccination is enhanced in chicks that have fasted for short periods of time (12–24 h), presumably the result of a permissive endocrine climate for these responses (36,37). Consequently, a short period (4–8 h) of feed withdrawal is sometimes used to increase humoral responses to vaccines in the poultry industry. Chronic feed restriction (usually at about 20% below voluntary intake) is commonly used in rearing and managing broiler breeders (38–40) and gilts (41) as a way to enhance productive life-span. These restrictive-feeding regimens improve resistance to a variety of infectious diseases. In addition to enhanced humoral immune responses, some of the improvement may be the result of inhibition of the involution of the thymus that is normally associated with aging.

Several intake-related situations are deleterious to immunocompetence. It is well known that long periods of fasting result in greatly elevated corticosterone levels and, eventually, impair both antibody- and cell-mediated immune responses. For example, chicken fasted for 14 d have decreased peripheral blood CD4+ helper T lymphocytes, impaired cell-mediated immunity, and increased susceptibility to *Salmonella enteritis* challenges (42,43). Conversely, overconsumption of a balanced diet is also immunomodulatory and results in impaired antibody responses (44). Similarly, chickens fed diets with very high nutrient density have inferior antibody responses to vaccination and increased lesions and morbidity following an infection with *E. coli* (45).

REGULATION BY AVAILABILITY OF SUBSTRATES   The cells of the immune system require nourishment in order to carry out their functions. Animal nutritionists would like to determine the total nutritional cost of maintaining the immune system, the additional cost of an immune response, and the priority of the immune system for nutrients when their supply is diminished by inadequate intake. If the immune system has an especially high demand for nutrients or if the immune system is unable to compete with other tissues for nutrients when they are limiting, then nutritionists must consider immunity when setting dietary requirements. Several lines of evidence provided below indicate that the immune system's needs for nutritional substrates are sufficiently small and of high priority that they are not of major concern when setting requirements of growing or reproducing animals. In other words, the levels of most nutrients that maximize growth and reproduction usually provide adequate substrates for the immune system to carry out its functions. It should be noted that animal nutritionists are not usually concerned with dietary requirements for animals at maintenance because in animal agriculture, animals are not typically kept if they are not either growing, producing, or reproducing.

Nutritional Costs of Immunity   The nutritional costs of a vigorous immune response have not been accurately quantified for any species, including humans and rodents. From a nutritional viewpoint, substrates (e.g., amino acids, glucose, fatty acids, enzyme cofactors) are needed to support the clonal proliferation of lymphocytes, the recruitment of new monocytes and heterophils from bone marrow, the synthesis of effector molecules (e.g., immunoglobulins, nitric oxide, lysozyme, complement), and communication molecules (e.g., eicosanoids, cytokines). Furthermore, most immune responses to pathogens are accompanied by a systemic inflammatory response, including the secretion of significant amounts of acute-phase proteins by the liver.

Estimation of the size of the immune system including bone marrow components reveals that a little less than 0.5% of the body is made up of leukocytes and their progenitors (46). Accessory cells such as reticular, dendritic, and stromal cells should also be charged to the immune system, but accurate quantitative estimates of their contribution are not yet available. Even if these accessory cells contribute similar mass to the immune system as leukocytes, the cellular components of the immune system probably do not exceed 1% of the body weight. Inclusion of the extracellular fluids and collagen and other structural components found in lymphoid organs brings the contribution of the immune system to the body weight up to 3–4%. In other words, the immune system represents a small organ relative to others such as the intestines, skeletal muscles, or the nervous system.

Nutritional costs of the immune system must also consider turnover rates of cells and macromolecules. In adults, leukopoiesis in bone marrow occurs at a rate of 0.03% of body weight per day (47) and lymphocytes in other tissues (e.g., thymus, spleen) contribute almost twice this amount for the purpose of replacing losses resulting from normal immunosurveillance (48). Rates of leukopoiesis in the bone marrow increase by about twofold during acute systemic infections. Normal rates of immunoglobulin synthesis in a young chicken is less than 0.02% of body weight per day (49). Although the rate of synthesis of specific antibodies increases dramatically during a disease challenge, the rate of synthesis of total antibodies increases only moderately. Hyperimmunization, for example, results in about a 25% increase in serum immunoglobulin. Based on serum concentrations and half-life estimates, other humoral components, such as complement, contribute an order of magnitude less to daily synthesis than do immunoglobulins.

Although accurate information on the nutritional demands of a vigorous immune response are clearly imperfect, it is apparent that the amount of substrate resources (nutrients) needed by the immune system is very low relative to needs for growth or milk or egg production. For example, the weight of new leukocytes and immunoglobulins normally produced each day (about 800 mg/kg body weight) appears to be less than 1% of the total increase in body weight of a 2-wk-old broiler chick. In fact, it is even less than 10% of the amount of the two pectoralis major (breast) muscles synthesized each day. Even if an infectious challenge increases the rate of leukopoiesis by considerably more than the twofold estimates that have been reported, it is doubtful that the immune system would be a significant consumer of nutritional resources in a growing animal. It is often stated that the depression in growth and reproductive performance associated with an immune response is the result of the diversion of nutrients away from anabolic process (e.g., growth) for use by the immune system. However, this conclusion is not supported by a quantitative analysis of the processes involved (Fig. 2).

Many infections are accompanied by an acute-phase response, which is characterized by increases in synthesis of acute-phase proteins, whole-body protein turnover, gluconeogenesis, and body temperature. The acute-phase response is characterized by nutrient

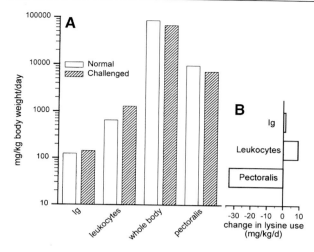

Fig. 2. (A) Mass on immunoglobulins (Ig) and leukocytes synthesized daily relative to the rate of accretion of pectoralis muscle and total-body tissue in a young chicken kept in pathogen free (Normal) conditions or during an infectious challenge (Challenged). See ref. *102* for references and assumptions. (B) The additional amount of lysine required during a challenge for the synthesis of new immunoglobulins and for additional leukocytes is easily met by the decrease in lysine use by a single large muscle (pectoralis major).

fluxes in several organ systems, especially the liver and muscle. Although descriptive information on the acute-phase response of poultry and livestock has been detailed (50,51), a quantitative evaluation of the nutritional demands of this response is needed. Clearly, the acute-phase response is a process that is both nutrient liberating (skeletal muscle catabolism) and nutrient consuming (acute-phase protein synthesis, fever). Given the marked increase in hepatic demand for amino acids to support gluconeogenesis and for acute-phase protein synthesis (52–54), it is likely that the amino acid costs of an acute-phase response are considerably greater than the relatively minute needs of leukocytes that respond to an infectious challenge. For several nutrients (e.g., zinc, copper, threonine), it is known that the amount liberated is sufficient to meet the needs of both acute phase and the immune responses (55–57). Given that the acute-phase response is likely to be a much larger consumer of nutrients during an infectious challenge than leukocytes, future studies on the impact of nutrition on resistance of animals should include measures of this process, such as production of acute-phase proteins.

Priority of the Immune System for Nutrients The priority of a cell type for nutrients can be inferred by the concentration and binding affinities of transport proteins on its cell membrane. For example, there are at least five types of glucose transporters, each conferring differing transport kinetics onto cells in the body. Lymphocytes utilize a transporter similar to that of neurons and erythrocytes (58). Furthermore, this transporter is constitutively expressed and is not sensitive to insulin or IGF-1, permitting the use of glucose even during periods of starvation. These transport characteristics indicate that lymphocytes have the highest priority for glucose relative to other cell types, such as muscle, liver, or fibroblasts. Similarly, pig lymphocytes constitutively express the ACS transporter for neutral amino acids (59). This system has a K_m that is almost a magnitude lower than the K_m of the A system, which is expressed on skeletal muscle and many other tissues.

Following stimulation with mitogen, activity of the ACS system of lymphocytes is induced and the A system is also expressed, permitting lymphocytes to transport large quantities of neutral amino acids across a wide range of tissue amino acid concentrations.

Additionally, the acute-phase response that accompanies most infectious challenges mobilizes large quantities of nutrients from other tissues, especially skeletal muscle and bone (see below). The catabolic response in these tissues not only releases amino acids but also trace nutrients. Thus, the immune system orchestrates the liberation of nutrients of other tissues to buffer transient deficiencies.

The high priority of the immune system for nutrients is further supported by the observation that moderate restriction of either total feed or protein that are sufficient to impair growth rate do not impair, and often improve, indices of immunocompetence (38,39,60). Thus, when considering nutrients as substrates, immunocompetence may not be a reliable index of nutrient requirements and sensitive indicators such as growth rate, efficiency of feed conversion, or the production of eggs, wool, or milk are usually more appropriate. In fact, the use of indices of immunocompetence as an indication of the requirement for macronutrients, such as energy or amino acids, results in a severe underestimate relative to the requirement for anabolic processes such as growth or reproduction.

It must be emphasized that the above discussion pertains to animals fed diets that are generally adequate in nutrients for maximal growth and reproduction. Animal nutritionists have not been particularly interested in the impact of severe nutrient deficiencies because these situations are assiduously avoided due to their severe economic impact. Clearly, deficiencies of many nutrients that are sufficiently severe to markedly decrease growth or reproduction impair crucial components of the immune system. Severe deficiencies are especially damaging during embryogenesis and the neonatal period when the expansion of leukocyte populations is rapid, the lymphoid organs are populated, and genetic recombination and selection events occur, which give unique clones of lymphocytes that mediate immunity later in life. In general, research in poultry and livestock has confirmed rodent studies showing that chronically severe deficiencies of micronutrients are more debilitating to the development and maturation of the immune system than macronutrients such as energy and protein. Severe nutrient deficiencies that are especially damaging during this period include linoleic acid, vitamin A, iron, selenium, and several of the B vitamins (13,61,62)

IMPACT ON THE PATHOLOGY CAUSED BY AN IMMUNE RESPONSE The effector functions of cytotoxic T cells, natural-killer cells, macrophages, and neutrophils result in the elaboration of a wide variety of destructive molecules into the surrounding microenvironment, including reactive oxygen intermediates, nitrous oxide, and catabolic enzymes. These defensive agents are cytotoxic and kill bacteria, parasites, and infected host cells, but they can also injure normal host cells and result in various pathologies. LPS injection into steers or *Eimeria maxima* infection of chickens causes sufficient production of nitric oxide that its concentration not rises only in the local area of challenge but also in the blood (33,63). Similarly, indices of oxidized PUFAs increase markedly during an inflammatory response to endotoxin (64). Widespread damage due to reactive oxygen and nitrogen intermediates may be minimized by a variety of mechanisms,

including reinforcement of antioxidant mechanisms of host cells resulting from local and systemic stress signals and the protective effects of several of the acute-phase proteins secreted from the liver. Local antioxidant defense is presumably facilitated by adequate vitamin E in cell membranes and by high levels of vitamin C in the cell cytosol. A deficiency of vitamin E or selenium results in peroxidation of lipids in the cell membranes and increased signs of functional damage during the inflammatory response induced by *S. minnesota* LPS (64). In poultry, dietary vitamin C reduces the lesions associated with an infection with Newcastle disease virus, *Mycoplasma gallisepticum*, or *E. coli* (65). β-Carotene is an effective antioxidant molecule in cell membranes of ruminants and may provide protection during a mastitis challenge in dairy cows (18,66). In that stressed host cells release cytokines and eicosanoids that downregulate the immune response, minimizing their injury would theoretically permit more sustained and vigorous immune responses and increased resistance. In practice, dietary vitamin E is supplemented in the diets of all animal species at several times its required level, partly because of reduced pathology observed during infectious episodes. Similarly, vitamin C is included in the diet of many animals, even though it is not a required nutrient.

Pro-inflammatory cytokines, including interleukin-1 (IL-1), interleukin-6 (IL-6), interleukin-8 (IL-8), and tumor necrosis factor-α (TNF-α), released during an immune response can exert tissue damage through hemodynamic changes, direct cytotoxicity, and increased release of free radicals and other oxidative molecules. Morbidity and mortality resulting from a wide range of infectious diseases has been attributed to excessive release of pro-inflammatory cytokines (67). Nutritional factors that dampen the release of pro-inflammatory cytokines such as n-3 PUFAs and dietary protein level appear to prevent pathology associated with some types of inflammatory and infectious challenges (4,33,68,69).

NUTRITIONAL IMMUNITY Pathogens require a host source of nutrients for their replication and virulence. The host animal can sometimes decrease the rate of replication of bacteria and parasites by withholding nutrients. Iron is the first limiting nutrient for the growth of many pathogens in extracellular fluids (70,71). During the acute phase of an immune response a variety of iron- and heme-binding proteins (e.g., lactoferrin, haptoglobin, hemopexin) are produced by the liver and by macrophages in an effort to remove iron from the body fluids. Circumventing an animal's innate ability to limit nutrients increases the susceptibility to many types of infections (72,73). Practices that neutralize nutritional immunity include injecting nutrients, feeding forms of nutrients that bypass controls of intestinal absorption, and preventing the anorexia that accompanies the acute-phase response.

Pig producers have been faced with a difficult dilemma in their effort to provide iron supplementation to newborn pigs and not impair nutritional immunity. Because of the sow's morphology at the endometrial–placental interface, the transfer of iron to the fetus is insufficient to sustain the neonate for more than a few weeks. Milk is deficient in iron and, in nature, baby pigs obtain their iron from the soil. Pig production in modern facilities does not permit this route of supplementation and artificial supplementation is required. Both research and practical experience have shown that oral supplementation of iron overcomes the nutritional immunity-based protective system in the intestine and promotes the growth of enterically pathogenic *Escherichia coli* (74). Consequently, iron supplementation is almost always done by the injection of slowly released iron dextran. Even this route of supplementation has been shown to overcome the baby pigs ability to withhold iron from pathogens, and oversupplementation causes increased proliferation of pathogenic strains of *E. coli* both systemically and enterically *(75,76)*.

IMPACT OF AN IMMUNE RESPONSE ON NUTRIENT REQUIREMENTS

Stimulation of the immune system causes a stress response that has important implications for an animal's nutrient requirements and its productivity. Specific shifts in cellular and metabolic processes, as well as change in behavior, are orchestrated by the immune system in response to a variety of stimuli. These changes are most obvious during the acute phase of an immune response but may become persistent if the immune response is chronic. The magnitude of the changes depends on the nature of the triggering immunogen and the amount and location of the response. The systemic manifestations induced by an immune response, and especially the inflammatory response, are highly conserved through the evolution of vertebrates and are observed in lizards, fish, birds, pigs, sheep, cattle, and horses. These alterations are expressed as decreased productivity (e.g., growth) and have significant implications on the nutritional needs of the animal. This section briefly considers the mechanisms through which the immune system takes command of intermediary metabolism and then explores the quantitative impact on energy and protein requirements of growing animals.

COMMUNICATION BETWEEN THE IMMUNE SYSTEM AND OTHER SYSTEMS

There are at least three general mechanisms through which an immune response located at an isolated site in the body can influence normal physiology throughout the body: release of pro-inflammatory cytokines, release of hormones, and neural communication. First, during most immune responses, monocytes and macrophages release the pro-inflammatory cytokines IL-1, IL-6, and TNF. Each of these cytokines has a specific role in the regulation of the immune response by acting in the local area of the challenge. If an immune response is sufficiently large, these cytokines increase in concentration in the blood and act systemically *(77)*. Cells in virtually of all tissues have receptors for these cytokines and respond to them (Table 1). Second, stimulated leukocytes produce releasing hormones that induce an endocrine (e.g., corticosterone) response *(29)*. For example, stimulated T-lymphocytes release ACTH, which increases the release of corticosterone. Third, there is extensive innervation of immune tissues such as the spleen and lymph nodes. Immune responses occurring in these tissues trigger neurologic responses that communicate this activity to the brain *(78,79)*. The above three mechanisms mediate cellular, metabolic, and behavioral changes that alter the partitioning of dietary nutrients away from growth, skeletal muscle accretion, or reproduction in favor of metabolic processes that support the immune response and disease resistance. As the immune system and its cytokines orchestrate this stress response, it is sometimes referred to as "immunologic stress" to differentiate it from other homeostatic stress responses.

During actual infectious challenges, the immune system adjusts the type and size of its response to the immunogenic and antigenic characteristics of the pathogen. Responses can be predominantly inflammatory or they may have variable cell-mediated and humoral components. The amounts and types of leukocytic cyto-

Table 1
Nutritionally Important Effects of
Proinflammatory Cytokines IL-1, IL-6, and TNF

Behavioral
    Decreased voluntary intake
    Increased sleep
    Decreased activity

Energetics
    Increased resting energy expenditure
    Increased body temperature (fever)
    Decreased activity, growth, eggs, milk

Protein Metabolism
    Increased synthesis of acute-phase proteins
    Increased whole-body protein turnover
    Increased muscle protein degradation
    Increased amino acid oxidation

Glucose Metabolism
    Increased oxidation
    Increased gluconeogenesis

Lipid Metabolism
    Decreased lipoprotein lipase activity
    Decreased lipolysis in adipocytes
    Increased hepatic triglyceride synthesis
Hypertriglyceridemia

Mineral Metabolism
    Increased hepatic metallothionein synthesis
    Increased lactoferrin synthesis
    Increased hepatic ceruloplasmin synthesis

Hormone Release
    Corticosteroid—increased
    Thyroxin—decreased
    Glucagon—increased
    Insulin—increased
    Growth hormone—increased (species dependent)

kines that are released reflect the type of immune response elicited by the challenging organism or agent. Studies that dissect the importance of these various arms of the immune system in modulating nutrition-related physiology are needed. Model systems using purified pro-inflammatory cytokines or maximally potent inflammatory agents such as LPS circumvent this question by inducing or mimicking potent inflammatory immune responses. Whether adaptive T- and B-cell-mediated responses contribute to altered animal productivity and nutrient requirements needs to be explored. Recent characterization of T-helper (Th) cell populations into Th_1 and Th_2 subpopulations and the regulation of this dichotomy by various interleukins *(80)* provides a starting point for understanding correlations between immune response types and nutrient needs. Th_1 cells promote a cell-mediated immune response by secreting interferon-γ, lymphotoxin, and TNF-α. These cytokines activate macrophages to increase their release of additional TNF-α and IL-1β. A Th_1 response is induced by IL-12 and inhibited by IL-10 and IL-4. Alternately, Th_2 cells promote a humoral response by secreting IL-4, IL-5, IL-10, and IL-13. These cytokines direct B cells to switch immunoglobulin isotypes to IgG-1 and IgE and inhibit macrophage activation. Thus, Th_2 responses would not be expected to cause nutritional disturbances that are as large as Th_1 and inflammatory responses. This scenario is complicated by the fact that macrophage populations and the cytokine profiles that they produce are also heterogeneous *(81)*. A thorough understanding of the contribution of different types of macrophage and lymphocyte responses to immunologic stress is clearly needed and the following discussion pertains to responses that include a vigorous inflammatory component.

NUTRITIONAL IMPLICATIONS Animal scientists have been especially concerned with the decreased growth and efficiency of utilization of feed nutrients for growth that accompanies immunologic stress. Reduced feed intake accounts for about 70% of the decreased growth; the remainder is the result of metabolic inefficiencies caused by the immune response *(82)*. Particularly disconcerting for animal producers is that the rate of skeletal muscle accretion is impaired more than that of most other organ systems, such as adipose, liver, and intestines, resulting in lower yields of edible meat *(83–85)*. The effect of these immune-mediated adjustments on the nutrient needs of animals has become a central research theme in animal nutrition and is described in the following subsections.

Food Intake Nutritionally, anorexia is, by far, the most important impact of the stress response orchestrated by the immune system. Many leukocytic cytokines are potentially anorexigenic, including IL-1α, IL-1β, IL-6, TNF-α, IL-8, and interferons; however, Il-1 is the most potent *(86)*. IL-1β acts on the central nervous system and gastrointestinal tract to impair appetite *(87)*. The reduction in the number and size of meals induced by IL-1 is augmented synergistically if TNF-α levels increase *(88)*. Cooperatively, these central and peripheral actions of leukocytic cytokines can decrease food intake by more than 50% during the acute phase of an infectious challenge.

A basal metabolic rate that is high relative to food intake and activity level accompanies an immune response and is measurable as an increase in body temperature (fever). Leukocytic cytokines act on the central nervous system to cause fever by inducing an increase in the temperature setpoint, invoking thermoregulatory responses similar to those of a hypothermic state *(89)*. Although an important contributor to the energetics of the catabolic state that accompanies immunologic stress, quantitative aspects of the altered basal metabolic rate have received very little direct research. In animal production, the increased metabolic rate because of infectious challenges is probably responsible for a considerable diminution of efficiency of feed conversion. Baracos et al. *(90)* estimated that heat production increases 33% in shorn sheep during an inflammatory response to LPS. However, the quantitatively large increase in the basal metabolism induced by leukocytic cytokines may be partially offset by decreases in activity resulting from the lethargy and sleepiness induced by these cytokines *(91)*. In growing animals, the energy requirement is further reduced because of a decreased rate of growth (net energy for growth) induced by inflammatory cytokines.

Animal nutritionists have attempted to alter dietary energy density or energy source (e.g., increasing dietary fat) to overcome the anorectic effect of immunologic stress. In general, these attempts have been largely unsuccessful. Increasing dietary energy density has little effect on caloric intake in immunologically stressed turkeys *(92)* or pigs *(93,94)*, but in some circumstances, it is beneficial in chickens *(83)*. Providing chickens with a nutrient-dense diet that is very high in carbohydrates ameliorates the change in caloric intake resulting from immunologic stress. However, the partitioning of nutrients between skeletal muscle and other tissues is still distributed, as reflected in changes in body composition.

Amino Acids Requirements During immunologic stress, skeletal muscle is mobilized to supply nutrients for use by other tissues *(51,95)*. Muscle catabolism is the result of a reciprocal increase in protein degradation and decrease in protein synthesis and is mediated by the synergistic effects of IL-1 and TNF-α. Released amino acids are used by the liver for the synthesis of acute-phase proteins and glucose, by the immune system to support the clonal proliferation of responding leukocytes, and for oxidation by leukocytes and other tissues. Additionally, many tissues increase both their rates of protein synthesis and protein degradation, resulting in increased protein turnover *(96)*. Enhanced protein degradation supplies peptides for major histocompatability complex presentation to lymphocytes. Thus, increased protein turnover in tissues also represents increased vigilance in the search for infected host cells.

The impact of immunologic stress on amino acid requirements of growing pigs and chickens has been investigated. A sustained immune response in young growing pigs decreases the lysine requirement by about 20% when expressed as percentage of the diet required to maximize growth. Because feed intake is decrease by chronic immune stimulation, the lysine requirement is decreased by 40% when expressed as grams required per day *(84)*. Similarly, the requirement for either lysine or methionine is decreased by immunologic stress in young broiler chicks *(97)*. These lower requirements suggests that slower growth rate and decreased skeletal muscle accretion induced by the immunologic stress spares more essential amino acids than are needed for anabolic processes in the liver and the immune system. This explanation is supported by the quantitative information shown in Fig. 2. Another conclusion of these studies is that the dietary protein requirement decreases more than the dietary energy requirement during immunologic stress.

Following a period of immune activation, young animals often undergo a period of compensatory growth *(98)*. In chickens, the enhanced rate of growth, particularly skeletal muscle accretion, increases the lysine requirement beyond that of chicks that have not undergone a response *(99)*. If additional dietary amino acids are not supplied, the compensatory growth period is prolonged or may not occur.

Other Nutrients Quantitative changes in the requirement of vitamins and minerals as the result of a sustained immune response have not been subjected to detailed study in poultry or livestock. Fortification of animal diets with trace nutrients represents less than 0.5% of the cost of a diet. Consequently, all of the trace minerals and vitamins are typically fortified to diets at levels that are at least 50% greater than the known requirement to provide a "margin of safety." It is generally thought that good trace nutrient stores prior to the disease challenge are important to permit the characteristic redistribution of these nutrients during an immune response. For example, during an acute-phase response, large amounts of copper and zinc are used by the liver for the synthesis of the acute-phase proteins ceruloplasmin and metallothionein *(55,56)*. This metabolic demand is fulfilled by copper and zinc stored in the liver or released from other tissues such as skeletal muscle. Because these metabolic changes represent redistributions within existing body pools, they do not represent an increase in the dietary requirement. However, intestinal absorption of many trace nutrients is decreased during immunologic stress as an integral part of nutritional immunity *(100)*. Furthermore, during the acute phase of an immune response, there is an increase in excretion of many nutrient from endogenous sources *(101)*. Presumably, there are increased requirements following the resolution of the immune response in order to compensate for these expenses; however, little quantitative information on these needs is available.

It should be noted that the above discussion considers the impact of a sustained immune response on nutrient needs. Usually, the agent that triggers an immune response (e.g., microorganism, autoantigen, food antigen) causes pathology to specific organs, which modifies the generic response. For example, many enteric infections cause substantial damage to the intestinal epithelium, which cause major disruptions in nutrient absorption. Thus, the total impact of an enteric infection on metabolism and nutrition is the sum of generalized effects of the immune system responding plus specific effects due to the destructive actions of the pathogen itself.

SUMMARY

Animal diets are scientifically formulated to exacting standards that have been determined by intense research over the years. Dietary requirements have been set at levels that maximize growth in young animals and reproduction or milk production in mature animals. More recently, research has been directed toward identifying nutritional factors that modulate the immune response and influence an animal's susceptibility to diseases prevented by or caused by the immune system. The complexity of the multitude of nutrient by immunity interactions has prompted animal nutritionists to base dietary management for the purposes of influencing immunocompetence on five mechanistic categories:

1. Nutrients such as polyunsaturated fatty acids and vitamins E, A, and D have direct regulatory actions on leukocytes by modifying intercellular or intracellular communication pathways.
2. The amount of calories consumed and the protein-to-calorie ratio indirectly impact immunity by influencing the levels of hormones that modulate the immune system.
3. Nutrients are needed as substrates for anabolic processes required for the development of the immune system and for an immune response. Chronic deficiencies of many trace nutrients cause impairments in the development of the immune system. However, moderate deficiencies in the diet of juvenile animals are usually not detrimental to the immune system because of its high priority for substrates when they become limiting in body fluids.
4. Some nutrients, especially those that serve as antioxidants, limit the pathology that results from effector functions of leukocytes.
5. The immune system orchestrates a decrease in the concentration of some nutrients in the blood and other body fluids in order to impair the replication of pathogens. Iron and possibly other trace minerals are important in this response.

Nutritionists concerned with animal production are also interested in the impact of an immune response on dietary requirements. The immune system is central to homeostasis and serves as both a sensory system that detects insults to homeostasis and a control system that orchestrates local and systemic responses directed toward reestablishing homeostasis. The cellular and metabolic sequelae that accompanies an immune response redirects nutrients away from physiological processes important for growth and reproduction toward processes important in host defense. Alterations in nutrient requirements because of a sustained immune response have at least two components. First, the requirement for energy and amino acids is decreased during the challenge when growth or reproduction is slowed and the immune system is responding vigorously. Second, requirements are increased following resolution of the challenge when pathologic insults are repaired and compensatory growth typically occurs.

REFERENCES

1. Sommer MH, Xavier MH, Fialho MB, Wannmacher CM, Wajner M. The influence of amino acids on mitogen-activated proliferation of human lymphocytes in vitro. Int J Immunopharmacol 1994; 16:865–72.
2. Fritsche KL, Cassity NA. Dietary N-3 fatty acids reduce antibody-dependent cell cytotoxicity and alter eicosanoid release by chicken immune cells. Poultry Sci 1992; 71:1646–7.
3. Fritsche KL, Huang SC, Misfeldt M. Fish oil and immune function. Nutr Rev 1993; 51:24.
4. Korver DR, Klasing KC. Dietary fish oil alters specific and inflammatory immune responses in chicks. J Nutr 1997; 127:2039–46.
5. Korver DR, Wakenell P, Klasing KC. Dietary fish oil or Lofrin, a 5-lipoxygenase inhibitor, decrease the growth-suppressing effects of coccidiosis in broiler chicks. Poultry Sci 1997; 76:1355–63.
6. Schenk H, Vogt M, Droge W, et al. Thioredoxin as a potent costimulus of cytokine expression. J Immunol 1996; 156:765–71.
7. Lander HM. An essential role for free radicals and derived species in signal transduction. FASEB J 1997; 11:118–24.
8. Sen CK, Packer L. Antioxidant and redox regulation of gene transcription. FASEB J 1996; 10:709–20.
9. Packer L, Suzuki YJ. Vitamin E and alpha-lipoate: role in antioxidant recycling and activation of the NF-κβ transcription factor. Mol Asp Med 1993; 14:229–239.
10. Grimble RF. Nutritional antioxidants and the modulation of inflammation: theory and practice. New Horizons 1994; 2:175–85.
11. Suzuki YJ, Packer L. Inhibition of NF-κβ activation by vitamin E derivatives. Biochem Biophys Res Commun 1993; 193:277–83.
12. Blumberg JB. Vitamins. In: Forse RA, ed, Diet, Nutrition, and Immunity, pp. 237–47. CRC, Boca Raton, FL, 1994.
13. Cook ME. Nutrition and the immune response of the domestic fowl. Crit Rev Poultry Biol 1991; 3:167–90.
14. Feng L, Xia Y, Garcia GE, Hwang D, Wilson CB. Involvement of reactive oxygen intermediates in cyclooxygenase-2 expression induced by interleukin-1, tumor necrosis factor-α, and lipopolysaccharide. J Clin Invest 1995; 95:1669–75.
15. Meydani SN, Blumberg JB. Vitamin E and the immune response. In: Cunningham-Rundles S, ed, Nutrition Modulation of the Immune Response. Marcel Dekker, New York, 1993.
16. Boren B, Bond P. Vitamin E and immunocompetence. Broiler Ind 1996; 11:26–33.
17. Leshchinsky TV, Klasing KC. Effect of vitamin E on the immunity of chicken. FASEB Meeting, San Francisco, 1998.
18. Chew BP. Antioxidant vitamins affect food animal immunity and health. J Nutr 1995; 125:1804S–8S.
19. Tengerdy RP, Nockels CF. Vitamin E or vitamin A protects chickens against E. coli infection. Poultry Sci 1975; 54:1292–6.
20. Nockels CF. Protective effects of supplemental vitamin E against infection. Fed Proc. 1979; 38:2134–8.
21. Sell JL, Trampel DW, Griffith RW. Adverse effects of Escherichia coli infection of turkeys were not alleviated by supplemental dietary vitamin E. Poultry Sci 1997; 76:1682–7.
22. Kennedy DG, Rice DA, Bruce DW, Goodall EA, McIlroy SG. Economic effect of increased vitamin E supplementation of broilers

diets on commercial broiler production. Br Poultry Sci 1992; 33:1015–23.

23. McIlroy SG, Goodall EA, Rice DA, McNulty NS, Kennedy DG. Improved performance in commercial broiler flocks with subclinical infectious bursal disease when fed diets containing increased concentrations of vitamin E. Avian Pathol 1993; 22:81–94.

24. Romach EH, Kidao S, Sanders BG, Kline K. Effects of RRR-alpha-tocopheryl succinate on Il-1 and PGE2 production by macrophages. Nutr Cancer 1993; 20:205–14.

25. Woods C, Domenget C, Solari F, Gandrillon O, Lazarides E, Jurdic P. Antagonistic role of vitamin D3 and retinoic acid on the differentiation of chicken hematopoietic macrophages into osteoclast precursor cells. Endocrinology 1995; 136:85–95.

26. Sklan D, Melamed D, Friedman A. The effect of varying levels of dietary vitamin A on immune response in the chick. Poultry Sci 1994; 73:843–7.

27. Friedman A, Sklan D. Effects of retinoids on immune responses in birds. Worlds Poultry Sci 1997; 53:186–95.

28. Lessard M, Hutchings D, Cave NA. Cell-mediated and humoral immune responses in broiler chickens maintained on diets containing different levels of vitamin A. Poultry Sci 1997; 76:1368–78.

29. Weigent DA, et al. Associations between the neuroendocrine and immune systems. J Leuk Biol 1995; 57:137–44.

30. Marsh JA. The integration of the neuroendocrine and immune system: a marriage of convenience of necessity? In: Davison TF, Morris TR, Payne LN, eds, Poultry Immunology, pp. 357–74. Carfax Publishing, Oxfordshire, 1996.

31. Johnson RW, Arkins S, Dantzer R, Kelley KW. Hormones, lympho-hemopoietic cytokines and the neuroimmune axis. Comp Biochem Physiol A: Physiol 1997; 116:183–201.

32. Elsasser TH, Richards M, Collier R, Hartnell GF. Physiological responses to repeated endotoxin challenge are selectively affected by recombinant bovine somatotropin administration to calves. Domest Anim Endocrinol 1996; 13:91–103.

33. Kahl S, Elsasser TH, Blum JW. Nutritional regulation of plasma tumor necrosis factor-alpha and plasma and urinary nitrite/nitrate responses to endotoxin in cattle. Proc Soc Exp Biol Med 1996; 215:370–6.

34. Elsasser TH, Kahl S, Steele NC, Rumsey TS. Nutritional modulation of somatotropic axis-cytokine relationships in cattle: a brief review. Comp Biochem Physiol A: Physiol 1997; 116:209–21

35. Myers MJ, Farrell DE, Evock-Clover CM, McDonald MW, Steele NC. Effect of growth hormone or chromium picolinate on swine metabolism and inflammatory cytokine production after endotoxin challenge exposure. Am J Vet Res 1997; 58:594–600.

36. Klasing KC. Influence of acute starvation or acute excess intake on immunocompetence of broiler chicks. Poultry Sci 1988; 67:626–34.

37. BoaAmponsem K, Yang A, Praharaj NK, Dunnington EA, Gross WB, Siegel PB. Impact of alternate-day feeding cycles on immune and antibacterial responses of white Leghorn chicks. J Appl Poultry Res 1997; 6:123–7.

38. Katanbaf MN, Dunnington EA, Siegel PB. Restricted feeding in early and late-feathering chickens. 1. Growth and physiological responses. Poultry Sci 1989; 68:344–51.

39. O'Sullivan NP, Dunnington EA. Growth and carcass characteristics of early- and late-feathering broilers reared under different feeding regimens. Poultry Sci 1991; 70:1323–32.

40. Praharaj NK, Gross WB, Dunnington EA, Nir I, Siegel PB. Immunoresponsiveness of fast-growing chickens as influenced by feeding regimen. Br Poultry Sci 1996; 37:779–86.

41. von Borell E, Morris JR, Hurnik JF, Mallard BA, Buhr MM. The performance of gilts in a new group housing system: endocrinological and immunological functions. J Anim Sci 1992; 70:2714–21.

42. Holt PS. Effect of induced molting on B cell and CT4 and CT8 T cell numbers in spleens and peripheral blood of white leghorn hens. Poultry Sci 1992; 71:2027–34.

43. Holt PS, Buhr RJ, Cunningham DL, Porter RE. Effect of two differ-

ent molting procedures on a Salmonella enteritidis infection. Poultry Sci 1994; 73:1267–75.

44. Klasing KC, Austic RE. Changes in protein degradation in chickens due to an inflammatory challenge. Proc Soc Exp Biol Med 1984; 176:292–6.

45. Praharaj NK, Dunnington EA, Gross WB, Siegel PB. Dietary effects on immune response of fast-growing chicks to inoculation of sheep erythrocytes and Escherichia coli. Poultry Sci 1997; 76:244–7.

46. Klasing KC. Nutritional modulation of resistance to infectious diseases. Poultry Sci 1998:1119–1125.

47. Elgert KD. Immunology. Wiley–Liss, New York, 1996.

48. Rocha B, Penit C, Baron C, Vasseur F, Dautigny N, Freitas AA. Accumulation of bromodeoxyuridine-labeled cells in central and peripheral lymphoid organs: minimal estimates of production and turnover rates of mature lymphocytes. Eur J Immunol 1990; 20:1697–1708.

49. Leslie GA, Clem LW. Chicken immunoglobulins: biological half-lives and normal adult serum concentrations of IgM an IgY. PSEBM 1970; 134:195–8.

50. Klasing KC, Johnstone BJ. Monokines in growth and development. Poultry Sci 1991; 70:1781–9.

51. Spurlock ME. Regulation of metabolism and growth during immune challenge: an overview of cytokine function. J Anim Sci 1997; 75:1773–83.

52. Hunter EAL, Grimble RF. Cysteine and methionine supplementation modulate the effect of tumor necrosis factor alpha on protein synthesis. Glutathione and zinc concentration of liver and lung in rats fed a low protein diet. J Nutr 1994; 124:2319–28.

53. Reeds PJ, Fjeld CR, Jahoor F. Do the differences between the amino acid compositions of acute-phase and muscle proteins have a bearing on nitrogen loss in traumatic states. J Nutr 1994; 124:906–10.

54. Grimble RF. Interaction between nutrients, pro-inflammatory cytokines and inflammation. Clin Sci 1996; 91:121–30.

55. Klasing KC. Effect of inflammatory agents and interleukin 1 on iron and zinc metabolism. Am J Physiol 1984; 247:R901–4.

56. Koh TS, Peng RK, Klasing KC. Dietary copper level affects copper metabolism during lipopolysaccharide-induced immunological stress in chicks. Poultry Sci 1996; 75:867–72.

57. MacDougall E. The effects of dietary threonine supplementation on growth and immunocompetence in chicks. FASEB J 1998; 12:AB73.

58. Bushart GB, Vetter U, Hartmann W. Glucose transport during cell cycle in IM9 lymphocytes. Horm Metab Res 1993; 25:210–3.

59. Borghetti AF, Tramacere M, Ghiringhelli P, Severini A, Kay JE. Amino acid transport in pig lymphocytes. Enhanced activity of transport system asc following mitogenic stimulation. Biochim Biophys Acta 1981; 646:218–30.

60. van Heugten E, Spears JW, Coffey MT. The effect of dietary protein on performance and immune response in weanling pigs subjected to an inflammatory challenge. J Anim Sci 1994; 72:2661–9.

61. Latshaw DJ. Nutrition—mechanisms of immunosuppression. Vet Immunol Immunopathol 1991; 30:111–20.

62. Dietert RR, Golemboski KA, Austic RE. Environment-immune interactions. Poultry Sci 1994; 73:1062–76.

63. Allen PC. Production of free radical species during eimeria maxima infections in chickens. Poultry Sci 1997; 76:814–21.

64. Sword JT, Pope AL, Hoekstra WG. Endotoxin and lipid peroxidation in vivo in selenium- and vitamin E-deficient and -adequate rats. J Nutr 1991; 121:251–7.

65. Gross WB, Bailey CA. Effects of ascorbic acid on stress and disease in chickens. Avian Dis 1995; 36:688–92.

66. Chew BP, Wong TS, Shultz TD, Magnuson NS. Effects of conjugated dienoic derivatives of linoleic acid and beta-carotene in modulating lymphocyte and macrophage function. Anticancer Res 1997; 17:1099–106.

67. Grimble RF. Malnutrition and the immune response. 2. Impact of nutrients on cytokine biology in infection. Trans Roy Soc Trop Med Hyg 1994; 88:615–9.

68. Schoenherr WD, Jewell DE. Nutritional modification of inflammatory diseases. Semin Vet Med Surg (Small Anim) 1997; 12:212–22.

69. Wander RC, Hall JA, Gradin JL, Du SH, Jewell DE. The ratio of dietary (n-6) to (n-3) fatty acids influences immune system function, eicosanoid metabolism, lipid peroxidation and vitamin E status in aged dogs. J Nutr 1997; 127:1198–205.

70. Ward CG, Bullen JJ, Rogers HJ. Iron and infection—new developments and their implications. J Trauma-Injury Infect Crit Care 1996; 41:356–64.

71. Kontoghiorghes GJ, Weinberg ED. Iron—mammalian defense systems, mechanisms of disease, and chelation therapy approaches. Blood Rev 1995; 9:33–45.

72. Murray MJ, Murray AB. Anorexia of infection as a mechanism of host defense. Am J Clin Nutr 1979; 32:593–6.

73. Kluger MJ, Rothenburg BA. Fever and reduced iron: their interaction as a host defense response to bacterial infection. Science 1979; 203:374–6.

74. Klasing KC, Knight CD, Forsyth DM. Effects of iron on the anti-coli capacity of sow's milk in vitro and in ligated intestinal segments. J Nutr 1980; 110:1914–21.

75. Knight CD, Klasing KC, Forsyth DM. E. coli growth in serum of iron dextran-supplement pigs. J Anim Sci 1983; 57:387–95.

76. Kadis S, Udeze FA, Planco J, Dreesen DW. Relationship of iron administration to susceptibility of newborn pigs to enterotoxic colibacillosis. Am J Vet Res 1984; 45:255–9.

77. Webel DM, Finck BN, Baker DH, Johnson RW. Time course of increased plasma cytokines, cortisol, and urea nitrogen in pigs following intraperitoneal injection of lipopolysaccharide. J Anim Sci 1997; 75:1514–20.

78. Deleplanque B, Vitiello S, Le Moal M, Neveu PJ. Modulation of immune reactivity by unilateral striatal and mesolimbic dopaminergic lesions. Neurosci Lett 1994; 166:216–20.

79. Besedovsky HO, del Rey A. Immune–neuro–endocrine interactions: facts and hypotheses. Endocr Rev 1996; 17:64–102.

80. Fearon DT, Locksley RM. Elements of immunity—the instructive role of innate immunity in the acquired immune response. Science 1996; 272:50–4.

81. Henson PW, Riches DWH. Modulation of macrophage maturation by cytokines and lipid mediators: a potential role in resolution of pulmonary inflammation. In: Chignard M, Pretolani M, Renesto P, Vargaftig B, eds, Cells and Cytokines in Lung Inflammation, pp. 298–311. The New York Academy of Sciences, New York, 1994.

82. Klasing KC, Laurin DE, Peng RK, Fry DM. Immunologically mediated growth depression in chicks: influence of feed intake, corticosterone and interleukin-1. J Nutr 1987; 117:1629–37.

83. Benson BN, Calvert CC, Roura E, Klasing KC. Dietary energy source and density modulate the expression of immunologic stress in chicks. J Nutr 1993; 123:1714–23.

84. Williams NH, Stahly TS, Zimmerman DR. Effect of chronic immune system activation on the rate, efficiency, and composition of growth and lysine needs of pigs fed from 6 to 27 kg. J Anim Sci 1997; 75:2463–71.

85. Williams NH, Stahly TS, Zimmerman DR. Effect of level of chronic immune system activation on the growth and dietary lysine needs of pigs fed from 6 to 112 kg. J Anim Sci 1997; 75:2481–96.

86. Plata-Salaman CR. Anorexia during acute and chronic disease. Nutrition 1996; 12:69–75.

87. Johnson RW. Inhibition of growth by pro-inflammatory cytokines: an integrated view. J Anim Sci 1997; 75:1244–55.

88. Yang ZJ, Koseki M, Meguid MM, Gleason JR. Synergistic effect of rhTNF-a and rhIL-1a in inducing anorexia in rats. Am J Physiol 1994; 267:R1056–61.

89. Kluger MJ. Fever: role of pyrogens and cryogens. Physiol Rev 1991; 71:93–7.

90. Baracos VE, Whitmore WT, Gale R. The metabolic cost of fever. Can J Physiol Pharmacol 1987; 65:1248–54.

91. Dantzer R, Bluth RM, Kent S, Goodall G. Behavioral effects of cytokines: an insight into mechanisms of sickness behavior. In: De Souza EB, ed. Nerobiology of Cytokines, pp. 130–43. Academic, San Diego, 1993.

92. Piquer FJ, Sell JL, Sotosalanova MF, Vilaseca L, Palo PE, Turner K. Effects of early immune stress and changes in dietary metabolizable energy on the development of newly hatched turkeys. 1. Growth and nutrient utilization. Poultry Sci 1995; 74:983–97.

93. van Heugten E, Coffey MT, Spears JW. Effects of immune challenge, dietary energy density, and source of energy on performance and immunity in weanling pigs. J Anim Sci 1996; 74:2431–40.

94. Spurlock ME, Frank GR, Willis GM, Kuske JL, Cornelius SG. Effect of dietary energy source and immunological challenge on growth performance and immunological variables in growing pigs. J Anim Sci 1997; 75:720–6.

95. Klasing KC, Korver DR. Leukocytic cytokines regulate growth rate and composition following activation of the immune system. J Anim Sci 1997; 75(suppl 2):58–68.

96. Breuille D, Rose F, Arnal M, Melin C, Obled C. Sepsis modifies the contribution of different organs to whole-body protein synthesis in rats. Clin Sci 1994; 86:663–9.

97. Klasing KC, Barnes DM. Decreased amino acid requirements of growing chicks due to immunologic stress. J Nutr 1988; 118:1158–64.

98. Samuels SE, Baracos VE. Tissue protein turnover is altered during catch-up growth following Escherichia coli infection in weanling rats. J Nutr 1995; 125:520–30.

99. Klasing KC, Roura E. Interaction between nutrition and immunity in chickens. Cornell Nutrition Conference, Proceedings 1991, pp, 94–101.

100. Sell JL, Angel RC. Nutritional aspects of selected enteric disorders with emphasis on young poultry. Crit Rev Poultry Biol 1990; 2:277–98.

101. Beisel WR. Metabolic and nutritional consequences of infection. In: Draper HH, ed, Advances in Nutritional Research, pp. 125–33. Plenum, New York, 1977.

102. Klasing KC. Interactions between nutrition and infectious disease. In: Calnek BW, ed, Diseases of Poultry, pp. 73–80. Iowa State University Press, Ames, 1997.

31 Cancer and Nutrition

Carolyn K. Clifford

INTRODUCTION

Cancer, a major cause of death that in the developed world is exceeded only by cardiovascular disease, remains an important public health concern (1,2). In the United States, it is estimated that, in 1998, about 1,228,600 new cases of cancer will be diagnosed and 564,800 Americans can be expected to die of cancer (1). The most common cancers likely will continue to be cancers of the prostate, breast, lung and bronchus, and colon/rectum. For Americans, the lifetime probabilities of developing these cancers are high—prostate (1 in 5), breast (1 in 8), lung and bronchus (men 1 in 12; women, 1 in 18), and colon/rectum (1 in 17) (1).

It is generally agreed that physiologic aging of the immune system, primarily manifested as changes in cell-mediated immunity, results in a decline in immune function that has been linked to the development of cancer and autoimmune diseases, as well as increased susceptibility to infection (3,4). Cancer, in fact, is considered to be a disease of aging. Sixty percent of all cancers occur in persons aged ≥65 yr, and persons in this age group have a risk 11 times greater than persons aged <65 yr (5).

Although it is recognized that interactions among nutrition, the immune system, and cancer development in all probability influence cancer risk, such interactions are not clearly understood (6). The relationship between diet and nutrition and cancer is well documented in the scientific literature (2,7), as are the effects of nutrition and diet-related factors on immune response (8–14). Untangling the likely complex interactions among diet and nutrition, immune response, and cancer development, however, remains a daunting task, and one that is of increasing interest to the medical research community (6,15).

Although many of the components of diet and lifestyle that appear to alter cancer risk also may affect immune function, it is not known to what extent the mechanisms involved in modulating both carcinogenesis and immune response by any specific component may overlap or influence each other. Some general properties, such as the ability to act as an antioxidant or an antiproliferative agent, may serve as common mechanisms. In contrast, some components may act in a manner that is unique to that component.

Changes in patterns of cancer with time, as well as cross-cultural and migrant studies, support the suggestion that as developing countries become more urbanized, the patterns of cancer incidence, especially for cancers associated with diet and lifestyle, tend to move toward patterns of the more economically developed countries, which generally have high incidence rates for cancer overall and cancers most affected by diet and/or lifestyle (2,7). For example, in Japan, cancer has become the leading cause of death over the last 50 yr, a period during which average daily per capita fat intake rose from 18.0 g (1950) to 56.6 g (1987), and average daily per capita fiber intake decreased from 27.4 g (1947) to 15.3 g (1987) (16). Such changes in patterns of cancer incidence provide clear evidence that environmental factors, including dietary and other lifestyle choices, play a definite role in determining risk for some cancers. Although conclusive evidence is not yet available, a large, consistent body of epidemiologic evidence and corroborating experimental studies strongly support associations between dietary constituents and the risk of specific cancers, suggesting that, in general, vegetables and fruits, dietary fiber, and certain micronutrients appear to be protective against cancer, whereas dietary fat, excessive calories, and alcohol seem to increase cancer risk (2,7,17). The effects of these dietary factors possibly build on individual genetic susceptibilities (18).

Some of the same components of normal healthful diets that influence cancer risk also may modulate immune system components and function. For example, a small excess of dietary antioxidants such as vitamins E and C, β-carotene, and selenium may be associated with an enhanced immune response (8,19), whereas dietary fat may either impair or enhance immune response, depending on total amount and type of fat intake, possibly by modifying macrophage function with regard to effectiveness in killing tumor cells (8,20,21). Caloric restriction (CR) can impair immune function responses if adequate intake of essential nutrients and protein is not maintained (22,23). Also, physical activity appears to modulate immune function; regular, moderate activity can stimulate the immune system, whereas overtraining may actually suppress the immune system (24).

This chapter presents evidence regarding the possible roles of diet and diet-mediated changes in the immune system as they relate to cancer prevention and considers likely mechanisms by which diet and diet-related immune responses may bring about cancer-protective effects. Discussion of the interactions among

From: *Nutrition and Immunology: Principles and Practice* (ME Gershwin et al. eds.), © Humana Press, Inc., Totowa, NJ

diet, nutrition, and the immune system in the treatment of cancer is beyond its scope.

CURRENT RESEARCH STATUS

The considerable body of evidence that links nutrition and cancer as well as nutrition and immunity includes data from epidemiologic, experimental, and clinical intervention studies. A brief summary of the evidence linking dietary fat, micronutrients, caloric restriction, and physical activity with cancer risk and with the immune system is presented here, including a discussion of possible mechanistic links among dietary factors, immune response, and cancer development.

DIETARY FAT

Association with Cancer Risk   A large body of international epidemiologic evidence and experimental data suggests that the amount and type of dietary fat consumed influence risk of cancer at several sites, most predominantly the breast, colon/rectum, and prostate (7,17,25,26). Diet and cancer studies show that, in general, diets low in animal fat and red meats tend to protect against cancer, whereas diets high in fat, especially saturated fat, seem to increase cancer risk. Although the exact relationship between total fat intake and cancer risk continues to be debated, evidence suggests that the primary link between fat and risk for some cancers may be the result of the type of fat consumed rather than or in addition to total fat intake.

Breast Cancer   Findings from epidemiologic studies regarding the association of fat and breast cancer are inconsistent (27). International correlations support a direct relationship between fat intake and breast cancer risk (25–27). Migrant studies similarly support an increased risk for breast cancer as eating patterns shift from a low-fat, high-fiber diet to a high-fat, low-fiber "Western" diet (28,29). Most case-control studies suggest modest positive associations between fat intake and risk for breast cancer (27). Meta-analyses of case-control studies in postmenopausal women that compared the highest and the lowest quintiles of consumption found a significant relative risk (RR) of 1.46 between breast cancer and saturated-fat intake (30) and an RR of 1.21 between breast cancer and total fat intake (31). In contrast, large cohort studies generally have failed to demonstrate a link between dietary fat intake and breast cancer risk (27). Two separate meta-analyses reported RRs of 1.01 (31) and 1.05 (32) for cohort studies investigating the effect of dietary fat on breast cancer risk.

International comparisons indicate that diets high in n-6 polyunsaturated fatty acids (PUFAs) (as found in corn oil) are associated with increased breast cancer risk (26). In contrast, consumption of oleic acid, a monounsaturated fatty acid found in olive oil, and n-3 PUFAs, present in certain fish and fish oils, does not increase and may even reduce risk of breast cancer (26,33–35). Some studies suggested no association between breast cancer and saturated fat intake (RR = 0.95), compared with PUFAs (RR = 0.70), oleic acid (RR = 0.81), and olive oil (RR = 0.87), each of which showed an inverse relationship with breast cancer risk (36,37). One case-control study of primarily postmenopausal breast cancer patients found direct associations between increased breast cancer risk and the concentrations of trans fatty acids (RR = 1.4, $p < 0.001$) and PUFAs (RR = 1.26) in gluteal adipose tissue. The specific roles of various types of fat and fatty acids in altering breast cancer risk in humans, however, have not yet been clearly established. It has been suggested that n-6 PUFAs may enhance

breast cancer invasion and metastasis via eicosanoid production, whereas n-3 PUFAs may have a suppressive effect via the same mechanism (38).

Several factors may explain the inconclusive nature of the epidemiologic data on dietary fat and breast cancer, including inaccuracy in dietary assessment methods, insufficient variation in fat intake within a study population, interactions of correlated variables, differences in data collection and analysis methods, inaccuracy in dietary assessment, an insufficient follow-up period, failure to distinguish between premenopausal and postmenopausal women, and the importance of diet before adulthood (27).

Colorectal Cancer   International correlation studies demonstrate strong, positive associations between colorectal cancer incidence and consumption of red meat and animal fats (2,7,17,26,39). A number of case-control and cohort studies, including investigations using adenomatous polyps as markers of risk, also support the associations with red meat, with data from fat intake being less convincing (40–43). Data from international correlation and case-control studies do not support an association with vegetable fat (2,7,17,40,42). Epidemiologic data suggest a protective effect of the consumption of fish or fish oil, calculated as a proportion of total or animal fat, on colorectal cancer risk (33,44).

Prostate Cancer   Numerous case-control and cohort studies suggest an inverse relationship between risk for prostate cancer and consumption of either animal fat or high-fat foods, especially red meat (45). Polyunsaturated fats, however, do not appear to be associated with cancer of the prostate (45). International and ethnic differences in prostate cancer incidence indicate that the effects of dietary factors may vary across populations. A study of the role of diet in prostate cancer development in blacks, whites, and Asians in the United States and Canada reported an overall significant, direct relationship with saturated fat; the highest risk (RR = 4.1, highest versus lowest quintiles of intake) was reported for Japanese-Americans, and the lowest risk (RR = 0.91) was for whites (46).

Data from a large cohort study suggested that α-linolenic acid increased risk for prostate cancer (RR = 3.43), in contrast with saturated fat (RR = 0.95), monounsaturated fat (RR = 1.58), and linoleic acid (RR = 0.64) (47). α-Linolenic acid also appeared to enhance prostate cancer risk in a smaller case-control study (48). A recent review of epidemiologic and experimental evidence suggested that n-3 PUFAs may retard prostate cancer progression (38).

The Immune System Connection   There is strong evidence that both the type and amount of dietary fat consumed influence immune function (49–53). The effect of fat intake on several components of the immune system may, in turn, promote or inhibit tumor growth. As outlined briefly in this section, there are several different types of cytotoxic interactions between tumor cells and the defense system of the host. Key to these interactions are lymphocyte proliferation, cytotoxic T-cell (CTL) activity, natural-killer (NK) cell activity, and macrophage and cytokine function and activity (10,11,54). Also of interest is the extent of the nonspecific immune responses of the host (55). Research suggests that the predominant type of fat in the diet has a more precise effect on immune response than total fat intake. Clarifying the exact role of specific dietary fats in modulating immune response thus appears to be fundamental to understanding how the composition of the diet connects immune function with cancer risk. One type of fatty acid, n-3 PUFAs, has been studied extensively for its proposed cancer-protective and immunomodulating activities.

Lymphocyte Proliferation   In general, ex vivo lymphocyte proliferation is lower in animals fed a high-fat diet than in those given a low-fat diet *(10)*. The type of fat in the diet also has an impact on lymphocyte proliferation. In his review, Calder *(10)* ranks the relative potencies of specific dietary fats to suppress lymphocyte proliferation in the context of a high-fat diet (i.e., for animals, 90+ g total fat or type of fat/kg body weight); this ranking is in order of increasing ability to suppress proliferation: saturated fat < n-6 PUFA-rich oils < oleic acid < linseed oil < n-3 PUFA-rich fish oils.

NK Cell and CTL Activity   Animals fed high-fat diets exhibit lower activity of both NK cells and CTLs when compared with animals on low-fat, no-fat, or saturated-fat diets *(10)*. With regard to type of fat, the sum of experimental data suggests that inhibition of NK cell and CTL activities is greatest for n-3 PUFA-rich fish oils, followed by linseed oil, olive oil, n-6 PUFA-rich oils, and, finally, saturated fat *(10)*. The impact of specific dietary fats on human NK cell activity has not been reported. However, reducing dietary fat intake to below 30% of total calories appears to increase the activity of natural-killer cells *(10)*. Thus, diets high in fat may reduce an individual's NK cell response.

Cytotoxic T cells and NK cells move through a series of steps before destroying the appropriate target cells *(49)*. This process likely involves contact between the plasma membrane of the CTL of NK cell and the membrane of its target cell. Experimental data suggest that incorporation of unsaturated fatty acids into plasma membranes enhances cytolytic behavior of T cells, whereas incorporation of saturated fatty acids inhibits this action *(49)*. The lipid profile of tumor cell membranes similarly affects the tumor cell's susceptibility to lysis. In vitro studies indicate that tumor cells in which the plasma membrane has a higher PUFA content are more likely to lyse than those with lower PUFA levels; in vivo studies have not consistently produced the same results, however *(51)*.

Macrophage and Cytokine Function and Activity   The results of animal studies investigating the effect of dietary fats on macrophage activity and macrophage-related cytokine production are mixed. For example, both enhanced and inhibited tumor necrosis factor (TNF)-α production in rodents fed n-3 PUFAs, fish oil, or safflower oil has been reported *(10,55)*. These differences may be due, at least in part, to varying test conditions *(10)*. In humans, consumption of either fish oil or linseed oil has been shown to reduce the production of TNF-α, interleukin (IL)-1α, IL-1β, and IL-2 *(10)*. Although results vary by study, there is growing evidence from experimental studies that dietary fish oils and/or n-3 PUFAs can selectively alter macrophage function and activity. Studies in rodents demonstrate that dietary fish oil decreases the ability of activated macrophages to produce TNF-α and kill tumor targets when compared with macrophages from animals given safflower oil *(55)*. In these experiments, the fish oil appeared to block TNF-α transcription. In contrast, other studies indicate that by enhancing the platelet-activating factor (PAF) signaling pathway, dietary fish oil appeared to stimulate TNF-α-mediated tumoricidal activity of macrophages to a much greater extent than safflower oil *(55)*. The role of PUFAs in modulating tumoricidal activity of macrophages may be related to plasma membrane structure and content. Specifically, as with CTLs, changes in the fatty acid content of the plasma membrane of

macrophages appear to alter these cells' functional activity *(49)*. Overall, these data, although seemingly contradictory, support the suggestion that dietary fatty acids may selectively alter the tumoricidal activity of macrophages.

n-3 PUFAs and Fish Oils   A large body of data suggests that long-chain PUFAs are the fats most likely to be involved in the modulation of immune function. The beneficial effects of these dietary fats generally are attributed to eicosapentanoic acid (EPA) and docosahexaenoic acid (DHA), both n-3 PUFAs. Research consistently demonstrates that EPA and DHA affect the production of certain eicosanoids—including PGE_2, thromboxane (TXA_2), prostacyclin, and leukotrienes (e.g., LTC_4, LTD_4)—from arachidonic acid (AA) *(53)*. The eicosanoids are important in maintaining or regulating a variety of normal biological functions, including immune function. The prostaglandins, primarily PGE_2, show both inhibitory and stimulatory effects toward the effector cells considered to be important in the immune defense against cancer *(56)*. As noted earlier, dietary fish oil and n-3 PUFAs appear to affect the production and function of macrophages and macrophage-derived cytokines, including ILs, TNFs, and colony-stimulating factors (CSFs) *(51,53)*. Such changes may be mediated through PGE_2 *(21,57,58)*.

Data from both animal and human studies suggest that production of eicosanoids and cytokines is reduced by increased intake of fish oils and n-3 PUFAs such as EPA and DHA *(49–53)*. It has been hypothesized that by affecting the synthesis of eicosanoids and cytokines, consumption of EPA and DHA also influences the effectiveness of these immune system components. Supplementing the diet with n-3 PUFAs or fish oil has been shown to enhance several indices of immune response in healthy humans in both short-term and longer-term (up to 12 wk) studies *(52,53)*. Also, using n-3 PUFAs or fish oil to treat conditions resulting from or aggravated by an impaired immune system—such as rheumatoid arthritis, inflammatory bowel disease, and psoriasis—generally has brought about at least modest improvement *(51,53)*. Not all studies report an immuno-enhancing or -protective role for n-3 PUFAs, however *(51–53)*. For example, consumption of fish oil supplements has been shown to suppress immune response, as indicated by decreases in helper T cells, depressed mitogen response, and inhibited delayed-type hypersensitivity (DTH) response *(53)*.

Several factors may explain the inconsistent effects of n-3 PUFAs on immune response *(10,11,51,52)*. Both total fat intake and the amount of other types of fat in the diet, relative to n-3 PUFA intake, may affect the action of n-3 PUFAs with regard to factors such as membrane fluidity, oxidative stress, and the distribution and concentration of serum lipoproteins *(49,52)*. Also, research suggests that high total fat intake inhibits immune function in both humans and animals, whereas consumption of n-6 PUFAs suppresses immune response in animals *(52,53)* but appears to have no notable adverse immunologic effects in healthy individuals *(52)*. Furthermore, the specific effects of fat intake on the role of prostaglandins—and PGE_2 in particular—in immune function are not yet clear *(49,52,59)*. Finally, the use of antioxidants by an individual and the overall health, nutritional status, and age of the individual may influence the action of fats on immune function *(53)*.

At a certain level of intake, PUFAs may favorably influence the impact of eicosanoids and cytokines on immune function by modulating their synthesis. However, overproduction of or an imbalance in the different types of eicosanoids and cytokines, as mediated through elevated PUFA consumption, can lead to disease. Of course, dramatic reductions of eicosanoids and cytokines (e.g., in the presence of a deficiency of essential fatty acids) also can impair normal functioning of the immune system (49,51–53). It follows that although consumption of certain fats can be beneficial and, in some cases, is essential (e.g., linoleic acid), excessive intakes may adversely affect health, possibly in part by suppressing, rather than stimulating, immune function.

Evidence that certain fats, consumed at appropriate levels, may protect or enhance immune response seems compelling, but defining a specific role for dietary fat in immune function is challenging, in part because of the highly complex nature of the immune system. Furthermore, although research on the immune-modulating effects of fat has focused largely on the regulation of eicosanoid (prostaglandin) metabolism, a more comprehensive approach that integrates the role of lipids in membrane structure and function, peroxidation and generation of free radicals, eicosanoid production, and cell activation processes warrants further investigation (51).

MICRONUTRIENTS

Association with Cancer Risk Epidemiologic studies have demonstrated cancer-protective relationships for foods high in antioxidant micronutrients such as vitamin C, β-carotene, vitamin E, and selenium, as well as the micronutrients vitamin A, calcium, and folate (2,7,60–63). It is likely that several rather than single micronutrients contribute to the observed overall protective effects. For example, a cohort study by Yong and colleagues recently reported that a combination of vitamins E and C and carotenoids was more protective (RR = 0.48) than any of them individually (RRs = 0.82, 0.49, 0.55, respectively) (64). Furthermore, micronutrients may, in fact, be markers for other constituents of plant foods that have preventive properties (65).

Vitamin E Epidemiologic studies that have investigated associations of cancer risk and diets high in vitamin E are limited in number and show inconsistent results—possibly because estimation of dietary vitamin E is difficult (60). A review of 10 studies of vitamin E intake and 8 measuring serum vitamin E levels in relation to breast cancer risk reported an overall inconclusive relationship (66). Another review found significant regression of premalignant lesions in the oral cavity for vitamin E alone and in combination with β-carotene (67). In the Alpha-Tocopherol, Beta-Carotene Cancer Prevention Study (ATBC), conducted in Finland with more than 29,000 male cigarette smokers at high risk for lung cancer, a 32% decrease in clinical prostate cancer incidence and a 41% decrease in prostate cancer mortality were observed among men who received daily vitamin E supplements (68). Also, 16% fewer cases of colorectal cancer were diagnosed in the same study (69). Although these results suggest a protective effect of vitamin E, prostate and colon cancers were not primary study endpoints; other controlled trials are needed to confirm the ATBC findings.

Vitamin A/β-Carotene Vitamin A influences cell differentiation, and a deficiency of this micronutrient leads to hyperplastic changes in epithelial tissues—such as are observed in certain precancerous conditions; thus, vitamin A is believed to be most effective in the promotion stage of carcinogenesis (70). In the 1960s and early 1970s, vitamin A was a research focus with regard to the inhibition of carcinogenesis; the considerable body of data

resulting from these studies, however, was somewhat inconsistent (2,7).

Published reviews of epidemiologic studies have consistently reported strong support for a significant protective effect of dietary β-carotene on lung cancer (61,71,72). One review noted that associations of either high intakes of β-carotene-rich vegetables and fruits or high blood concentrations of β-carotene with reduced cancer risk were most consistent for lung and stomach cancer. Esophageal cancer showed limited but promising risk reduction (61). Reported findings for the effects of both β-carotene and vitamin A are equivocal for prostate cancer (45) and indicated a possible protective effect of β-carotene for breast cancer (73) and colon cancer (61). Two trials in high-risk individuals found no evidence of reduction in colorectal polyp incidence—and no evidence of harm—after 4 yr of intervention using β-carotene (74,75).

Vitamin C Epidemiologic evidence for a protective effect of diets high in vitamin C-containing vegetables and fruits is strong and consistent for cancers of the oral cavity, esophagus, and stomach, but moderate and less consistent for colon and lung cancers. Data do not support an association with prostate cancer and the evidence for breast cancer is conflicting (60,76,77). A review of more than 50 case-control and cohort studies that investigated intakes of vegetables and fruits and vitamin C and E reported that, across studies, individuals in the highest category of vegetable and fruit intake had approximately 40% less risk of gastrointestinal and respiratory tract cancers than those in the lowest intake category (60). Indices of vitamin C computed from vegetable and fruit intakes also were associated with lower risk in these studies.

Selenium Cancer mortality in international correlation studies suggest an inverse association between selenium status and cancer incidence (78). Data from case-control and cohort studies, however, have not been convincing for cancer sites investigated, including lung, breast, and stomach (72,73,79). A recent randomized, controlled clinical intervention showed significant reductions in total cancer mortality (RR = 0.5), total cancer incidence (RR = 0.63), and incidences of lung (RR = 0.54), colorectal (RR = 0.42), and prostate (RR = 0.37) cancers for individuals who received selenium supplements, compared with controls (80). These positive findings support the cancer-protective effect of selenium but must be confirmed in independent intervention trials.

The Immune System Connection The importance of specific micronutrients to the immune system is demonstrated most clearly in cases of moderate to severe, single- or multiple-nutrient deficiencies in which immune responses are impaired (14,19,22). A growing body of research suggests, however, that even marginal deficiencies may compromise immune function (14). Furthermore, although deficiency is the most commonly encountered state in which the immune system is affected adversely, excessive intakes of some micronutrients also may impair immune function (81). Defining the balance across adequate versus optimal versus excessive intakes of nutrients, as they relate to maintaining health and especially to disease prevention, remains a challenge.

Vitamins and minerals likely affect the immune system through a variety of mechanisms that may serve to connect immune function with cancer risk. Research suggests that in maintaining or supporting immune function, vitamins E and C, β-carotene, and selenium (an essential component of glutathione peroxidase) may (1) act as antioxidants that help control pro-oxidative activities of the abundant phagocytes in the body, which, in turn, prevents oxidative tissue damage in the absence of a threat to the host

(14), (2) provide a more general antioxidant defense through, for example, sequestering of free radicals *(82)*, and (3) stimulate the synthesis of cytokines (e.g., ILs, TNFs) in response to mitogen exposure, which, in turn, promotes clonal expansion of lymphocytes involved in normal immune function and tumor inhibition (e.g., helper T cells, cytotoxic T cells) and rejuvenates immune function *(82,83)*. Vitamin E, in particular, is critical for preventing the oxidation of PUFAs and, consequently, for maintaining cell membrane stability *(84,85)*. Also, through its antioxidant effects, vitamin E may limit the activity of cyclooxygenase, which results in decreased production of the immune suppressor PGE_2 *(86)* and thus may confer a benefit with regard to cancer risk.

Deficiencies in vitamins E, C, and A and β-carotene are associated with signs of a compromised immune system *(19,22)*. The factors affected by such deficiencies that also are likely to be related to tumor development include reduced NK cell activity, decreased lymphocyte response to mitogens, impaired macrophage activity, reduced phagocytic activity, and suppressed cytokine production (e.g., interleukins, TNF-α) *(22,83,87)*. Impairment of these immune functions and components is reversed through adequate intakes of the deficient nutrient(s) *(83,87)*.

Vitamin E. The antioxidative and immunoprotective properties of vitamin E may underlie the proposed epidemiologic associations between vitamin E intake and reduced risk for diseases of aging, including cardiovascular disease and cancer *(11,84,85,88)*. By preventing damage from free radicals and products of lipid peroxidation, vitamin E helps maintain the structural integrity of cells, including immune cells *(11,85)*; these actions, in turn, may retard or prevent the initiation or promotion of some cancers. Although a deficiency in vitamin E disrupts the stability of cell membranes, supplementation restores cell structure and function *(88)*. To illustrate, in one study of elderly hemodialysis patients, 300 mg vitamin E/d (via oral supplementation for 15 d) increased vitamin E concentrations in peripheral blood mononuclear cells and decreased the amount of fatty acid oxidative products in the membranes of red blood cells *(86)*.

Vitamin E deficiency in animals has been shown to suppress B-cell function, immunoglobulin production, T-lymphocyte response, phagocytic function, and cytokine and lymphokine function and production *(11,22)*. Supplementing the diets of animals with vitamin E enhanced immune response by suppressing or decreasing prostaglandin synthesis *(85,89,90)*, stimulating helper T-cell activity *(91)*, and improving macrophage function and mitogen-induced lymphocyte responsiveness *(92)*. In these studies, the decline in immune function normally observed in aging animals was reversed at least partially through vitamin E supplementation.

Experimental studies further demonstrate that dietary vitamin E supplementation protected against transplantation of virus-transformed K3T3 tumor cells *(85)* and that treatment of K3T3 tumor cells with vitamin E prior to transplantation facilitated the rejection of transplantation of these cells in mice *(85)*. In these studies, the cancer-protective activity of vitamin E appeared to be linked at least in part to its effects on immune function. Additional studies suggested that vitamin E inhibited the transplantation of K3T3 cells by increasing the expression of antibody receptor-mediated phagocytosis and Ia antigen and decreasing the expression of cell-surface molecules that are important in the tumorigenic and metastatic potential of tumor cells (e.g., glycolipids) *(85)*.

The impact of vitamin E intake on immune function also has been examined in humans, especially older persons, who, as a group, are at increased risk for reduced immune function, cancer, and vitamin E deficiency *(85,88)*. Two such studies—placebo-controlled, double-blind trials in healthy individuals at least 60 yr old—support the proposed immuno-enhancing capabilities of vitamin E and suggest a benefit for supplementation among the elderly *(93,94)*. In one study, a daily oral supplement of 800 international units (IU) vitamin E for 30 d improved three measures of T-cell function: DTH skin test, immune response to concanavalin A, and IL-2 production *(93)*. Lymphocyte vitamin E concentrations increased threefold and were correlated with enhanced immune function. Also, PGE_2 synthesis by monocytes and concentrations of plasma lipid peroxides were reduced. Further, no clinical, physiologic, or metabolic side effects were reported, suggesting that short-term vitamin E supplementation at 800 IU/d in healthy elderly individuals is safe *(95)*. The second study examined dose-related changes in T-cell function among healthy, older adults given a 60-, 200-, or 800-IU vitamin E supplement daily for 30 d *(94)*. T-Cell function improved following supplementation, with the greatest increase in immune response observed among those receiving 200 IU vitamin E/d.

Vitamin A/β-Carotene. Both deficiencies and excesses of vitamin A may adversely affect immune function *(19,22)*. Animals deficient in vitamin A exhibit clear signs of a compromised immune system: decreased thymus and spleen sizes, reduced NK cell activity, reduced interferon and antibody production, impaired DTH, less effective fat macrophage activity, depressed lymphocyte response to mitogens, reduced phagocyte activity, and greater susceptibility to infection *(19,22,96)*. Impaired immune function in vitamin A-deficient animals usually is partially to fully recovered following compensatory supplementation or administration *(96)*.

Although severe deficiencies of vitamin A clearly have adverse consequences in humans in terms of morbidity and mortality, particularly for infants and children *(22,96)*, the impact of marginal to moderate vitamin A deficiencies on immune status in humans, particularly adults, is less clearly defined. Extremely high intakes of vitamin A, however, appear to impair immune function *(19,96)*. To illustrate, in one study of two infants with clinical evidence of vitamin A deficiency, a single megadose of vitamin A (90 mg all-*trans*-retinol) caused a dramatic, immediate drop in the ability of lymphocytes to respond to phytohemagglutinin; this depressed lymphocyte function persisted for 10 d before starting to return to pretreatment response levels *(19)*. In the general population, excessive vitamin A intake, which usually occurs via oversupplementation, can have serious consequences that include and extend beyond the immune system (e.g., increased susceptibility to infection, severe liver damage) *(96,97)*. In animals, vitamin A supplementation beyond levels necessary for health have been reported to increase the rate of rejection of autologous skin grafts, suppress induction of T-cell cytolysis, and increase, in a dose-dependent fashion, macrophage-mediated tumoricidal activity, phagocytosis, and DTH *(96)*. Although moderate increases in the latter group of immune responses may be beneficial to the host, overproduction or overstimulation of these same responses may adversely affect the host defense system *(96)*. Thus, whereas slightly elevated intakes of vitamin A may enhance some immune system components, the broader risks associated with hypervitaminosis A must be considered when studying the impact of large doses of vitamin A on immune function.

In brief, vitamin A-altered immune function may have a role in cancer prevention and development, with hypovitaminosis A suppressing and mild hypervitaminosis A sometimes promoting immune function and response *(96)*. Although a clear and convincing mechanism linking vitamin A intake with immune function and tumor growth or inhibition is lacking, several hypotheses have been suggested *(14,98)*. Studies indicate that vitamin A (which is not a strong antioxidant) and its analogs augment the tumoricidal activity of alveolar macrophages *(12,99)* and suppress the generation of superoxide anions by polymorphonuclear leukocytes *(100)*. The role of vitamin A in maintaining epithelial integrity and other mechanical barriers also may link immune function and cancer risk *(14,98)*. A deficiency in vitamin A inhibits δ-interferon production and NK cell activity *(82)*, whereas an excess may interfere with normal functioning of the vitamin by downregulating nuclear retinoid receptors *(12,96)*.

β-Carotene, a vitamin A precursor that is converted to vitamin A in the body, is a strong antioxidant without the toxic potential of vitamin A. A variety of immunoenhancing effects have been reported for β-carotene, including increased resistance to immunogenic tumors *(96,101)*. In experimental feeding studies, β-carotene stimulated rat lymphocyte mitogenesis (T and B cells) *(102)*, increased thymic weight, stimulated allograft rejection, and inhibited virally induced tumor growth in mice *(102)*. β-Carotene also enhanced tumor immunity and markedly reduced tumor growth in mice exposed to tumor cells and rechallenged with the same tumor *(103)*. β-Carotene also has been shown to stimulate NK cell activity *(22,96)* and—in contrast with other retinoids—enhance tumor cytolytic factors against a variety of tumor cell lines when added to human lymphatic cultures *(96)*.

Findings from several studies suggest that β-carotene enhances the production and/or activity of IL-1α and/or TNF-1α in monocytes collected from hamsters *(104)* or healthy human subjects *(105,106)*. In one study using human cells, concentrations of these factors were significantly higher ($p < 0.05$, IL-1; $p < 0.01$, TNF) in β-carotene-exposed cells compared with control cells *(106)*. In a second human study, TNF levels were significantly higher ($p < 0.05$) in ex vivo stimulated cells obtained from healthy adult men given 15 mg β-carotene/d (via supplements) for 28 d when compared with cells from men in the placebo group *(105)*. Other studies have monitored β-carotene-induced alterations in immune function. An increase was reported in the frequency or number of lymphocytes with CD3+ (total T cells) and CD4+ (T helper cells) but not CD8+ (T suppressor/cytotoxic cells) in healthy human volunteers given 180 mg β-carotene/d for 2 wk *(107)*. Also, increased concentrations of surface markers of NK cells were found within 72 h after peripheral blood mononuclear cells (PBMCs) from healthy adults were exposed to β-carotene *(108)*. Similar findings were reported following administration of at least 30 mg β-carotene/d for 2 mo to 10 men and 10 women *(109)*.

For β-carotene, the interplay between immune function and inhibition of carcinogenesis appears to rest, at least in part, with the ability of β-carotene to stimulate cellular immunity. For example, β-carotene increases the number and activity of NK cells, T helper cells, and macrophages, relative to other lymphoid cells; the compound also promotes the differentiation of lymphoid precursors to T helper and NK cells *(83,96,109)*. This selective immunomodulatory effect of β-carotene provides another mechanism, in addition to its antioxidant and antiproliferative functions, for its proposed anticancer activity *(106)*. The broad immune-enhancing activities of β-carotene, combined with its ability to modulate specific components of the immune system that are targeted against

tumor development and its low toxicity, suggest an interesting intersection between chemoprevention and immunoprotection that warrants further study.

Vitamin C. A series of studies in guinea pigs (which, like humans, do not synthesize vitamin C) found that vitamin C-deficient animals had decreases in T lymphocyte response, DTH, phagocytic function, complement formation or function, and epithelial integrity *(22,110,111)*. These animals also appear to be more susceptible to infection and were less likely to accept skin allografts than animals given adequate amounts of the vitamin *(99,110)*. Further investigations in irradiated mice and guinea pigs suggest that vitamin C is required for the production and/or activity of thymic humoral factors *(110)*, and studies in laboratory animals stressed through administration of steroids indicate that ascorbate may be essential to the differentiation of lymphoid tissue *(110)*.

Results of both experimental and clinical studies of vitamin C-mediated T-cell responses are equivocal *(110)*. In animals, vitamin C deficiency has been shown to increase circulating B cells and decrease T cells, whereas high doses (250 mg/d) have the opposite effect on these lymphocyte populations *(110)*. The number of splenic T cells does not appear to be affected by a deficiency in vitamin C, thus suggesting a sequestering or compartmentalizing of these cells during deprivation. Clinical studies, in which marginal vitamin C deficiency or scurvy was induced experimentally, found normal lymphocyte stimulation in response to T-cell mitogens but no change in other lymphocyte subpopulations among elderly persons *(110,112)*. High oral doses of vitamin C (1–5 g/d) stimulated the mitogenic responses of lymphocytes in healthy young adults *(113,114)*. Similar results were reported in subjects over 70 yr old who were given daily intramuscular injections of 500 mg vitamin C for 30 d *(115)*, but not in elderly individuals taking megadose supplements of the vitamin *(110)*. Vitamin C may affect lymphocyte function (and cancer risk) indirectly, through its ability to regenerate vitamin E from a tocopherol free radical, which is produced as a result of scavenging by vitamin E for reactive oxygen molecules *(110,111)*. Results of studies in guinea pigs suggest further that the primary impact of vitamin C deficiency on mitogen-stimulated B- and T-cell responses may be a result of vitamin C-related depletion of vitamin E *(110)*.

Vitamin C markedly and consistently affects phagocyte activity *(110,111)*, and numerous in vitro experiments support a direct relationship between vitamin C concentration and phagocytic function *(110,111,116)*. In the guinea pig, phagocyte motility appears to be dependent on vitamin C status *(110,111)*. In adult volunteers, experimentally induced vitamin C depletion retarded phagocyte function and decreased bactericidal capacity of neutrophils and macrophages *(117)*, whereas doses of at least 2 g vitamin C/d increased neutrophil motility and chemotaxis *(110,111)*. Studies of cancer patients have reported markedly reduced leukocyte levels of vitamin C, which are reversed with supplementation *(110)*. Vitamin C likely acts as an antioxidant to protect phagocytes against oxidative damage caused by the generation of highly reactive free radicals and other oxygenated products resulting from phagocytic activity *(111)*.

A very small number of studies have examined the impact of vitamin C on cytokine production. These experiments found that dietary vitamin C enhanced interferon production both in vivo and in vitro—following exposure to murine leukemia virus in mice and in culture with murine L cells or embryonic fibroblasts *(110)*. In vitro studies suggest that vitamin C may act in part by modulating cytokine production, specifically, IL-2 activation of lymphocytes *(110)*. These limited data suggest a specific mechanism by which vitamin C may modulate tumor growth through its effects on immune response.

Although studied extensively over the past decades, the impact of vitamin C intake on immune function remains undefined *(110,116)*. The sum of data regarding whether vitamin C deficiency consistently impairs cell-mediated or humoral immunity in humans is still somewhat uncertain *(22)*. Similarly, evidence that high intakes of vitamin C (usually through supplementation) stimulate immune response is countered by equivocal results of studies investigating the ability of pharmacologic doses of ascorbic acid to prevent infection *(22,116)*. One challenge to this area of research is the lack of studies with acceptable experimental designs and methods that can either confirm or refute the findings of prior reports *(81,110,116)*.

Selenium. Studies in a variety of animal species suggest that depletion of selenium leads to impaired immune function, whereas supplementation with low doses of selenium restore or enhance immunologic activity *(83,116,118)*, demonstrating a role for selenium in immune responses that may influence tumor development or progression *(83,118)*.

The effects of selenium deficiency on the immune system of animals are extensive and include reduced resistance to microbial and viral infections, inhibited neutrophil function, decreased antibody production, reduced mitogen-stimulated proliferation of T and B lymphocytes, and inhibited cytotoxicity of T cells and NK cells *(118)*. Selenium supplementation in animals overcomes these effects and also has been shown to (1) stimulate DTH reactions and allograft rejection, (2) enhance the ability of animals to reject transplanted malignant tumors, (3) restore glutathione peroxidase activity, and (4) stimulate the production of lymphokines, chemicals produced and released by T cells that attract macrophages to sites of infection or inflammation *(118,119)*. Selenium also appears to be essential to the synthesis of prostacyclin, which possesses antimetastatic activity *(99)*.

In contrast with the many studies of the impact of selenium intake on immunologic health and disease in animals, only a limited number of studies in humans have been conducted. In one report, 40 healthy volunteers with low serum selenium levels received either a supplement of 200 μg selenium/d or a placebo for 11 wk, followed by assessment of immune function using a series of in vitro tests of lymphocyte and granulocyte activity *(120)*. Results showed no differences between the two groups with respect to phagocytosis, chemotactic factor generation, antibody or leukocyte production, or mitogen-induced proliferative responses. A recent review suggests that this level of supplementation may have been too low to produce any remarkable results; supplementation of up to 1 mg selenium/d, which more closely approximates the doses used in animal studies, may be necessary *(83)*.

Selenium appears to act in concert with vitamin E, as suggested by reports that selenium-deficiency-associated impairments in immune function can be corrected with vitamin E supplementation *(116)* and that impaired immune responses are magnified when the diet is deficient in selenium plus vitamin E (compared with a complete diet or a diet deficient in only one of these nutrients) *(82)*. In addition to its antioxidative properties, selenium appears to enhance T-cell clonal expansion and NK cell activity by inducing posttranscriptional expression of the IL-2R receptor on the α-chain of IL-2 *(83,118)*. High doses of selenium also may, via various methylated metabolites or their derivatives, indirectly enhance DNA repair mechanisms *(83,121)*. The immunostimulant effects of subtoxic levels of selenium, however, do not appear to be mediated either by such mechanisms or via selenium-dependent enzymes *(83,121)*.

CALORIC RESTRICTION

Association with Cancer Risk Animal studies demonstrate that marked reductions in caloric intake (between 20% and 40% below usual intake), without a deficiency in any essential nutrients, lowers the incidence and delays the onset of most spontaneous and induced tumors *(2,122–125)*. A striking demonstration of this effect is the ability of caloric restriction (CR) to delay spontaneous tumorigenesis in mice carrying a null mutation in the p53 tumor suppressor gene *(126)*.

Numerous case-control and cohort studies have investigated the association between caloric intake and cancer risk in adults through the assessment of either relative body weight or body size (as measured through body mass index [BMI]); relative body weight reflects caloric intake in relationship to energy expenditure *(2,122)*. The strongest direct associations of BMI and cancer risk have been found with breast and colon cancer *(2)*. It should be noted that diets high in fat and/or calories contribute to weight gain and obesity, as does little or no regular physical activity. It is postulated that all of these factors most likely work in concert to influence cancer risk.

Breast Cancer. Based on epidemiologic data, weight and body size appear to influence breast cancer risk, particularly in relation to menopausal status *(127–131)*. Findings indicate that obesity prior to menopause appears to protect against breast cancer, whereas postmenopausal obesity is associated with increased risk *(130,132)*. Gaining weight after age 18 and being overweight during the premenopausal years, however, appear to ultimately increase risk for breast cancer after menopause *(131–133)*. In contrast, weight loss prior to and after menopause is associated with reduced risk *(132)*. With the onset of menopause, estrogen derived from the conversion of androgens in adipose tissue predominates. Obese postmenopausal women, when compared with their leaner counterparts, may have an elevated risk for breast cancer owing to reduced levels of sex-hormone-binding globulin and higher levels of circulating estrogen secondary to the increased metabolic activity in adipose tissue *(128,134)*.

Colorectal Cancer. Leanness has been associated with reduced risk, and obesity with increased risk, for colorectal cancer in men and, in many cases, women *(2,39,135,136)*. This protective effect has been observed for both adenomas and cancer and appears to be strongest for lesions of the colon *(137,138)*. Data from the Nurses' Health Study indicated an increased risk for colon cancer (RR = 1.45) in women with a BMI greater than 29 kg/m², compared with women with a BMI less than 21 kg/m² *(136)*.

Prostate Cancer Current data do not support a relationship between obesity in adults and prostate cancer *(45,139)*. However, a recent study of nearly 48,000 men participating in the Health Professionals Follow-Up Study found that obesity during childhood (age 10 or under) had a strong inverse association with prostate cancer *(140)*. Lean body mass and high percent muscle mass in adult men increase the risk of prostate cancer, possibly as a result of elevated levels of circulating androgens *(45,139)*.

The Immune System Connection The impact of caloric restriction on immune function depends in part on the nutrient(s) being restricted. For example, protein-calorie malnutrition has consistently been shown to impair immune function in both animals and humans, leading to an increased risk for infection and compromising overall health *(15,19,22,81,141)*. Severe protein-calorie malnutrition, which almost always is accompanied by deficiencies in other nutrients, has a significant adverse effect on all aspects of immune response *(141)* and, consequently, dramatically impairs the ability to use immune defenses to fight against tumor development *(15)*. Specifically, severe protein-calorie malnutrition markedly impairs cell-mediated immune responses, production of secretory IgA antibody, phagocyte function, antibody activity, and cytokine production *(22,141,142)*.

In contrast, normal immune function may be maintained or even enhanced if caloric restriction is accompanied by adequate intake of other essential nutrients. CR in animals has been shown to slow the immunologic alterations that normally accompany aging *(13)*; CR also inhibits age-related decreases in IL-2 production and responsiveness, enhances NK cell function, and retards the age-related decrease in DNA repair by lymph cells *(13)*. Furthermore, in animals, caloric restriction—in the presence of adequate consumption of other essential nutrients—appears to confer compensatory or reserve immunologic function that is stimulated when challenged, for example, when exposed to tumor cells or tumor tissue *(23)*. Such findings suggest that the immune response in calorie-restricted animals is highly adapted to the environment and to environmental stimuli in a way that benefits the host *(23,143,144)*. In sum, the overall beneficial outcomes of CR in rodents include reduced mortality from chronic diseases, extended life-span, and delayed onset of illness, including cancer and diseases of impaired immune function *(13,23,143,144)*.

The proposed immunologic reserve under conditions of caloric restrictions is suggested by a series of animal studies. Rodents fed restricted-calorie diets have lower numbers of cells in the spleen and lymph nodes and lower unstimulated NK cell activity than animals fed *ad libitum*. However, these same calorie-restricted animals exhibit a greater level of lymphocyte proliferation, poly(I-C)-induced NK cell activity, production of and response to IL-2, and T-cell killing of tumor cells *(23)*. Also, a marked restriction in caloric intake (40–45% below usual intake) has been associated with an improved proliferative response of blood lymphocytes (considered to be an index of improved host immunity), as well as increased cytolytic activity of peritoneal macrophages and elevation in serum immunoglobulins *(145)*. These data support other studies in which calorie-restricted animals exhibit a burst of protective immune responses when physiologically challenged.

Whether such findings, which are well established in mice and rats, also apply to other animals, including nonhuman primates, is not entirely clear. One study under way in 30 adolescent Rhesus monkeys suggests some limited adverse effects on immune function after up to 4 yr of CR (18% fewer calories than the usual diet), including overall reductions in NK cell activity and antibody response following administration of a trivalent influenza vaccine *(146,147)*. Cell-surface antigens and peripheral blood lymphocyte counts were unaffected. At least two other ongoing studies in nonhuman primates are investigating the impact of CR on immune response in conjunction with the development of diabetes and atherosclerosis *(147–149)*.

The benefits of reduced-caloric intake likely occur via several metabolic mechanisms, through reduced free-radical production,

increased free-radical detoxification, increased rate of apoptosis (programmed cell death), enhanced enzyme-mediated DNA repair, and reduced cellular proliferation at a variety of sites (e.g., within the epithelial layer of the gastrointestinal tract, colonic mucosa, thymus, liver, and spleen) *(13,23,122,141,150,151)*. Such mechanisms, individually and collectively, can provide strong protection against progressive diseases such as cancer, which ordinarily develop with age.

The connection between CR, immune function, and cancer development also is demonstrated in studies in which calorie-restricted animals exposed to viral-associated cancers such as the mouse mammary tumor virus (MMTV) or murine leukemia virus (MuLV) have fewer tumors and/or delayed latency to onset of cancer than animals fed *ad libitum* *(23)*. In such cases, expression of the cancer-related virus and proliferation of cells in the target tissue are much lower in calorie-restricted animals than in controls. Thus, low-calorie diets may protect the host against "infection" by tumor-related viruses. Furthermore, components of the immune system that protect against tumor development, including lymphocyte proliferation, mitogen-induced NK cell activity, IL-2, and tumor-targeted T-cell cytotoxicity, are enhanced in animals fed low-calorie diets compared with animals allowed to eat freely *(23,143,144)*.

PHYSICAL ACTIVITY

Association with Cancer Risk   Data from the first National Health and Nutrition Examination Study (NHANES I) indicated that physical inactivity at work and low levels of recreational activity were related to an increased overall cancer risk in both men and women *(152)*. Numerous cohort and case-control studies have investigated the roles of physical activity (energy expenditure) in relation to cancer risk. The strongest association has been found with colon cancer; high levels of physical activity also may protect against breast cancer *(2,153)*.

Breast Cancer.   Although promising, the results from case-control and cohort studies of either leisure-time or total physical activity and breast cancer risk are not entirely consistent *(153)*. Some studies suggest that approximately 4 hr or 4000 kcal of physical activity or exercise per week, either on the job or during leisure time, or both, can markedly reduce the risk for breast cancer *(154–156)*. Several studies, however, reported no relationship between physical activity and breast cancer risk *(152,157,158)*. a few studies suggest that physical activity in adolescence and young adulthood may be protective against later development of breast cancer *(153)*. Sustained physical activity, although leading to weight loss as well as loss of body fat, generally helps reduce circulating levels of estrogen and progesterone, and possibly breast cancer risk.

Colorectal Cancer.   Regular physical activity, whether recreational or occupational, has been associated with reduced risk for colorectal cancer in men and women *(39,136,159–161)*. A review of 11 case-control studies and 9 cohort studies that examined the association between physical activity and colon cancer reported that at high physical activity levels, risk is approximately 60% below that of sedentary people *(2)*. Some data are consistent with an interaction between activity and body mass such that the highest risk is seen in those with the lowest level of physical activity and the highest body mass *(162)*. Physical activity may modulate colon cancer risk by any one or more of several proposed mechanisms, including stimulation of immune function, bile acid metabolism, colonic peristalsis, and reduction in intestinal transit time *(39)*.

The Immune System Connection The current body of evidence generally supports a beneficial role of regular exercise in cancer prevention, with exercise possibly modulating cancer risk through its effects on immune function *(163,164)*. Research suggests that the intensity, duration, and frequency of physical activity or exercise, as well as fitness level of the exerciser, all affect components of the immune system that may, in turn, influence cancer risk. Comprehensive reviews indicate that exercise can induce favorable changes in the function of macrophages and NK cells, as well as lymphokine activator killer (LAK) cells and related cytokines such as IL-1, IL-2, interferons, and TNFs, that could check the growth and enhance the lysis of tumor cells *(9,165)*. In humans, regular, moderate exercise (e.g., 5 d/wk, 40–50 min/d, at 60–85% heart rate reserve) generally enhances immune function by increasing resting NK cell activity, increasing mitogen-induced lymphocyte proliferation, and raising circulating T cell (e.g., CD4+) counts *(166–168)*. Furthermore, when elevated slightly, as with moderate physical activity, cytokines (e.g., IL-2, interferon-α, interferon-γ) stimulate NK cell activity *(163,168)*. The ability of moderate physical activity to affect these parameters and to stimulate the production and activity of NK cells either directly or indirectly boosts one of the body's first-line defenses against the development and progression of malignancies *(9,163,164)*.

Although moderate training generally tends to enhance immune function, single bouts of intense physical activity and chronic overtraining can suppress immune response and appear to increase susceptibility to infection, inflammation, and possibly cancer and autoimmune diseases *(168)*. The adverse effects of overtraining or exhaustive activity on the immune system are exacerbated further in the presence of nutrient deficiencies. This may be a result, in part, of the tremendous oxygen demand—and subsequent generation of free radicals—that physical activity places on the body *(169)*. A general profile of the responses of certain components of the immune system at the end of and during recovery from a single exercise session or intense physical activity is as follows: leukocyte, monocyte, lymphocyte, and NK cell counts increase, then drop, especially if the workout is exhaustive; the ratio of helper to suppressor cells drops, whereas the number of cytotoxic cells increases; lymphocyte proliferation rates are suppressed; circulating levels of immunoglobulins (and their synthesis in vitro) decrease; and factors such as C reactive protein, IL-1, and interferon increase *(168,170)*. For single bouts of exercise, these responses usually are transient and return to preworkout status within 2 h *(166,168)*. Adverse effects of an exhaustive, 90-min (or longer) workout (e.g., reduced NK cell counts), however, can persist for a week or more, thereby increasing susceptibility to infection or tissue damage. The effects of chronic overtraining thus mirror those of single bouts of exhaustive exercise but are sustained for longer periods *(168)*.

Several mechanisms whereby regular, moderate physical activity may protect against cancer have been proposed. One review suggests that exercise exerts its anticancer effect by stimulating those components of the monocyte–macrophage lineage that are capable of inhibiting tumor growth and destroying cancer cells *(164)*. Physical activity appears to (1) draw such immune cells into various tissues in response to an inflammatory challenge, (2) increase the release of macrophage-generated cytokines with antitumor properties (e.g., TNF-α), (3) increase the cytotoxic activity of macrophages against tumors, and (4) stimulate the production and activity of tumor-derived macrophages (which can either attack or stimulate the tumor). Results of animal studies indicate that these effects are influenced by both exercise "dose" (i.e., duration, frequency, and intensity of the activity) and functional status of the macrophage at the time of exercise *(163,164)*. Specific studies demonstrated that moderate (not defined) daily exercise in animals inoculated with tumor cells caused a significant increase in the number and activity of tumor-infiltrating cells, most of which were macrophages; the effect was greatest when macrophages were fully active. Slowed progression of growth of certain tumors in moderately exercised animals also has been reported. Although studies of exhaustive exercise have produced mixed results *(163,164)*, the evidence generally suggests that the overproduction of cytokines that stimulate NK activity—an outcome of excessive training—adversely affects the NK system *(168)*. Furthermore, when exercise leads to tissue damage (e.g., through the generation of free radicals), as would occur most commonly with overtraining or exercising to exhaustion, PGE_2 levels increase, causing a drop in the cytolytic activity of NK cells *(163)*.

FUTURE DIRECTIONS

It is evident that the scope of research required to examine the possible roles of diet-related factors and changes in the immune system mediated by these factors–as they relate to influencing both overall cancer risk and risk for specific cancers—will be multidisciplinary, complex, and extremely challenging. Within this framework, numerous research areas can be identified that will benefit from focused efforts by the scientific community and that have potential for cancer prevention. Examples of such areas include identification of genetic susceptibility factors and gene/nutrient interactions and clarification of their significance for immune function; elucidation of the underlying mechanisms by which diet- or lifestyle-related factors exert a biological and clinical effect to help determine any existing relationship among cancer, immune function, and the factor in question; and investigation of possible interactions among diet- or lifestyle-related factors and their subsequent effects on immune function and cancer risk.

Much remains to be learned about the effects of genetic susceptibility and gene–nutrient interactions with regard to cancer risk. Genetic susceptibilities (which include germline mutations in tumor-associated genes, as well as inheritable variations in carcinogen-metabolizing enzymes [polymorphisms], DNA adduct formation, and DNA repair mechanisms) may significantly influence response to environmental exposures, including dietary and lifestyle factors, and, consequently, affect cancer risk *(171)*. To illustrate, polymorphisms in the DNA repair enzyme O^6-alkyldeoxyguanine-DNA transferase (which reverses DNA-damage caused by *N*-nitroso compounds [NOCs], commonly found in the diet and cigarette smoke *(18)*) might markedly influence the burden on the immune system, as well as the need for vitamins E and C, which may inhibit the formation of endogenous NOCs *(172)*. Humans display significant interindividual variability, as much as 180-fold, in the activity of this repair enzyme *(18)*. As another example, polymorphisms in the genes that encode glutathione *S*-transferases and *N*-acetyl transferases—enzymes important in the detoxification of activated metabolites of carcinogens *(18)*—could influence both immune function and the degree of cancer risk possibly associated with dietary components that either induce or inhibit these enzymes. Studies are needed that identify susceptible populations and begin to define the role of genetic susceptibility in investigations of diet, nutrition, and cancer as well as its relationship to immune function. Such studies will contribute to a better understanding of the true relationships between diet-related factors and cancer risk and of the underlying mechanisms that affect cancer development.

In reality, cancer is a complex group of different diseases, and the mechanisms primarily associated with various types of cancer may understandably differ to some extent; thus, the operating mechanisms in the diet–immune system connection also may differ for various cancers. Furthermore, some dietary factors may act through numerous mechanisms. For example, although the exact mechanism(s) by which dietary fat promotes mammary tumorigenesis in animal models is not known, evidence supports a number of possibilities, including alteration in immune responsiveness, modulation of eicosanoid production, changes in membrane fluidity, production of peroxides, alterations in cellular interaction, and alterations in hormone secretion (20). Also, dietary fat, which can increase the endogenous production of PGE_2, may thus indirectly interact with an antiproliferative gene whose expression is enhanced by PGE_2. This gene may play a role in PGE_2-mediated inhibition of macrophage proliferation, with implications for enhanced cancer risk (20). In general, there is a need for further research that focuses on the possible mechanistic linkages between specific effects on the immune system and modulation of cancer risk by diet-related factors.

Many gaps in knowledge exist concerning the possible interactions of diet- and lifestyle-related factors with regard to their effects on the immune system and cancer risk. Given the widespread enthusiasm of some people for dietary supplementation with high levels of nutrients, it is important to have a better understanding of how such supplementation might affect the overall balance of nutrients and what the consequences might be for cancer risk as well as for overall health. To illustrate, researchers are increasingly debating whether current dietary recommendations for vitamin E—12 IU for adult women and 15 IU for adult men—and other nutrients are adequate (14,84). These recommended levels for vitamin E fall far below those suggested to improve immune response in the elderly (200 IU/d) (94), protect smokers against depletion of circulating leukocytes (75 IU/d) (14), and inhibit (40 IU/d) (84) or significantly reduce (400 IU/d) (88) susceptibility to oxidation of low-density lipoproteins. In addition, studies indicate that for diets rich in long-chain PUFAs, fish, and fish oils, which are readily oxidized, vitamin E consumption should be approximately 2.7 IU/d/1 g PUFA (84). Further research, however, is needed to better define vitamin E requirements as related to specific physiological effects, especially for the elderly, and to determine any consequences, either beneficial or adverse, of vitamin E interaction with other dietary factors. This same argument can be made for other micronutrients. Although the majority of research efforts have focused on specific dietary nutrients, consideration of the whole foods that contain these specific factors also is important with regard to reducing cancer risk. Vegetables and fruits, for example, in addition to antioxidant nutrients, contain numerous phytochemical constituents that have demonstrated cancer-protective effects (2,7) and that also may affect immune function; these constituents may act either individually or in combination.

SUMMARY

A convincing body of experimental, epidemiologic, and clinical evidence strongly supports the existence of a causal link between diet and cancer. In general, certain micronutrients, dietary fiber, vegetables and fruits, and moderate physical activity appear to be protective against cancer, whereas dietary fat, excessive calories, and alcohol seem to increase cancer risk. Dietary factors that contribute to cancer risk can be influenced by individual genetic susceptibilities, which may, in turn, contribute to some of the inconsistencies observed across epidemiologic studies.

Physiologic aging of the immune system results in a decline in immune function that has been linked to cancer development; cancer, in fact, is considered to be a disease of aging. Many components of normal healthy diets and lifestyle that appear to alter cancer risk, however, also may modulate immune response. Dietary antioxidants may enhance immune response, whereas caloric restriction can impair immune response if adequate intake of protein and essential nutrients is not maintained. Dietary fat can either impair or enhance immune response, depending on total and type of fat intake. Similarly, physical activity appears to either stimulate (regular, moderate activity) or suppress (overtraining) immune response.

It is unclear to what extent the mechanisms involved in modulation of carcinogenesis and immune response by any specific diet-related factor may overlap or influence each other. Some factors may have certain mechanisms in common, such as the ability to act as an antiproliferative agent or an antioxidant. Many results from investigations of the interplay among individual diet-related factors, immune function, and cancer risk are equivocal. The lack of conclusive findings likely stems from possible interactions among several factors; thus, the totality of and balance among effects of various diet- and lifestyle-related factors must be considered. In reality, these effects may be difficult to separate.

Definitive proof that diet- and/or lifestyle-related factors influence cancer development through specific effects on the immune system does not yet exist. Continued comprehensive research efforts that encompass experimental, epidemiologic, and clinical studies—including randomized clinical trials designed to evaluate intervention effects on both measures of cancer development and associated immune response—will be required to expand knowledge in this area and to provide clear direction for planning more refined cancer prevention strategies.

ACKNOWLEDGMENTS

The author would like to thank Ms. Sharon McDonald and Ms. Mary Cerny of The Scientific Consulting Group, Inc., for their expert editorial assistance.

REFERENCES

1. Landis SH, Murray T, Bolden S, Wingo PA. Cancer statistics, 1998. CA Cancer J Clin 1998; 48:6–29.
2. World Cancer Research Fund. Food, Nutrition and the Prevention of Cancer: A Global Perspective. American Institute for Cancer Research, Washington, DC, 1997.
3. Fernandes G. Nutritional factors: modulating effects on immune function and aging. Pharmacol Rev 1984; 36:123–8.
4. Lesourd BM. Nutrition and immunity in the elderly: modification of immune responses with nutritional treatments. Am J Clin Nutr 1997; 66:478–84.
5. Yancik R. Cancer burden in the aged: an epidemiologic and demographic view. Cancer 1997; 80:1273–83.

6. Sanders BG, Kline K. Nutrition, immunology and cancer: an overview. In: Longenecker JB, ed, Nutrition and Biotechnology in Heart Disease and Cancer, pp. 185–94. Plenum, New York, 1995.

7. National Academy of Sciences, National Research Council, Commission on Life Sciences, Food and Nutrition Board. Diet and Health. Implications for Reducing Chronic Disease Risk. National Academy Press, Washington, DC, 1989.

8. Grimble RF. Interactions between nutrients and the immune system. Nutr Health 1995; 10:191–200.

9. Hoffman-Goetz L. Influence of physical activity and exercise on innate immunity. Nutr Rev 1998; 56:126–30.

10. Calder PC. Dietary fatty acids and the immune system. Nutr Rev 1998; 56:70–83.

11. Meydani SN, Beharka AA. Recent developments in vitamin E and immune response. Nutr Rev 1996; 56:49–58.

12. Semba RD. The role of vitamin A and related retinoids in immune function. Nutr Rev 1998; 56:38–48.

13. Lorenz E, Good RA. Nutritional indications for cancer prevention—calorie restriction. In: Cunningham-Rundles S, ed, Nutrient Modulation of the Immune Response, pp. 481–90. Marcel Dekker, New York, 1993.

14. Anderson R, Van Antwerpen VL. Vitamins in the maintenance of optimum immune functions and in the prevention of phagocyte-mediated tissue damage and carcinogenesis. Bibliothecca Nutricia Dicta 1995; 52:66–74.

15. Chandra RK. Nutrition and immunoregulation significance for host resistance to tumors and infectious diseases in humans and rodents. Am J Clin Nutr 1992; 122:754–7.

16. Tsuji K, Harashima E, Nakagawa Y, Urata G, Shirataka M. Time-lag effect of dietary fiber and fat intake ratio on Japanese colon cancer mortality. Biomed Environ Sci 1996; 9:223–8.

17. U.S. Department of Health and Human Services. The Surgeon General's Report on Nutrition and Health. Public Health Service, U.S. Government Printing Office, Washington, DC, 1988, NIH Publication No. 88-50210.

18. Perera FP. Molecular epidemiology: insights into cancer susceptibility, risk assessment, and prevention. J Natl Cancer Inst 1996; 88:496–509.

19. Chandra RK. 1990 McCollum Award Lecture. Nutrition and immunity: lessons from the past and new insights into the future. Am J Clin Nutr 1991; 53:1087–101.

20. Erickson KL, Hubbard NE. A possible mechanism by which dietary fat can alter tumorigenesis: lipid modulation of macrophage function. In: Diet and Breast Cancer, pp. 67–81, American Institute for Cancer Research, Plenum, New York, 1994.

21. Erickson KL, Hubbard NE. Dietary fish oil modulation of macrophage tumoricidal activity. Nutrition 1996; 12:34–8.

22. Scrimshaw NS, San Giovanni JP. Synergism of nutrition, infection, and immunity. Am J Clin Nutr 1997; 66:464–72.

23. Engelman RW, Day NK, Good RA. Calories, cell proliferation, and proviral expression in autoimmunity and cancer. Proc Soc Exp Biol Med 1993; 203:13–7.

24. Newsholme EA. Biochemical mechanisms to explain immunosuppression in well-trained and overtrained athletes. Int J Sports Med 1994; 15:142–7.

25. Rose DP, Boyar AP, Wynder EL. International comparisons of mortality rates for cancer of the breast, ovary, prostate, and colon and per capita food consumption. Cancer 1986; 58:2363–71.

26. Hursting SD, Thornquist M, Henderson MM. Types of dietary fat and the incidence of cancer at five sites. Prevent Med 1990; 19:242–53.

27. Wynder EL, Cohen LA, Muscat JE, Winters B, Dwyer JT, Blackburn G. Breast cancer: weighing the evidence for a promoting role of dietary fat. J Natl Cancer Inst 1997; 89:766–75.

28. Parkin DM. Studies of cancer in migrant populations. IARC Sci Publ 1993; 23:1–10.

29. Ziegler RG, Hoover RN, Hildesheim A, et al. Migration patterns and breast cancer risk in Asian-American women. J Natl Cancer Inst 1993; 85:1819–27.

30. Howe GR, Hirohata T, Hislop TG, et al. Dietary factors and risk

of breast cancer: combined analysis of 12 case-control studies. J Natl Cancer Inst 1990; 82:561–9.

31. Boyd NF, Martin LJ, Noffel M, Lockwood GA, Tritchler DL. A meta-analysis of studies of dietary fat and breast cancer risk. Br J Cancer 1993; 68:627–36.

32. Hunter DJ, Spiegelman D, Adami H-O, et al. Cohort studies of fat intake and the risk of breast cancer—a pooled analysis. N Engl J Med 1996; 334:356–61.

33. Caygill CPJ, Charlett A, Hill MJ. Fat, fish, fish oil and cancer. Br J Cancer 1996; 74:159–64.

34. Willett WC. Specific fatty acids and risks of breast and prostate cancer: dietary intake. Am J Clin Nutr 1997; 66:1557–63.

35. Lipworth L, Martinez ME, Angell J, Hsieh C-C, Trichopoulos D. Olive oil and human cancer: an assessment of the evidence. Prevent Med 1997; 26:181–90.

36. Franceschi S, Favero A, Decarli A, et al. Intake of macronutrients and risk of breast cancer. Lancet 1996; 347:1351–6.

37. La Vecchia C, Netri E, Franceschi S, Decarli A, Giacosa A, Lipworth L. Olive oil, other dietary fats, and the risk of breast cancer (Italy). Cancer Causes Control 1995; 6:545–50.

38. Rose DP. Dietary fatty acids and cancer. Am J Clin Nutr 1997; 66:998–1003.

39. Kune GA. Diet. In: Causes and Control of Colorectal Cancer: A Model for Cancer Prevention, pp. 69–115. Kluwer Academic, Boston, 1996.

40. Giovannucci E, Rimm EB, Stampfer MJ, Colditz GA, Ascherio A, Willett WC. Intake of fat, meat, and fiber in relation to risk of colon cancer in men. Cancer Res 1994; 54:2390–7.

41. Giovannucci E, Willett WC. Dietary factors and risk of colon cancer. Am Med 1994; 26:443–52.

42. Potter JD, Slattery ML, Bostick RM, Gapstur SM. Colon cancer: a review of the epidemiology. Epidemiol Rev 1993; 15:499–545.

43. Potter JD. Nutrition and colorectal cancer. Cancer Causes Control 1996; 7:127–46.

44. Hill MJ. Diet and cancer: a review of scientific evidence. Eur J Cancer Prev 1995; 4:3–42.

45. Kolonel LN. Nutrition and prostate cancer. Cancer Causes Control 1996; 7:83–94.

46. Whittemore AS, Kolonel LN, Wu AH, et al. Prostate cancer in relation to diet, physical activity, and body size in blacks, whites, and Asians in the United States and Canada. J Natl Cancer Inst 1995; 87:652–61.

47. Giovannucci E, Rimm EB, Colditz GA, et al. A prospective study of dietary fat and risk of prostate cancer. J Natl Cancer Inst 1993; 85:1571–9.

48. Gann PH, Hennekens CH, Sacks FM, Grodstein F, Giovannucci EL, Stampfer MJ. Prospective study of plasma fatty acids and risk of prostate cancer. J Natl Cancer Inst 1994; 86:281–6.

49. Hwang D. Essential fatty acids and immune response. FASEB J 1989; 3:2052–61.

50. Goodwin JS, Ceuppens J. Regulation of the immune response by prostaglandins. J Clin Immunol 1983; 3:295–315.

51. Peck MD. Interactions of lipids with immune function II: experimental and clinical studies of lipids and immunity. J Nutr Biochem 1994; 5:514–21.

52. Kelley DS, Daudu PA. Fat intake and immune response. Prog Food Nutr Sci 1993; 17:41–63.

53. Meydani SN, Dinarello CA. Influence of dietary fatty acids on cytokine production and its clinical implications. Nutr Clin Pract 1993; 8:65–72.

54. Guillou PJ, Monson JR, Sedman PC, Brennan TG. Modification of lymphocyte function by fatty acids—biological and clinical implications. In: Cunningham-Rundles S, ed, Nutrient Modulation of the Immune Response, pp. 369–91. Marcel Dekker, New York, 1993.

55. Erickson KL. Dietary fat, breast cancer, and nonspecific immunity. Nutr Rev 1998; 56:99–105.

56. Young MRI. Eicosanoids and the immunology of cancer. Cancer Metastasis Rev 1994; 13:337–48.

57. Ben-Efraim S, Bonta IL. Modulation of antitumor activity of macro-

phages by regulation of eicosanoids and cytokine production. Int J Immunopharmacol 1994; 16:397–9.

58. Somers SD, Erickson KL. Alteration of tumor necrosis factor-α production by macrophages from mice fed diets high in eicosapentaenoic and docosahexaenoic fatty acids. Cell Immunol 1994; 153:287–97.

59. Waymack JP, Klimpel G, Haithcoat J, Rutan RL, Herndon DN. Effect of prostaglandin E on immune function in normal healthy volunteers. Surg Gynecol Obstet 1992; 175:329–32.

60. Byers T, Guerrero N. Epidemiologic evidence for vitamin C and vitamin E in cancer prevention. Am J Clin Nutr 1995; 62:1385S–92S.

61. van Poppel G, Goldbohm RA. Epidemiologic evidence for β-carotene and cancer prevention. Am J Clin Nutr 1995; 62:1393S–402S.

62. Lipkin M, Newmark H. Calcium and the prevention of colon cancer. J Cell Biochem 1995; 22(suppl):65–73.

63. Dorgan JF, Schatzkin A. Antioxidant micronutrients in cancer prevention. Hematol Oncol Clin North Am 1991; 5:43–68.

64. Yong L-C, Brown CC, Schatzkin A, et al. Intake of vitamins E, C, and A and risk of lung cancer. Am J Epidemiol 1997; 146:231–43.

65. Rock CL, Jacob RA, Bowen PE. Update on the biological characteristics of the antioxidant micronutrients: vitamin C, vitamin E, and the carotenoids. J Am Diet Assoc 1996; 96:693–702.

66. Kimmick GG, Bell RA, Bostick RM. Vitamin E and breast cancer: a review. Nutr Cancer 1997; 27:109–17.

67. Garewal HS, Meyskens FL Jr, Killen D, et al. Response of oral leukoplakia to beta-carotene. J Clin Oncol 1990; 8:1715–20.

68. Heinonen OP, Albanes D, Virtamo J, et al. Prostate cancer and supplementation with α-tocopherol and β-carotene: incidence and mortality in a controlled trial. J Natl Cancer Inst 1998; 90:440–6.

69. Alpha-Tocopherol Beta-Carotene Cancer Prevention Study Group, Heinonen OP, Huttunen JK, Albanes D. The effect of vitamin E and beta carotene on the incidence of lung cancer and other cancers in male smokers. N Engl J Med 1994; 330(15):1029–35.

70. Gerster H. β-carotene, vitamin E and vitamin C in different stages of experimental carcinogenesis. Eur J Clin Nutr 1995; 49:155–68.

71. Ziegler RG. Vegetables, fruits, and carotenoids, and the risk of cancer. Am J Clin Nutr 1991; 53:251s–9s.

72. Ziegler RG, Mayne ST, Swanson CA. Nutrition and lung cancer. Cancer Causes Control 1996; 7:157–77.

73. Hunter DJ, Willett WC. Nutrition and breast cancer. Cancer Causes Control 1996; 7:56–68.

74. Greenberg ER, Baron JA, Tosteson TD, et al. A clinical trial of antioxidant vitamins to prevent colorectal adenoma. N Engl J Med 1994; 331:141–7.

75. MacLennan R, Macrae F, Bain C, et al. Randomized trial of intake of fat, fiber, and beta carotene to prevent colorectal adenomas. J Natl Cancer Inst 1995; 87:1760–6.

76. Daviglus ML, Dyer AR, Persky V, et al. Dietary beta-carotene, vitamin C, and risk of prostate cancer: results from the Western Electric Study. Epidemiology 1996; 7:472–7.

77. Block G. Vitamin C and cancer prevention: the epidemiologic evidence. Am J Clin Nutr 1991; 53:270s–82s.

78. Schrauzer GN, White DA, Schneider CJ. Cancer mortality correlations studies III: statistical associations with dietary selenium intakes. Bioinorg Chem 1977; 7:23–34.

79. Kono S, Hirohata T. Nutrition and stomach cancer. Cancer Causes Control 1996; 7:41–55.

80. Clark LC, Combs GF Jr, Turnbull BW, et al. Effects of selenium supplementation for cancer prevention in patients with carcinoma of the skin. JAMA 1996; 276:1957–63.

81. Chandra RK. Graying of the immune system: can nutrient supplements improve immunity in the elderly? JAMA 1997; 277:1398–9.

82. Grimble RF. Malnutrition and the immune response: 2. Impact of nutrients on cytokine biology in infection. Trans Roy Soc Trop Med Hyg 1994; 88:615–9.

83. McCarty MF. Promotion for interleukin-2 activity as a strategy for "rejuvenating" geriatric immune function. Med Hypotheses 1997; 48:47–54.

84. Weber P, Bendich A, Machlin LJ. Vitamin E and human health: rationale for determining recommended intake levels. Nutrition 1997; 13:450–60.

85. Meydani SN, Blumberg JB. Vitamin E and the immune response. In: Cunningham-Rundles S, ed, Nutrient Modulation of the Immune Response, pp. 223–38. Marcel Dekker, New York, 1993.

86. Anonymous. Vitamin E supplementation enhances immune response in the elderly. Nutr Rev 1992; 50:85–7.

87. Grimble RF. Nutritional antioxidants and the modulation of inflammation: theory and practice. New Horiz 1994; 2:175–85.

88. Meydani M, Meisler JG. A closer look at vitamin E. Postgrad Med 1997; 102:199–207.

89. Meydani SN, Meydani M, Verdon CP, Shapiro AA, Blumberg JB, Hayes KC. Vitamin E supplementation suppresses prostaglandin E 1/2 synthesis and enhances the immune response of aged mice. Mech Ageing Dev 1986; 34:191–201.

90. Beharka AA, Wu D, Han SN, Meydani SN. Macrophage prostaglandin production contributes to the age-associated decrease in T cell function which is reversed by the dietary antioxidant vitamin E. Mech Ageing Dev 1997; 93:59–77.

91. Tanaka H, Hirose M, Kawabe M, et al. Post-initiation inhibitory effects of green tea catechins on 7,12-dimethylbenz[a]anthracene-induced mammary gland carcinogenesis in female Sprague–Dawley rats. Cancer Lett 1997; 116:47–52.

92. Sakai S, Moriguchi S. Long-term feeding of high vitamin E diet improves the decreased mitogen response of rat splenic lymphocytes with aging. J Nutr Sci Vitaminol 1997; 43:113–22.

93. Meydani SN, Barklund MP, Liu S, et al. Vitamin E supplementation enhances cell-mediated immunity in healthy elderly subjects. Am J Clin Nutr 1990; 52:557–63.

94. Meydani SN, Meydani M, Blumberg JB, et al. Vitamin E supplementation and in vivo immune response in healthy elderly subjects: a randomized controlled trial. JAMA 1997; 277:1380–6.

95. Meydani SN, Meydani M, Rall LC, Morrow F, Blumberg JB. Assessment of the safety of high-dose, short-term supplementation with vitamin E in healthy older adults. Am J Clin Nutr 1994; 60:704–9.

96. Watson RR, Earnest DL, Prabhala RH. Retinoids, carotenoids, and macrophage activation. In: Cunningham-Rundles S, ed, Nutrient Modulation of the Immune Response, pp. 63–74. Marcel Dekker, New York, 1993.

97. Chandra RK. Trace element regulation of immunity and infection. J Am Coll Nutr 1985; 4:5–16.

98. Ross AC. Vitamin A status: relationship to immunity and the antibody response. Proc Soc Exp Biol Med 1992; 200:303–20.

99. Das UN. Nutrients, essential fatty acids, and prostaglandins interact to augment immune responses and prevent genetic damage and cancer. Nutrition 1989; 5:106–10.

100. Witz G, Goldstein BD, Amoroso M. Retinoid inhibition of superoxide anion radical production by human polymorphonuclear leukocytes stimulated with tumor promoters. Biochem Biophys Res Commun 1980; 97:883.

101. Bendich A. β-carotene and the immune response. Proc Nutr Soc 1991; 50:263–74.

102. Bendich A, Shapiro SS. Effect of β-carotene and canthaxanthin on the immune responses on the rat. J Nutr 1986; 116:2254–62.

103. Tomita Y, Himeno K, Nomoto K, Endo A, Hirohata T. Augmentation of tumor immunity against syngenic tumors in mice by beta-carotene. J Natl Cancer Inst 1987; 78:679–80.

104. Bendich A. Carotenoids and the immune response. J Nutr 1989; 119:112–5.

105. Hughes DA, Finglas PM, Wright AJA, et al. Dietary beta-carotene supplementation modulates the production of tumour necrosis factor-α by human monocytes. Biochem Soc Trans 1996; 24:387S.

106. Abdel-Fatth G, Watzl B, Huang D, Watson RR. Beta-carotene in vitro stimulates tumor necrosis factor alpha and interleukin 1 alpha secretion by human peripheral blood mononuclear cells. Nutr Res 1993; 13:863–71.

107. Alexander M, Newmark H, Miller RG. Oral beta-carotene can increase the number of OKT4+ cells in human blood. Immunol Lett 1985; 9:221–4.

108. Prabhala RH, Garewal HS, Meyskens FL Jr, Watson RR. Immuno-modulation in humans caused by beta-carotene and vitamin A. Nutr Res 1990; 10:1473–86.

109. Watson RR, Prabhala RH, Plezia PM, Alberts DS. Effects of β-carotene on lymphocyte subpopulations in elderly humans: evidence for a dose-response relationship. Am J Clin Nutr 1991; 53:90–4.

110. Cunningham-Rundles WF, Berner Y, Cunningham-Rundles S. Inter-action of vitamin C in lymphocyte activation: current status and possible mechanisms of action. In: Cunningham-Rundles S, ed, Nutrient Modulation of the Immune Response, pp. 91–103. Marcel Dekker, New York, 1993.

111. Muggli R. Vitamin C and phagocytes. In: Cunningham-Rundles S, ed, Nutrient Modulation of the Immune Response, pp. 75–90. Marcel Dekker, New York, 1993.

112. Kay NE, Holloway DE, Hutton SW, Bone ND, Duane WC. Human T-cell function in experimental ascorbic acid deficiency and sponta-neous scurvy. Am J Clin Nutr 1982; 36:127–30.

113. Yonemato RH, Chretien PB, Fehninger TF. Enhanced lymphocyte blastogenesis by oral ascorbic acid. Proc Am Assoc Cancer Res 1976; 17:228.

114. Anderson R, Oosthuizen R, Maritz R, Theron A, Van Rensberg A. The effects of increasing weekly doses of ascorbate on certain cellular and humoral immune functions in normal volunteers. Am J Clin Nutr 1980; 33:71–6.

115. Kennes B, Dumont I, Brohee D, Hubert C, Neve P. Effect of vitamin C supplements on cell-mediated immunity in old people. Gerontol-ogy 1983; 29:305–10.

116. Beisel WR. Single nutrients and immunity. Am J Clin Nutr 1982; 35:417–68.

117. Jacob RA, Kelley DS, Pinalto FS, et al. Immunocompetence and oxidant defense during ascorbate depletion of healthy men. Am J Clin Nutr 1991; 54:1302–9.

118. Kiremidjian-Schumacher L, Stotzky G. Selenium and immune responses. Environ Res 1987; 42:277–303.

119. Kiremidjian-Schumacher L, Roy M, Wishe HI, Cohen MW, Stotzky G. Supplementation with selenium augments the functions of natural killer and lymphokine-activated killer cells. Biol Trace Element Res 1996; 52:227–39.

120. Arvilommi H, Poikonen K, Jokinen I, et al. Selenium and immune functions in humans. Infect Immun 1983; 41:185–9.

121. Ip C, Hayes C, Budnick RM, Ganther HE. Chemical form of sele-nium, critical metabolites, and cancer prevention. Cancer Res 1991; 51:595–600.

122. Weindruch R, Albanes D, Kritchevsky D. The role of calories and caloric restriction in carcinogenesis. Hematol Oncol Clin North Am 1991; 5:79–89.

123. Albanes D. Total calories, body weight, and tumor incidence in mice. Cancer Res 1987; 47:1987–92.

124. Macrae FA. Fat and calories in colon and breast cancer: from animal studies to controlled clinical trials. Prevent Med 1993; 22:750–66.

125. Freedman LS, Clifford CK, Messina M. Analysis of dietary fat, calories, body weight, and the development of mammary tumors in rats and mice: a review. Cancer Res 1990; 50:5710–9.

126. Hursting SD, Perkins SN, Phang JM. Calorie restriction delays spontaneous tumorigenesis in p53-knockout transgenic mice. Proc Natl Acad Sci USA 1994; 91:7036–40.

127. Albanes D. Energy balance, body size, and cancer. Crit Rev Oncol Hematol 1990; 10:283–303.

128. Ballard-Barbash R, Swanson CA. Body weight: estimation of risk for breast and endometrial cancers. Am J Clin Nutr 1996; 3:437S–41S.

129. Kuller LH. The etiology of breast cancer—from epidemiology to prevention. Public Health Rev 1995; 23:157–213.

130. La Vecchia C, Negri E, Franceschi S, et al. Body mass index and post-menopausal breast cancer: an age-specific analysis. Br J Cancer 1997; 75:441–4.

131. Brinton LA, Swanson CA. Height and weight at various ages and risk of breast cancer. Ann Epidemiol 1992; 2:597–609.

132. Trentham-Dietz A, Newcomb PA, Storer BE, et al. Body size and risk of breast cancer. Am J Epidemiol 1997; 145:1011–9.

133. Radimer K, Siskind V, Bain C, Schofield F. Relation between anthro-pometric indicators and risk of breast cancer among Australian women. Am J Epidemiol 1993; 138(2):77–89.

134. Potischman N, Swanson CA, Siiteri P, Hoover RN. Reversal of relation between body mass and endogenous estrogen concentrations with menopausal status. J Natl Cancer Inst 1996; 88:756–8.

135. Sandler RS. Epidemiology and risk factors for colorectal cancer. Gastroenterol Clin North Am 1996; 25:717–35.

136. Martinez ME, Giovannucci E, Spiegelman D, Hunter DJ, Willett WC, Colditz GA. Leisure-time physical activity, body size, and colon cancer in women. J Natl Cancer Inst 1997; 89:948–55.

137. Giovannucci E, Ascherio A, Rimm EB, Colditz GA, Stampfer MJ, Willett WC. Physical activity, obesity, and risk for colon cancer and adenoma in men. Ann Intern Med 1995; 122:327–34.

138. Giovannucci E, Colditz GA, Stampfer MJ, Willett WC. Physical activity, obesity, and risk of colorectal adenoma in women (United States). Cancer Causes Control 1996; 7:253–63.

139. Andersson S-O, Wolk A, Bergstrom R, et al. Body size and prostate cancer: a 20-year follow-up study among 135,006 Swedish construc-tion workers. J Natl Cancer Inst 1997; 89:385–9.

140. Giovannucci E, Rimm EB, Stampfer MJ, Colditz GA, Willett WC. Height, body weight, and risk of prostate cancer. Cancer Epidemiol Biomark Prevent 1997; 6:557–63.

141. Woodward B. Protein, calories, and immune defenses. Nutr Rev 1998; 56:84–92.

142. Chandra RK, Kumari S. Nutrition and immunity: an overview. J Nutr 1994; 124:1433–5.

143. Weindruch R, Walford RL, Fligiel S, Guthrie D. The retardation of aging in mice by dietary restriction: longevity, cancer, immunity and lifetime energy intake. J Nutr 1986; 116:641–54.

144. Licastro F, Weindruch R, Davis LJ, Walford RL. Effect of dietary restriction upon the age-associated decline of lymphocyte DNA repair activity in mice. AGE 1988; 11:48–53.

145. Mukhopadhyay P, Das Gupta J, Sanyal U, Das S. Influence of dietary restriction and soyabean supplementation on the growth of a murine lymphoma and host immune function. Cancer Lett 1994; 78:151–7.

146. Kemnitz JW, Weindruch R, Roecker EB, Crawford K, Kaufman PL, Ershier WB. Dietary restriction of adult male rhesus monkeys: design, methodology, and preliminary findings from the first year of study. J Gerontol Biol Sci 1993; 48:17–26.

147. Roecker EB, Kemnitz JW, Ershler WB, Weindruch R. Reduced immune responses in rhesus monkeys subjected to dietary restriction. J Gerontol 1996; 51A:276–9.

148. Ingram DK, Cutler RG, Weindruch R, et al. Dietary restriction and aging: the initiation of a primate study. J Gerontol Biol Sci 1990; 45:148–63.

149. Hansen BC, Bodkin NL. Primary prevention of diabetes mellitus by prevention of obesity in monkeys. Diabetes 1993; 42:1809–14.

150. Warner HR, Fernandes G, Wang E. A unifying hypothesis to explain the retardation of aging and tumorigenesis by caloric restriction. J Gerontol 1995; 50A(3):B107–9.

151. Steinbach G, Heymsfield S, Olansen NE, Tighe A, Holt PR. Effect of caloric restriction on colonic proliferation in obese persons: impli-cations for colon cancer prevention. Cancer Res 1994; 54:1194–7.

152. Albanes D, Blair A, Taylor PR. Physical activity and risk of cancer in the NHANES I population. Am J Public Health 1989; 79:744–50.

153. U.S. Department of Health and Human Services. Physical Activity and Health: A Report of the Surgeon General. U.S. Department of Health and Human Services, Centers for Disease Control and Prevention, National Center for Chronic Disease Prevention and Health Promotion, Atlanta, GA, 1996.

154. Bernstein L, Henderson BE, Hanisch R, Sullivan-Haley J, Ross RK. Physical exercise and reduced risk of breast cancer in young women. J Natl Cancer Inst 1994; 86:1403–8.

155. Thune I, Benn T, Lund E, Gaard M. Physical activity and the risk of breast cancer. N Engl J Med 1997; 336:1269–75.

156. Freidenreich CM, Rohan TE. Physical activity and risk of breast cancer. Eur J Cancer Prevent 1995; 4:145–51.

157. Taioli E, Barone J, Wynder EL. A case-control study on breast cancer and body mass. Eur J Cancer 1995; 31A(5):723–8.

158. Paffenbarger RS Jr, Hyde RT, Wing AL. Physical activity and incidence of cancer in diverse populations: a preliminary report. Am J Clin Nutr 1987; 45:312–7.

159. Neugut AI, Terry MB, Hocking G, et al. Leisure and occupational physical activity and risk of colorectal adenomatous polyps. Int J Cancer 1996; 68:744–8.

160. Enger SM, Longnecker MP, Lee ER, Frankl HD, Haile RW. Recent and past physical activity and prevalence of colorectal adenomas. Br J Cancer 1997; 75:740–5.

161. Colditz GA, Cannuscio CC, Frazier AL. Physical activity and reduced risk of colon cancer: implications for prevention. Cancer Causes Control 1997; 8:649–67.

162. Slattery ML, Potter J, Caan B, et al. Energy balance and colon cancer—beyond physical activity. Cancer Res 1997; 57:75–80.

163. Shephard RJ, Shek PN. Cancer, immune function, and physical activity. Can J Appl Physiol 1995; 20:1–25.

164. Woods JA, Davis JM. Exercise, monocyte/macrophage function, and cancer. Med Sci Sports Exerc 1994; 26:147–56.

165. Shephard RJ, Shek PN. Heavy exercise, nutrition and immune function: is there a connection? Int J Sports Med 1995; 16:491–7.

166. Pedersen BK, Tvede N, Klarlund K, et al. Indomethacin in vitro and in vivo abolishes post-exercise suppression of natural killer cell activity in peripheral blood. Int J Sports Med 1990; 11:127–31.

167. Shinkai S, Shore S, Shek PN, Shephard RJ. Acute exercise and immune function: relationship between lymphocyte activity and changes in subset counts. Int J Sports Med 1992; 13:452–61.

168. Shephard RJ, Rhind S, Shek PN. Exercise and the immune system. Sports Med 1994; 18:340–69.

169. Giuliani A, Cestaro B. Exercise, free radical generation and vitamins. Eur J Cancer Prevent 1997; 6:55–67.

170. Mackinnon LT. Exercise and natural killer cells: what is the relationship? Sports Med 1989; 7:141–9.

171. Ishibe N, Kelsey KT. Genetic susceptibility to environmental and occupational cancers. Cancer Causes Control 1997; 8:504–13.

172. Helser MA, Hotchkiss JH, Roe DA. Influence of fruit and vegetable juices on the endogenous formation of N-nitrosoproline and N-nitrosothiazolidine-4-carboxylic acid in humans on controlled diets. Carcinogenesis 1992; 13(12):2277–80.

32 AIDS

WILLIAM R. BEISEL

INTRODUCTION

The AIDS (acquired immunodeficiency syndrome) epidemic, which appeared suddenly in the early 1980s, has largely stabilized in countries where antiretroviral drugs are widely available. However, in underdeveloped countries, especially those in Africa and Asia, the epidemic rages on at a frightening rate. The causative Human Immunodeficiency Virus (HIV) was first identified in 1983, a time when published reports *(1,2)* were beginning to describe AIDS-related cachexia and the fundamental role of malnutrition in the pathogenesis of AIDS. Unexplained weight loss remains an important criterion in the diagnosis of AIDS *(3)*.

Nutritional status plays a cardinal role in the gradual progression of HIV infections to full-blown AIDS. Although combinations of antiretroviral drugs greatly reduce the HIV burden and delay the decline in T-helper (CD4+) lymphocytes, optimal nutrition plays a prophylactic role by supporting helper-cell proliferation and by ensuring the maintenance of other immune system activities as well as innate, nonspecific aspects of host defense. The asymptomatic period of HIV infections is not nutritionally benign, for it is accompanied by production of pro-inflammatory cytokines, body hypermetabolism *(4)*, and an accelerated metabolic degradation of many essential micronutrients *(5,6)*. Body energy expenditure increases as the viral burden increases. These facts must be taken into account when providing prophylactic nutritional support.

Eventually, secondary infections and/or malignancies develop in HIV-positive individuals. These illnesses are accompanied by a release of additional pro-inflammatory cytokines, by cytokine-induced cachexia, as well as by reductions in both food intake and the intestinal absorption of nutrients (*see* Fig. 1). As described throughout this book, various forms of malnutrition lead to dysfunctions of the immune system and impair other host defensive mechanisms as well. These Nutritionally Acquired Immunodeficiency Syndromes (NAIDS) that result are intensely synergistic with AIDS *(7)*. This synergism permits the development of severe, protracted immune suppression, and the secondary infections which lead to additional losses of body weight and nutrient stores, and to early death. Intensive use of aggressive nutritional therapy during symptomatic AIDS can slow, and sometimes reverse, this downward spiral and can greatly improve the quality and duration of life.

The important prophylactic and therapeutic roles of nutritional support have gained increasing attention, as evidenced by publications of original data, reviews, and by AIDS conferences with a nutritional focus *(8–10)*. It is to be hoped that the growing success of combined antiretroviral therapy and its ability to prolong the asymptomatic period of HIV infections will not cause therapists to forget lessons already learned about the benefits of aggressive nutritional support throughout the full course of HIV infections.

PATHOGENESIS AND PATHOPHYSIOLOGY OF HIV INFECTIONS

Two HIV types (type 1 in America and most of the world, and type 2 in some parts of Africa) produce similar human illnesses. Both HIV retroviruses are spherical and exhibit two identical RNA strands within a cone-shaped core surrounded by viral proteins. After cellular infection, viral RNA is converted by the action of reverse transcriptase enzymes to pro-virus DNA, which then moves to the nucleus, where it becomes incorporated into host cell genomes. The bilayered outer envelope of HIV is composed of host-derived phospholipids which support protruding virally encoded glycoproteins, gp41 and gp120. HIV penetration into CD4+ helper lymphocytes, macrophages, and follicular dendritic cells (in lymph nodes) requires initial binding of gp120 to cell-wall receptors. In T helper cells, the HIV receptor is the CD4+ molecule itself. Because viral envelope proteins contain highly variable amino acid sequences, HIV has an innate ability to resist the immune system as well as experimental vaccines.

Infection is followed by rapid, continuous viral replication and dissemination. The resulting viral burden (or load) can be quantitated by commercially available assays (which employ competitive reverse transcription chain reactions, or nucleic acid sequence-based amplification) expressed as HIV-1 copies/mL of plasma or serum. Within 3 mo, anti-HIV antibodies are formed that partially curtail plasma viremia and induce the sequestration of HIV in lymphoid tissues (*see* Fig. 2).

The human immunodeficiency virus is transmitted to other persons via blood, semen, or other body fluids when the virus contacts open lesions or traumatized mucosa in the recipient's body. Preinfection risk factors include sexual orientation, an HIV-infected partner, intravenous drug use, contact (including transfusions) with whole blood or products derived from human blood,

From: *Nutrition and Immunology: Principles and Practice* (ME Gershwin et al. eds.), © Humana Press, Inc., Totowa, NJ

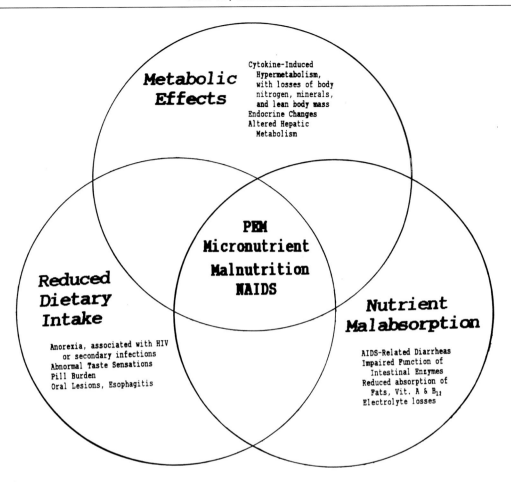

Fig. 1. Schematic portrayal of the three major factors (alone or in varying combinations) that lead to malnutrition. The pro-inflammatory cytokines induce major metabolic effects associated with the induction of body hypermetabolism and the loss of lean body mass. In patients with HIV infections, these effects begin early in the asymptomatic stage and continue throughout the illness. Reduced dietary intake and nutrient malabsorption begin much later, often in concert with secondary infections or malignancies. PEM = protein-energy malnutrition; NAIDS = nutritionally acquired immunodeficiency syndrome.

breast-feeding, and open lesions of the mouth or genitalia, the latter often resulting from other sexually transmitted diseases.

The CDC Classification System *(3)* for Patients with HIV infection (Table 1) was introduced as a consistent guideline for recognizing specific stages in the ensuing clinical progression of infection. It is also useful for discussing the pathogenesis and pathophysiology of HIV infections.

ACUTE HIV INFECTION   Acute, transient signs and symptoms (headache, malaise, slight fever, sore throat, rashes) sometimes develop 2–6 wk after the initiation of HIV infection. However, this inconsistent illness may be absent or ignored, despite the fact that the HIV is becoming abundant in both blood and spinal fluid.

Risk Factors   Variable risk factors, involving both virus and host, will then influence the subsequent course of illness. Viral factors include the virulence and cytopathogenicity of the infecting strain, the expression of regulatory and structural genes (activated, in part, by pro-inflammatory cytokines) that influence replication rates, and the magnitude of viral spread to macrophages and lymph nodes throughout the body. The viral burden, when assayed every

3–4 mo, is an invaluable guide to progression of infection *(see* Fig. 2).

A larger variety of risk factors involves the host. These risks include genetic predisposition, age, sex, lifestyle, coexisting disease conditions acquired either before or during HIV infection, the specific stimulatory or inhibitory cytokines generated by secondary infections, the use of tobacco, alcohol, and drugs, and, importantly, the pre-existing and ensuing nutritional status (as influenced by the daily intake of dietary and supplemental nutrients), as well as the presence of anorexia, malabsorption, and/or diarrhea *(10)*.

One recently identified deletion of an allele from the human CKR5 structural gene (a defect present in approximately 10% of American Caucasians) appears to interfere with HIV attachment to CD4+ cells. This genetic defect may markedly delay the progression of HIV-1 infections to symptomatic AIDS *(11)*.

ASYMPTOMATIC HIV INFECTION   Several months after the initial infection, serum antibodies against various HIV components begin to develop. However, antibodies produced against HIV-1 components may not interact with those of HIV-2, and

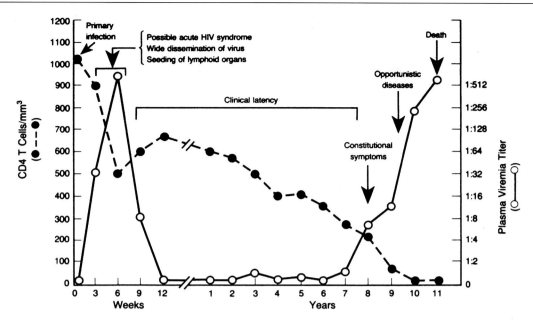

Fig. 2. Schematic portrayal of a typical, multiyear course of HIV infection, as shown by sequential changes in CD4 T helper cells and the changing viral burden, as measured in plasma. (From Pantaleo G, Graziosi C, Fauci AS, The immunopathogenesis of human immunodeficiency infection. N Engl J Med 1993; 328:327–35; reproduced with permission.)

vice versa. The asymptomatic stage can persist for many years (*see* Fig. 2), during which time body weight and the daily intake of food nutrients remain normal *(10)*. The asymptomatic period may be greatly extended by effective, combined antiviral therapy.

Depletion of T Helper Lymphocytes Measurable losses of CD4+ cells (from normal counts of 1000/mm³) during the asymptomatic stage provide clinical evidence of the progression of infection toward AIDS (*see* Fig. 2), as do measurements of viral burden. Exaggerated losses of body weight *(12)*, a declining

production of interferons *(13)*, and a disappearance of delayed dermal hypersensitivity responses *(14)* can also serve as independent predictors of the progression of HIV infections. Secondary infections generally begin when CD4+ counts fall below 500/mm³.

In this unrelenting war between HIV and the immune system, transcription of HIV genes within CD4+ helper cells is undoubtedly influenced by activation of infected lymphocytes by antigens and/or cytokines. Cytokines also stimulate HIV gene expression in macrophage/monocytes and may serve to activate HIV synthesis

Table 1
Centers for Disease Control (CDC) Classification System for Patients with HIV Infection

Group I   *Acute HIV Infection:* The early, transient signs and symptoms of acute infection, sometimes manifested shortly after initial infection by the human immunodeficiency virus.

Group II   *Asymptomatic HIV Infection:* The variably long (often years) period following initial infection during which virus–body cell interactions progress without inducing symptoms or lymphadenopathy.

Group III   *Persistent Generalized Lymphadenopathy:* The period in which the patient develops lymphadenopathy (nodes larger than 1 cm in diameter, in two or more extrainguinal sites, and lasting more that 3 mo.

Group IV   *Other HIV Disease Subgroups*

    IV A   *Constitutional Disease:* Patients with one or more of the following: more than a month of fever or diarrhea, more than 10% involuntary weight loss.

    IV B   *Neurological Disease:* Patients with dementia, myelopathy, or peripheral neuropathy.

    IV C   *Secondary Infectious Disease:* Patients with one of the following HIV-related secondary infections:

        Category C-1: Infections listed in the CDC definition of AIDS (i.e., *Pneumocystis carinii* pneumonia, chronic cryptosporidosis, toxoplasmosis, extraintestinal strongyloidiasis, isosporiasis, candidiasis (esophageal, bronchial, or pulmonary), cryptococcosis, histoplasmosis, mycobacterial infections with *M. avium* complex or *M. kansasii,* cytomegalovirus infection, chronic mucocutaneous or disseminated herpes simplex virus infection, and progressive multifocal leukoencephalopathy).

        Category C-2: Symptomatic or invasive disease with oral, hairy leukoplakia, multidermatomal herpes zoster, recurrent salmonella bacteremia, nocarditis, tuberculosis, or oral candidiasis.

    IV D   *Secondary Cancers:* HIV-related Kaposi's sarcoma, non-Hodgkin's lymphoma, or primary lymphoma of the brain.

    IV E   *Other Conditions (Clinical Findings That May Be the Result of HIV Disease):* Chronic lymphoid interstitial pneumonia, constitutional findings, infections, or cancers not listed in Subgroups A, C, or D.

in latently infected body cells. Thus, HIV replication is stimulated by the same mechanisms that promotes growth of host T cells. Not only do CD4+ helper cell populations fall during HIV infections, but their subpopulations may be altered, with a gradual decline in Th1 helper cells, which secrete interleukin (IL)-2, IL-12, and gamma interferon, and a proportional increase in Th2 cells, which secrete IL-4, IL-5, IL-6, and IL-10.

A number of mechanisms, including antibody-mediated cytotoxicity, actions of natural-killer cells, and apoptosis (cell suicide) (15), have been postulated to explain the continuing destruction of HIV-infected CD4+ helper cells. Losses of these multifunctional lymphocytes also impair the functions of other cell-mediated and humoral immune mechanisms, as well as the competence of non-specific host defenses (including innate defenses provided by macrophages and natural-killer lymphocytes). Secondary dysfunctions of humoral immunity include abnormalities in B cell activation, an impaired humoral response to newly introduced antigens, and a paradoxical increase in total plasma IgG concentrations. It should be noted that many of the immunological dysfunctions that characterize protein-energy malnutrition (PEM)-induced NAIDS resemble those caused by HIV infections. However, dysfunctions caused by NAIDS are preventable, or reversible, by nutritional support and rehabilitation. This fact also emphasizes the need for maintaining optimal nutrition throughout the asymptomatic stage of HIV infections.

Hypermetabolic Effects of HIV Infection As noted previously, the asymptomatic period is not quiescent but is characterized by an intense competition between the generation of additional HIV copies and the maintenance of immune cell numbers and functions, particularly those involving CD4+ helper T lymphocytes. In light of this continuing virus–host interplay and laboratory evidence of an accelerated metabolic degradation of vitamins (5), it is not surprising that patients are hypermetabolic during asymptomatic stages of HIV infection (4). Resting energy expenditures and fat-oxidation rates are increased during this asymptomatic period, even before CD4+ cell counts begin to decline (4). Generalized body hypermetabolism is not an unexpected finding, for it is a commonly seen response to pro-inflammatory cytokines released during generalized infections and after trauma (16). Although 10% losses of body weight have diagnostic significance during HIV infections, 5% losses predict the onset of opportunistic infections and progression of the disease to AIDS.

PERSISTENT GENERALIZED LYMPHADENOPATHY Generalized, persistent lymphadenopathy occurs in about 20% of HIV-infected patients. This lymphadenopathy is defined as unexplained lymph node enlargements, involving two or more groups of nodes (excluding femoral and inguinal regions), lasting 3–6 mo. It often includes nodes located in the neck and axilla. Generalized lymphadenopathy can occur in 35% HIV seropositive subjects of all ages. Although lymphadenopathy is considered a component of the AIDS-related complex, its development provides evidence for the progressive worsening of the patients condition. On the other hand, prominent lymphadenopathy does not seem to be necessary for the progression of HIV illness to full-blown AIDS.

Lymph nodes throughout the body are primary sites of HIV replication. The predominant pathophysiological effects of HIV infection on T cells occurs within the lymph nodes, with resultant lymphadenopathy. Lymph node infection is eventually followed by the destruction of nodal architecture and by nodal atrophy.

AIDS-Related Complex This complex is a clinically recognizable syndrome seen in HIV-infected patients, but one somewhat less severe than the various forms of diagnosable AIDS. The AIDS-related complex includes generalized lymphadenopathy, fatigue, weight loss, fevers, diarrhea, and minor opportunistic infections, such as thrush or herpetic dermatitis. The AIDS-related complex may persist for years without progressing to full-blown AIDS. Some patients exhibit a "softer" form of the complex which, in addition to chronic lymphadenopathy, including fatigue, malaise, sensations of undocumented fever, and mild or sporadic diarrheas.

AIDS MANIFESTED BY CONSTITUTIONAL DISEASE
The HIV infection can progress to AIDS without the occurrence of secondary infectious illnesses or malignancies. After a prolonged asymptomatic period, this form of AIDS may become manifest by the development of chronic fever, with or without concomitant diarrhea, and by more that a 10% involuntary loss of body weight.

Role of Pro-inflammatory Cytokines Production of pro-inflammatory cytokines (IL-1, IL-6, IL-8, tumor necrosis factor [TNF], and gamma interferon) is a cardinal feature of most infectious illnesses (7,16). These cytokines initiate fever by inducing the release of prostaglandins within the hypothalamic temperature-regulating center (16). Pro-inflammatory cytokines also enhance the proliferation of HIV (17,18). These mechanisms thus contribute to the losses of body weight in AIDS patients, as do metabolic effects by which pro-inflammatory cytokines lead to direct losses of body nutrient stores (Fig. 1) (16). Alpha interferon may also play a contributory role in the generation of malnutrition (19).

Cytokines can function in different body locations as apocrines, paracrines, or endocrines. Thus, they do not need to reach the plasma in order to induce cellular responses. For this reason, measured concentrations of individual cytokines in plasma do not necessarily reflect their true activity during HIV infections.

Pro-inflammatory cytokines are also subject to numerous checks and balances, including the release of cell-wall receptors, which can inactivate them, the synthesis of receptor antagonists (blockers), which prevent them from initiating target-cell responses, and the synthesis of other cytokines (such as IL-10) or cortisol, which can inhibit their synthesis. Losses of body weight appear to correlate with serum concentrations of the IL-1 receptor antagonist (20).

Pro-inflammatory cytokines trigger a broad array of acute-phase reactions, as listed in Table 2. Although these diverse, generalized, cytokine-induced responses are believed to represent beneficial host defensive mechanisms, they also incur large nutritional costs (see Fig. 1). Such losses of body nutrients can lead to damaging immunosuppressive consequences.

The nutritional costs of cytokine-induced acute-phase reactions include losses of energy stores resulting from hypermetabolism, losses of lean body mass and body weight (21), direct (measurable) losses from the body of nitrogen, phosphorus, magnesium, zinc, and potassium, losses of amino acids because of their metabolic degradation and exaggerated rates of conversion into glucose, and hypermetabolic degradation or direct losses of vitamins (16). Furthermore, such losses occur at a time when nutrient intake is generally diminished (see Fig. 1).

Cytokine-induced nutritional losses develop in rough proportion to the magnitude of fever, to its duration, and to closely spaced recurrent fevers (16). Losses of body energy, protein,

Table 2
Pathophysiological Responses in the Acute-Phase Reactions Initiated by Pro-inflammatory Cytokines
(IL-1, IL-6, IL-8, TNF, gamma-INF)

Fever and generalized body hypermetabolism.

Anorexia, with depressed nutrient intake.

Headache and somnolence.

Myalgias and arthralgias.

Catabolism of skeletal muscle proteins with loss of lean body mass. Newly released branched-chain acids can be oxidized *in situ* to generate energy. Their nitrogenous components are then synthesized into new gluconeogenic amino acids. This altered combination of muscle amino acids is released into the plasma for use elsewhere in the body.

Accelerated hepatic uptake of amino acids, iron, and zinc with sizable declines in their plasma values.

Accelerated hepatic synthesis of many proteins, including:

    Numerous hepatocyte enzymes

    Acute-phase reactant plasma proteins, including C-reactive protein, haptoglobin, ceruloplasmin, fibrinogen, alpha 1 acid glycoprotein (orosomucoid), amyloid A factor, alpha 1 antitrypsin, alpha 1 antichymotrypsin, complement components. Increased ceruloplasmin concentrations in plasma are accompanied by increased copper values.

    Zinc-binding metallothionein.

    Lipoproteins.

Accelerated synthesis of many other proteins, including cytokines, complement and kinin components, fibronectin, and immunoglobulins.

Decreased synthesis of plasma albumin and retinol binding protein.

Markedly accelerated hepatic glyuconeogenesis, with increased size of the extracellular glucose pool, and evidence for impaired cellular responsiveness to insulin.

Endocrine gland responses, including

    Activation of the pituitary/adrenal axis, with increased secretion of ACTH, cortisol, other gluconeogenic steroids, and aldosterone.

    Increased pituitary secretion of growth hormone and vasopressin.

    Diminished thyroid gland activity, and altered metabolism of circulating thyroid hormones.

    Increased pancreatic secretion of both insulin and glucagon.

    Decreased gonadal secretion of sex hormones.

Generation of nitric oxide from arginine, its only substrate.

Activation of the immune system and phagocytic cell functions.

minerals, and essential micronutrients, in combination, lead to the development of NAIDS, with its diverse combination of immunological dysfunctions. Millions of children throughout the Third World suffer from NAIDS, as do some aged individuals and many seriously ill patients in our most modern hospitals *(16)*. NAIDS also develops subsequent to losses of weight and body nutrients associated with AIDS. As previously noted, synergistic interactions between NAIDS and AIDS combine to further compromise immune system functions *(7)*. The combination of AIDS and NAIDS thereby leads to an early death.

AIDS-Related Diarrheas Chronic diarrhea is frequently observed in association with AIDS. Diarrheas cause direct losses of sodium, potassium, and bicarbonate, and possibly proteins and unabsorbed fats as well. Diarrheas can also be associated with chronic mucosal inflammation (with detectable HIV in both mucosal lymphatic tissues and stools). Increased concentrations of plasma TNF *(21,22)* may be detected during AIDS-related diarrheas, as may varying degrees of villus shortening and the malabsorption of nutrients *(10)*, including those of vitamin A and B_{12} (*see* Fig. 1). Lactose intolerance may also contribute to some pathogen-negative diarrheas, as may adverse reactions to antibiotics and other drugs being consumed.

However, most diarrheas in AIDS patients are caused by secondary infectious agents such as cryptosporidia, microsporidia, clostridia, salmonella, campylobacter, giardia, amoeba, cytomegalovirus, and *Mycobacterium avium (10,23)*. These agents localize in different areas of the gastrointestinal tract. Organism isolation may therefore require a variety of diagnostic manipulations

(endoscopy, flexible sigmoidoscopy, colonoscopy), biopsies, and cultures. However, some AIDS-related diarrheas are found to be pathogen negative *(23)*.

Diminished Intake of Nutrients Although dietary food intake may be normal or even increased during the asymptomatic period of HIV infections, the weight loss associated with AIDS is generally accompanied by reductions in nutrient consumption. These reductions are often multifactorial (*see* Fig. 1), with causes including anorexia, abnormal taste sensations, a huge daily consumption of medications, oral lesions, and esophagitis.

Anorexia and abnormal taste sensations may be associated with progressive HIV infection, with other secondary infections, or the presence of central nervous system (CNS) involvement. The sheer number of pills and capsules prescribed for HIV-infected patients and their specified consumption schedules (i.e., on an empty stomach or with meals) often interfere with normal eating patterns, especially in children *(24)*.

The AIDS patients can be afflicted with a variety of oral lesions that interfere with food consumption. These lesions include oral thrush, hairy leukoplakia, Kaposi's sarcoma, gingivitis, aphthous ulcerations, dental infections, and intraoral warts *(25)*.

In addition, esophagitis can become a major nutritional factor by preventing the swallowing of foods and fluids. Ulcerative esophagitis in AIDS patients is often caused by candida, herpes, or cytomegalovirus, alone or in combination. Therapeutic feedings by nonoral routes will then be required.

AIDS MANIFESTED BY NEUROLOGICAL DISEASE The HIV infections involve the brain or peripheral nervous system in almost one-third of all patients who develop AIDS. There is an increased expression of TNF receptors in brain macrophages and microglial cells of patients with AIDS, along with an upregulation of IL-I, IL-6, TNF, and reverse transcriptase enzyme activity in brain tissues (26,27). Cytokines may also stimulate the release of nitric oxide by brain cells (28). All of these biologically active molecules may function as mediators of CNS damage.

Neurological diseases are manifest by diverse findings, including AIDS–dementia complex, myelopathies, or peripheral neuropathies. Many of these neurological complications can be attributed directly to invasion of the nervous system by HIV and the fundamental role of cytokines in propagating the virus (29).

However, secondary invaders can also play a role by causing focal or diffuse subacute encephalitis, multifocal leukoencephalopathy, and/or meningitis. These invaders may include toxoplasma, cryptococci, candida, and mycobacterial species. Secondary neoplasms can also involve the central nervous system in AIDS patients, with primary, meningeal, or epidural lymphomas being the usual culprits, although plasmacytomas may also occur. In addition, vascular pathology can lead to cerebral arteritis, thromboses, or hemorrhage. CNS pathology is more common than peripheral neuropathy.

Like other forms of AIDS, neurological diseases can also be associated with malnutrition, but by somewhat different mechanisms. These include the development of anorexia and altered taste perceptions, the reduced ability of a patient to feed himself, and the previously described detrimental effects of cytokine production.

AIDS ASSOCIATED WITH SECONDARY INFECTIOUS DISEASES
As CD4+ counts begin to fall and the viral burden begins to rise (Fig. 2), HIV-infected patients become especially susceptible to a large group of primarily commensal, opportunistic microorganisms (see Table 1). These specific secondary infections develop with great frequency in AIDS patients. Infections involving the urinary tract may also occur, especially in older patients (30). Some anticipated infections can be prevented or reduced in severity by the prophylactic administration of organism-specific antibiotics or vaccines (31). Successful elimination of a secondary infection can sometimes allow a patient to return to the asymptomatic phase. More often, however, each secondary infection is followed by another, with the AIDS illness taking a progressively downhill spiral.

Effects on the Lean Body Mass   Secondary infections often generate a large additional outpouring of pro-inflammatory cytokines and the nutritional costs that go with them. Thus, secondary infections play a major role in initiating the wasting syndrome in AIDS, with weight loss progressing to severe cachexia (32). Losses of lean body mass are especially important, especially losses greater than 10%, for they deplete the body of its major storage banks for labile, readily available, properly balanced, amino acid mixtures. Nutritional depletion of lean body mass can, at times, be accompanied by histologic evidence of myopathy (AIDS polymyositis) in skeletal muscle (33). Quantitative losses of lean body mass can be measured and followed by the use of bioelectrical impedance analysis (34).

Therapeutic nutritional repletion of the lean body mass is especially difficult in the face of continuing, smoldering secondary infections, and almost impossible if a patient's HIV burden is on the rise. As previously noted, depletion of protein energy and other body nutrients gives rise to NAIDS and its synergistic immunological interactions with AIDS (7).

Endocrine Responses   A large number of hormonal changes are induced by cytokines during acute-phase reactions. Such hormonal responses can also develop during the secondary infections associated with AIDS. Cytokine-stimulated release of corticotropin within the hypothalamus causes pituitary/adrenal activation with increased secretions of ACTH, cortisol, and other glucocorticoid hormones (35). Cortisol, in turn, has an inhibitory effect on cytokine production. However, some degree of adrenal insufficiency (possibly associated with blunted pituitary and adrenal responses to corticotropin-releasing hormone (35)) develops in about 20% of patients with advanced AIDS, usually within 6 mo after secondary infections begin (36). This insufficiency is manifested by depressed cortisol concentrations in plasma and a reduced response to adrenal stimulation. AIDS patients who develop adrenal insufficiency usually suffer an early demise.

During acute-phase reactions, growth hormone values are generally elevated in plasma, but these increases may be reversed in the face of AIDS-related malnutrition. Epinephrine/norepinephrine secretions may also increase, especially during gram-negative sepsis. However, neither thyroid gland responses nor circulating thyroid hormones appear to play significant roles in the ongoing, cytokine-induced hypermetabolism. The thyroid gland reacts sluggishly to the actions of thyrotropin-releasing factor and thyroid-stimulating hormone. Degradation rates for circulating thyroid hormones may be slowed, and there is an increased conversion of plasma T_4 to reverse T_3 rather than to T_3 itself (16).

Carbohydrate metabolism is markedly altered during acute-phase reactions, during which the production of both insulin and glucagon are increased. In fact, the oxidation of glucose supplies much of the energy needed to sustain a hypermetabolic state. Increased rates of hepatic glycogen synthesis from amino acids and substrates such as lactate and pyruvate are abetted by insulin, and an increased conversion of glycogen to glucose is stimulated by glucagon. Despite these hormonal responses, patients develop adult-onset types of diabetic glucose tolerance curve within hours after the onset of infectious fevers. Glucose intolerance is accompanied by sizable increases in the peripheral glucose pool and by evidence for a peripheral cell resistance to action of insulin (16).

Hypogonadism generally develops during AIDS-induced cachexia. This is accompanied by a markedly reduced synthesis of gonadal steroids, especially testosterone, in both men and women. Low testosterone values contribute importantly to difficulties in reversing the losses of lean body mass by nutritional therapy.

AIDS ASSOCIATED WITH SECONDARY CANCERS
The HIV infection often leads to the development of certain secondary malignancies (as listed in Table 1). Their progression, localization, and/or therapy can also contribute to a severe depletion of body nutrients, as often occurs during malignancies in non-HIV patients. Cancer-induced malnutrition will also be magnified by the advent of secondary infections and the development of NAIDS.

HIV INFECTIONS IN NEONATAL INFANTS AND CHILDREN
The human immunodeficiency virus can be transmitted to fetal and neonatal infants born to HIV-infected mothers. Placental transfer of the virus can occur in utero or infection can occur during delivery. Mother's milk can also serve a source of HIV, as proven by the transmission of HIV to infants by mothers who

did not become infected until after they were already nursing. This fact creates a dilemma in impoverished lands where sanitation is primitive, infectious diseases are rife, and suitable alternatives to breast-feedings are nonexistent. In such situations, the risks of HIV transmission by milk seem far less than the almost certain early deaths of babies taken off the breast. An alternate possibility is breast-feeding by a surrogate HIV-negative woman.

The HIV infections in infants and children are somewhat different from those in adults, although children also have an asymptomatic period of variable length before they develop immunological defects and AIDS-like illnesses. The incubation period is shorter in children, and the infection is characterized by a failure to thrive (21), reductions of lean body mass (37), which may even include the myocardium, and often by retarded cerebral development, which may have a nutritional component (38). Infants with HIV encephalopathy can progress to microcephaly. In contrast to HIV-infected adults, parotid gland swelling is frequent in infants and children.

Secondary infections in children also tend to be different, with gram-negative sepsis and lymphotrophic interstitial pneumonitis (as a result of the Epstein–Barr virus) being common. Chronic chest infections occur more frequently in HIV-infected children than in adults. Persistent diarrheas are accompanied by fecal shedding of retroviral nucleic acids (39). Secondary intestinal infections with cytomegalovirus and herpes simplex virus are seen, but *Pneumocystis carinii* are more frequent pathogens, which often can resist immunoprophylactic regimes directed at their prevention (40).

Malnutrition in infants and children was noted quite early in the AIDS epidemic (1). A decline in weight and decreased linear growth may begin before 6 mo of age (41). Infected children commonly suffer from recurrent infections, protracted diarrheas, and malabsorption, all of which contribute to malnutrition. Childhood malnutrition is manifest by PEM as well as by a depletion of essential single nutrients. Vitamin A deficiency appears to be far more important in the progression of HIV infections in children than in adults (21,42). Long-chain PUFAs (polyunsaturated fatty acids) are depressed in the plasma of children with AIDS, as they are during severe PEM in HIV-uninfected patients (43,44).

Early and aggressive nutritional support is of great importance in HIV-infected children (45). Micronutrient deficiencies involving vitamins A and E, copper, and PUFAs all occur during the asymptomatic stages of HIV infections (44). An adequate caloric intake can improve weight, but often has little effect on linear growth or lean body mass (41). Gastrostomy tube supplementation can improve body weight and fat mass when other oral intake methods fail, and this can lead to a prolongation of life (46).

DOCUMENTED ALTERATIONS IN BODY NUTRITION DURING HIV INFECTIONS

PROTEIN-ENERGY MALNUTRITION   On a worldwide basis, PEM is the most common form of malnutrition, being seen predominantly in Third World children, in the aged, and in patients with serious medical and surgical diseases. Clinically evident PEM is rarely "pure," for it is typically accompanied by varying shortages of other essential macronutrients and micronutrients. PEM, as previously noted, is also the most common precursor of NAIDS and diverse secondary infections. All of these facts hold true for the malnutrition seen in AIDS patients.

In patients with HIV infections, all three major factors in the genesis of malnutrition (Fig. 1) do contribute. Of these, cytokine-induced malnutrition, with its many metabolic components, plays the major role by far, especially in the early development of both progressive disease and malnutrition. Conversely, diminished food intake and malabsorption are late participants.

As previously noted, pro-inflammatory cytokines contribute to body hypermetabolism during HIV infections, and the increased expenditures of body energy stores that must support it. Metabolic rates increase 7% for every degree Fahrenheit rise in body temperatures (16). Pro-inflammatory cytokines also act directly on skeletal muscle proteins, causing a catabolic release of free amino acids and the loss of lean body mass. Branch-chain amino acids are then oxidized to supply muscle energy, with their nitrogen skeleton being resynthesized to gluconeogenic amino acids. Large quantities of newly released free amino acids are taken up by the liver, where they are used for the synthesis of proteins necessary for host defenses. At the same time. hepatic synthesis of albumin and retinol-binding proteins is reduced.

Thus, in AIDS, as in other generalized infections, protein catabolism and protein anabolism are stimulated concurrently, as confirmed by ^{40}K (47) and leucine kinetic studies (48). Nitrogen components from amino acids sacrificed for gluconeogenesis are then synthesized into urea and excreted from the body. Clinically, the catabolic effects (as evidenced by falling body weight, loss of lean body mass, and low albumin values) are far more evident than the simultaneously ongoing anabolic responses.

LIPIDS AND ESSENTIAL PUFAS   Although body fat depots play an obvious role in energy generation, excess serum concentrations of various lipids are generally immunosuppressive. Significant increases in serum PUFA and triglyceride values are present in patients with advanced AIDS (49), but it is not known if these increases contribute to immune system dysfunctions in these patients. Hypertriglyceridemia may be induced by TNF and other cytokines in AIDS patients (44,49), as it is during other infections, especially the gram-negative ones (16).

Cytokines trigger the conversion of cell-wall PUFA to arachidonic acid (from n-6 PUFA) or eicasapentenoic acid (from n-3 PUFA), and then to biologically active eicosanoids, including the prostaglandins, thromboxanes, and leukotrines (16). Prostaglandin actions in the temperature-regulating center induce fever. Severe PEM in children with AIDS can retard this conversion of PUFA to eicosanoids (43).

FAT-SOLUBLE VITAMINS   Fat-soluble vitamins in serum may be reduced in concentration in patients with AIDS because of the combined effects of hyperutilization, increased excretion, decreased intake and intestinal absorption, cytokine-induced effects (21), as well as a diminished production of carrier proteins.

Vitamin A   Vitamin A and carotenoids have been most widely studied during HIV infections (5,6,21,42,44,50–53), with the greatest deficiencies being noted in infants and children. HIV-infected women with the lowest serum vitamin A values are the most frequent transmitters of the virus to their infants (42). Vitamin A deficiencies contribute to the various secondary infections seen in these children (51). Vitamin A deficiency during advancing AIDS is also an excellent predictor of mortality (50).

Vitamin E   Values for vitamin E, an antioxidant, show only minimal reductions in patients with AIDS (5,6,52–54). However, both free oxygen radical production and lipid peroxidation are increased during AIDS *(54)*.

WATER-SOLUBLE VITAMINS

B-Group Vitamins Many B-group vitamins appear unaffected by HIV infection, but declines may occur in riboflavin (B_2), pyridoxine (B_6), folate, and cobalamine (B_{12}) *(5,6,52,55)*. Of these, B_6, B_{12}, and folate are of greatest importance for supporting immune system functions *(16)*, although B_{12} deficiency is the only one that seems to adversely influence the course of HIV infections. Patients with low B_{12} values are 3.4 times more likely to progress rapidly from an asymptomatic state to a full AIDS *(55)*.

Vitamin C Ascorbic acid has important functions as an antioxidant in the production of adrenal glucocorticoid hormones and in the locomotion of phagocytic cells *(16)*. Its concentrations generally decline during infectious illnesses. Little has been reported about the nutritional status of vitamin C in HIV infections, but depressed concentration in the brain have been postulated to permit damage from oxidative stress and to the development of dementia.

TRACE AND ULTRATRACE ELEMENTS

Iron As a result of cytokine actions during generalized infectious illnesses, iron is quickly removed from the plasma and sequestered in storage depots. The sequestered iron is not used for incorporation into the hemoglobin of new red blood cells. Thus, in chronic infections, an anemia may develop that is both hypochromic and microcytic, although it is unlike the usual form of iron-deficiency anemia, because body iron stores remain high and plasma ferritin values are elevated *(16)*. This same pattern of iron sequestration appears to hold true for patients with advancing HIV infections, for iron accumulates in their bone marrow and livers, in macrophages, and in cells of the brain and muscle *(56)*.

On the other hand, anemia associated with a deficiency of iron has been described in HIV-infected children, in an apparent association with intestinal malabsorption of iron *(57)*. In these children, oral or parenteral iron therapy resulted in an improved production of hemoglobin.

Because iron is essential for the growth of many microorganisms and parasites, controversy exists as to whether to administer iron or to withhold it in patients with infectious diseases. This question is still an unsettled one in HIV-infected patients *(56,57)*.

Zinc Zinc is undoubtedly the most important trace element with respect to its role in supporting immune system functions. In addition to its presence in scores of important enzymes, zinc is the activating element that allows thymic hormones to play a stimulatory role in bodywide T-lymphocyte functions. Unfortunately, there are no reliable methods to measure zinc deficiency in a given patient and no body site where zinc is stored. Hair zinc measurements are unreliable for demonstrating body deficiencies and serum values can change dramatically during severe illness. Serum zinc values decline abruptly, by as much as 50%, during acute-phase reactions, in which zinc enters the liver and becomes bound to newly synthesized metallothionein *(16)*. However, such abrupt sequestrations of zinc do not indicate that the body is deficient in zinc.

In HIV-infected patients, serum zinc values generally decline progressively as the disease advances in severity *(54,58,59)*. This decline usually occurs in association with a heightened incidence of secondary infections *(60)*. Although declining zinc values are undoubtedly caused by acute-phase reactions, it is equally possible that actual zinc malnutrition develops concomitantly with the PEM cachexia of advancing AIDS.

Copper Copper values in the serum of patients with HIV infection have been found to be normal *(58)* or elevated *(60)*. Serum copper values typically become elevated during acute-phase responses because of the increased hepatic production of ceruloplasmin, the copper-transporting protein *(16)*.

Selenium Selenium in the most important antioxidant trace element, appearing to act in synergy with both vitamin C and E. Selenium also plays a role in supporting the immune system. Concentrations of selenium in serum are significantly reduced in patients with HIV infections, even during asymptomatic stages *(54,58,61)*. Such low values can be corrected by low-dose selenium supplementation *(61)*.

MANAGEMENT OF HIV INFECTIONS, WITH EMPHASIS ON THE ROLE OF NUTRITIONAL PROPHYLAXIS AND THERAPY

As with all generalized infectious diseases, the primary aim of therapy is to bring infecting microorganisms under control. Prevention or elimination of concomitant malnutrition is usually a secondary concern, one that can eventually be resolved after the infection is cured. However, the persistence of HIV, despite the best available antiretroviral therapy, makes concomitant malnutrition a very important issue, especially because malnutrition and HIV infections are intensely synergistic. The following steps are suggested for preventing, or managing, both infections and malnutrition during progressive stages of HIV disease.

MANAGEMENT DURING ASYMPTOMATIC AND LYMPHOADENOPATHIC PHASES

- Establish an unequitable serological diagnosis of HIV infection.
- Determine the viral burden at the onset of management (two assays separated by a 2- to 4-wk period) and at 3- to 4-mo intervals thereafter. Use viral burden assays to evaluate the effectiveness of antiretroviral therapy, including any necessary changes in drug combinations *(31)*.
- Measure CD4+ cell counts at baseline and at 3- to 4-mo intervals.
- If CD4+ counts/mm are greater than 500 and the viral burden is less than 10,000 copies/mL, antiretroviral therapy may be delayed until these indices are exceeded *(31)*.
- Otherwise, initiate antiretroviral therapy with at least three drugs (*see* Table 3), including two nucleotide analogs plus one protease inhibitor or one non-nucleoside reverse transcriptase inhibitor *(31)*.
- Based on viral burdens and CD4+ counts, consider the use of available prophylactic measures or drugs, in an attempt to block anticipated secondary infections by organisms frequently encountered in AIDS patients (*see* Table 3).
- Obtain an accurate initial body weight (without shoes or heavy clothing). Inform patients about their baseline body weights and about the exact weights that will indicate 5% and 10% declines. Stress to each patient the prognostic implications of these declines.
- Initiate prophylactic nutritional support by consultations with knowledgeable dieticians, if possible. Diets should include balanced amounts of energy, protein, and all other essential nutrients. Attempt to maintain a stable ideal body weight, with lean body mass at optimal levels. Ensure the adequacy of all nutrients known to support immunological functions.

Table 3
Pharmacologic Agents Used in the Complex Treatment of HIV Infections (generic name [trade name])

1. Antiretroviral Drugs. A combination of three drugs is now considered optimal, taking care not to combine drugs that react adversely with each other.
   A. Nucleoside Analogs
      Zidovudine [Retrovir]
      Didanosine [Videx]
      Zalcitabine [HIVID]
      Stavidine [Zerit]
      Lamivudine [Epivir]
   B. Protease Inhibitors
      Saquinavir [Invirase]
      Ritonavir [Norvir]
      Indinavir [Crixivan]
      Nelfinavir [Viracept] (approval pending)
   C. Non-nucleoside Reverse Transcriptase Inhibitors
      Nevirapine [Viramune]
      Delaviridine [Rescriptor] (approval pending)
2. Prophylactic agents used to decrease the chance of contracting specific secondary infections, listed in order of preference.
   A. Against *Pneumocystis carinii*—trimethoprim–sulfamethoxazole [Bactrim], dapsone, pentamidine (aerosolized) [NebuPent]
   B. Against *Mycobacterium tuberculosis*—isoniazid [INH] plus pyridoxine (vitamin B_6), Rifampin [Rifadin]
   C. Against *Mycobacterium avium*—clarithromycin [Biaxin], azithromycin [Zithromax]
   D. Against *Streptococcus pneumoniae*—pneumococcal vaccine
   E. Against *Toxoplasma gondii*—Trimethoprim–sulfamethoxazole [Bactrim], dapsone plus leucovorin, or plus pyrimethamine [Daraprim], or plus both
3. Appetite stimulants, for possible use in advanced AIDS
   A. Megestrol [Megace], normally used for the palliative treatment of advanced malignancies
   B. Dronabinol [Marinol], a bioactive substance derived from marijuana
4. Anabolic hormones, for helping rebuild lean body mass
   A. Testosterone, long acting, [DEPO-testosterone], useful in both sexes
   B. Growth hormone, nonvirilizing in women
   C. Synthetic androgens, may further depress testosterone production Nandrolone [Deca-durabolin, Durabolin]

Consider additional daily supplementation with a complete multivitamin/multimineral preparation but do now allow the daily intake of zinc to exceed 15 mg/d.

- Emphasize the need for a healthy lifestyle and the importance of prophylactic measures that may delay the progression of infection.
- Recommend a program of daily physical training, within the patients exertional limits (i.e., one that will help maximize lean body mass).
- Although the CDC diagnostic standards (*see* Table 1) require a 10% unexplained los of body weight for establishing diagnoses regarding the progression of HIV infections to AIDS, a 5% loss of body weight should trigger intensive nutritional intervention by the therapist.
- Attempt to provide the nutritional support and virological control measures necessary to allow normal growth and development in HIV-infected infants and children.

MANAGEMENT AFTER HIV INFECTIONS HAVE PROGRESSED TO FULL-BLOWN AIDS

- Continue use of three antiretroviral drugs. If a drug combination becomes ineffective, change therapy by the simultaneous substitution of at least two different antiretroviral drugs *(31)*.
- Continue surveillance of CD4+ counts, viral burden, and body weight.
- Continue to emphasize the importance of nutrition in slowing the progression of AIDS. If it seems useful in individual patients, plan additional small meals each day, making sure

that they do not interfere with the timing of prescribed drugs. Encourage the patient not to skip meals, especially breakfast.
- Emphasize the continuing importance of physical exercise, again within the limits of individual patients.
- Whenever fever develops in HIV-infected patients, especially those with advanced disease, a diagnostic search is required to determine if the fever is caused by advancing HIV infection *per se* or by the onset of a new, secondary, opportunistic infection.
- Establish exact diagnoses of intercurrent infections or malignancies and initiate appropriate therapy.
- Establish the etiologic diagnosis of any persistent diarrhea, if possible, and employ appropriate therapeutic measures to minimize losses or malabsorption of body nutrients.
- Provide whatever nutritional support is necessary in patients with neurological manifestations of AIDS.
- Treat developing malnutrition vigorously, attempting to restore adequate body nutrition and normal body composition. Use supplements whenever indicated, paying special attention to those that impact strongly on immune system functions and lean body mass. As noted earlier, weight loss must be managed aggressively if it reaches 5%.
- Consider the use of select nutritional supplements, especially those that support immune system functions. These supplements are particularly valuable in the treatment of AIDS. These include the following:

Vitamin A. Supplementation with vitamin A and/or beta-carotene have been recommended for patients with HIV infection *(50,51)*. In children born to HIV-infected mothers, supplementation reduced overall morbidity, especially that caused by diarrheas *(51)*. Doses should be aimed at preventing deficiencies but not at overloading storage depots that engenders vitamin A toxicity. The intake of vitamin A and the rate of progression to AIDS appears to be U-shaped, with patients in both the lowest and the highest quartiles of intake doing most poorly and those in the middle two quartiles showing the slowest progression of disease *(62)*.

B-Group Vitamins. Although all members of the B group of vitamins play some role in supporting the immune system, vitamin B$_6$, folate, and vitamin B$_{12}$ are especially important. The same may hold true in patients with HIV infections, where low plasma values are common. Vitamin B$_6$ benefits on CD4+ counts and mortality were evident at doses higher than two times the RDA, whereas vitamins B$_1$ and B$_2$ benefits became evident at doses five times normal *(63)*. Vitamin B$_{12}$ deficiencies, like body weight, are predictive of AIDS progression.

Vitamin C. Supplemental increases of vitamin C are often recommended in AIDS patients, although the value (or potential danger) of megadose intakes have never been established. In fact, from data generated by Tang et al. (in 281 carefully followed patients, over an 8-yr period), the largest dietary intakes of vitamin C caused a marginally significant increase in the progression of illness to full-blown AIDS *(62)*.

Vitamin E. Like vitamin C, tocopherols function as important antioxidants. Supplemental doses of 400 mg/d appear to have no harmful effects. In fact, supplementation with a combination of both vitamins C and E may have synergistic effects.

Iron. As noted earlier, different opinions have been expressed concerning whether to administer iron supplements to HIV-infected patients, to withhold them, or to administer chelators designed to reduce body iron stores. In a controlled study of dapsone (given to HIV-infected patients in a prophylactic attempt to prevent *P. carinii* pneumonia), a preparation that contained iron as well as dapsone was used *(64)*. Test patients actually received 30 mg/d of iron and showed a quickened mortality *(64)*. Based on these data *(64)*, iron supplementation is contraindicated during HIV infections. In contrast, true iron-deficiency anemia is often seen in children with AIDS, and for them, iron therapy has proven to be beneficial rather that harmful *(57)*.

Zinc. As with uncertainties about iron supplementation, questions have been raised about the value and safety of zinc supplements in patients with AIDS. Depressed serum zinc concentrations are typical in patients with AIDS and are said to be of prognostic importance. Because low serum zinc values typify cytokine-induced acute-phase reactions, their diagnostic importance must be questioned, for low plasma zinc values could indicate active ongoing secondary infections rather than a depletion of body zinc. Nevertheless, the use of zinc supplements has often been recommended. Zinc supplements may serve as adjuncts of zidovuline antiretroviral therapy and may help reduce the risk of secondary *Candida* and *P. carinii* infections *(59)*.

On the other hand, detailed lengthy studies of zinc supplementation in HIV-infected patients, conducted by Tang et al. *(62,63)*, showed that any zinc supplementation was associated with poorer survival. In their first study, the survival of patients who took zinc supplements became longer than that of other HIV patients, beginning at about 2000 d postdiagnosis. Survival in the two groups were markedly different by d 3000, with more rapid deaths among the zinc-supplemented group *(62)*.

In the second Tang et al. study *(63)*, HIV patients whose zinc intake was greater than 20.2 mg/d showed a decreased survival rate beginning at about 1000 d, when compared with HIV patients whose zinc intake was less than 14.2 mg/d. Survival differences between these groups continued to increase throughout 2500 d of observation. Survival of patients who consumed zinc in the 14.2- to 20.2-mg/d range was intermediate between the low and high zinc intake groups *(63)*. Increased dietary intakes of zinc are also known to be immunosuppressive in normal subjects *(16)*. Based on the excellence and long-term follow-ups in the studies by Tang et al. *(62,63)*, it can be recommended that dietary zinc intakes of HIV patients should not exceed the Recommended Daily Allowance, with zinc supplementation excluded at all times.

Selenium. Low-dose selenium supplementation in HIV-infected patients is effective in returning depressed serum values to normal *(61)*. However, the value of these supplements in supporting the immune system, in controlling antioxidant toxicity, or in prolonging the life of AIDS patients have yet to be established.

Amino Acids. Two amino acids, glutamine and arginine, have shown promise in improving the immunological functions of seriously ill surgical patients. Glutamine also plays an important role in maintaining the structure and function of the intestinal mucosa. These amino acids may also be of value in AIDS patients, as illustrated by the supplemental administration of arginine (*see* Fig. 3). Arginine has an additional unique value in infected patients, in that it is the sole source of nitric oxide, an important antimicrobial agent.

- Pay very close attention to declines in lean body mass, as best measured by bioelectrical impedance analysis. Restoration of lean body mass should be the primary goal of nutritional rehabilitation, but it can seldom be accomplished if infections are progressing. Antiviral control of HIV and elimination of secondary infections is mandatory. Thus, infection control has considerable nutritional value, in that it is necessary in order to allow concomitant dietary therapy to restore body weight and fat depots. Unfortunately, such weight gains are seldom accompanied by a meaningful correction of deficits in lean body mass.

- Additional pharmacologic measures may be necessary in an attempt to restore muscle protein deficits. These steps could include the use of growth hormone and/or androgenic steroids (Table 3), especially in patients with low serum testosterone concentrations and CD4+ cell counts below 200.

- Consider the use of appetite stimulants, such as megestrol (Megace) or dronabinol (Marinol) (Table 3) in patients with wasting illness. Megestrol, widely used as an adjunct in cancer therapy, has a secondary effect of weight gain caused by a stimulation of appetite. In AIDS patients, it is generally well tolerated in doses twice as large as those used in cancer

PHA, Stimulation Index

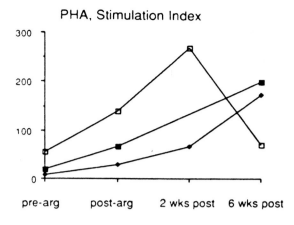

Con A, Stimulation Index

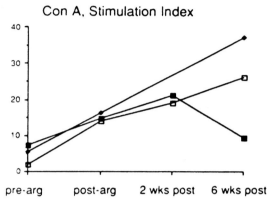

Fig. 3. Effects on the averaged mitogenic responsiveness (to PHA and Con A) of peripheral blood lymphocytes from three asymptomatic HIV-infected subjects to a 2-wk period of arginine supplementation. (From Barbul A, Cunningham-Rundels S, eds, Nutrient modification of the immune response. In: The Role of Arginine as an Immune Modulator, pp. 47–61. Marcel Dekker, New York, 1993; reproduced with permission.)

patients, but still within its safety limits. Dronabinol may have side effects such as confusion and somnolence because it includes a marijuana-like component.

- In the event of severe esophagitis or intestinal malabsorption, the use of aggressive alternatives to oral feedings may become necessary. These include gastrotomy tube feedings or total parenteral nutrition *(46)*.

- Anorexia, nausea, and vomiting are common components of the secondary infections seen in AIDS patients, especially children. These problems have a serious negative effect on all attempts to maintain an optimal nutritional status. If secondary infections can be brought under control, every effort must then be made, after appetite is regained, to reverse the depletion of body nutrients that accompanied these infections.

ADDITIONAL DISCUSSION

The maintenance, or restoration, of body nutrient stores must be regarded as one of the basic foundations for the management of HIV infections. Optimal HIV management demands that every patient be informed in full about the importance of maintaining

body weight, about the detailed steps that must be accomplished BY THE PATIENT to achieve this goal, and about the prognostic risks generated by falling body weights.

The huge daily pill burden and the timing of pill consumption required by HIV-infected patients has been recognized for its adverse consequences on food consumption, especially in infants and children. Consultation with dieticians to plan meal composition, timing, and/or the need for extra small meals can be of great importance in maintaining a full intake of nutrients.

Despite a lack of nutritional training for most practitioners, the nutritional side of HIV management cannot be shifted to dieticians, however knowledgeable they may be. The primary therapist must personally attend to nutritional issues in a very positive way, and at every follow-up visit. Hopefully, successful long-term reductions in viral load brought about by combined antiretroviral therapy will not lull patients or therapists into a reduced sense of importance about the value of prophylactic and therapeutic nutritional measures. Rather, although the years of asymptomatic illness may grow longer, body nutrition and losses of weight remain unchanged in their importance.

SUMMARY

The progression of HIV infections to AIDS is intimately linked to nutritional status. Optimal nutrition, involving protein energy, minerals, and essential micronutrients, serves to strengthen and protect the immune system as well as the many generalized (antigen nonspecific) aspects of host defense.

At all times during HIV infections, proper nutrition and aggressive nutritional support play an essential role, but one that is secondary to the primary use of antiviral and antimicrobial therapies given to minimize HIV replication and to eliminate secondary infections which typify the AIDS phase of illness. Combinations of three antiviral drugs, each aimed at a different phase of the HIV replicatory cycle, when given concurrently, can markedly reduce HIV burdens and the destruction of CD4+ T helper lymphocytes. Combined antiviral therapy markedly lengthens the asymptomatic phase of HIV infections and delays the onset of AIDS. Present success should be intensified further by improved antiviral drugs currently under development and testing. Antimicrobial therapies (or prophylaxis) for the secondary infections seen during AIDS are also of primary importance for helping to prevent or minimize the loss of body nutrients that accompany generalized febrile infections.

Infections caused by the HIV and secondary invaders stimulate production of pro-inflammatory cytokines such as IL-1 and TNF. These cytokines cause fever, various signs and symptoms of illness, and the catabolism of skeletal muscle protein and exaggerated losses of body nutrients. Losses of body nutrients, in turn, lead to the development of NAIDS and impaired body defenses. NAIDS and AIDS are intensely synergistic and lead to a rapid demise. However, aggressive nutritional support can reverse NAIDS and prolong survival.

Patients should be taught to participate fully in maintaining optimal body nutrition. A proper balance of nutrients is essential, but excess iron and zinc should be avoided. Supplements with vitamin A, the B-group vitamins, and antioxidants are recommended. Appetite stimulants and exercise regimens may help in regaining muscle mass after secondary infections have been treated. In advanced AIDS, total parenteral nutrition or gastrotomy tube feedings may become necessary.

REFERENCES

1. Goudsmit J. Malnutrition and concomitant herpesvirus infection as a possible cause of immunodeficiency syndrome in Haitian infants. N Engl J Med 1983; 309:54.

2. Lapointe N, Chad Z, Delage G, et al. To the editor. N Engl J Med 1983; 309:55.

3. Centers for Disease Control and Prevention. Revised classification system for HIV infection and expanded surveillance case definition for AIDS among adolescents and adults. Morb Mort Wkly Rep 1992; 41(RR-17):1–19.

4. Hommes MJT, Romi FA, Endert E, Sauerwein HP. Resting energy expenditure and substrate oxidation in human immunodeficiency virus (HIV)-infected asymptomatic men: HIV affects host metabolism in the early asymptomatic stage. Am J Clin Nutr 1991; 54:311–5.

5. Beach RS, Mantero-Atienza E, Shor-Posner G, et al. Specific nutrient abnormalities in asymptomatic HIV-infection. AIDS. 1992; 6:701–8.

6. Baum MK, Sher-Posner G, Lu Y, et al. Micronutrients and HIV-1 disease progression. AIDS 1995; 9:1051–6.

7. Beisel WR. Nutrition and immune function: overview. J Nutr 1996; 126(suppl 10):2611S–5S.

8. Watson RR, ed. Symposium: nutrition, immunomodulation and AIDS: an overview. J Nutr 1992; 122:715–57.

9. Raiten DJ, Talbot JM, eds. Nutrition in pediatric HIV infections: setting the research agenda. N Nutr 1996; 126(suppl 10):2597S–696S.

10. American Gastroenterological Association. AGA Technical Review: Malnutrition and cachexia, chronic diarrhea, and hepatobiliary disease in patients with human immunodeficiency virus infection. Gastroenterology 1996; 111:1724–52.

11. Dean M, Carrington M, Winkler C, et al. Genetic restriction of HIV-1 infection and progression of AIDS by a deletion allele of the CKR5 structural gene. Science 1996; 273:1856–61.

12. Stuttmann U, Ockenga J, Selberg O, et al. Incidence and prognostic value of nutrition and wasting in human immunodeficiency virus-infected patients. J Acquir Immun Defic Syndr Hum Retrovirol 1995; 8:239–46.

13. Rossol S, Voth R, Lauberstein HP, et al. Interferon production in patients infected with HIV-1. J Infect Dis 1989; 159:813–23.

14. Gordin FM, Hartigan PM, Kilmas NG, et al. Delayed-type hypersensitivity skin tests are an independent predictor of human immunodeficiency virus disease progression. J Infect Dis 1994; 169:893–7.

15. Laurent-Crawford AG, Krust B, Muller S, et al. The cytopathic effects of HIV is associated with apoptosis. Virology 1991; 185:829–39.

16. Beisel WR. Nutrition and infection. In: Linder MC, ed, Nutritional Biochemistry and Metabolism. 2nd ed, pp. 507–42. Elsevier, New York, 1995.

17. Esser R, Glienke W, von Briesen H, et al. Differential regulation of proinflammatory and hematopoietic cytokines in human macrophages alter infection with human immunodeficiency virus. Blood 1996; 88:3474–81.

18. Dondrop AM, Veenestra J, van der Poll T, Mulder JW, Reiss P. Activation of the cytokine network in a patient with AIDS and the recalcitrant erythematous desquamating disorder. Clin Infect Dis 1994; 18:942–5.

19. Constans J, Pellegin JI, Peuchant E, et al. Plasma interferon α and the wasting syndrome in patients infected with the human immunodeficiency virus. Clin Infect Dis 1995; 20:1069–70.

20. Rimaniol AC, Zylberberg H, Zavala F, Viard JP. Inflammatory cytokines and inhibitors of HIV infection: correlation between interleukin-1 receptor antagonist and weight loss. AIDS 1996; 10:1349–56.

21. Cunningham-Rundles S, Kim SH, Dnistrian A, et al. Micronutrients and cytokine interaction in congenital pediatric HIV infection. J Nutr 1996; 126(suppl 10):2674S–9S.

22. Kelly P, Summerbell C, Ngwenya B, et al. Systemic immune activation as a potential determinant of wasting in Zambians with HIV-related diarrhea. Quart J Med 1966; 89:831–7.

23. Lambi BB, Federman M, Pleskow D, Wanke CA. Malabsorption and wasting in AIDS patients with microsporidia and pathogen-negative diarrhea. AIDS 1996; 10:739–44.

24. Oleske JM, Rothpletz-Puglia PM, Winter H. Historical perspectives on the evolution in understanding the importance of nutritional care in pediatric HIV infection. J Nutr 1996; 126(suppl 10):2616S–9S.

25. Farthing CF, Brown SE, Staughton RCD. Color Atlas of AIDS and HIV Disease. 2nd ed. Yearbook Med, Publ, Chicago, 1988.

26. Sippy BD, Hofman FM, Wallach D, Hinton DR. Increased espression of tumor necrosis factor alpha receptors in the brains of patients with AIDS. J Acquir Immun Defic Syndr Hum Retrovirol 1995; 15:511–21.

27. Pulliam L, Gascon R, Stubbiebine M, McGuire D, McGrath MS. Unique monocyte subset in patients with AIDS dementia. Lancet 1997; 349:692–5.

28. Kong LY, Wilson BC, McMillian MK, et al. The effects of the HIV-1 envelope protein gp120 on the production of nitric oxide and pro-inflammatory cytokines in mixed glial cell cultures. Cell Immunol 1996; 172:77–83.

29. Yoshioka M, Bradley WG, Shapshak P, et al. Role of immune activation and cytokine expression in HIV-1-associated neurological diseases. Adv Neuroimmunol 1995; 5:335–8.

30. Kwan DJ, Iowe FC. Genitourinary manifestations of the acquired immunodeficiency syndrome. Urology 1995; 45:13–27.

31. The Johns Hopkins University AIDS Service. Update on HIV management: recommendations. Hopkins HIV Rep 1997; 9(suppl):1–12.

32. Weinroth SE, Parenti DM, Simon GL. Wasting syndrome in AIDS: pathophysiologic mechanisms and therapeutic approaches. Infect Agents Dis 1995; 4:76–94.

33. Gherardi R, Chariot P, Authier PJ. Muscular involvement in HIV infection. Rev Neurol Paris 1995; 151:603–7.

34. Ott M, Fischer H, Polat H, et al. Bioelectrical impedance analysis as a predictor of survival in patients with the human immunodeficiency virus infection. J Acquir Immun Defic Synd Hum Retrovirol 1995; 9:20–5.

35. Biglino A, Limone P, Forno B, et al. Altered adrenocorticotropin and cortisol response to corticotropin-releasing hormone in HIV-1 infection. Eur J Endocrinol 1995; 133:173–9.

36. Piedrola G, Casado JL, Lopez E, et al. Clinical features of adrenal insufficiency in patients with acquired immunodeficiency syndrome. Clin Endocrinol (Oxford) 1966; 45:97–101.

37. Miller TI, Evans SJ, Orav EJ, et al. Growth and body composition in children with the human immunodeficiency virus-1. Am J Clin Nutr 1993; 57:588–92.

38. Brouwers P, Decarli C, Heyes MP, et al. Neurobehavioral manifestations of symptomatic HIV-1 disease in children: can nutritional factors play a role? J Nutr 1966; 126(suppl 10):2651S–62S.

39. Yolken RH, Li S, Perman J, Viscidi R. Persistent diarrhea and fecal shedding of retroviral nucleic acids in children infected with human immunodeficiency virus. J Infect Dis 1991; 164:61–6.

40. Ramos-Soriano AG, Saavedra JM, Wu TC, et al. Enteric pathogens associated with gastrointestinal dysfunction in children with HIV infection. Mol Cell Probes 1996; 10:67–73.

41. Winter H. Gastrointestinal tract function and malnutrition in HIV-infected children. J Nutr 1996; 126(suppl 10):2620S–2S.

42. Semba RD, Miotti PG, Chiphangwl JD, et al. Maternal vitamin A deficiency and mother-to-child transmission of HIV-1. Lancet 1994; 343:1593–7.

43. Decsi T, Zakun D, Zakun J, Sperl W, Koletzko B. Long-chain polyunsaturated fatty acids in children with severe protein-energy malnutrition with and without human immunodeficiency virus-1 infection. Am J Clin Nutr 1995; 62:1283–8.

44. Periquet BA, Jammes NM, Lambert WE, et al. Micronutrient levels in HIV-1-infected children. AIDS 1995; 9:887–93.

45. Henderson RA, Saavedra JM. Nutritional considerations and management of the child with human immunodeficiency virus infection. Nutr 1995; 11:121–8.

46. Miller TL, Awnetwant EL, Evans S, et al. Gastrostomy tube supplementation in HIV-infected children. Pediatrics 1995; 96:696–702.

47. Kotler DP, Wang J, Pierson RN Jr. Body composition studies in

patients with the acquired immunodeficiency syndrome. Am J Clin Nutr 1985; 42:1255–65.

48. Macallan DC, McNurlan MA, Milne E, et al. Whole-body turnover from leucine kinetics and the response to nutrition in human immunodeficiency virus infection. Am J Clin Nutr 1995; 61:818–26.

49. Grunfeld C, Feingold KR. The role of the cytokines, interferon alpha and tumor necrosis factor in the hypertriglyceridemia and wasting of AIDS. J Nutr 1992; 122:749–53.

50. Semba RD, Caiaffa WT, Graham NH, Cohn S, Vlahov D. Vitamin A deficiency as predictors of mortality in human immunodeficiency virus-infected injection drug users. J Infect Dis 1995; 171:1196–202.

51. Coutsoudis A, Bobat RA, Coovadia HM, et al. The effects of vitamin A supplementation on the morbidity of children born to HIV-infected women. Am J Public Health 1995; 85:1076–81.

52. Coodley GO, Coodley MK, Nelson HD, Loveless MO. Micronutrient concentrations in the HIV wasting syndrome. AIDS 1993; 7:1595–600.

53. Coodly GO, Coodly MK. Serum carotenoids, vitamin A and vitamin E in HIV infected patients. J Nutr Immunol 1996; 4:25–37.

54. Favier A, Sappey C, Leclerc P, Faure P, Micoud M. Antioxidant status and lipid peroxidation in patients infected with HIV. Chem Biol Interact 1994; 91:165–80.

55. Tang AM, Graham NMH, Chandra RK, Saah AJ. Low serum B-12 concentrations are associated with faster human immunodeficiency virus type 1 (HIV-1) disease progression. J Nutr 1997; 127:345–51.

56. Boelaert JR, Weinberg CA, Weinbeerg ED. Altered iron metabolism in HIV infection: mechanisms, consequences, and proposals for management. Infect Agents Dis 1996; 5:36–46.

57. Castaldo A, Tarallo L, Palomba E, et al. Iron deficiency and intestinal malabsorption in HIV disease. J Pediat Gastroenterol Nutr 1996; 22:359–63.

58. Allavena C, Dousset B, May T, et al. Relationship of trace element, immunological markers, and HIV1 infection progression. Biol Trace Element Res 1995; 47:133–8.

59. Mocchegiani E, Veccia S, Ancarani F, Scalise G, Fabris N. Benefit of oral zinc supplementation as an adjunct to zidovudine (AZT) therapy against opportunistic infection in AIDS. Int J Immunopharm 1995; 17:719–27.

60. Graham NM, Sorensen D, Odaka N, et al. Relationship of serum copper and zinc levels to HIV-1 seropositivity and progression to AIDS. J Acquir Immun Defic Syndrome 1991; 4:976–80.

61. Cirelli A, Ciardi M, de Simone C, et al. Serum selenium concentration and disease progression in patients with HIV infection. Clin Biochem 1991; 24:211–4.

62. Tang AM, Graham NMH, Kirby AJ, et al. Dietary micronutrient intake and the risk of progression to acquired immunodeficiency virus type 1 (HIV)-infected homosexual men. Am J Epidemiol 1993; 138:937–51.

63. Tang AM, Graham NMH, Saah AJ. Effects of micronutrient intake on survival in human immunodeficiency virus type 1 infection. Am J Epidemiol 1996; 143:1244–56.

64. Jacobus DP. Randomization to iron supplementation of patients with advanced human immunodeficiency virus disease—An inadvertent but controlled study with results important for patient care. J Infect Dis 1996; 153:1044–5.

33 Aging

Nutrition and Immunity

SIMIN NIKBIN MEYDANI AND MICHELLE SCHELSKE SANTOS

STATEMENT OF THE PROBLEM

According to the final 1994 data released by the National Center for Health Statistics, life expectancy at birth in the United States for all races and both sexes is 76 yr *(1)*. Future projections indicate that increases in the population sector of individuals age 65 yr and over will continue into the second millennium. Age-associated changes in physiological, psychological, social, and economic factors may adversely affect the nutritional and immunological status of older individuals; these changes are often reflected in poor health and reduced quality of life. Incidence of infections and diseases such as cancer, atherosclerosis, and autoimmunity have been shown to increase with age.

Correction of nutritional deficiencies can restore compromised immune function and aid in the maintenance of health during aging. In addition, supplementation of some micronutrients may boost the immune responses of healthy elderly and aid in the establishment of optimal health and extension of a youthful, more vigorous lifestyle.

INTRODUCTION

Humans age at different rates, which are influenced by a wide range of factors *(2)*. Interactions of a multifactorial nature contribute to the aging process and include such variables as lifestyle, nutrition, physical activity, family and social support, education, genetic predisposition, monetary resources, mental ability, and culture. Because of the heterogeneity of variables among individuals, chronological age is not necessarily equal to biological age *(2)*. For example, one 75-yr-old individual may enjoy roller-skating with her great-grandchildren, whereas another 75-yr-old individual may be in the intensive care ward of a hospital after major cardiac surgery waiting for her great-grandchildren to visit her. These two women are of the same chronological age, yet they differ greatly in their biological age, with the roller-skating grandmother being effectively younger in her ability to maintain the physical vigor and quality of life she possessed decades earlier. Evidence is accumulating that emphasizes the importance of maintaining good nutritional and immunological status for the preserva-

tion and maximization of a youthful biological status during chronological aging.

Recognizing that different types or categories of aging exist, how, then, can "aging" be defined? Two major categories of the theories of aging have been proposed *(3,4)*. The first describes aging as a genetically programmed series of events that occur as the years pass; the second category describes aging as a progressive accumulation of defective and/or disruptive molecules resulting in the dysregulation of cell processes and subsequent death *(3,4)*. It is this second theory of aging that can best describe the differences between chronological and biological aging, and to which interventions can best be applied for the preservation and maximization of good health.

Physiological changes associated with aging may produce outcomes that alter the nutritional and immune status of older individuals. Increases in illness and chronic diseases result in physical weakness, dependence on others, decreased mobility, and isolation. These physical changes and impediments can, in turn, result in psychological repercussions such as lowered self-esteem and sense of worthlessness as well as depression, at least in part because of the loss of independence. Increased financial burdens because of lowered income in retirement years and concomitant increases in health care costs add to feelings of distress. Together, these age-associated changes in physiological, psychological, social, and economic conditions contribute to a reduction in the quality of the diet of many older individuals, which can have quantifiable repercussions on their immune and health status (Fig. 1).

On the other hand, immune dysregulation resulting from environmental factors or aging itself may be found at the root of the physical ailments that contribute to a reduction in the quality of diet among older individuals. Dysregulation of immune function may be a result of the reduction in beneficial immune responses, such as innate and acquired immunity, or increases in harmful immune responses such as the production of antibodies against one's own body (Fig. 1).

Incidence of infections *(5)* and diseases such as cancer, atherosclerosis, and autoimmunity *(6)* have been shown to increase with age, reflecting, in part, alterations in immune function seen in the aged. Oxidative stress is an important factor in both aging and the onset and progression of disease. Oxidative stress is postulated to be an important contributor to the age-associated decline in

From: *Nutrition and Immunology: Principles and Practice* (ME Gershwin et al. eds.), © Humana Press, Inc., Totowa, NJ

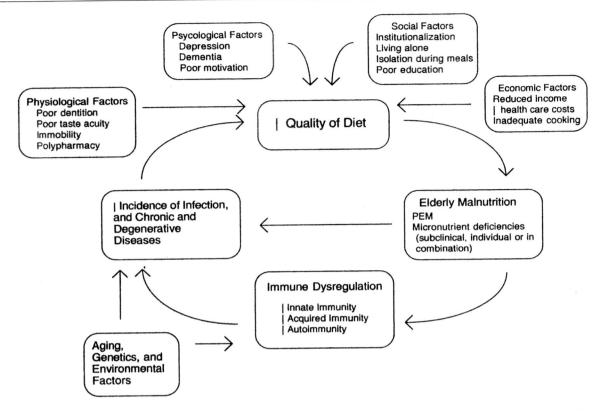

Fig. 1.   Relationship between factors associated with aging, nutrition, immune function, and health status in elderly individuals.

different immune responses and to the progression of various diseases such as cancer, atherosclerosis, autoimmunity, and amyloidosis (6,7).

The human body's ability to combat and clear foreign invaders or "non-self" antigens is an important part of health maintenance and contributes to decreased incidences of infection and illness. Healthy immune function has also been linked to greater lifespans. There are two main branches of immunity: innate or natural immunity and acquired immunity (8). Innate immunity involves immune surveillance and killing mechanisms, which do not require a previous encounter with foreign substance by immune cells. Examples of innate immunity include phagocytosis by neutrophils and macrophages (Mφ) and the tumoricidal and virucidal activities of natural killer (NK) cells. On the other hand, acquired immunity necessitates the encounter of an antigen for the priming of a specific immune response. Acquired immunity involves Mφ, T cells, and B cells and includes cell-mediated functions and humoral immunity or antibody production.

Dysregulation of immune function with aging has been well established (9,10) and contributes to higher incidence of as well as morbidity and mortality from cancer and infectious, autoimmune, and neoplastic diseases. A decrease in T-cell mediated function, including thymus involution and in vivo decreases in the delayed-type hypersensitivity (DTH) skin response, the graft-versus-host reaction, resistance to tumors, viruses, and parasites, T-cell-dependent primary and secondary antibody responses, and the proportion of T-cell subsets with naive cell-surface markers encompasses a large part of the overall decline (11). In addition, in vitro mitogen-stimulated lymphocyte proliferation, interleukin (IL)-2 production, and responsiveness to IL-2 have also been

shown to decline with age. It appears that decreases and dysfunctions in cell function occur largely as a result of the aging cell's decreased ability to receive and respond to cell signals (12–16). Some decline is also seen in humoral immune function, particularly in the loss of high-affinity cell-surface receptors for antigen and for cytokines. Proliferation of B cells is fairly well maintained; however, old animals show impaired response to antigens that stimulate CD5⁻ B cells (foreign antigens). On the other hand, the ability of CD5⁺ B cells to respond to autoantigens remains intact (17). Thus, whereas the ability to respond to foreign antigens declines with age, autoantibody formation increases with age, which may contribute to autoimmune disease (18–20). This "dysregulated" immune response is also observed in T cells in which production of Th_1 cytokines is decreased and the production of Th_2 cytokines is reported to be increased with age (21). Furthermore, increased production of suppressive factors such as prostaglandin (PG) E_2 by Mφ has been reported to contribute to the dysregulation of T-cell function (22,23). However, there is no clear consensus on age-related changes in NK activity. Reviews on research in NK activity (24,25) summarize reports of decreases, stasis, and increases in NK activity with aging. Differences in sample size, criteria used for the inclusion of "healthy elderly," and age range, as well as contamination by other cell types are possible contributing factors to these wide-ranging results (26).

CHANGES IN NUTRITIONAL STATUS WITH AGING

Specific nutrient requirements during the life cycle, including old age, are discussed in Part II of this book; therefore, in this section, only the age-related changes in the intake, absorption, and metabolism of nutrients that have been shown to play a part in the regulation of immunity in older individuals are summarized.

Intake of antioxidant nutrients lower than the Recommended Dietary Allowance (RDA) has been reported for the elderly. For example, Garry et al. *(27)* reported that 50% of the elderly (mean age 60 yr) have less than two-thirds of the RDA intakes of vitamin E, vitamin C, and zinc. Ryan et al. *(28)* conducted a national household survey of food consumption practices of individuals 65 yr of age and older and reported that more than 40% of men and women had intakes of vitamin E and zinc below two-thirds of the RDA. Panemangalore and Lee *(29)* recently showed that 37% of elderly (average age 73 yr) had tocopherol intake below the RDA.

The low intake and poor nutritional status of vitamin C among the elderly in Great Britain have been suggested as significant contributory factors to the high disease prevalence among individuals in this age group *(30,31)*. Burr et al. *(32)* studied the residents of a British village who were over 65 yr of age; the researchers found that women had higher plasma and leukocyte ascorbate contents than men and that subjects over 75 yr of age, regardless of sex, had significantly lower plasma and leukocyte vitamin C levels. These values were also found to decline with advancing age. The lower plasma and leukocyte levels appeared to be caused by a lower dietary intake of ascorbate, as there was a significant correlation between frequency of fruit of green vegetable consumption and plasma and leukocyte ascorbate concentration.

In contrast to many antioxidant nutrients, there is no RDA established for β-carotene. Therefore, it is difficult to evaluate changes in dietary intake of β-carotene with age. In addition, there is a limited amount of data available on elderly β-carotene levels in plasma and blood cells *(33–36)*. These limited studies indicate no age-related differences in β-carotene levels, nor do they indicate age-related differences in response to β-carotene supplementation.

Dietary intake of vitamin B$_6$ among the elderly has been shown to fall well below established RDAs, including free-living healthy individuals as well as the institutionalized elderly *(37)*. In addition, plasma levels of pyridoxal phosphate (PLP) diminish with aging, and some age-related differences in vitamin B$_6$ metabolism, including tryptophan loading, urinary excretion of pyridoxic acid, and enzyme activation may also contribute to age-associated changes in vitamin B$_6$ status *(37)*. Because a large quantity of corporal PLP is found in muscle and is involved in glycogen phosphorylase activity and because decreases in this enzyme and in overall muscle mass are associated with aging, these factors likely play an additional role in the age-associated reduction in vitamin B$_6$ levels *(38)*.

Marginal and clinical zinc deficiencies occur at a high frequency among the elderly population; this may be partially the result of the fact that intake of dietary zinc in the elderly is affected by social and economic factors, including total calorie intake, food selection, and amount of money spent on food (the main sources of zinc—meats, fish, and poultry—are expensive menu items) *(39)*. Marginal and clinical zinc deficiencies may also occur in the elderly, particularly when they are challenged with illness and infection and/or are hospitalized *(40)*. Clinical symptoms of zinc deficiency include impairment of a wide variety of cell-mediated immune responses, particularly T-cell-dependent and NK-cell-mediated functions *(41)*, in addition to impaired taste acuity and wound healing.

The varied soil content of selenium is a major contributing factor in its availability in the food supply at different geographical locations; this makes it difficult to establish usual intakes. Limited information is available on selenium intake among the elderly, but it has been postulated that reductions in selenium intake may contribute to reduced levels of plasma selenium seen in the elderly *(42)*. Dietary selenium from grain products is usually reduced in conjunction with a reduced intake of total kilocalories, which is often observed among the elderly. Reduced selenium intake among the elderly may be a result of the consumption of fewer good sources of selenium: reduced intake of grain products, coupled with reduced intake of seafood because of economic constraints *(43)*.

EFFECTS OF NUTRIENTS ON IMMUNITY WITH AGING

The last two and a half decades of immunogerontological investigation have focused more and more on nutrition as an important component in the process of aging. Consequently, micronutrient and macronutrient supplementation in frail and healthy elderly has been considered in order to develop optimal immune function for the promotion of health during chronological aging *(44–46)*.

It is important to establish that "immune function" and "immune response" are not all-inclusive terms; nor does an increase in a specific parameter always mean that the clinical outcome will be positive. For these reasons, the literature must be carefully interpreted both by the investigators as well as by the readers of the publications. There are many branches of immunity that require different tools for assessment of function. To date, there is not a single micronutrient that has been able to enhance all parameters of immune function tested. It is more common to see a single micronutrient affect a specific branch or area of immunity, which, in the case of the aged "dysregulated" immune response, could be advantageous.

Some of the effects of macronutrient and micronutrient supplementation in the elderly result in the restoration of immune response after correction of subclinical or marginal nutrient deficiencies, whereas some immunostimulatory effects are observed in healthy elderly in the absence of deficiencies, at least as determined by the classic definition of "deficiency." This immunostimulatory effect restores a phenotypically young, more vigorous immune response.

MACRONUTRIENTS

Protein and Calories Many elderly are at high risk of malnutrition because of their limited income, limited food preferences, and overall health status resulting from chronic disease. Linn and Jensen *(47)* studied the prevalence of malnutrition in young (<65 yr) and old (>65 yr) outpatients of an ambulatory care unit, excluding those with infection, autoimmune diseases, and major medical diseases. Malnutrition was more prevalent in the older than in the younger group. Malnourished subjects in both age groups had less lymphocyte response to allogenic cells and to phytohemagglutinin (PHA) but greater response to pokeweed mitogen (PWM) and higher IgA levels. Polymorphonuclear cells (PMN) from malnourished elderly patients had lower stimulated chemotaxis than those from well-nourished individuals, as assessed by migration of neutrophils through a Boyden chamber with or without zymosan-activated serum.

Chandra and Puri *(48)* showed that nutritional supplementation of 30 malnourished elderly men aged 70–84 yr improved their antibody response to influenza vaccine. Hamm et al. *(49)* examined the effect of protein levels (6% vs 25%) in the diet on Fc and C3b receptor-mediated phagocytosis of elicited peritoneal Mφ of young (6 mo) and old (24 mo) C57BL/6NIA mice. They found that Fc receptor-mediated phagocytosis was depressed after 5 wk of feeding a 6% protein diet in 24-mo-old mice but not in 6-mo-old animals. Furthermore, old mice fed the 25% protein diet had augmented C3b receptor-mediated phagocytosis. These effects were not explained by changes in membrane fluidity.

The respiratory burst activity of neutrophils, as well as the level of the various neutrophil enzymes secreted during degranulation, from elderly individuals is decreased in response to a wide variety of stimuli (50–52). These changes in function were not sufficient to cause a measurable decrease in the ability of neutrophils from the elderly subjects to phagocytize or kill bacteria. Nonetheless, infections are more common among the elderly, especially when they are malnourished (53). Lipschitz and Udupa (54) examined the combined effect of aging and protein deficiency on neutrophil function in mice. Six-mo-old or 24- to 26-mo-old C57BL/6NIA mice were fed isocaloric diets containing 2% or 20% casein for 3 wk, respectively. The old mice fed the 20% protein diet had significantly less phorbal myrestate acetate (PMA)-induced superoxide generation than young mice fed the same diet. Neutrophils from both young and old mice fed the 2% protein diet produced less superoxide than those from mice fed the 20% protein diet. Neutrophils from old mice also had significantly lower baseline and PMA-stimulated lysozyme, myeloperoxidase, and glucoronidase levels than those from young mice. Lower levels of these enzymes were detected in the mice fed the 2% protein diet compared with those fed the 20% protein diet. There was no difference in phagocytic or bactericidal activity between young and old mice fed the 20% protein diet. However, neutrophils from young mice fed the 2% protein diet killed a higher percentage of the ingested bacteria than those from old mice fed the same diet. Thus, although neutrophil activity is compromised by aging, in the absence of additional environmental stress such as protein deficiency, these changes do not necessarily affect their functional capacity. These studies emphasize the importance of protein-calorie malnutrition on changes in host-defense mechanisms in the elderly.

Lesourd (55) studied the effect of protein-calorie undernutrition in three populations as defined by the SENIEUR Protocol (56): healthy young adults (20–50 yr), healthy elderly subjects (78.7±7 yr), and healthy elderly subjects (79.4±7.5 yr) with low nutritional status as defined by a serum albumin level between 30 and 35 g/L. Several indices of immune response were evaluated; the authors noted that whereas certain indices of immune response (percent CD3+ cells, mitogenic response, IL-2 production, and antibody response to influenza vaccine) were lower in both elderly groups compared to the younger group, other indices (e.g., percent CD4+ cells and DTH response) were lower only in the undernourished elderly group compared with the young group. Furthermore, in almost all indices examined, the age-related difference was more pronounced in the undernourished group. Lesourd (55) also demonstrated that the magnitude of the decrease in nutritional status, as determined by serum albumin levels, was important in determining the immune response in the elderly (i.e., the lower serum albumin levels the lower the immune response). It is important to note that in these studies, the low albumin level was not the result of the presence of disease; rather, it reflected low nutritional status. These studies clearly demonstrate that undernutrition contributes to the decline of immune responsiveness with aging. This is further supported by the observation that the immune response in undernourished elderly supplemented with 500 kcal/d of ready-to-use complete nutritional supplement was significantly higher than in the nonsupplemented undernourished elderly (55). From these studies, however, it is not clear how much of the effect is the result of protein-calorie undernutrition and how much is the result of micronutrient deficiencies present under these conditions.

Lipids Changes in the fatty acid composition of the diet are known to modulate membrane phospholipid fatty acid composition (57,58), resulting in alteration in the oxygenated products of arachidonic acid (AA) (59–63). Eicosanoids originated from AA are the most abundant as well as, in most cases, the most active mediators. The n-3 polyunsaturated fatty acids (PUFAs) can interfere with arachidonic acid (AA) metabolism at the cyclooxygenase and lipoxygenase levels. Increased intake of n-3 PUFAs decreases the generation of eicosanoids from AA (60,63) and promotes the generation of the 3-series PG (59,61,62) and 5-series leukotrienes (LT) (64–66).

The AA metabolites, including PG, LT, and hydroxyeicosatetraenoic acid (HETE), can be produced by immune cells in response to different stimuli. In general, cellular and humoral immune responses are negatively regulated by cyclooxygenase products. PGE_2 has been shown to inhibit lymphocyte proliferation (67,68), cytokine production (69), the generation of cytotoxic cells (70), and NK activity (71). Lipoxygenase products of AA (i.e., LT and HETE) also affect these immune functions (72,73). Because PGE_2 production has been shown to increase with age (23,74) and contributes to the decline in T-cell proliferation and IL-2 production (75), we investigated the effect of n-3 PUFA supplementation on inflammatory cytokine production and T-cell-mediated function of heathy young and elderly subjects (76).

Six healthy young (23–33 yr) and six healthy older (51–68 yr) women were recruited after they were screened for their disease history, health status, and drug use. Each subject's usual diet was supplemented with n-3 PUFAs contained in Pro-Mega capsules, providing 1.68 g eicosapentaenoic acid (EPA), 0.72 g docosahexaenoic acid (DHA), 0.6 g other fatty acids, and 6 IU vitamin E per day for 3 mo. Blood was collected at baseline and at the end of 1, 2, and 3 mo of supplementation with fish oil. Peripheral blood mononuclear cells (PBMC) were separated from blood and cultured in the presence or absence of mitogens for measurement of lymphocyte proliferation, cytokine, and PGE_2 production.

The results showed that n-3 PUFA supplementation for 3 mo significantly increased plasma levels of EPA and DHA in both young and older subjects; however, the increase in EPA and DHA was greater in older than in young subjects. AA was significantly decreased in older subjects, whereas it did not change in young subjects, resulting in a lower ratio of AA/EPA in older than in young subjects. There was no significant age-associated difference in the production of inflammatory cytokines. n-3 PUFA supplementation decreased the production of all the inflammatory cytokines tested in both young and older subjects, with a greater decrease observed in the older subjects. IL-1β synthesis was reduced 48% in young subjects and 90% in older subjects; TNF was reduced by 58% in young and 70% in older subjects; and IL-6 was reduced by 30% in young and 60% in older subjects.

Interleukin-2, a T-cell growth factor necessary for lymphocyte activation, was produced in a significantly lower amount in older subjects than in young subjects at baseline and after 1 mo of n-3

PUFA supplementation. Consumption of n-3 PUFA tended to reduce IL-2 production, but only the reduction in older subjects reached significance. Proliferation response of PBMC to T-cell mitogens was significantly lower in older subjects at all time points compared to that in young subjects. n-3 PUFA supplementation inhibited lymphocyte to proliferation significantly in old subjects (36% reduction after 3 mo) but not in young subjects. PGE_2, a suppressive factor of T-cell function, was found decreased by 57% in older subjects and by 40% in young subjects after 3 mo of n-3 PUFA supplementation. However, the decrease seen in young subjects did not reach statistical significance. Similar results were observed by Endres et al. (77,78), who demonstrated that n-3 PUFA supplementation (4.69 g/d) in healthy men for 6 wk reduced IL-1β, TNF, and IL-2 production, as well as lymphocyte proliferation.

It is interesting to note the age-associated difference in the suppressive effect of n-3 PUFA on these parameters. Although the mechanism of this age difference was not determined, the more dramatic changes in older subjects were associated with a larger increase in plasma EPA and DHA and a greater decrease in AA in older subjects compared to young subjects. This difference in the magnitude of n-3 PUFA-induced changes in plasma fatty acid might be a result of age-associated differences in fatty acid absorption (79).

Prostaglandin E_2 has been shown to suppress IL-1 and IL-2 production and lymphocyte proliferation (80,81). We showed that a decrease in PGE_2 production by tocopherol supplementation enhances IL-2 production and lymphocyte proliferation in old mice (82) and elderly human subjects (83). Contrary to the presumption that reduced production of PGE_2 should lead to enhanced IL-2 production and lymphocyte proliferation, n-3 PUFA supplementation resulted in suppressed T-cell-mediated function. Similarly, Meydani et al. (63) showed a decrease in both PGE_2 production and NK activity in mice fed a fish-oil-supplemented diet, although PGE_2 has been reported to inhibit NK activity (71,84). These results indicate that mechanisms other than those mediated through PGE_2 may exist and may play a dominant role in the n-3 PUFA-induced effect on immune function.

Excessive production of lipid peroxides, such as hydrogen peroxide (H_2O_2), has been shown to suppress lymphocyte proliferation (85). Meydani et al. (86) showed that n-3 PUFA supplementation increased plasma malonaldehyde levels, with older women exhibiting a greater increase than younger women. IL-2 is a key cytokine in cell-mediated immune response, and its production may be affected directly by PUFA independent of the changes in eicosanoid production as indicated by Santoli and Zurier (87). Furthermore, Hughes et al. showed, in both in vivo (88) and in vitro (89,90) studies, that n-3 PUFA supplementation can inhibit the antigen-presenting function of human blood monocytes by reducing the expression of related cell-surface molecules, such as major histocompatibility complex (MHC) class II, intercellular adhesion molecule-1 (ICAM-1), leukocyte function associated antigen (LAF)-1, and LAF-3. A recent study (91) showed that feeding mice a low-fat diet enriched in n-3 PUFA (EPA and DHA) for a short term (10 d) suppressed concanavalin (Con) A-induced lymphocyte proliferation and IL-2 production, which was accompanied by a reduction in the production of lipid second messengers, diacylglycerol (DAG), and ceramide. DAG and ceramide play an important role in murine T-cell proliferation (92). In vitro supplementation with EPA and DHA was also shown to inhibit phospholipase C

activity in mouse splenocytes (93) and in rat peritoneal Mφ (94). These results indicate that the n-3 PUFA-induced effects on T cells might be mediated through a change in signal transduction.

In order to determine if the suppressive effects observed were specific to n-3 PUFAs or not, we investigated the effect of long-term feeding on the National Cholesterol Education Panel (NCEP) Step-2 diet high in n-3 PUFAs or in plant-derived n-6 and n-3 PUFA on the immune response of healthy adults (95). Twenty-two healthy volunteers over the age of 40 were divided into two groups and fed NCEP Step-2 diets enriched with either 1.23 g/d EPA and DHA (high fish) or 0.27 g/d EPA and DHA (low fish); the remaining n-3 PUFAs in the two diets was provided as plant-derived linolenic acid, 18:3n-3. After 6 mo of supplementation, the high-fish group had a small but significant decrease in the percentage of helper T cells, whereas the percentage of suppressor T cells was increased. This change was accompanied by a significant reduction in DTH response and proliferative response of PBMC to T-cell mitogen Con A. A significant correlation between changes in DTH and plasma EPA levels was observed. As reported in previous studies, IL-1β, TNF-α, and IL-6 produced by PBMC from subjects fed the high-fish diet were significantly reduced. In addition, an insignificant decrease in IL-2 and granulocyte Mφ growth factor (GM-CSF) was observed in this group. In contrast, the low-fish group showed increased PBMC proliferative response to Con A as well as production of IL-1β and TNF-α, but no significant effect on DTH, IL-6, GM-CSF, or PGE_2 production. These results indicated that the suppressive effect of n-3 PUFAs is not observed with plant-derived n-6 and n-3 PUFA. When expressed as a ratio to PUFAs (per double bonds), plasma tocopherol was significantly decreased in the high-fish group but not in the low-fish group. Because a decrease in tocopherol level has been shown to suppress T-cell-mediated function, these results indicate that n-3 PUFA may in part exert their effect indirectly through a reduction in tocopherol level. Reduction in tocopherol status has also been observed following fish oil consumption in animals (96–99).

As discussed earlier, decreased PGE_2 production after n-3 PUFA consumption does not result in an enhanced immune response as expected; rather, n-3 PUFAs in most studies were shown to suppress immune response. Increased lipid peroxidation (86,99–102) and compromised vitamin E status (96–99) have been implicated as contributing factors to the immunological effects of marine-derived n-3 PUFAs. Further support for this was provided by animal studies in which the provision of adequate tocopherol prevented the suppressive effect of n-3 PUFAs on T-cell function (103,104).

This is consistent with the studies reported by Kramer et al. (105) in which supplementation of humans with 15 g/d of fish oil for 10 wk suppressed the mitogenic responsiveness of PBMC to Con A, and supplementation with 200 mg tocopherol for 8 wk reversed the depressed mitogenic response induced by feeding fish oil. They further showed a positive correlation between plasma α-tocopherol concentrations and responsiveness of PBMC to Con A. Further well-designed human studies are needed to determine the appropriate levels of n-3 PUFA and vitamin E supplementation to optimize the beneficial anti-inflammatory effect of n-3 PUFA and minimize their suppressive effect on T-cell function of the elderly.

MICRONUTRIENTS Several vitamins and minerals have been shown to play a regulatory role in the immune response.

Marginal and severe deficiencies of some of these nutrients are associated with impairment of T-cell-mediated function similar to those observed with aging. With decreases in immunity associated with aging and increases in malnutrition among the elderly established, the question was asked whether a multivitamin/mineral supplement could remedy the multifactorial etiology of immunosenescence. In a landmark study, Chandra analyzed the immunomodulating and clinical effects of a 1-yr supplementation of a multivitamin/mineral supplement that contained close to RDA levels of a variety of micronutrients; the only exceptions were vitamin E and β-carotene (as provitamin A), which were included at levels four times greater than the RDA *(106).*

This was a randomized, double-blind, placebo-controlled trial of 96 men and women over the age of 65-yr who had no known chronic or serious illnesses and/or were taking no known medications that might alter immunological or nutritional status. It is interesting to note that those characterized as healthy elderly had a variety of micronutrient deficiencies, defined as blood concentrations below the 95% confidence interval (CI). One year after supplementation had begun, significant reductions in deficiencies of vitamin A, β-carotene, vitamin B_6, vitamin C, iron, and zinc were seen among those taking the supplement; however, no differences in deficiencies were seen among those taking placebo. Significantly greater levels of total T cells (CD3+), as well as T-cell subsets (CD3+/CD25 [IL-2R], CD4+) and NK cells (but not B cells or T-cell subsets CD4+/CD45RA+ or CD8+) were observed in the supplemented group. Lymphocyte function was also improved in all three branches of peripheral immunity. Significant increases in lymphocyte proliferation in response to PHA, in production of IL-2, and IL-2 receptor release (cell-mediated immunity), NK activity (natural or innate immunity), and antibody response to influenza vaccination (humoral immunity) were all observed *(106).*

These indices of immune function also proved to be clinically relevant. Those receiving the micronutrient supplements were significantly less likely to suffer infection-related illnesses compared to those receiving placebo.

In 1994, a 1-yr, placebo-controlled, double-blind trial tested the effectiveness of a daily micronutrient formulation to augment the delayed-type hypersensitivity skin response to seven recall antigens in apparently healthy older individuals (59–85 yr; $n =$ 56) *(46).* No significant differences in DTH responses were seen among those older individuals receiving placebo, and they were more likely to have micronutrient deficiencies, measured as nine blood micronutrient values, than those who received the daily micronutrient supplement. Midpoint analysis after 6 mo supplementation revealed significant increases in circulating blood micronutrient ascorbate, β-carotene, folate, and vitamin B_6; however, significant increases in the DTH skin response were not identified until after the full year of supplementation. This enhancement in the skin response was reflected by significant increases in both the number of positive antigens and the total diameter of induration. After the year's supplementation, significant increases in circulating α-tocopherol levels were identical in addition to the increases in the above-mentioned micronutrients. Weak but significant correlations between increases in DTH response and increases in blood levels of ascorbate, β-carotene, folate, and α-tocopherol were also found.

The micronutrient content differed in the vitamin/mineral supplements utilized in the two studies discussed, with the formulation used by Bogden et al. *(46)* containing the additional micronutrients pantothenic acid, biotin manganese chromium, molybdenum, and phosphorus and the formulation used by Chandra *(106)* containing higher levels of β-carotene, vitamin E, selenium, and calcium than that of Bogden *(46).* Nonetheless, both 1-yr studies *(46,106)* point to amelioration of micronutrient deficiencies in apparently healthy older individuals as the potential mechanism of immunomodulation. Enhancement in immune indices and immune cell functions were identified in those receiving active supplements when compared to those receiving placebo. In the case of Chandra's study, this immunomodulation was translated into improvements in the clinical outcome of lower frequency of infection-related illnesses. In a subsequent study, Pike and Chandra *(107)* evaluated the effect of the same supplement on the immune response of another apparently healthy group of elderly subjects. Particular attention was given to initial health status through clinical and laboratory investigations. However, no significant improvement in functional assays of immune response as a result of supplementation was observed. Thus, multivitamin/mineral supplements using the approximate RDA level of nutrients might be more effective in improving immune response of less healthy elderly with a lower nutritional status.

The question, however, still remains as to the source of effectiveness of the micronutrient supplement: Could the immunoenhancement be attributed to specific individual nutrients, and which micronutrients are responsible for modulating different immune indices and functions? For example, Penn et al. *(108)* showed that short-term (28 d) supplementation with vitamins A, C, and E (800 IU, 100 mg, and 50 mg, respectively) significantly improved the number of T cells, T helper cells, the ratio of T helper to T suppressor cell, and the PHA-induced proliferation of lymphocytes in the elderly. Furthermore, as will be discussed, single-micronutrient supplementation has been shown to enhance the immune response in the aged. Studies analyzing the immunological effects of individual micronutrients will shed light on these questions.

Vitamin B_6   Animal studies reporting the detrimental effects of vitamin B_6 deficiency and restoration of immune responses with repletion have been summarized elsewhere *(38,109),* and although not focused on aspects of aging immunity, they provided useful information on which clinical trials to develop for testing the effects of vitamin B_6 supplementation on the elderly, who are known to have poor vitamin B_6 status *(see* Section 3).

Two studies have examined the effects of vitamin B_6 supplementation on elderly immune responsiveness, although study designs and purposes were distinct. The first study by Talbott et al. *(110)* was a 2-mo supplementation trial of 50 mg pyridoxine hydrochloride (PN) or placebo in 14 elderly women (and 1 man) who lived independently and ate their normal diets. Fourfold to eightfold increases in plasma PLP were seen in the supplemented group. Proliferation of both T lymphocytes (PHA stimulation, but not Con A) and B lymphocytes (PWM, SAC) was significantly enhanced after 2 mo of PN supplementation. Those subjects who began the study with the lowest levels of plasma PLP had the greatest lymphoproliferative responses to PN supplementation, suggesting that restoration of marginal vitamin B_6 deficiency produced more prominent immune responses than enhancement of immunity during a nondeficient state of vitamin B_6 nutriture. Preliminary analyses of total T cells and T-cell subsets by flow cytometry from a subset of subjects ($n = 5$) revealed significant increases in percentages of total T cells (CD3+) and T helper cells (CD4+) and a trend (not significant) for greater percentages of CD8+ T cells (110). The dose of pyridoxine used in this study was 25 times the RDA (adults +51 yr: 1.6 mg/d for women and 2.0 mg/d for men), and although no toxic side effects were reported in this study, sensory neuropathies have been documented after ingestion of gram quantities of vitamin B_6 for prolonged periods (111). Therefore, results of this study must be considered carefully and applied cautiously (38).

The second study, which examined the effects of vitamin B_6 supplementation on immune responsiveness in elderly men ($n = 8$), involved a depletion period (less than or equal to 20 d) followed by three-wk repletion phases (3.00, 15.00, 22.50, and 33.75 μg B_6/kg body wt), and a final 4 d of 50 mg B_6 supplementation (112). Vitamin B_6 deficiency resulted in significantly impaired T (Con A and PHA stimulated) and B (SAC stimulated) lymphocyte proliferation and IL-2 production (Fig. 2), which correlated with decreased levels of plasma PLP, in addition to reduced percentages of lymphocytes. Repletion of vitamin B_6 (to 1.9 mg/d in women and 2.88 mg/d in men) partially restored immune function to levels similar to those of baseline values; however, measures of immune function in over half of the subjects were not completely restored to baseline levels at the end of the repletion period (or final period). These results suggest that the levels of vitamin B_6 necessary to restore declines in the numbers of lymphocytes and depression in their proliferative and secretory (IL-2) functions in the elderly are greater than those dietary levels currently recommended (112).

Although not addressed directly in either of the studies presented, potential mechanisms through which vitamin B_6 may be operating to maintain sufficient numbers and immune responsiveness of lymphocytes may resolve around the importance of vitamin B_6 in the utilization of single carbon units from serine for the synthesis of DNA and RNA (113). Nucleic acid synthesis is vital for the replication of lymphocytes, both in maintenance of cell numbers and in the proliferative response to antigenic challenge. Decreases in numbers of lymphocytes, particularly CD4+ T helper cells, resulting from insufficient synthesis of nucleic acids, could explain decreased production of IL-2. Because IL-2 is an important T-cell growth factor, lowered levels of this cytokine could also have negative repercussions on the ability of lymphocytes to proliferate (112).

Vitamin C Kennes et al. (114) examined the effect of intramuscular injections of vitamin C (500 mg/d for 1 mo) on proliferative response of lymphocytes to PHA and Con A and DTH response to tuberculin in 20 elderly subjects over the age of 70. A significant increase in [³H]-thymidine incorporation stimulated by PHA and Con A was observed after 30 d of supplementation. Vitamin C-supplemented subjects also had an increase in the mean DTH induration diameter to tuberculin relative to placebo-treated subjects. As vitamin C status was not determined, it is not clear whether the observed improvement was caused by correction of a vitamin C deficiency state or by a direct immunostimulatory action of injected vitamin C. An immunostimulatory effect of vitamin C has been claimed in young people with presumably normal vitamin C levels (115).

Delafuente et al. (116) studied a group of elderly patients over

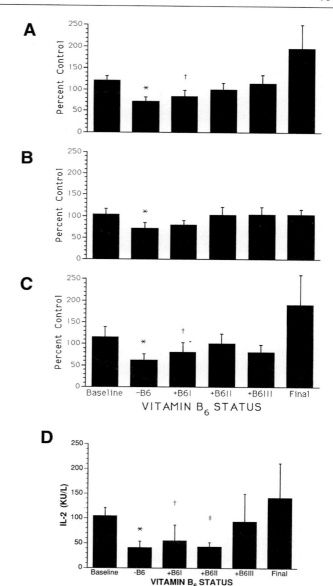

Fig. 2. Effect of vitamin B_6 status on mitogenic response and IL-2 production of PBMC from healthy elderly adults to optimal doses of Con A **(A)**, PHA **(B)**, and SAC **(C)**. IL-2 production **(D)** was measured in response to Con A. Data in (A), (B), and (C) are expressed as percent of response of control subjects tested in the same day as experimental subjects. Data represent mean ± SEM.*†‡ Significantly different from baseline at *$p < 0.01$,†‡$p < 0.05$. (Data reprinted from ref. 111 with permission.)

65 yr of age with chronic cardiovascular diseases receiving a variety of medication and examined the effect of in vitro and in vivo supplementation of vitamin C on lymphocyte proliferation and DTH to *Candida albicans* and mumps skin test antigen. They found that although in vitro addition of vitamin C to lymphocytes from elderly subjects increased their Con A-stimulated proliferation to levels comparable to those of young subjects, in vivo supplementation with 2 g/d vitamin C for 3 wk did not significantly affect mitogenic responses or reverse anergy. These in vivo results are in contrast to those of Kennes et al. (114) described earlier,

who employed healthy elderly subjects receiving 500 mg/d of vitamin C intramuscularly with no other medication and found improvement in the immunologic parameters measured following supplementation. Unfortunately, plasma or white blood cell vitamin C levels were not measured in these studies.

Ziemlanski et al. *(117)* found significantly increased IgG, IgM, and complement C3 levels in 158 women over 78 yr of age receiving 400 mg ascorbic acid supplements. Goodwin and Ceuppens *(118)* found that the healthy elderly subjects within the top 10% for plasma vitamin C concentrations had significantly fewer anergic subjects in response to four different antigens and higher mean DTH scores. However, no difference in mitogenic response to PHA was observed between those with high and low vitamin C status.

Several studies have indicated that a low vitamin C intake *(119)* or blood level *(120,121)* is associated with increased risk of death. However, in two randomized, controlled trials, vitamin C supplementation of elderly people with low blood ascorbate levels did not decrease the mortality rate *(121,122)*. The failure of supplementation trials to show any beneficial effect may be because irreversible damage had occurred as a result of a long-standing vitamin C deficiency, and supplementation should have started earlier in life. On the other hand, low vitamin C status may have occurred as a consequence of poor health, which ultimately caused death.

The mechanism of the immunostimulatory effect of vitamin C is not known. However, the serum level of lipid peroxides rises in healthy subjects with increasing age *(123,124)*, suggesting that the immunostimulatory effect of vitamin C might be mediated through its antioxidant function. The concentration of certain antioxidants such as vitamin C, selenium, and superoxide dismutase decreases with advancing age *(125)*. Supplementation of elderly women with vitamin C or vitamin E for 12 mo decreased serum peroxide levels by 13% and 26%, respectively *(126)*. On the other hand, vitamin C has been reported to increase in vivo generation of cyclic GMP *(127)*, a signal cell for cell commitment into the S phase *(128)*.

In summary, lower plasma and leukocyte levels of vitamin C and age-related increases in serum lipid peroxides have been reported in the elderly. Compromised vitamin C status appears to contribute to the decreased immune responsiveness observed in the elderly, although conflicting reports on the beneficial effects of high-dose supplementation with this vitamin makes an unequivocal recommendation impossible.

Vitamin E   Vitamin E is the most effective chain-breaking, lipid-soluble antioxidant in biologic membranes of all cells, but it is found in especially high concentrations in the membranes of immune cells because their high polyunsaturated fatty acid content puts them at especially high risk for oxidative damage *(129,130)*. Free-radical damage to immune cell membrane lipids may ultimately impair the ability of immune cells to respond normally to challenge. Several animal and human studies have shown that vitamin E deficiency is associated with an inadequate immune response, whereas higher than recommended amounts have, in some instances, improved immunity.

Vitamin E supplementation has been successfully used to improve some aspects of the age-related decline in laboratory animal immune function *(131)*. Meydani et al. *(82)* showed that increasing the level of dietary vitamin E from 30 to 500 ppm significantly increases plasma vitamin E levels, DTH, lymphocyte

Table 1
Effects of Vitamin E on Immune Response of 24-mo-Old Mice

Parameters	30 ppm[a]	500 ppm[a]
Serum α-tocopherol	71	194[b]
DTH skin test	36[b]	75
T-cell lymphocyte proliferation	5[b]	38
B-cell lymphocyte proliferation	24[b]	85
Interleukin-2	44[b]	85
Ex vivo splenic PGE$_2$ synthesis	123[b]	89

[a]All values expressed as a percentage of 3-mo-old control group (fed 30 ppm vitamin E).
[b]Significantly different from control and other experimental group, $p \leq 0.05$.

proliferation to Con A, and IL-2 production in old mice; this effect of vitamin E was associated with a decrease in PGE$_2$ production (Table 1). Vitamin E-supplemented animals from this study also had a lower incidence of kidney amyloidosis than control (30 ppm vitamin E) animals *(132)*. Another recent study confirmed these findings *(133)*. Sakai et al. *(133)* reported that vitamin E supplementation (585 mg/kg diet) for 12 mo significantly improved T-cell-mediated function compared with rats fed a control diet containing 50 mg vitamin E/kg. In another study, Meydani et al. *(76)* showed that although vitamin E supplementation did not have an effect on natural killer cell activity of unchallenged young or old mice, it was effective in preventing sheep red blood cell (SRBC)-induced suppression of NK activity in old mice.

Relatively few controlled clinical studies have been conducted to determine the effect of vitamin E on the immune response of elderly persons. Vitamin E supplementation has been shown to enhance immunity in elderly populations. Ziemlanski and co-workers *(117)* supplemented institutionalized healthy elderly women with 100 mg vitamin E twice daily and assessed serum proteins and immunoglobulin concentrations after 4 and 12 mo. Vitamin E increased total serum protein with the principal effect seen in the α2- and β2-globulin fractions occurring at 4 mo. No significant effects were noted in the levels of either immunoglobulins or complement C3 after 12 mo, although there was a significant increase in serum protein concentration. However, another group that was supplemented with vitamin C along with vitamin E displayed significant increases in IgG and complement C3 levels.

Harman and Miller *(134)* supplemented 103 elderly patients from a chronic care facility with 200 or 400 mg/d α-tocopherol acetate but did not see any beneficial effect on antibody development against influenza virus vaccine. Unfortunately, data on the subjects' health status, medication use, antibody levels, and other relevant parameters were not reported.

In a double-blind, placebo-controlled study, Meydani and co-workers *(135)* supplemented 34 healthy men and women (> 60 yr of age) with either a soybean oil placebo or 800 mg dl-α-tocopherol for 30 d. The study evaluated the subjects' DTH, mitogenic response, and IL-1, IL-2, and PGE$_2$ production. Vitamin E supplementation was associated with increases in plasma vitamin E, DTH score, mitogenic response to Con A, and IL-2 production (Fig. 3). Vitamin E supplementation was associated with decreases in PHA-stimulated PGE$_2$ production by PBMC as well as plasma lipid peroxide levels. IL-1 production and PHA-induced proliferation of PBMC were not affected by vitamin E supplementation.

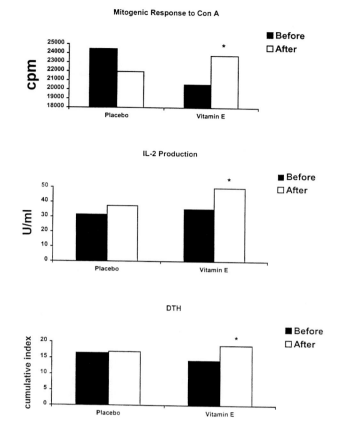

Fig. 3. Effect of vitamin E supplementation on mitogen response, IL-2 production, and DTH in elderly humans. Thirty-four elderly men and women were supplemented with either placebo or 800 IU α-tocopherol for 30 d. (Data reprinted from ref. *208* with permission.)

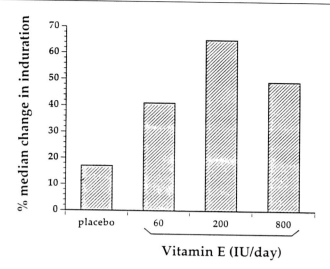

Fig. 4. Effect of vitamin E supplementation on DTH of healthy elderly. Subjects were supplemented with placebo, 60, 200, or 800 IU/d of vitamin E for 4.5 mo. DTH was assessed before and after supplementation using Multi-test CMI (Pasteur Mérieux Connaught, Lyon, France). Data represent the sum of induration of all positive responses. (Data reprinted from ref. *208* with permission.)

In a recent study, Meydani et al. *(136)* supplemented healthy elderly (>65 yr old) with placebo, 60 mg/d, 200 mg/d, or 800 mg/d of dl-α-tocopherol for 235 d using a double-blind, randomized design. All three vitamin E doses significantly enhanced DTH. Subjects consuming 200 mg/d vitamin E had the highest percent increase in DTH. The median percent change in DTH in the subjects supplemented with 200 mg/d vitamin E (65%) was significantly higher than that of the placebo group (17%) (Fig. 4). Although the median percent change in the groups supplemented with 60 and 800 mg/d vitamin E (41% and 49%, respectively) were similar to the 65% change observed in the 200 mg/d group, these changes did not reach statistical significance compared with those of the placebo group. There was no significant effect of supplementation with 60 mg/d in response to hepatitis B or tetanus and diphtheria vaccines. However, a significant increase in antibody response to hepatitis B was observed in subjects consuming 200 or 800 mg/d (Table 2). Those consuming 200 mg/d also had a significant increase in antibody response to tetanus toxoid vaccine. There was no effect of vitamin E supplementation on the level of two autoantibodies, anti-DNA and antithyroglobulin, or the ability of neutrophils to kill *C. albicans*. These data suggest that although supplementation with 60 mg/d vitamin E might enhance DTH, it is not adequate to cause a significant increase in antibody titer against hepatitis B or tetanus toxoid. Supplementation with 200 mg/d vitamin E, however, caused a significant

increase in DTH and antibody response, and the magnitude of response for both indices was higher than those observed in the two other vitamin E groups. Thus, it was concluded that 200 mg/d represents the optimal level of vitamin E for the immune response of the elderly. The observation that the optimal response was detected in the 200-mg/d group suggests that there may be a threshold level for the immunostimulatory effect of vitamin E. Interestingly, vitamin-E-supplemented subjects had a 30% lower incidence of self-reported infections, indicating that the immunostimulatory effect of vitamin E might have clinical significance for the elderly.

This is supported by studies conducted in laboratory animals. Hayek et al. *(137)* fed young and old mice either 30 or 500 ppm vitamin E for 8 wk, at which time they were infected with influenza virus. Old mice fed 30 ppm of vitamin E had higher viral titer than young mice fed 30 ppm vitamin E. Influenza lung viral titers were lower in old mice fed 500 ppm vitamin E compared with the age-matched mice fed 30 ppm vitamin E. The authors suggested that the effect of vitamin E may be the result, in part, of preservation of antioxidant status and NK cell activity because old mice fed 500 ppm vitamin E maintained a higher antioxidant index than age-matched controls, and the age-associated decline in NK activity was prevented by feeding old infected mice 500 ppm vitamin E. Furthermore, vitamin E supplementation at 500 ppm did not affect secondary splenic cytotoxic T-cell activity or primary pulmonary cytotoxic T lymphocytes (CTL) activity in this study. However, the mechanism for the effect of vitamin E on reducing influenza viral titer is still unclear. In a subsequent study, Han et al. *(138)* showed that the preventive effect of vitamin E was not observed following supplementation with other antioxidant compounds such as glutathione (GSH), melatonin, or strawberry extract. Furthermore, vitamin E prevented the weight loss associated with influenza infection; other dietary antioxidant treatments did not have an effect on weight loss.

No adverse effects because of short-term, high-dose vitamin

Table 2
Effect of Vitamin E (E) Supplementation on Antibody Titer to Hepatitis B in Elderly Subjects

Group	Geometric mean (IU/mL)					% with detectable Hep B Titer[b]
	Baseline	Post 1	Post 2	Post 3	P[a]	
Placebo (n = 16)	4.0	4.0	4.6	7.3	0.2	19
60 mg E (n = 18)	4.0	4.0	6.2	10.4	0.12	28
200 mg E (n = 18)	4.0	7.2	12.1	23.9	0.05	41
800 mg E (n = 18)	4.0	4.0	4.4	9.2	0.03	42

Note: A standard dose of hepatitis B was administered on d 156 of the study. Two additional hepatitis B booster doses were administered on d 186 and 216 of the study. Blood for serum antibody level measurement was collected before, 1 mo after vaccination, and 1 mo following the second and third hepatitis B booster administration. Sera with undetectable levels were assigned 4 units/mL for the purpose of calculating geometric means.
[a]Post 3 compared with baseline using Wilcoxon signed rank test followed by Bonferroni correction for multiple comparisons.
[b]Greater than or equal to 8 IU/mL as detected by RIA after third hepatitis B (Hep B) booster.
Source: ref. *136* with permission.

E supplementation were observed on the immune indices tested. Recently, the safety of 4 mo of supplementation with 60, 200, and 800 IU/d of dl-α-tocopherol on general health, nutrient status, liver enzyme function, thyroid hormones, creatinine levels, serum autoantibodies, killing of *Candida albicans* by neutrophils, and bleeding time in elderly subjects was assessed. Supplementation with vitamin E at these levels and for this period of time had no adverse effects on these parameters *(139)*.

In another study, Cannon et al. *(140)* supplemented young (22–29 yr) and old (55–74 yr) subjects with 400 IU dl-α-tocopherol twice daily for 48 d before undergoing eccentric exercise (downhill running). They reported that young subjects consuming placebo capsules had a significantly greater neutrophilia and plasma creatine kinase in response to eccentric exercise compared with old subjects consuming placebo. Vitamin E supplementation eliminated the age difference in neutrophilia and creatine kinase. In a subsequent report, Cannon et al. *(141)* demonstrated that although vitamin E supplementation did not affect production of IL-1 or TNF, it prevented the eccentric exercise-induced rise in IL-1. Vitamin E supplementation, however, inhibited the production of another cytokine, IL-6. Because IL-1 and IL-6 have been implicated in the inflammatory process and the acute-phase response and IL-1 has been found to be involved in exercise-induced muscle proteolysis and damage, their inhibition by vitamin E during damaging exercise could have practical implications. These studies indicated that in addition to its enhancement of cell-mediated immunity, vitamin E, by its modulation of cytokine production, can affect the catabolic consequences of the inflammatory process and acute-phase response.

Several epidemiologic studies have investigated the interaction between vitamin E supplementation and immune function of free-living elderly. Goodwin and Ceuppens *(118)* studied a population of healthy adults (65–94 yr old) consuming high doses of vitamin E and did not find any correlation between vitamin E intake and DTH, mitogen-stimulated lymphocyte proliferation, serum antibodies, or circulating immune complexes. In this study, subjects taking supplemental doses of vitamin E greater than five times the RDA had lower absolute circulating lymphocyte counts than the rest of the population. Unfortunately, the results from this study are confounded by the fact that the subjects were consuming high doses of several vitamin supplements in addition to vitamin E.

Chavance et al. *(142,143)* conducted a community-based sur-vey on the relationship between nutritional and immunological status in 100 healthy subjects over 60 yr of age. They reported that plasma vitamin E levels were positively correlated with positive DTH responses to diphtheria toxoid, *C. albicans,* and trichophyton. In men only, positive correlations were also observed between vitamin E levels and the number of positive DTH responses. Subjects with tocopherol levels greater than 135 mg/L were found to have higher helper-inducer/cytotoxic-suppressor ratios. Blood vitamin E concentrations were also negatively correlated with the number of infectious disease episodes in the preceding year.

Payette et al. *(144)* reported a negative correlation between dietary vitamin E and ex vivo IL-2 production in free-living elderly Canadians. This result is suspect, however, because 70% of the presumably "healthy" elderly in this study had undetectable IL-2 levels. Others have reported that although IL-2 production in healthy older adults is about one-half to two-thirds that of young subjects, it is still detectable *(83,145,146)*. The study is further complicated because dietary vitamin E intake rather than plasma vitamin E level was used as the indicator of a subject's tocopherol status. Nutrient databases for vitamin E are incomplete and do not necessarily represent the actual tocopherol status of a given individual.

The mechanism behind the immunostimulatory effect of vitamin E has eluded scientists to this day. However, there is compelling evidence suggesting that vitamin E exerts its immunoenhancing effect by reducing prostaglandin synthesis *(82,83)* and/or decreasing free-radical formation *(147)*.

Increased free-radical formation, whether the result of aging, environmental pollutants, or diet, damages the components of the immune system. Oxygen metabolites, especially H_2O_2, produced by activated Mφ depress lymphocyte proliferation *(148)*. Tocopherol has been shown to decrease H_2O_2 formation by neutrophils *(149)*. Additionally, the immunosuppressive effect of vitamin E deficiency appears to be the result of increased free-radical reactions that result in increased non-enzyme-catalyzed lipid peroxidation as well as enzyme-catalyzed lipid peroxidation (i.e., formation of PGE_2). Mφ from vitamin E-deficient rats showed a threefold increase in chemiluminescence and increase in membrane viscosity compared with those from control rats *(150)*.

Vitamin E supplementation may provide protection for the cells of the immune system against oxidative damage. Villa et al. *(151)* reported that vitamin E supplementation in vitro caused a concentration-dependent inhibition of arachidonic acid-induced aggregation of PMN and mononuclear leukocytes. They suggested that this may have been the result of interference with lipoxygenase activity. Topinka et al. *(152)* found that the addition of α-tocopherol (0.2 μmol/L) to human lymphocytes in vitro suppressed lipid peroxidation and oxidant damage to DNA when induced by the catalytic system of Fe^{2+}–sodium ascorbate. Sepe and Clark *(153)* studied neutrophil lysis in liposome target vesicles, demonstrating that stimulated neutrophils secrete myeloperoxidase and H_2O_2, which combine with extracellular lipids to form a membrane lytic system. In vitro addition of α-tocopherol to the liposomes increased their resistance to the myeloperoxidase–H_2O_2 system.

In addition to its reduction of nonenzymatic products of lipid peroxidation, vitamin E may also modulate immune responsiveness through its effect on the synthesis of arachidonic acid metabolites. At low concentrations, PGE_2 is believed to be necessary for certain aspects of cellular immunity; however, at higher concentrations, PGE_2 has a suppressive effect on several indices of cellular and humoral immunity, such as antibody formation, DTH, lymphocyte proliferation, and cytokine production. Vitamin E deficiency was shown to increase the production of eicosanoids, whereas vitamin E supplementation decreased their formation *(82)*. Beharka et al. *(75)* used an in vitro coculture system in which purified Mφ and T cells from young and old mice were cultured together to demonstrate that Mφ from old mice were inhibitory to T cells from young mice resulting, at least in part, from increased Mφ production of PGE_2. Vitamin E improved T-cell responsiveness in this system by reducing Mφ PGE_2 production, although a direct effect of vitamin E on T cells was also observed. Furthermore, Wu et al. *(154)* demonstrated that vitamin E supplementation of old mice decreased the age-associated increase in PGE_2 production and inducible cyclooxygenase (COX)-2 activity in Mφ from old mice *(74)*. Although it appears that vitamin E enhancement of the aged immune system is mostly mediated through a decrease in PGE_2 production, further studies are needed to determine the direct effect of vitamin E on T cells and its contribution to the immunostimulatory effect of vitamin E.

β-Carotene The human trials investigating the immunological effects of β-carotene supplementation in elderly individuals have been reviewed *(155)*. The first documented trial was a variable-dose β-carotene supplementation (0, 15, 30, 45, 60 mg/d) trial in a mixed-gender, older population (mean age = 56 yr) of a very limited sample size (four subjects per group) *(156)*. A significant increase in the percentage of T helper (CD4+) cells, NK cells (CD16+), and cells expressing IL-2R (CD25+) and TFR was reported for subjects taking 30, 45, and 60 mg/d β-carotene when compared to those receiving placebo. However, no significant changes in total T cells or T suppressor/cytotoxic (CD8+) cells were reported as a result of β-carotene supplementation. Because of the small per group sample size and the lack of measurements of immune cell function, it is difficult to evaluate the significance of the findings of this study.

Two distinct β-carotene trials of short and long duration were presented together in support of similar conclusions. The short-term effect of β-carotene (90 mg/d for 3 wk) on T-cell mediated immunity was assessed in a randomized, double-blind, placebo-controlled longitudinal comparison of healthy elderly women (60–80 yr; n = 23) *(157)*. The long-term effect of β-carotene (50 mg every other day for 10–12 yr) on T-cell-mediated immunity was assessed in a randomized, double-blind, placebo-controlled longi-

Table 3
Effect of β-Carotene Supplementation on the Lytic Activity of NK Cells

Treatment group	Lytic activity ($LU^{30}/10^6$ $PBMC^2$)[a]
Placebo	
Middle-aged (n = 17)	156.3 ± 37.7[b]
Elderly (n = 13)	39.8 ± 6.7
β-Carotene	
Middle-aged (n = 21)	102.1 ± 23.8
Elderly (n = 8)	63.5 ± 7.4[b]

[a]Lytic unit (LU) = the number of PBMC required to cause 30% target cell lysis.
[b]X ± Sem. Greater than elderly placebo group; $p < 0.05$, unpaired t-test on log-transformed data.
Source: ref. *158*, with permission.

tudinal comparison of men (51–86 yr; n = 59) enrolled in the Physicians' Health Study *(157)*. Subjects from both the short- and long-term studies who were taking β-carotene had significantly greater plasma β-carotene levels than subjects from respective studies taking placebo. The change in delayed-type hypersensitivity skin responses from baseline to follow-up between β-carotene and placebo groups were not significantly different in the short- or long-term study. There were no significant effects of β-carotene supplementation on in vitro lymphocyte proliferation and production of interleukin-2 or prostaglandin E_2 as a result of short- or long-term β-carotene supplementation. In addition, there were no differences in the profiles of lymphocyte subsets (total T cells, CD3+; T helper cells, CD4+; T cytotoxic/suppressor cells, CD8+; B cells, CD19+) as a result of short- or long-term β-carotene supplementation, nor were there differences in percentages of CD16+ NK cells or activated lymphocytes (cells expressing IL-2 receptor, or transferrin receptor) because of long-term β-carotene supplementation. Consistent results from these two distinct trials demonstrate that β-carotene supplementation does not have an enhancing or suppressive effect on the T-cell-mediated immunity of healthy elderly individuals.

The potential chemopreventive effect of β-carotene is of particular importance to the elderly, whose cancer incidence is greatest. In a recent study, the effects of long-term β-carotene supplementation on a healthy aging population were investigated, focusing on NK cell activity as a potential immunological link between β-carotene and cancer prevention *(158)*. Natural-killer-cell activity among 59 (38 middle-aged, 51–64 yr; 21 elderly, 65–86 yr) Boston area participants in the Physicians' Health Study, a randomized, double-blind, placebo-controlled trial of β-carotene (50 mg on alternate days) for prevention of cancer and cardiovascular disease, was evaluated after a 10- to 12-y β-carotene supplementation. No significant difference was seen in NK cell activity resulting from β-carotene supplementation in the middle-aged group. The elderly had significantly lower NK cell activity than the middle-aged. β-Carotene supplementation eliminated the age difference in NK cell activity. β-carotene-supplemented elderly had significantly greater NK cell activity when compared to the elderly receiving placebo (Table 3); this was not the result of an increase in the percentage of NK cell cells, in IL-2R expression, or in IL-2 production *(158)*.

In a subsequent study designed to further explore the mechanisms of β-carotene-induced enhancement of elderly NK cell activity *(159)*, Boston area participants in the Physicians' Health Study (men 65–88 yr, mean age 73 yr) who had supplemented with β-carotene (50 mg on alternate days) for an average of 12 y participated. It was confirmed that long-term β-carotene supplementation significantly enhances NK cell activity in elderly men in the absence of differences in percentages of NK cells (CD16⁺ CD56⁺). Production of cytokines interleukin-12, interferon-α, or interferon-γ, all of which possess NK-cell-enhancing properties, was not significantly different between β-carotene-supplemented elderly and elderly taking placebo. This enhancement in NK cell activity is not explained by upregulation of individual NK-cell-stimulatory cytokines interferon-α, Con A-stimulated interferon-γ, interleukin-12, or interleukin-2 *(158)*, nor by downregulation of NK-cell-suppressive factor prostaglandin E₂ *(158)*. Although the exact mechanisms have not been delineated, potential upregulation of tumor necrosis factor-α, or synergism between two cytokines that act to costimulate NK cells and subsequently upregulate NK cell activity might contribute to the higher NK cell activity of β-carotene-supplemented elderly men.

β-Carotene supplementation is not an effective immunomodulator for the T-cell-mediated branch of immunity in the elderly; however, long-term β-carotene supplementation may be beneficial for enhancing NK cell activity (innate immunity), potentially increasing viral and tumoral surveillance in older individuals and providing one possible link between β-carotene intake and prevention of certain cancers *(105)*.

Results from two large, randomized, placebo-controlled trials, whose subjects were primarily cigarette smokers, have raised questions concerning the safety of β-carotene supplementation. Because primary outcomes of these studies include incidences of cancer and cardiovascular disease, diseases that may involve T-cell-mediated and innate immunity, it is important to consider potential negative effects of β-carotene supplementation on immune responses. Both the Alpha-Tocopherol, Beta Carotene (ATBC) Cancer Prevention Trial *(160)* and the Beta Carotene and Retinol Efficacy Trial (CARET) *(161)* reported no benefits of supplementation with regard to cancer or cardiovascular disease, but, instead, reported higher rates of lung cancer and cardiovascular disease in subjects supplemented with β-carotene. On the other hand, results of the Physicians' Health Study (the cohort from which the immunological substudies described above were derived) have indicated no benefit nor any harm for an average of 12-yr β-carotene supplementation among male physicians followed for endpoints of malignant neoplasms, cardiovascular disease, and death *(162)*. These results held for nonsmokers, former smokers, and current smokers.

Zinc The effects of zinc supplementation on elderly immune function were thoroughly reviewed by Beisel in 1991 *(163)*. One of the first studies measuring the effects of zinc supplementation on elderly immune responses was carried out in healthy institutionalized elderly (*n* = 38; 70 yr and older) for 1 mo with a dose of 440 mg zinc sulfate/d (176 mg zinc/d) *(164)*. Significant increases among in vivo measures of immunity included increases in DTH cutaneous response to several recall antigens and in the IgG antibody response to tetanus vaccination. The numbers of T cells were also elevated with zinc supplementation. However, in vitro measurements of T- and B-lymphocyte proliferation and the numbers of total circulating lymphocytes did not change. The investigators concluded that the large quantity of zinc was acting pharmacologically (versus physiologically) to produce some beneficial

immunostimulatory effects *(164)*. Because zinc status was not monitored in the plasma or blood cells, it was difficult to interpret whether the increase in immune response was the result of the correction of a latent zinc deficiency or a clear immunostimulatory effect *(165)*.

A 3-mo, double-blind, randomized, placebo-controlled trial of zinc (25 mg zinc sulfate/d) and/or vitamin A (800 μg retinal palmitate/d) supplementation in 118 elderly people (mean age 80 yr) from a home for older people was recently reported *(166)*. Dietary analysis showed that approximately 80% of the subjects had zinc intakes below 7 mg (RDA = 15 mg for men and 12 mg for women). The zinc-supplemented group showed a slight significant improvement in the lymphocyte proliferative response to T-cell mitogen Con A (not PHA) when compared to baseline values, and they showed trends for greater T helper and cytotoxic T cells. When the data were reanalyzed to compare those who received zinc (alone or in combination with vitamin A) to those who did not receive zinc (placebo or vitamin A), significantly greater numbers of CD4+/DR+ T cells, and CD3+/CD16+/CD56+ cytotoxic T cells were seen in those supplemented with zinc. In contrast, significantly lower numbers of CD3+ and CD4+ T cells were seen among those elderly supplemented with vitamin A compared to those who received no vitamin A. Results from this reanalysis were confirmed to be statistically robust after multiple adjustments for baseline immune status and prognostic factors (body mass index, depression, chronic disease, smoking, and acute respiratory diseases) and after comparison of regression coefficients. No significant immunological effects were reported for the zinc/vitamin A combination *(166)*.

When zinc-deficient elderly (65–78 yr) were deliberately selected for a 4.5-mo study, supplementation with 60 mg zinc/d in the form of zinc acetate resulted in a significant improvement in the number of positive antigens in the DTH response *(167)*. Significantly greater levels of zinc in plasma and lymphocytes were also documented *(167)*.

In vitro addition of zinc was found in one study to correct impaired NK cell activity in the elderly *(168)*.

In contrast to studies showing some immunomodulatory effects by zinc supplementation in the elderly, other studies showed no effects. Elderly subjects (mean age = 74 yr) supplemented for 1 mo with zinc (50 mg ionic zinc/d) in the elderly showed no significant difference in antibody response to influenza vaccine when compared to placebo *(169)*. Other investigators later documented a similar lack of effect of zinc supplementation on antibody response to influenza vaccination in the elderly *(170)*.

Additional studies of immunity in zinc-deficient elderly, for which results are difficult to interpret or apply at large as a result of the study design and/or limited sample sizes, reported enhanced DTH responses *(171,172)*, whereas others reported no effect of zinc on lymphocyte proliferation, DTH cutaneous responses, or NK activity *(173,174)*.

Mildly zinc-deficient elderly subjects had significantly lower IL-2 production compared with zinc-adequate elderly and young subjects *(175)*. Zinc supplementation for the elderly deficient in the mineral may act to modulate or restore lowered levels of T-cell mediated immunity through its antioxidant- and membrane-stabilizing ability, or by increasing levels of the thymic hormone thymulin, which is normally reduced in the elderly as a result of age-associated thymic atrophy *(176)*. An improvement in plasma thymulin activity (as well as increased production of IL-1) was seen among zinc-deficient elderly ($n = 13$) who were supplemented with 30 mg zinc for 6 mo (177). Differences in the effects of zinc supplementation on the humoral branch of immunity in elderly individuals may vary depending on the antigen, in addition to the status of zinc nutriture at the time the antibody response was induced. An immunostimulatory effect of zinc supplementation beyond correction of impaired immunity because of zinc deficiency has not been clearly documented and might cause impairment of the immune response (178).

Selenium Selenium has been shown to be an essential nutrient for the maintenance of the immune response. Recent animal studies have indicated that Se supplementation might improve the immune response in the aged. Kiremidjian-Schumacher and Roy (179) showed that 24-mo-old mice supplemented with 2.0 ppm Se for 8 wk had higher mitogenic response to PHA and cytolytic T-lymphocyte activity against malignant cells. This effect was not the result of increases in IL-1, IL-2, or INF-γ production; it was related to the ability of Se to enhance the expression of α(p55) and/or β(p70/75) subunits of the IL-2R on the surface of activated cells.

A 6-mo, double-blind, placebo-controlled trial of selenium supplementation (100 μg/d as selenium-enriched yeast) in institutionalized elderly (mean age 78 yr; $n = 22$) revealed significantly greater lymphocyte proliferation in response to PWM (180). This increase in proliferative response was limited to B cells and was not exhibited in proliferative responses to T-cell mitogens PHA or OKT3. No significant correlations between plasma selenium levels and lymphoproliferative responses were established, although it is interesting to note that the greatest increases in B-cell proliferation occurred in subjects who had the lowest plasma selenium levels at baseline. Based on this, the authors concluded that Se supplementation enhances immune response in the elderly. This conclusion, however, is not supported by the data presented. As mentioned earlier, the main age-related difference occurs in T-cell-mediated function. Selenium supplementation did not improve mitogenic response to T-cell mitogens; thus, Se supplementation in this study was not effective in changing the age-associated defect in T cells.

Potential mechanisms through which selenium may enhance lymphocyte proliferation may revolve around selenium being an integral component of the enzyme glutathione peroxidase, a member of the antioxidant enzyme system. Glutathione peroxidase is involved in reducing the oxygen metabolites H_2O_2, which has been shown to impair lymphocyte proliferation and lipid hydroperoxides (LOOH), which can be deleterious to cellular membranes and also lead to impaired immune responses (181). A reduction in the activity of erythrocyte glutathione peroxidase has been reported with aging, which may be the result of significantly lower plasma levels of selenium with aging (42); therefore, restoration of selenium pools through supplementation could work to restore glutathione peroxidase activity and, in turn, restore some measures of immune function. Why the restoration of lymphocyte proliferation would be selective to B cells is not known and remains to be explored. Additional studies among the elderly are warranted to determine if the aging immune response will benefit from additional selenium supplementation.

OTHER SUBSTANCES

Glutathione Glutathione is the most abundant intracellular nonprotein thiol. This ubiquitous tripeptide is known to be involved in numerous cellular functions, including DNA and protein synthesis, transport of amino acids, metabolism of various

endogenous compounds (182), enzyme activation (183), and protection of cells from harmful effects of radiation, oxygen intermediates, and free radicals. Since the early 1980s, numerous studies have shown the association of glutathione with immune function. Intracellular glutathione has been proven to be essential for lymphocyte activation and proliferation. Altered glutathione status results in a corresponding change in cell-mediated immune response.

It has been suggested that GSH status is inversely related to aging and may be a predictor of morbidity and mortality (184). Lower GSH levels were observed in the brain, liver, lens, lung, and spleen of old mice compared with young mice (185–188). Lang et al. (184) showed that about half of healthy human subjects over 60 yr of age had lower blood GSH levels compared to young subjects. A positive correlation between the tissue GSH levels and the life-span in mice (189) and mosquitoes (190) has been demonstrated. These changes occur as a function of age and have been suggested to be responsible in part for the progression of aging process. GSH status might also be related to increased incidence of tumors in the aged. It is well known that the incidence and mortality rates from most cancers increase with age. GSH plays an important role in the detoxification of a wide variety of exogenous and endogenous carcinogens and free radicals, as well as in the maintenance of immune function. Administered GSH reduced the tumor burden of oral cancer in hamsters (191) and inhibited hepatocellular carcinoma growth in humans (192). Therefore, decreased GSH status with age might contribute to increase incidence of tumors in the aged.

A limited number of studies have been performed to investigate the effect of GSH on the immune response of the aged. We conducted a study to find if the decline in immune response with age can be reversed by GSH supplementation (185). In this study, young (4 mo), middle-aged (17 mo), and old (24 mo) C57BL/6NIA mice were fed diets containing different amounts of GSH (0, 0.1, 0.5 1.0%) for 4 wk. The results revealed a lower GSH level and decreased in vivo (as indicated by DTH test) and in vitro (as indicated by mitogenic response of splenocytes) T-cell-mediated immune responses in old mice compared to young mice. Dietary GSH supplementation reversed the age-associated decline in GSH level while significantly improving their immune response. Franklin et al. (193) reported that in vitro addition of GSH to splenocytes from young and old rats significantly enhanced their mitogenic response; a higher percentage increase was seen in old (eightfold) as compared to young animals (threefold). Liang et al. (194) found that GSH magnified the effect of IL-2 on the proliferation of IL-2-dependent cytotoxic T cells, increased the amount of IL-2 bound to high affinity receptors, and shortened its internalization and degradation time.

To further extend these findings to humans, we conducted an in vitro GSH supplementation study (195). A wide range of GSH supplementation levels was used to determine the optimal level of GSH. At concentrations between 2 and 10 mmol/L, GSH enhanced mitogenic response of PBMC from both young and old subjects, with maximal enhancement occurring at 5 mmol/L, which was, therefore, considered the optimal level. It is interesting to note that this optimal level is about or slightly higher than the physiological level of GSH found in most body tissues. At lower concentrations (0.5 and 1.0 mmol/L) however, GSH significantly decreased mitogenic response of PBMC from both young and old subjects.

Similar to the observation in rats *(193)*, we noticed that glutathione-induced enhancement of proliferative response to the T-cell mitogens Con A and PHA was greater in lymphocytes from old subjects than in those from young subjects. This increased responsiveness of lymphocytes was accompanied by an elevated cellular glutathione concentration. GSH significantly increased IL-2 production while decreasing PGE_2 production, both of which can contribute to immunostimulatory effect of GSH.

We examined the effects of GSH supplementation on production of eicosanoids and IL-2 by the lymphocytes from young and old subjects. PGE_2, a cyclooxygenase product of AA, is an important suppressive factor in immunoregulation *(73)*, and AA lipoxygenase product LTB_4 has been reported to inhibit lymphocyte proliferation *(196)*. We observed that the addition of 5 mmol/L GSH inhibited calcium ionophore A23187-stimulated PGE_2 and LTB_4 synthesis in the lymphocytes from young and old subjects. IL-2 production, on the other hand, was found to be enhanced by 197% and 140% in young subjects versus 306% and 372% in old subjects for PHA and Con A, respectively. A GSH-induced decrease in PGE_2 and LTB_4 as well as increase in IL-2 production can contribute to the stimulatory effect of GSH on mitogenic proliferation. It is interesting to note that the age-associated difference in immunostimulatory effect of GSH was observed despite equal reduction by GSH in PGE_2 production in young and old subjects. This can be the result of the fact that the cells from old subjects are more sensitive to inhibitory effect of PGE_2. The addition of PGE_2 at 0.1 µmol/L significantly inhibited lymphocyte proliferation in old subjects (36%, $p < 0.01$), but only a marginally significant inhibition (19%, $p < 0.07$) was seen in young subjects. This altered sensitivity with age to PGE_2 inhibition has also been observed by other investigators in humans *(197)* and rats *(198)*. In these experiments, the PGE_2-induced inhibition of lymphocyte proliferation was totally reversed by adding 5 mM GSH.

Glutathione may also regulate immune function by affecting transmembrane signal transduction and activation of nuclear transcription factors. Depletion of GSH results in reduced $[Ca^{2+}]$ mobilization and impaired tyrosine phosphorylation of several proteins, including phospholipase C-γ1 in lymphocytes following stimulation of the CD3 receptor *(199)*. GSH was shown to protect signal transduction from impairment induced by oxidant stress in pulmonary type II epithelial cells *(200)*. Nuclear transcription factors have also been shown to be sensitive to the intracellular thiol level. It is interesting to note that NF-κB activation was recently shown to be impaired in T cells from old subjects *(201)*.

Functional Foods   To date, very few studies have evaluated the effect of "functional foods" on the immune response of the aged, yet it has been speculated that several of these "foods" have antiaging and immunoenhancing effects. In two separate studies, we evaluated the effect of two such food components—mushroom extract and conjugated linoleic acid (CLA)—on the immune response of young and old mice.

Protein-bound polysaccharides (PSP) are a class of compounds found in abundance in certain mushrooms. They have been widely used as biological response modifiers to enhance immune response and reduce tumor burden *(202)*. There are, however, few published, well-controlled studies, particularly in unchallenged and healthy hosts, to substantiate the immunostimulatory claims attributed to these compounds. Therefore, we examined the effect of dietary supplementation with a mushroom extract containing PSP on in vitro and in vivo immune function of old (23 mo) and young

(5 mo) C57BL/6NCrlBR mice. Animals were fed purified diets containing extract derived from the mycelia of *Coriolus versicolor* with either 0%, 0.1%, 0.5%, or 1.0% PSP. After 1 mo of this supplemented diet, indices of immune function were measured. PSP supplementation had no significant effect on mitogenic response to Con A, PHA, or lipopolysaccharide (LPS) nor any significant effect on the production of IL-1, IL-2, IL-4, or PGE_2. Of the in vivo indices of immune function tested, old mice fed 1% PSP had significantly higher DTH response than those fed 0% PSP. No significant effect of PSP on the DTH response of young mice was observed. These results suggest that PSP-containing mushroom extract might have a modest immunoenhancing effect in aged mice but not in young mice.

Conjugated linoleic acid is a naturally occurring substance originally described as an anticarcinogenic agent in grilled ground beef *(203)*. CLA added in vitro to porcine lymphocyte cultures increased mitogen-induced lymphocyte blastogenesis, lymphocyte cytotoxic activity, and murine Mφ killing ability *(204)*. An increase in PHA-stimulated blastogenesis was also noted in CLA-fed chicks challenged with LPS *(205)*. The immunostimulatory effect of CLA has been attributed to its antioxidant properties and its ability to interfere with arachidonic acid metabolism (e.g., PGE_2 *(203,206)*). We, therefore, evaluated the effect of CLA supplementation on the immune response of young and old mice *(207)*. Young (4 mo) and old (24 mo) C57BL/6NCrlBR mice were fed semipurified diets containing either 0% or 1% CLA for 8 wk. In vitro and in vivo indices of the immune responses were evaluated. CLA supplementation significantly increased all CLA isomers measured in hepatic neutral lipids and phospholipids. Young mice fed 1% CLA had greater proliferative response to Con A and PHA than those fed 0% CLA. No effect of CLA supplementation on mitogenic response of old mice to PHA was observed. However, old mice fed 1% CLA had significantly higher mitogenic response to Con A compared with those fed 0% CLA. Old mice fed 0% CLA had significantly lower IL-2 production than young mice. In addition, IL-2 production in old mice fed 1% CLA was not significantly different from that of young mice. CLA supplementation had no effect on NK cell cytotoxicity, DTH, antibody response to SRBC, or PGE_2 production. Thus, CLA supplementation appears to enhance in vitro T-cell-mediated function, but it has no effect on the in vivo indices of the immune response. It is, therefore, not clear if CLA supplementation would be of clinical significance to the aged.

There is great interest in determining the health benefits of other (than essential nutrients) components of foods, especially in the aged. The immune system provides a clinically relevant, easily accessible biological system to determine the health benefits of these components. Very few studies have addressed the immunological effects of these compounds. Further studies are needed in this area.

SUMMARY

Dysregulation of the immune response with age has been observed in all species studied, including humans. These changes contribute to increased incidence of tumors as well as infectious and neoplastic diseases. Decreased intake and/or serum levels of several nutrients with known immunoregulatory functions have been reported in the elderly. This has led to the proposal that the age-related immunological changes could be, in part, the result of deficiencies and/or increased utilization of certain nutrients. This is supported by the results of interventional studies using single-nutrient or multinutrient cocktails, which have shown improvement in certain aspects of the aged immune response. Several studies have indicated that in malnourished elderly individuals, a general nutritional supplement will improve their immune response. A few studies have also shown that supplementation with higher than currently recommended levels of a single nutrient can improve the immune response in healthy elderly subjects. This raises the question of whether higher than currently recommended levels of certain nutrients are needed to maintain an optimal immune response in the elderly. Studies in which clinical significance of nutrient-induced immunoenhancement in the aged has been determined will help address this question. Further studies are also needed to determine the effect and mechanisms of action of specific nutrients on the immune response of the aged. Such information will shed light on our understanding of the etiology of age-related immune dysregulation, which, in turn, should result in the design of more effective nutritional interventions to maintain optimal immune response in the elderly. This information would also be useful in determining the specific nutrient requirements for the elderly.

ACKNOWLEDGMENTS

The authors' work has been funded at least in part with federal funds from the U.S. Department of Agriculture, Agricultural Research Service under contract number 53-K06-01 as well as funds from NIA Grant AG09140, USDA Grant 94-37200-0489, and Hoffmann LaRoche, Inc. The contents of this publication do not necessarily reflect the views or policies of the U.S. Department of Agriculture nor does mention of trade names, commercial products, or organizations imply endorsement by the U.S. Government.

The authors would like to thank Timothy S. McElreavy, M.A., for preparation of this manuscript.

REFERENCES

1. Singh GK, Kochanek KD, MacDorman MF. Advance report of final mortality statistics, 1994. Monthly vital statistics report. 1996; 45:19.
2. Kerstetter JE, Holthausen BA, Fitz PA. Malnutrition in the institutionalized older adult. J Am Diet Assoc 1992; 92:1109–16.
3. Laughrea M. On the error theories of aging. A review of the experimental data. Exp Gerontol 1982; 17:305.
4. Sharma R. Theories of aging. In: Timiras PS, ed. Physiological Basis of Aging and Geriatrics, pp. 37–46. CRC, Boca Raton, FL, 1994.
5. Crossley KB, Peterson PK. Infections in the elderly. Clin Infect Dis 1996; 22:209–15.
6. Cross CE, Halliwell B, Borish ET, Pryor WA, Ames BN, Saul RL, et al. Oxygen radicals and human disease. Ann Intern Med 1987; 107:526–45.
7. Halliwell B. Oxidants and human disease: some new concepts. FASEB J 1987; 1:358–64.
8. Abbas AK, Lichtman AH, Pober JS. Cellular and Molecular Immunology. W. B. Saunders, Philadelphia, 1991.
9. Makinodan T, Hirokawa K. Normal aging of the immune system. In: Johnson HA, ed, Relations Between Normal Aging and Disease, pp. 117–32. Raven, New York, 1985.
10. Green-Johnson J, Wade AW, Szewczuk MR. The immunobiology of aging. In: Cooper EL, Nisbet-Brown E, eds, Developmental Immunology, pp. 426–51. Oxford University Press, New York, 1993.
11. Miller RA. Cellular and biochemical changes in the aging mouse immune system. Nutr Rev 1995; 53(suppl):S14–7.
12. Schwab R, Weksler ME. Cell biology of the impaired proliferation of T cells from elderly humans. In: Goidl EA, ed, Aging and the Immune Response, pp. 67–80. Marcel Dekker, New York, 1987.
13. Gottesman SRS. Changes in T-cell-mediated immunity with age: an update. Rev Biol Res Aging 1987; 3:95–127.
14. Chopra RK. Mechanisms of impaired T-cell function in the elderly. Rev Biol Res Aging 1990; 4:83–104.
15. Makinodan T. Patterns of age-related immunologic changes. Nutr Rev 1995; 53:S27–S31.
16. Miller RA, Garcia G, Kirk CJ. Early activation defects in T lymphocytes from aged mice. Immun Rev 1997; 160:79–90.
17. Weksler ME. Immune senescence: Deficiency or dysregulation? Nutr Rev 1995; 53:S3–S7.
18. Wade AW, Szewczuk MR. Changes in the mucosal-associated B-cell response with age. In: Goidl EA, ed, Aging and the Immune Response, pp. 95–121. Marcel Dekker, New York, 1987.
19. Nagel JE, Proust JJ. Age-related changes in humoral immunity, complement, and polymorphonuclear leukocyte function. Rev Biol Res Aging 1987; 3:147–59.
20. Ennist DL. Humoral immunosenescence: an update. Rev Biol Res Aging 1990; 4:105–20.
21. Ernst DN, Weigle O, Hobbs MV. Aging and lymphokine gene expression by T cell subsets. Nutr Rev 1995; 53(suppl):S18–S25.
22. Beharka AA, Wu D, Santos MS, Meydani SN. Increased prostaglandin production by murine macrophages contributes to the age-associated decrease in T cell function. FASEB J 1996; 9:A754.
23. Hayek MG, Meydani SN, Meydani M, Blumberg JB. Age differences in eicosanoid production of mouse splenocytes: effects on mitogen-induced T-cell proliferation. J Gerontol 1994; 49:B197–B207.
24. Bender BS. Natural killer cells in senescence: analysis of phenotypes and function. Rev Biol Res Aging 1987; 3:129–38.
25. Bloom ET. Natural killer cells, lymphokine-associated killer cells, and cytolytic T lymphocytes: compartmentalization of age-related changes in cytolytic lymphocytes? J Gerontol 1994; 49:B85–B92.
26. Krishnaraj R, Blandford G. Age-associated alterations in human natural killer cells: 1. Increased activity as per conventional and kinetic analysis. Clin Immunol Immunopathol 1987; 45:268–85.
27. Garry PJ, Goodwin JG, Hunt WC, Hooper EM, Leonard AG. Nutritional status in a healthy elderly population: dietary and supplemental intakes. Am J Clin Nutr 1982; 36:319–31.
28. Ryan AS, Craig L, Finn SC. Nutrient intakes and dietary patterns of older Americans: a national study. J Gerontol 1992; 47:M145–50.
29. Panemangalore M, Lee CJ. Evaluation of the indices of retinol and alpha-tocopherol status in free-living elderly. J Gerontol 1992; 47:B98–B104.
30. Kataria MS, Rao DB, Curtis RC. Vitamin C levels in elderly. Gerontol Clin 1965; 7:189–90.
31. Taylor G. Diet of elderly women. Lancet 1966; 1:926.
32. Burr ML, Elwood PC, Hole DJ, Hurley RJ, Hughes RE. Plasma and leukocyte ascorbic acid levels in the elderly. Am J Clin Nutr 1974; 27:144–51.
33. Meydani M, Martin A, Ribaya-Mercado JD, Gong J, Blumberg JB, Russell RM. β-Carotene supplementation increases antioxidant capacity of plasma in older women. J Nutr 1994; 124:2397–403.
34. Murata T, Tamai H, Morinobu T, Manago M, Takenaka H, Hayashi K, et al. Effect of long-term administration of β-carotene on lymphocyte subsets in humans. Am J Clin Nutr 1994; 60:597–602.
35. Murata T, Tamai H, Morinobu T, Manago M, Takenaka A, Takenaka H. Determination of beta-carotene in plasma, blood cells, and buccal mucosa by electrochemical detection. Lipids 1992; 27:840–43.
36. Norkus EP, Bhagavan HN, Nair PP. Relationship between individual carotenoids in plasma, platelets and red blood cells. FASEB J 1990; 4:A1174.
37. van den Berg H, Bode W, Mocking JAJ, Lowik MRH. Effect of aging on vitamin B$_6$ status and metabolism. Ann NY Acad Sci 1990; 585:96–105.
38. Rall LC, Meydani SN. Vitamin B$_6$ and immune competence. Nutr Rev 1993; 51:217–25.
39. Sandstead HH, Henriksen LK, Greger JL, Prasad AS, Good RA. Zinc nutriture in the elderly in relation to taste acuity, immune response and wound healing. Am J Clin Nutr 1982; 26:1046–59.
40. Beisel WR. Impact of infectious disease upon fat metabolism and immune functions. Cancer Res 1981; 41:3797–8.
41. Good RA, Gajjar AJ. Diet, immunity, and longevity. In: Hutchinson

ML, Munro HN, eds. Nutrition and Aging, pp. 235–49. Academic, Orlando, FL, 1986.

42. Olivieri O, Stanzial AM, Girelli D, Trevisan MT, Guarini P, Terzi M, et al. Selenium status, fatty acids, vitamins A and E, and aging: the Nove Study. Am J Clin Nutr 1994; 60:510–7.

43. Schlenker ED. Nutrition in Aging. Mosby, St. Louis, MO, 1984.

44. Meydani SN, Blumberg JB. Nutrition and immune function in the elderly. In: Munro HN, Danford DE, eds, Nutrition, Aging, and the Elderly, pp. 61–87. Plenum, New York, 1989.

45. Chandra RK. Nutrition is an important determinant of immunity in old age. In: Prinsley DM, Sandstead HH, eds, Nutrition and Aging, pp. 321–34. Alan R. Liss, New York, 1990.

46. Bogden JD, Bendich A, Kemp FW, Bruening KS, Skurnick JH, Denny T, et al. Daily micronutrient supplements enhance delayed-hypersensitivity skin test responses in older people. Am J Clin Nutr 1994; 60:437–47.

47. Linn BS, Jensen J. Malnutrition and immunocompetence in older and younger outpatients. South Med J 1984; 77:1098–102.

48. Chandra RK, Puri S. Nutritional support improves antibody response to influenza virus vaccine in the elderly. Br Med J Clin Res Ed 1985; 291:705–6.

49. Hamm MW, Winick M, Schachter D. Macrophage phagocytosis and membrane fluidity in mice: the effect of age and dietary protein. Mech Ageing Dev 1985; 32:11–20.

50. McLaughlin ME, Kao R, Liener IE, Hoida JR. A quantitative in vitro assay of polymorphonuclear leukocyte migration through human amnion membrane utilizing 111in-oxine. J Immunol Method. 1986; 95:89–98.

51. Nagel JE, Pyle RS, Chrest FJ, Adler WH. Oxidative metabolism and bactericidal capacity of polymorphonuclear leukocytes from normal young and aged adults. J Gerontol 1982; 37:529–34.

52. Suzuki H, Kurita T, Kakinuma K. Effects of neuraminidase on O_2 consumption and release of O_2 and H_2O_2 from phagocytosing human polymorphonuclear leukocytes. Blood 1982; 60:446–53.

53. Gladstone JL, Recco A. Host factors and infectious diseases in the elderly. Med Clin North Am 1976; 60:1225–40.

54. Lipschitz DA, Udupa KB. Influence of aging and protein deficiency on neutrophil function. J Gerontol 1986; 41:690–4.

55. Lesourd BM. Protein undernutrition as the major cause of decreased immune function in the elderly: clinical and functional implications. Nutr Rev 1995; 53(suppl):S86–S94.

56. Ligthart GJ, Corberand JX, Fournier C, Galanaud P, Hijmans W, Kennes B, et al. Admission criteria for immunogerontological studies in man: the SENIEUR Protocol. Mech Ageing Dev 1984; 28:47–55.

57. Huang CJ, Cheung NS, Lu VR. Effects of deteriorated frying oil and dietary protein levels on liver microsomal enzymes in rats. JAOCS 1988; 65:1796–803.

58. Clandinin MT, Cheema S, Field CJ, Garg ML, Venkatraman J, Clandinin TR. Dietary fat: exogenous determination of membrane structure and cell function. FASEB 1991; 5:2761–9.

59. Leaver HA, Howie A, Wilson NH. The biosynthesis of the 3-series prostaglandins in rat uterus after alpha-linolenic acid feeding: mass spectroscopy of prostaglandins E and F produced by rat uteri in tissue culture. Prostagland Leuk Essential Fatty Acids 1991; 42:217–24.

60. Huang DH, Boudreau M, Chanmugan P. Dietary linolenic acid and longer-chain n-3 fatty acids: comparison of effects on arachidonic acid metabolism in rats. J Nutr 1988; 118:427–37.

61. Davits FA, Nugteren A. The urinary excretion of prostaglandin E and their corresponding tetranor metabolites by rats fed a diet rich in eicosapentaenoate. Biochim Biophys Acta 1988; 958:289–99.

62. Knapp HR. Prostaglandins in human semen during fish oil ingestion: evidence for in vivo cyclooxygenase inhibition and appearance of novel trienoic compound. Prostaglandins 1990; 39:407–23.

63. Meydani SN, Stocking LM, Shapiro AC, Meydani M, Blumberg JB. Fish oil- and tocopherol-induced changes in ex vivo synthesis of spleen and lung leukotriene B4 (LTB4) in mice. Ann NY Acad Sci 1988; 524:395–7.

64. Lee TH, Hoover R, Williams JD, Sperling J, Raralese J, Spur BW, et al. Effect of dietary enrichment with eicosapentaenoic and docosahexaenoic acids in vitro neutrophil and monocyte leukotriene generation and neutrophil function. N Engl J Med 1985; 312:1217–24.

65. Leitch AG, Lee TH, Ringel EW, Prickett JD, Robinson WR, Pyme SG, et al. Immunologically induced generation of tetraene and pentaene leukotrienes in the peritoneal cavities of menhaden-fed rats. J Immunol 1985; 132:2559–65.

66. Whelan KS, Broughton B, Lokesh B, Kinsella JE. In vivo formation of leukotriene E5 by murine peritoneal cells. Prostaglandins 1991; 41:29–41.

67. Webb DR, Rogers TJ, Nowowiejski E. Endogenous prostaglandin synthesis and the control of lymphocyte function. Proc NY Acad Sci 1980; 332:260–70.

68. Goodwin JS, Messner RP, Peake GT. Prostaglandin suppression of mitogen stimulated leukocytes in culture. J Clin Invest 1974; 4:368–78.

69. Gordon D, Bray M, Morley J. Control of lymphokine secretion by prostaglandins. Nature 1976; 262:401–2.

70. Plaunt M. The role of cyclic AMP in modulating cytotoxic T lymphocytes. J Immunol 1979; 123:692–701.

71. Roder JC, Klein M. Target–effector interaction in the natural killer cell system. J Immunol 1979; 123:2785–90.

72. Goodman MG, Weigle WO. Modulation of lymphocyte activation I. Inhibition of an oxidation product of arachidonic acid. J Immunol 1980; 125:593–600.

73. Rola-Plezczunski M. Immunoregulation by leukotrienes and other lipoxygenase metabolites. Immunol Today 1985; 6:302–7.

74. Hayek MG, Mura CV, Paulson KE, Beharka AA, Hwang D, Meydani SN. Enhanced expression of inducible cyclooxygenase with age in murine macrophages. J Immunol 1997; 159:2445–51.

75. Beharka AA, Wu D, Han S-N, Meydani SN. Macrophage prostaglandin production contributes to the age-associated decrease in T cell function which is reversed by the dietary antioxidant vitamin E. Mech Ageing Dev 1997; 94:157–65.

76. Meydani SN, Endres S, Woods MN, Goldin RD, Soo C, Morrill-Labrode A, et al. Oral (n-3) fatty acid supplementation suppresses cytokine production and lymphocyte proliferation: comparison between young and older women. J Nutr 1991; 121:547–55.

77. Endres S, Cannon JG, Ghorbani R, Dempsey RA, Sisson SD, Lonnemann G, et al. In vitro production of IL-1β, IL-1α, TNF and IL2 in healthy subjects: distribution, effect of cyclooxygenase inhibition and evidence of independent gene regulation. Eur J Immunol 1989; 19:2327–33.

78. Endres S, Meydani SN, Ghorbani R, Schindler R, Dinarello CA. Dietary n-3 fatty acids suppress interleukin-2 production and mononuclear cell proliferation. J Leuk Biol 1993; 54:599–603.

79. Hollander D, Dadufabza VD, Sletten EG. Does essential fatty acid absorption change with age? J Lipid Res 1984; 25:129–34.

80. Goodwin JS, Webb DA. Regulation of the immune response by prostaglandins. Clin Immunol Immunopathol 1980; 15:106–22.

81. Knusden PJ, Dinarello CA, Strom TB. Prostaglandins posttranscriptionally inhibit monocyte expression of interleukin 1 activity by increasing intracellular cyclic adenosine monophosphate. J Immunol 1986; 137:3189–94.

82. Meydani SN, Meydani M, Verdon CP, Shapiro AC, Blumberg JB, Hayes KC. Vitamin E supplementation suppresses prostaglandin E_2 synthesis and enhances the immune response of aged mice. Mech Ageing Dev 1986; 34:191–201.

83. Meydani SN, Barklund MP, Liu S, Meydani M, Miller RA, Cannon JG, et al. Vitamin E supplementation enhances cell-mediated immunity in healthy elderly subjects. Am J Clin Nutr 1990; 52:557–63.

84. Brunda MJ, Heberman RB, Holden HT. Inhibition of natural killer cell activity by prostaglandins. J Immunol 1980; 124:2682–7.

85. Zoschke DC, Messner RP. Suppression of human lymphocyte mitogenesis mediated by phagocyte-released reactive oxygen species, comparative activities in normal and chronic granulomatous disease. Clin Immunol Immunopathol 1984; 32:29–40.

86. Meydani M, Natiello F, Goldin B, Free N, Woods M, Schaefer E,

et al. Effect of long-term fish oil supplementation on vitamin E status and lipid peroxidation in women. J Nutr 1991; 121:484–91.

87. Santoli D, Zurier RB. Prostaglandin E precursor fatty acids inhibit human IL-2 production by a prostaglandin E-dependent mechanism. Immunology 1989; 143:1303–9.

88. Hughes DA, Pinder AC, Piper Z, Johnson IT, Lund EK. Fish oil supplementation inhibits the expression of major histocompatibility complex class II molecules and adhesion molecules on human monocytes. Am J Clin Nutr 1996; 63:267–72.

89. Hughes DA, Pinder AC. Influence of n-3 polyunsaturated fatty acids (PUFA) on the antigen-presenting function of human monocytes. Biochem Soc Trans 1996; 24:389S.

90. Hughes DA, Southon S, Pinder AC. (n-3) Polyunsaturated fatty acids modulate the expression of functionally associated molecules on human monocytes in vitro. J Nutr 1996; 126:603–10.

91. Jolly CA, Jiang Y-H, Chapkin RS, McMurray DN. Dietary (n-3) polyunsaturated fatty acids suppress murine lymphoproliferation, interleukin-2 secretion, and the formation of diacylglycerol and ceramide. J Nutr 1997; 127:37–43.

92. Jolly CA, Laurenz JC, McMurray DN, Chapkin RS. Diacylglycerol and ceramide kinetics in primary cultures of activated T-lymphocytes. Immunol Lett 1996; 49:43–8.

93. VanMeter AR, Ehringer WD, Stillwell W, Blumenthal EJ, Jenski LJ. Aged lymphocyte proliferation following incorporation and retention of dietary omega-3 fatty acids. Mech Ageing Dev 1994; 75:95–114.

94. Tappia PS, Man WJ, Grimble RF. Influence of unsaturated fatty acids on the production of tumor necrosis factor and interleukin-6 by rat peritoneal macrophages. Mol Cell Biol 1995; 143:89–98.

95. Meydani SN, Lichtenstein AH, Cornwall S, Meydani M, Goldin BR, Rasmussen H, et al. Immunologic effects of National Cholesterol Education Panel (NCEP) Step-2 diets with and without fish-derived n-3 fatty acid enrichment. J Clin Invest 1993; 92:105–13.

96. Farwer SR, der Boer BC, Haddeman E, Kivits GA, Wiersma A, Danse BH. The vitamin E nutritional status of rats fed diets high in fish oil, linseed oil, or sunflower oil. Br J Nutr 1994; 72:127–45.

97. Fritsche KL, Cassity NA, Huang S-C. Dietary (n-3) fatty acid and vitamin E interactions in rats: effects on vitamin E status, immune cell prostaglandin E production and primary antibody response. J Nutr 1992; 122:1009–18.

98. Meydani SN, Shapiro AC, Meydani M, Macauley JB, Blumberg JB. Effect of age and dietary fat (fish, corn and coconut oils) on tocopherol status of C57BL/6NIA mice. Lipids 1987; 22:345–50.

99. Wander RC, Hall JA, Gradin JL, Du SH, Jewell DE. The ratio of dietary n-6 to n-3 fatty acids influences immune system function, eicosanoid metabolism, lipid peroxidation, and vitamin E status in aged dogs. J Nutr 1997; 127:1198–205.

100. Piche A, Draper HH, Cole PD. Malondialdehyde excretion by subjects consuming cod liver oil versus a concentrate of n-3 fatty acids. Lipids 1988; 23:370–1.

101. L'Abbe MR, Trick KD, Beare-Rogers J. Dietary (n-3) fatty acids affect rat heart, liver and aorta protective enzyme activities and lipid peroxidation. J Nutr 1991; 121:1331–40.

102. Wander RC, Du SH, Ketchum SO, Rowe KE. Alpha-tocopherol influences in vivo indices of lipid peroxidation in postmenopausal women given fish oil. J Nutr 1996; 126:643–52.

103. Shapiro AC, Wu D, Hayek MG, Meydani M, Meydani SN. Role of eicosanoids and vitamin E in fish oil-induced changes to splenocyte proliferation to T cell mitogens in mice. Nutr Res 1994; 14:1339–54.

104. Wu D, Meydani SN, Meydani M, Hayek MG, Huth P, Nicolosi RJ. Immunological effects of marine-and plant-derived (n-3) polyunsaturated fatty acids in non-human primates. Am J Clin Nutr 1996; 63:273–80.

105. Kramer TR, Schoene N, Dougless LW, Judd JT, Ballard-Barbash R, Taylor PR, et al. Increased vitamin E intake restores fish-oil-induced suppressed blastogenesis of mitogenic-stimulated T lymphocytes. Am J Clin Nutr 1991; 54:896–902.

106. Chandra RK. Effect of vitamin and trace-element supplementation on immune responses and infectious disease in elderly subjects. Lancet 1992; 340:1124–27.

107. Pike J, Chandra RK. Effect of vitamin and trace element supplementation on immune indices in healthy elderly. Int J Vit Nutr Res 1995; 65:117–21.

108. Pen ND, Purkins L, Kelleher J, Heatley RV, Mascie-Taylor BH, Belfield PW. The effect of dietary supplementation with vitamins A, C, and E on cell-mediated immune function in elderly long-stay patients: a randomized controlled trial. Age Aging 1991; 20:169–74.

109. Chandra RK, Sudhakaran L. Regulation of immune responses by vitamin B₆. Ann NY Acad Sci 1990; 585:404–23.

110. Talbott MC, Miller LK, Kerkvliet N. Pyridoxine supplementation: effect of lymphocyte response in elderly persons. Am J Clin Nutr 1987; 46:569–664.

111. Council NR. Recommended Dietary Allowances. 10th ed. National Academy Press, Washington, DC, 1989.

112. Meydani SN, Ribaya-Mercado JD, Russell RM, Sahyoun N, Morrow FD, Gershoff SN. Vitamin B-6 deficiency impairs interleukin-2 production and lymphocyte proliferation of older adults. Am J Clin Nutr 1991; 53:1275–80.

113. Axelrod AD, Trakatellis AC. Relationship of pyridoxine to immunological phenomena. Vitam Horm 1964; 22:591–607.

114. Kennes B, Dumont I, Brohee D, Hubert C, Neve P. Effect of vitamin C supplementation on cell-mediated immunity in old people. Gerontology 1983; 29:305–10.

115. Anderson R, Oosthuigen R, Maritz R, Theron A, Van Rensburg A. The effect of increasing weekly doses of ascorbate on certain cellular and humoral immune functions in normal volunteers. Am J Clin Nutr 1980; 33:71–6.

116. Delafuente JC, Prendergast JM, Modigh A. Immunological modulation by vitamin C in the elderly. Clin Immunol Immunopathol 1986; 8:205–11.

117. Ziemlanski S, Wartanowicz M, Klos A, Raczka A, Klos M. The effect of ascorbic acid and alpha-tocopherol supplementation on serum proteins and immunoglobulin concentration in the elderly. Nutr Int 1986; 2:1–5.

118. Goodwin JS, Ceuppens J. Regulation of immune response by prostaglandins. J Clin Immunol 1983; 3:295–315.

119. Hodkinson HM, Exton-Smith AN. Factors predicting mortality in the elderly in the community. Age Aging 1976; 5:110–15.

120. Wilson TS, Weeks MM, Mukheyee SK, Murrell JS, Andrews CT. A study of vitamin C levels in the aged and subsequent mortality. Gerontol Clin 1972; 14:17–24.

121. Wilson TS, Datta SB, Murrell JS, Andrews CT. Relationship of vitamin C to mortality in a geriatric hospital: A study of the effect of vitamin C administration. Age Aging 1973; 2:163–71.

122. Burr ML, Hurley RJ, Sweetnam PM. Vitamin C supplementation of old people with low blood levels. Gerontol Clin 1975; 17:236–43.

123. Satoh K. Serum lipid peroxides in cerebrovascular disorders determined by a new calorimetric method. Clin Chim Acta 1978; 90:37–43.

124. Svematsu T, Kamada T, Abe H, Kikudzi S, Yagi K. Serum lipoperoxide level in patients suffering from liver disease. Clin Chim Acta 1977; 79:267–71.

125. Leibovitz BE, Siegel BV. Aspects of free radical reactions in biological systems. Aging J Gerontol 1980; 7:45–56.

126. Wartanowicz M, Panczenko-Kresowska B, Ziemlanski S, Kowalska M, Okolska G. The effect of alpha-tocopherol and ascorbic acid on the serum lipid peroxide level in elderly people. Am Nutr Metab 1984; 28:186–91.

127. Atkinson J, Kelly J, Weiss A, Wedner H, Parker C. Enhanced intracellular cGMP concentrations and lectin-induced lymphocyte transformation. J Immunol 1978; 121:2282–91.

128. Katz S, Kierszenbaum F, Waksman B. Mechanism of action of lymphocyte activating factor, III. Evidence that LAF acts on stimulated lymphocytes by raising cyclic GMP in G1. J Immunol 1978; 126:2386–91.

129. Coquette A, Vray B, Vanderpas J. Role of vitamin E in the protection

of the resident macrophage membrane against oxidative damage. Arch Int Physiol Biochem 1986; 94:529–34.

130. Hatman LJ, Kayden HJ. A high-performance liquid chromatographic method for the determination of tocopherol in plasma and cellular elements of the blood. J Lipid Res 1979; 20:639–45.

131. Harman D. Free radical theory of aging: Beneficial effect of antioxidants on the lifespan of male NZB mice; role of free radical reactions in the deterioration of the immune system with age and in the pathogenesis of systemic lupus erythematosus. Age 1980; 3:64–73.

132. Meydani SN, Cathcart ES, Hopkins RE, Meydani M, Hayes KC, Blumberg JB. Antioxidants in experimental amyloidosis of young and old mice. In: Glenner GG, Asserman EP, Benditt E, et al. eds, Fourth International Symposium on Amyloidosis, pp. 683–92. Plenum, New York, 1986.

133. Sakai S, Moriguchi S. Long-term feeding of high vitamin E diet improves the decreased mitogen response of rat splenic lymphocytes with aging. J Nutr Sci Vitaminol 1997; 43:113–22.

134. Harman D, Miller RW. Effect of vitamin E on the immune response to influenza virus vaccine and the incidence of infectious disease in man. Age 1986; 9:21–23.

135. Meydani SN, Barklund PM, Liu S, Meydani M, Miller RA, Cannon JG, et al. Vitamin E supplementation enhances cell-mediated immunity in healthy elderly subjects. Am J Clin Nutr 1990; 52:557–63.

136. Meydani SN, Meydani M, Blumberg JB, Leka LS, Siber G, Loszewski R, et al. Vitamin E supplementation enhances in vivo immune response in healthy elderly subjects: a randomized controlled trial. JAMA 1997; 277:1380–6.

137. Hayek MG, Taylor SF, Bender BS, Han SN, Meydani M, Smith DE, et al. Vitamin E supplementation decreases lung virus titers in mice infected with influenza. J Infect Dis 1997; 176:273–6.

138. Han SN, Wu D, Ha WK, Smith DE, Beharka AA, Martin KR, et al. Vitamin E (E) supplementation increases splenocyte IL-2 and interferon-γ production of old mice infected with influenza virus. FASEB J 1998; 12:A819.

139. Meydani SN, Meydani M, Blumberg J, Leka L, Pedrosa M, Stollar BD, et al. Safety assessment of long-term vitamin E supplementation in healthy elderly. Am J Clin Nutr, in press.

140. Cannon JG, Orencole SF, Fielding RA, Meydani M, Meydani SN, Fiatarone MA, et al. The acute phase response in exercise: interaction of age and vitamin E on neutrophils and muscle enzyme release. Am J Physiol 1990; 259:R1214–9.

141. Cannon JG, Meydani SN, Fielding RA, Fiatarone MA, Meydani M, Orencole SF, et al. Acute phase response in exercise. II. Associations between vitamin E, cytokines, and muscle proteolysis. Am J Physiol 1991; 260:R1235–40.

142. Chavance M, Brubacher G, Herbeth B, et al. Immunological and nutritional status among the elderly. In: De Wick AL, ed, Lymphoid Cell Functions in Aging, pp. 231–7. Eurage, Interlaken, 1984.

143. Chavance M, Brubacher G, Herbert B, Vernhers G, Mistacki T, Dete F, et al. Immunological nutritional status among the elderly. In: Chandra RK, ed, Nutritional Immunity and Illness in the Elderly, pp. 137–42. Pergamon, New York, 1985.

144. Payette H, Rola-Pleszczynski M, Ghadriran P. Nutritional factors in relation to cellular and regulatory immune variables in a free-living elderly population. Am J Clin Nutr 1990; 33:606–8.

145. Meydani SN, Meydani M, Blumberg JB. Antioxidants and the aging immune response. Adv Exp Med Biol 1990; 262:57–68.

146. Nagel JE, Chorpa RK, Chrest FJ, Chrest FJ, McCoy MT, Schneider EL. Decreased proliferation, interleukin 2 synthesis, and interleukin 2 receptor expression are accompanied by decreased mRNA expression in phytohemagglutin-stimulated cells from elderly donors. J Clin Invest 1988; 81:1096–102.

147. Corwin LM, Shloss J. Role of antioxidants on the stimulation the mitogen response. J Nutr 1980; 110:2497–505.

148. Metzger Z, Hoffeld JT, Oppenheim JJ. Macrophage-mediated suppression I. Evidence for participation of both hydrogen peroxide and prostaglandin in suppression of murine lymphocyte proliferation. J Immunol 1980; 124:938–88.

149. Baehner RL, Boxer LA, Allen JM, Davis J. Autooxidation as a

basis for altered function by polymorphonuclear leukocytes. Blood 1977; 50:327–35.

150. Sharmanov AT, Aidarkhanov BB, Kurmangaliev SM. Effect of vitamin E on oxidative metabolism of macrophages. Bull Exp Biol Med 1986; 101:723–5.

151. Villa S, Lorico A, Morazzoni G, de Gaetano G, Semerano N. Vitamin E and vitamin C inhibit arachidonic-induced aggregation of human peripheral blood leukocytes in vitro. Agents Actions 1986; 19:127–31.

152. Topinka J, Binkovaa B, Sram RJ, Erin AN. The influence of alpha-tocopherol and pyritinol on oxidative DNA damages and lipid peroxidation in human lymphocytes. Mutat Res 1989; 225:131–6.

153. Sepe SM, Clark RA. Oxidant membrane injury by the neutrophil myeloperoxidase system. II. Injury by stimulated neutrophils and protection by lipid-soluble antioxidants. J Immunol 1985; 134:1896–901.

154. Wu D, Han SN, Meydani SN. Vitamin E (E) supplementation inhibits macrophage (Mϕ) cyclooxygenase (COX) activity of old mice. Am J Physiol, in press.

155. Meydani SN, Wu D, Santos MS, Hayek MG. Antioxidants and immune response in the aged: overview of present evidence. Am J Clin Nutr 1995; 62 (suppl):1462S–76S.

156. Watson RR, Prabhala RH, Plezia PM, Alberts DS. Effect of beta-carotene on lymphocyte subpopulations in elderly humans: evidence for a dose-response relationship. Am J Clin Nutr 1991; 53:90–4.

157. Santos MS, Leka LS, Ribaya-Mercado JD, Russell RM, Meydani M, Hennekens CH, et al. Short- and long-term β-carotene supplementation do not influence T cell-mediated immunity in healthy elderly. Am J Clin Nutr, in press.

158. Santos MS, Meydani SN, Leka L, Wu D, Fotouhi N, Meydani M, et al. Natural killer cell activity in elderly men is enhanced by β-carotene supplementation. Am J Clin Nutr 1996; 64:772–7.

159. Santos MS, Gaziano JM, Leka LS, Beharka AA, Hennekens CH, Meydani SN. β-carotene-induced enhancement of natural killer cell activity in elderly men is not explained by upregulation of individual cytokines. Am J Clin Nutr 1998; 67.

160. The Alpha-Tocopherol BCCPSG. The effect of vitamin E and beta carotene on the incidence of lung cancer and other cancers in male smokers. N Engl J Med 1994; 330:1029–35.

161. Omenn GS, Goodman GE, Thornquist MD, Balmes J, Cullen MR, Glass A, et al. Effects of a combination of β-carotene and vitamin A on lung cancer and cardiovascular disease. N Engl J Med 1996; 334:1150–5.

162. Hennekens CH, Buring JE, Mason JE, Stampfer M, Rosner B, Cook NR, et al. Lack of effect of long-term supplementation with β-carotene on the incidence of malignant neoplasms and cardiovascular disease. N Engl J Med 1996; 334:1145–9.

163. Beisel WR. Evaluation of publicly available scientific evidence regarding certain nutrient-disease relationships: 2. Zinc and immune function in the elderly. Life Sciences Research Office, Baltimore, Maryland, 1991.

164. Duchateau J, Delpesse G, Vrijens R, Collet H. Beneficial effects of oral zinc supplementation on the immune response of old people. Am J Med 1981; 70:1001–4.

165. Meydani SN. Micronutrients and immune function in the elderly. In: Bendich A, Chandra RK, eds, Micronutrients and Immune Functions, pp. 196–207. New York: New York Academy of Science, New York, 1990.

166. Fortes C, Forastiere F, Agabiti N, Fano V, Pacifici R, Virgili F, et al. The effect of zinc and vitamin A supplementation on immune response in an older population. J Am Geriatr Soc 1998; 46:19–26.

167. Cossack ZT. T-lymphocyte dysfunction in the elderly associated with zinc deficiency and subnormal nucleoside phosphorylase activity: effect of zinc supplementation. Eur J Cancer Clin Onco 1989; 25:973–6.

168. Ventura MT, Crollo R, Lasaracine E. In vitro zinc correction of natural killer activity in the elderly. Clin Exp Immunol 1986; 54:223–4.

169. Bracker MD, Hollingsworth JW, Saltman PD, Strause LG, Klauber

MR, Lugo NJ. Failure of dietary zinc supplementation to improve the antibody response to influenza vaccine. Nutr Res 1988; 8:99–104.

170. Remarke EJ, Witkamp L, Masure N, Lithgart GJ. Zinc supplementation does not enhance antibody formation to influenza virus vaccine in the elderly. Aging Immunol Immunopathol 1993; 4:17–23.

171. Wagner PA, Jernigan JA, Bailey LB, Nickens C, Brazzi GA. Zinc nutriture and cell-mediated immunity in the aged. Int J Vitam. Nutr Res 1983; 53:94–101.

172. Soltesz KS, Williford JJ, Renker LP, Meserve LA. Zinc nutriture and cell mediated immunity in institutionalized elderly. J Nutr Elder 1988; 8:3–17.

173. Bogden JD, Oleske JM, Lavenhar MA, Munves EM, Kemp FW, Bruening KS, et al. Zinc and immunocompetence in elderly people: Effects of zinc supplementation for 3 months. Am J Clin Nutr 1988; 48:655–63.

174. Bogden JD, Oleska JM, Lavenhar MA, Muneves EM, Kemp FW, Bruening KS, et al. Effects of one year of supplementation with zinc and other micronutrients on cellular immunity in the elderly. J Am Coll Nutr 1990; 9:214–25.

175. Kaplan J, Hess JW, Prasad AS. Impaired interleukin-2 production in the elderly: association with mild zinc deficiency. J Trace Elements Exp Med 1988; 1:3–8.

176. Meydani SN. Micronutrients and immune function in the elderly. Ann NY Acad Sci 1990; 587:196–207.

177. Prasad A, Fitzgerald JT, Hess JW, et al. Zinc deficiency in elderly patients. Nutrition 1993; 218–24.

178. Chandra RK. Excessive intake of zinc impairs immune responses. J Am Med Assoc 1984; 252:1443–6.

179. Kiremidjian-Schumacher L, Roy M. Selenium and immune function. Z Ernahrungswiss 1998; 37:50–6.

180. Peretz A, Neve J, Desmedt J, Duchateau J, Dramaix M, Famaey J-P. Lymphocyte response is enhanced by supplementation of elderly subjects with selenium-enriched yeast. Am J Clin Nutr 1991; 53:1323–8.

181. Bendich A. Antioxidant micronutrients and immune responses. Ann NY Acad Sci 1990; 587:168–80.

182. Meister A, Anderson ME. Glutathione. Ann Rev Biochem 1983; 52:711–60.

183. Fanger MW, Hart DA, Wells JV, Nisondoff A. Enhancement of reducing agents of the transformation of human and rabbit peripheral lymphocytes. J Immunol 1970; 130:362–4.

184. Lang CA, Naryshkin S, Schneider DL, Mills EJ, Linderman RD. Low blood glutathione levels in healthy aging adults. J Lab Clin Med 1992; 120:720–5.

185. Furukawa T, Meydani SN, Blumberg JB. Reversal of age-associated decline in immune responsiveness by dietary glutathione supplementation in mice. Mech Ageing Dev 1987; 38:107–17.

186. Chen TS, Richie JR, Lang CA. Life span profiles of glutathione and acetaminophen detoxification. Drug Metab Dispos 1990; 18:882–7.

187. Liu J, Mori A. Age-associated changes in superoxide dismutase activity, thiobarbituric acid reactivity, and reduced glutathione level in brain and liver senescence-accelerated mice (SAM): a comparison with ddY mice. Mech Aging Dev 1993; 71:23–30.

188. Uejima Y, Fukuchi Y, Teramoto S, Tabata R, Orimo H. Age changes in visceral content of glutathione in the senescence accelerated mouse (SAM). Mech Ageing Dev 1993; 67:129–39.

189. Abraham EC, Taylor JF, Lang CA. Influence of mouse age and erythrocyte age on glutathione metabolism. Biochem J 1978; 176:819–25.

190. Hazelton GA, Lang CA. Glutathione levels during the mosquito life span with emphasis on senescence. Proc Soc Exp Biol Med 1984; 176:249–56.

191. Trickler D, Shklar G, Schwartz J. Inhibition of oral carcinogenesis by glutathione. Nutr Cancer 1993; 20:139–44.

192. Dalhoff K, Ranek L, Mantoni M, Poulsen HE. Glutathione treatment of hepatocellular carcinoma. Liver 1992; 12:341–3.

193. Franklin RA, Li YM, Arkins S, Kelley KW. Glutathione augments in vitro proliferative responses of lymphocytes to Concanavalin A to a greater degree in old than in young rats. J Nutr 1990; 120:1710–17.

194. Liang CM, Lee N, Cattell D, Liang SM. Glutathione regulates interleukin-2 activity on cytotoxic T-cells. J Bio Chem 1989; 264:13,519–23.

195. Wu D, Meydani SN, Sastre J, Hayek M, Meydani M. In vitro glutathione supplementation enhances interleukin-2 production and mitogenic response of peripheral blood mononuclear cells from young and old subjects. J Nutr 1994; 124:655–63.

196. Shapiro AC, Wu D, Meydani SN. Eicosanoids derived from arachidonic and eicosapentaenoic acids inhibit T cell proliferative response. Prostaglandins 1993; 45:229–40.

197. Goodwin JS. Increased sensitivity to prostaglandin E_2 in old people. Prostagland Med 1979; 3:395–400.

198. Franklin RA, Arkins S, Li YM, Kelley KW. Macrophages suppress lectin-induced proliferation of lymphocytes from aged rats. Mech Ageing Dev 1993; 67:33–46.

199. Kavanagh TJ, Grossmann A, Jinneman JC, Kanner SB, White CC, Eaton DL, et al. The effect of 1-chloro-2,4-dinitrobenzene exposure on antigen receptor (CD3)-stimulated transmembrane signal transduction in purified subsets of human blood lymphocytes. Toxicol Appl Pharmacol 1993; 119:91–9.

200. Brown LAS. Glutathione protects signal transduction in type II cells under oxidant stress. Am J Physiol 1994; 266:L172–7.

201. Uken G. Immune dysregulation in aging: Role of NFkB. FASEB J 1994; 8:A753.

202. Jong SC, Birmingham JM. Medicinal and therapeutic value of the Shiitake mushroom. Adv Appl Microbiol 1993; 39:153–84.

203. Ha YL, Grimm NK, Pariza MW. Anticarcinogens from fried ground beef: heat-altered derivatives of linoleic acid. Carcinogenesis 1987; 8:1881–7.

204. Michal JJ, Chew BP, Schultz TD, Wong TS, Magnuson NS. Interaction of conjugated dienoic derivatives of linoleic acid with β-carotene on cellular host defense. FASEB J 1992; 6:A1102.

205. Cook ME, Miller CC, Park Y, Pariza M. Immune modulatyion by altered nutrient metabolism control of immune-induced growth depression. Poultry Sci. 1993; 72:1301–5.

206. Ha YL, Storkson J, Pariza MW. Inhibition of benzo(a)pyrene-induced mouse forestomach neoplasia by conjugated dienoic derivatives of linoleic acid. Cancer Res 1990; 50:1097–101.

207. Hayek MG, Han SN, Wu D, Watkins BA, Meydani M, Dorsey JL, et al. Dietary conjugated linoleic acid influences the immune response of young and old C57BL/6NIA mice, in preparation.

208. Meydani SN, Hayek MG, Wu D, Meydani M. Vitamin E and the Aging Immune Response. Recent Advances in Canine and Feline Nutrition. Volume II. 1998 Iams Nutrition Symposium Proceedings, 1998, pp. 295–303.

34 Role of Nutrition in Common Oral Diseases

CECILIA GORREL AND TIFFANY L. BIERER

INTRODUCTION

Oral diseases are extremely common in man and animals. In fact, animal dentistry is a rapidly expanding specialist area within veterinary medicine. The two most common conditions seen in man are dental caries and periodontal disease. Developmental lesions of the teeth (e.g., enamel hypoplasia) are not uncommon and have a multitude of causes. In our domesticated pets, the pathology seen encompasses the whole spectrum of problems as seen in man. Periodontal disease is, however, the most common oral condition seen in dogs and cats. Indeed, it is probably the single most common disease in small animal practice *(1)*.

Nutrition plays an important role in tooth formation and development, as well as in bone development and metabolism. It may also be involved in disease processes affecting the tooth and its supporting structures. It is well documented that an increased consumption of fermentable carbohydrates, especially simple sugars, plays an important role in the etiology and pathogenesis of caries. Although there is currently no known single nutrient, or combination of nutrients, that will prevent the development of periodontal disease, deficiencies of many nutrients are thought to be linked to the development and progression of both gingivitis and periodontitis.

This chapter will discuss the etiology and pathogenesis of common oral conditions and discuss the potential effects of nutritional factors on these conditions.

THE DENTITION

The dentition of the dog and cat resembles that seen in man. There are differences in tooth number and shape, but the basic anatomy is similar. Each tooth has a crown (above the gum) and one or more roots (below the gum). The bulk of the tooth is composed of dentine, which is covered by enamel on the crown and by cementum on the roots. The center of the tooth contains the pulp or endodontic system. Figure 1 depicts the basic structure of a tooth.

The crowns of dog and cat have teeth have a more tapered shape with sharp cutting edges and fewer chewing surfaces as

compared to human teeth. Also, the teeth are spaced further apart and where there is contact between teeth, the contact area is smaller and not as tight.

Man, dog and cat are diphyodont (i.e., primary [deciduous] teeth are followed by a permanent dentition). The respective dental formulas of the primary and permanent dentitions of man, dog and cat are depicted in Fig. 2.

The formation of the crown of both primary and permanent teeth occurs within the alveolar bone. Enamel formation is completed before the tooth erupts. Once the enamel has been formed, the ameloblasts (the cells that produce the enamel matrix) are lost and further development of enamel does not occur. The only natural form of repair that can occur to enamel after eruption is surface mineralization (i.e., through deposition of minerals, mainly from saliva, into the superficial enamel layer). Thus, when the tooth erupts, enamel formation is completed but dentine production is just beginning. Moreover, root development (i.e., growth in length and formation of a root apex) is by no means complete at the time of eruption. Figure 3 depicts maturation of a permanent tooth following eruption.

In man, tooth formation and maturation occurs over a prolonged period of time. The formation of the crowns of the primary teeth starts *in utero* and root development commences shortly after birth. The primary teeth start erupting during the first year of life, and by 2 yr of age, most children have a full set of primary teeth. However, root development of the primary teeth is not completed until 3 yr of age. The crowns of the permanent dentition start forming in the alveolar bone at around the time of birth. Between the age of 5.5 and 8.5 yr of age, the primary teeth start to exfoliate and are replaced by the permanent teeth. Permanent teeth eruption, with the exception of the third molar (wisdom tooth), is usually complete by 12 yr (± 18 mo) of age. The third molar tooth commonly erupts later in life. In some instances, one or more of the wisdom teeth do not erupt. Congenital absence of one or more wisdom teeth is also not uncommon.

In the dog and cat, tooth formation and maturation occurs over a much shorter period of time. The primary teeth start forming *in utero* and erupt between 3 and 12 wk of age. The permanent crowns start forming at or shortly after birth and mineralization of the crowns is complete by around 11 wk of age. Exfoliation of the primary teeth and replacement by the permanent dentition

From: *Nutrition and Immunology: Principles and Practice* (ME Gershwin et al. eds.), © Humana Press, Inc., Totowa, NJ

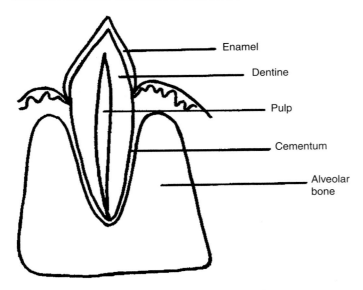

Fig. 1.   Basic structure of the tooth.

Man: Temporary teeth 2 ($I\frac{2}{2}$ $C\frac{1}{1}$ $P\frac{2}{2}$)   = 20

Permanent teeth 2 ($I\frac{2}{2}$ $C\frac{1}{1}$ $P\frac{2}{2}$ $M\frac{2(3)}{2(3)}$)   = 28-32

Dog: Temporary teeth 2 ($I\frac{3}{3}$ $C\frac{1}{1}$ $P\frac{3}{3}$)   = 28

Permanent teeth 2 ($I\frac{3}{3}$ $C\frac{1}{1}$ $P\frac{4}{4}$ $M\frac{2}{3}$)   = 42

Cat: Temporary teeth 2 ($I\frac{3}{3}$ $C\frac{1}{1}$ $P\frac{3}{2}$)   = 26

Permanent teeth 2 ($I\frac{3}{3}$ $C\frac{1}{1}$ $P\frac{3}{2}$ $M\frac{1}{1}$)   = 30

'I' represents incisors, 'C' represents canines, 'P' represents premolars, 'M' represents molars

Fig. 2.   Dental formulas of man, dog, and cat. Teeth can be recorded as a dental formula, which shows the number of teeth in the upper and lower jaws of one side of the head.

occurs between 3 and 7 mo of age in the dog and between 3 and 5 mo of age in the cat. Once the crowns of the permanent teeth have erupted, root development continues for several months.

ANATOMY OF THE TOOTH

As already mentioned, the tooth consists of enamel, dentine, cementum, and pulp. The detailed structure of these tissues will be discussed in the following subsections.

ENAMEL   Enamel is the hardest and most mineralized tissue in the body. It does not have a nerve or a blood supply. The inorganic content of mature enamel amounts to 96–97% by weight, the remainder being organic material and water *(2)*. The inorganic material consists of calcium hydroxyapatite crystals arranged in an orderly fashion at right angles to the tooth surface. The organic content is made up of soluble and insoluble proteins and peptides.

The enamel of dog and cat teeth is thinner than that of humans, generally being 0.2 mm in the cat and 0.5 mm in dogs, rarely exceeding 1 mm even at the tips of the teeth *(3)*, compared with up to 2.5 mm in man *(4)*.

DENTINE   The bulk of the tooth is made up of dentine, which is continuously deposited throughout life by odontoblasts lining the pulp system. The primary dentine is the layer that is present at tooth eruption. Throughout life, there is a slow continuous physiologial deposition of dentine, which is called secondary dentine. In response to trauma, dentine is laid down rapidly and in a less organized fashion. This type of dentine is called reparative or tertiary dentine.

The composition of dentine on a wet weight basis is 70% inorganic material, 18% organic material, and 12% water *(5)*. Because of the normal and progressive mineralization of dentine after the tooth is fully formed, the composition will vary depending on the age of the tooth. The inorganic portion of dentine consists mainly of calcium hydroxyapatite crystals, which are similar to those seen in cementum and bone, but smaller than the hydroxyapatite crystals in enamel. Other inorganic calcium salts, as well as trace elements such as fluoride, copper, zinc, and iron are also present. The organic portion consists mainly of collagen. Fractions of lipids, mucopolysaccharides, and other proteins are also present, as well as citric acid.

Dentine has a tubular structure. The tubules traverse the entire width of dentine, from the pulpal tissue to the dentino-enamel junction (DEJ) in the crown or the dentino-cementum junction (DCJ) in the root. They contain dentinal fluid and the cytoplasmic processes of the odontoblasts. The dentine tubules are more numerous and have a wider diameter closer to the pulp than toward the enamel or cementum surface. Exposed dentine tubules thus allow communication between the pulp and the external environment. The number of dentine tubules (20,000–40,000/mm^2) and diameter (tapering from 3 to 4 μm near the pulp to under 1 μm in the outer layer of dentine) are similar in cats, dogs, monkeys, and humans *(6)*. Dentinal tubules make up 20–30% of the volume of dentine.

CEMENTUM   Cementum, although part of the tooth, is classified as part of the periodontium and is discussed later in this chapter.

PULP   The pulp is composed of connective tissue liberally interspersed with tiny blood vessels, lymphatics, myelinated and unmyelinated nerves, and undifferentiated mesenchymal cells. As already mentioned, the pulp system is lined by odontoblasts, which produce dentine.

In the crown, the section containing the pulp is called the pulp chamber, and in the root(s), it is called in the root canal(s). The root canal opens into the periapical tissues at the root apex. The apical foramen of immature teeth is a single wide opening. As the individual ages, closure of the apex (apexogenesis) occurs by continuous deposition of dentine and cementum (Fig. 3) until, in mature teeth, the root apex consists of numerous small openings or foramina, allowing the passage of blood vessels, lymphatics, and nerves.

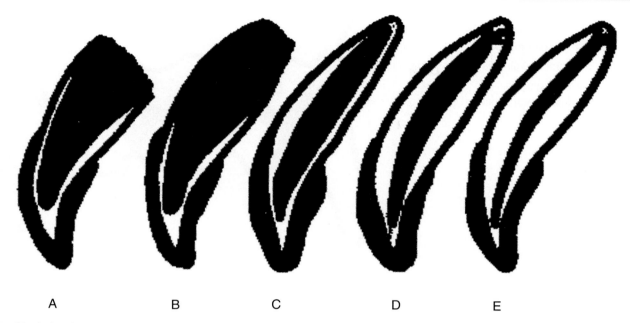

A   B   C   D   E

Fig. 3. Tooth development of an upper canine tooth in a dog. At 4 months (A), the crown has formed, with its full complement of enamel, but is usually still unerupted or just beginning to come through the gingiva. By 7 months (B), the root has elongated, which contributes to tooth eruption. The apex closes at approximately 12 months. Dentine deposition then continues throughout life, resulting in a progressively narrower pulp system. Cementum deposition also occurs throughout life, but at a much slower rate. C = 1.5 years of age; D = 2 years; E = 3.5 years.

ANATOMY OF THE PERIODONTIUM

The periodontium is an anatomical unit whose main functions are to attach the tooth to the jaw and provide a suspensory apparatus resilient to normal functional forces. It is made up of the gingiva, periodontal ligament, cementum, and alveolar bone (Fig. 4).

THE NORMAL GINGIVA   The normal gingiva surrounds the teeth and the marginal parts of the alveolar bone, forming a cuff around each tooth.

The gingiva (Fig. 5) can be divided into the free gingiva, which is closely adapted to the tooth surface, and the attached gingiva, which is firmly attached to the underlying periosteum of the alveolar bone. The attached gingiva is delineated from the oral mucosa by the muco-gingival line except in the palate where no such delineation exists. An interdental papilla is formed by the gingival tissues in the spaces between the teeth (the interproximal spaces).

The margin of the free gingivia is rounded in such a way that a small invagination or sulcus is formed between the tooth and the gingiva. The gingival sulcus is thus a shallow groove surrounding each tooth. The depth of the sulcus can be assessed by gently inserting a graduated periodontal probe until resistance is encountered. This resistance is taken to be the base of the sulcus. The depth from the free gingival margin to the base of the sulcus can thus be measured (Fig. 6a). In the periodontally healthy individual, the sulcus is 1–3 mm deep in man and dog and 0.5–1 mm in cats. Measurements in excess of these values usually indicates the presence of periodontitis when the periodontal ligament has been destroyed and alveolar bone resorbed, thus allowing the probe to be inserted to a greater depth. The term used to describe this situation is periodontal pocketing (Fig. 6b). Gingival inflammation resulting in swelling or hyperplasia of the free gingiva

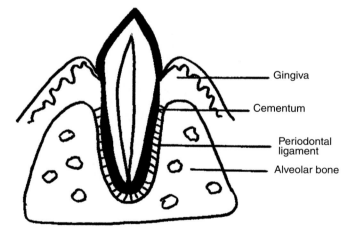

Fig. 4.   Anatomy of the periodontium.

will, of course, also result in measuring sulcus depths in excess of normal values. In these situations, the term pseudo-pocketing is used because the periodontal ligament and bone are intact and the increase in measurement is the result of swelling or hyperplasia of the gingiva (Fig. 6c).

The oral surface of the gingiva is lined by a parakeratinized squamous cell epithelium, the oral gingival epithelium. The gingival sulcus is lined by the oral sulcular epithelium. In addition to the sulcular epithelium closely apposed to the tooth surface but not attached to it, there is a thin layer of highly permeable epithelium adherent to the tooth surface called the epithelial attachment or

MGJ = Mucogingival junction or line.

AM = Alveolar mucosa

AG = Attached gingiva

FG = Free gingiva

IP = Interdental papilla

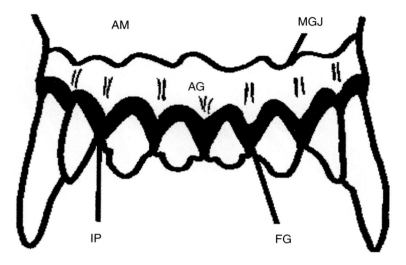

Fig. 5. The visible landmarks of clinically normal gingiva.

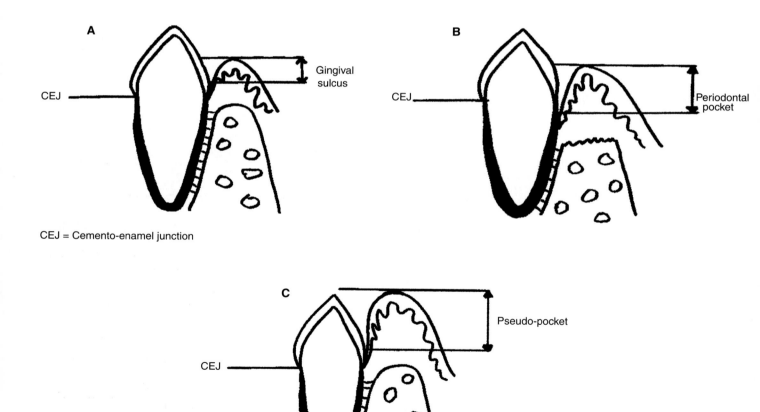

CEJ = Cemento-enamel junction

Fig. 6. **(A) Gingival sulcus.** The gingival sulcus is the narrow space between the sulcular epithelium and the enamel of the tooth. It can be measured using a periodontal probe. Note that the base of the junctional epithelium is normally at the cemento-enamel junction (CEJ). **(B) Periodontal pocket.** The junctional epithelium has migrated apically and now attaches on the root surface well below the CEJ. **(C) Pseudo-pocket.** The gingiva is hyperplastic, but the junctional epithelium is in its normal position.

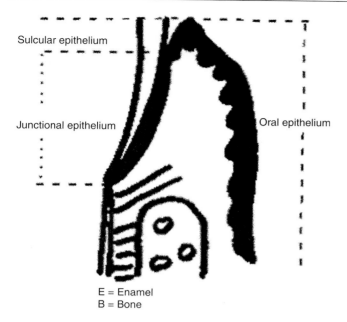

E = Enamel
B = Bone

Fig. 7. Anatomy of the gingival cuff.

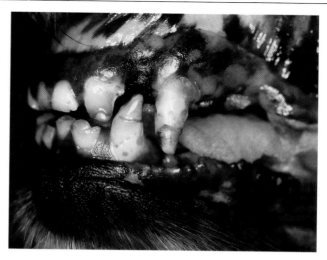

Fig. 8. Enamel hypoplasia in a dog. A number of factors may affect amelogenesis resulting in the formation of defective enamel. In this instance, the dog has a history of fever of unknown origin when it was around 4 wk of age, resulting in enamel hypoplasia of the cusps of several teeth. In the dog and cat, amelogenesis of the permanent dentition is completed by around 11 wk of age.

junctional epithelium (Fig. 7). Both the oral sulcular epithelium and the junctional epithelium are nonkeratinized squamous cell epithelia and have a very rapid cell turnover (5–8 d).

The gingival connective tissue is densely fibrous and firmly attached to the periosteum of the alveolar bone.

PERIODONTAL LIGAMENT The periodontal ligament is the connective tissue that attaches the root cementum to the alveolar bone. It acts as a suspensory ligament for the tooth and is in a continual stage of physiologic activity.

The collagen fibers within the ligament are arranged in functional groups. Individual fibers do not span the entire distance between bone and cementum; they branch and reunite in an interwoven pattern. All fibers follow a wavy course that allows for slight movement of the tooth and will absorb mild impact to the tooth.

CEMENTUM The cementum is an avascular bone-like tissue that covers the root surfaces. It does not contain Haversian canals and is, therefore, denser than bone. It is less calcified than enamel or dentine, but like dentine, cementum deposition is continuous throughout life. The initial thin layer of cementum is acellular. The continuous deposition is more marked at the apical area (toward the tip of the root) and is comprised of cellular cementum. Cementum is a very important component involved in tooth support, as it is capable of both resorptive and reparative processes. Resorption and apposition phenomena are, however, slower than in bone.

ALVEOLAR BONE The alveolar bone is composed of the ridges of the jaw that support the teeth. The roots of the teeth are contained in deep depressions, the alveolar sockets, in the bone. The alveolar bone develops during tooth eruption and undergoes atrophy with tooth loss. It responds readily to external and systemic influences. The usual response to stimuli results in resorption, but this may be accompanied by apposition in some situations.

Alveolar bone consists of four layers. In addition to the three layers found in all bones, namely periosteum, dense compact bone, and cancellous bone, there is a fourth layer, the cribriform plate,

that lines the alveolar sockets. Radiographically, this appears as a fine radiodense line called the lamina dura. The alveolar crest is normally located around 1 mm below the cemento-enamel junction (Fig. 4). Vessels and nerves run through the alveolar bone and perforate the cribriform plate. The majority of these blood and nerve vessels supply the periodontal ligament.

ENAMEL HYPOPLASIA

Enamel hypoplasia may be defined as an incomplete or defective formation of the organic enamel matrix of teeth.

In man, two basic types exist:

1. A hereditary type (many subclassifications based on the different modes of inheritance and clinical appearance). Both the primary and permanent dentition is affected and the defect is usually limited to the enamel. Some types show hypocalcification as well as hypoplasia of the enamel matrix.
2. A type caused by environmental factors. Either dentition may be involved, sometimes only a single tooth; both enamel and dentine are usually affected, at least to some degree.

Enamel hypoplasia results only if the injury occurs during the formative stage of enamel development (i.e., during amelogenesis). In animals, as well as in man, disease or trauma may affect amelogenesis. Affected teeth may appear normal at the time of eruption, but the porous enamel soon becomes discolored and flakes off sometimes. In more severe cases, the enamel is visibly deficient, discolored in patches, or partly missing already at the time of eruption (Fig. 8). The clinical significance of these defects is that exposed dentine is painful, particularly in young individuals in whom the dentine is relatively thin and the pulp thus proportionally larger than in mature teeth. These teeth do become less sensitive with increasing age as secondary dentine is lain down continuously by the pulp tissue, thus reducing the communication of the pulp with the external environment.

Environmental factors known to cause enamel hypoplasia in man are nutritional deficiency (vitamins A, C, and D, calcium, zinc, magnesium), exanthematous diseases (measles, scarlet fever, chicken pox), hypocalcemia, birth injury (permaturity, Rh hemolytic disease), local infection or trauma, ingestion of chemicals (chiefly fluoride), and idiopathic causes *(7)*.

There has been considerable controversy as to whether there is any relationship between enamel hypoplasia and dental caries. Clinical reports have given conflicting results. Most authors assume that the two are not related, although hypoplastic teeth do appear to decay at a more rapid rate once decay has started *(7)*.

DENTAL PLAQUE—THE PROBLEM

Plaque deposition on the tooth surfaces is the primary cause of periodontal disease and caries. Dental plaque is composed of aggregates of bacteria and their by-products, salivary components, oral debris, and occasional epithelial and inflammatory cells. The initial accumulation of plaque occurs supragingivally (on the tooth surfaces above the gingiva margin) but will extend into the sulcus and populate the subgingival region if left undisturbed.

The microbiota of the oral cavity is a complex ecological system. Nutrients and microbes are repeatedly introduced into and removed from the oral cavity. The flow of saliva is so high that the only organisms that can colonize the oral cavity are those that can adhere to surfaces within the cavity or that are in some other way retained. In addition to salivary flow, the flow of gingival fluid in the gingival sulcus, chewing, oral hygiene procedures, and desquamation of epithelial cells from the mucous membranes serve to remove bacteria from the oral surfaces. Some bacteria may be retained simply by obtaining refuge in pits and fissures of the teeth; others need to rely on specific mechanisms of adherence. The oral cavity contains several sites that will each support the growth of a particular type of microbial community. Enormous differences thus exist between the composition of the microbiota on the mucous membranes, the tongue, the teeth, and in the gingival sulcus.

The tooth surfaces are initially covered by the pellicle, which is a highly structured organic film derived from salivary glycoproteins (mucins). The pellicle alters the charge and free energy of the tooth surface, which increases the efficiency of bacterial adhesion. The bacterial flora together with salivary glycoproteins form the major components of plaque, which rapidly covers the tooth surface when no oral hygiene measures are performed.

Calculus (tartar) is mineralized plaque. Both supragingival and subgingival plaque become mineralized. Supragingival calculus is not thought to exert an irritant effect on the gingival tissues. In fact, it has been shown that under certain circumstances, a normal attachment may be seen between the junctional epithelium and calculus *(8)*. It has also been shown that sterilized calculus may be encapsulated in connective tissue without causing marked inflammation *(9)*. The main importance of calculus in periodontal disease seems to be its role as a retention surface for plaque; however, subgingival calculus may be more directly involved in the pathogenesis of periodontitis.

PERIODONTAL DISEASE

Periodontal disease is a collective term for a number of plaque-induced inflammatory reactions that affect the periodontium of the tooth. Gingivitis is inflammation of the gingiva (Fig. 9), which is reversible. Periodontitis is the term used when the inflammatory

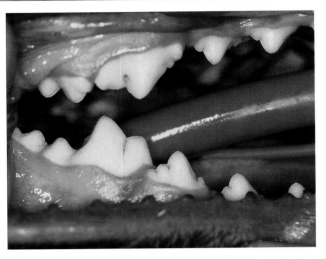

Fig. 9.   Generalized gingivitis in an 8-mo-old dog. This dog has never received any oral hygiene measures. The gingivae are inflamed (erythema and swelling) as a result of the undisturbed plaque accumulation. Note that plaque is not readily visible to the naked eye unless disclosed with a dye.

reactions also involve the periodontal ligament, root cementum, and alveolar bone (Fig. 10). The end result of periodontitis is loss of the tooth due to progressive destruction of its attachment apparatus.

Periodontal disease is one of the most common oral diseases seen in man and the most common oral disease in the dog and cat. The disease can cause discomfort to affected individuals. Moreover, there is mounting circumstantial evidence that periodontitis could lead to development of disease in other organs and tissues *(10)*. Consequently, prevention of periodontal disease is of importance for the general health and welfare of both man and companion animals.

ETIOLOGY AND PATHOGENESIS OF PERIDONTAL DISEASE   The primary cause of gingivitis and periodontitis is accu-

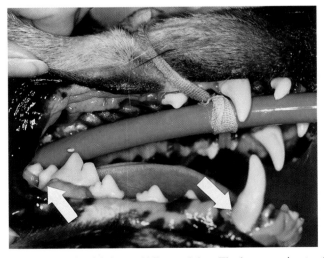

Fig. 10.   Periodontitis in a middle-aged dog. The lower canine tooth and the distal root of the lower first molar tooth (arrows) exhibit marked destruction of the periodontal ligament and alveolar bone in combination with gingival recession, thus exposing the root surfaces. These teeth could be maintained with regular oral hygiene measures.

mulation of plaque on the tooth surfaces. Calculus (tartar) is a secondary etiologic factor.

The pathogenesis of periodontal disease is by no means fully elucidated. The plaque bacteria and their products, as well as the inflammatory and immune reactions of the host, contribute to the destruction of the periodontium. The pathogenic mechanisms involved in periodontal disease include the following:

1. Direct injury by plaque micro-organisms
2. Indirect injury by plaque micro-organism via inflammation

Although numerous microbiological studies have been performed, the association between specific periopathogens and periodontitis remains to be conclusively proven, and it is not yet possible to state whether the microbiota found in deep periodontal pockets, where supporting structures have been destroyed, are the cause or an effect of periodontitis.

Many microbial products have little or no direct toxic effect on the host; instead, they possess the potential to activate nonimmune and immune inflammatory reactions. It is these inflammatory reactions that actually cause the tissue damage.

In many instances, disease progression may be an episodic occurrence rather than a continuous process. Tissue destruction occurs as acute bursts of disease activity followed by relatively quiescent periods. The acute burst is clinically characterized by rapid deepening of the periodontal pocket as a consequence of detachment of periodontal ligament fibers from root cementum and loss of alveolar bone. The quiescent phase is not associated with clinical or radiographic evidence of disease progression. Complete healing does not occur during this quiescent phase because subgingival plaque remains on the root surfaces and inflammation persists in the connective tissue. The inactive phase often lasts for extended periods of time.

Other conditions, such as physical or psychological stress and malnutrition, may impair protective responses, such as the production of antioxidants and acute-phase proteins, and can, as such, aggravate periodontitis but not cause destructive tissue inflammation *per se*. The effect of nutritional factors on periodontal disease is reviewed in detail as a separate section later in this chapter.

In summary, it is not yet possible to entirely account for the pathogenesis of periodontal disease. The dog has for the last 30 yr been used as the experimental model for human periodontal disease. Despite this, we still do not fully understand the mechanisms involved in disease development in either species. It is now well accepted, however, that *it is the host's response to the plaque bacteria rather than microbial virulence* per se *that directly causes the tissue damage (11).*

CLINICAL CONSIDERATIONS Undisturbed plaque accumulation will result in gingivitis. However, all animals with untreated gingivitis will not progress to periodontitis.

Clinically healthy gingivae (Fig. 11) can be maintained by frequent, usually daily, plaque removal. Animals with clinically healthy gingivae will not develop periodontitis. Untreated gingivitis will, in some individuals, progress to periodontitis. At our current level of knowledge, we cannot predict which individuals with gingivitis will develop periodontitis.

Conservative or cause-related periodontal therapy consists of professional periodontal therapy followed by the daily maintenance of oral hygiene. In individuals with clinically healthy periodontal tissues the goal is to prevent all gingivitis and, consequently, periodontitis. In individuals with gingivitis, the aim is

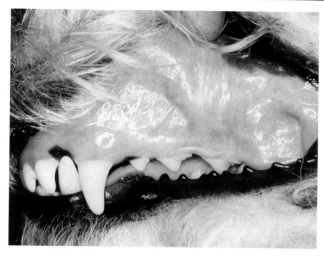

Fig. 11. Clinically healthy gingivae in a 9-yr-old dog. This dog has better periodontal health and hygiene than many human patients. The gingivae are pale pink and firmly attached to underlying structures. There is no sign of erythema, swelling, or bleeding on examination. This dog has had its teeth brushed daily since it was 5 mo of age. Thus, maintaining periodontal health in our pets is possible!

to restore the tissues to clinical health, and in individuals with established periodontitis lesions, the aim of therapy is to prevent progression of disease. Mechanical plaque control is the mainstay of periodontal disease prevention and therapy with adjunctive chemical plaque control being indicated in some situations.

CONTROL OF DENTAL PLAQUE Periodontal disease can be prevented by means of meticulous plaque control. Plaque control is also an integral part of caries prevention. In man, the single most effective means of removing plaque is frequent, preferably daily, toothbrushing. This has also been shown to hold true for the dog *(12,13)*.

Several recent studies have investigated mechanical means of reducing accumulation of dental deposits (plaque and calculus) via dietary texture *(14–17)* in the dog. These modified dry diets and dental hygiene chews do reduce the accumulation of plaque and calculus and also the severity of gingivitis. They do not maintain clinically healthy gingivae in the absence of toothbrushing. Moreover, it has yet to be demonstrated that reducing the severity of gingivitis will necessarily prevent the development of periodontitis. The relationship between dietary texture and the accumulation of plaque and development of gingivitis has not been clearly demonstrated in humans, although a link has been determined in dogs *(14–18)*. Several workers have investigated the effect of the daily addition of raw apples or carrots to the diet on gingival health in man. With the exception of one study *(19)* that showed a reduction in gingivitis, others showed no beneficial effect being derived from the addition of these foods *(20–22)*. It has been proposed that differences seen between studies in man and dogs may be the result of the different tooth anatomy (i.e., dog teeth are more tapered, which may allow for more efficient cleaning of the tooth surface through chewing). Although fibrous foods may help to remove plaque from chewing surfaces, the area around the gingival margin (the important area for the initiation of periodontal disease) is not efficiently cleansed by chewing.

Aside from mechanically cleaning the teeth, food that encourages chewing will also stimulate salivary flow. Saliva contains antibacterial agents that help keep the mouth clean. It has also been speculated that chewing helps strengthen the alveolar bone and periodontal ligament, thus reducing the risk of developing periodontitis. However, the evidence to support this theory is lacking.

Another point to consider concerning texture of the diet is the stickiness of a food product and the risk of developing caries. Foods like potato chips, which are high in starch carbohydrates and tend to stick to the teeth when eaten, provide a readily accessible substrate for cariogenic bacteria once the starches are broken down into sugars through enzymatic activity by the saliva.

Numerous chemical agents have been evaluated for the supplementation of patient-dependent mechanical plaque control. Clinically effective antiplaque agents are characterized by a combination of intrinsic antibacterial activity and good oral retention properties. Agents that have been evaluated include chlorhexidine, essential oils, triclosan, sanguinarine, fluorides, oxygenating agents, quaternary ammonium compounds, substituted amino alcohols, and enzymes. Of the above, the greatest effect on the reduction of plaque and gingivitis can be expected from chlorhexidine, essential oils, triclosan, and substituted amino alcohols. Antiplaque agents delivered from toothpastes, gels, or mouthrinses can augment mechanical oral hygiene to control the formation of supragingival plaque and the development of early periodontal disease. It must be emphasized that none of these agents will prevent gingivitis on their own (i.e., in the absence of mechanical plaque removal) (23,24). Moreover, all these agents are associated with adverse side effects. These effects vary according to the chemical agent and include poor taste, a burning and/or numbing of oral mucous membranes, staining of teeth and soft tissues, and allergic reactions. The use of chemical antiplaque agents should be seen as adjunctive to the mechanical removal of plaque by means of toothbrushing.

The incorporation of fluoride into toothpaste (as well as other means of delivering fluoride) has been of paramount importance in reducing the incidence of caries in man. The mechanisms of action of fluoride are discussed later in the chapter.

NUTRITIONAL INFLUENCES The primary cause of periodontal disease is the accumulation of plaque on the tooth surfaces. However, possible nutritional influences on the development and progression of disease may occur at several points, as shown in Fig. 12. The role of dietary texture as a mechanical means of plaque reduction has been discussed in **Subheading 7.3**. Other mechanisms by which nutrition may affect periodontal disease include the following:

1. *Antimicrobial action.* Many nutrients have antimicrobial activity. These may alter the quantity and/or quality of dental plaque, and thus be associated with a reduction in gingival inflammation.
2. *Anti-inflammatory effect.* Nutrients that decrease the host response to injury may result in a reduction in the severity of gingivitis and/or development and progression of periodontitis. These work by affecting the enzymes involved in the production of the anti-inflammatory compounds or by altering which compounds are actually produced.
3. *Immune system modification.* Some nutrients are thought to act as immune system modifiers in that they optimize the host's immune response so that the protective immune reactions outweigh the self-destructive ones. This could

also be accomplished by alteration of the permeability of the gingival epithelium, thus changing host resistance to bacterial products.
4. *Antioxidant effect.* Nutrients with an antioxidant action help maintain cell integrity by reducing the free-radical damage to host tissues that is initiated by the host's inflammatory and immune reactions. They also serve to protect the host from bacterial damage.

In the following, the most common nutrients and their possible role in periodontal disease will be discussed.

Protein/Energy Malnutritions Protein/energy malnutritions (PEM) are the most common nutritional diseases found in man and occur quite frequently in underdeveloped countries. Chronic, severe PEM can eventually lead to the development of other nutritional deficiencies. It has been noted in man and in other animals that PEM can result in a decrease in the quantity as well as the antibacterial properties of saliva, leading to increases in plaque accumulation on the tooth surfaces (25,26). Insufficient protein in the diet will also reduce the production of essential components of the immune system, resulting in an increased susceptibility to infections, which may include periodontal disease. Protein deficiencies have also been associated with increased loss of the periodontal ligament, osteoporosis of the alveolar bone, and delayed wound healing (27). However, experiments looking at the effects of protein supplementation on the development and progression of periodontal disease have been inconclusive (28).

Whereas the initial host responses in early periodontal disease are protective to the host and need to be maintained, the host's inflammatory and immune reactions in more advanced periodontal disease are actually self-destructive. Research with immune-compromised individuals suggests that although these individuals have a decreased ability to mount an adequate immune response to fight infections, this may actually provide a protective effect against developing periodontitis (29). The complicated balance between essential protective and self-destructive components of the host response makes modulation of the immune response as a method of reducing periodontal disease a difficult and perhaps impossible task.

Fats Evidence exists that nonsteroidal anti-inflammatory drugs (NSAIDS) can aid in reducing periodontal disease through reductions in gingival inflammation as well as decreases in alveolar bone loss (30,31). This effect is accomplished through inhibition of the cyclooxygenase fatty acid metabolic pathway, which, in normal metabolism of some essential fatty acids, can produce a series of prostaglandins that are inflammatory and can trigger bone resorption. Some polyunsaturated fatty acids (PUFAs), among which are the omega-3 fatty acids, can also affect inflammation through the cyclooxygenase pathway by production of an alternate series of prostagandins, which are, in general, less inflammatory. The effects of these fatty acids or other naturally occurring anti-inflammatory nutrients on gingival inflammation and alveolar bone loss warrant further investigation.

Vitamin C (Ascorbic Acid) Although deficiencies of several vitamins exhibit oral manifestations, only vitamin C deficiency is directly associated with the development of a specific form of peridontal disease, namely scorbutic gingivitis. It is characterized by swollen, bluish colored, bleeding gums and tooth loss. One of the main functions of ascorbic acid in the body is in the area of collagen synthesis. Defects in collagen synthesis are thought to be

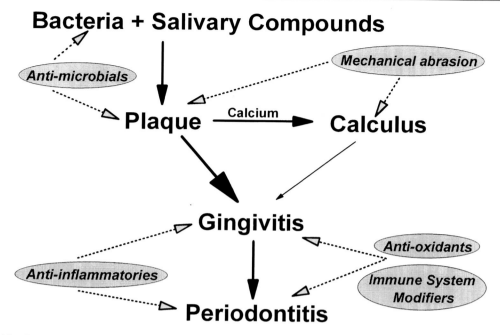

Fig. 12. Potential targets for nutritional influences on the progression and development of periodontal disease.

one of the main factors in the development of scorbutic gingivitis. Inverse relationships have also been seen between levels of vitamin C in gingival sulcular epithelium and permeability of that tissue *(32,33)*. Although adequate vitamin C intake will prevent scorbutic gingivitis, supplemental intakes above recommended levels, while shown to raise gingival sulcular epithelial vitamin C levels, have not been shown to prevent or reduce other forms of gingivitis or periodontitis *(34)*.

Vitamin A   Vitamin A deficiency is one of the most common nutritional deficiencies in the world. Vitamin A plays an integral role in vision and is also an important player in the maintenance and differentiation of epithelial cells, making it critical for those cells with a rapid turnover rate.

There are several factors that indicate that vitamin A may be important for the prevention of periodontal disease. First, the gingival sulcular epithelium and the junctional epithelium, which play a critical role in the initiation and progression of the disease, both have a very rapid turnover rate and adequate levels of vitamin A would be important for their maintenance and differentiation. Of further importance is that the vitamin also plays a role in the differentiation of immune cells, and deficiency is often associated with a decreased resistance to infection. Vitamin A also plays a role in normal bone metabolism and deficiencies have been associated with alveolar bone loss *(35)*. Finally, there is evidence to indicate that the vitamin has a coenzyme role in the formation of glycoproteins which contribute to the formation of dental plaque.

Epidemiological studies in man have seen a possible weak association between serum vitamin A levels and periodontal disease *(36)*. The main problem with many of these studies is that serum vitamin A levels are a poor indicator of vitamin A status unless the individual is severely deficient. However, in animals with severe vitamin A deficiency, increases in both gingivitis and periodontitis have been recorded *(35)*, although the methods used to diagnose disease have not always been strictly accurate. As with vitamin C,

supplemental intakes above recommended levels have not been shown to prevent or reduce gingivitis or periodontitis.

Folic Acid   Folic acid plays a role in the synthesis of DNA. It is therefore, like vitamin A, a particularly important nutrient for those cells in the body that have a high rate of turnover, such as the gingival sulcular epithelium and junctional epithelium. Such cells would theoretically be more sensitive to a mild folic acid deficiency.

Studies in man and animals have shown that deficiencies in folic acid may increase the permeability of the oral mucosa and, more specifically, the gingival sulcular epithelium *(37,38)*. This would affect the animal's exposure to plaque bacteria and their products on the tooth surfaces.

Women who are pregnant or taking oral contraceptives are reported as having an increased incidence and severity of gingivitis. This has been attributed to an increased permeability of the gingiva sulcular epithelium, possible the result of decreases in folate levels also associated with these conditions. However, the nutritional status of other nutrients such as vitamin A, zinc, and vitamin C can also be affected by oral contraceptive use and pregnancy. Supplementation of women with folic acid during pregnancy and when taking oral contraceptives has shown improvements in gingivitis even though most of these women exhibited serum folacin levels within normal ranges *(37,39)*. This suggests a possible end-organ deficiency of folic acid in the gingival tissues of women in these conditions. The use of folic acid supplementation for periodontal disease prevention warrants further investigation.

Vitamin D, Calcium, and Phosphorus   Adequate intake of calcium, phosphorus, and vitamin D are essential for the development and maintenance of bone, including alveolar bone. In man and animals, a calcium-deficient diet will result in low extracellular calcium levels and hypocalcemia. This triggers release of parathyroid hormone, which promotes resorption of calcium from the

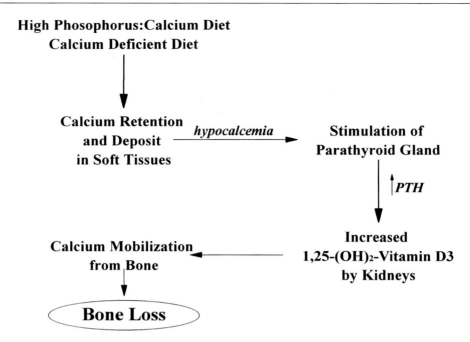

High Phosophorus:Calcium Diet
Calcium Deficient Diet

Calcium Retention   *hypocalcemia*   **Stimulation of**
and Deposit   **Parathyroid Gland**
in Soft Tissues

                                                          ↑*PTH*

Calcium Mobilization   **Increased**
from Bone   **1,25-(OH)₂-Vitamin D3**
                                                         by Kidneys

Bone Loss

Fig. 13. Nutritional secondary hyperparathyroidism. A low calcium or a high phosphorus : calcium ratio in the diet can result in nutritional secondary hyperparathyroidism. A rise in parathyroid hormone (PTH) coupled with 1,25-(OH)²-vitamin D3 induces calcium resorption from bone. Alveolar bone will also be lost in this condition.

bone in an attempt to raise extracellular calcium levels. In the dog, alveolar bone has been shown to be especially susceptible to resorption *(40)*. This condition is classified as nutritional secondary hyperparathyroidism and can also be induced by a deficiency of vitamin D (Fig. 13).

Excess phosphorus in the diet can also result in secondary hyperparathyroidism. The optimal ratio of calcium to phosphorus is believed to be approximately 1 : 1. A low ratio, as with a high-phosphorus diet, has been shown in animals to cause increases in bone resorption. In humans, a high-phosphorus diet has not been conclusively shown to cause increased bone resorption as long as calcium intake is adequate *(41)*.

In dogs and cats with hyperparathyroidism, a distinct pattern of bone loss is consistently seen. The first bone affected is the mandible, followed by the maxilla, then the other bones of the skull, the axial skeleton, and then, finally, the long bones of the limb. Before the rest of the skeleton is affected, the bones of the jaws may be severely demineralized, which is evident clinically as softening, hence commonly referred to as "rubber jaw." The bone will remineralize if the nutritional deficiency is corrected. Hyperparathyroidism does not cause periodontitis. It will, however, exacerbate bone loss and exfoliation of teeth in animals with plaque-induced periodontitis.

Antioxidants   As discussed in previous chapters in this book, the intake and serum levels of antioxidant nutrients have been associated with reduced risks of many diseased states. Although there is no evidence to suggest that increased intakes of these nutrients are associated with a decreased risk of periodontal disease, it is known that several antioxidant nutrients and enzymes are present in the sulcular epithelium and gingival crevicular fluid. Some of the nutrients that influence an individual's oxidative status include vitamin C, vitamin E, zinc, copper, manganese, and selenium. Antioxidant enzymes include glutathione peroxidase

and superoxide dismutase. It is not surprising that these antioxidants are found in the oral epithelium and secretions considering the responses elicited by the host against pathogenic oral bacteria. These antioxidant compounds are essential for helping to maintain cell integrity by reducing free-radical damage to the gingival tissues that is initiated by the host's inflammatory and immune responses. In PEM, antioxidant levels in the serum have been shown to be dramatically decreased *(42)*, which may result in increased tissue damage throughout the body. The role and supplemental use of antioxidant nutrients in the maintenance of oral health warrants further investigation.

Essential Oils, Herbs, and Other Phytonutrients   There are several oils (tea tree, eucalyptus, and clove) that have known antimicrobial properties, and their use is currently being promoted in dental hygiene products. Although they may be efficacious as antimicrobial agents, there is limited knowledge about the true efficacy and safety of these compounds in the oral cavity. Even less information is available about their safety and efficacy than in animals other than humans. This is also true in regard to the vast majority of herbs (yucca, echinacea) and phytonutrients (polyphenols, carotenoids, tannins) which are thought to have immune modifying or antioxidant properties. Basic research investigating the effectiveness and especially the safety of these compounds is required before they can be justified for use in the prevention or treatment of periodontal disease.

Summary   Research to date shows that deficiencies of several nutrients have an effect on the development and progression of periodontal disease. On the other hand, there is no conclusive evidence that supplementation of any nutrient above and beyond required levels has an effect on the development of periodontal disease. Interestingly, the development of periodontal disease can have a profound effect on nutritional status of the individual. Pain and loss of teeth can affect the emotional well-being of the individual and will also affect the food choices made. This can, in itself, result in the development of nutritional deficiencies and/or severe malnutrition, which are even more detrimental to the affected individual.

It should be emphasized that there is no known nutritional intervention that can be used as a substitute for daily toothbrushing and regular dental checkups. Balanced nutrition should be used in conjunction with an effective dental hygiene program to reduce the risk of developing periodontal disease.

CARIES

Caries or dental decay is also primarily caused by plaque accumulation on the tooth surfaces. The disease is common in man. It does occur, but is less common, in the dog and it has not been reported in the cat. Dental caries can occur on any exposed tooth surface (i.e., crown and/or root).

ETIOLOGY AND PATHOGENESIS In simple outline, dental caries occurs as plaque bacteria (notably *Streptococcus* and *Lactobacillus* species) and metabolizes fermentable carbohydrates, producing organic acids such as lactic, acetic, and proprionic acids. These acids diffuse through the plaque into the enamel and dissolve mineral (calcium and phosphate). If mineral diffuses out of the tooth and into the oral environment, then demineralization occurs. If the process is reversed, the mineral goes back into the tooth and the damaged crystals are rebuilt; then we have remineralization. Caries occurs when demineralization exceeds remineralization. Frequent consumption of a diet rich in easily fermentable carbohydrates, in combination with inadequate plaque control, will result in a situation in which demineralization dominates and enamel substance is progressively lost. Once the dentine becomes involved, the process is irreversible and accelerates as an organic decay and will eventually involve the pulp tissue. Inflammation of the pulp is called pulpitis. Untreated chronic pulpitis often progresses to pulpal necrosis. Both chronic pulpitis and pulpal necrosis can induce a variety of inflammatory lesions in the alveolar bone surrounding the apex (the periapical region). These periapical lesions (Fig. 14) include granuloma, cyst, or abscess formation. In some instances, osteomyelitis of the jaw bone can occur as a consequence of a chronically inflamed or necrotic pulp.

Dental decay can occur on any exposed tooth surface. Most research has concentrated on enamel caries. Caries does, however, also occur on exposed root surfaces. Research into the etiology, epidemiology, and pathogenesis of root caries is rather limited. Bacterial penetration of the dentine tubules occurs early but tends not to extend deeply into the tissue and only progresses slowly with minor accompanying inflammatory reactions in the pulp. No specific micro-organism species, such as *Streptococcus* and *Lactobacillus* species implicated in enamel caries, has been incriminated convincingly in root caries, although the *Actinomyces* species have attracted considerable interest. The optimal preventive measures have not been determined, although as with enamel caries prevention, the importance of plaque removal has been cited. It has been shown that frequent professional cleaning, coupled with a high standard of plaque control, is capable of almost totally preventing the development of root surface caries.

CLINICAL CONSIDERATIONS The initial inorganic demineralization of the enamel can be halted as long as the process has not reached the enamel–dentine junction. Meticulous dental hygiene in combination with topical fluoride treatment can lead to remineralization of the initial defect.

In the dog, caries is very rarely diagnosed at the early enamel demineralization stage. Moreover, the type of dental care required to halt the process is not usually practically feasible. Consequently, diagnosed caries in the dog is usually an indication for restorative dentistry. If pulpal pathology is present (Fig. 15), then endodontic therapy prior to restoration is required, but if too much tooth structure has been lost, extraction may be necessary.

DIETARY AND NUTRITIONAL INFLUENCES The role of diet and nutrition in the etiology and pathogenesis of caries may be viewed as systemic and local effects.

Systemic Effects Nutritional factors may have an effect on the following:

1. The morphology of the teeth
2. The quality of the dental hard tissues
3. The quality of saliva

It is well known that teeth with deep, narrow fissures and marked pits and grooves are more susceptible to caries than those with fewer plaque-retentive areas. The morphology of the tooth is largely determined by genetic factors, but animal studies have shown that they can be influenced by gross nutritional imbalances of protein, fat, and carbohydrate (43). In man, there are no such data available and it seems unlikely that changes in the anatomy of the teeth caused by nutritional imbalances of protein, fat, or carbohydrate play a significant role in the etiology or pathogenesis of caries.

As already mentioned, nutritional deficiencies result in enamel hypoplasia. However, hypoplastic teeth have not been shown to be more prone to caries than normal teeth.

The quality of the hard tissues of the tooth can be influenced by nutrition. These changes may be of importance for caries development and progression. In animal studies, it has been shown that feeding the females a diet high in sugar during pregnancy and lactation will result in changes in the offspring's dental tissues, namely higher levels of carbonate, mucopolysaccharides, and carbohydrates in the enamel, which later in life made them more susceptible to caries. Feeding a diet high in protein to females during pregnancy and lactation resulted in offspring with lower levels of carbonate, mucopolysaccharides, and carbohydrates in the enamel. These animals were found to be more resistant to caries (43).

Studies have linked the dietary changes in Europe during World War II with a drastic reduction in the incidence of caries during those years (44,45). The main dietary changes during the war were a marked reduction in per capita calorie intake, a marked decrease in the ingestion of protein, fat, and milk products, an increase in the consumption of vegetables, especially root crops such as turnips and beets, and a reduction in sugar and sweet consumption. In the years immediately after the war, the caries incidence in children whose teeth had been developing during the times of these dietary changes remained low (45) despite the fact that their diet returned to prewar status. In man, a low carbonate content in the enamel is also associated with decreased susceptibility to caries. The fact that the carbonate content of the enamel of teeth mineralized during the war was low has been used by some investigators to explain the lag in the increase of the caries frequency seen after the war.

Thus, in man and animals, nutrition will affect the composition

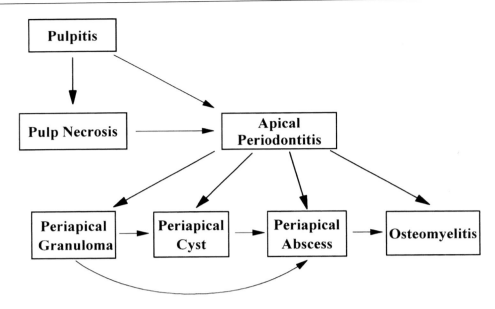

Fig. 14.   Summary of pulp and periapical pathophysiology.

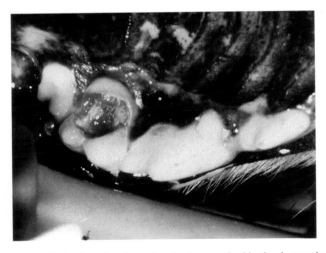

Fig. 15.   Caries in a dog. Dental caries has resulted in the destruction of most of the occlusal surface of the upper first molar. The process has invaded the pulp, which is exposed and inflamed. Treatment at this stage is extraction of a periodontally sound tooth.

of the dental hard tissues. However, these changes are considered to be of secondary importance to other factors involved in caries development and progression.

Nutrition may also affect the quality of the saliva. The main influence is the effect on the buffering capacity of saliva. It has been shown in man that individuals on a lacto-vegetarian, high-protein, or high-fat diet produce saliva with a high buffering capacity, whereas individuals on a high-carbohydrate diet produce saliva with a lower buffering ability *(43)*. This reduction in buffering capacity is associated with a reduction in the carbonate content of the saliva with high carbohydrate ingestion. The significance

of these nutritional effects on salivary quality in the etiology of caries are unclear.

Local Effects   The local effects of diet and nutrition are more important in the development and progression of caries than the systemic effects. Numerous studies have shown that frequent consumption of rapidly diffusing and easily fermentable sugars, primarily sucrose, leads to the formation of large quantities of a plaque, which is rich in polyglycans and contains large numbers of acid-producing *Streptococci, Lactobacillus,* and yeasts *(46–50)*. The frequent intake of meals and snacks rich in sucrose will favor colonization of the tooth surfaces by the most aggressive of the cariogenic bacteria, namely *Streptococcus mutans.* Under these circumstances, *Streptococcus mutans* will not only colonize retention surfaces on the tooth such as occlusal fissure but also the smooth surfaces that are otherwise less readily colonized by oral bacteria.

The critical pathogenic mechanism in human caries is the rapid acid production by plaque bacteria while fermenting various food substrates. This acid production causes a drop in pH in the dental deposits and an acid attack on the tooth surface. During the acid attack, the enamel is demineralized. The severity and duration of the acid attack is more extensive if the plaque accumulation is thick and rich in bacteria. It also increases in severity and duration in direct relation to a rising concentration of sugar in plaque and saliva. Thus, a frequent intake of sugars will induce a prolonged and intense acid attack on the tooth surfaces. Moreover, the time available for remineralization is thus decreased.

The texture of the diet is also important, both for salivary secretion and elimination of fermentable carbohydrates from the oral cavity. A diet that requires thorough chewing will result in the secretion of large amounts of saliva with a high pH and a strong buffering capacity. The same effect on salivary flow and composition can be achieved with sour or bitter substances. In contrast, a finely textured diet that requires little mastication tends to be retained in the oral cavity and eliminated slowly.

In contrast to many other health problems associated with a high-fat diet, an inverse relationship between percentage of fat in the diet and the development of caries has been identified. High levels of fat in the diet binds to various sugars in the diet, thus reducing their solubility *(51)*. The result is a lower drop in pH and weaker acid attacks. Fat is also thought to have a local protective effect on the tooth surfaces.

In addition to fluoride, which has a strong anticaries effect, other trace elements and organic compounds such as theobromine, vanilline, phytates, and polyphenols have been reported to have a protective effect against dental caries.

In Summary The microflora of the oral cavity and the local effects of diet are the two most important aspects in the etiology and pathogenesis of dental caries. Local nutritional effects influence the quantity and quality of the dental plaque formed, as well as its microflora. The frequent intake of sucrose results in the formation of a thick plaque, rich in cariogenic bacteria. The replacement of sucrose by nonfermentable or slowly fermentable sweetening agents (e.g., under experimental conditions, sorbitol has drastically reduced the incidence of caries in both man and animals) *(52–54)*.

THE ROLE OF FLUORIDE Fluoride is used extensively in human dentistry mainly because of its anticaries effect. To achieve this effect, it has been administered either systemically (water fluoridation, fluoride tablets) or topically (fluoride toothpastes, varnishes, gels). It must, however, be remembered that fluoride is a potentially hazardous substance. Systemic intake of large doses, or chronic ingestion of smaller doses, can result in a variety of side effects such as acute gastric and renal disturbances, dental and skeletal fluorosis, or even death *(55,56)*. The main source of fluoride is in the drinking water, but various portions of the fluoride applied for topical uses are, however, swallowed and subsequently absorbed.

For many years, it was thought that the incorporation of fluoride into the apatite-like enamel crystals during their development, making the crystal more resistant to subsequent acid attack after the tooth had erupted, was the most important mode of action. Today, we know that caries reduction in humans is not dependent on systemic fluoride administration or having high levels of fluoride in sound enamel. It is now well accepted that the caries reduction is predominantly affected by fluoride being present during active caries development at the plaque–enamel interface where it will directly alter the dynamics of mineral dissolution and reprecipitation (i.e., reduce/inhibit demineralization and enhance remineralization) *(57)*. A regime using high-frequency topical application of low fluoride concentrations is, therefore, the present recommendation.

Fluoride treatment will not, of itself, arrest caries lesion development and progression of every caries-susceptible site in all individuals. The causative agent, the microbial plaque, has to be removed and patients made to understand the importance of proper oral hygiene. If oral hygiene is combined with dietary modification (reduction in the frequency of easily fermentable carbohydrate intake) and a selective use of fluoride therapy (frequent topical application of a low concentration of fluoride), a total arrest of caries can be achieved in most, otherwise healthy individuals.

The role of fluorides in prevention and treatment of root caries remains unclear, although its cariostatic effect can be ascribed almost entirely to its topical effect on the ongoing caries processes *(57)*. It is possible to reharden even extensive active root caries

lesions and so avoid the need to restore such surfaces by means of topical fluoride application.

There is no conclusive evidence that the fluoride ion has any benefit in preventing gingivitis. Stannous fluoride is an exception to this and does possess an antiplaque effect *(58)*. This effect is almost certainly derived from the stannous rather than the fluoride ion. Other metal ions, including zinc and copper also have a moderate quantitative effect on plaque accumulation, although additional qualitative effects on plaque may occur *(59)*.

In veterinary dentistry, fluoride administration has been recommended for the treatment of a number of conditions ranging from caries to periodontal disease. Topical application of fluoride preparations in the treatment of caries is certainly beneficial. There is, however, no good evidence that fluoride plays a useful role in the management of periodontal disease. Thus, although topical fluoride is theoretically of benefit in veterinary dentistry, there is the complication that our pets will swallow the fluoride-containing agents and have a variable and relatively uncontrolled systemic administration, which may result in fluoride toxicity. The use of professionally applied varnishes and gels associated with a moderate rise in plasma fluoride concentrations may well be safer than daily use of fluoride-containing toothpastes in the dog and cat.

SUMMARY

Periodontal disease is one of the most common diseases in man and pets. It is a collective term for plaque-induced inflammatory conditions affecting the periodontium. Gingivitis is a reversible inflammation of the gingiva, whereas periodontitis results in irreversible destruction of the supporting structures and eventual tooth loss. The primary cause of periodontal disease is accumulation of plaque on the tooth surfaces, resulting in inflammatory responses by the host. Toothbrushing is the most effective means of regular plaque removal. Dietary texture has been shown to influence accumulation of dental deposits in the dog, although such a link has not been established in man. Nutritional deficiencies have been shown to affect periodontal disease primarily by altering the host response to plaque, but no nutrient will prevent disease development or progression. Supplementation of nutrients has not been shown to affect disease, although several, including folic acid and vitamin C, warrant further investigation.

Caries is common in man and does occur in the dog. The development of caries is directly linked with the frequent consumption of a diet containing easily fermentable carbohydrate (notably simple sugars) in combination with poor oral hygiene. Frequent plaque removal, reduction in the frequency of consumption of easily fermentable carbohydrates, and frequent topical application of low concentration fluoride preparations will prevent caries in most individuals.

Thus, although diet alone marginally affects common oral diseases, the combination of a well-balanced diet, regular dental examinations and cleanings, and a good home dental hygiene program will reduce the risk of developing periodontal disease and caries in man and animals.

REFERENCES

1. Gorrel C, Robinsonn J. Periodontal therapy and extraction technique. In: Crossley, DA, Penman S, eds, Manual of Small Animal Dentistry, pp. 139–49. British Small Animal Veterinary Association, U.K., 1995.
2. Fejerskov O, Thylstrup A. Dental enamel. In: Mjör IA, Fejerskov O,

eds, Histology of the Human Tooth, 2nd ed, pp. 75–103. Munksgaard, Copenhagen, 1979.

3. Crossley DA. Results of a preliminary study of enamel thickness in the mature dentition of domestic dogs and cats. J Vet Dent 1995; 12(3):111–3.

4. Schroeder HE. Oral Structural Biology. Thieme, New York, 1991.

5. Mjör IA. Dentin and Pulp. In: Mjör IA, Fejerskov O, eds, Histology of the Human Tooth, 2nd ed, pp. 43–74. Munksgaard, Copenhagen, 1979.

6. Ahlberg K, Brännström M, Edwall L. The diameter and number of dentinal tubules in rat, cat, dog and monkey. A Comparative Scanning Electron Microscope Study. Acta Odont Scand 1975; 33:234.

7. Shafer WG, Hine MK, Levy BM. Developmental disturbances of oral and paraoral structures. In: Shafer WG, Hine MK, Levy BM, eds, A Textbook of Oral Pathology 3rd ed, pp. 2–80. W.B. Saunders, Philadelphia, 1974.

8. Fitzgerald R.J., McDaniel EG. Dental calculus in the germ free rat. Arch Oral Biol 1960; 2:239–40.

9. Allen DL, Kerr DA. Tissue response in the guinea pig to sterile and non-sterile calculus. J Periodontol 1965; 36:121–6.

10. DeBowes LJ, et al. Association of periodontal disease and histologic lesions in multiple organs from 45 dogs. J Vet Dent 1996; 13(2):57–60.

11. Kinane DF, Lindhe J. Pathogenesis of periodontitis. In: Lindhe J, Karring T, Lang NP, eds, Clinical Periodontology and Implant Dentistry, 3rd ed, pp. 189–225. Munksgaard, Copenhagen, 1997.

12. Troomp JA, Jansen J, Pilot T. Gingival health and frequency of tooth-brushing in the beagle dog model. Clinical findings. J Clin Periodontol 1986; 13:164–8.

13. Tromp JA, van Rijn LJ, Jansen J. Experimental gingivitis and frequency of tooth-brushing in the beagle dog model. Clinical findings. J Clin Periodontol 1986; 13:190–4.

14. Logan EI. Oral cleansing by dietary means: results of six-month studies. Proceedings of a Conference on Companion Animal Oral Health, University of Kansas, 1996.

15. Gorrel C, Rawlings JM. The role of a "dental hygiene chew" in maintaining periodontal health in dogs. J Vet Dent 1996; 13(1):31–4.

16. Gorrel C, Rawlings JM. The role of tooth-brushing and diet in the maintenance of periodontal health in dogs. J Vet Dent 1996; 13(3):139–43.

17. Gorrel C, Rawlings J, Markwell P. Effect of two dietary regimens on gingivitis in the dog. J Small Anim Pract 1997; 38:147–51.

18. Egelberg J. Local effect of diet on plaque formation and development of gingivitis in dogs. I: effect of hard and soft diets. Odont Rev 1965; 16:31–41.

19. Slack GL, Martin WJ. Apples and dental health. Br Dent J 1958; 105:366–71.

20. Lindhe J, Wicen PO. The effects on the gingivae of chewing fibrous foods. J Periodontol Res 1969; 4:193–201.

21. Reece JA, Swallow JN. Carrots and dental health. Br Dent J 1970; 128:535–9.

22. Longhurst P, Berman DS. Apples and gingival health; repeat on a feasibility study. Br Dent J 1973; 134:475–9.

23. Matsson L, Klinge B, Willard LO, Attstrom R, Edwardsson S. The effect of Octapinol on dento-gingival plaque and development of gingivitis. II. Long term studies in beagle dogs. J Periodontal Res 1983; 18:438–44.

24. Hamp SE, Lindhe J, Joe H. Long term effect of chlorhexidine on developing gingivitis in the Beagle dog. J Periodont Res 1973; 8:63–70.

25. Johansson I, Ericson T. Biosynthesis of a salivary bacteria-agglutinating glycoprotein in the rat during protein deficiency. Caries Res 1992; 21:7–14.

26. Johansson I, Ericson T, Steen L. Studies of the effect of diet on saliva secretion and caries development; the effect of fasting on saliva composition of female subjects. J Nutr 1984; 114:2010–20.

27. Chawla TN, Glickman I. Protein deprivation and the periodontal structures of the albino rat. Oral Surg Oral Med Oral Pathol 1951; 4:578–602.

28. Cheraskin E, Ringsdorf WM Jr, Setyaadmadja ATSH, Barrett RA. An ecologic analysis of gingival state: effect of prophylaxis and protein supplementation. J Periodont 1968; 39:316–20.

29. Alfano MC. Controversies, perspectives and clinical implications of nutrition in periodontal disease. Dent Clin North Am 1976; 20:519–48.

30. Offenbacher S, Williams RC, Jeffcoat MK, et al. Effects of NSAIDs on beagle crevicular cyclo-oxygenase metabolites and periodontal bone loss. J Periodont Res 1992; 27:207–13.

31. Howell TH, Williams RC. Nonsteroidal anti-inflammatory drugs as inhibitors of periodontal disease progression. Crit Rev Oral Biol Med 1993; 177–95.

32. Alvares O, Siegel I. Permeability of the gingival sulcular epithelium in the development of scorbutic gingivitis. J Oral Pathol 1981; 10:40–48.

33. Mallek H. An investigation of the role of ascorbic acid and iron in the etiology of gingivitis in humans. Doctoral theses, Institute archives, Massachusetts Institute of Technology, 1978.

34. Woolfe SN, Kenney EB, Hume WR, Carranza FA. Relation between ascorbic acid levels in blood and ginngival tissue with response to periodontal therapy. J Clin Periodont 1984; 11:159–65.

35. Shaw JH. The relation of nutrition to periodontal disease. J Dent Res 1962; 41:264–74.

36. Russell AL. International nutrition surveys; a summary of preliminary dental findings. J Dent Res 1963; 42:233–44.

37. Vogel RI, Deasy M, Alfano M, Schneider L. The effect of folic acid on gingival health in women taking oral contraceptives. J Prev Dent 1980; 6:221–31.

38. Dreizen S, Levy B, Bernick S. Studies on the biology of the periodontium of marmosets. VIII. The effect of folic acid deficiency on marmoset oral mucosa. J Dent Res 1970; 49:616–20.

39. Pack A, Thomson M. Effects of topical and systemic folic acid supplementation and gingivitis in pregnancy. J Clin Periodont 1980; 7:402–14.

40. Henrickson PA. Periodontal disease and calcium deficiency. An experimental study in the dog. Acta Odont Scand 1968; 26(50):1–132.

41. Spencer H, Kramer L, Osis D. Do protein and phosphorus cause calcium loss? J Nutr 1988; 118:657–60.

42. Huang CJ, Fwu ML. Degree of protein deficiency affects the extent of the depression of the anti-oxidant enzyme activities in the enhancement of tissue lipid peroxidation in rats. J Nutr 1993; 123:803–10.

43. Frostell G. Kost och karies. In: Kariologiska Principer, Nordisk Larobok i Kariologi (Nutrition and caries: In: Principles of Cariology, Nordic Textbook of Cariology), 5th ed, pp. 187–215. Tandläkarförlaget, Stockholm, 1980.

44. Sognnaes RF. Analysis of wartime reduction of dental caries in European children. Am J Dis Child 1948; 75:792.

45. Toverud G. The influence of war and postwar conditions on the teeth of Norwegian school children. Milbank Mem Fund Quart 1957; 33:2.4.

46. Frostell G. Dental plaque pH in relation to intake of carbohydrate products. Acta Odont Scand 1969; 27:3.

47. Guggenheim B, Konig KG, Herzog E, Muhlemann HR. The cariogenicity of different dietary carbohydrates tested on rats in relative gnotobiosis with a Streptococcus producing extracellular polysaccharide. Helv Odont Acta 1966; 10:101.

48. Jay P. The role of sugar in the aetiology of dental caries. J Am Dent Assoc 1940; 27:393.

49. Weiss RL, Trithart AH. Between-meal eating habits and dental caries experience in preschool children. Am J Public Health 1960; 50:1097–104.

50. Winholt AS. Sucrose content and plaque formation in extracts from various food products. Odont Rev 1970; 21:301.

51. Stralfors A. Inhibition of hamster caries by substances in chocolate. Arch Oral Biol 1967; 12:982.

52. Newbrun E, Frostell G. Sugar restriction and substitution for caries prevention. Caries Res 1978; 12(suppl 1):65.

53. Frostell G, et al. Substitution of sucrose by Lycasin in candy. "The Roslagen Study." Acta Odont Scand 1974; 32:235.

54. Frostell G. The caries reducing effect of carbamide in hamsters and rats. Svensk Tandläk-Tidskr (Swed Dent J) 1970; 63:475.

55. Whitford GM, Ekstrand F. Fluoride toxicity. In: Ekstrand J, Fejerskov O, Silverstone LM, eds, Fluoride in Dentistry, pp. 171–89. Munksgaard, Copenhagen, 1988.

56. Fejerskov O, Kragstrup F, Richards A. Fluorosis of teeth and bone. In: Ekstrand J, Fejerskov O, Silverstone LM eds, Fluoride in Dentistry, pp. 190–228. Munksgaard, Copenhagen, 1988.

57. Featherstone FDB, ten Cate FM. Physicocemical aspects of fluoride-enamel interactions. In: Ekstrand J, Fejerskov O, Silverstone LM, eds, Fluoride in Dentistry, pp. 125–49. Munksgaard, Copenhagen, 1988.

58. Svatun B, Gjermo P, Eriksen HM, Rølla G. A comparison of the plaque inhibiting effect of stannous fluoride and chorhexidine. Acta Odont Scand 1977; 35:247–50.

59. Geddes DAM, Røla G. Fluoride in saliva and dental plaque. In: Ekstrand J, Fejerskov O, Silverstone LM, eds, Fluoride in Dentistry, pp. 60–76. Munksgaard, Copenhagen, 1988.

35 The Anti-Inflammatory Effects of Chinese Herbs, Plants, and Spices

Christopher Chang and M. Eric Gershwin

The Yellow Emperor said, "Man is afflicted when he cannot rest and when his breathing has a sound (is noisy)—or when he cannot rest and his breathing is without sound. He may rise and rest (his habits of the day may be) as of old and his breathing is noisy; he may have his rest and his exercise and his breathing is troubled (wheezing, panting): or he may not get any rest and be unable to walk about and his breathing is troubled. . . .

Huang Ti Nei Ching Su Wen *(1)*

INTRODUCTION

Of all the herbal pharmacopoeias of the many ancient civilizations, those from China have the longest history and form perhaps the most complex and intricate systems of all forms of empiric medicine. The Chinese pharmacopoeia is a treasure chest of pharmacological products, derived from plants, animals and minerals, which have been used to treat patients for over 5000 yr. In contrast to drugs used in Western medicine, which go through rigorous scientific study before being presented to the public, most of the herbal preparations or animal products used in Chinese medicine were developed by trial and error and have been handed down from physician to student, generation after generation. The enormity of this experience should not be lost on the reader. Thousands of products have been identified that have beneficial effects in thousands of diseases, without the help of the fundamental biochemical and biophysical knowledge and without the benefit of a double-blinded, placebo-controlled study method. Over the entire planet, other ancient civilizations have undergone the same evolution, from the Egyptians, to the Greeks, the Romans, Hindus, and American Indians. All of these cultures have their own collection of pharmaceutical and herbal products used in folklore medicine. Oftentimes, the same plant has been independently identified to work in the same disease states by cultures thousands of miles apart, separated in time by thousands of years, with completely different medical theories and doctrines.

From: *Nutrition and Immunology: Principles and Practice* (ME Gershwin et al. eds.), © Humana Press, Inc., Totowa, NJ

CHINESE MEDICINE AND THE IMMUNE SYSTEM: YIN AND YANG

Although Traditional Chinese Medicine (TCM) does not even identify the existence of an "immune system," the concepts of *Yin* and *Yang* may be thought of as analogous to Western ideas of self and non-self. One finds that many original herbal preparations from the Chinese pharmacopoeia may significantly modulate the human immune system. The extent of this modulation is currently the subject of extensive research in Europe, Asia, and the Americas.

AN IMMUNOLOGICAL COMPARISON BETWEEN EAST AND WEST
Chinese medicine addressed self and non-self issues in terms of internal and external forces. *Yin* and *Yang* are the most popular terms derived from Chinese medicine, familiar though poorly understood concepts to the Western world. *Yin* and *Yang* represent two opposite poles, which are in balance during periods of good health, but when one is in excess over the other, the balance is upset and sickness ensues. The Chinese character for *Yang* was originally calligraphied to represent the sun, whereas the character for *Yin* represents the shade (Fig. 1).

Yin is often described as the negative or female principle, representing the structure or composition of an organ, and *Yang* represents the positive pole or the active or functional component of the organ *(2)*. Of course, this is an oversimplification and, as will be shown later, this is but one of the many representations of *Yin* and *Yang*.

As we will discuss later, heat and cold are also important principles in Chinese medicine, manifested clinically by fever or chills. *Yin* represents cold, hypofunction, or internal forces, whereas *Yang* can represent hyperfunction, heat, or external forces. These two forces must be in balance in order for good health to be maintained. The two poles may augment or oppose one another, and descriptions of this are illustrated by the following translations from Chinese medical theory. In general, "the growth of *Yin* depends on the normal development of *Yang*" and "impairment of *Yin* would impede the generation of *Yang* and vice versa." Medications also have "hot" and "cold" properties. Often a medication with "cold" properties is used to treat a disease where there

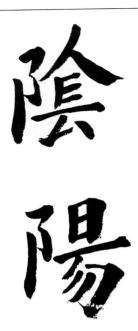

Fig. 1. Chinese characters representing *Yin* and *Yang*.

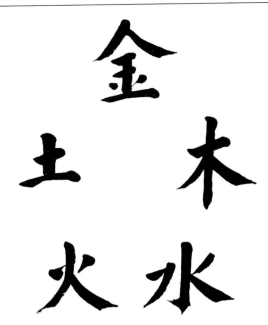

Fig. 2. Chinese characters representing the five elements; starting from the top and proceeding clockwise: metal, wood, water, fire, and earth.

is too much "heat" and vice versa. Properties of cold and hot medications are shown in Table 1.

In order to begin to understand what the scholars and medical professionals of ancient China meant by these concepts, it is also important to introduce several other concepts. The first of these is the theory of the five elements, where each element represents an organ system or a combination of organ systems. The five elements are metal, wood, water, fire, and earth (Fig. 2). They represent the lung, liver, kidney, heart, and spleen, respectively. Indeed, the relationship between water (kidney) and fire (heart) and the need for these two elements to complement and balance

each other makes fundamental biological sense to those trained in Western medicine, when one considers the close relationship between the kidney and the heart in classical anatomy and physiology. What is more interesting is the complex relationship between the five elements. This network of relationships was derived over thousands of years ago. Within the five elements, there is a pattern of evolution in which one element is derived from another. At the same time, one element may act opposite to the other (3).

Another important concept in traditional Chinese medicine is the *qi* (pronounced *chi*), which is an inner strength that can be summoned from the deepest part of the human body. It is not something physical or tangible. Rather, it is a type of vital energy. There are several types of *qi*, relating to either inner forces or outer forces. There must be balance in *qi* for good health to be sustained. There are a series of exercises, called *qigong*, which helps to keep that balance in place.

In Western medicine, all of the above major organ systems are also related, and we have nerves and other conduits in the body, which transmit signals similar to the way Chinese medicine explains the meridians. However, these systems are, at the same time, superficially different from one another. Therefore, we cannot always seek to find an analogous system between the two disciplines. Yet, the human body is fundamentally nonvariant, and no matter what tool one uses to understand it, the empirical experience that one gains leads to either continued use of a medication or its dismissal as an effective agent. As an example, some of the medications, which we now use in Western medicine to treat asthma, have been actually used for centuries by Chinese physicians in their native forms of herbs (Table 2).

Another important aspect of Chinese medicine that is important to note is the emphasis that Chinese medicine places on health maintenance and disease prevention. Chinese medicine seeks to preserve the equilibrium between internal and external forces and this involves correcting problems before disease strikes. Treating

Table 1
Characteristics of "Cold" and "Warm" Medications

Cold	Mild	Warm
Damp heat clearing	Latent heat clearing	Qi stimulant
Anti-helminthic	Antipyretic	Spleen invigorative
Anti-inflammatory	Antirheumatic	Digestant
Antirheumatic	Vital-energy stimulant	Damp clearing
Analgesic		Mucolytic
Expectorant		Antitussive
Antitussive		Lung demulcent
Antipyretic		Antiasthmatic
Antiasthmatic		Spasmolytic
Blood stimulant		Blood stimulant
Astringent		Antihelminthic
Hemostatic		Anti-inflammatory
		Antiarrythmic
		Antiemetic
		Diuretic
		Liver restoring
		Stasis eliminating
		Muscle relaxant
		Laxative
		Hemostatic

Table 2
Similarities Between Western and Chinese Medications

Western medicine	Chinese medicine
Bronchodilators	
B-adrenergic	Ma Huang
Theophylline/caffeine	
Anticholinergics	
Anti-inflammatory agents	
Steroids	Zu Huang
Cromolyn	Dai Ling
Steroid-sparing agents	Steroid precursors
Others	
Platelet-activating factor inhibitors	Common spices
Leukotriene receptor antagonists	Gingko

the disease is frequently considered a failure and requires that the physician restore the natural energy balance and harmony among the body's organ systems and external agents.

Western medicine has identified many types of immunological disorders, ranging from autoimmune disorders, such as systemic lupus erythematosis, to inflammatory disorders, such as asthma, to delayed hypersensitivity conditions like allergic contact dermatitis. In addition, there are many disorders that lead to the recruitment of inflammatory cells such as infections, cancer, and so forth. All of these disorders are also described in Chinese medicine. The way these disorders are thought of philosophically may be very different, but oftentimes the treatments are very similar.

The definition of asthma in Western medicine is a reversible obstruction of the airways resulting from inflammatory processes, including cell infiltration and mucus production, leading to the clinical symptomatology of wheezing, cough, and respiratory distress. One definition in Chinese medicine is as follows: "if evil air enters the nose during the accumulation of disease in the heart or lungs, nasal disease develops, either of chill lung or fever type lung." It is in some ways a very vague definition, but it does provide an early link between allergic rhinitis and asthma.

HISTORY

The use of herbal medications in inflammatory conditions dates back many centuries. The first recorded history of medicine can be found in the Huang Ti Nei Ching Su Wen (The Yellow Emperors Canon of Internal Medicine) (1) (Fig. 3). This text contains many of the concepts and practices of 4–5 thousand years ago, although the book was probably compiled during the Zhou dynasty between 475 and 221 BC. There are many descriptions of illnesses that resemble inflammatory conditions, such as arthritis, asthma, and lupus erythematosis. Along with descriptions of the clinical presentation of these diseases, there are also synopses of methods of treatment, including medicinal herbs, animal extracts, and how to combine them to achieve maximum effect. As early as 2000 BC, the emperor Shen Nong was credited with introducing herbal medications. Indeed, many of the medications described do seem to have had benefit in modulating the immune system, most in ways as yet not understood or accepted by Western science.

Other resources can be found in the many ancient Chinese texts of pharmacology that have been handed down throughout the ages, such as the Pen Ts'ao Kang Mu or Chinese Materia

Medica, written during the Ming dynasty (AD 1368–1644 by Li Shih-chen) and spanning 52 volumes listing 1892 medical substances, including illustrations. The Shen Nong Ben Cao Jing, or Shen Nong's herbal encyclopedia, written in the first century BC is the world's earliest Materia Medica.

Other well-known Chinese physicians and pharmacologists include Li Zhong-zi, who lived during the Ming dynasty and who wrote the "Essentials of Internal Classic." Ge Qian-sun also lived during the Ming dynasty and wrote on the treatment of pulmonary tuberculosis.

Other cultures also have a rich history of using herbal products for maintaining good health and treating disease. Some examples of these are shown in Table 3. Some products have been discovered independently by more than one ancient culture for either the same or different conditions. For example, blackberry has been used in the Middle East for bleeding gums and in China to improve stamina and vigor.

THE BENEFICIAL EFFECTS OF HERBS, SPICES, AND OTHER FOODS

Although there are many exotic herbs known to contain medications useful in asthma, we need not go too far from the kitchen to find some which have been in use by Chinese physicians. These include such plants as alfalfa, astragalus, bee pollen, dong quai, garlic, schizandra (Wu Wei Zi), capsicum, and licorice. Other familiar herbs also thought to have anti-inflammatory effects include gingko and ginseng.

Other common household products that have beneficial effects in inflammatory diseases include cinnamon, capsicum (or red peppers), and orange peel. In general, according to traditional Chinese medicine, any food substance that enhances the moisture (or Yin) of the lung will help asthma. These include garlic, onion, leek, grapes, apricots, almonds, lychee, and mustard green. Foods that are thought to decrease inflammation are collard greens, garlic, onion, turnips, apricots, cherries, green vegetables, sprouted seeds, turnips, raw nuts and seeds, and elderberries (4).

CHINESE MEDICINAL PLANTS

Ginger (Zingiber officinale) Ginger grows perennially in warm climates. The active ingredients are thought to be a group of compounds called gingerols. Other components are zingerone, phellandrene, camphene, citral, borneol, and cineol. Ginger has been used in the treatment of motion sickness. It also improves digestion and is used to treat colds, chills, and other respiratory problems (5). Ginger (in Chinese, gan jiang) or dried ginger is used for flavoring in Chinese cooking. It is considered a warm medication in Chinese medication. It dissolves phlegm and is, therefore, useful in treating colds and chills, as well as coughs. It also has found frequent usage in Europe for its beneficial effects on the digestive system.

Honey Honey has been used by many ancient cultures for many uses, including as an expectorant and in asthma. One of the side effects known to practitioners of Western medicine includes botulism. Honey has also been used in wartime to counter wound infections.

Peppers Capsicum peppers are also a common food substance among Chinese, although it has not had a wide use as a medicinal product in the Orient. Rather, it has been used for medicinal purposes in other areas of the world, including the United States, Africa, and India. In these areas, it has been used widely as a gastrointestinal stimulant. Of interest are its uses as

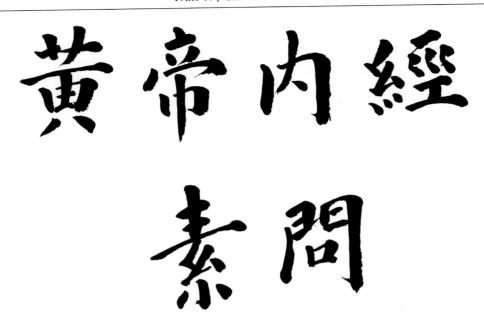

Fig. 3.   Chinese characters representing Huang Ti Nei Ching Su Wen or The Yellow Emperor's Canon of Internal Medicine.

a warming agent for the feet and as a therapy for topical neuritis. It is also known to inhibit histamine reactions of the skin and decrease sneezing, congestion, and running nose by inhalation of a solution containing capsicum *(6)*.

Rose Hips   Rose hips have been used in Europe. Rose hips are one of the richest sources of vitamin C, and the beneficial effect of vitamin C is a subject that has been considered for decades. Vitamin C is thought to augment the immune system and prevent viral infections. The rose hips are the mature ovaries found on the branches of *Rosa canina* and other rose species. Other constituents of rose hips include citric acids, polyphenols, pectin, and carotenoids. Other common plants with a high concentration of vitamin C include the Barbados cherry, *Terminalia ferdinandiana,* guavas, and other tropical vegetables *(7)*.

Astragalus   Astragalus is thought to be a very important and potent immune system booster; this plant also possesses significant antiviral effects. Astragalus is one of the herbs studied extensively by Western science. Some of the mechanistic effects that this medication possesses include stimulation of interferon production and inhibition of T-cell-suppressor activity. It also may possess anticancer activity. From a TCM standpoint, it is considered a "warm" medication. Astragalus is prepared from the root of the plant *Astragalus hoantchy* or *huang chi (8)*. It is often used in combination with other immune-enhancing medications, such as ginseng or schizandra.

Rosemary   Rosemary is another of those common food products used in ancient cultures throughout the world. In Greece, it was used as a memory enhancer, in Europe to treat headaches and wound infections, to improve memory, and to treat colds. In China, it was used to treat stomach disorders and headaches. It has also been known to be used as a mild antimalarial agent in China. Rosemary also has been indicated for treating skin problems caused by allergies such as eczema. Typically, the whole plant is used to prepare either a tea or a tonic. Rosemary has also been found to prevent hair loss.

Basil   In TCM, basil is used as an expectorant for the treatment of coughs and colds. It also has antibacterial properties and is used in the treatment of hymenoptera stings and venomous bites.

Cinnamon (Cinnamomum zeylanicum, C. Assia, or rou qui)   Cinnamon is commonly used in the treatment of fatigue in TCM. It is native to Southeast Asia and the bark of the plant is used for medicinal purposes. It is considered very warming and is used along with ephedra in the treatment of colds and viral infection. It has a stimulating effect on perspiration, which "chases away" the undesirable energies of viral upper respiratory infections. The plant contains an essential oil, cinnamon aldehyde, said to have antiviral effects.

Alfalfa (Medicago sativa)   Alfalfa is a common food substance, with worldwide use as a medication as well. The Columbians used it for cough and native American Indians for earaches. The Egyptians used it in beverages and the English used it for stomach disorders. The Chinese also used alfalfa to treat asthma and allergies, among other illnesses. Alfalfa is also supposed to have a significant immune boosting activity. Alfalfa contains a high concentration of chlorphyll, vitamins, and minerals, including beta-carotene, vitamins C, D, E, and K, calcium, potassium, phosphorus, and iron.

Aloe Vera   Aloe vera is well known to the Western world; aloe is used in shampoos, soaps, and other skin products. Aloe is a very "cold" medicine. Its Chinese name is *Lu Hui*. The part of the plant used is typically the juice of the leaves, and it has been found to be beneficial when used alone or in combination to treat eczema and psoriasis. Aloe has been suggested to possess anticancer activity. Dosages range from 0.1 to 1.0 g. It is sold as a juice in Chinese pharmacies. It is also used for digestive tract disorders, including constipation, heartburn, and intestinal parasites.

Angelica (Angelica anomala)   Angelica is a perennial herb native to China and Japan. The Chinese name of the plant is *bai zhi*. The root of the plant is used and made into a powder, pills, or capsules. Three grams a day are taken to treat nasal congestion,

Table 3
Herbal Remedies Used by Ancient Cultures

Herb	Remedy
Greeks	
Agrimony	Eye ailments
Aloe	Constipation, burns, kidney ailments
Amaranth	Immune booster
Anise	Coughs
Coltsfoot	Coughs
Comfrey	Bleeding, body tissue repair
Thyme	Antispasmodic, whooping cough, wound healing, asthma attacks
Rosemary	Memory enhancement
Nutmeg	Digestive stimulant
Romans	
Bee propolis	Antibiotic, immune booster
Chicory	"Blood purifier"
Coltsfoot	Cough
Walnut	Parasites, anti-inflammatory
Americas	
Alfalfa—Columbians	Coughs, earaches
Barberry—American Indians	Jaundice
Birch bark—American Indians	Headaches, abdominal cramps
Echinacea	Immune deficiency, viral infections
European	
Sage—American Indians	Healing skin sores
Alfalfa—English	Upset stomachs
Agrimony—Anglo-Saxons	Wounds, gout, fevers, rheumatism
Parsley—Middle Ages	Anti-asthmatic, expectorant, stimulant
Rosemary—France	To kill germs, used in WWII to counter wound infection, bleeding gums
Lavender	Wound infection
Arabs	
Senna	Cathartic
Lavender	Expectorant, antispasmodic
Blackberry	Bleeding gums
Hindus	
Datura	Asthma
Egyptians	
Barberry	Hypertension, plague
Juniper	Cholera, thyphoid, dysentery, and tapeworms
South Africans	
Buchu	Stimulant

itchy skin rashes, and bronchitis. It is also used to treat eye allergies and headaches. In Chinese medicine, it is used to treat problems caused by excessive wind. It is considered a warm medication. The English used a concoction of "Angelica water" mixed with nutmeg and made into a tea to treat the plague. However, caution should be exercised because angelica, if taken in large quantities, can cause complications. Angelica should not be taken during pregnancy, as large amounts can cause uterine contractions.

Jasmine Jasmine is a component of tea leaves and the Chinese have known the flowers for centuries. There are more than one species of Jasmine, including *J. officinale* and *J. Sambac*. Though native to China, it is currently also grown in the Mediterranean.

Parsley (Petroselinum sativu) Parsley was used by the Greeks and Romans as a food product, but in the second millennium in Europe, it was also used as an antiasthmatic and expectorant. It is truly ubiquitous, having been used in many cultures. In China, parsley is also used as a food substance. It is considered an immune booster and used to treat arthritis and other rheumatologic conditions.

Turmeric (Curcuma longa) Tumeric is a common household spice used in India, China, and the Pacific Islands not only as a food substance but also to fight ringworm, bruises, sores, and menstrual problems. It has been known as the yellow cancer fighter. It is commonly used in foods, but it has been thought to have anticancer properties and anti-infammatory activity.

Cumin (Cuminum cyminum) Cumin is also used as a food substance and may possess antiviral properties. It has been used in Asia. The active ingredient is an aldehyde.

Blackberry Blackberry is noted for its *Yin* properties. It improves stamina and vigor.

Schizandra (Wu Wei Zi) Schizandra can be literally translated to five flavor seeds. It is a popular herbal preparation used in China as an antitussive and as an astringent. The plant contains a lot of essential oils and is believed to help digestion and to act as an antibiotic. The berries of the plant are desiccated and made into a decoction of 2–6 g/dose, or a powder, which can be placed in tablet or capsule form. It can also be produced in a drinkable form and is taken as a tea. In TCM, schizandra is considered a warm medication with predominant effects on the kidneys and the lung. It is indicated for asthma and helps to moisturize the airways. Other uses include its effects as an aphrodesiac *(9)*. In Western medicine, schizandra has been used for its antihepatotoxic effects as well as its effects on the centra nervous system. In addition, the antioxidant effects of schizandra have been extensively studied *(10)*.

Garlic (Allium sativum) Garlic has been used by various cultures, including the Chinese, Greeks, Egyptians, and Europeans, as an antibiotic and immune booster. It has been suggested that garlic possesses antimicrobial activity against fungi, bacteria, and viruses. A popular proposed mechanism is that garlic increases body defenses against mutation by inhibiting nitrosamine formation. This has not been scientifically proven. Garlic was used in World War I to treat wound infection and, indeed, has been labeled the "Russian penicillin" in some circles. It has been also used to treat asthma, colds, and coughs. Garlic is rich in minerals and antioxidant vitamins. In recent years, garlic has undergone a great deal of research with regard to its antitumor activity. It has been shown that garlic intake in Chinese people protects against lung and stomach cancers. However, these were epidemiological studies and not double-blinded, placebo-controlled studies. In fact, the antitumor effect of garlic may be related to the high selenium content in garlic *(11)*.

Ginseng Ginseng is known as the "root of life." There are many forms of ginseng, including American Ginseng, Siberian

Table 4
The Four Types of Ginseng

Common name	Scientific name	Use
American Ginseng	*Panax qinquefolius*	Qi tonic, cardiotonic, immunostimulant, aphrodisiac
White Ren Shen	*Panax pseudoginseng*	Immuno-stimulant, cell proliferant
Red Ren Shen	*Panax schin-seng*	Asthma, bronchitis, blood disorders, impotence, chronic fatigue
Siberian Ren Shen	*Eleuthercoccus senticosus*	Antispasmodic, antirheumatic

Ginseng, White Ginseng, and Red Ginseng (*see* Table 4). In Chinese, ginseng is called *Ren Shen*. Ginseng is commercially available worldwide as a dried root, which can be made into a decoction or a powder encased in capsule or pill form. It has "warm" properties, the degree of which is dependent on the species. It is useful in treating colds, pneumonia, and bronchitis. In TCM, it is also an immune stimulant or tonic, an aphrodisiac, and an antihypertensive. Although it has undergone extensive study, it is very difficult to analyze the effects of ginseng in an objective way. Suggested effects of ginseng range from anticancer activity to stimulation of interferon production *(12)*. The antimetastatic effects of ginseng root extract have been demonstrated in vivo in B16-BL6 melanoma cells in syngeneic mice, but it was the intestinal bacterial metabolite M1 formed from protopanaxadiol saponin of ginseng that inhibited in vitro tumor cell invasion and migration *(13)*. Ginseng is also believed to regulate blood sugar and hematological parameters. Other proposed effects include antioxidant effects, relief from stomach aches, and stimulation of adrenal glands, liver function, and memory. It has also been suggested that ginseng prevents heart attacks and heals corneal lesions. Ginseng has so many proposed beneficial uses that in TCM it approaches the status of a panacea. That one substance can have all these effects seems rather far-fetched. Whereas ginseng probably does have positive health effects, one must be objective about the data. Like many other herbal products, the studies are of dubious quality.

ANIMAL PRODUCTS   Not all Chinese pharmaceuticals are products of plants. Animal products also have been used to treat asthma. Di Long, which is dried earthworm, has been found to be an antipyretic with antiasthmatic properties as well. It is considered a heat clearing medicine and is used in conjunctivitis, headache, convulsion, high fever, tachypnea, and pharyngitis. Other animal products used in Chinese medicine include hornet's nest (Feng Fang), cockle shell (Wa Leng Zi), praying mantis egg case (Sang Piao Xiao), gecko (Ge Jie), cuttle fish bone (Hai Piao), and abalone shell (Shi Jue Ming). Minerals are also used, including pumice (Fu Hai Shi), Glauber's salt (Mang Xiao), Oyster shell (Mu Li), amber (Hu Po), talcum (Hua Shi), indigo (Da Quing Ye), kaolin (Ci Shi), and frankincense (Ru Xiang).

HERBAL PREPARATIONS USED IN ASTHMA

Chinese medications can be grouped into warm and cold categories, reflecting their properties based on *Yin* and *Yang*. Each disease is considered to be an excess of either too much heat or too much cold, resulting in an imbalance that can be treated by the contrary properties of Chinese herbal or animal preparations. Table 5 lists Chinese medicines used for asthma grouped according to their properties of heat and cold. In practice, many of the medications sold in Chinese medicine shops contain a combination of plant and/or animal products (Table 6).

As a result of 2000 yr of trial and error, there are many combinations of herbs that practitioners have concocted that may have synergistic effects in the reversal of airway obstruction. These medications can be prepared and administered in many ways, including decoctions, soups, creams, and ointments.

Asthma is an example of an inflammatory condition, although it was not thought to be an inflammatory condition until fairly recently. In Western medicine, asthma is treated by medications ranging from bronchodilators, which act on the smooth muscle lining the bronchial tubes, to anti-inflammatory medications such as steroids, which provide preventative benefits by their actions on the cells lining the respiratory tract. It is only recently that this strategy of preventing inflammation was introduced in Western medicine.

The inflammatory process in asthma results in pathological changes in the tissues, including bronchial constriction, mucus secretion, and increased airway resistance, and leads to clinical symptoms of wheezing, dyspnea, hypercapnia, and, sometimes, death. Many Western medications developed in the past century have been synthesized or isolated to counteract these changes and restore the patient to health. However, many of these medications, or their analogs, are derivatives of herbal and animal products that have been in use much longer in Chinese medicine. Some of the medications used in Western medicine whose roots can be traced to Chinese medicine include β_2-adrenergics, such as Ma Huang, anti-inflammatory agents such as disodium cromoglycate, and medications containing anticholinergic agents such as atropine, scopolamine, and others. However, there are many more Chinese medications, the constituents of which are vaguely described as a combination of oils or volatile oils, that are used in asthma and allergy. With greater study, many of these may turn out to be useful adjuncts for asthma therapy in Western medicine.

In Chinese medicine, asthma was first described in the *Yellow Emperor's Classic of Internal Medicine (1)*. It has been called *shen-sou, hsiao-chuan, pa'o-hsiao,* and *ke-ni-shang-chi,* which are Chinese terms to describe the clinical symptoms of the asthmatic patient.

The most widely known Chinese herb used to treat asthma is Ma Huang *(14)*. Ma Huang is the Chinese name for Ephedra Herba, which represents a collection of plants of the genus *Ephedra,* containing the drug ephedrine. Some of the species include *Ephedra vulgaris, E. altissimia, E. distachya, E. helvetica,* and *E. major.* Common names of the ephedra include sea-grape, mahuang, yellow horse, yellow astringent, joint fir, squaw tea, Mormon tea, popotillo, and teamster's tea. These herbs are evergreen shrubs with horse-shaped yellow flowers. They have a strong pine odor. The name Ma Huang comes from the numbing effect, which the herb has on the tongue (Ma), and the yellow color of the flowers (Huang).

Ephedrine was isolated from these plants in the late part of

Table 5
Herbal Medications or Preparations Used
in Asthma by Practitioners of Chinese Traditional Medicine

Cold	Mild	Warm
Shanglu	Jinjier	YinYangHuo
Qinpi	Jiujiefeng	Kuandonghua
Shandougen		Baibu
Huzhang		Chenpi
Maqianzi		Yunmuxiang
Kushen		Shidiaolan
Zhudan		Zangqie
Longkui		Xuanfuhua
DiLong		Lingzhi
Cebaiye		Qingpi
		Mianhuagen
		Mianzi
		Yunxiangcao
		Kuxingren
		Dong Chongxiacao
		Shuichangpu
		Foshou
		Chansu
		Chuanshanlong
		Hancai
		Guizhi
		Ai
		Mahuang

Table 6
Components of Little Green Dragon Concoction:
An Example of Combination Drug Therapy

Joint fir	*Pinella ternata*
Psoralea corylifolia	White peony
Licorice	Schisandra
Asarum sieboldi	Horny goat weed
Cinnamon	Balloon flower
Almond	Earthworm

the nineteenth century. Subsequently, ephedrine was used to treat asthma in the Western hemisphere from about the 1920s. Later, many more derivatives with activity more specific to bronchial musculature have been synthesized. Medications such as albuterol and terbutaline fall into this class of medications. In current TCM practice, ephedrae are still widely used for a variety of bronchial disorders and as a stimulant and diuretic.

The active ingredients of Ephedrae Herba include 0.03–1.5% alkaloids, including ephedrine, pseudoephedrine, norephedrine, norpseudoephedrine, N-methylephedrine, N-methlepsuedoephedrine, ephedradines A, B, and C, and the essentials oils 1-α-terpineol, nonacosan-10-ol, tricosan-1-ol, and nonacosane. The natural form of ephedrine is the levorotatory form.

Although Ma Huang is generally safe, we know that all β_2-adrenergics have potential side effects. Indeed, Chinese physicians have also known of the side effects of ephedrine. Side effects of ephedra include hypotension, hypertension, hypoglycemia, hyperglycemia, nervousness, headache, insomnia, dizziness, palpitations, skin flushing, tingling, vomiting, anxiety, restlessness, toxic psychosis, and skin reactions.

Another well-known herb used in the treatment of asthma is licorice (15). Licorice is also known as sweetwood. Licorice, or *glycyrrhiza glabra,* is a herb used for a great number of years, not just by the Chinese but also by the Romans, including Hippocrates and Pliny the Elder. Pliny the Elder actually recommended it as an expectorant. It was later used in Britain, having been introduced by black friars. In addition to its beneficial effects in asthma, it also has been used to treat ulcers, seborrheic dermatitis, and arthritis. Several glycyrrhic analogs have been found to inhibit prostaglandin E2 (PGE_2), a fact which may play some role in the anti-inflammatory characteristics of licorice. Licorice is, however, not without side effects. Ingestion of large amounts can produce

hypokalemia, resulting in lethargy, flaccid weakness, and dulled reflexes. Licorice, along with nine other components, has been incorporated into a Japanese herbal medicine called Saiboku-to. The components of Saiboku-to have been found to inhibit platelet-activating factor (PAF) activity, which may translate into anti-inflammatory effects in asthma.

Production of gingko is a major industry in Europe, where the incorporation of Chinese medicine into their culture has been more successful than in the United States. The Gingko tree (also known as the maidenhair tree or kew tree) is one of the oldest known living species. Individual trees live to be over a thousand years old. Their fan-shaped leaves distinguish the trees. The Chinese used gingko to treat asthma in ancient times. In addition, other beneficial effects attributed to gingko over the years have been improved mental facilities and improved circulation to the brain and other organs. It has been used to treat short-term memory loss and tinnitus and to prevent stroke and transient ischemic attacks. It is very popular in Europe, representing a $500 million a year industry. Gingko leaves have been found to contain a number of terpenes, pro-anthrochyanidines, hertosides, and biofavones, including sciapitysin, ginkgetin, isoginkgetin, bilobetin, and ginkgolic acid. Isolation of flavonoids included a substance called gingkolide B. This is thought to be the active component, but the exact mechanism is still under investigation. The amount of these substances in the gingko leaf seems to depend on the time of the year, the highest amounts being in autumn. Ginkgo extracts, like vitamins C and E, have been found to be excellent scavengers of oxygen free radicals. Clinical effects of gingko extracts include a dilation of blood vessels and inhibition of platelet aggregation. It has been shown that antagonists ginkolide B platelet-activating factor (PAF) can inhibit eosinophil and neutrophil chemotaxis (16). PAF derived from ginkolides have also been shown to inhibit IGE production in the laboratory (17).

The mechanism of action of gingko leaves in asthma may be that it inhibits PAF-induced bronchspasm. Side effects of ginkgo leaves include headaches, gastrointestinal disturbances, allergic reactions, contact allergy, loss of consciousness, and seizures (18).

Another anti-inflammatory agent of plant origin used in asthma is cromolyn. Cromolyn, or disodium cromoglycate (DSCG), is a derivative of the plant Khellin (*Ammi visinaga*). The seed of the plant is the part that contains the inflammatory medication. Khellin itself has side effects, which render it virtually useless in the clinical setting, but cromolyn is a well-studied alternative that has been used for decades in the treatment of allergic and asthmatic disorders.

An analog of DSCG, called Scute, is a component of many Chinese herbal combinations used to treat asthma (19). Scute contains a variety of flavinoids, including baicalein, which supposedly has mast cell degranulation inhibition activity. Other herbs that have similar activity include cinnamon, pueraria, magnolia, asarum, jujube, and Ma Huang. Scute also inhibits phosphodiesterase, as do santine derivatives, perilla leaves, and the Western medications theophylline and caffeine.

Other Chinese herbal medications with derivatives now used in Western medicine include the anticholinergics. Datura stramonium is an anticholinergic used by the Hindu to treat asthma.

Echinacea is now one of the most popular herbal products on the market. *Echinacea augustifolia* is not a Chinese medication; it is a Native American herb that has been used to boost immunity and treat infection. It has been known as the "King of the Blood Purifiers." Significant research has been done on Echinacea leading to claims that it has antibiotic activity, antiviral activity, cancer-suppression activity, wound healing activity, immune stimulation, and stimulation of phagocytosis. Some sources even suggest that Echinacea blocks viral recognition sites on cell membranes. One must, however, be fairly skeptical of the study methodology used to obtain these results. Unfortunately, with such a broad range of suggested effects, a fad has recently occurred with the notion that Echinacea can cure many, if not all illness, leading to a sense of well-being. The reality is that one still has no idea how Echinacea works and whether or not its apparent effects are partially or completely a placebo effect. Echinacea may have some immune system effects, but what dose is needed to produce what effect is certainly not known at this time.

Whereas the origins of ephedrine and other pharmaceuticals addressed earlier are clearly elucidated, many of the other herbs used in asthma are less well studied. It is difficult to make sense of all the various combinations and formulations used in Chinese medication. Indeed, we have large gaps in our knowledge of the constituents of these herbs and whether these constituents have any therapeutic effect, or even if they are safe. It is difficult to place this tremendous wealth of information into a format, which is easily understandable.

Many of these herbs have suggested active ingredients that do not have known activity in Western medicine. For example, the active ingredients of many herbal products are listed as essential oils. Essential oils, also known as aromatic oils, are isolated from various plants by extraction and have their roots in the old discipline known as alchemy *(20)*. Another example of substances thought to be beneficial in Chinese medicine and not yet well studied in Western medicine involve steroid precursors. For example, the sapoginens are known to be precursors of steroids in the human body, but it is unknown if administering sapogenins to an asthmatic leads to production of steroids as a metabolite.

In TCM, various parts of the plant can have different actions. Leaves, roots, flowers and stems, and fruits have been prepared in various forms such as decoctions, soups, teas, ointments, pills, powders, and capsules.

Many roots are known to have anti-inflammatory properties. *Yun Mu Xiang* is a *qi* stimulant and is used in India to treat bronchial asthma *(21)*. In Arabia, it is used to treat rheumatism, and it does appear to have some benefit as an antihelminthic. It is the root of *Auklandia lappa* and it has a bitter taste and acrid smell. It is considered a warm pharmaceutical. It is composed of 0.3–3% volatile oils, including apltaxene, *a*-costene, *b*-costene, costus lactone, dihydrocostus lactone, 12-methoxy-dihydrocostus lactone, costus acid, costol, and saussurine. One of the activities of the lactones is that they inhibit the bronchoconstricting effect of histamine. The saussurine component is known to have bronchodilator effects.

Baibu is the root of *Stemona japonica* and it also has warm properties *(22)*. It is used as a antitussive and antihelminthic. The constituents of Baibu include stemonine, stemonidine, and isostemonidine. The action of Bailbu is thought to be on the respiratory center, where it inhibits stimulation. Another root used to treat asthma is Xiangfu *(23)*, obtained from *Cyperus rotunda*. In addition to its effects on inflammation, Xiangfu is also used as a digestive medicine and for menstrual problems in China and India. The preparation consists of volatile oils, which vary depending on where it is produced. It also contains akaloids, cardiac glycosides, and flavonoids.

Huzhang, isolated from the root and rhizome of *Polygonom cuspidatum*, contains anthraquinones (emodin, chrysophaol, rheic acid, emodin monomethyl ether, polygonin, physcion-8-β-D-glycoside and tannins) *(24)*. It has antiviral, antibacterial, antiasthmatic, and antitussive properties and is used to treat acute inflammatory diseases, chronic bronchitis, hepatitis, neonatal jaundice, leukopenia, and arthritis. Its side effects are mild and include serosomia, bitter aftertaste, nausea, vomiting, and diarrhea.

Dong Quai, also known as oriental angelica or *Angelica polymorpha*, is an herb used to treat allergic attacks, but it is also used in menstrual problems, as an antihypertensive, and to treat ulcers, constipation, and anemia. It has been found to inhibit experimentally induced IgE titers *(25)*. It contains six coumarin derivatives and the oil also contains safrole, cadinene, and *n*-butylphthalide *(26)*.

Kuan Dong Hua is a flower that is used to treat chronic and acute asthma. It has antitussive, mucolytic, and antiasthmatic action. It is the flower bud of *Tusilago farfara*. In Western nomenclature, it is known as coltsfoot, cough wort, or horsehoof. It has also been used as a folk medicine in Europe for the above-noted conditions. Unfortunately, coltsfoot has been shown to be carcinogenic in rats, an observation that has been attributed to the component senkirkine *(27)*.

Lingzhi is the fruit of *Ganoderma lucidum*. It has been found to possess significant antitussive and expectorant actions. It also has effects on the central and autonomic nervous system and coronary circulation. The components of Lingzhi include ergosterol, fungal lysozyme, and acid protease.

Occasionally, the whole plant is used, as in the case with Yin Yang Huo *(28)*. Yin Yang Huo is the whole plant of *Epimedium sagittatum*, which is considered a warm medicine and is used to treat asthma, cough, rheumatism, impotence, low back pain, amnesia, and hypertension. The above-ground part of the plant contains icariin, des-*O*-methylicariin, *b*-anhydroicaritin, and magnoflorine. The root contains des -*O*-methyl-*b*-anhydroicaritin, and icariins A, B, C, and D.

Pinellia ternata or *Pinellia tuberifera* is a common herb used in asthma. It is native to southern and central China. TCM describes it as a warm medication that expels dampness. The herb is prepared as a decoction and is sometimes combined with ginger juice. This combination is commonly used for asthma. A typical dose is 5–12 g. Commercial preparations in pill form are available. Other components of the pill include essential oils.

Kan Lin *(29)* and Wen Yang Pill *(30)* are combination herbal preparations that have also been found to be useful in asthma.

Table 7
Combination Therapy Used in Eczema

Name of combination	Major components of combination product
Tang-kuei and peony formula	Peony, hoelen, alisma, scute
Ephedra decoction	Ephadra, almond, cinnamon, licorice
Angelica restorative decoction	*Angelica sinensis,* cinnamon ginger, Chinese jujube, White peony, licorice
Bupleurum and Artemisia decoction	White peony, *Artemisia capillaris,* Hare's ear, Tuckahoe, licorice, American ginseng, *Angelica sinensis, Atractylodes chinesis, Peucedanum decursivum, Scutellaria macrantha*
Ma Huang and asarum combination	Joint fir, *Asarum sieboldi, Aconitum fischeri*
Angelica and White Peony decoction	*Alisma plantago, Angelica sinensis,* White peony, Tuckahoe, *Atractylodes macrocephala, Ligusticum wallichii*
Major Bupleurum decoction	Hare's ear, *Pinellia ternata, Scutellaria macrantha,* Chinese jujube, rhubarb, ginger, White peony, trifoliate orange
Ginseng and Rehmannia Pills	Ginseng, *Rehmannia glutinosa,* broomrape, *Atratylodes macrocephala, Dendrobruim nobile, Thuja orientalis,* Dodder, *Eleutherococcus gracilistylus,* Morinda root, chrysanthemum
Alisma and Hoelen Sixteen Combination	Stephania root, Morus root bark, astragalus root, atractylodes rhizome, polyporus plant, chaenomeles fruit, Hoelen plant, Akebia stem, *Pinellia rhizome,* ginger rhizome, citrus peel, cinnamon twig, areca peel, licorice root, Magnolia bark

HERBAL MEDICATIONS USED IN ECZEMA

Eczema is described in Chinese medicine as a blistering rash consisting of sores that occur on various parts of the body in response to insults from wind, heat, and moisture. The rash has also been described as dry. The treatment of eczema by TCM depends on whether the rash is chronic or acute *(31)*. Pruritis is present in both forms of the rash. The acute rash is more red and blistery, containing yellow fluid or crusts. One of the formulations used to treat the acute phase is Gentian Combination in combination with Calcite and Phellodendron Formula. This serves as a moisturizing agent. Hoelen and Magnolia combination are also used as moisturizing agents. Other combination therapies for eczema is shown in Table 7. In the case of chronic eczema, the rash is described as being coarse and hyperpigmented with dermal thickening. Of interest is that the treatment also depends on the site of the eczema. Eczema above the waist is treated with a combination of mulberry leaves, wild chrysanthemum, and cicada. Eczema in the middle part of the body is treated additionally with gentiana and gardenia.

ACUPUNCTURE

The ancient art of acupuncture relies on accessing the major points of *qi,* or the vital energy, which flows along channels known as meridians. There are 12 such channels in the body. Of these 12 channels, 6 correspond to *Yin* organs and 6 to *Yang* organs. The *Yin* channels include the lung, heart, pericardium, liver, kidney, and spleen. The *Yang* channels include the large and small intestines, gallbladder, bladder, stomach, and San Jiao, which has no anatomic analog in Western medicine. *Qi* circulates throughout these 12 meridians and have periods of peak and trough. The times during the day that each channel attains its maximum and minimum levels varies according to the organ system. These channels communicate with each other throughout the body. There are points along these channels that one can access via acupuncture needles to revitalize the *qi,* which flows through these channels.

Unfortunately, meridians are not anatomically definable and there is no analog in Western medicine. However, studies have been undertaken over the years to "find" the anatomical meridians.

Most of these studies are not well designed, and results are not consistent. In 1970, a study was done to relate skin resistance and electrical conductance with acupuncture points. Other epidemiological studies have demonstrated a possible beneficial effect on the clinical severity of bronchial asthma *(35–38)*.

Acupuncture has been sanctioned by the World Health Organization for the treatment of asthma. The needle points for the treatment of asthma, cough, and sore throat, as identified by the Standard International Acupuncture Nomenclature, follow the lung channel, the points of which are along the arm. These points start at Zhongfu (Lu.1) in the chest and, from proximal to distal, include Chize (Lu.5), Kongzui (Lu.6), Lieque (Lu.7), Taiyuan (Lu.9), and Shaoshang (Lu.11), located near the thumbnail.

In addition, studies on the efficacy of acupuncture have shown that there is, indeed, some benefit of acupuncture to allergic rhinitis *(39)*. The effects of acupuncture on the immune system has been evaluated *(40–44)*.

FACT OR FICTION:
THE SCIENTIFIC STUDY OF CHINESE MEDICINES

Chinese herbs have been used for centuries to treat all ailments known to humans. To those educated in the Western world, it is still a mystery. This is partly the result of the paucity of valid scientific studies on these herbs, and partly the result of a reluctance to accept alternative medicine. In addition to this, most of the herbal treatments are unproven and controversial and have been abused or misused over the years by Western practitioners who know very little about TCM.

The question of regulation of this industry arises; more specifically, whether the dispensing of these herbs should be regulated at all. These preparations are obviously available and they can be obtained from Chinese medicine shops, which are usually located in or around the Chinatowns of the larger metropolitan areas. One can order Chinese herbal medications from wholesalers or distributors, most of whom are located in San Francisco, Los Angeles, Portland, and New York. Other sources include the health food stores or herbal stores, where more of the everyday household spices, such as ginger, garlic, or peppers are readily available.

Table 8
Sources of Information About Natural Products

The Lawrence Review of Natural Products
American Herbal Products Association
American Foundation of Traditional Chinese Medicine
Centers for Disease Control
Herb Research Foundation
National Council Against Health Fraud
National Nutritional Foods Association
World Association of Natural Medicine
The Internet

Internet sites:

http://altmed.od.nih.gov/	Office of Alternative Medicine (NIH)
http://www.actcm.org/	American College of Traditional Chinese Medicine
http://www.eucm.org/sinobiology/	European University of Chinese Medicine
http://www1.btwebworld.com/lcta/	London College of Traditional Acupuncture and Oriental Medicine
http://www.acchs.edu/	Academy of Chinese Culture and Health Sciences
http://www.demon.co.uk/acupuncture/index.html	Foundation for Traditional Chinese Medicine
http://www.wp.com/icm/home.html	Institute of Chinese Medicine
http://www.qi-journal.com/	Qi-The Journal of Traditional Eastern Health and Fitness
http://www.halcyon.com/niaom/	Northwest Institute of Acupuncture and Oriental Medicine
http://www.holistic.com/listings/aom.html	Academy of Oriental Medicine
http://Acupuncture.com/	Acupuncture.com
http://www.acaom.edu/	American College of Acupuncture and Oriental Medicine
http://www.holistic.com/listings/06811ch1.html	Healing Arts Center
http://www.njutcm.edu.cn/	Nanjing University of Traditional Chinese Medicine
http://members.aol.com/medchina/group.htm	East West Institute

These herbs are not considered pharmaceuticals, which means that they are not subject to the stringent regulation that the pharmaceutical industry is. Anyone can purchase or use these preparations, and there is, at present, only loose regulation regarding practicing as a doctor of Chinese medicine. One of the governing bodies for these such licenses is the National Commission for the Certification of Acupuncturists. Another is the American Association of Acupuncture and Oriental Medicine.

One can obtain information on these issues from a variety of sources, some of which are listed in Table 8. The World Health Organization (WHO) and the Center for Disease Control and Prevention (CDC), as well as an assortment of private corporations can provide information on TCM. In addition, the Internet contains a vast ocean of information on TCM, and the websites directed to this field are increasing daily (Table 8).

ALTERNATIVE MEDICINE STUDIES AND CENTERS

There has been an explosive growth in recent years in the field of alternative medicine, to the extent that major medical centers of Western medicine are establishing their own alternative medicine departments.

One of the areas of greatest resource, and, indeed, one that has been significantly tapped into by the public at large, is the area of TCM. TCM encompasses a wide range of herbal remedies, as well as empirically derived combinations of animal and plant products (and unclassifiable modalities of treatment such as acupuncture). Many of these therapies have been demonstrated to be beneficial simply by observation over many centuries. Some of them have even been studied by researchers in the West, using Western scientific method. In recent years, the Western public

has been more eager to accept the use of alternative medicine than are Western medical practitioners. The health industry has also been quick to take advantage of this enthusiasm, as can be seen from the wide variety of commercial products on the market.

The Office of Alternative Medicine at the National Institutes of Health is conducting ongoing monitoring of the resources and experiments being done to bring alternative medicine to a more acceptable status among health professionals. In general, the principles of traditional Chinese medicine are difficult for those trained in Western medicine to grasp (45). They tend to be abstract and can be thought of as almost more religion than science, for one cannot always find an objectively observable mechanism by which the concepts relate to the human body. The concepts have been handed down from teacher to apprentice over the generations and the practices are consistent and engrained, without serious quest for explanations as to why and how.

SUMMARY

In summary, alternative medicine offers unorthodox methodology in the treatment of immune dysfunction, including allergies and asthma (46–48). Traditional Chinese medicine includes herbal preparations, acupuncture, and qigong. Some common food substances such as turmeric, garlic, ginger, and cumin have been used by the Chinese not only as spices but also as immune boosters or stimulants, anti-inflammatory agents, and anti-infectives. The importance of nutrition in maintenance of good health has been stressed by TCM over the years. Agents used in asthma include Ma Huang, licorice, schizandra, ginseng, and gingko. There is a lot of information available in TCM that is potentially valuable to Western practitioners, provided they keep an open mind about alternative medicine and if they knew how to tap into this information source. Unfortunately, it is often difficult to remain open-minded because of the lack of scientific data to support any therapeutic value of most of these herbal preparations. In fact, Chinese traditional medicine has indeed been experiencing a sort of fad culture in recent years. What is disturbing is that although there are potential benefits to some of the herbs, the hype is significantly more than the truth, and many more studies will need to be conducted before all therapeutic indices and side effects are known. Moreover, there are always subsets of physicians or laypersons who will seek to take advantage of the current hype for their personal financial gain, with very little knowledge or reservation regarding patient safety. In the meantime, it is doubtful that the common spices used nowadays, such as garlic or ginger, are dangerous to our health. In the absence of such negative concerns, it is probably not inappropriate to accept, if not support, the use of such herbs by our patients. Ongoing studies will have to be undertaken to delineate the true value of such substances.

For those Western practitioners who are unable to at least consider this exciting new area of research, an old adage that seems to have been proven in medicine over and over again must be remembered, that what is considered alternative, or inappropriate, or even "dead wrong" today may one day be considered to be mainstream practice.

REFERENCES

1. Huang Ti, Huang Ti Nei Ching Su Wen: The Yellow Emperor's Canon of Internal Medicine, Veith I, trans. University of California Press, Berkeley, 1949.
2. Hardy L. Asian Healing Secrets. The Complete Guide to Asian Herbal Medicine. Crown Publishers, New York, 1996.
3. Williams T. The Complete Illustrated Guide to Chinese Medicine, Barnes and Nobles Books, New York, 1996.
4. Reid D. A Handbook of Chinese Healing Herbs, Shambhala Publications, Boston, 1995.
5. Ody P. The Complete Medicinal Herbal, p. 115. Dorling Kindersley Ltd, London, 1993.
6. Ritchason J. The Little Herb Encyclopedia. Woodland Health Books, Pleasant Grove, CA, 1995.
7. Burnham T, ed. The Lawrence Review of Natural Products. Facts and Comparisons, St. Louis, MO, 1995.
8. Yen KY. The Illustrated Chinese Materia Medica—Crude Drugs, p. 32. Southern Materials Center, Taipei, 1984.
9. Yen KY. The Illustrated Chinese Material Medica—Prepared Drugs, p. 109. Southern Materials Center, Taipei, 1980.
10. Li XJ, Zhao BL, Liu GT, Xin WJ. Scavenging effects on active oxygen radicals by schizandrins with different structures and configurations. Free Radical Biol Med 1990; 9(2):99–104.
11. Ip C, Lisk DJ. Efficacy of cancer prevention by high-selenium garlic is primarily dependent on the action of selenium. Carcinogenesis 1995; 16(11):2649–52.
12. Beijing Institute of Medical and Pharmaceutical Industry. Chin Tradit Herbal Drugs Commun 1970; 1:14.
13. Wakabayashi C, Hasegawa H, Murata J, Saiki I. In vivo antimetastatic action of ginseng protopanaxadiol saponins is based on their intestinal bacterial metabolites after oral administration. Oncol Res 1997; 9(8):411–7.
14. Yen KY. The Illustrated Chinese Material Medica—Prepared Drugs, p. 53. Southern Materials Center, Taiwan, 1980.
15. Ody P. The Complete Medicinal Herbal, p. 65. Dorling Kindersley Ltd, London, 1993.
16. Kurihara K, Wardlaw AJ, Moqbel R, Kay AB. Inhibition of platelet-activating factor (PAF)-induced chemotaxis and PAF binding to human eosinophils and neutrophils by the specific ginkgolide-derived PAF antagonist, BN 52021. J Allergy Clin Immunol 1989; 83(1):83–90.
17. Gilfillan AM, Wiggan GA, Hope WC, Patel BJ, Welton AF. Ro 19-3704 directly inhibits immunoglobulin E-dependent mediator release by a mechanism independent of its platelet-activating factor antagonist properties. Eur J Pharmacol 1990; 176(3):255–62.
18. Bauer U. Six month double blind randomized clinical trial of ginkgo biloba extract versus placebo in two parallel groups in patients suffering from peripheral arterial insufficiency. Arzneim Forsch 1984; 34:716.
19. But P, Chang C. Chinese herbal medicine in the treatment of asthma and allergies. Clin Rev Allergy Immunol 1996; 14:253–69.
20. Lawless J, ed. The Illustrated Encyclopedia of Essential Oils. Barnes and Nobles Books, New York, 1996.
21. Yen KY. The Illustrated Chinese Material Medica—Crude Drugs, p. 73. Southern Materials Center, Taipei, 1984.
22. Yen KY. The Illustrated Chinese Material Medica—Prepared Drugs, p. 57. Southern Materials Center, Taipei, 1980.
23. Yen KY. The Illustrated Chinese Material Medica—Prepared Drugs, p. 71. Southern Materials Center, Taipei, 1980.
24. Luo ZH. The use of Chinese traditional medicines to improve impaired immune functions in scald mice. Chung Hua Cheng Hsing Shao Shang Wai Ko Tsa Chih 1993; 9(1):56–8.
25. Sung CP, Baker AP, Holden DA, Smith WJ, Chakrin LW. Effect of extracts of Angelica polymorpha on reaginic antibody production. J Natl Prod 1982; 45(4):398–406.
26. Ivie GW. Natural toxicants in human foods: psoralens in raw and cooked parsnip root. Science 1981; 213(4510):909–10.
27. Hirono I, Mori H, Culvenor CC Gann. Carcinogenic activity of coltsfoot. Tussilago farfara 1 1976; 67(1):125–9.
28. Reid D. The Complete Book of Chinese Health and Healing, p. 414. Barnes and Noble Books, New York, 1994.
29. Wang JS, Lai DI, Chen HC, Tsai HY. Clinical trial of Kan-Lin in the treatment of pediatric asthma. Proceedings of the 4th International Congress of Oriental Medicine, 1986, pp. 110–6.
30. Shen ZY, Hu GR, Shi SZ, Zhang LJ, Wu BS, Chen WH, et al. Prevention of seasonal attack of bronchial asthma by Wen Yang Pill and study on its mechanism. Proceedings of the 4th International Congress on Oriental Medicine, 1986, pp. 117–21.
31. Hsu HY. Chinese herb therapy for eczema. Bull Orient Healing Art Inst USA 1983; 8(6):30–6.
32. Morishima A. The use of the Minor Blue Dragon Combination (Hsiao-Ching-Lung-Tang) in the treatment of children with bronchial asthma. Bull Oriental Heal Art Inst USA 1982; 7(2):1–16.
33. Tani T. Treatment of type 1 allergic disease with Chinese herbal formulas Minor Blue Dragon Combination and Minor Bupleurum Combination. Int J Orient Med 1989; 14(3):155–66.
34. Keigo N. Treatment of asthma with Chinese formulas. Bull Orient Heal Art Inst USA 1983; 8(2):1–8.
35. Adrian AP. The acupunctural treatment of bronchial asthma in the base of workers exposed to silicon dust. Proceedings of the 4th International Congress of Oriental Medicine, 1986, pp. 3758.
36. Pontinen PJ. Acupuncture in bronchial asthma. Proceedings of the 4th International Congress on Oriental Medicine, 1986, p. 132.
37. Takashima T, Mue S, Tamura G, Ishihara T, Watanabe K. The bronchodilating effect of acupuncture in patients with acute asthma. Ann Allergy 1982; 48(1):44–9.
38. Tandon MK, Soh PF. Comparison of real and placebo acupuncture in histamine-induced asthma. A double-blind crossover study. Chest 1989; 96(1):102–5.
39. Chari P, Biwas S, Mann SB, Sehgal S, Mehra YN. Acupuncture therapy in allergic rhinitis. Am J Acupunct 1988; 16(2):143–7.
40. Bianchi M, Jotti E, Sacerdote P, Panerai AE. Traditional acupuncture increases the content of beta-endorphin in immune cells and influences mitogen induced proliferation. Am J Chin Med 1991; 19(2):101–4.
41. Chao WK, Loh JW. The immunological responses of acupuncture stimulation. Acupunct Electrother Res 1987; 12(3–4):282–3.
42. Cheng XD, Wu GC, He QZ, Cao XD. Effect of continued electroacupuncture on induction of interleukin-2 production of spleen lymphocytes from the injured rats. Acupunct Electrother Res 1997; 22(1):1–8.
43. Kasahara T, Amemmiya M, Wu Y, Oguchi K. Involvement of central

opioidergic and non opioidergic neuroendocrine systems in the suppressive effect of acupuncture on delayed type hypersensitivity in mice. Int J Immunopharmacol 1993; 15:501–8.

44. Chin TF, Lin JG, Wang SY. Induction of circulating interferon in humans by acupuncture. Am J Acupunct 1988; 16(4):319–22.

45. White AR, Resch KL, Ernst E. Complementary medicine: use and attitudes among GPs. Fam Pract 1997; 14(4):302–6.

46. Toyohiko K. Treatment of bronchial asthma with oriental medicine. Bull Orient Heal Art Inst USA 1983; 8(2):9–14.

47. Chen MF. Allergic rhinitis. Int J Orient Med 1991; 16(2):124–7.

48. Hsu HY. Chinese herb therapy for chronic rhinitis. Bull Orient Heal Art Institute USA.

36 The Influence of Probiotic Organisms on the Immune Response

Stephanie blum, Yves Delneste, Anne Donnet,
and Eduardo Jorge Schiffrin

INTRODUCTION

Mucosal surfaces represent extensive areas of interface between the host and its external environment. They are the site at which most of the host's infectious processes begin. Physiologically, they can be relatively sterile (i.e., the distal pulmonary track) or colonized (even highly colonized), as the distal gastrointestinal tract (GIT).

Mucosal mechanisms of defense have evolved with common strategies for all mucosal surfaces (1), but striking differences exist depending on the local level of colonization. A major physiological feature of the intestinal mucosa is its capacity to mount an energetic response against invasive pathogens and, at the same time, remain nonresponsive or hyporesponsive to food antigens or indigenous bacteria. The lack of response is an active process, based on various mechanisms, which are globally called oral tolerance. Thus, gut mucosal defenses are able to cope with environmental antigens, including infectious agents, without triggering a constant and severe inflammatory reaction that, in itself, would induce an important tissue damage. Certainly, the integrity of the mucosal barrier is a basic requirement for the host survival, both from the nutritional and defensive points of view.

The above-mentioned dichotomy requires a fine-tuning of responses to maintain a continuous low-grade activation of the GIT immune system. Both endogenous mediators as well as luminal factors (in the case of colonized surfaces, bacterial factors) may contribute to this homeostatic system (2).

The main focus of our work is to understand how luminal signals in the intestine, delivered by nutrients, can modify the status of immune activation during physiological and pathological conditions.

COMPARTMENTS OF THE MUCOSAL IMMUNE SYSTEM

The most sophisticated and probably best understood defensive system of the intestinal mucosa is the production of secretory immunoglobulins against intestinal damaging agents such as toxins, pathogenic bacteria, and viruses. Other immunological mechanisms are present and are also important for mucosal defenses.

The anatomical compartments of the mucosal immune system may be analyzed bearing in mind that in the mucosal immune response, a clear compartmentalization of inductive and effector sites exists.

LYMPHOID AGGREGATES The humoral mucosal immune response starts in a well-defined anatomical compartment where antigens have a facilitated access to the host. The afferent limb of the mucosal immune response takes place at lymphoid aggregates, called Peyer's patches, in the small bowel and solitary follicles in the colon (3). They are covered by a specialized epithelium that contains the M cell, adapted for sampling the intestinal content (4). The underlying lymphocytes are arranged in prominent follicles that contain T- and B-cell compartments. The prominent germinal centers (GC) of the gut-associated lymphoid tissue (GALT) are the main lymphopoietic sites for mucosal B cells, with a preferential commitment to immunoglobulin A (IgA) production. GC development depends on antigenic challenge, mainly of microbial origin. The B cells migrate into the follicles and GC according to their affinity for specific antigens. The B cells then undergo somatic mutation of their antigen receptors (immunoglobulins), which leads to increased affinity for the specific epitopes. Follicular dendritic cells in the GC retain immune complexes on their surfaces exposed in such a way that B cells, with the correct mutations, are stimulated and, consequently, rescued from deletion. In contrast, low-affinity B cells are deleted by apoptosis. Immunoglobulin isotype switching then occurs predominantly toward the IgA isotype. CD4+ T cells (T helper lymphocytes) expressing CD40 ligand and producing interleukin (IL)-4, IL-10, IL-5 colocalise with GC centrocytes (B cells in maturation) that are undergoing isotype switching and participate actively in this process (5).

LAMINA PROPRIA The B and T lymphocytes activated at the afferent sites of the mucosal immune system, leave the Peyer's patches and migrate through lymph and blood to finally come back into mucosal tissues. Although B cells remain in the lamina propria (LP), T lymphocytes migrate into the lamina propria and

From: *Nutrition and Immunology: Principles and Practice* (ME Gershwin et al. eds.), © Humana Press, Inc., Totowa, NJ

the epithelial layer. The B and T cells participate in the efferent limb of the mucosal immune response.

The specific homing of mucosal primed lymphocytes into mucosal effector sites takes place through downregulation of L-selectin and induction of α4 β7 integrin expression, the latter recognizing the mucosal addressing cell-surface molecule (MAd-CAM-1) expressed on mucosal blood vessels (6).

After homing into the lamina propria, B and T lymphocytes complete their differentiation and participate in the effector mechanisms of mucosal immunity, the best known of which is the production of secretory IgA (1). IgA is secreted by lamina propria plasmacytes, terminally differentiated B lymphocytes, and is transported through the epithelial layer toward the intestinal lumen by the polymeric Ig receptor or secretory component. When secretory IgA (sIgA) reaches the intestinal lumen, it reacts with specific antigens, preventing the physical interaction of noxious agents with the mucosal surface. This process is called immune exclusion and that does not imply activation of inflammatory processes. Production and secretion of IgA is further regulated at the LP by (1) endogenous environmental mediators, such as T-cell growth factor (TGF)-β and IL-5, mainly produced by regulatory T cells (7–9), and (2) intestinal bacterial colonization (10).

The LP contains a large number of B and T cells, plasma cells, and accessory immune cells. In contrast to intraepithelial lymphocytes, LP T lymphocytes are exclusively of thymic origin. They leave the thymus as naïve cells to repopulate the paracortical areas of the lymphoic follicles (i.e., at Peyer's patches), where antigenic stimulation takes place. Antigen-committed T cells leave the lymphoid follicles to recirculate and home back into the lamina propria, similar to B cells. In contrast to the predominance of CD8+ T lymphocytes in the intraepithelial compartment, in the LP CD4+ and CD8+ T cells are found in a proportion similar to that of the peripheral blood. In addition, the γδ+ T-cell-receptor (TCR) subpopulation is not as high as is found in the intraepithelial compartment and it reproduces the proportion found in peripheral blood.

A remarkable feature of CD4+ LP T cells is the high amount of memory cells and the abundant expression of activation markers. With regard to cytokine production, LP CD4+ cells are predominantly of the TH2 type (IL-4, IL-5), although this can be shifted to TH1 (IL-12, interferon (IFN)-γ) in some pathologies such as inflammatory bowel disease (IBD). Indeed, it was shown that both clinical and experimental enteropathies are associated with an increased production of the TH1 cytokines IFN-γ and IL-12 (2).

An important physiological feature of helper LP T cells is their capacity to induce IgA secretion (11). This demonstrates a dual function of T cells in IgA production, which is performed at the level of different mucosal compartments: in fact, they participate in (1) switching events in the PP GC and (2) later on, IgA synthesis and secretion in the LP.

EPITHELIAL COMPARTMENT   The epithelial compartment is a very important microenvironment of the mucosal immune system and involves at least two types of immunocompetent cells: the intraepithelial lymphocytes (IEL) and the intestinal epithelial cells (IEC).

Intraepithelial lymphocytes are an important component of the mucosal immune system and are located within the intestinal compartment, in close association to the basal and lateral membranes of the IEC. Constitutively or upon stimulation, they are capable of modifying the epithelial immune phenotype and its

immunological or defensive functions (12). These effects could be mediated by cell-to-cell interactions implying surface molecules, such as αE β7/E-cadherin interactions and through secreted products like cytokines, mainly IFN-γ.

Human and murine IELs are enriched for T cells that express γδ TCR. In humans, IEL express a limited array of TCR αβ and, to a lesser extent, TCR γδ, indicating that they recognize a restricted range of antigens in the context of MHC class I-related molecules (13–15). The γδ TCR+ IEL is a population that seems to be less dependent on bacterial antigenic challenge than the αβ TCR IEL, as colonization of germ-free mice preferentially induce the appearance or expansion of the later.

Most of the IELs are mature T cells (CD3+) of the CD8+ (suppressor/cytotoxic) phenotype, which express the homodimeric form of the CD8 molecule (CD8αα). The predominant expression of CD8αα is considered as an evidence of their extrathymic origin, because peripheral blood CD8+ T cells exclusively express the CD8 αβ heterodimer (16). It is commonly accepted that TCR/CD3-mediated signals in IELs are diminished compared to peripheral T lymphocytes (17). This functional characteristic seems to contribute to the local homeostasis that is achieved through specific bidirectional cross-talk with neighboring IECs and LP T cells, therefore controlling the level of immune stimulation within the microenvironment. Moreover, IEL may influence functional aspects of adjacent IEC, such as barrier functions and ion transport, probably by secretion of soluble factors.

The specific homing of IEL into mucosal sites seems to depend on the expression of αE β7 integrin found on all IELs. Its ligand, E-cadherin, is expressed on the basolateral membrane of the enterocyte (18). These integrins can function as accessory molecules in TCR-mediated responses (19,20). Because αE β7 expression is upregulated by TGF-β (21), mainly derived from enterocytes, it will be of great interest to understand how luminal signals can modulate IEC-dependent TGF-β production. Therefore, nutrients with the capacity to modulate TGF-β production could have a major impact on mucosal mechanisms of defence.

Intraepithelial lymphocytes show high cytolytic (CTL) activity in vitro, suggesting that one of their main functions in vivo could be the elimination of infected or highly damaged cells. It was shown that a fraction of IELs contains intracytoplasmic perforin and granzyme-containing granules and exerts immediate cytolytic activity upon TCR stimulation. Furthermore, IELs express Fas-ligand and are able to kill Fas-bearing targets (22). To date, it is not clear which cytolytic pathway, Fas or perforin mediated, is preferentially used by IEL (23).

INTESTINAL EPITHELIAL CELLS   Intestinal epithelial cells (IEC) are considered to be a constitutive component of the mucosal immune system. They are the first host cell in contact with luminal antigens and micro-organisms and were proven to be antigen-presenting cells (24). Upon stimulation they are able to produce a wide range of immunomodulatory cytokines (25). In addition, they can actively participate in the local reaction against pathogens, exerting a form of innate immunity (26).

In contrast, very little is known about the modulation of epithelial immunocompetence by nonpathogenic bacteria and their role in the physiology of mucosal mechanisms of defense. The use of specific bacterial strains in foods (functional nutrients), which provide the consumer with health benefits, particularly for the control of gastrointestinal infections, makes this a field of high interest (27).

INDIGENOUS MICROFLORA AND MECHANISMS OF DEFENSE

At the colonized mucosal surfaces, the host entertains a symbiotic relation with the commensal microflora that implies both nutritional and defensive aspects.

With regard to the defensive function, the resident microflora prevents colonization of the gut by pathogens, the so-called "barrier effect" of the microflora or colonization resistance. The exclusion of exogenous micro-organisms by commensals involves the competence for mucosal-specific niches or nutrients and the productions of bactericidal or bacteriostatic products. These aspects will not be discussed in this chapter.

Moreover, the endogenous microflora seems to have a modulatory effect on the mucosal immune homeostatis and, therefore, on the mucosal mechanisms of defense. To better understand the functional role of bacteria in gut homeostasis, the underlying molecular mechanisms have to be elucidated at different compartmental levels.

BACTERIAL MODULATION OF DISCRETE COMPONENTS OF THE MUCOSAL IMMUNE SYSTEM

NONPATHOGENIC INTESTINAL MICROFLORA AND THE EPITHELIAL COMPARTMENT

As mentioned earlier, activation of the IEL by bacteria (or bacterial products) can lead to modifications of the IEC phenotype (12). It was demonstrated that IFN-γ derived from activated IEL can induce the expression of immune markers such as MHC class II on IEC (28). Moreover, the lack of MHC class II expression during the neonatal period (29) or in germ-free animals (30) strongly suggests a role for the normal microflora in the immune regulation at the epithelial compartment.

Bacterial colonization of germ-free mice induces a rapid expansion of the IEL population, suggesting activation through specific antigens or a polyclonal type of stimulation, something that so far is not clear (31).

A function that has been consistently detected for the small-bowel IEL is their constitutive cytolytic activity (32). Interestingly, cytolytic activity is highly dependent on the colonization of the gut, because it is lower in the germ-free animals (33). Paradoxically, murine studies have shown that IEL numbers are higher in the small bowel than in the highly colonized colon (31,34). In addition, the colonic IEL phenotype is closer to peripheral blood lymphocytes and colonic IEL do not express spontaneous cytolytic activity (35).

Our group has been working for the last years on the influence of nonpathogenic bacteria on the biology of the enterocyte. The assumption being that nonpathogenic bacteria normally do not invade or translocate into the host and, therefore, the signal for modulation of mucosal immune homeostasis has to be "processed" by the IEC.

With this hypothesis in mind, it was demonstrated that lactic acid bacteria and gram-negative bacteria, both components of the resident microflora, exert a different pattern of IEC phenotype modulation (36). This observation is of great interest, because lactic acid bacteria constitute a group of micro-organisms that are introduced as probiotics in fermented foods to provide heath benefits to the host.

Relevant IEC immune markers can be grouped in molecules involved in the following: (1) antigen presentation (MHC class II, Cd1), an early event of the immune response; (2) cross-talk between IEC and lymphocytes (ICAM-1, Fas, IFN-γ receptor), crucial for homeostatic regulation, and, finally, (3) soluble mediators such as cytokines and chemokines (IL-8, TNF-α, MCP-1), promoting the recruitment and activation of immune cells in the different intestinal microenvironments.

Stimulation of the human intestinal cell line HT-29 in vitro using a nonpathogenic E. coli increased the basal expression of ICAM-1 (CD54) and IFN-γR (CD119). Furthermore, when E. coli was combined with IFN-γ, constitutively produced by IEL, a synergistic effect was detected for the expression of MHC class II molecules (HLA-DR), ICAM-1, Fas, and IFN-γR. In addition, pro-inflammatory cytokines such as TNF-α, IL-8, MCP-1, and GM-CSF were induced by the gram-negative bacteria and the induction was significantly increased when the E. coli was combined with IFN-γ. Lactic acid bacteria (LAB), in contrast, did not show any agonistic effect with respect to the onset of pro-inflammatory cytokines. However, the combination of LAB and IFN-γ increased the expression of IFN-γ R (36). The molecular basis of this LAB-potentiating effect is not understood and is the subject of current research.

The fact that LAB alone or in combination with IFN-γ did not induce any of the pro-inflammatory cytokines suggests that LAB could participate in tissue protection against the deleterious effect of an ongoing inflammatory process. Bacterial–epithelial cell contact was a prerequisite in this system for induction of IEC phenotypic changes, giving support to an important selection criteria for probiotic bacteria, namely adherence to the intestinal epithelium (37).

LAMINA PROPRIA

It has been repeatedly observed that germ-free animals have a lower number of immune cells than the lamina propria when compared to conventional (normally colonized) genetically identical counterparts. Experimental evidence clearly shows that the indigenous bacterial flora is the major stimulus for the development of IgA-secreting plasma cells (38). Some authors have found increased numbers of lamina propria cells in intestinal bacterial overgrowth, whereas others have found more subtle changes such as a shift from IgA1- to IgA2-producing plasma cells (10).

LYMPHOID AGGREGATES

Lymphoid aggregates of germ-free animals are devoid of germinal centers (GC). The development of this B-cell compartment depends on a specific immune response against colonizing bacteria. In a monocolonized animal model, GC appear soon after bacterial colonization and disappear some weeks later, although IgA-specific response persists for a longer time (39).

Recently, it has been reported that the human indigenous microflora is only partially covered by IgA-specific antibodies and even less so by IgG and IgM (40). An important proportion of the microflora, close to 50%, is not covered by antibodies at all.

Both findings seem to show that the partial unresponsiveness to the autochthonous microflora may appear after a transient immune response took place, which, in fact, is suggested by the gnotobiotic animal model. As yet, the effect of exogenous ingested bacteria, such as probiotics, for sustaining activation at the GC level is not known, but, conceivably, they could contribute to it and thereby promote an IgA response that is not only specific against bacterial antigens but also against bystander antigens sampled through the follicular-associated epithelium (FAE) containing the M cells.

THE MUCOSAL IMMUNE SYSTEM AND ITS REGULATION BY LUMINAL FACTORS: NEW PERSPECTIVES

It has been shown that IEC may be participants in the initiation of the mucosal immune response as suggested by antigen presentation in vitro (24); however, this function is not confirmed in vivo. On the other hand, antigen (Ag) presentation by IEC could involve, in addition to MHC class II molecules (41), specific restriction molecules such as CD1d (13) or other nonpolymorphic class-1 molecules such as thymus leukemia (TL) antigens. In addition to the IEC accessory function for Ag presentation, they produce cytokines under physiological conditions (25) and in response to pathogenic bacteria. The differentially expressed cytokines then promote the recruitment and activation of effector immune cells for clearance of the pathogens (26).

Our experimental contribution using a reductionist IEC in vitro model puts forward further support for both functions. Moreover, the regulation of the immune phenotype with regard to specific molecules involved in cell-to-cell interactions, playing a key role in the homeostasis of the immune system, seems to suggest a role for the regulation of the cellular environment at the intraepithelial compartment and at the lamina propria. Interestingly enough, the IEC are in permanent interactions with the luminal content, including comensal microflora, and the endogenous cellular network of professional immune cells. The appropriate function of IEC can adapt the physiological reactivity of the host tissues to a highly changing intestinal content. A dysfunction of this interphase could promote a discordance between the luminal signal and the initiated response. This could be the origin of pathological conditions resulting from exaggerated responses to nondangerous signals, like food antigens, resulting in food allergy or in chronic inflammation (i.e., inflammatory bowel disease). In fact, the specific systemic unresponsiveness to oral antigens is an important physiological characteristic of the mucosal immune system and has been called oral tolerance.

On the other extreme, a weak communication of a harmful luminal signal could be associated with a lack of appropriate response for controlling luminal pathogens or potential pathogens, as can be observed in some cases of intestinal immunological disorders. The fine-tuning of this dynamic interphase is probably not only dependent on the IEC but also on an intricate cell-to-cell cross-talk, where IEL and LP immune cells are further participants. This is the subject of current research activities. However, there is a strong evidence that the IEC plays a central role in delivering early signals to the neighboring cells. The knowledge about the downstream cascade of events will give us unique possibilities to modify the gut homeostasis by nutritional interventions.

Finally, it is possible that the IEC play an effector role in the clearance or very basic defense mechanisms against pathogens. These functions may be, in turn, regulated by the immune cells in the vicinity.

CONCLUSION

Intestinal bacterial signaling of the mucosal mechanisms of defense can cover a wide range, from the physiological interactions between the resident microflora and the host cells in the superficial mucosal microenvironment, to the inflammatory, exudative reaction promoted by invasive pathogens, which implies the recruitment of blood leukocytes. Both types of reaction are adaptive mechanisms of defense adequate for the triggering signal. Nevertheless, it is obvious that the second type of response implies inflammatory tissue damage of the mucosal barrier and a response that can lead to systemic inflammatory reactions. Therefore, the understanding of how commensal bacteria or other nutritional strategies (e.g., probiotics) can improve pro-inflammatory mechanisms of defense is of major interest. The strengthening of this mechanisms will diminish the interactions between virulent microorganisms and the mucosal surface.

The first level of defense takes pace at the intestinal lumen–mucosa interface and is represented mainly by secretory immunity (sIgA) and, possibly, other components of innate immunity secreted into the intestine. There is growing experimental evidence that the epithelial layer also participates in local mechanisms of defense as an effector cell by altering its immune phenotype and as part of a local control against infections.

SUMMARY

The intestinal mucosal surface is colonized by the comensal microflora that attains very high numbers of bacterial cells in the distal intestine and more specifically in the colon. At the same time, these extensive areas are the interface with the external environment, through which most pathogens initiate infectious processes in mammals. Intestinal mechanisms of defense need to discriminate accurately between comensal, symbiotic microflora and exogenous pathogens. Today, we do not fully understand the essence of the mechanism of discrimination. However, it is known that comensal microflora helps the host to better mount defensive mechanisms against exogenous pathogens. These mechanisms imply both bacterial–bacterial antagonisms, and, in addition, the comensal microflora modulate the host's reactivity against the infectious agents. Since some years ago, it is known that the commensal microflora can be improved in their functions, by giving exogenous beneficial bacteria in foods. They have been called probiotics. Probiotics specific for the improvement of mucosal defensive mechanisms have been our main research area for some years. The purpose of this chapter was to give an explanation of immunomodulatory activities of bacteria on well-defined compartments of the mucosal immune system and to approach the modulation of immune markers of the mucosal surface by this food-borne beneficial bacterial called probitics.

REFERENCES

1. Underdown BJ, Schiff JM. Strategic defense initiative at the mucosal surfaces. Annu Rev Immunol 1986; 4:389–417.
2. Klapproth JM, Donnenberg MS, Abraham JM, Mobley HLT, James SP. Products of enteropathogenic Escherichia coli inhibit lymphocyte activation and lymphokine production. Infect Immun 1995; 63: 2248–54.
3. Abreu-Martin MT, Targan SR. Regulation of immune responses of the intestinal mucosa. Crit Rev Immunol 1996; 16:277–309.
4. Neutra MR, Frey A, Kraehenbuhl JP. Gateways for mucosal infection and immunization. Cell 1996; 86:345–8.
5. Liu YJ, Arpin C. Germinal centre development. Immunol Rev 1997; 156:11–26.
6. Berlin C, Berg EL, Briskin MJ, Andrew DP, Kilshaw PJ, Holzmann B, et al. Alpha-4 beta-7 intefrin mediates lymphocyte binding to the mucosal addressin MAdCAM-1. Cell 1993; 74:158–95.
7. Lebman DA, Lee FD, Coffman RL. Mechanism for transforming growth factor beta and IL-2 enhancement for IgA expression in liposaccharide-stimulated B cell cultures. J Immunol 1990; 144: 952–9.

8. Stavnezer J, Shocket P. Effects of cytokines on switching to IgA and alpha germline transcripts in the B lymphoma 1.29. Transforming growth factor-beta activates transcription of the unrearranged C alpha gene. J Immunol 1991; 147:4374–83.

9. Coffman RL, Lebman DA, Shrader B. Transforming growth factor beta specifically enhances IgA production by liposaccharide-stimulated murine B-lymphocytes. J Exp Med 1989; 170:1039–44.

10. Kett K, Baklein K, Bakken A, Kral JG, Fausa O, Brandtzaeg P. Intestinal B-cell isotype response in relation to bacterial load: evidence for immunoglobulin A subclass adaptation. Gastroenterology 1995; 109:819–25.

11. Smart CJ, Trejdosiewicz LK, Badr-el-Din S, Heatley RV. T lymphocytes of the human colonic mucosa: functional and phenotypic analysis. Clin Exp Immunol 1988; 73:63.

12. Cerf-Benussan N, Quaroni A, Kurnick JT, Bhan AK. Intraepithelial lymphocytes modulate 1a expression by intestinal epithelial cells. J Immunol 1984; 132:2244–52.

13. Blumberg RS, Terhorst C, Bleicher P, McDermott FV, Allan CH, Landau SB, et al. Expression of a nonpolymorphic MHC class I-like molecule, CD1d, by human intestinal epithelial cells. J Immunol 1991; 147:2518–24.

14. Tanaka Y, Morita CT, Nieves E, Brenner MB, Bloom BR. Natural and synthetic nonpeptide antigens recognized by human gd T cells. Nature 1995; 375:155–8.

15. Panja A, Blumberg RS, Balk S, Mayer L. Cd1d is involved in T cell-intestinal epithelial cell interactions. J Exp Med 1993; 178:1115–9.

16. Guy-Grand D, Cerf-Benussan N, Malissen B, Malasssis-Seris M, Briottet C, Vasalli P. Two gut intraepithelial CD8+ lymphocyte populations with different T cell receptors: a role for the gut epithelium in T cell differentiation. J Exp Med 1991; 173:471–8.

17. Christ AD, Colgan SP, Balk S, Blumberg RS. Human intestinal epithelial cell lines produce factor(s) that inhibit CD3-mediated T lymphocyte proliferation. Immunol Lett 1997; 58:159–65.

18. Cepek KL, Shaw SK, Parker CM, Russell GJ, Morrow RS, Rimm D, et al. Adhesion between epithelial cells and lymphocytes is mediated by E-cadherin and the alpha E beta-7 integrin. Nature 1994; 372:190–3.

19. Sarnacki S, Begue B, Buc H, Le Deist F, Cerf-Benussan N. Enhancement of CD3-induced activation of human intestinal intraepithelial lymphocytes by stimulation of the b7-containing integrin defined by HLM-1 monoclonal antibody. Eur J Immunol 1992; 22:2887–92.

20. Lefrançois L, Barrett TA, Havran WL, Puddington L. Developmental expression of aIELb7 integrin on T cell receptor gd and T cell receptor ab. Eur J Immunol 1994; 24:635–40.

21. Parker CM. A family of b7 integrin on human lymphocytes. Proc Natl Acad Sci USA 1992; 89:1924–8.

22. Rocha B, Guy-Grand D, Vasalli P. Extrathymic T cell differentiation. Curr Opin Immunol 1995; 7:235–42.

23. Gelfanov V, Lai YG, Liao NS. Activated ab-CD8+ but not aa-CD8+, TCR-ab+ murine intestinal intraepithelial lymphocytes can mediate perforin-based cytotoxicity whereas both subsets are active in Fas-based cytotoxicity. J Immunol 1996; 157:35–41.

24. Bland PW, Warren LG. Antigen presentation by epithelial cells of the rat small intestine. Immunology 1986; 58:1–7.

25. Eckmann L, Jung HC, Schürer-Maly C, Panja A, Morzycka-Wrobleska E, Kagnoff MK. Differential cytokine expression by human intestinal epithelial cell lines: regulated expression of interleukin 8. Gastroenterology 1993; 105:1689–97.

26. Jung HC, Eckmann L, Yang SK, Panja A, Fierer J, Morzycka-Wrobleska E, et al. A distinct array of pro-inflammatory cytokines is expressed in human colon eoithelial cells in response to bacterial invasion. J Clin Invest 1995; 95:55–65.

27. Brassart D, Schiffrin EJ. The use of probiotics to reinforce mucosal defence mechanisms. Trends Food Sci Tech 1997; 8:321–6.

28. Ishikawa H, Li Y, Abeliovich A, Yamamoto S, Kaufman SH, Tonegawa S. Cytotoxic and IFNg producing activities of gd T cells in the mouse intestinal epithelium are strain dependent. Proc Natl Acad Sci USA 1993; 90:8204.

29. Hughes A, Block KJ, Bhan AK, Gillen D, Giovino VC, Harmatz PR. Expression of MHC class II (Ia) antigen by the neonatal enterocyte: the effect of treatment with IFNg. Immunology 1991; 72:491–6.

30. Barclay AN, Mason DW. Induction of Ia antigen in rat epidermal cells and gut epithelium by immunological stimuli. J Exp Med 1982; 156:1665–9.

31. Link H, Rochat F, Saudan KY, Schiffrin EJ. Immunomodulation of the gnotobiotic mouse through colonization with lactic acid bacteria. In: Mestecky J, ed, Advances in Mucosal Immunity, pp. 465–7. Plenum, New York, 1995.

32. Guy-Grand D, Malasssis-Seris M, Briottet C, Vasalli P. Cytotoxic differentiation of mouse gut thymodependent and independent intraepithelial T lymphocytes is induced locally. Correlation between functional assays, presence of perforin and granzyme transcripts, and cytoplasmic granules. J Exp Med 1991; 173:1549–52.

33. Lefrançois L, Goodman T. In vivo modulation of cytolytic activity and Thy-1 expression in TCR-gd+ intraepithelial lymphocytes. Science 1989; 243:1716–8.

34. Beagly KW, Fujihashi K, Lagoo AS, Lagoo-Deenadaylan S, Black CA, Murray AM, et al. Differences in the intraepithelial lymphocyte T cell subsets isolated from murine small versus large intestine. J Immunol 1995; 154:5611–9.

35. Camerinin V, Panwala C, Kronenberg M. Regional specialization of the mucosal immune system. Intraepithelial lymphocytes of the large intestine have a different phenotype and function than those of the small intestine. J Immunol 1993; 151:1765.

36. Delneste Y, Donnet-Hughes A, Schiffrin EJ. Functional foods: mechanisms of action on immunocompetent cells. Nutr Rev 1998; 56:S93–8.

37. Bernet MF, Brassart D, Nesser JR, Servin AL. Gut 1994; 35:483–9.

38. Crabbe PA, Bazin H, Eyssen H, Heremans JF. The normal microbial flora as a major stimulus for proliferation of plasma cells synthesizing IgA in the gut. Int Arch Allergy 1968; 34:362–75.

39. Shroff KE, Meslin K, Cebra JJ. Commensal enteric bacteria engender a self-limiting humoral mucosal response while permanently colonizing the host. Infect Immun 1995; 63:3904–13.

40. Van der Waaij LA, Lindburg PC, Mesander G, van der Waaji D. In vivo IgA coating of anaerobic bacteria in human faeces. Gut 1996; 38:348–54.

41. Kaiserlian D, Vudal K, Revillard JP. Murine enterocytes can present soluble antigen to specific class II-restricted CD4+ T cells. Eur J Immunol 1989; 19:1513.

37 Nutritional Effects on the Pathogen Genome and Phenotypic Expression of Disease

Melinda A. Beck

INTRODUCTION

Infectious disease has long been known to be associated with poor nutrition *(1)*. Indeed, throughout history, periods of famine are often followed by epidemics of infectious disease. Both animal and human studies have demonstrated this association. For example, rotavirus-induced diarrhea is much more severe in malnourished children *(2)* and a deficiency in vitamin A in children is associated with increased severity of measles *(3)*. In animal models, a deficiency in a wide range of nutrients from generalized protein malnutrition to specific deficiencies such as zinc or vitamin E results in increased susceptibility to a number of pathogens, both viral and bacterial *(4,5)*.

The association between malnourishment and increased susceptibility to infectious disease is thought to be related to the immune response of the host; that is, malnourishment leads to decreased immunity, which, in turn, leads to increased susceptibility to disease. This relationship is diagrammed in Fig. 1. In this model, the increased susceptibility to disease rests exclusively on the inability of an impaired immune response (resulting from malnutrition) to protect the host from infectious agents. However, one must remember that the pathogen itself is also replicating in a malnourished environment. Viruses that require the cellular machinery of their host in order to replicate may also be susceptible to a less than optimal environment in a malnourished host. This chapter will discuss recent evidence that demonstrates that the oxidative stress status of the host, imposed by a nutritional deficiency, can have a profound influence on the phenotypic expression of disease, in some cases, through changes in the pathogen genome, such that a normally avirulent virus can become virulent. Both animal models and human diseases will be presented.

MALNUTRITION AND VIRAL DISEASE

A number of studies have examined the effect of host nutrition on immune function and this volume provides many examples of immune modulation with varying nutritional deficiencies. Rather

From: *Nutrition and Immunology: Principles and Practice* (ME Gershwin et al. eds.), © Humana Press, Inc., Totowa, NJ

than repeat these studies, this chapter will focus on the effects of host nutrition on the viral pathogen. Several examples of the impact of host nutrition on viral pathogenesis will be provided. The idea that the pathogen itself may be directly influenced by the nutritional status of the host has just begun to be studied.

Diarrhea caused by rotavirus is a much more serious problem in developing countries when compared with developed countries. Over 18 million cases of severe diarrhea caused by rotavirus occurs in developing countries each year, with an estimated 873,000 deaths occurring in children under the age of 4 yr. In an animal model of rotavirus infection, more severe and longer persisting diarrhea occurred in protein-deficient mice *(6)*. Another animal study found that pups born to malnourished dams were also more susceptible to rotavirus-induced diarrheal disease *(7)*.

Similarly, respiratory disease caused by viruses is also more severe in developing countries and malnutrition clearly contributes to the increase in susceptibility. Acute respiratory tract infections, in which viruses are the most likely infecting agents, are responsible for 4.5 million deaths among children a year, predominantly in developing countries *(8)*. Other risk factors associated with an increase in severity and mortality are also present in developing countries, including poor sanitation, crowding, low birth rate, and so forth, but malnutrition also plays an important role. Not only does malnutrition reduce the effectiveness of the immune response, but weakness in the muscles which control breathing can also be affected, as well as normal lung development *(9,10)*. Studies have found that underweight children have an increased likelihood of developing pneumonia following an infection than normal-weight children, which then leads to increased mortality *(11)*.

Malnutrition has long been associated with the development of severe measles. In developed countries, measles is generally a mild disease in an unvaccinated host and rarely results in complications. However, in developing countries, infection with the measles virus can result in severe complications associated with a high mortality rate. This increase in severity has been shown to be associated with a deficiency in vitamin A *(12)*. Several studies have shown that children given supplements of vitamin A have a decreased risk of developing severe measles. Therefore, the World Health Organization has recommended treatment with vita-

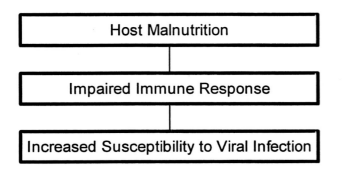

Fig. 1. Outline of standard model commonly used to describe the relationship between host nutritional status and infectious disease. Note that the response is unidirectional.

min A of all measles virus-infected children in developing countries.

Vitamin A deficiency has also been associated with an increase in severity of respiratory syncytial virus infection (RSV). RSV causes lower-respiratory-tract infections and is responsible for worldwide epidemics every year. Several studies have demonstrated decreased vitamin A levels in children hospitalized with RSV-associated illness *(13)*.

Zinc has also been associated with protection from infection. Clinical volunteers who consumed zinc gluconate lozenges prior to exposure to rhinovirus had fewer cold symptoms than those who were given a placebo *(14)*. In animal models, mice treated with zinc acetate survive for longer periods of time when infected with either yeast or Semliki Forest virus *(15)*. An interesting experiment by Grimstad and Haramis *(16)* found that female mosquitoes reared under conditions of malnourishment were more susceptible to La Crosse virus and were able to transmit more La Crosse virus when biting, when compared with mosquitoes raised under normal dietary conditions. Thus, not only are vertebrate hosts affected by malnutrition, but insect vectors can be affected as well. This finding has important implications for the spread of arthropod-borne diseases in areas of widespread malnutrition.

As mentioned in the Introduction, malnutrition is thought to affect susceptibility to viral infection by inhibiting immune function. However, a series of experiments by Beck et al. *(17–19)* examined not only the relationship between nutritional deficiency and the host but also the relationship between nutritional deficiency and the viral pathogen. This work began as a study of Keshan disease, a nutritional-deficiency disease that was suspected to have a viral etiology.

KESHAN DISEASE

In the early 1930s, a disease characterized by cardiomyopathy was identified in specific regions in China. Later termed Keshan disease, after Keshan County, Heilongjiang Province in northeast China where the disease was first identified, Keshan disease was found to affect mainly women of childbearing age and older children *(20)*. The heart pathology was characterized by areas of necrosis throughout the heart muscle with both cellular infiltration and calcification. Epidemiological studies found that Keshan disease was distributed in specific band-like areas in China. These areas were found to have low concentrations of the trace element selenium (Se) in the soil. Thus, grains grown in Se-deficient soils would also be Se deficient. Because food was grown and consumed

locally, individuals living in areas with Se-deficient soils had low blood Se levels as a consequence of eating Se-deficient grains. Selenium is an essential nutrient for humans and is a cofactor for glutathione peroxidase, an enzyme with antioxidant properties. Selenium is also a component of several other Se-containing proteins, including iodothyrodine deiodinase, thioredoxin reductase, and selenoprotein P and W.

Because of the association of Keshan disease with low Se status, the Chinese government began a randomized, placebo-controlled intervention trial with sodium selenite in Keshan endemic areas. A significant drop in Keshan disease in the Se-treated group was noted before the scheduled end of the trial, which led to the discontinuation of the study and supplementation of all individuals at risk of Keshan disease with sodium selenite.

Supplementation with Se has essentially prevented Keshan disease in China. However, there were several aspects of the disease that could not be wholly attributed to a lack of Se. Keshan disease was found to have both a seasonal and annual incidence, and not every individual with low Se status developed the disease. Thus, the epidemiological data suggested that an infectious cofactor might also be required along with a deficiency in Se. Scientists in China examined the blood and tissues from Keshan disease victims for the presence of infectious agents and found enteroviruses in many of the samples. Enteroviruses, and particularly the coxsackieviruses, are known to infect heart muscle and cause inflammation (myocarditis).

A coxsackievirus B4 isolated from a Keshan disease victim was found to cause severe heart damage when used to infect Se-deficient mice *(21)*. Selenium-adequate mice infected with the same virus had much less pathology. In one study, 87.5% of myocardial samples from Keshan disease patients were positive for enteroviral RNA using the technique of reverse-transcriptase polymerase chain reaction (RT-PCR), whereas only 3% of controls (myocardial samples from non-Keshan disease tissue) were positive *(22)*. Thus, it appears that an infectious cofactor may be involved in the development of Keshan disease, a Se-responsive cardiomyopathy.

SELENIUM DEFICIENCY AND COXSACKIEVIRUS B3 INFECTION

In order to further understand the relationship between a deficiency in Se and its impact on a viral infection, a well-characterized mouse model of coxsackievirus B3-induced myocarditis, which closely mimics the human disease, was utilized to probe the effect of specific nutritional deficiencies on a viral infection.

Two strains of coxsackievirus B3 were utilized in these studies: CVB3/20, which is a myocarditic strain, and CVB3/0, which is an amyocarditic strain. Both strains will replicate to essentially identical titers in the heart tissue of mice; however, only the myocarditic CVB3/20 strain induces myocarditis, or inflammatory heart disease. The virulent strain of coxsackievirus, CVB3/20, causes an acute inflammation in the heart characterized by an infiltration of inflammatory cells and subsequent necrosis and calcification of the heart muscle. This inflammation is similar to what occurs in infected humans.

Coxsackievirus B3 is a single-stranded RNA virus of approximately 7400 nucleotides. Four structural capsid proteins make up the outer shell, which protects the viral RNA as well as providing the site for attachment to and subsequent entry into a host cell. There are only seven nucleotide differences between the myocar-

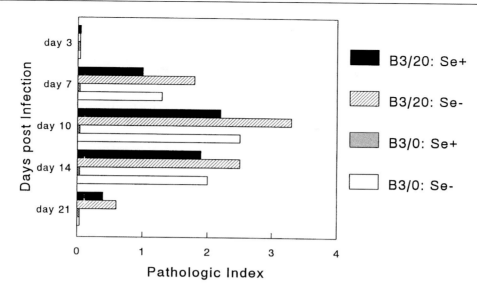

Fig. 2. Anatomically similar portions of the left ventricle were graded for inflammation. Inflammation was graded on a scale of 0 to 4+. Pathologic scores: 0, no lesions; 1+, foci of mononuclear cell inflammation associated with myocardial cell reactive changes without myocardial cell necrosis; 2+, inflammatory foci clearly associated with myocardial cell reactive changes; 3+, inflammatory foci clearly associated with myocardial cell necrosis and dystrophic calcification; 4+, extensive inflammatory infiltration, necrosis, and dystrophic calcification. Each bar represents the mean score of 15 mice.

ditic strain of CVB3, CVB3/20, and the amyocarditic strain, CVB3/0. These seven nucleotides are not clustered in one area of the genome, rather they are scattered throughout, both in structural and nonstructural regions of the virus. This is not unusual for this group of viruses, as another closely related enterovirus, poliovirus, can become avirulent by very few mutations in the viral genome.

ALTERED PATHOGENESIS IN CVB3-INFECTED SE-DEFICIENT MICE Mice were fed a diet deficient in Se for 4 wk prior to viral infection. Gutathione peroxidase levels, as a biomarker of Se status, were fivefold lower in the mice fed the Se-deficient diet as compared with control mice fed the Se-adequate diet. Following infection with the myocarditic strain CVB3/20, the hearts of the Se-deficient mice were found to have much more severe inflammation and necrosis when compared with mice fed the Se-adequate diet (Fig. 2). Thus, the Se-deficient mice were more susceptible to the cardiovirulent properties of the myocarditic virus. Cardiopathology occurred earlier and was more severe at each time-point postinfection.

Of particular interest, the Se-deficient mice infected with the avirulent CVB3/0 virus also developed myocarditis, whereas the CVB3/0 infected Se-adequate mice did not develop any myocarditis (Fig. 2). Thus, the Se-deficient mice became vulnerable to the pathogenic effects of a normally avirulent virus.

Was the change in pathology related to increased amounts (titers) of virus in the Se-deficient mice? To answer this question, hearts from viral-infected Se-deficient and Se-adequate mice were screened for virus. The Se-deficient mice infected with either CVB3/20 or CVB3/0 had approximately 100-fold higher viral titers in the heart when compared with infected Se-adequate mice (Fig. 3). Although the titers were higher in the Se-deficient mice, the kinetics of the response was similar to the Se-adequate mice; that is, virus was first detected in the hearts of the Se-adequate and Se-deficient mice at an identical time-point, and both groups

were able to remove the virus in a similar time period. Thus, Se-deficient mice had higher viral titers, although clearance of the virus was not affected.

IMMUNOLOGICAL EFFECTS OF SE DEFICIENCY The fact that the amount of virus was elevated in the infected Se-deficient mice suggested that the immune response of the Se-deficient mice was impaired. An inadequate immune response would be unable to prevent the increased replication of the virus. In order to determine if this was the case, both humoral and cellular aspects of the immune response were tested.

Both CVB3/20- and CVB3/0-infected Se-deficient mice were found to have equivalent levels of a specific CVB3-neutralizing antibody when compared with infected Se-adequate mice. Thus, the ability of B cells to produce antibodies that can inactivate the virus was not affected by a deficiency in Se. However, the ability of splenic T cells to proliferate in response to both mitogen (Con A) and specific CVB3 antigen exposure were decreased in the Se-deficient mice when compared with Se-adequate mice. Natural-killer cell activity was identical between Se-adequate and Se-deficient mice, demonstrating no effect of the Se deficiency on this component of the immune response. Although antibody production and NK active was not affected by a deficiency in Se, the fact that the T-cell proliferative response was greatly diminished suggests that immune dysfunction may be responsible for the increase in viral titers found in the Se-deficient mice. The cause of the decrease in T-cell proliferation may be due to a number of different possibilities, including decreased cytokine production required for proliferation. The observation that antibody responses are intact suggests that an imbalance may have occurred, such that TH2 cells, which provide signals for B-cell production of antibody are favored over TH1 cells, which secrete cytokines important for proliferation.

VIRAL GENOMIC CHANGES The increase in virulence of both the myocarditic and the amyocarditic viruses in the Se-

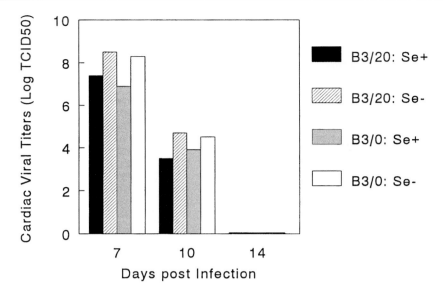

Fig. 3. Viral titers (expressed as log tissue culture infectious dose 50 per gram of heart tissue) of heart at various times post inoculation. Each bar represents the mean of 15 animals.

deficient mice may have been the result of a compromised immune response. This hypothesis would postulate that the increased pathogenicity of the viruses was the result of a less than optimal immune response, which resulted in increased viral replication and, hence, increased pathogenicity. However, a second hypothesis can be postulated that takes into account the pathogen itself, rather than just the host. This hypothesis would suggest that the virus itself may be altered as a consequence of replicating in a Se-deficient animal. To differentiate between these possibilities, a passage experiment was devised (Fig. 4).

Mice were fed a diet either deficient or adequate in Se for 4 wk prior to infection with CVB3/0, the amyocarditic strain of virus. At 10 d postinfection, the mice were killed and the virus was isolated from the heart tissue. This virus was renamed CVB3/0Se– to distinguish it from the CVB3/0 parent strain. Similarly, virus obtained from the hearts of infected Se-adequate mice was renamed CVB3/0Se+. Following isolation, CVB3/0Se– and CVB3/0Se+ were passed back into Se-adequate mice and the histopathology of the heart was examined 10 d later. If Se-deficiency primarily affects the host, then Se-adequate mice infected with virus isolated from a Se-deficient animal will not develop myocarditis because the virus is avirulent in a Se-adequate host. However, if the virus itself is affected, thus altering the phenotypic expression of disease, then the Se-adequate animal may be at risk for developing myocarditis.

As shown in Table 1, Se-adequate mice infected with virus isolated from CVB3/0– infected Se-deficient mice (CVB3/0Se–) developed mycarditis. Control mice in which virus isolated from Se-adequate mice (CVB3/0Se+) and passed back into Se-adequate mice did not develop myocarditis, demonstrating that passage of virus alone did not induce a change in virulence. Thus, a phenotype change occurred in the virus that was replicated in a Se-deficient host, changing a normally avirulent virus to a virulent one.

The most logical explanation for the phenotype change of the CVB3/0Se– virus is a change in the viral genome. In order to confirm this possibility, virus obtained from both Se-adequate

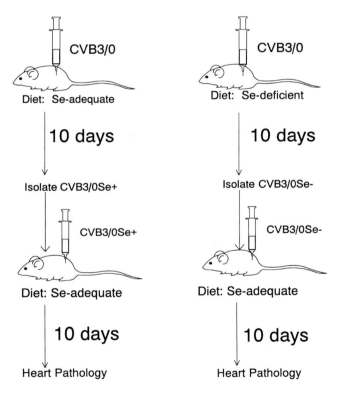

Fig. 4. Diagram of passage experiment used to determine if host factors or viral factors are responsible for the change in virulence of CVB3/0 in Se-deficient mice.

(CVB3/0Se+) and Se-deficient (CVB3/0Se–) mice was sequenced. Comparison of the CVB3/0Se+ and CVB3/0Se– viruses revealed six nucleotide changes between the two viruses *(23)*. The sequence of the CVB3/0Se+ virus was identical to the sequence of the original CVB3/0 input virus. Thus, the change in virulence of the CVB3/0Se– virus was the result of a change in the viral genome.

Table 1
Heart Pathology 10 d
Post CVB3/0Se+ and CVB3/0Se– Inoculation

Virus[a]	Recipient diet	Heart pathology[b]	Viral genome change?
CVB3/0Se+	Se adequate	0	No
CVB3/0Se–	Se adequate	2–3+	Yes
CVB3/0 (parental strain)	Se adequate	0	No

[a]Ten mice were inoculated with indicated virus. CVB3/0Se+ virus was isolated from a CVB3/0 infected mouse fed a Se-adequate diet. CVB3/0Se– virus was isolated from a CVB3/0-infected mouse fed a Se-deficient diet. Recipient mice were fed the Se-adequate diet.
[b]Heart histopathology was scored as for Fig. 2.

The six nucleotide changes seen in the CVB3/0Se– virus were all identical to nucleotides found in known virulent strains of CVB3. Thus, out of the seven nucleotides that distinguish an avirulent virus from a virulent one, six nucleotides of the avirulent virus mutated to nucleotides found in the virulent virus. Nucleotide 2690, which is an adenosine in the avirulent virus, remained a cytosine in the CVB3/0Se– virus, which is the same as the parent CVB3/0 virus. The sequence of four CVB3/0Se– isolates from four separate mice were identical in that they all carried the same six mutations. This suggests that these sites are more susceptible to mutation or that these sites convey a fitness advantage to the virus. The mutated nucleotides are spread throughout the genome, two in nontranslated regions of the virus, two in the capsid regions, and two in the nonstructural protein regions. Which of these mutations, or if all of these mutations, are required for the change to virulence is not known.

These results were the first to demonstrate that the nutritional status of the host could have an affect on the genome of a pathogen, changing a normally avirulent virus into a virulent one. Once the genomic changes occurred, now even hosts with normal nutritional health became vulnerable to the mutated virus.

GLUTATHIONE PEROXIDASE AND COXSACKIEVIRUS INFECTION

Selenium is an essential component of glutathione peroxidase. There are four isozymes of glutathione peroxidase that catalyze the degradation of hydroperoxides using glutathione as the hydrogen donor. Glutathione peroxidase 1 (GPX-1) is the most abundant selenoprotein and appears to be present in all cell types, with high levels in heart, liver, and kidney tissue. The enzyme is found in cytosol and mitochondria. The glutathione peroxidases are thought to play an important role in the defense of the organism against oxidative injury. Although many cell culture studies have demonstrated a role for GPX-1 as an antioxidant, less is known about its role in whole animals.

In order to determine if the increased virulence of CVB3 infection in Se-deficient mice was the result of a decrease in GPX-1 activity, a Gpx1 knockout mouse was utilized. Mice with a disrupted *Gpx1* gene (*Gpx1⁻* or Gxp1-KO) *(24)* were inoculated with the avirulent CVB3/0. At 10 d postinfection, a little over half of the Gpx1-KO mice developed myocarditis, whereas none of the wildtype mice developed any pathology. The heart histopathology of the Gpx1-KO mice was similar to that seen in Se-deficient

mice. Thus, it appeared that the susceptibility of the Se-deficient mice to CVB3-induced myocarditis was mediated through decreased GPX-1 activity.

Interestingly, the immune response of the Gpx1-KO mice was dissimilar to the Se-deficient mice. Whereas Se-deficient mice had normal antibody responses, but decreased T-cell proliferative responses to both mitogen and antigen, the Gpx1-KO mice had decreased antibody responses and normal T-cell proliferative responses when compared with the wild-type mice. This would seem to suggest that the immune response is independent of the viral pathogenesis. The amount of virus present in the heart of Gpx1-KO mice was equivalent to wild-type mice. This is in contrast to Se-deficient mice, which had higher viral titers in the heart when compared with Se-adequate mice. Thus, although increased pathogenicity of the CVB3/0 virus occurs in both Se-deficient and Gpx1-KO mice, the immune response to the virus is very different, as well as the titer of replicating virus in the heart, suggesting that components of the immune response other than the antibody response may be required for viral clearance.

To determine if viral genomic changes similar to what was seen in the Se-deficient mice also occurred in virus obtained from Gpx1-KO mice, virus isolated from both wild-type and Gpx1-Ko mice was sequenced. The same six nucleotide changes identical to the ones found in virus recovered from Se-deficient mice were found in virus isolated from Gpx1-KO mice. In addition, a seventh nucleotide at position 2690 was also altered in the Gpx1-KO mice, which was not found in the Se-deficient mice. This nucleotide changed from cytosine to adenosine in the Gpx1-KO mice. As for virus isolated from Se-deficient mice, virus isolated from Gpx1-KO mice also mutates to a more virulent genotype. This result demonstrates the importance of GPX-1 activity in protection from oxidative stress and, thus, vulnerability to viral infection.

VITAMIN E DEFICIENCY AND COXSACKIEVIRUS B3 INFECTION

Vitamin E is a fat-soluble vitamin that acts as an antioxidant. Under certain conditions, vitamin E and Se can spare one another's activity. Similar to what was found for Se-deficient mice, vitamin E-deficient mice develop more severe myocarditis when infected with the myocarditic strain, CVB3/20. In addition, vitamin E-deficient mice also develop myocarditis when infected with the avirulent CVB3/0 strain. Of particular interest, vitamin E-deficient diets using menhaden oil as a fat source rather than lard exacerbate the pathology beyond the lard-based vitamin E-deficient diet. Menhaden oil provides a source of readily peroxidizable, highly unsaturated fatty acids. In addition, menhaden oil antagonizes vitamin E by a mechanism that is not entirely clear. It may be that the lower concentration of α-tocopherol in serum of mice fed menhaden oil may be the result of destructive interaction of the oil and vitamin E in the gastrointestinal tract or may be due to an accelerated post absorptive utilization of vitamin E in the tissues.

Similar to Se-deficient mice, the amount of virus present in the hearts of vitamin E-deficient mice is elevated when compared with vitamin E-adequate mice. However, in contrast to Se-deficient mice, virus persists longer in the vitamin E-deficient mice, although the deficient mice are able to clear the virus from the heart 3 wk following the infection.

The immune response of the viral-infected vitamin E-deficient mice was similar to what was found for Se-deficient mice. The antibody response was unaffected, but the T-cell proliferative response to both mitogen and antigen was greatly reduced. In addition, natural-killer (NK) cell activity was unaffected by the diet, unless the diet contained menhaden oil as the fat source, either with or without vitamin E. Both menhaden-oil-containing diets suppressed NK activity. Natural killer activity has been previously shown to be suppressed by a fish-oil-rich diet. Thus, both Se and vitamin E deficiency can adversely affect the immune response.

The observation that both Se- and vitamin E-deficient mice develop more severe myocarditis post CVB3 infection suggests that the oxidative stress status of the host is the common element. To further test the hypothesis that oxidative stress played a role in the increase in pathology post viral infection, N,N'-diphenyl-p-phenylenediamine (DPPD) was added to the vitamin E-deficient diet. DPPD is a synthetic antioxidant structurally unrelated to vitamin E, which mimics its antioxidant properties. Mice fed vitamin E-deficient diets supplemented with DPPD had serum α-tocopherol levels (0.8 ± 0.1 μmol/L) similar to unsupplemented vitamin E-deficient diets (0.6 μmol/L). This is in contrast to mice fed a vitamin E-adequate diet in which the levels of α-tocopherol are nine times higher (4.5 ± 0.1 μmol/L). Following infection with CVB3/20, mice fed a vitamin E-deficient diet supplemented with DPPD were protected from the increased myocarditis seen in the mice fed the unsupplemented vitamin E-deficient diet.

Thus, several lines of evidence suggest that the mechanism of enhanced pathogenesis post CVB3 infection is dependent on increased oxidative stress of the host animal:

1. Selenium deficiency enhances CVB3-induced myocarditis.
2. Mice deficient in Gpx-1 activity are more susceptible to CVB3-induced myocarditis.
3. Vitamin E-deficient mice are more susceptible to CVB3-induced myocarditis.
4. Consumption of menhaden oil, a peroxidizable fat, increases the pathogenesis of CVB3 infection.
5. A synthetic antioxidant, DPPD, can prevent the increased myocarditis seen in CVB3-infected vitamin E-deficient mice.

CHEMOKINES AND NUTRITIONALLY INDUCED OXIDATIVE STRESS

Chemokines are small molecules involved in leukocyte trafficking. They are produced by a variety of cell types and many have overlapping functions and receptors by in vitro analysis. The chemokine macrophage inflammatory protein-1α (MIP-1α) induces chemotaxis of monocytes, CD8+ T cells, and B cells in vitro. Cook et al. *(25)* demonstrated that mice deficient in MIP-1α (MIP-1α knockout mice) are completely protected from developing myocarditis when inoculated with the virulent strain of CVB3, CVB3/20. This result demonstrates that other members of the chemokine family, including those chemokines that share the same receptor with MIP-1α, cannot functionally substitute for MIP-1α in vivo.

To determine if nutritionally induced oxidative stress can have an effect on the MIP-1α-driven inflammatory response, MIP-1α knockout mice were fed a diet deficient in both Se and vitamin E prior to infection with CVB3/20. Although MIP-1α knockout mice fed an adequate diet did not develop any myocarditis, approx-

imately 50% of MIP-1α KO mice fed the deficient diet developed myocarditis. Thus, the protective effect of a lack of MIP-1α could be overcome by inducing oxidative stress in the host by feeding an antioxidant-deficient diet.

Chemokines such as MIP-1β, RANTES, and MCP-1 which have activities similar to MIP-1α, are not elevated in the MIP-1α KO mice fed the deficient diet, suggesting that overcompensation by other chemokines is not the explanation for the change in pathogenesis. At this point, it is not known how the oxidative stress affects the chemokine response.

Cardiac virus titers in the MIP-1α KO mice fed the deficient diet were significantly lower than the virus titers of mice fed an adequate diet. This could be explained by the presence of inflammation in the oxidatively stressed MIP-1α KO mice which could then contribute to viral clearance. Neutralizing antibody titers are not effected, but the T-cell proliferative responses are decreased to both mitogen and antigen in both MIP-1α KO and wild-type mice fed the deficient diet.

EPIDEMIC OF OPTIC AND PERIPHERAL NEUROPATHY IN CUBA

In the early 1990s, an epidemic of optic and peripheral neuropathy affected more than 50,000 people in Cuba. Extensive epidemiologic studies carried out with international cooperation *(26)* revealed that the disease was associated with an unbalanced diet low in animal proteins, fats, and B-group and other vitamins, and an increased consumption of sugar. In particular, the investigative team suggested an impairment of protective antioxidant pathways because patients had lower levels of riboflavin, vitamin E, Se, and α- and β-carotenes and especially the carotenoid lycopene when compared to matched controls. Smoking of cigars was also a risk factor that intensified the effects of the nutritional deficiencies and is thought to increase the production of oxygen radicals.

The number of cases reached 50,466 by the end of 1993, an incidence of 462 per 100,000 population. Most patients responded to parenteral vitamin therapy, and the epidemic began to subside when oral vitamin supplementation with B complex vitamins, vitamin A, and folate was begun for the entire population in 1993. New cases have continued to accumulate at a low rate.

In order to rule out the possibility of an infectious agent, virus isolation attempts from cerebrospinal fluid (CSF) was begun in 1993. Unexpectedly, viruses resembling enteroviruses were found in 105 of 125 (84%) CSF samples cultured. Five of those isolated were typical strains of coxsackievirus A9, identified by neutralization. The other 100 isolates produced an atypical pattern of replication in cell culture. Analysis of viral proteins revealed a lack of the typical outer capsid proteins characteristic of enteroviruses. Rather than four individual proteins of varying size, one large protein was found. By neutralization, the viruses were related to both coxsackievirus A9 and B4 *(27)*.

In order to further understand the phenotypic difference between CVA9 and the atypical Cuban isolates, one isolate, 44/93 IPK, was sequenced and compared with the sequence of CVA9 and other known enteroviruses. Although a number of nucleotide differences between CVA9 and 44/93 IPK were identified, the most interesting finding concerns the active site of the 2A proteinase. The 2A proteinase is responsible for initiating the cleavage of the viral polyprotein into the four capsid proteins that make up the viral shell. The enterovirus 2A proteinase is structurally similar to cellular serine proteinases, which characteristically fold to form a catalytic triad of histidine, aspartic acid, and serine. In the enteroviruses, however, the catalytic site contains cysteine instead of serine, and the enzyme is inhibited by compounds known to inhibit thiol proteinases. Zinc also plays an essential structural role in this enzyme.

The Cuban isolate, 44/93 IPK, resembles other enteroviruses in that it contains the three amino acids of the 2A catalytic triad: His21, Asp39, and Cys110. However, unlike CVA9 or any of the other known enterovirus sequences, 44/93 IPK has a mutation that introduces another cysteine four residues away from the active site, at position 25. CVA9 strains that have been studied all have histidine or arginine at this locus: Coxsackievirus B strains have histidine, arginine, or serine. The introduction of another cysteine so close to the essential cysteine of the catalytic site suggests the possibility of dimerization to form cysteine, thus leading to inactivation of the enzyme, especially under oxidizing conditions. The 44/93 IPK isolate has two other amino acid substitutions within five positions of the 2A catalytic site, neither of which occurs in any of the CA9 or CB strains studied: lysine for threonine at position 26 and isoleucine for valine at position 17. Impairment of the function of the 2A proteinase would prevent appropriate cleavage of the polyprotein, thus leading to an absence of viral capsid proteins. This may explain the apparent absence of the normal capsid proteins and the appearance instead of a high-molecular-weight protein, which may be the uncleaved capsid protein precursor.

POSSIBLE MECHANISMS FOR VIRAL GENOMIC CHANGE IN NUTRITIONALLY DEFICIENT ANIMALS

DIRECT OXIDATIVE DAMAGE TO VIRAL RNA Damage to DNA by oxygen radicals has been widely documented. Indeed, the mammalian antioxidant system is highly developed in order to decrease damage that can occur by the presence of oxygen radicals. Reactive oxygen species (ROS), produced when oxygen undergoes a series of univalent reductive steps rather than forming water through reductive pathways in the mitochondrial respiratory chain, are highly reactive and can cause damage to DNA as well as to cellular membranes. Thus, the organism strives to have a balance between oxidants and antioxidants, and oxidative stress results when an imbalance occurs that favors the oxidants. Currently, the application of dietary interventions to affect the oxidative stress status of mammalians is under intense study.

Although oxidative damage to DNA has been accepted, less is known about oxidative damage to RNA. Several studies have shown that RNA can be oxidatively damaged. For example, RNA can be damaged oxidatively by dye photosensitization, and ultraviolet A radiation of skin fibroblasts increases the levels of guanine hydroxylation. Rats treated with a hepatocarcinogen develop 8-hydroxyguanosine as well as 8-hydroxydeoxyguanosine, resulting from oxidative damage to RNA and DNA. In *E. coli,* the muT protein (which has mammalian homologs) protects transcriptional fidelity by hydrolyzing oxidized guanine, which mispairs with adenine.

Thus, although there is more information on DNA damage by ROS, it is also possible that direct oxidative damage to viral RNA can occur as well in an oxidatively stressed animal. CVB3 is a single-stranded RNA virus, and single-stranded RNA has been suggested to be more susceptible than double-stranded DNA to damage by free radicals. Guanine has a high oxidative potential

and this nucleotide is the site of mutation at 3/7 sites in the CVB3 virus obtained from oxidatively stressed mice. During DNA replication, unrepaired oxidized bases can cause DNA mispairing and mutation. Mutations resulting from oxidized bases may also occur in RNA genomes, particularly because RNA viruses lack efficient proofreading and postreplicative repair activities. Thus, RNA viruses have at least a 100-fold higher mutation rate in general than the mutation rate for cellular DNA. Therefore, in an individual virus population, individual genomes that differ in one or more nucleotides will form the average or consensus sequence of the population, which have been termed quasispecies. A high mutation rate coupled with a lack of antioxidant protection increases the likelihood of an accelerated mutation rate, thus leading to the genomic changes found in the nutritionally deficient mice.

SELECTION OF VIRULENT VIRUS: QUASISPECIES
Because of the high mutation rate of RNA viruses (*see* Section 9.1), any individual RNA virus will form a collection of closely related mutants, termed quasispecies. Rather than a single RNA genome, any particular RNA virus will represent a consensus or average sequence. It is believed that this heterogeneous pool of RNA viruses allows for rapid adaptation to changes in the environment that would convey a survival advantage.

If the RNA virus is replicating in an oxidatively stressed host because of dietary deficiency, then the selection of a pre-existing mutant from the quasispecies pool, which is more suited for growth under conditions of increased host cellular oxidative stress, may occur. In the case of coxsackievirus, the selected mutant or quasispecies is more virulent than the original quasispecies. Thus, the nutritional status of the host may play a large (and until recently, unstudied) role in determining the evolutionary development of a viral disease.

In addition, the oxidative stress status of the host also affects the immune response. A dysfunctional immune response would also be expected to have an effect on the virus by allowing the virus to escape normal immune clearance mechanisms. This, in theory, would allow for the expansion of viral clones and potentially increase the mutational rate of the virus, leading to the selection of a quasispecies with altered phenotypic properties. Based on the current knowledge of quasispecies and oxidative damage, the following hypothesis can be put forward to explain the transformation of a benign coxsackievirus into a virulent one by genomic mutations. First, oxidative damage occurs to the viral genome because of the presence of ROS in nutritionally deficient mice. This damage in viral RNA leads to an increased incidence of mutation from a lack of proofreading enzymes as well as a lack of an efficient immune response to clear the mutated virus. Once these changes have occurred, the virus now has an altered expression of virulence. This work clearly demonstrates the important role antioxidant nutrition plays in protection of the host from viral pathogens.

HUMAN IMMUNODEFICIENCY VIRUS AND ANTIOXIDANT NUTRIENTS

The virus responsible for acquired immunodeficiency disease syndrome (AIDS), the human immunodeficiency virus (HIV), is similar to other RNA viruses in that it has a high mutation rate and it occurs as a quasispecies. Therefore, one could hypothesize that this virus, like coxsackievirus, may be susceptible to genetic changes when the oxidative stress status of the host is increased.

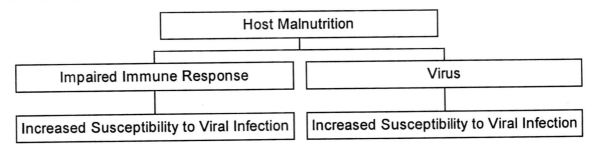

Fig. 5. Revised model based on recent data demonstrating that host nutritional status can directly affect the virus, as well as the host immune response.

Indeed, several investigators have looked at the role of antioxidants during infection with HIV.

Infection with HIV is often associated with weight loss and chronic oxidative stress. As the disease progresses, levels of several antioxidants decrease, glutathione is consumed and the survival of AIDS patients can be correlated with a deficiency in glutathione of CD4+ T cells and low serum thiol levels.

One study showed that HIV-1-related mortality could be correlated with a deficiency in Se: Lower Se levels were associated with increased mortality. Serum Se, plasma glutathione, and red cell glutathione are decreases as HIV-1 infection progresses. It has been suggested that supplementation with Se of HIV-infected patients may improve symptoms and prolong life.

In vitro studies have demonstrated that Se supplementation can suppress HIV-1 replication by decreasing tumor necrosis factor (TNF) induction of NF-κB activation replication. Thus, the selenium status of the HIV-1-infected individual and, hence, their oxidative stress status may have an influence on the progression of AIDS, perhaps by altering the development of quasispecies. HIV-1-infected individuals who experience rapid CD4+ T-cell decline have a quasispecies virus population that is relatively stable, whereas those with less T-cell loss have virus populations still evolving. Perhaps the pro-oxidant–antioxidant balance of the host contributes to this process.

POTENTIAL NEW VIRAL GENES VIA SELENOCYSTEINE

Nutritional status of the host can also influence the genome of the virus in other ways. Because the amount of coding in a particular virus is constrained by size limitations, viruses must maximize the information contained in their genes. One possibility for maximizing that information is to place overlapping genes in different reading frames. Thus, the coding regions are expanded without having to increase the total number of nucleotides.

Using the idea of the possibility of overlapping reading frames, Taylor et al. (28) explored the possibility that a normal stop codon, UGA, could be read as a selenocysteine and, thus, translation would continue. In order for the normal stop codon UGA to be used for selenocysteine incorporation, a SECIS element (a structural signal in the mRNA-3′-untranslated region) must be present. In searching for potential new genes, a computer method was used to translate the coxsackievirus genome in all 3 reading frames, assuming that UGA was seen as selenocysteine. If an overlap was found with a known coding region, then a frameshift sequence was looked for and, if found, the secondary structure of the RNA was examined for RNA stems or pseudoknots close to the frame-

shift. If these conditions were found, then the new sequence was translated and protein databases searched for homology.

Using this technique, two potential selenoproteins genes in CVB3 can be identified. One potential gene has a strong homology with a family of proteins that contains epidermal growth factor. Novel genes were also found in HIV using the computer algorithm. These results are intriguing, especially in light of the finding that the virus molluscum contagiosum codes for a protein with high homology to the selenoenzyme glutathione peroxidase (29). The authors speculate that this virus may carry this gene in order to reduce the local presence of oxidative stress in the tissue. Thus, it appears that, at least for this virus, preventing localized oxidative stress conveys a survival advantage.

SUMMARY

The results presented in this chapter point to the importance of oxidative stress in modulating the response of the host to the virus. In addition, the virus itself is affected by the host oxidative stress status, such that the genome of the virus itself is altered. This is possible due to the high mutation rate of RNA viruses in general. Thus, RNA viruses are continually changing and rapidly adapting to their environment. Rather than a unidirectional model of host nutritional status impacting the immune response, which, in turn, leads to increased susceptibility to viral infection (Fig. 1), a revised model can be constructed that incorporates the finding that host nutritional status can directly affect the virus (Fig. 5).

The fact that changes in host nutrition that affect the antioxidant pathways of the host can have profound effects on a virus suggests that limiting oxidative stress in the host may be beneficial, both by preventing decreases in the immune response as well as by limiting the potential adverse mutations that can occur in the virus. Although emerging infectious diseases are often thought of as arising because of a number of factors, including increased global travel, changes in agricultural practices, cutting down rain forests, and so forth, little attention has been focused on the impact of nutrition. It remains to be seen how many emergent infectious diseases are the result of an interplay between host nutritional status and the infecting virus. Continued interdisciplinary research in the fields of nutrition, immunology, and virology are required to further investigate these questions.

REFERENCES

1. Scrimshaw NS, Taylor CE, Gordon JE. Interactions of Nutrition and Infection, WHO Monograph Series No. 57. World Health Organization, Geneva, 1968.

2. Dagan R, Bar-David Y, Sarov B, Katz M, Kassis I, Greegerg D, et al. Rotavirus diarrhea in Jewish and Bedouin children in the Negev region of Israel: epidemiology, clinical aspects, and possible role of malnutrition in severity of illness. Pediatr Infect Dis J 1990; 9:314–21.

3. Frieden TR, Sowell AL, Henning KJ, Huff DL, Gunn RA. Vitamin A levels and severity of measles: New York City. Am J Dis Child 1992; 146:182–6.

4. Beck MA. The role of nutrition in viral disease. J Nutr Biochem 1996; 7:683–90.

5. Bendich A, Chandra RK. Micronutrients and immune functions. Ann NY Acad Sci 1990; 587:168–80.

6. Riepenhogg-Talty M, Offor E, Kossner K, Kowalski E, Carmody PJ, Ogra PL. Effect of age and malnutrition on rotavirus infection in mice. Pediatr Res 1985; 19:1250–3.

7. Noble RL, Sidwell RW, Mahoney AW, Barnett BB, Spendlove RS. Influence of malnutrition and alterations in dietary protein on murine rotaviral disease. Proc Soc Exp Bio Med 1983; 173:417–26.

8. Gwatkin DR. How many die? A set of demographic estimates of the annual number of infant and child deaths in the world. Am J Public Health 1980; 70:1286–9.

9. Christie CD, Heikens GT, Black FL. Acute respiratory infections in ambulatory malnourished children: a serological study. Trans Roy Soc Trop Med Hyg 1990; 84:160–1.

10. Brussow H, Sidoti J, Dirren H, Freire WB. Effect of malnutrition in Ecuadorian children on titers of serum antibodies to various microbial antigens. Clin Diagn Lab Immunol 1995; 2:62–8.

11. Berman S. Epidemiology of acute respiratory infections in children of developing countries. Rev Infect Dis 1991; 13:S454–62.

12. Hussey GD, Klein M. A randomized, controlled trial of vitamin A in children with severe measles. N Engl J Med 1990; 323:160–4.

13. Quinlan KP, Hayani KC. Vitamin A and respiratory syncytial virus infection. Serum levels and supplementation trial. Arch Pediatr Adolesc Med 1996; 150:25–30.

14. Al-Nakib W, Higgins PG, Barrow I, Batstone G, Tyrrell DA. Phrophylaxis and treatment of rhinovirus colds with zinc gluconate lozenges. J Antimicrob Chemother 1987; 20:689–901.

15. Singh KP, Zaidi SIA, Raisuddin S, Saxena AK, Murphy RC, Ray PK. Effect of zinc on immune functions and host resistance against infection and tumor challenge. Immunopharmacol Immunotoxicol 1992; 14:813–40.

16. Grimstad PR, Haramis LD. Aedes triseriatus (Diptera: Culicidae) and La Crosse virus. III. Enhanced oral transmission by nutrition-deprived mosquitos. J Med Entomol 1984; 21:249–256.

17. Beck MA, Kolbeck PC, Rohr LH, Shi Q, Morris VC, Levander OA. Amyocarditic coxsackievirus becomes myocarditic in selenium deficient mice. J Med Virol 1994; 43:166–70.

18. Beck MA, Kolbeck PC, Rohr LH, Shi Q, Morris VC, Levander OA. Increased virulence of a human enterovirus (coxsackievirus B3) in selenium-deficient mice. J Infect Dis 1994; 170:351–7.

19. Beck MA, Kolbeck PC, Rohr LH, Shi Q, Morris VC, Levander OA. Vitamin E deficiency intensifies the myocardial injury of coxsackievirus B3 infection of mice. J Nutr 1994; 124:345–58.

20. Li Y, Wang F, Kang D, Li C. Keshan disease: an endemic cardiomyopathy in China. Hum Pathol 1985; 16:602–9.

21. Bai J, Wu S, Ge K, Deng X, Su C. The combined effect of selenium deficiency and viral infection on the myocardium of mice. Acta Acad Med Sinica 1980; 2:31–3.

22. Li Y, Zhang H, Yang Y, Chen H, Archard LC. High prevalence of enteroviral genomic sequences in an endemic cardiomyopathy (Keshan disease) detected by nested polymerase chain reaction. Progress in Clinical Virology 1995 Joint Meeting 1995, p. 172 (abstract).

23. Beck MA, Shi Q, Morris VC, Levander OA. Rapid genomic evolution of a non-virulent Coxsackievirus B3 in selenium-deficient mice results in selection of identical virulent isolates. Nat Med 1995; 1:433–6.

24. Ho Y-S, Magnenat JL, Broonson RT, Cao J, Gargano M, Sugawara M, et al. Mice deficient in cellular glutathione peroxidase develop normally and show no increased sensitivity to hypoxia. J Biol Chem 1997; 272:16,644–51.

25. Cook DN, Beck MA, Coffman TM, Kirby SL, Sheridan JF, et al. Requirement of MIP-1α for an inflammatory response to viral infection. Science 1995; 269:1583–5.

26. Cuba Neuropathy Field Investigation Team. Epidemic optic neuropathy in Cuba–clinical characterization and risk factors. N Engl J Med 1995; 333:1176–82.

27. Mas P, Pelegrino JL, Guzman MG, Comellas MM, Resik S, et al. Viral isolation from cases of epidemic neuropathy in Cuba. Arch Pathol Lab Med 1997; 121:825–33.

28. Taylor EW, Ramanathan CS, Jahari RK, Nadimpalli RG. A basis for new approaches to the chemotherapy of AIDS: novel genes in HIV-1 potentially encode selenoproteins expressed by ribosomal frameshifting and termination suppression. J Med Chem 1994; 37:2637–54.

29. Shisler JL, Senkevich TG, Berry MS, Moss B. Ultraviolet-induced cell death blocked by a selenoprotein from a human dermatotropic poxvirus. Science 1998; 279:102–5.

FUTURE DIRECTIONS   V

38 Whither Nutrition and Immunology Interactions Toward the Next Millennium? What Is Past Is Prologue

Noel W. Solomons

WHEN NUTRITION MEETS IMMUNOLOGY

What is the purpose and target of a handbook? Usually, it is to synthesize the most relevant and current information on a topic and to provide a resource for that relevant and current information or to provide a manual for instruction in that information to be consulted by students, teachers, and research professionals. Our present collection of 38 chapters attempts to address such a mission. However, most of the chapters contribute only a piece to a larger jigsaw puzzle. Now that all the pieces have been laid into place, I have been given the task to step back and survey the overall image in the assembled portrait of nutrition and immunology in the context of the *future*. In this respect, what we know today and know how to do today are the prologue for the next decade into the next millennium.

Both Nutritional Sciences and Immunology are mature academic and scientific disciplines. A forerunner of the present textbook is undoubtedly the thoughts and insights of Nevin Scrimshaw, Carl Taylor, and John Gordon in their *Interaction of Nutrition and Infection (1,2)*. Hence, it was 40 yr ago that the first incarnation was published. The present book is yet another reincarnation in that tradition, one that brings many more insights from the clinical and molecular domain of immunologists. A very helpful intellectual tool to keep the labyrinth of complexity from becoming a morass is the five-tiered outline of mechanisms of interaction of nutrition and immunity provided by Klasing and Leshchinsky *(3)*:

1. Direct regulation by nutrients;
2. Indirect modulation mediated by the endocrine system;
3. Regulation by availability of substrates;
4. Modulation on the pathology caused by an immune response; and
5. Nutritional immunity.

Recently, the issue of vitamin A deficiency and childhood mortality, introduced to the world by Sommer and colleagues

From: *Nutrition and Immunology: Principles and Practice* (ME Gershwin et al. eds.), © Humana Press, Inc., Totowa, NJ

(4,5), may epitomize the issue of nutrition and immunity. With respect to vitamin A deficiency, we are confronted with an extraordinary lethal reality. It has been estimated that upwards of 2 million children between 6 mo and 5 yr of age die annually as a consequence of hypovitaminosis A *(6)*. Obviously, an equal number would be saved if vitamin A deficiency were eliminated. However, as the foregoing chapters have pointed out with exhausting frequency, the facts that emerge present us with paradoxes and unresolved inconsistencies. So, one is forced immediately to focus on the immunity, given this paradox of equivalent incidence of infections but an apparently reduced severity and lower case-fatality rate of those who do get infected.

In the final overview, however, although infection has been the highest lightning rod for interests in immunity (and nutrition and immunity), the immune system is the center of issues related to cancer, allergy, autoimmune diseases, and aging as well. If the bottom line of medicine and public health is length of life, then we should note the following:

- Infection is the traditional killer of developing countries' children and adults.
- Neoplasia is the leading or second most important cause of mortality in industrialized countries.
- Systemic lupus erythematous, ulcerative colitis, Crohn's disease, bullous pemphigus, and a host of diseases of an autoimmune nature can shorten life both by chronic progression or acute crises.
- Anaphylaxis and asthmatic crises can also be life-threatening or lethal.

In this context, our attention can be focused like a laser on any insights and techniques that can lead the interaction of nutritional science and immunology to the resolution of the health problems to which they contribute.

NUTRITION AS IMBALANCE; IMMUNITY AS DYSREGULATION

In the synthesis of this book, we have the weaving of two disciplinary strands: nutrition and immunology. Any bringing together of the two discipines—either in a book such as this or in the context of collaborative investigation—would tend to highlight differences across the two. Placed into relief here has been a contrast of the underlying paradigm of nutrition, which has to do with the *external* balance of nutrient flows into and out of the organism, and immunology, which deals with an *internal* balance and harmony among degrees of expression in innate responses, acquired defenses, and autoimmunity.

NUTRITION: FEAST OR FAMINE The fields of animal nutrition and human nutrition, including clinical nutrition and public health nutrition, originated with concerns for *deficiencies*. This can be seen in the observations of Lind with citrus fruits and scurvy, or of Goldberger and the origins of pellagra. Livestock husbandry progressed only through the identification and redress of deficits of nutrients in the forages and fodders. With the close of World War II and a turning of attention to nutrition in developing countries, it was the "Protein Gap" and an obsession with protein-energy malnutrition that dominated the agenda of the United Nations' agencies and the bilateral assistance programs around the world. On the nutrition side of the ledger, the dominant paradigm of the last decade in human and public health nutrition has been "hidden hunger" *(7)* or micronutrient malnutrition. This was led by the vitamin A issue, but it has come to embrace those of iodine, iron, and zinc.

Meanwhile, over the last half century, an abundance of foods in the affluent countries of the postwar industrialization combined with a more sedentary lifestyle has led to nutrient *excess* becoming a problem with public health ramifications. This is highlighted in the pandemic of obesity in the developed nations. This dietary surfeit is associated with the etiology of circulatory diseases and neoplasia. Excess storage of iron is also associated with increased chronic disease risk. The manufacture and promotion of nutrients in dietary supplements allows those with the means to overstuff themselves with the whole range of micronutrients and phytochemicals with varying toxicological hazards for the overconsumer. With migration and urbanization in low-income developing countries, sedentarism and high-fat foods have made excess a concern for the health of the indigenous and poor populations, including the insulin-resistance syndrome (hyperinsulinemia with hypertension, glucose intolerance, and dyslipidemia) of Syndrome X.

To some extent, an organism has appetite regulation of intake to adjust consumption with respect to energy and hydration needs; we also have some mechanisms to excrete or metabolize unneeded quantities of energy or nutrients. However, in the main, it is not so much regulation but simply the balance sheet of income and outgo economics that define the variance in nutriture. Nutrition is fundamentally about deficiency and excess, feast or famine.

IMMUNITY: YIN AND YANG Given their grounding in this paradigm of too much or too little in relationship to intakes or losses (above), nutritionists might be tempted to see immunology in a parallel light, bolstered by terms such as immunodeficiency syndromes and allergic hyperreactivity. However, the message that comes through in booming decibels in this book is that immunity is all about delicate homeostatic regulation.

In Chapter 35 on Chinese herbal medicines, Chang provides the concept that sets the tone for an understanding of immune function *(8)*. It is *Yin* and *Yang*: the opposing—but complementing—elements of balance. We often talk about "enhancing" the immune response or "suppressing" it. However, just as a diminished response may leave the organism open to infection or cancer, too vigorous a response may deplete nutritional stores, generate

genetic damage, or be an allergic response or an autoimmune reaction. One cannot say that *more* is better. One cannot say that *less* is better. In fact, more and less are better at the same time. Hence, the modulation of the immune system by blood products and pharmacological agents—or by diet and nutritional status—should not be seen outside of the context of restoring an intricate and enduring *balance*.

This sets the stage for a consideration of how the host status with respect to nutrition and nutrient reserves is a determinant of immune status. Importantly, in the *Yin* and *Yang* concept, both undernutrition and overnutrition influence immune function and, generally, it is depressive (anti-inflammatory) at both extremes. The readership of this book will be divided into two polar spheres. If it is the personal, pubic health, or clinic setting in an affluent country, it will be *over*nutrition and excess that will dominate contemporary concern. If it is the practice of hospital medicine and surgery, geriatrics, or public health concerns of developing countries, then *under*nutrition will be the paradigm to pursue. Klasing and Leshchinsky's *(3)* analysis of a case in point with respect to supplementation with omega-3 fatty acids in a single feeding trial for the poultry industry is poetically illustrative. In the example, close to a million chicks were fed either a fish-oil-rich or an animal-fat-based feed. Those receiving the omega-3 fats "decreased the incidence of septicemia of all causes and the incidence of cellulitis ... by 18%," whereas "the incidence of tumors, both spontaneous and from Marek's disease virus, increased by 24%" *(3)*.

The question is again placed into relief when the question becomes the vigor of the body's defense against exogenous versus endogenous agents and antigens. In their chapter in this book, Jolly and Fernandes *(9)* state: "The immune system plays a leading role in fighting off the constant bombardment of our bodies by invading pathogenic organisms, such as bacteria, fungi, viruses, toxins, and allergic compounds." One can consider this the limb most commonly posed as concerns in clinical medicine and public health, that focusing on immune defense against *exogenous* factors. The Texas investigators have provided a comprehensive litany. Yet, there is another side to the actions of the immune response, which we might consider as against endogenous factors. In this, we would consider both vigilance against mutated cells that could become the precursors of cancer and autoimmune reactions that mediate damage to our own host tissues.

The issue of balance between stimulation and moderation of the immune response is typified by the conundrum of immunity and aging. There are theoretical reasons why one would want a more vigorous immune response in advanced age. Older organisms are more susceptible to both infectious morbidity and tumors. On the one hand, an *enhanced* antipathogen armamentarium and monitoring of cell mutation would auger for maintenance of general immune vigor. On the other hand, the increased risk of autoimmune disease with aging would militate in favor of a dampening down of the vigor of the inflammatory response. Moreover, calorie restriction has been found to extend longevity in experimental situations and it is associated with a diminution of the immune response. Literally, when one confronts that gerontologic immune system, it presents the question of whether it should be *Yin* or *Yang* or both.

From the standpoint of evolutionary biology, however, advanced age is not a "natural" condition. Having members of the herd or clan living beyond the reproductive span has only limited survival value for the species. Imagine if a butterfly were to acquire Teflon wings and try to make a go of it for a second season, or if a salamander became a newt, reproduced, and then sought to assume its terrestrial form again. Death shortly after the reproductive cycle is natural. One would argue from an evolutionary standpoint that dysregulation of the immune system in older animals is a favorable situation for the species, as it prunes the population of individuals who have expended their utility and represent only competition for the same space and food with younger, reproductively relevant adults. However, in veterinary and clinical medicine, we have made the practical and ethical decision to extend both life and good health and functioning. This places technology in the protagonistic position of counteracting what might be the scheme of Nature to weaken the defenses against infection and tumors and increase the attack on host tissue to shorten the span of life for those surviving through the reproductive cycle. If we accept the logic of an imperative in Nature *not* to defend the elderly organisms of a species, we might similarly explain the dysregulation of the immune protection scheme in other conditions that are out of bounds of normative health. As studied extensively and cited herein, obesity and cachexia would represent the passages beyond these boundaries. Natural Selection would disfavor procreation by those whose constitutions allow for severe underweight or gross overweight. It is not surprising that the immune system changes in ways that do not favor freedom from infection, autoimmune diseases, and malignancies when body weight transgresses the extremes.

When do health-adverse dysregulations of the immune system become determinant of nutritional status? The answer is in *numerous* circumstances. This is illustrated by the role of immunopathology in conditions of oral pathology, a situation in which eating becomes more difficult and selection of foods is conditioned by what can be tolerated in the oral cavity, chewed, and swallowed. Further along the alimentary tract, autoimmune conditions from celiac disease to inflammatory bowel conditions interfere with appetite and nutrient absorption, provoke proscriptive diets, and enhance transintestinal nutrient losses. To the extent that cancer is the result, in part, of the failure of immune vigilance, the myriad ways by which tumorous conditions produce undernutrition from psychic depression to intestinal obstruction become obvious. The role of cytokines in mediating the wasting cachexia in cancer as well as in inflammatory autoimmune conditions such as rheumatoid arthritis cannot be ignored in this immunity-on-nutrition survey of effects.

NUTRIENT INTAKE: TOO MUCH OR TOO LITTLE?

So many dietary situations cut in every direction when it comes to a desirable clinical outcome. Caloric restriction would be a case in point. Fraker *(10)* has given us a picturesque image in her chapter with its subsection "Dietary restriction: When less may be more for the immune system." To quote from her sage observations: "Regardless, . . . a variety of kinds of dietary restriction can have a positive impact on such diverse phenomena as aging, autoimmunity, and malignancy." Fasting, for instance, induces remission in Crohn's disease. Chronic caloric restriction in animals blunts the aging process and delays the formation of age-associated tumors *(11)*. Organ transplants do more poorly in underfed than in well-fed animals. One wonders, in weighing the evidence, whether the dietary restriction is acting directly on the immune response or on a common provocative mechanisms for aging, autoimmunity, and neoplasia, namely limiting tissue oxidation.

What a careful weighing of current—and future—evidence should be focused on is whether dietary restriction works by alleviating the load for the actions of our immune defenses or modulates these mechanisms toward appropriate control. Logically, the direction of immune response for avoiding autoimmune responses would be toward suppression, whereas that for defer malignancy would be toward enhancement.

Conversely, the primary thrust of the observations by Scrimshaw et al. *(1,2)* were to show how protein and energy deficiencies enhanced susceptibility to infectious pathogens. In a contemporary context, underconsumption is a devastating consequences of AIDS and, at the same time, an aggravant of clinical decline.

Finding the critical balance between too little and too much *iron* appears to be an issue in the appropriate functional outcome for the immune system. In HIV-infected patients, excess iron seems to accelerate progression *(12)*. In the elderly, too much iron in the stores may enhance the production of tissue free radicals with all of the consequences for chronic disease risk. The findings in the longitudinal follow-up of HIV seropositive men on the eastern coast of the United States *(13)* is illuminating, insofar as those consuming the highest dietary levels of zinc, or taking any zinc-containing supplements, had a more rapid progression to AIDS and an earlier mortality.

Nutritional status and dietary management issues of diseases or conditions that are *themselves* the consequences of altered immunity, such as AIDS, inflammatory bowel disease, and allografts (organ transplants) have been illustrated. In these instances, food and nutrients are not aimed directly at immunomodulation. The rationales are quite variable and interesting. In organ transplants, chronic rejection entails a process not dissimilar to primary atherosclerosis, and dietary manipulations similar to those ordered by cardiology dietitians are of potential value in slowing the vasculopathies in the allografts.

THE ACUTE-PHASE RESPONSE: WHERE THE RUBBER MEETS THE ROAD

It is probably in the context of the acute-phase response to injury that immunity and nutrition come into the most interesting and complex interaction. It was the studies of Beisel *(14)*, one of the contributors to this book, that identified the pattern and magnitude of nutrient wastage in the face of infection. It was highly associated with the interval of fever and its intensity. We have long understood the nature of fever and its role in the immune process; interestingly, it can both favor and oppose the control of proliferation of invading organisms. In fact, it was the search for and characterization of the "endogenous pyrogen," which became "leukocyte endogenous mediator," and, finally, "monokine," cum "cytokine" that has revealed to us the biology of the acute-phase response. Keusch *(15)* has characterized the issue thusly:

> . . . its discovery (IL-1) initiated a true revolution in biology, that is appreciation of the role of cytokine regulator peptides in biology, and a revolutionary way to look at nutrition–infection interactions as specifically regulated events. According to this view, infections were processes in which microbial products or products of the pathogen–host interaction were able to activate leukocytes to produce cytokine mediators which, in turn, acted as transcriptional regulators of a set of genes whose products initiate and mediate the acute-phase response during infection. With this as a framework, it became possible to ask specific questions to define the nature of

the regulatory events for the metabolic and immunologic responses to infection, ...

With respect to nutrition and the nutritional impact of the acute-phase reaction, it is not inconsequential that the original name for the cytokine now known as tumor necrosis factor-alpha was "cachetin," as it was named for the biological effect of producing emaciation (cachexia) in those producing it endogenously or injected with the peptide. Of course, the acute-phase response must be fed; it requires nutrients. Amino acids must be diverted from muscle and visceral proteins for the enhanced synthesis of acute-phase-reactant proteins. It is believed that the siphoning of zinc from the circulation is related to an enhanced need for acute-phase proteins.

IMPACT OF THE IMMUNE RESPONSE ON NUTRIENT REQUIREMENTS

A unique and underconsidered aspect of the immune response is its effect on nutrient requirements. Klasing and Leshchinsky's (3) use the elegance and control permitted by livestock husbandry and animal experimentation to demonstrate an influence of immune responses on nutrient requirements. This becomes obvious in the *aftermath* of an infection, where one expects bulk losses of nutrients (14) to be replaced. In a more specific reparative context, a recent comment by Grimble (16) is pertinent:

> Activation of the immune system will exert a stress upon the antioxidant defenses of the body as is evident from lipid peroxides. The oxidative damage is a by-product of attempts by the immune system to combat invading pathogens by production of oxidant molecules. Thus, activation of the system will lead to a degree of depletion of components of antioxidant defenses. . . .

During the infection itself, the issue of requirements diverges along two paths. In terms of requirements to mount a response, different immune cell types have different priorities for nutrients. Hepatic synthesis of acute-phase proteins during acute and chronic infections requires a pattern of amino acids, one distinct from that to proliferate the immune cells.

On the other hand, the chronically immunostimulated animal is not growing at a normal rate, being constrained by the overt or occult inflammatory agents. Hence, the requirements for intake to maintain the *retarded* growth rate are actually lower (3). In animal husbandry, this has implications for the projected and real costs for feed.

NUTRITIONAL STATUS OR DIETARY EXPOSURE?

It is said that "we are what we eat." In fact, the set-point of our immune response may be what we eat. Complete foods and beverages are considered in their abilities to modify the immune response in both appropriate (favorable, regulatory) and pathological (adverse, dysregulatory) ways. This would be most immediately understood as a paradigm when issues such as allergy, atopy, and asthma are considered: Specific food proteins triggering allergic responses from histamine release with urticaria and bronchospasm to tissue infiltrations mediated by a cellular inflammatory response. The concept of diet and immunity is not new or novel.

However, beyond food allergies, the discussion is often more related to nutrients because they influence our nutritional state. Speaking from the nutritional side of the ledger, we may still be too confined in our paradigms to nutritional *status,* the quantities of nutrients in functional sites or reserves in the body rather than

in the issues of the behavior that subtend nutriture, namely diet, cuisine, culinary practices, and eating behavior. My discipline has been very conservative in this respect, that is, to focus on nutrients. Harper (17) has commented: "Guidelines for healthy diets and guidelines for disease prevention are components of public health policy. They represent advice for the public that may be instituted, not only on scientific grounds, but for a variety of political considerations." Getting beyond the "nutrients" (i.e., the 13 vitamins and umpteen minerals considered to be essential) is a major challenge, perhaps with a major payoff.

One obvious exception to the restrictions to nutrients is the discussion of immunity and breast milk. Breast milk is a food, indeed a source of nutrients, but the whole context of lactation and immunity has to do with anti-infective cells and substances in the beverage and the lack of offending antigens to provoke allergies. Breast milk may represent, in part, the antithesis of the allergic paradigm, having the proteins of its prenatal uterine environment. Epidemiological evidence indicates decreased incidences of otitis media and other infections in breast-fed infants well into their childhoods.

In addition, another category of foods, edible plants, assumes importance on the dietary stage. The discussion on Chinese herbs covers ground that is refreshing both to the geographic context of where the people live and in breaking away from the straight-jacket of the specific nutrient. Specific plants, and a series of chemicals, have long been known for medicinal properties to influence what we now understand to be the allergic response. Moreover, Chinese herbs, plants, and spices, the botanic bounty of traditional medicine, are also modifiers of the immune response, primarily as anti-inflammatory agents.

Yogurt and other probiotic and prebiotic foods take a page out of the notebook of breast milk in terms of their expressed abilities to seed a certain flora (probiotics) and then to nourish and maintain it (prebiotics). Probiotic approaches have been observed to reduce the incidence of gastrointestinal infections. The immune mechanisms are presumed to be multiple, embracing competitive displacement of potential pathogenic coliform organisms by colonization of *Bifidobacteria* and *Lactobacillus* and reinforcing the responsiveness of the gut-associated lymphoid tissue (GALT).

Another deviation from nutrients is the role of phytochemicals and other non-nutrient compounds in the foods of our usual diets. Phytochemicals are molecules of plant origin that cannot be strictly classified as vitamins, but that exercise beneficial effects on human health. Two classes of phytochemicals can be singled out as modulators and modifiers of human immune function both in a stimulatory and suppressive dimension: carotenoids and flavonoids. Alpha-lipoic acid and its metabolite, dihydrolipoic acid, are compounds found in the diet and synthesized in the body that exercise an effect on the oxidant/antioxidant system of a magnitude to reflect on immune function.

The dietary sources of fats produce critical influences on the immune response. Lipids of different lengths and patterns of desaturation have profound effects on the inflammatory response. This is mediated in part by the predominance of immunosuppressive prostaglandins or immunostimulatory prostaglandins and allied compounds, derived from essential fatty acids. In general, the omega-3 fatty acids in fish are generally immunosuppressive in their modulation of the inflammatory process.

Reflecting on the inventory that has been made, it really may be more "Dietetics and Immunology," rather than Nutrition and

Immunology, because the effects of foods, beverages, and dietary patterns hold at least an equal footing with issues of nutritional status of the host.

"NUTRITIONAL IMMUNITY" AND ORIGINS OF AN "ANDROMEDA STRAIN"

The law of the jungle once prevailed for all of the species, and *homo sapiens* was part of the jungle. Birth and death were the elements of evolution. Birth and death were the elements of species survival. Hence, in certain ecosystems, certain nutrient deficiency states were taken advantage of to protect host species from the ravages of certain microbial pathogens in their environment *(18)*. This is the situation in which nutritional deficiency of the host is protective against infections, presumably by depriving the invading organisms of an essential nutrient or conditioning the host organism to deprive the pathogen of optimal conditions. For iron-requiring protozoa, such as the amoeba, an iron-deficient zone is a hostile environment. In theory, if antioxidant status is low in red cells, they become inadequate homes for the malaria *Plasmodia,* and parasitemias cannot develop.

This concept of *nutritional immunity,* introduced by Weinberg *(19)* and referred to by Klasing and Leshchinsky *(3)* as a manner by which "the host animal can sometimes decrease the rate of replication of bacteria and parasites by withholding nutrients." Specifically, with regard to iron, in the feeding of piglets in unsanitary environments and in the treatment of human infants with septicemia, iron administration has been documented to cause adverse infectious outcomes. Of course, in clinical medicine, the application of these principles is problematic. Technology and ethics have brought us beyond the law of the jungle in matters of care of humans and their domesticated animals. However, where both wild, roving animals and unacculturated human populations are concerned, the indiscriminate exposure to nutrient-rich foods may disrupt an *adaptation* between host nutriture and pathogen virulence that had evolved over time to the protective benefit of the host populations. This is the practical significance of the nutritional immunity concept.

An exciting and new facet of the story harkens to the images of Michaell Crichton's *Andromeda Strain.* Recent research suggests that a nutrient-deficient intracellular milieu may have given rise to the mutations of pathogens with greater virulence than the native strains. Specifically, in a system involving modification of the antioxidant status related to selenium and vitamin E, Beck *(20)* illustrates this potential to enhance the virulence of a murine Coxsackie virus through its passage through nutritionally deficient mice. The world's populations, specifically those with micronutrient deficiencies, may become the breeding ground for these "Andromeda strain" organisms; that is, mutation or adaptation to a virulent status for viruses that are otherwise commensal and innocuous may occur in the face of specific single-nutrient deficiencies. However, as further illustrated by the work of Beck *(20),* once established, the mutations are virulent for healthy, well-nourished individuals as well.

FUTURISTIC PERSPECTIVES

In the domain of population and public health, whither we go in the next millennium will be conditioned by a geographic context. The social and economic panorama portends more of a "rich get richer and a poor get poorer" scenario, both within societies and across nations. Thus, the challenges to *implement* the information in this book lie both in the salons of Soho and the slums of Dhaka.

NUTRITION AND IMMUNITY BEYOND 2000: THE RICH MAN'S VIEW For those with burgeoning affluence and technology, access to excesses of nutrients is the risk. As mentioned, too much iron accumulation in body stores has implications for the immune response because of increased free-radical generation. Overweight has implications for the vigor of the immune defenses. The pandemic of obesity in developed countries continues to extend with each cycle of national surveys. Eating too much of what our forbearers scrimped and saved to taste, however, may be only part of the problem of affluence.

Through the miracle of food technology, we can create molecules that were heretofore never seen, much less consumed and introduced to the human inner ecology. The sucrose-ester fat substitute olestra (Olean) is a much hyped illustration of an unlimited technological possibility. As we continue to make synthetic proteins and synthetic molecules for the "functional foods" of the future, we enter a Brave New World of novel exposures to challenge our immune system.

NUTRITION AND IMMUNITY BEYOND 2000: THE POOR MAN'S VIEW The population will reach 6 billion inhabitants shortly after the turn of the millennium. Of these, 70–80% will live in so-called developing or transitional nations, largely in the tropics and emerging or emerged from a colonial experience. The mantra of the United Nations' health-related organizations was "health for all in the year 2000." It might be safe to say that that goal will not be reached.

For those on the shorter end of the economic stick, deaths from childhood illnesses such as diarrhea, respiratory infections, malaria, measles, and others are the enduring reality for those of Third World regions. The anti-infective effectiveness of supplementation and fortification with vitamin A, zinc, and iron may provide a major tool for controlling death from these epidemic and pandemic problems. Safe motherhood and the reduction of death from childbirth-related infections may also have a public health solution in appropriate dietary and nutritional support to pregnant peasants and urban slum-dwellers. In the councils of the United Nations and of bilateral development-assistance agencies, with their mandates for service to the world's less fortunate, any anti-infective effects of restoring micronutrient nutriture have gained growing attention.

The AIDS epidemic arose within the last two decades of the millennium. Other novel virus diseases—Hanta, Ebola, Lasar, and higher alphabet hepatitides—emerged in this same era. In Africa, Asia, and Latin America, where access to an adequate nutrient intake is often denied by economic circumstances or crop failures, the vulnerability to these and other, novel infective agents will remain high. Already on the horizon is a massive change in the public health landscape of these less-developed zone by the pandemic of the HIV infection. The immunomodulating properties of dietary and supplemental nutrients will be enrolled to maximize the length and quality of life, avoiding high intakes of nutrients such as iron *(12)* and zinc *(13)* and looking for other adverse interactants.

NUTRITION AND IMMUNOLOGY BEYOND 2000: THE INVESTIGATIVE PERSPECTIVE To resolve the futuristic issues posed, the platform for research needs to reflect the essentials of this book. Investigation will have to be deep, but concepts and hypotheses will have to be broad. However, experimentation and clinical therapies must go into depth. The advance of technology in molecular biology in research and biotechnology in pharmaceutical therapeutics are the two axes to a deep probing of the nutrition and immunology interaction in the new millennium.

The future portends rapidly emerging concepts about diet and disease and equally rapid advances in technology to assess human nutritional status and the functional state of the various components of the human immune response. Progress can also be expected in the area of animal and in vitro models of human diseases. With a firm grasp on immunological technology with assays for both immune capacity and immune function, one can link alterations in dietary intake and nutritional status as the independent variables and immunity as the dependent component. Obviously, this requires the controlled manipulation of nutritional status, as that caused by disease already is confounded in the immune sphere. Nutrient deficiency, nutrient excess, and nutrient imbalances would be created in volunteers in the metabolic setting. How graded change in diet and nutrient status produces responses in inflammation and its mediators and cellular components, on the acute-phase response generation, on humoral immunity, on immune vigilance, and on the atopy pattern would be the focus of this first tier. It clarifies the causal limb of the *mechanism* that links diet and nutrition to disease. However, disease or physical incapacitation of the host is the bottom line of medical and personal concern. The link from immune function to clinical manifestation cannot be predicted on a priori grounds. Thus, the substance of this book most valuable in clinical management relates immunodetermined outcomes viewed in the pathological domain. This includes diet and nutrients with infectious diseases or allergy and asthma or cancer.

It was the technology of Edward Jenner that provided the first key to manipulation of the immune response in humans, the anti-small-pox vaccination. Immunization with natural—and then artificial—vaccines has advanced and is credited with the advance in longevity of the population worldwide. Furthermore, manipulation of the immune process is in sight, and to some extent in practice. Already in clinical trials are antibodies and other agents that block the effects of the cytokine mediators of the acute-phase reaction. The wisdom of the principle and the caveats of the application are unknown. For erythropoiesis failure, we now have recombinant genetic technology to support the red cell mass; similarly, immune-cell-targeted hormonal stimulation is not far beyond. The ultimate immune reconstitution, allogenic bone marrow transplantation, is routinely practiced to reconstitute congenital immunodeficiency.

With respect to the broad view, the solving of problems will have to fuse a diversity of disciplines among sciences and across science and technology. The contributors to this book present an interesting mixture of physician–clinician investigators and doctors of philosophy in the scientific disciplines. Some studious contributors are *both*. It would be interesting to make a VENN diagram of membership in the Federation of American Societies of Experimental Biology (or their regional equivalents) for the contributors to this book. How many are members only of the American Institute of Immunologists? How many only of the American Society for Nutritional Sciences? How many of both? Indeed, we shall have to go with—but also *beyond*—nutrition and immunology to address the present and future health issues emerging from either domain. Epidemiologists, nutritional biochemists, and dieticians will have to combine with infectious disease physicians, immunologists, and pathologists. Food science and technology will have to interface with rheumatologists and allergists and others. Only by taking a *holistic* grasp of the evidence presented in this book will the intersection of issues come into focus to guide such interdisciplinary efforts for the future.

REFERENCES

1. Scrimshaw NS, Taylor CE, Gordon JE. Interaction of nutrition and infection. Am J Med Sci 1959; 237:367–403.
2. Scrimshaw NS, Taylor CE, Gordon JE. Interaction of nutrition and infection. World Health Organization, Geneva, 1968.
3. Klasing KC, Leshchinsky TV. Interactions between nutrition and immunity: Lessons from animal agriculture. In: Gershwin ME, German B, Keen CL, eds, Nutrition and Immunology: Principles and Practice, pp. xx. Humana, Totowa, NJ, 1999 (this volume).
4. Sommer A, Tarwotjo I, Hussaini G, Susanto D. Increased mortality in children with mild vitamin A deficiency. Lancet 1993; 2:585–8.
5. Sommer A. New imperatives for an old vitamin (A). J Nutr 1989; 119:96–100.
6. Humphery JH, West K Jr, Sommer A. Vitamin A deficiency and attributable mortality among under 5-year olds. Bull WHO 1992; 70:232–9.
7. Maberly GF, Trowbridge FL, Yip R, Sullivan KM, West CE. Program against micronutrient malnutrition. Ending hidden hunger. Ann Rev Public Health 1994; 15:277–301.
8. Chang R. The anti-inflammatory effects of Chinese herbs, plants, and spices. In: Gershwin ME, German B, Keen CL, eds, Nutrition and Immunology: Principles and Practice, pp. xx. Humana, Totowa, NJ, 1999 (this volume).
9. Jolly and Fernandes Protein Energy Malnutrition and Infectious Disease: Synergistic Interactions. In: Gershwin ME, German B, Keen CL, eds, Nutrition and Immunology: Principles and Practice. pp. xx. Humana, Totowa, NJ, 1999 (this volume).
10. Fraker P. Impact of Nutritional Status on Immune Integrity. In: Gershwin ME, German B, Keen CL, eds, Nutrition and Immunology: Principles and Practice, pp. xx. Humana, Totowa, NJ, 1999 (this volume).
11. Masoro EJ, Yu BP, Bertrand HH. Action of food restrictions in delaying the aging process. Proc Natl Acad Sci USA 1982; 79:4239–41.
12. Jacobus DP. Randomization to iron supplementation of patients with advanced human immunodeficiency virus disease—an inadvertent but controlled study with results important for patient care. J Infect Dis 1996; 153:1044–5.
13. Tang AM, Graham NMH, Kirby AJ, McCall LD, Willett WC, Saah AJ. Dietary micronutrient intake and risk for progression to acquired immunodeficiency syndrome (AIDS) in human immunodeficiency virus type-1 (HIV-1) infected homosexual men. Am J Epidemiol 1993; 138:937–51.
14. Beisel WR. Metabolic response to infection. Annu Rev Med 1975; 26:9–20.
15. Keusch GT. Infection: nutritional interactions. In: Sadler M, Strain JJ, Caballero B, eds, Encyclopedia of Human Nutrition, pp. 1117–1120. Academic, London, 1998.
16. Grimble RF. Effect of antioxidant vitamins in immune function with clinical application. Int J Vitam Nutr Res 1997; 67:312–20.
17. Harper AE. Dietary standards and dietary guidelines. In: Brown ML, ed, Present Knowledge in Nutrition, 6th ed, pp. 491–501. ILSI—Nutrition Foundation, Washington, DC, 1990.
18. Solomons NW. Biological, ecological and social origins of trace element deficiencies in developing countries. In: Wahlqvist ML, Truswell AS, Smith R, Nestel PJ, eds, Nutrition for a Sustainable Environment. Proceedings of the XV International Congress on Nutrition, pp. 299–302. Smith-Gordon, London, 1994.
19. Weinberg E. Nutritional immunity. Physiol Rev 1984; 64:65–102.
20. Beck M. Nutritional effects on the pathogen genome and phenotypic expression of disease. In: Gershwin ME, German B, Keen CL, eds, Nutrition and Immunology: Principles and Practice, pp. xx. Humana, Totowa, NJ, 1999 (this volume).

Index